AF576818

Liver Cancer

Liver Cancer

Edited by

Kunio Okuda, M.D., Ph.D.
Professor Emeritus
First Department of Medicine
Chiba University School of Medicine
Chiba, Japan

Edward Tabor, M.D.
Director
Division of Transfusion Transmitted Diseases
Center for Biologics Evaluation and Research
Food and Drug Administration
Bethesda, Maryland

CHURCHILL LIVINGSTONE
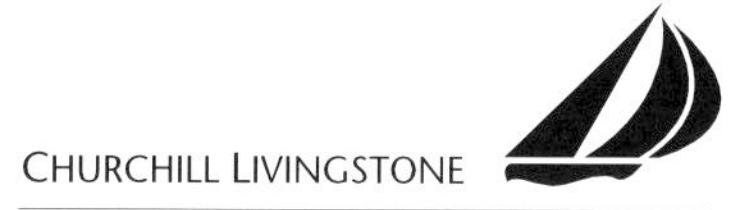
New York, Edinburgh, London, Madrid, Melbourne, San Francisco, Tokyo

CHURCHILL LIVINGSTONE

Medical Division of Pearson Professional Limited

Distributed in the United States of America by Churchill Livingstone Inc., 650 Avenue of the Americas, New York, N.Y. 10011, and by associated companies, branches, and representatives throughout the world

First published 1997

ISBN 0-443-05481-9

British Library Cataloguing in Publication Data
A catalogue record for this book is available from the British Library

Library of Congress Cataloging in Publication Data
A catalog record for this book is available from the Library of Congress

Medical knowledge is constantly changing. As new information becomes available, changes in treatment, procedures, equipment and the use of drugs become necessary. The editors/authors/contributors and the publishers have, as far as it is possible, taken care to ensure that the information given in this text is accurate and up to date. However, readers are strongly advised to confirm that the information, especially with regard to drug usage, complies with the latest legislation and standards of practice.

The Publishers have made every effort to trace the copyright holders for borrowed material. If they have inadvertently overlooked any, they will be pleased to make the necessary arrangements at the first opportunity.

Acquisitions Editor: *Sheila Khullar*
Production Editor: *Dave Terry*
Production Supervisor: *Sharon Tuder*
Cover Design: *Jeannette Jacobs*

Printed in the United States of America

CONTRIBUTORS

B. S. Anand, M.D., D.Phil.
Associate Professor, Department of Medicine, Baylor College of Medicine; Staff Physician, Digestive Diseases Section, Veterans Affairs Medical Center, Houston, Texas

Peter Bannasch, M.D.
Professor and Head, Division of Cell Pathology, German Cancer Research Center, Heidelberg, Germany

Oliver F. Bathe, M.D., M.Sc., F.R.C.S.(C)
Department of Surgery, University of British Columbia Faculty of Medicine, Vancouver, British Columbia, Canada

F. Xavier Bosch, M.D., M.P.H.
Chief, Epidemiology Service and Cancer Registry, Catalan Institute of Oncology, Barcelona, Spain

Jean-Pierre Bronowicki, M.D.
Department of Hepatology and Gastroenterology, University Hospital; Laboratory of Cellular Pathology in Nutrition, University Henri Poincaré, Nancy, France

Andrew Buczkowski, M.D.
Section of Hepatobiliary Surgery, Department of Surgery, University of British Columbia Faculty of Medicine, Vancouver, British Columbia, Canada

Nadine R. Caron, B.Sc.
University of British Columbia Faculty of Medicine, Vancouver, British Columbia, Canada

Ding-Shinn Chen, M.D.
Director, Division of Gastroenterology, Department of Internal Medicine, National Taiwan University College of Medicine; Professor and Director, Hepatitis Research Center, National Taiwan University Hospital; Taipei, Taiwan

Pei-Jer Chen, M.D., Ph.D.
Professor, Graduate Institute of Clinical Medicine, National Taiwan University College of Medicine; Consultant Physician, Division of Gastroenterology, Department of Internal Medicine, National Taiwan University Hospital, Taipei, Taiwan

Toshiya Chiba, M.D.
Department of Gastroenterology and Hepatobiliary Diseases, Institute of Clinical Medicine, University of Tsukuba Faculty of Medicine, Tsukuba, Japan

Byung Ihn Choi, M.D.
Professor, Department of Radiology, Seoul National University College of Medicine; Director, Division of Gastrointestinal Radiology and Abdominal Imaging, Department of Diagnostic Radiology, Seoul National University Hospital, Seoul, Korea

Massimo Colombo, M.D.
Professor, Department of Internal Medicine, University of Milan Faculty of Medicine; Director, University Research Unit for Liver Cancer, Maggiore Research Institute Hospital, Milan, Italy

Richard M. Conran, Ph.D., M.D.
Associate Professor, Department of Pathology, Uniformed Services University of the Health Sciences F. Edward Hébert School of Medicine, Bethesda, Maryland; Consulting Staff Pathologist, Department of Pediatric Pathology, Armed Forces Institute of Pathology, Washington, D.C.

John R. Craig, M.D., Ph.D.
Associate Clinical Professor, Department of Pathology, University of Southern California School of Medicine, Los Angeles, California; Medical Director, Oncology Services, St. Jude Medical Center, Fullerton, California

Yves Deugnier, M.D.
Professor, Department of Hepatology, National Institute of Health and Medical Research Faculty of Medicine; Consultant, Liver Unit, Pontchaillou Hospital, Rennes, France.

Michel Doffoel, M.D.
Professor, Department of Hepatology and Gastroenterology, University of Strasbourg; Chief Department of Hepatology and Gastroenterology, University Hospital, Strasbourg, France

Masaaki Ebara, M.D.
Associate Professor, First Department of Medicine, Chiba University School of Medicine, Chiba, Japan

Michael Geissler, M.D.
Molecular Hepatology Laboratory, Massachusetts General Hospital and Harvard Medical School, Boston, Massachusetts

Michael A. Gerber, M.D.
Professor and Chairman, Department of Pathology and Laboratory Medicine, Tulane University School of Medicine, New Orleans, Louisiana

Annette Gesien, M.D.
Molecular Hepatology Laboratory, Massachusetts General Hospital and Harvard Medical School, Boston, Massachusetts

F. Blaine Hollinger, M.D.
Professor, Departments of Medicine and Virology and Epidemiology, Baylor College of Medicine; Director, Eugene B. Casey Hepatitis and HIV Research Center and Diagnostic Laboratory, Houston, Texas

Masahiso Hoso, M.D.
Assistant Professor, Second Department of Pathology, Kanazawa University School of Medicine, Kanazawa, Japan

Kamal G. Ishak, M.D., Ph.D.
Chairman, Department of Hepatic and Gastrointestinal Pathology, Armed Forces Institute of Pathology, Washington, D.C.; Professorial Lecturer, Department of Pathology, Mt. Sinai School of Medicine of the City University of New York, New York, New York; Clinical Professor, Department of Pathology, Uniformed Services University of the Health Sciences F. Edward Hébert School of Medicine, Bethesda, Maryland

Gilbert Jay, Ph.D., D.Sc.
Professor, Department of Biochemistry and Molecular Biology, George Washington University School of Medicine, Washington, D.C.; Head, Department of Virology, Jerome H. Holland Laboratory, American Red Cross, Rockville, Maryland

Shuichi Kaneko, M.D.
Associate Professor, First Department of Internal Medicine, Kanazawa University Faculty of Medicine and Kanazawa University Hospital, Kanazawa, Japan

Michael C. Kew, Ph.D.,M.D., D.Sc., F.R.C.P.
Dora Dart Professor, Department of Medicine, and Director, Medical Research Council/University Molecular Hepatology Research Unit, Department of Medicine, University of the Witwatersrand Faculty of Medicine; Senior Physician, Department of Medicine, Johannesburg and Baragwanath Hospitals, Johannesberg, South Africa

Chang-Min Kim, M.D., Ph.D.
Chief, Third Department of Internal Medicine, Korea Cancer Center Hospital, Seoul, Korea

Kenichi Kobayashi, M.D.
Professor, First Department of Internal Medicine, Kanazawa University Faculty of Medicine and Kanazawa University Hospital, Kanazawa, Japan

Masamichi Kojiro, M.D.
Professor and Chairman, First Department of Pathology, Kurume University School of Medicine, Kurume, Japan

Yoichiro Kondo, M.D.
Professor, Department of Pathology, Chiba University School of Medicine, Chiba, Japan

Masatoshi Kudo, M.D.
Visiting Clinical Professor, Fourth Department of Medicine, Kobe University School of Medicine, Kobe, Japan; Visiting Clinical Professor, Department of Diagnostic Radiology, Shiga Medical School, Shiga, Japan; Chief, Section of Hepatology, Division of Gastroenterology, Department of Medicine, Kobe City General Hospital, Kobe, Japan

Tito Livraghi, M.D.
Chief, Department of Radiology, Civilian's Hospital,Vimarcate (Milano), Italy

Janice Main, M.B., Ch.B., F.R.C.P. (Edin and Lond)
Senior Lecturer, Department of Medicine, Imperial College School of Medicine at St. Mary's, London, England

Yashushi Matsuzaki, M.D., Ph.D.
Assistant Professor, Department of Gastroenterology and Hepatobiliary Diseases, Institute of Clinical Medicine, University of Tsukuba Faculty of Medicine, Tsukuba, Japan

Takamichi Murakami, M.D., Ph.D.
Assistant Professor, Department of Radiology, Osaka University Medical School; Assistant Professor, Radiology Clinic, Osaka University Hospital, Osaka, Japan

Peter Nagy, M.D., Ph.D.
Associate Professor, Department of Pathology and Experimental Cancer Research, Semmelweis University of Medicine, Budapest, Hungary

Hironobu Nakamura, M.D., Ph.D.
Professor and Chairman, Department of Radiology, Osaka University School of Medicine, Osaka, Japan; Professor and Director, Radiology Clinic, Osaka University Hospital, Osaka, Japan

Yasuni Nakanuma, M.D.
Professor, Second Department of Pathology, Kanazawa University School of Medicine, Kanazawa, Japan

Showgo Ohkoshi, M.D., Ph.D.
Assistant Professor, Third Department of Internal Medicine, Niigata University School of Medicine, Niigata, Japan

Shuichi Okada, M.D.
Head, Hepatobiliary and Pancreatic Oncology Division, National Cancer Center Hospital, Tokyo, Japan

Kunio Okuda, M.D., Ph.D.
Professor Emeritus, First Department of Medicine, Chiba University School of Medicine, Chiba, Japan

Toshiaki Osuga, M.D., Ph.D.
Professor Emeritus, Department of Gastroenterology and Hepatobiliary Diseases, Institute of Clinical Medicine, University of Tsukuba Faculty of Medicine, Tsukuba City, Japan

Pascal Pineau, M.D.
Genetic Recombination and Expression Unit, Pasteur Institute, Paris, France

Keith Rolles, M.A., M.S., F.R.C.S.
Consultant Surgeon and Director, Liver Transplant Unit, Royal Free Hospital, London, England

Zsuzsa Schaff, M.D., Ph.D., D.Sci.
Professor, Department of Pathology and Experimental Cancer Research, Semmelweis University of Medicine, Budapest, Hungary

Charles H. Scudamore, M.D., M.Sc., F.R.C.S.(C)(Ed)(Eng), F.A.C.S.
Associate Professor and Head, Section of Hepatobiliary and Pancreatic Surgery, Division of General Surgery, Department of Surgery, University of British Columbia Faculty of Medicine, Vancouver, British Columbia, Canada

Daniel Shouval, M.D.
Professor, Department of Medicine, Hadassah University Faculty of Medicine; Director, Liver Unit, Department of Medicine, Hadassah University Hospital, Jersusalem, Israel

J. Thomas Stocker, M.D.
Professor, Department of Pathology, Uniformed Services University of the Health Sciences F. Edward Hébert School of Medicine, Bethesda, Maryland; Clinical Professor, Department of Pathology, Georgetown University Medical School, Washington, D.C.

Edward Tabor, M.D.
Director, Division of Transfusion Transmitted Diseases, Center for Biologics Evaluation and Research, Food and Drug Administration, Bethesda, Maryland

Kenichi Takayasu, M.D.
Head, Department of Diagnostic Radiology, National Cancer Center Hospital, Tokyo, Japan

Zhao-You Tang, M.D.
Professor and Chairman, Liver Cancer Institute, Zhong Shan Hospital, Shanghai Medical University, Shanghai, China

Tadashi Terada, M.D.
Associate Professor, Second Department of Pathology, Kanazawa University School of Medicine, Kanazawa, Japan

Howard C. Thomas, B.Sc., Ph.D., F.R.C.P., F.R.C.Path.
Professor and Head, Department of Medicine, Imperial College School of Medicine at St. Mary's, London, England

Swan N. Thung, M.D.
Professor, Department of Pathology, Mount Sinai School of Medicine of the City University of New York, New York, New York

Pierre Tiollais, M.D.
Professor, Department of Retroviruses, Unit of Genetic Recombination and Expression, Pasteur Institute, Paris, France

Hirohiko Tsujii, M.D., Ph.D.
Professor, Proton Medical Research Center, University of Tsukuba Faculty of Medicine, Tsukuba, Japan; Director, Department of Radiation Medicine, Research Center of Charged Particle Therapy, National Institute of Radiological Sciences, Chiba, Japan

Bruno Turlin, M.D.
Assistant Professor, Department of Pathology, National Institute of Health and Medical Research Faculty of Medicine, Rennes, France

Hiroyuki Ueda, M.D., Ph.D.
Assistant Professor, Department of Obstetrics and Gynecology, Niigata University School of Medicine, Niigata, Japan

Masashi Unoura, M.D.
Director, Division of Gastroenterology, Department of Medicine, Toyama Prefectural Central Hospital, Toyama, Japan

Denis Vetter, M.D.
Professor, Department of Hepatology and Gastroenterology, University Louis Pasteur and University Hospital, Strasbourg, France

Jack R. Wands, M.D.
Associate Professor, Department of Medicine, Harvard Medical School; Director, Molecular Hepatology Laboratory, Massachusetts General Hospital Cancer Center, Charlestown, Massachusetts

Gerald N. Wogan, Ph.D.
Professor, Division of Toxicology, Massachusetts Institute of Technology, Cambridge, Massachusetts

Heide Zerban, Ph.D.
Division of Cell Pathology, German Cancer Research Center, Heidelberg, Germany

ACKNOWLEDGMENTS

The editors would like to acknowledge the continuing support for research in the areas described in this book that has been provided throughout the years by the National Institutes of Health and the Food and Drug Administration; the administrative assistance of Ms. Catherine Fox; and the cooperation of the staff of Churchill Livingstone.

CONTENTS

1

SECTION I
CLINICAL FEATURES OF HEPATOCELLULAR CARCINOMA

CLINICAL PRESENTATION AND NATURAL HISTORY OF HEPATOCELLULAR CARCINOMA AND OTHER LIVER CANCERS

KUNIO OKUDA

PRESENTATION OF HEPATOCELLULAR CARCINOMA

The clinical presentation of hepatocellular carcinoma (HCC) varies greatly depending on the coexisting liver disease. In southern Africa, Bantu patients with HCC typically present with malaise, a large hepatic mass, and abdominal discomfort and/or pain.[1,2] In contrast, Japanese patients more often come to the physician first with symptoms or signs due to liver cirrhosis such as pedal edema, ascites, or variceal bleeding (Table 1-1),[3] and an HCC is found by biochemical and imaging examinations. Currently, about 80% of HCC patients in Japan are diagnosed when they are found to have a small HCC in a screening program for chronic liver disease or at the time of a regular medical check-up. These patients have no HCC-specific complaint. In other countries, the presenting symptoms and signs are somewhere between these two extremes.

An HCC developing in a liver without advanced chronic disease, as is often the case with African blacks,[4,5] can grow to an enormous size before the patient succumbs, whereas an HCC developing in a liver markedly shrunk as a result of advanced cirrhosis has no time to grow large before the patient dies from hepatic failure or with end-stage cirrhosis. A comparison of liver weights between African black and Japanese HCC patients clearly demonstrates this point (Fig. 1-1). The vast majority of autopsied livers from Mozambican blacks weighed more than 3 kg, some up to 7 kg. Such a patient could be walking around the hospital with a huge protruding abdomen due to an enlarged liver. Even though the liver is almost totally replaced by HCC, leaving very little normal parenchyma, it can sustain life because the remaining tissue is not cirrhotic. In our series of autopsies in Japan, the majority of livers bearing HCC weighed less than 3 kg, the smallest being 600 g, and none weighed more than 6 kg; 88% of these HCC patients had cirrhosis or advanced chronic liver disease (for instance, with fibrosis).[6] Similar weight differences in HCC patients with and without liver disease have been reported by others.[4]

The complaints of the patient and clinical signs are often a mixture of those attributable to a large mass in the liver and those due to liver cirrhosis (Table 1-1). One important symptom is a dull abdominal pain, found in 46% of patients in Japan and 90% to 95% of patients in Africa. Cirrhotic patients without HCC do not have such pain. In other words, if a patient with cirrhosis has onset of upper abdominal pain or discomfort, HCC

TABLE 1-1. Early Symptoms and Signs in Hepatocellular Carcinoma

	Southern African Black[1,2]		Japan
Symptom	Berman (1951)[1] (n = 75)	Kew and Geddes (1982)[2] (n = 550)	Liver Cancer Study Group (1984–85) (n = 2300)
General malaise	86%		61%
Abdominal pain	90	95%	46
Full sensation in abdomen		43	45
Anorexia		25	45
Weight loss	83	34	29
Ascites	45	51	27
Palpable mass	100[a]	92	23
Pedal edema	30		17
Jaundice	45	28	17
Fever	38	35	17
Nausea, vomiting		8	16
Hematemesis		2	8
Dyspnea	25		
Anemia	34		
Bone pain		3	

[a] 96% had tender abdominal mass.

should be suspected. Loss of weight is clearly more noticeable in HCC patients without cirrhosis, and an enlarged liver (or a hepatic mass) is invariably palpable, sometimes with visible abdominal enlargement. The surface may not necessarily be uneven or irregular by palpation. Auscultation of the liver frequently elicits arterial bruit, which suggests extensive arterial neovasculature. A pedunculated HCC may be recognized grossly as a protruding lump in the upper abdomen (Fig. 1-2).

Berman[1] described five patterns of clinical presentation of HCC. In the major clinical type, *frank cancer*, the signs and symptoms are referred to the liver in patients previously in good health. The clinical findings are asthenia, loss of weight, abdominal pain and tenderness, and enlargement of the liver (Fig. 1-3). Less frequent signs are anemia, jaundice, ascites, peripheral edema, dilatation of the superficial abdominal veins, and dyspnea (from lung metastases). This type accounted for 63% of his cases. The liver weight ranged from 2 to 7.1 kg, averaging 4 kg. In Japan, before the early detection of HCC by screening became possible, frank cancer was common (Table 1-2). However, at that time, 23% of patients had clinical signs that were predominantly associated with cirrhosis without overt hepatomegaly (cirrhotic type).[3]

The second most frequent clinical type described by Berman was *occult cancer*, in which HCC was found during examination for complaints other than those attributable to the liver. It accounted for 16% of cases. Some were hospitalized for nonhepatic diseases, and in the oth-

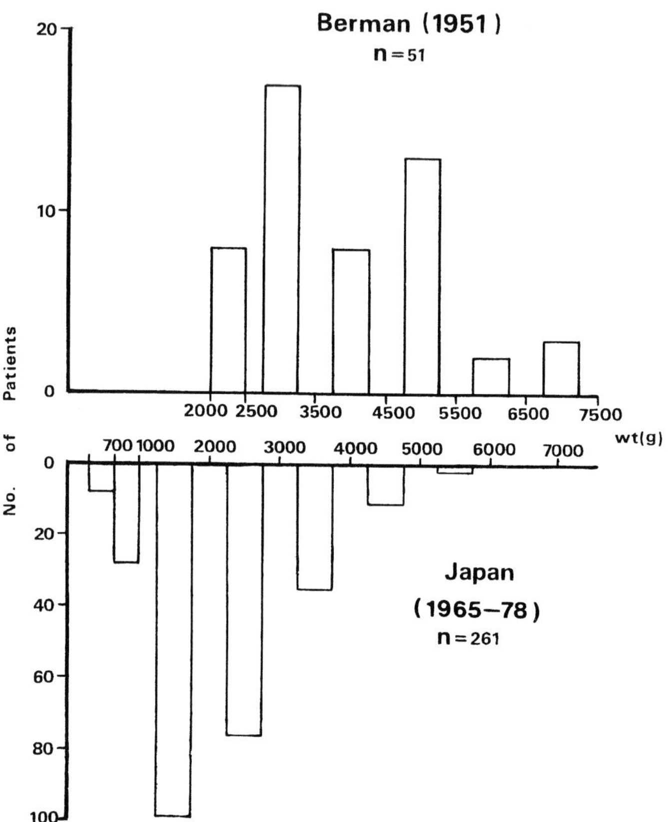

FIGURE 1-1. Comparison of liver weights at autopsy between HCC patients in southern Africa[1] and Japan.[6] Livers among Japanese patients are mostly cirrhotic, hence smaller in weight.

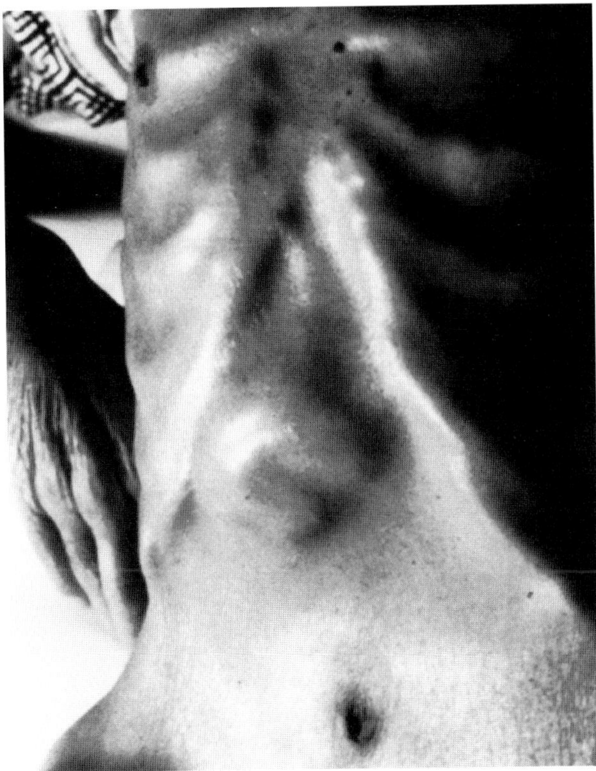

FIGURE 1-2. Pedunculated HCC developing in a cirrhotic liver. Dark skin discoloration and unrecognizable liver suggest advanced cirrhosis. Only a protruding mass is visible in the upper abdomen. (From Okuda,[7] with permission.)

ers HCC was an incidental finding at autopsy. In our series, only 4% were of this type.

The third type was *acute abdominal cancer*, which accounted for 8% in Berman's series and 3% in ours. Most patients were in good health and suddenly developed signs and symptoms pointing to an acute abdominal catastrophe. Abnormal muscular exertion would occasionally precipitate rupture of a latent cancer nodule in the liver surface. In two of our cases the rupture was deemed to have been caused by forceful palpation by a physician (Fig. 1-4). Unmistakable signs of severe loss of blood are noted; the patient is distressed and restless, the conjunctivae are pale, the skin is cold and clammy, and the pulse is rapid and feeble. The abdomen is distended, painful, tender, and rigid. Abdominal tap yields blood. Emergency ultrasonography may demonstrate the possible site of bleeding (Fig. 1-5). Immediate hepatic arteriography demonstrates the bleeding artery, and attempts should be made to occlude it with Gelfoam particles. Less acute bleeding is much more common in advanced HCC patients, and at the time of autopsy, about 80% of patients have blood in ascites. Immediate operation may result in an 18% survival rate,[9] but the outcome of acute bleeding of HCC is often fatal.

TABLE 1-2. Clinical Types of HCC: A Comparison of African and Japanese Patients

Clinical Type of HCC	South African Black Berman (1951)[1]	Japan Okuda (1979)[3]
	Number of Patients	Number of Patients
Frank	47 (62.7%)	229 (60.9%)
Cirrhotic		87 (23.1)
Occult	12 (16.2)	14 (3.7)
Febrile	6 (8.0)	8 (2.1)
Acute abdominal	6 (8.0)	11 (2.9)
Metastatic	4 (5.3)	11 (2.9)
Cholestatic		7 (1.9)
Hepatic		3 (0.8)
Unclassifiable		6 (1.6)
Total	75	376

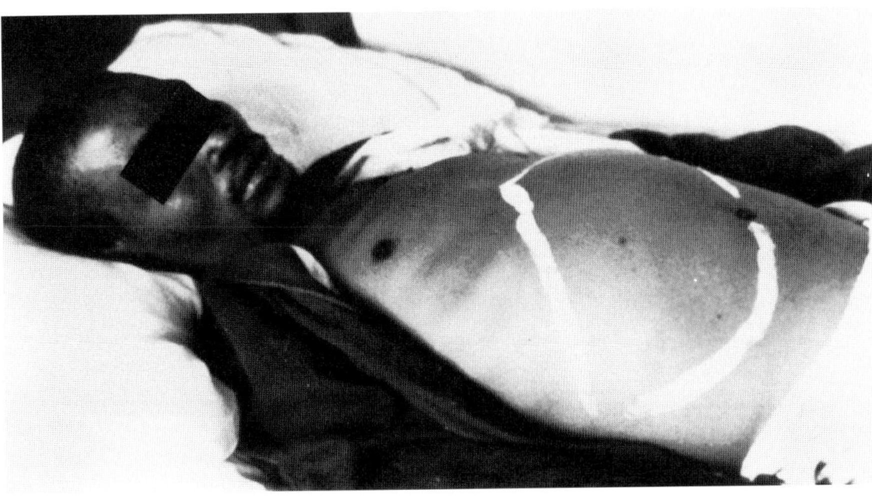

FIGURE 1-3. Typical frank cancer type HCC.[1]

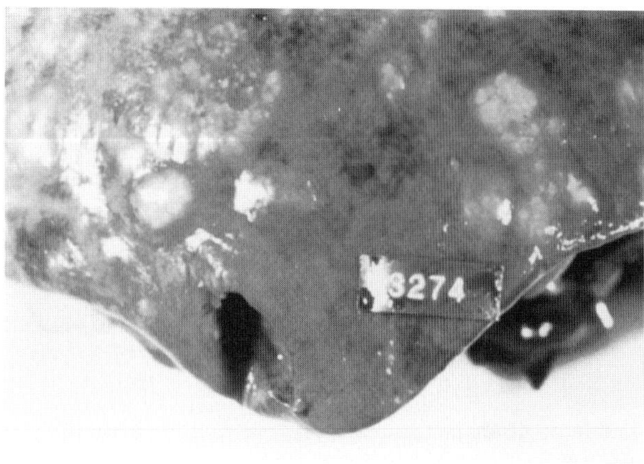

FIGURE 1-4. Bleeding site in a noncirrhotic liver bearing an HCC, believed to have been caused by a forceful palpation. (From Okuda,[8] with permission.)

FIGURE 1-5. The site of bleeding from the liver surface seen by ultrasound. The round mass in the liver surface and the surrounding ascites are apparent. The protrusion from the mass (arrow) may represent a blood clot. (From Okuda,[7] with permission.)

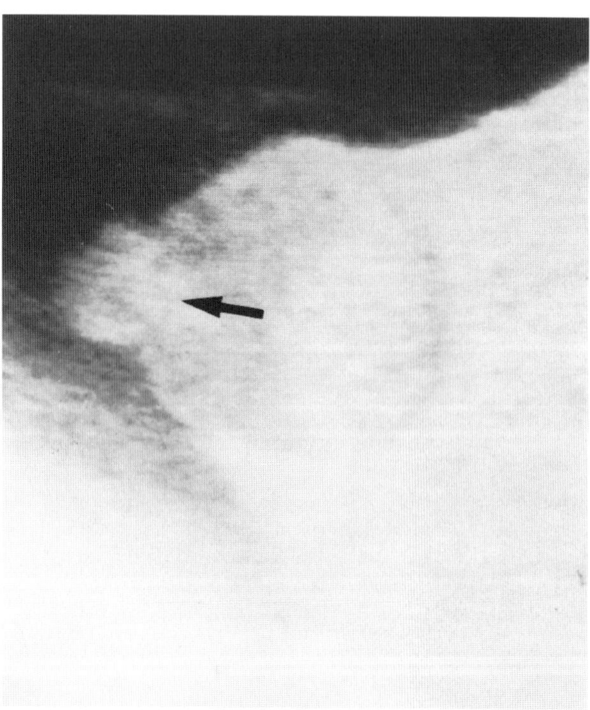

In the fourth clinical type, *febrile cancer*, the patient complains of severe pain and tenderness in the liver region accompanied by high fever and a toxemic syndrome. The clinical picture is that of liver abscess (Fig. 1-6). This type was found in 8% of Berman's patients[1] and 2.1% of ours. Patients had leukocytosis, an accelerated erythrocyte sedimentation rate, and a nodular abdominal mass with a tendency to central necrosis. We were able to study five such cases histologically (four by autopsy). The febrile cancer HCC is a poorly differentiated HCC with sarcomatoid features.[10] In two of our cases, the differential diagnosis from abscess was not possible, and exploratory laparotomy was carried out. The higher frequency of this type among African blacks probably reflects the more frequent poorly differentiated HCC as observed by Steiner.[4]

The fifth clinical type is *metastatic cancer*, in which symptoms due to metastases in remote organs completely overshadow those of the primary lesion in the liver, and may even be the only manifestation of otherwise symptomless or unsuspected liver cancer. In Berman's series, this type occurred in four (5%) patients; one presented with expectoration of blood and dyspnea due to lung metastases, one with headache due to brain metastasis, and two others with lumps over the occiput and a rib due to bone metastasis. In our autopsy series of 232 cases, clinically recognizable metastases were in the lung in 51.6% of cases, the bone in 5.8%, the meninges in 5.4%, the brain in 2.7%, the diaphragm in 10.2%, Douglas' pouch (lower pelvis) in 6.2%, and lymph nodes in the neck in 5.3% of cases. Dissemination to the lung in its early stage mimics miliary tuberculosis (Fig. 1-7). The only difference on the chest film is a heavier distribution of miliary lesions in the lower lung in HCC compared to heavier distribution in the upper lung in tuberculosis. We had a patient who coughed up a small piece of tissue, which on histologic examination turned out to be HCC (Fig. 1-8). A small lesion was subsequently found in the lung hidden behind the mediastinal shadow. Bone metastasis may be recognized as an obvious lump in the head (Fig. 1-9) or from neurologic signs due to a spinal lesion.

Besides these five types described by Berman, some patients (1.9% in our series) may develop symptoms similar to those due to bile duct obstruction, which are manifested by acute progressive jaundice, or which may mimic stone disease with pain as a result of intraductal HCC invasion. Ductal invasion has been reported in 10% of cases at autopsy.[11] Sometimes the pain is due to hemobilia. We have seen several patients who presented with an acute severe flare-up of chronic hepatitis accompanied by elevated aminotransferase levels, and on autopsy the liver was already cirrhotic, suggesting coexistent rapidly progressive hepatitis and HCC ("hepatitic type"). Muscular invasion by HCC as the first clinical sign is very uncommon. Although at autopsy tumor dissemina-

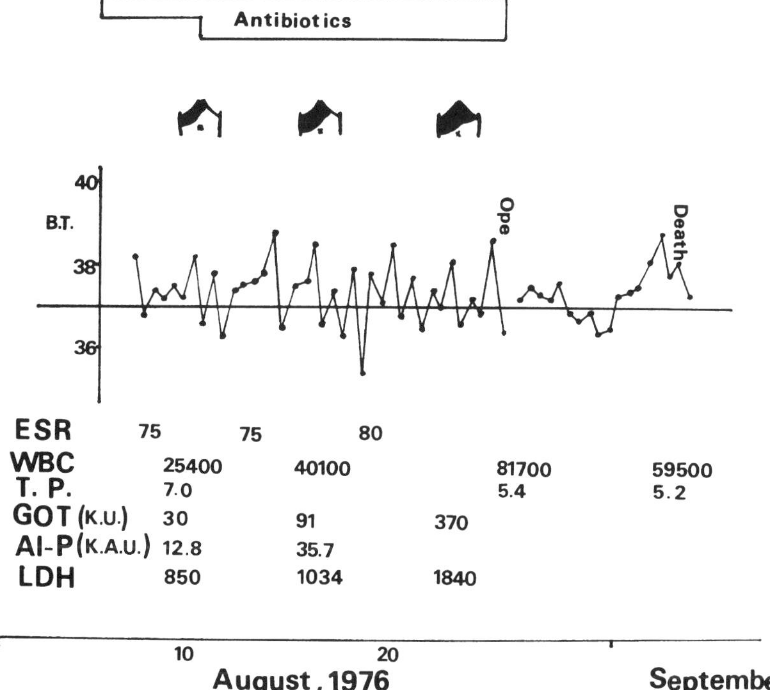

FIGURE 1-6. Course of disease in a 42-year-old man who presented with abdominal pain, a large liver, and high fever. The liver was enlarging very rapidly, and a tentative diagnosis of liver abscess was made because of marked leukocytosis and accelerated erythrocyte sedimentation rate. Exploratory laparotomy was carried out; the patient died 10 days later. Autopsy disclosed a large nodular HCC with central necrosis.

FIGURE 1-7. Miliary dissemintation of metastatic HCC in the lungs. Distribution of small densities is heavier in the lower lung, unlike miliary tuberculosis in which more lesions are seen in the upper lung. (From Okuda,[8] with permission.)

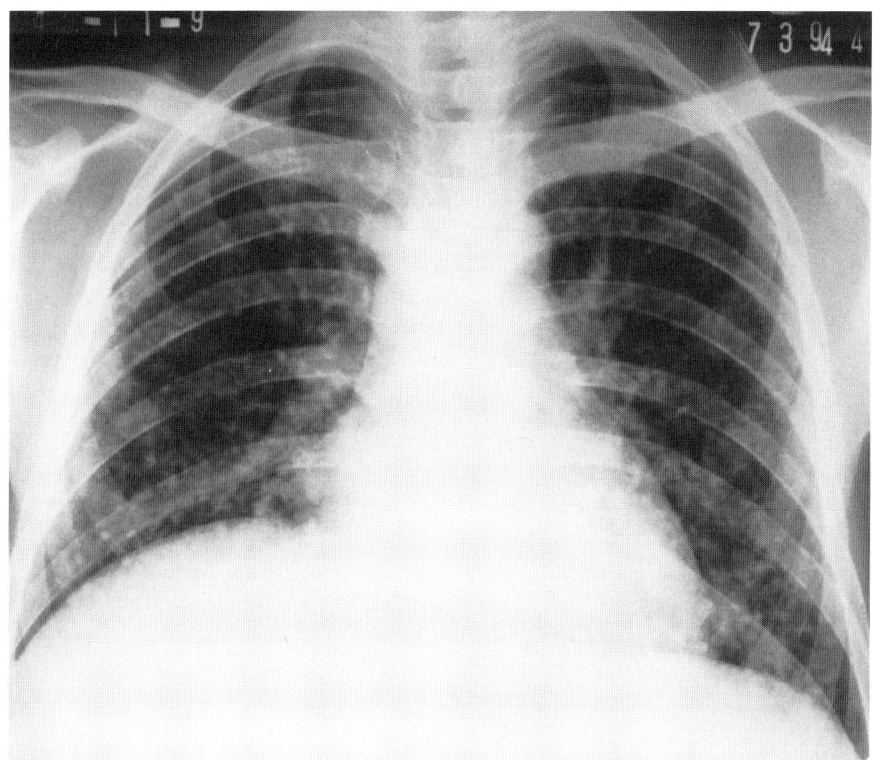

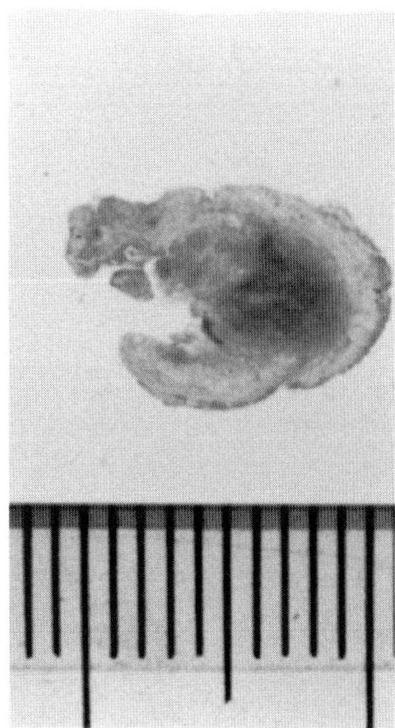

FIGURE 1-8. A small tissue fragment that was coughed up with blood by a 57-year-old patient who was otherwise healthy. The tissue on histologic examination proved to be HCC. Subsequent examination of the lung disclosed a small lesion in the right lung behind the mediastinal shadow; it was not seen in the anteroposterior projection. (From Okuda,[8] with permission.)

FIGURE 1-9. A computed tomography scan of the head of a 56-year-old man who noted a lump in the forehead (arrow) but had no abdominal symptoms; this was shown to be a typical case of metastatic cancer by the Berman classification.

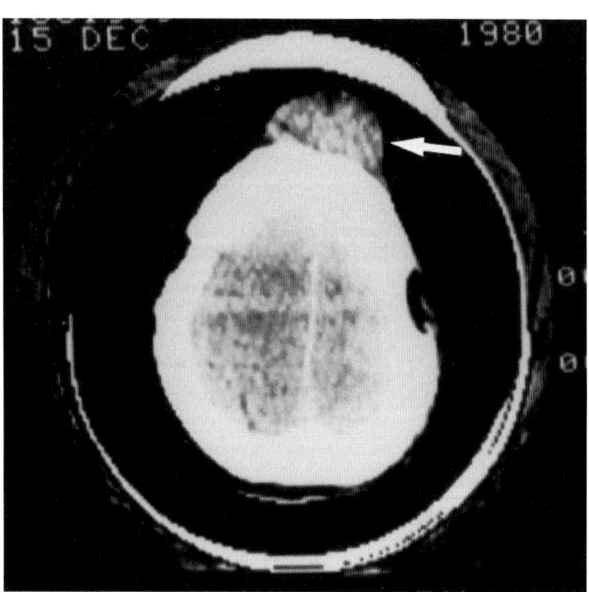

tion may be seen in Douglas' pouch in the pelvis, intraperitoneal dissemination is very uncommon.

CLINICAL COURSE AND OUTCOME OF HCC

Without treatment, HCC is relentlessly progressive. As already discussed, HCC in a noncirrhotic liver usually enlarges at a rapid pace, and the physician almost feels as if the tumor growth were visible. The speed of growth of HCC varies from case to case. Reports of HCC doubling time have ranged from 29 to 398 days in Taiwan[12] (no correlation with the histologic grading) and from 27 to 606 days in Italy (with histologic features and sonographic findings correlated with a doubling time).[13] The speed of growth remains constant in some patients and changes unpredictably in others. The patient eventually develops hepatic failure with prostration, emaciation, progressive jaundice, and disturbances of consciousness. In the absence of marked jaundice, the death may be called a "cancer death." Patients who present with predominantly cirrhosis signs, namely a small liver, small HCC, ascites, and signs of portal hypertension (varices, splenomegaly), hepatic failure is the likely cause of death. The patient dies before HCC attains a grossly recognizable size. In the survey conducted the Liver Cancer Study Group of Japan in 1990–1991,[14] (Tables 1-3 and 1-4), sudden deterioration of the patient often accompanied diffuse spread of the tumor within the liver (Fig. 1-10). In Japan, practically all livers with diffuse type HCC (Fig. 1-10) represent portal spread of HCC within a short time (Fig. 1-11); none of six such patients lived more than 7 weeks.[15] In the absence of portal spread, the clinical course of HCC in a cirrhotic liver is relatively slow, particularly if the HCC is encapsulated.[16] In the preterminal stage of the disease, the patient's condition may acutely deteriorate with a sudden sharp elevation of serum alanine aminotransferase (ALT) levels. It is due to ischemic necrosis of liver parenchyma as a result

TABLE 1-3. Size of Main HCC at Autopsy[14]

Main Tumor Size (cm)	No.	%
<1.9	55	7.7
2.0–4.9	174	24.3
5.0–9.9	245	34.2
10–14.9	116	16.2
15–19.9	55	7.7
20–24.9	18	2.5
<25	53	7.4
Total	716	

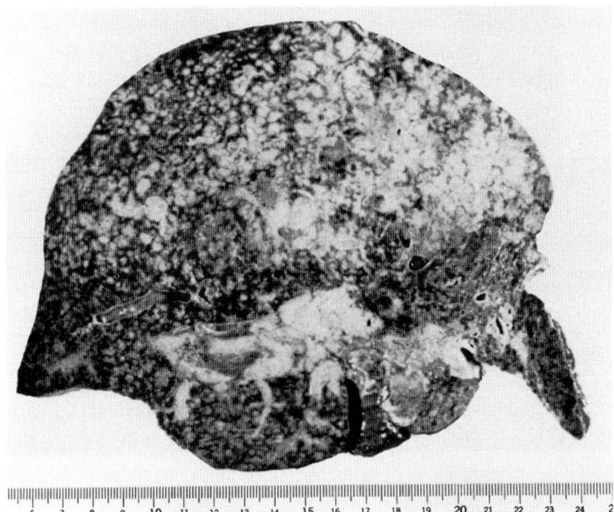

FIGURE 1-10. Diffuse type HCC. Numerous small cancer lesions are scattered throughout the liver as a result of intrahepatic portal spread. The clinical course was very rapidly downhill (see Fig. 1-11).

of portal hypotension in the presence of portal tumor thrombosis.[19] The patient in a terminal stage may complain of sudden dyspnea on changing the posture; this could be the sign associated with tumor growth into the right atrium from the vena cava.[8] There are only a few

TABLE 1-4. Cause of Death in HCC Patients[14]

Cause	No.	%
"Cancer death"	1,432	46.3
Hepatic failure	1,025	33.2
Tumor rupture	237	7.7
Variceal bleeding	195	6.3
G.I. bleeding	121	3.9
Operative death	82	2.7
Other cause	242	7.8
Total	3,092	

reports of spontaneous regression of HCC.[17,18] Considering the large number of HCCs as the denominator, spontaneous cure is totally unexpected even though the tumor sometimes undergoes necrosis.

After successful treatment, the patient's condition becomes stabilized, but if it deteriorates acutely, tumor recurrence or multiple metastases should be suspected. More often, serum α-fetoprotein (AFP) levels rise in such a situation. Following portal vein invasion, increase in portal venous pressure, hence increase in spleen size may be expected. Portal occlusion does not occur quickly, however, so it is not diagnosed clinically without imaging. Acute increase in serum bilirubin should arouse suspicion of intraductal invasion. Several paraneoplastic

FIGURE 1-11. The clinical course of a 54-year-old man who was admitted because of jaundice and ascites. The acute elevation of SGOT and SGPT levels was due to ischemic necrosis of the parenchyma secondary to portal vein occlusion and lowered blood pressure. (From Okuda,[1] with permission.)

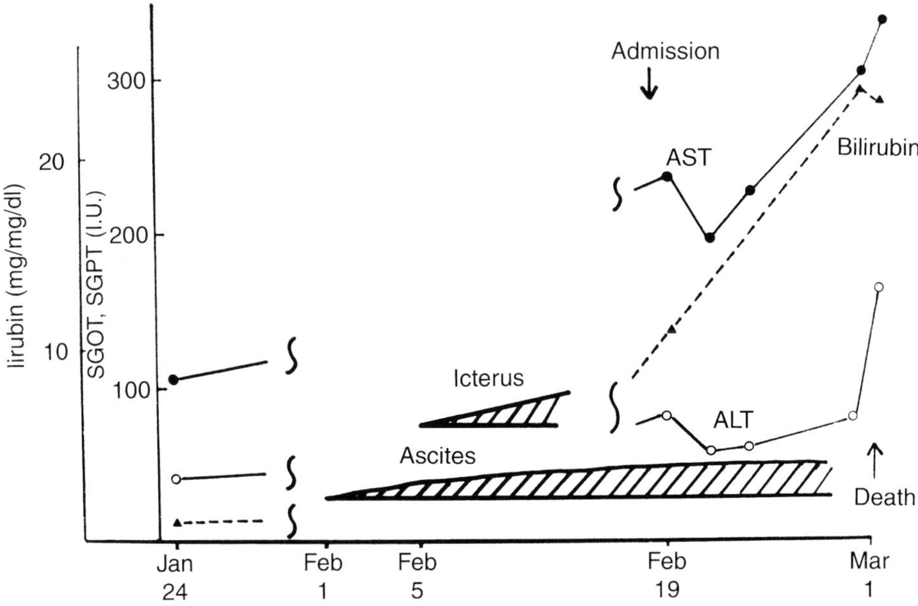

syndromes are known in association with HCC, such as hypoglycemia, polycythemia, and feminization, as discussed elsewhere in Chapter 20.

PROGNOSIS

When Primack et al.[20] analyzed 72 untreated patients with HCC in Uganda in the early 1970s, only 30% of patients were alive at one month (Fig. 1-12). Serum bilirubin greater than 2 mg/dl and weight loss greater than 25% of body weight were the poorest prognostic features. With better medical facilities in Hong Kong, the diagnosis may have been made earlier, yet the median survival of 104 untreated patients seen in the late 1970s was 3.5 weeks.[21] These figures are similar to the survival of untreated Okuda's stage 3 patients in Japan[22] and Spain.[23] In other words, patients with advanced HCC live on average only 1 month from the time of diagnosis, regardless of the geographic region. The median survival of untreated stage 1 patients was 8 months in Japan[22] (Fig. 1-13) and 12.8 months in Spain.[23] Prognosis is correlated with the stage of disease as shown in this figure, but is also correlated with the Child's score, because the majority of patients have cirrhosis.[13,23,24] Other factors that have been reported to be of predictive value include serum AFP values, age, tumor size, number of tumors, portal invasion, bilirubin, ascites, and presence of metastases.[13,14,24–26]

OTHER PRIMARY LIVER CANCERS INCLUDING VARIANT HCC

Fibrolamellar Carcinoma

Fibrolamellar carcinoma[27] is a variant of HCC that primarily affects young adults. It is relatively common among whites, accounting for 40% of HCC cases in those younger than 35 years,[28] but is nearly nonexistent in Asia. The presentation is not much different from that of HCC, but intrahepatic and extrahepatic metastases are relatively late events, accounting for its better prognosis. Successful resection affords more than 5 years of disease-free living in 25% of patients.[29] The early observation of high vitamin B_{12} levels in blood led to the subsequent elucidation of production of transcobalamin-1 by this variant of HCC.[30]

Sclerosing Hepatic Carcinoma

Sclerosing hepatic carcinoma, another variant of HCC, consists of abundant fibrosis and an epithelial component that is ductlike but has eosinophilic cytoplasm. It occurs in 3% to 4% of primary liver malignancies[31] (Fig. 1-14). It is often (70%) associated with hypercalcemia,[31,32] and patients often have drowsiness and lethargy.

Cholangiocarcinoma

Cholangiocarcinoma may be divided into the peripheral and hilar types based on differences in clinical presentation and course.[33] In the hilar type, obstructive jaundice is usually the first presentation. Klatskin[34] emphasized the exaggerated clinical signs for the small size of the mass and observed that palliation usually occurs with biliary drainage. Hilar carcinoma may be included in primary liver cancer.[35] Because of obstruction, biliary infection commonly occurs and, if not managed well, adversely affects the clinical course, shortening the life span. Although jaundice is manageable with biliary drainage, the prognosis is usually poorer in the hilar type than in the peripheral type. Table 1-5 compares the initial symptoms and chief complaints on admission between the peripheral and hilar bile duct carcinoma. The clinical course of peripheral type cholangiocarcinoma is somewhat similar to HCC that is not associated with cirrhosis, but the tumor growth is relatively slow. The

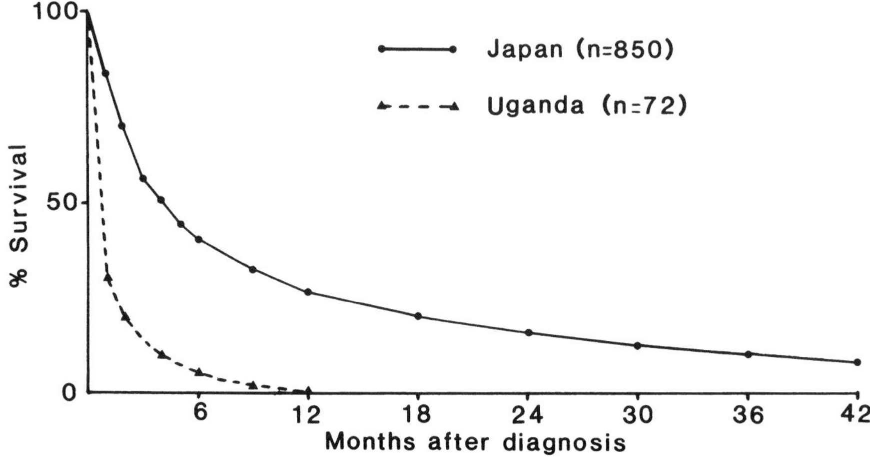

FIGURE 1-12. Life-table analysis of survival of patients with HCC in Uganda[19] and Japan.[21] The latter included patients of stages 1, 2, and 3, and the former perhaps only stage 3 patients. The survival curve for stage 3 patients in the Japanese series (see Fig. 1-13) is the same as that for the Ugandan patients.

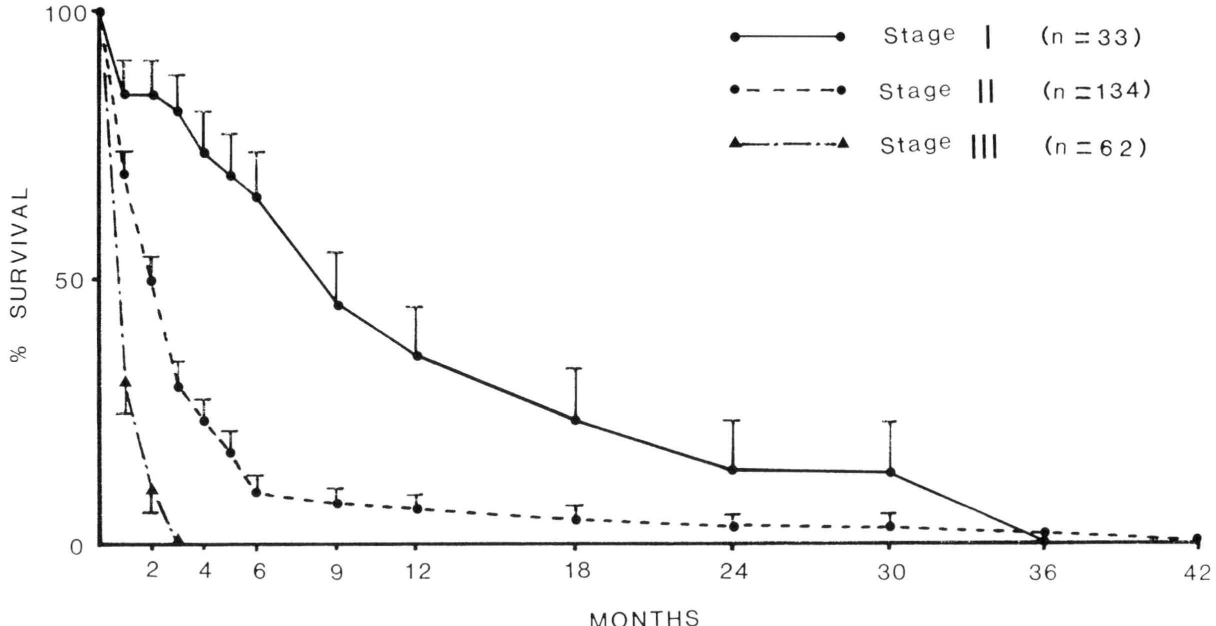

FIGURE 1-13. The actuarial survival curves for 229 HCC patients in Japan who did not receive specific treatment. The median survival of stage 3 patients was only 1 month, whereas that of stage 1 patients was 8 months. (From Okuda,[22] with permission.)

overall survival in 57 cases of intrahepatic bile duct carcinoma was 6.5 months (range of 1 to 44.5 months).[33] If biliary drainage is carried out effectively, the patient with hilar carcinoma can live quite long. In our series, two such patients lived for more than 2 years. Lymphatic metastasis is more frequent in the hilar carcinoma than in HCC, and distant metastasis is more common with the peripheral type because of the longer survival rate.[36]

Combined Hepatocholangiocarcinoma

Combined hepatocholangiocarcinoma is an uncommon cancer in which histologic components of both HCC and cholangiocarcinoma coexist. It comprises 2% of primary liver malignancies in Japan.[37] The clinical presentation and subsequent course are more like those of HCC than cholangiocarcinoma, although features of both cancers are recognizable. Depending on the site of the cholangiocarcinoma component, the disease may behave like cholangiocarcinoma, with more frequent jaundice than in HCC. However, cirrhosis frequently precedes the disease with edema, ascites and gastrointestinal bleeding (Table 1-6), serologic markers of the hepatitis B virus,[38] and elevated AFP levels (which are usually lower than in HCC).[37] Thus, the diagnosis of combined hepatocholangiocarcinoma is difficult to make without imaging and biopsy.

Hepatoblastoma

Hepatoblastoma is primarily a tumor of young children and occurs only rarely in adults.[39] The presenting symptom is usually an enlarging abdomen. The patient has anorexia, weight loss, nausea, and vomiting and may complain of abdominal pain. Jaundice is uncommon. Physical examination shows a firm, large right upper abdominal mass of irregular surface that extends to the left and down to the pelvic brim. Some patients exhibit a paraneoplastic syndrome such as precocious puberty with genital enlargement, pubic hair, and deepening voice, due to increased levels of serum and urinary human chorionic gonadotropin produced by the tumor. Some tumors also produce cystathionine with increased urinary excretion.

The tumor is usually solitary and therefore amenable to surgical resection. Even though the mass may occupy nearly the entire liver, the remaining parenchyma may support life. In about half of patients, however, the diagnosis is delayed, and the tumor is unresectable, or operative morbidity is high.[40] Some recommend preoperative chemotherapy to reduce the tumor size and make resection possible.

The prognosis largely depends on the resectability and histologic type of the tumor. Long-term survival ranges from 15% to 37%.[40] Children with the pure fetal cell histologic type of hepatoblastoma, in whom resec-

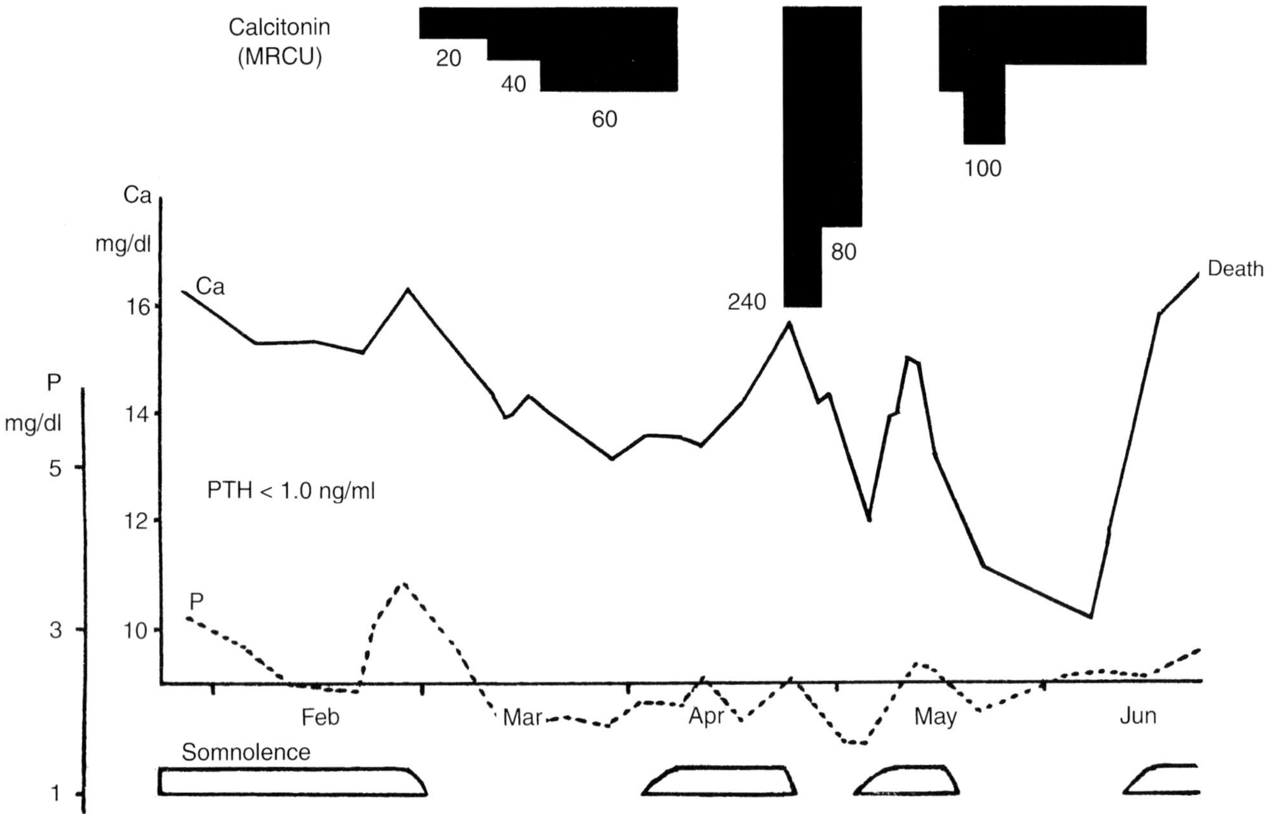

FIGURE 1-14. Clinical course of a 51-year-old woman who presented with drowsiness and hepatomegaly. Autopsy showed a whitish firm "sclerosing" type HCC with marked fibrous tissue and malignant epithelial cells. P, phosphorus; PTH, parathyroid hormone.

TABLE 1-5. Early Symptoms in 57 Cases of Intrahepatic Bile Duct Carcinoma[33]

	Number of Patients with Symptoms Initial Symptom		Number of Patients with Symptoms Chief Complaint on Admission	
Symptom	Peripheral Type (n = 28)	Hilar Type (n = 29)	Peripheral Type (n = 28)	Hilar Type (n = 29)
Abdominal pain	10	0	15	7
General malaise	7	13	1	8
Jaundice	5	10	10	23
Anorexia	8	5	1	4
Pruritus	0	3	1	2
Fever	0	3	6	4
Abdominal mass	0	3	0	2
Nausea	2	0		
Weight loss	2	0	1	1
Change in bowel movements	1	1		
Abdominal distention and fullness			3	4

TABLE 1-6. Comparison of Initial Symptoms and Signs Between HCC, Cholangiocarcinoma, and Combined Hepatocholangiocarcinoma[a]

Initial Symptoms	HCC (n = 2,502)	Cholangiocarcinoma (n = 133)	Combined form (n = 20)
Abdominal pain	45%	55%	62%
Abdominal fullness	43	35	40
Palpable mass	22	21	20
Anorexia	44	54	40
General malaise	59	55	40
Weight loss	26	36	50
Jaundice	15	32	27
Fever	15	26	17
Nausea, vomiting	15	17	10
Edema	14	1	8
Ascites	23	9	25
Hematemesis, melena	5	3	17

[a] Primary Liver Cancer Study Group of Japan, Report 9 (1986–1987).

tion was successfully carried out, have the best prognosis. The anaplastic histologic type of hepatoblastoma is almost always fatal regardless of treatment.

Epithelioid Hemangioendothelioma

This recently characterized malignant tumor of the liver occurs more frequently in women.[41] The symptoms and signs include weakness, anorexia, nausea, vomiting, upper abdominal pain, jaundice, and hepatosplenomegaly. The growth of this tumor is slow. Metastasis occurs in 28%, but 12 of 17 patients reported by Ishak et al.[41] lived more than 3 years (range, 3 to 28 years; average, 9.8 years). In another series, 9 of 10 patients who underwent transplantation were alive 5 to 134 months after surgery.[42]

Sarcomas

Angiosarcoma is perhaps the most malignant of liver sarcomas.[43,44] Most patients die within 6 months of diagnosis. Kaposi's sarcoma in the liver is one of the complications of acquired immunodeficiency syndrome (AIDS), but the patient usually dies of other causes.[44] Embryonal rhabdomyosarcoma arises in the extrahepatic bile duct and may also involve the intrahepatic biliary system. It affects mostly children. The prognosis depends on the treatment, but a long period of survival after treatment has been reported. Embryonal sarcoma (undifferentiated sarcoma, malignant mesenchymoma) occurs more commonly in children between the ages of 6 to 10 years.[45] The prognosis is generally poor. Other sarcomas include primary malignant lymphoma of the liver, fibrosarcoma, and leiomyosarcoma.

REFERENCES

1. Berman C. Primary Carcinoma of the Liver. Lewis Co, London, 1951, pp. 49–59
2. Kew MC, Geddes EW. Hepatocellular carcinoma in rural southern African blacks. Medicine 1982;61:98–108
3. Okuda K, Suzuki N, Kubo Y, Obata H. Clinical aspects of hepatocellular carcinoma. In Thatcher N (ed): Advances in Medical Oncology, Research and Education. Pergamon, Oxford, 1979, pp. 133–140
4. Steiner PA. Cancer of the liver and cirrhosis in trans-Saharan Africa and the United States of America. Cancer 1960;13:1085–1166
5. Okuda K, Peters RL, Simson IW. Gross anatomical features of hepatocellular carcinoma from three disparate geographic areas. Proposal of new classification. Cancer 1984;54: 2165–2173
6. Nakashima T, Okuda K, Kojiro M et al. Pathology of hepatocellular carcinoma in Japan. 232 consecutive cases autopsied in ten years. Cancer 1983;51:863–877
7. Okuda K. The patient with a suspicious liver mass. In Terblanche T (ed): Hepatobiliary Malignancy. Edward Arnold, London, 1994, pp. 27–49
8. Okuda K. Clinical aspects of hepatocellular carcinoma—analysis of 134 cases. In Okuda K, Peters RL (eds): Hepatocellular Carcinoma. Wiley, New York, 1976, pp. 387–436
9. Ong GB, Chan PKW. Primary carcinoma of the liver. Surg Gynecol Obstet 1976;143:31–38
10. Okuda K, Kondo Y, Nakano M et al. Hepatocellular carcinoma presenting with pyrexia and leukocytosis: report of five cases. Hepatology 1991;13:695–700
11. Kojiro M, Kawabata K, Kawano Y et al. Hepatocellular carcinoma presenting as intrabile duct tumor growth. A clinicopathologic study of 24 cases. Cancer 1982;49:2144–2147

12. Sheu JC, Sung JL, Chen DS et al. Growth rate of asymptomatic hepatocellular carcinoma and its clinical implications. Gastroenterology 1985;89:259–266
13. Barbara L, Benzi G, Galani S et al. Natural history of small untreated hepatocellular carcinoma in cirrhosis: a multivariate analysis of prognostic factors of tumor growth rate and patient survival. Hepatology 1992;16:132–137
14. Liver Cancer Study Group of Japan. Survey and follow-up of primary liver cancer in Japan—Report 11. Shinko Press, Kyoto, 1992
15. Okuda K, Noguchi T, Kubo Y et al. A clinical and pathological study of diffuse type hepatocellular carcinoma. Liver 1981;1:280–289
16. Okuda K, Musha H, Nakajima Y et al. Clinicopathological features of encapsulated hepatocellular carcinoma. Cancer 1977;40:1240–1245
17. Gottfried EB, Steller R, Paronetto F, Lieber CS. Spontaneous regression of hepatocellular carcinoma. Gastroenterology 1981;82:770–774
18. Gaffey MJ, Joyce JP, Carlson GS, Esteban JM. Spontaneous regression of hepatocellular carcinoma. Cancer 1990;65: 2779–2783
19. Okuda K, Musha H, Kanno H et al. Localized submassive liver cell necrosis as a terminal event of liver carcinoma. Cancer 1976;37:1965–1972
20. Primack A, Vogel CL, Kyalwazi SK et al. A staging system for hepatocellular carcinoma: prognostic factors in Ugandan patients. Cancer 1975;35:1357–1364
21. Lai CL, Lam KC, Wong KP et al. Clinical features of hepatocellular carcinoma: review of 211 patients in Hong Kong. Cancer 1981;47:2746–2755
22. Okuda K, Ohtuki T, Obata H et al. Natural history of hepatocellular carcinoma and prognosis in relation to treatment. Study of 850 patients. Cancer 1985;56:918–928
23. Calvet X, Bruix J, Bru C et al. Natural history of hepatocellular carcinoma in Spain. Five years' experience in 249 cases. J Hepatol 1990;10:311–317
24. Rosellini SR, Arienti V, Nanni O et al. Hepatocellular carcinoma. Prognostic factors and survival analysis in 135 Italian patients. J Hepatol 1992;16:6–72
25. Nomura F, Ohnishi K, Tanabe Y. Clinical features and prognosis of hepatocellular carcinoma with reference to serum alpha-fetoprotein levels. Analysis of 606 patients. Cancer 1989;64:1700–1707
26. Calvet X, Bruix J, Gines P et al. Prognostic factors of hepatocellular carcinoma in the West: a multivariate analysis in 206 patients. Hepatology 1990;12:753–760
27. Craig JR, Peters RL, Edmondson HA, Omata M. Fibrolamellar carcinoma of the liver: a tumor of adolescents and young adults with distinctive clinicopathologic features. Cancer 1980;46:372–279
28. Farhi DC, Shikes RH, Murari PJ, Silverberg SG. Hepatocellular carcinoma in young people. Cancer 1983;52: 1516–1525
29. Rolfes DB. Fibrolamellar carcinoma of the liver. In Okuda K, Ishak KG (eds): Neoplasms of the Liver. Springer, Tokyo, 1987, pp. 137–142
30. Waxman S, Gilbert HA. A tumor-related vitamin B_{12} binding protein in adolescent hepatoma. N Engl J Med 1973; 289:1053–1056
31. Craig JR, Peters RL, Edmondson HA. Tumors of the Liver and Intrahepatic Bile Ducts. Armed Forces Institute of Pathology, Washington DC, 1989, pp. 186–190
32. Omata M, Peters RL, Tatter D. Sclerosing hepatic carcinoma: relationship to hypercalcemia. Liver 1981;1:33–49
33. Okuda K, Kubo Y, Okazaki N et al. Clinical aspects of intrahepatic bile duct carcinoma including hilar carcinoma. A study of 57 autopsy-proven cases. Cancer 1977;39:232–246
34. Klatskin G. Adenocarcinoma of the hepatic duct at its bifurcation within the porta hepatis. An unusual tumor with distinctive clinical and pathological features. Am J Med 1965; 38:241–256
35. Edmondson HA, Steiner PE. Primary carcinoma of the liver. A study of 100 cases among 48,900 necropsies. Cancer 1954; 7:462–503
36. Sugihara S, Kojiro M. Pathology of cholangiocarcinoma. In Okuda K, Ishak KG (eds): Neoplasms of the Liver. Springer, Tokyo, 1987, pp. 143–158
37. Kojiro M, Nakashima T. Pathology of hepatocellular carcinoma. In Okuda K, Ishak KG (eds): Neoplasms of the Liver. Springer, Tokyo, 1987, pp. 81–104
38. Tomimatsu M, Ishiguro N, Taniai M et al. Hepatitis C virus antibody in patients with primary liver cancer (hepatocellular carcinoma, cholangiocarcinoma, and combined hepatocellular-cholangiocarcinoma) in Japan. Cancer 1993;72: 693–698
39. Okuda K, Liver Cancer Study Group of Japan. Primary liver cancers in Japan. Cancer 1980;45:2663–2669
40. Stocker JT, Ishak KG. Hepatoblastoma. In Okuda K, Ishak KG (eds): Neoplasms of the Liver. Springer, Tokyo, 1987, pp. 127–136
41. Ishak KG, Sesterhenn IA, Goodman ZD et al. Epithelioid hemangioendothelioma of the liver: a clinicopathologic and follow-up study of 32 cases. Hum Pathol 1984;15:839–852
42. Kelleher MB, Iwatsuki S, Sheahan DG. Epithelioid hemangioendothelioma of liver: clinicopathologic correlation of 10 cases treated by orthotopic liver transplantation. Am J Surg Pathol 1989;13:999–1008
43. Ishak KG. Mesenchymal tumors of the liver. In Okuda K, Peters RL (eds): Hepatocellular Carcinoma. New York, Wiley, 1976, pp. 247–307
44. Ishak KG. Malignant mesenchymal tumors of the liver. In Okuda K, Ishak KG (eds): Neoplasms of the Liver. Springer, Tokyo, 1987, pp. 159–176
45. Stocker JT, Ishak KG. Undifferentiated embryonal sarcoma of the liver. Cancer 1978;42:336–348

2

GLOBAL EPIDEMIOLOGY OF HEPATOCELLULAR CARCINOMA

F. XAVIER BOSCH

LIVER CANCER IN THE WORLD

Progress has been made at the international level in recording cases of liver cancer and in the identification of several of the key risk factors. The recognition of the role played by chronic hepatitis B virus (HBV) infections and the development of safe and highly immunogenic HBV vaccines led to the recommendation in the early 1980s to vaccinate all newborns regardless of the country of birth and the HBV status of the mother.[1,2] When HBV vaccination becomes universally applied, it should contribute to a reduction in cases of liver cancer in Africa and Asia. In low-risk countries in Europe and the Americas, HBV vaccination may have an impact in reducing acute and chronic liver disease but will have no direct effect on cases of liver cancer related to HCV and alcohol.

This chapter reviews the available data on cancer incidence and mortality and generally discusses its variations in occurrence in terms of the distribution of some of the risk factors in different populations. Unless otherwise specified, the term *liver cancer* is used throughout the text and largely corresponds (80% to 85%) to the histopathologic diagnosis of hepatocellular carcinoma (HCC). This oversimplification is necessary because cancer registries and mortality statistics do not usually report on histologic types. The code "liver" (ICD 9th: 155) used in the Cancer Registry data corresponds to malignant neoplasms of the liver and intrahepatic bile ducts.

ESTIMATED NUMBER OF CASES

It has been estimated that in 1985, some 315,000 new cases of primary liver cancer became apparent worldwide, accounting for 4.1% of all human cancer cases. In the same year, 312,000 patients died as a consequence of the disease. Both estimates, however, are strikingly different when analyzed by sex and geographic area. Among men, the estimated incidence is close to 214,000 cases (5.6% of all cancer cases) and among women it is 101,000 cases (2.7% of all cancers). The largest concentration of cases is found in Asia; these represent 70% of all liver cancer cases in the world (154,000 cases of liver cancer in Asia in men and 64,600 cases in women). China accounts for close to 100,000 cases in men and 40,000 cases among women. Japan accounts for close to 23,000 cases per year. As a continent, Africa is second in terms of number of cases, accounting for 26,000 cases among men and 11,600 among women.

In North America (based on data from the United States and Canada) close to 7,000 cases per year occur; there are 30,000 cases in Europe and 12,000 cases in the

This chapter is dedicated to the memory of the late Calum S. Muir (1930–1995), who inspired most of the current knowledge on geographic variation in cancer incidence.

countries of the former Soviet Union. Australia, New Zealand, and the Pacific Islands account for fewer than 1,000 cases per year (estimated 500 cases among men and 200 among women).

In terms of relative frequencies over the estimated total number of cancer cases, liver cancer ranks eighth in frequency in the world, sixth among men and eleventh among women. The ranking of the proportions hold true if colon and rectum cases are grouped together and mouth and pharynx are grouped together. However, if each primary site is taken separately, liver cancer would rank fifth (fourth in males), accounting for 4% to 5% of the global cancer burden, at the same level as colon cancer (4.6%), rectal cancer (4.3%), esophageal cancer (4.0%), and the lymphomas (4.2%). In the developing countries, liver cancer is, by all estimates, the third most common cancer among men after stomach and lung cancers.[3,4]

INCIDENCE RATES: STANDARDIZED CANCER REGISTRIES

Cancer incidence rates are useful parameters to establish estimates and comparisons of risk between populations of different sizes. Age adjustments further correct the estimates for the different age structures within populations and are widely used. However, the resulting age-adjusted incidence rates (AAIRs) are abstract values, heavily dependent on the standard population used to adjust. Using the world standard population, adjusted rates in developing countries become significantly higher than crude rates (i.e., in China estimated rates increase from a crude of 17.7 to an AAIR of 21.8 per 100,000). The opposite is true for the developed populations where the fraction of individuals in older age groups is high. For example, in Japan, the crude rates of 27.8 are reduced to an adjusted estimate of 22.9 per 100,000. Cumulative risk is another indicator that expresses the probability (in percent) of developing liver cancer up to a given age.

Tables 2-1 to 2-5 show the AAIRs and the cumulative risks to age 74 of liver cancer from standardized and internationally reviewed cancer registries.[5] National summaries have been computed for some countries by pooling the results from all available registries, keeping the age adjustment.

In Europe, relatively high incidence and mortality rates (AAIRs between 5 and 10 per 100,000 in men) are seen in certain areas of Switzerland, northern Italy, Rumania, Spain, Greece, and in certain regions of France and Poland. A threefold to sixfold North-South gradient is observed between the low-risk countries in the North and the high-risk areas in parts of central Europe and the Mediterranean basin.

In North America, the highest incidence rates (> 10 per 100,000 among men) are seen among migrants from high-risk countries, notably China and Korea. Incidence rates in blacks are about twice as high as those in whites. In Latin America, moderately high incidence rates (> 5 per 100,000 among men) are reported from Trujillo, Peru, and from French Martinique.

TABLE 2-1. Liver Cancer Registration in Europe (1982–1988)

	Age-Adjusted Incidence Rates		Cumulative Rate (0–74)	
Country	Males	Females	Males	Females
Belarus	4.34	1.96	0.58	0.25
Czechoslovakia[a]	5.74	2.40	0.72	0.28
Denmark	4.02	2.09	0.48	0.24
Estonia	4.29	1.62	0.56	0.21
Finland	4.71	2.32	0.58	0.25
France[b]	5.89	0.99	0.80	0.12
Germany[c]	3.94	1.53	0.51	0.18
Hungary[d]	4.13	1.59	0.55	0.21
Iceland	2.41	1.66	0.27	0.15
Ireland, Southern	1.07	0.95	0.14	0.11
Italy[e]	8.41	3.08	1.06	0.34
Latvia	3.08	1.50	0.40	0.19
Netherlands[f]	1.17	0.54	0.16	0.06
Norway	2.06	1.02	0.23	0.11
Poland[g]	5.15	3.62	0.63	0.42
Portugal, V N de Gaia	3.12	2.25	0.34	0.26
Romania, County Cluj	9.68	4.64	1.24	0.58
Russia, St. Petersburg	5.80	2.45	0.71	0.30
Slovenia	3.37	1.55	0.43	0.18
Spain[h]	5.78	2.46	0.72	0.24
Sweden	4.54	2.61	0.51	0.27
Switzerland[i]	6.26	1.49	0.74	0.18
UK, England, and Wales	1.71	0.84	0.20	0.09
UK, Scotland	2.94	1.15	0.35	0.12

[a] Bohemia and Moravia, Slovakia

[b] Bas-Rhin, Calvados, Doubs, Isère, Somme, Tarn

[c] GDR, Saarland

[d] Szabolcs, Vas

[e] Florence, Genoa, Latina, Varese, Parma, Ragusa, Romagna, Torino, Trieste

[f] Eindhoven, Maastricht

[g] Cracow City, Lower Silesia, Nowy Sacz, Opole, Warsaw City, Warsaw Rural

[h] Basque country, Tarragona, Granada, Murcia, Navarra, Zaragoza

[i] Basel, Geneva, Neuchatel, St Gall, Vaud, Zurich

TABLE 2-2. Liver Cancer Registration in Central and South America (1982–1989)

Country	Age-Adjusted Incidence Rate		Cumulative Incidence Rate (0–74)	
	Males	Females	Males	Females
Brazil (Goiania, Porto Alegre)	2.83	2.97	0.29	0.32
Colombia (Cali)	2.34	1.59	0.32	0.21
Costa Rica	3.98	2.58	0.45	0.28
Cuba	3.61	3.63	0.40	0.38
Ecuador (Quito)	3.13	4.10	0.32	0.54
Martinique	4.99	1.19	0.61	0.15
Paraguay (Asuncion)	1.08	1.50	0.11	0.19
Peru (Trujillo)	7.41	5.07	0.78	0.49
Puerto Rico	3.21	1.34	0.39	0.16

In Africa, very high rates (> 45 per 100,000 among men) are observed in some of the few cancer registries from the sub-Saharan countries, in contrast with low rates in the Mediterranean area of Setif, Algeria.

In Asia, the highest rates in the world (occasional AAIRs > 90 per 100,000 among men) have been observed in registries in the southeastern countries and in parts of China. In these large populations, viral hepatitis and related chronic diseases including liver cancer are common conditions and affect young age groups in both sexes.

INCIDENCE RATES: OTHER CANCER REGISTRIES

In addition to established cancer registries, developing registries have occasionally provided relevant data. From these, it is recognized that liver cancer is the most common cancer among men in Harare, Zimbabwe (AAIR = 34.6 in men and 19.2 in women),[6] in southwestern Zimbabwe (AAIR = 52.1 in men and 20.6 in women),[7] in Mozambique (AAIR = 112.9 in men and 30.8 in women),[8] and in Dakar, Senegal (AAIR = 25.6 in men).[9] Intermediate incidence rates have been reported from Uganda (AAIR = 7.5 in men)[10] and Ibadan, Nigeria (AAIR = 10.4 in men).[11]

TABLE 2-3. Liver Cancer Registration in Africa (1986–1989)

Country	Age-Adjusted Incidence Rate		Cumulative Incidence Rate (0–74)	
	Males	Females	Males	Females
Algeria (Setif)	3.87	5.49	—	—
The Gambia	36.00	12.11	—	—
Mali (Bamako)	47.91	21.45	5.60	2.56

TABLE 2-4. Liver Cancer Registration in North America (1983–1987)

Country	Age-Adjusted Incidence Rate		Cumulative Incidence Rate (0–74)	
	Males	Females	Males	Females
Bermuda	0.93	0.63	0.06	0.09
Canada	2.58	0.97	0.31	0.11
US, White[a]	2.39	1.02	0.28	0.11
US, Black[a]	4.85	1.58	0.62	0.18
US, Japanese[b]	5.86	2.42	0.76	0.27
US, Chinese[b]	11.68	3.76	1.25	0.48
US, Filipino[b]	6.25	2.04	0.60	0.25
US, Los Angeles: Spanish surname White	4.79	1.68	0.50	0.19
US, Los Angeles: Korean	20.06	3.92	1.90	0.42
US, Hawaii: Hawaiian	8.14	1.70	1.02	0.15
US, New York City	3.50	1.39	0.41	0.16

[a] SEER (Alameda, Bay Area, Connecticut, Atlanta, Hawaii, Iowa, Detroit, New Mexico, Utah, Seattle), Los Angeles, New Orleans

[b] Los Angeles, Hawaii

In Asia, two cancer registries in the Philippines (Manila and the province of Rizal) reported AAIR of 20.7 and 20.0 among men and 6.8 and 8.1 among women, respectively.[12] In Hanoi, Vietnam, the AAIRs were 14.0 among men and 3.7 among women.[13] Liver cancer is also relatively common in some less investigated areas, such as far eastern Siberia (AAIR = 14.9 in men and 8.0 in women).[14]

MORTALITY FROM LIVER CANCER

The mortality/incidence ratio reported by the cancer registries is close to or greater than 1, indicating that the majority of cases do not survive 1 year. This is confirmed by most clinical series, particularly in developing countries.

Mortality statistics on liver cancer have serious limi-

TABLE 2-5. Liver Cancer Registration in Asia (1983–1987) and Oceania (1986–1989)

Country	Age-Adjusted Incidence Rate		Cumulative Incidence Rate (0–74)	
	Males	Females	Males	Females
China (Qidong, Shanghai, Tianjin)	33.67	11.42	3.90	1.37
Hong Kong	39.25	9.65	4.55	1.12
India (Ahmedabad, Bangalore, Bombay, Madras)	2.77	1.28	0.33	0.14
Israel	2.85	1.23	0.34	0.14
Japan (Hiroshima, Miyagi, Nagasaki, Osaka, Saga, Yamagata)	32.79	8.00	4.07	0.97
Kuwait	9.36	3.35	1.17	0.38
Kyrgyzstan	8.39	4.44	1.06	0.54
Philippines (Manila, Rizal)	22.37	8.12	2.71	0.94
Singapore	23.48	6.81	2.93	0.79
Thailand (Chiang Mai, Khon Kaen)	42.81	19.18	5.13	2.33
Australia (Capital territory, New South Wales, South, Tasmania, Victoria, Western)	2.06	0.66	0.25	0.08
New Zealand	2.72	1.04	0.30	0.11

tations; a proportion of cases are reported as "liver cancer unspecified" and the coding recommendations concerning metastatic disease have changed from ICD 8 and ICD 9.[15,16] The probability of misclassifying primary liver cancer with liver metastasis is paradoxically high in developed countries where liver cancer is rare among patients presenting with a liver mass.

Wherever it is possible to examine mortality data, a similar pattern is seen. In Europe, relatively high rates (> 5.0 per 100,000) are seen in Italy, Spain, France, Switzerland, and some Eastern European countries. The highest mortality rates are seen in Greece (16.1 and 7.8 per 100,000 in men and women, respectively), a country without established cancer registries.

LIVER CANCER INCIDENCE: GLOBAL ESTIMATES FOR 24 AREAS IN THE WORLD

Worldwide estimates of AAIRs of liver cancer have been obtained by combining all available data on incidence, mortality, and relative frequencies by international region (Fig. 2-1 and 2-2).[3,17] The areas at higher risk are the coastal areas of South East Asia, China, Japan, the sub-Saharan African countries, and Melanesia. Areas at intermediate risk are the northern Mediterranean countries and the lowest risk are recorded in countries in northern Europe, most of the Americas and Australia.

VARIABILITY IN THE INCIDENCE OF LIVER CANCER WITHIN HOMOGENEOUS POPULATIONS

In Europe, twofold to fourfold differences in AAIR are observed in France, Italy, Switzerland, and Spain (Fig. 2-3). These ranges are observed in both sexes, although they tend to be of lesser amplitude among women. For example, the registry in Bas Rhin (northeast France) reports an AAIR of 8.90 among men in contrast with the registry in Tarn (southern France), which reports an equivalent AAIR of 2.21. The fourfold difference in men is paralleled by a moderate 2.5-fold difference in the AAIRs of liver cancer among women in the same registry. In Italy, the registry in Trieste (North East) reports AAIRs of 14.49 in men in contrast with the Registry in Florence (slightly south of Trieste), reporting an AAIR of 5.70. However, among women, the AAIRs are similar in both registries (2.45 in Trieste and 2.94 in Florence). The cancer registries in Romagna and Latina (both in central Italy) report similar AAIRs among men (6.56 and 6.27) and a threefold difference in AAIRs among women (1.52 and 4.72, respectively). Cancer registries in the United Kingdom report consistently low rates of liver cancer.

Some registries (but not all) report a high rate of histologic confirmation of the diagnosis (i.e., France, 65.3%; Italy, 40.4%; Spain, 40.5%; Switzerland, 85.4%). Likewise, coding and reporting of liver cancer in death certificates have been standardized at the national level in the period considered by most of the data summarized

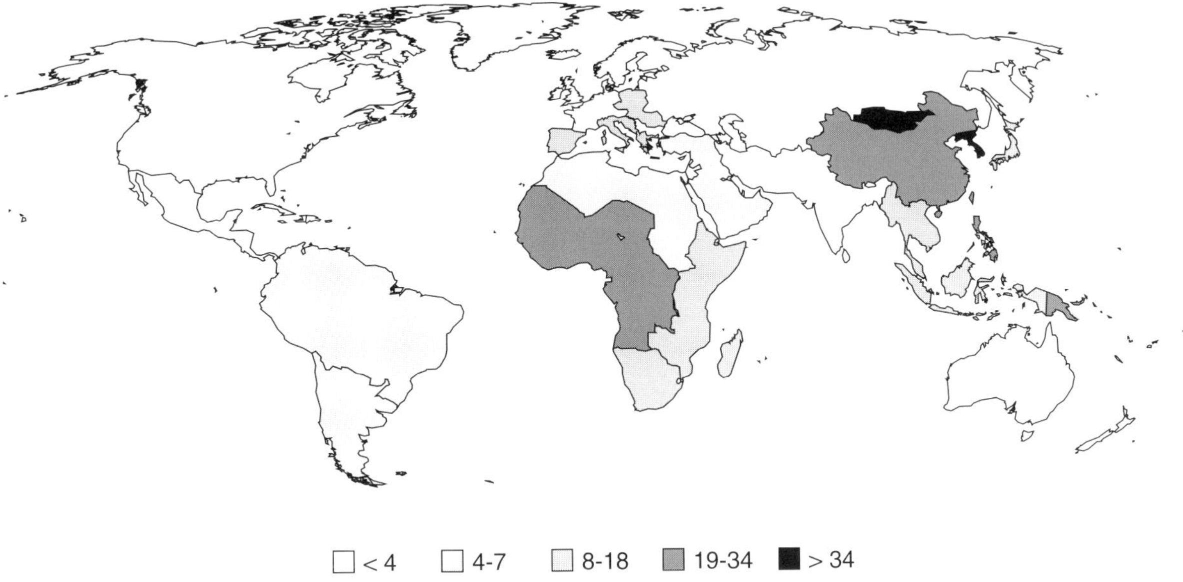

FIGURE 2-1. Age-adjusted incidence rates of liver cancer in men by world area.

here (1983–1987), and the registration practices have been centrally and independently reviewed. It seems likely that (1) differences in exposure to risk factors are capable of modulating the incidence of liver cancer even in fairly homogeneous populations in developed countries and (2) that these modifying factors affect men more than women.

In the United States, the range of AAIR among men is consistently wider than that observed among women (Fig. 2-4). In North America, the highest incidence rates are seen in migrants from high-risk countries, notably China and Korea (Table 2-4). Chinese in the United States show the widest range, reflecting perhaps their place of origin within China. However, rates are up to six-fold lower than the rates among Chinese in China (see scales in Figs. 2-3 and 2-4). For example, the highest rates observed among the male Chinese population in Los Angeles (14.65) are similar to the rates observed in the Italian population in Trieste (14.49) and close to those observed in Torino (10.44) or Varese (10.28). AAIRs among

FIGURE 2-2. Age-adjusted incidence rates of liver cancer in women by world area.

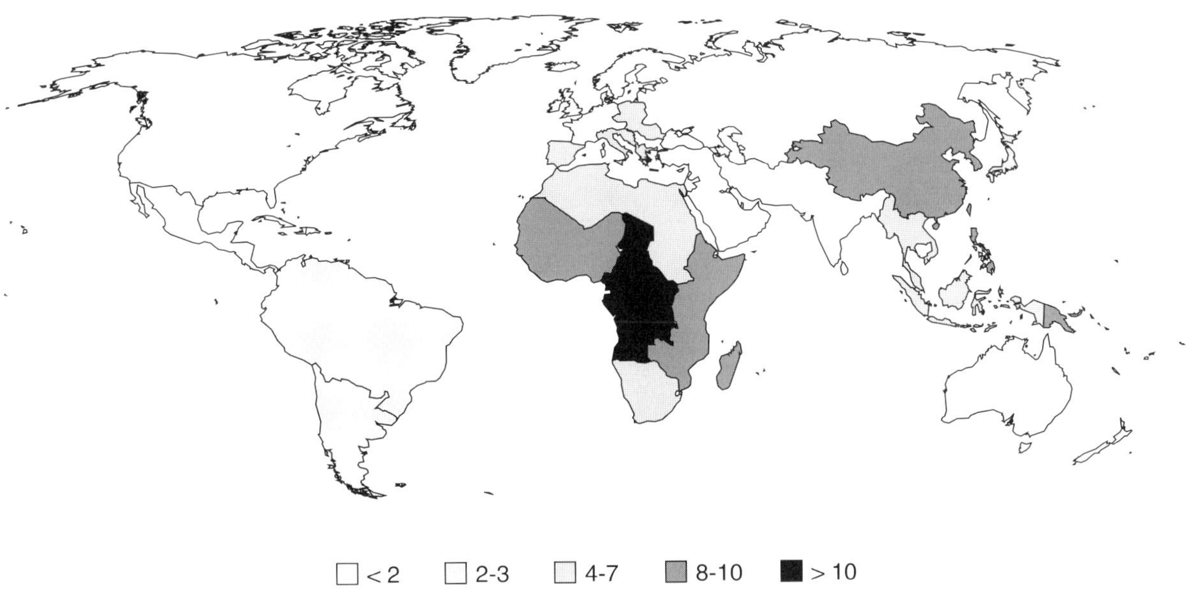

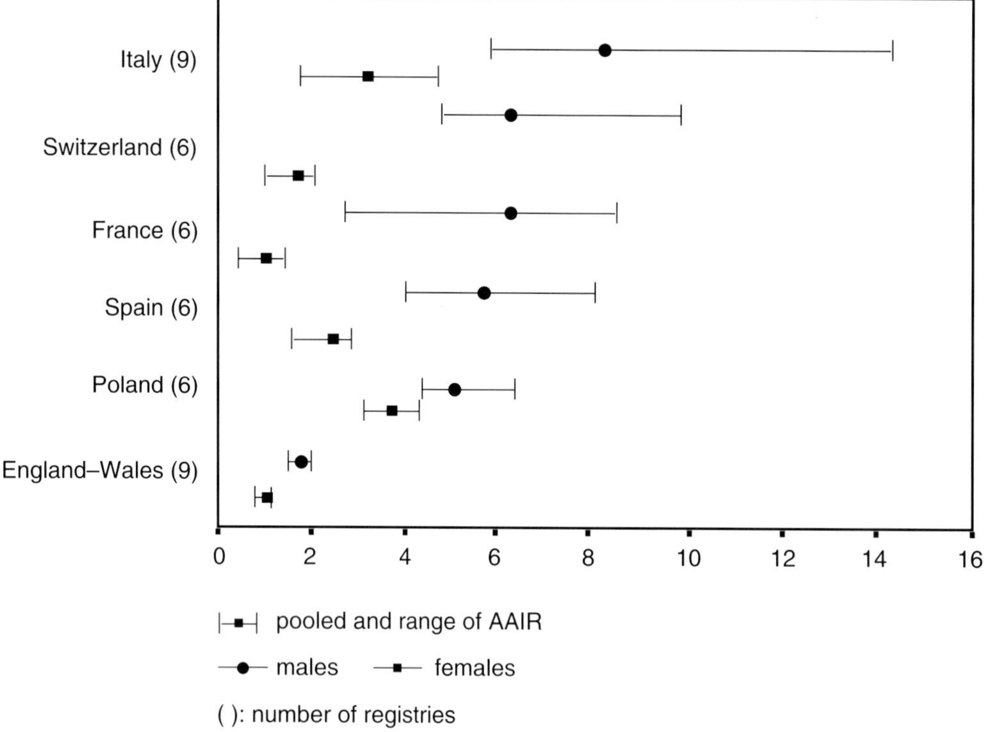

FIGURE 2-3. Age-adjusted incidence rates of liver cancer in six European countries, 1982–1988.

FIGURE 2-4. Age-adjusted incidence of liver cancer in the United States by ethnic group, 1983–1987.

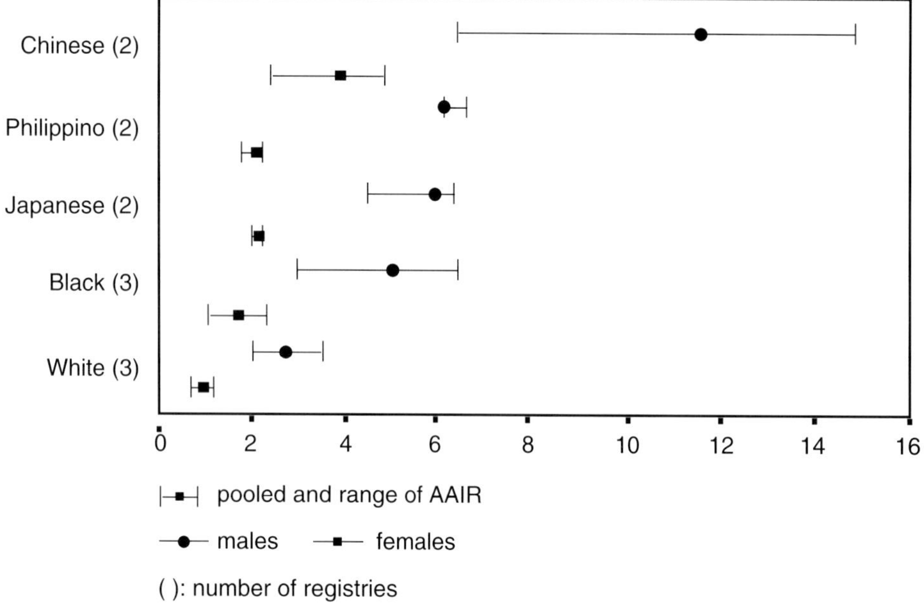

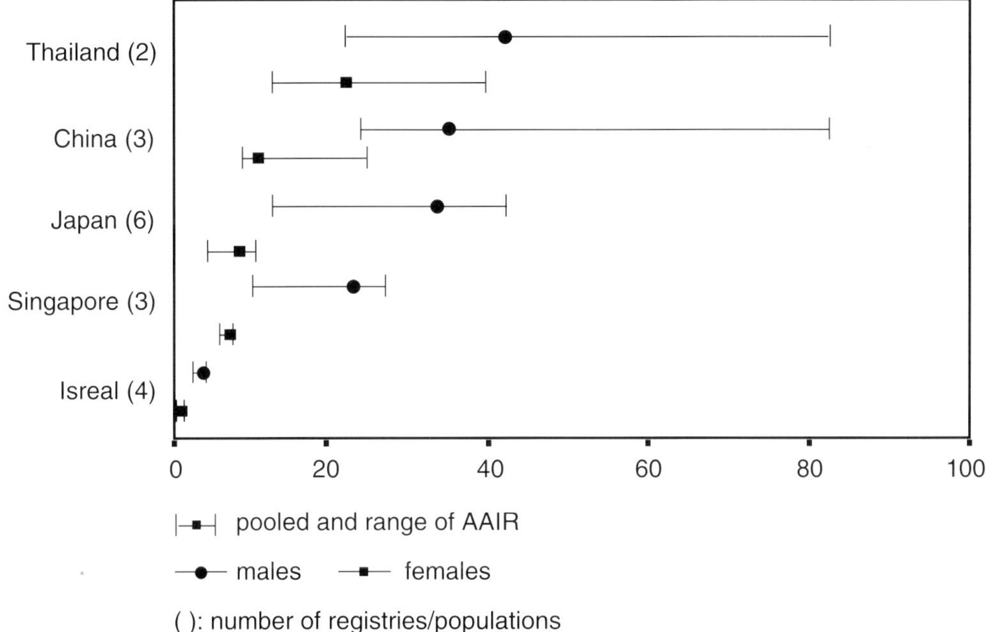

FIGURE 2-5. Age-adjusted incidence rates of liver cancer in five countries in Asia, 1983–1987.

Chinese men in China range from 23.61 to 89.92. This suggests that migrants from Asian countries retain rates of liver cancer higher than host populations but also that within the life span of one to three generations, the new environment can reduce significantly the occurrence of liver cancer.

There is variation by country reported by registries in Asia (Fig. 2-5). In Thailand, a fourfold to fivefold difference has been reported between the registry in Chiang Mai (AAIR in men = 19.76) in the far north and the registry in Khon Kaen in the not-so-distant northeast (AAIR in men = 90.01). More recent data (1988–1991) from these and a third new registry in Songkhla in the south indicate that the differences are still more pronounced (AAIR in males = 10.7 in Songkhla, 27.9 in Khon Kaen, and 94.8 in Chiang Mai).[18] The strong gradient in liver cancer in Thailand has been investigated extensively, which is largely attributable to the variation in the occurrence of cholangiocarcinoma. This rare tumor is in turn related to exposure to liver flukes, a fresh water parasite that is acquired by humans through dietary consumption of contaminated raw fish.[18,19]

In China, the marked geographic differences in liver cancer incidence have been correlated with differences in the prevalence of hepatitis B surface antigen (HBsAg) and to the consumption of moldy corn, which is interpreted as a surrogate marker of exposure to aflatoxin (AF). In a large study involving 65 counties, direct measurements of aflatoxin metabolites in urine did not correlate with liver cancer mortality, however.[20,21]

The internal variation observed in the Singapore Cancer Registry is related to the ethnic composition of the population. Chinese comprise 77% of the total population and display high rates of liver cancer (AAIR in men = 26.8) as compared to Malays (15% of the population) and Indians (6% of the population) who have incidence rates among men twofold to threefold lower (AAIR = 13.24 and 9.43, respectively).[5,22]

OTHER POPULATIONS OF EPIDEMIOLOGIC INTEREST

Eskimos

Eskimos constitute circumscribed populations. Studies among Eskimos were among the earliest to show (1) the high prevalence of HBV infections (55% exposure rates and 14% HBsAg carrier rates) and the intrafamilial clustering of HBV,[23] (2) the association of the HBV and liver cancer,[24] (3) the risk of liver cancer among HBsAg-positive persons,[25] (4) the value of screening those with HBsAg for early detection of liver cancers,[26] and (5) the efficacy of the new HBV vaccines.[27] Not all the evidence, however, is consistent. At least one early study among Eskimos in Greenland reported low incidence rates of liver cancer in a population with high HBsAg prevalence.[28] The observation deserves follow-up because Eskimos may represent one of the few populations in which hepatitis B virus is common, and exposure to aflatoxin in the diet is unlikely.

Drug Addicts

Intravenous drug addicts are exposed to multiple viral infections including HBV, hepatitis D virus (HdV), hepatitis C virus (HCV), human T-cell lymphotropic virus type I (HTLV-I), and human immunodeficiency virus (HIV). They are also often exposed to smoking and alcohol, potential liver carcinogens, as well as hepatotropic drugs. Some evidence of liver disease is frequent among most drug addicts, but an excess of liver cancer has not been reported.[29] Long-term follow-up of addicts who are carriers of several hepatotropic viruses may provide an opportunity to evaluate interactions among viruses in the origin of cirrhosis and liver cancer.

Immunosuppressed Transplantation Recipients and HIV Infected Patients

It has been postulated that immunosuppression is a risk factor for viral-related cancers. In a study involving more than 16,000 renal transplant recipients, a 30-fold increased risk over the expected rate for cancers of the hepatobiliary tract (OR = 30.4; 95% CI: 12.2, 62.6) was observed. The risk among transplant recipients was also increased for non-Hodgkin's lymphoma (OR = 32.0; 95% CI: 24.0, 42.1), cervical cancer (OR = 4.7; 95% CI: 1.9, 9.7), lung cancer (OR = 2.4; 95% CI: 1.2, 4.2), bladder cancer (OR = 5.5; 95% CI: 2.5, 10.5), malignant melanoma (OR = 3.9; 95% CI: 1.4, 8.5), and thyroid cancer (OR = 4.0; 95% CI: 1.1, 10.2).[30]

Patients who have been exposed to hemodialysis and probably received multiple transfusions may have an excess incidence of liver cancer and hepatitis. It is difficult to evaluate the independent contribution of immunosuppression to the observed excess of liver cancer over and above the expected excess attributable to HBV and HCV. Studies on HIV patients have not shown an excess of hepatocellular carcinoma, although other cancers have been found in excess.[31–33]

Migrant Populations

Several studies have shown that migrants from high- to low-risk countries for liver cancer retain the high rates of their country of origin. The finding has been reported among migrants to Australia from Asia, the Middle East, and Southern Europe[34] and migrants to the United Kingdom from Africa and the Caribbean[35] and to Israel from Africa and eastern Europe.[36]

West and central Africans migrating to France have a 2.5 to 6.6-fold increased risk of liver cancer compared to the French-born population.[37] Published reports on the mortality of Chinese populations migrating to either the United States, Canada, or Australia show a 3- to 11-fold excess of mortality due to liver cancer and a rapid decline in second generations.[38] These studies illustrate how HBV exposure acquired in infancy in the country of origin conveys a subsequent risk of liver cancer that is maintained for several decades after migration. Nevertheless, migration to a new environment with a lower prevalence of hepatitis viruses reduces the lifetime risk of liver cancer as additional births in the population escape infection. These studies will accumulate years of observation among descendants and will provide more reliable estimates of the decline in risk after migration.

TRENDS IN LIVER CANCER INCIDENCE

International variation in coding and registration practices for primary and secondary liver cancer makes difficult the interpretation of long-term time trends. In 96 cancer registries, two recent time intervals (1978 to 1982 and 1983 to 1986) have been chosen to evaluate trends while limiting the variability induced by registration and diagnostic practices (Table 2-6).[5,39] In Europe, an increase for both males and females in Scandinavia, notably in Norway and Finland, has been reported and partially attributed to an increase in the autopsy rate (with increased detection) and to an increase in alcohol consumption.[40] In Japan, there is a 15% to 20% increase in the recorded incidence of liver cancer, which is consistent for both sexes and across age groups. The increasing trend in Japan has been documented since the early 1970s[41] and has been largely attributed to massive exposure of the population to HCV through transfusion or contaminated needles in the early 1960s.[42] Other registries suggesting increasing trends include those in Australia, Canada (males), and several ethnic groups in the United States. Moderate increases, particularly among men, have been recorded in France, Italy, and some registries in the United Kingdom. A decrease in the liver cancer AAIRs has been reported in several registries in India, Israel, Spain, and Latin America.

AGE AND SEX DISTRIBUTION

In most developed countries, the incidence of liver cancer is very low before 40 years of age and increases progressively between ages 40 and 80 years. In high-risk areas in Africa and China, cases of HBV-related liver

TABLE 2-6. Percent Change in the Age-Adjusted Incidence Rates (AAIR) of Liver Cancer in Selected Countries in 1978–1986

Registries or Groups of Registries	Men			Women		
	AAIR 1978–82	AAIR 1983–86	% Change	AAIR 1978–82	AAIR 1983–86	% Change
Australia	1.57	2.06	31.21	0.52	0.66	26.92
Canada	2.08	2.58	24.04	1.04	0.97	−6.73
China	32.63	33.67	3.19	11.22	11.42	1.78
France	5.41	5.89	8.87	0.91	0.99	8.79
India	3.54	2.77	−21.75	1.94	1.28	−34.02
Israel	3.29	2.84	−13.68	1.80	1.22	−32.22
Italy	7.59	8.41	10.80	3.01	3.08	2.33
Japan	26.75	32.79	22.58	6.96	8.00	14.94
Spain	7.27	5.78	−20.50	4.89	2.46	−49.69
Switzerland	6.35	6.26	−1.42	1.55	1.49	−3.87
U.K.	1.76	1.85	5.11	0.85	0.88	3.53
US, white	2.33	2.63	12.88	1.05	1.02	−2.86
US, black	4.92	5.26	6.91	1.54	1.73	12.34
US, Japanese	5.31	5.86	10.36	1.75	2.42	38.29
Latin America	4.41	3.41	−22.68	2.39	2.27	−5.02
Scandinavian	3.87	3.99	3.10	2.17	2.16	−0.50

cancer may occur as early as 15 years of age (Figs. 2-6 and 2-7).

The registry in Qidong, China, shows a deviation from the general pattern, with very high rates in men at age 30, decreasing steadily after age 55. The male Chinese populations in urban Shanghai have lower rates before 65 and higher rates after age 70. The contrast between Qidong and Shanghai deserves further attention in subsequent reports from these registries. If this contrast is confirmed, it would suggest that different factors are affecting the occurrence of liver cancer in these two populations. Some time trend analyses from the registry in Shanghai indicate that the cancer incidence pattern is evolving toward a western model, including an overall decrease in the incidence of liver cancer in both sexes.[43] The Chinese population in Los Angeles had the lowest rates, with an age distribution closer to the model in Shanghai.

The registry in The Gambia, West Africa, shows increasing trends with age up to age 40 to 45 years and a plateau after age 50 among men. The registry in Mali does not show a plateau but rather a steady increase in incidence with age, suggesting that in these evolving health systems, underdiagnosis and reporting of liver cancer may be occurring, particularly in the older age groups.

In most developed countries, the average age at onset of HBV-related liver cancer is several years younger than that of HCV-related liver cancer.[44] In Japan, where HCV-related liver cancer cases now predominate, the average age at diagnosis of liver cancer has shifted from 57.8 years in the period from 1973 to 1977 to an average of 61.7 years in the period from 1983 to 1987 (calculated from references 5 and 9).

Rates are higher for males than for females in most populations, with male:female ratios (sex ratios) between 1.5 and 3.0. In high-risk countries, sex ratios tend to be higher, and the male excess is more pronounced around 40 to 50 years of age. In populations with low incidence rates, the sex ratio peak occurs at about 60 to 70 years of age. This difference is clearly illustrated by the peak in Japanese populations in Japan (45 years) and in Japanese populations migrating to the United States (65 years).[45]

Several factors probably contribute to the peculiar patterns of the age- and sex-specific incidence of liver cancer. Exposure to HBV in early life in high-risk countries (largely from infected mothers) may account for the early onset and rise in incidence, as well as the early occurrence of the male excess. Other risk factors, such as HCV, alcohol, oral contraceptives, and tobacco, may account in part for the late onset cancers, the progressive increase in incidence with age, and the later peak in the male excess.

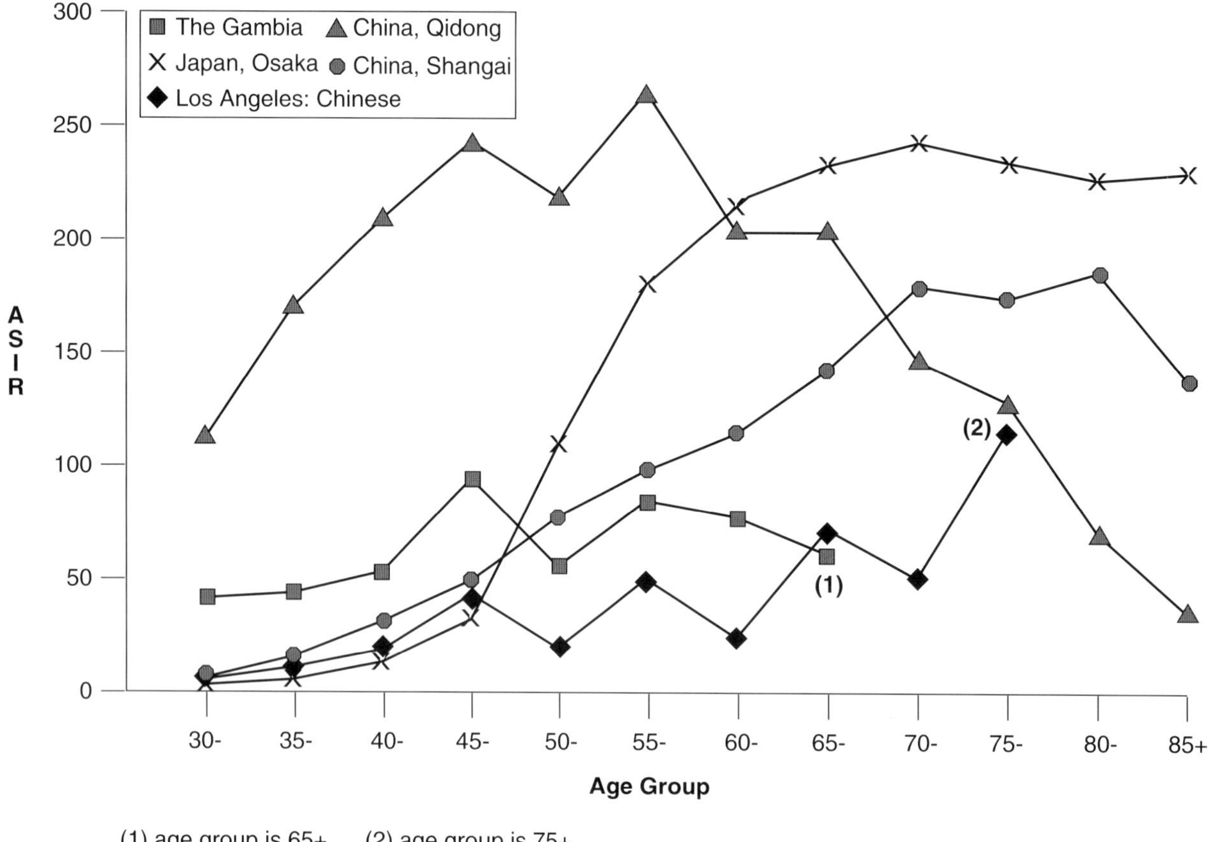

FIGURE 2-6. Age-specific incidence rates (ASIR) of liver cancer in men in selected populations.

CORRELATIONS OF LIVER CANCER INCIDENCE

Correlations of AAIRs between cancer sites have been explored to develop hypotheses about common risk factors. Correlation coefficients in men (CCm) and women (CCw) weighed by the size of each registry were computed using the data from the 157 registries (Tables 2-1 to 2-5).

Liver cancer incidence in men is strongly correlated with the incidence of esophageal cancer (CCm = 0.451 p = 0.000; CCw = 0.194, p = 0.015) and gastric cancers (CCm = 0.579, CCw = 0.570, p = 0.000) and negatively correlated with colorectal cancers in both sexes (CCm = −0.267, CCw = −0.303, p = 0.000), breast cancer in women (CCw = −0.506, p = 0.000) and cancer of the corpus uteri (CCw = −0.488, p = 0.000). The pattern is similar if the liver cancer incidence among women is taken as the reference.

Globally, risk factors for liver cancer are the same for both sexes, with remarkably little variation.[46] The correlation between liver cancer in males and females in 157 registries worldwide is extremely high (CC = 0.953, p = 0.000) as shown in Figure 2-8A. Correlations were also derived to explore consistency within more homogeneous populations (Fig. 2-8B). The association persisted, although the magnitude of the coefficients was reduced among populations of Caucasian ancestry (CC = 0.758, p = 0.000 corresponding to 70 cancer registries in North America and Europe) and in North America in black and white patients (partial CC white = 0.421, p = 0.056; partial CC black = 0.421, p = 0.018).[46]

In western industrial populations, the variability in the correlation is greater (reduced magnitude of the CC), suggesting an impact of sex-specific risk factors. Oral contraceptives in particular have been strongly related to liver cancer, and the association appears to be independent of the effect of HBV.[47,48] Alcohol and tobacco are risk factors to which men have been more exposed than women in most cultures. Their role as causal factors of liver cancer can explain the increased variability of the correlation between the sex-specific AAIRs among Caucasians (Fig. 2-8B) and the twofold to threefold male excess of liver cancer in all geographic areas.

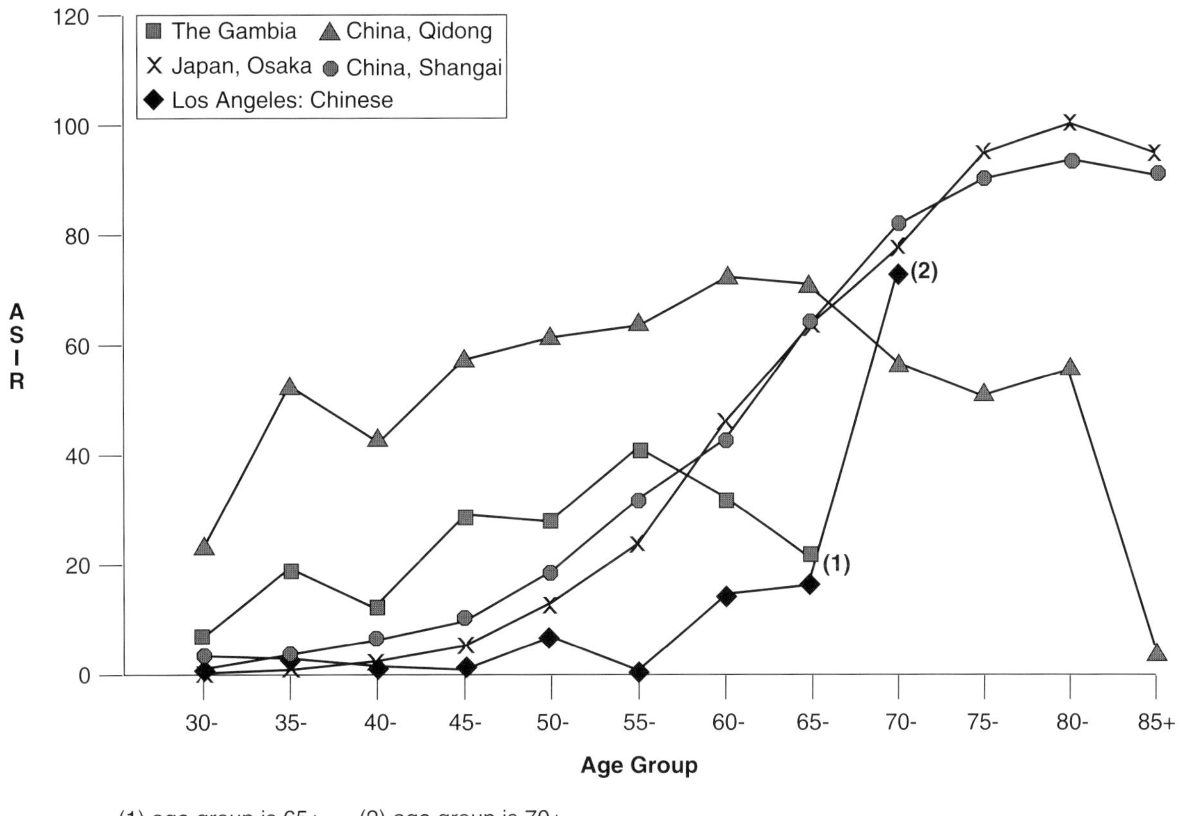

FIGURE 2-7. Age-specific incidence rates (ASIR) of liver cancer in women in populations.

SUMMARY OF RISK FACTORS AND CONSISTENCY WITH THE UNEVEN DISTRIBUTION OF LIVER CANCER

Viral Factors

In developed populations at low risk for liver cancer in the United States, Europe, and Japan, HBV and HCV may account for 70% to 75% of liver cancer cases. In high-risk countries in southeast Asia, China and sub-Saharan Africa, HBV is highly prevalent and responsible for more than 60% of the liver cancer cases. HCV may play a minor role in these areas, perhaps in fewer than 10% of cases (Table 2-7).

The majority of the epidemiologic studies on HBV and liver cancer have been conducted using the one-time detection of HBsAg by conventional radioimmunoassay as the marker of persistent HBV infection. These measurements may underestimate chronic HBV infection. Studies using polymerase chain reaction (PCR) methods to detect HBV DNA in serum or liver tissues and Southern blots investigating integrated HBV DNA have documented that some of the HCC tissues from HBsAg-negative HCC cases contained HBV DNA.[49–51] The probability of misclassification seems to be higher among alcoholics and drug addicts showing unusual HBV profiles.[29,52] Finally, HBV variants have been described that may escape the protection conferred by vaccine-induced antibodies. These variants theoretically could be related to some HCC cases erroneously labeled as unrelated to HBV.[53,54]

Likewise, tests to detect exposure to HCV have been in constant development since they were first reported in 1989.[55] HCV RNA detection by PCR can be intermittent, and repeated testing may be necessary.[56] Technical details in the definition of the cut-off values, length of storage, and preparation of the serum specimen may grossly distort the estimates of the attributable fractions.[57] Analysis of sequence variation allowed the description of at least six distinct genotypes of HCV,[58,59] with different geographic prevalences.[60,61]

Alcohol and Tobacco

Alcohol is a risk factor for cirrhosis and for liver cancer. In western countries, cirrhosis is viewed as a liver cancer precursor. Cigarette smoking has shown inconsistent as-

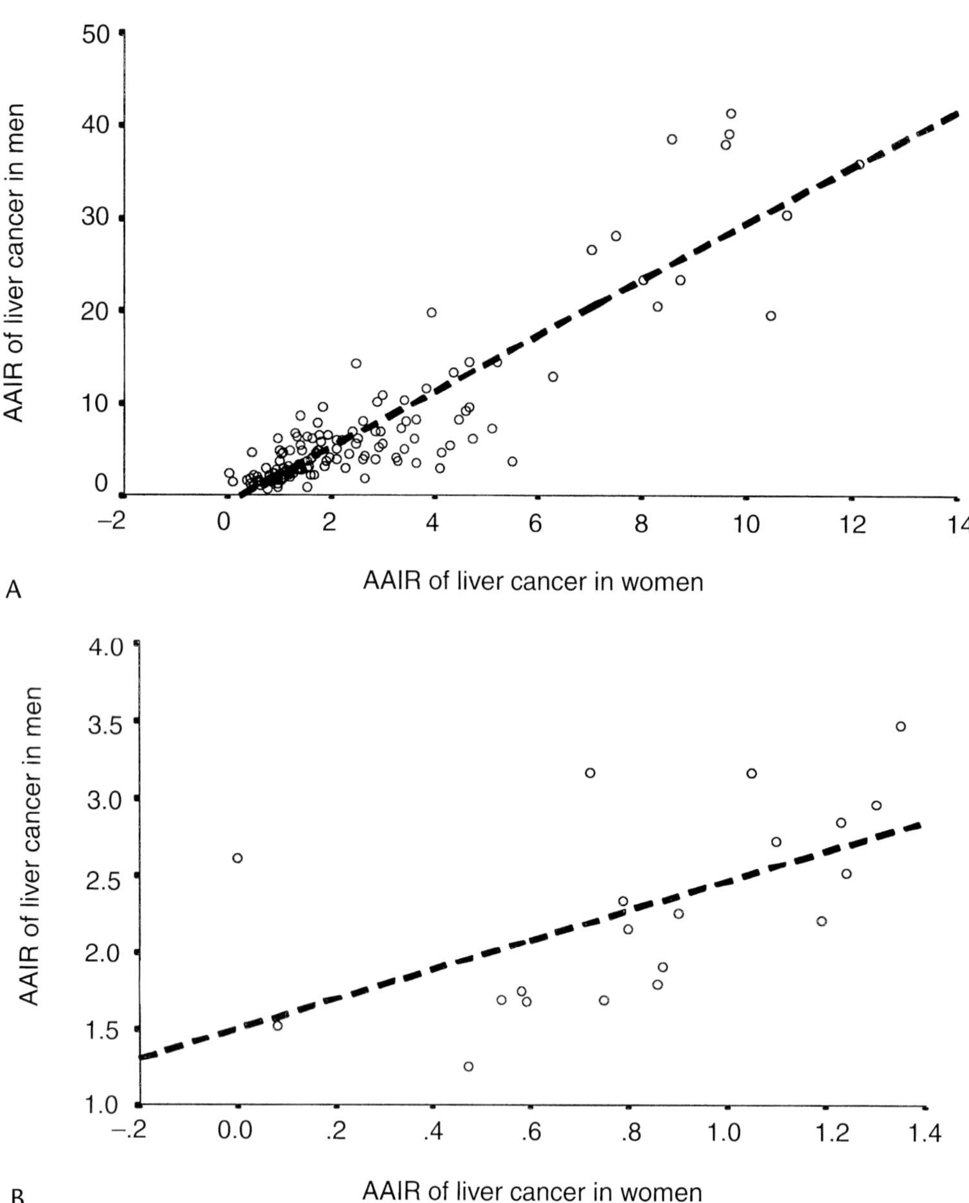

FIGURE 2-8. Correlation between the age-adjusted incidence rates of liver cancer (AIRR) in males and females. Correlation coefficient (CC) weighted by registry size (*A*) Data from 157 cancer registries. CC = 0.953; *P* = 0.000. (*B*) Data from 19 cancer registries (whites from United States and Canada). CC = 0.421; *P* = 0.056.

sociations with liver cancer. The associations of liver cancer with alcohol and tobacco are in the range of 1.2- to 2-fold.[62] The lack of a significant correlation between the AAIR of liver and lung cancers (CCm = −0.154, p = 0.054; CCw = −0.062, P = 0.443) suggests that cigarette smoking provides only a minor contribution to the geographic variation in the incidence of liver cancer.

Oral Contraceptives

Case-control studies in developed countries show a twofold to fivefold risk of liver cancer with oral contraceptive use.[47] In populations with widespread use and where HBV is rare, this may represent perhaps half of the liver cancer cases among women attributable to long-term use of oral contraceptives. This estimate is not entirely supported by the time trends in incidence (Table 2-6) or mortality[63,64] and suggest that oral contraceptives may act as a co-factor or a promoter of the carcinogenic process. The independence of oral contraceptives as a risk factor for HCC, although likely, has not been unequivocally assessed with regard to possible roles of HCV and HBV in the populations studied.

TABLE 2-7. Causal Factors of Liver Cancer and Estimates of the Attributable Fractions[46,62,63,73,74]

	Low Risk Countries in Europe and the US		Japan		High Risk Countries in Africa and Asia	
Factor	Estimate	Range	Estimate	Range	Estimate	Range
Hepatitis B Virus	<15%	4–50%	20%	18–44%	60%	40–90%
Hepatitis C Virus[a]	60%	12–64%	50%	40–80%	<10%	NE
Aflatoxin	limited exposure		limited exposure		important exposure[b]	
Alcohol	<15%[c]		<20%	11–30%	NE	
Tobacco	<12%[c]		40%	38–51%	NE	
Oral contraceptives		10–50%[d]	NE		NE	
Other	<5%				<5%	

[a] not including double infections with HBV and HCV. Very few studies available using second-generation assays.

[b] attributable risk not quantified.

[c] estimates for the US.

[d] restricted to liver cancer in women.

NE: nonevaluated.

Note: attributable fractions do not necessarily add to 100% because of multiple exposures and possible interactions between risk factors.

Aflatoxin

In Africa and some areas of China and southeast Asia, liver cancer incidence correlates with estimates of aflatoxin (AF) consumption at the population level.[65] However, lack of reliable techniques to assess individual exposure over long periods still limits our ability to quantify the risk. The presence of AF-specific mutations in the genome of liver cancer cells was suggested.[66] Liver cancer biopsies from patients in 14 countries showed that among 72 liver cancer specimens from South Africa and southeast Asia (assumed to have been exposed to AF), 12 (17%) showed a specific G to T mutation at codon 249 of the p53 gene. The mutation was not found in any of 95 liver cancer specimens from countries where AF exposure is rare. An additional analysis restricted to 27 HBV-exposed liver cancer patients from Mozambique showed that the frequency of the mutation was 53%, compared to 8% in patients from low-AF areas in the Transkei. The estimated food contamination levels with AF was four-fold higher in Mozambique.[67] Other reports indicated high rates (i.e., 50%) of the p53 codon 249 mutations in liver cancer specimens from Qidong, China,[68] and South Africa,[69] but lower frequencies were reported from Thailand, where AF contamination of foods has been documented.[70] As in many other cancer models, the genetic changes indicated a multistep process that is complex.[71]

A word of caution should be raised about these pioneer studies with regard to (1) their small sample size and limited methodology and (2) inadequate adjustment of the correlations for key risk factors, viral and nonviral, at an individual level.

Nevertheless, studies using these biologic markers may represent a real breakthrough in the field of liver cancer epidemiology. In particular, the genetic markers may help to quantify the role of AF as an independent cause of liver cancer and can be used to evaluate the likely interactions with the hepatitis viruses in humans as has been shown recently in the woodchuck model.[72]

ACKNOWLEDGMENTS

The author is grateful to Mireia Diaz (SERC) for assistance in the preparation of tables and graphs and to Montse Balagué (SERC) for the analysis of the correlations between cancer incidence rates.

Dr. Jaume Galceran (Tarragona Cancer Registry) assisted in the preparation of the maps and Pilar Martinez (SERC) helped in the edition of the manuscript.

This work has been partially supported by the Fondo de Investigacíon Sanitaria (FIS) of the Spanish Government (FIS 94/1635) and the Fundació August Pi i Sunyer (FAPS 1995).

REFERENCES

1. Prevention of Liver Cancer, Technical Report Series, vol 691. World Health Organization, Geneva, 1983
2. ACIP. Hepatitis B virus: a comprehensive strategy for eliminating transmission in the United States through universal childhood vaccination: recommendations of the Immunization Practices Advisory Committee. MMWR 1991;40:1–25

3. Parkin DM, Pisani P, Ferlay J. Estimates of the worldwide incidence of eighteen major cancers in 1985. Int J Cancer 1993;54:1–13
4. Pisani P, Parkin DM, Ferlay J. Estimates of the worldwide mortality from eighteen major cancers in 1985. Implications for prevention and projections of future burden. Int J Cancer 1993;55:891–903
5. Parkin DM, Muir CS, Whelan SL et al. Cancer incidence in five continents. Vol. VI. IARC Scientific Publications, Lyon, No. 120, 1992
6. Basset MT, Chokunonga E, Mauchaza B et al. Cancer in the African population of Harare, Zimbabwe, 1990–1992. Int J Cancer 1995; 63:29–36
7. Parkin DM, Vizcaino AP, Skinner MEG, Ndhlovu A. Cancer patterns and risk factors in the African population of Southwest Zimbabwe, 1963–1977. Cancer Epidemiol Biomarkers Prev 1994;3:537–547
8. Prates MD. Cancer incidence in Mozambique. Lourenço Marques 1956–1960. In Doll R, Payne P, Waterhouse J (eds): Cancer Incidence in Five Continents. A Technical Report. Geneva UICC, 1966
9. Waterhouse J, Muir C, Shanmugaratnam K et al (eds): Cancer Incidence in Five Continents, Vol. IV. International Agency for Research on Cancer, Lyon, 1982
10. Wabinga HR, Parkin DM, Wadwire-Mangen F, Mugerwa JW. Cancer in Kampala, Uganda, in 1989–91: changes in incidence in the era of AIDS. Int J Cancer 1993;54:26–36
11. Waterhouse J, Muir C, Correa P et al (eds): Cancer Incidence in Five Continents, Vol. III. International Agency for Research on Cancer, Lyon, 1976
12. Laudico AV, Esteban D, Parkin DM. Cancer in the Philippines. IARC Technical Report No. 5. International Agency for Research on Cancer, Lyon, 1989
13. Anh PTH, Parkin DM, Hanh NT, Duc NB. Cancer in the population of Hanoi, Vietnam, 1988–1990. Br J Cancer 1993;68: 1236–1242
14. Zaridze DG, Marochko A, Basieva T, Duffy SW. Cancer incidence in the native peoples of far eastern Siberia. Int J Cancer 1993;54:889–894
15. International Classification of Diseases, Eighth Revision, adapted for use in the United States. Public Health Service Publication No. 1693. Department of Health, Education and Welfare, Washington, DC, 1967
16. International Classification of Diseases, 9th Revision, Clinical Modification. DHHS No. (PHS) 80–1260), Department of Health and Human Services, Washington, DC, 1979
17. United Nations. World population prospects 1990. UN Department of International Economic and Social Affairs, New York, 1991
18. Vatanasapt V, Martin N, Sriplung H et al. Cancer incidence in Thailand, 1988–1991. Cancer Epidemiol Biomarkers Prev 1995;4:475–483
19. Parkin DM, Srivatanakul P, Khlat M et al. Liver cancer in Thailand. I. A case-control study of cholangiocarcinoma. Int J Cancer 1991;48:323–328
20. Junshi C, Campbell TC, Junyao L et al (eds): Diet, life-style and mortality in China. A study of the characteristics of 65 Chinese counties. Oxford University Press, Oxford, 1990
21. Hsing AW, Guo W, Chen J et al. Correlates of liver cancer mortality in China. Int J Epidemiol 1991;20:54–59
22. Lee HP, Day NE, Shanmugaratnam K (eds): Trends in cancer incidence in Singapore, 1968–1982. IARC Scientific Publications No. 91. International Agency for Research on Cancer, Lyon, 1988
23. Barrett DH, Burks JM, McMahon B et al. Epidemiology of hepatitis B in two Alaskan communities. Am J Epidemiol 1977;105:118–122
24. Lanier AP, McMahon BJ, Alberts SR et al. Primary liver cancer in Alaskan natives, 1980–1985. Cancer 1987;60: 1915–1920
25. McMahon BJ, Alberts SR, Wainwright RB et al. Prospective study in 1400 hepatitis B surface antigen-positive Alaska native carriers. Arch Intern Med 1990;150:1051–1054
26. McMahon BJ, Wainwright RW, Lanier AP. The Alaska native HCC screening program: a population-based screening program for hepatocellular carcinoma. In Tabor E, Di Bisceglie AM, Purcell RH (eds): Etiology, Pathology, and Treatment of Hepatocellular Carcinoma in North America. Portfolio, The Woodlands, Texas, 1991, pp. 231–242
27. McMahon BJ, Rhoades ER, Heyward WL et al. A comprehensive programme to reduce the incidence of hepatitis B virus infections and its sequelae in Alaskan natives. Lancet 1987;2:1134–1136
28. Melbye M, Skinhoj P, Nieisen NH et al. Virus-associated cancers in Greenland: frequent hepatitis B virus infection but low primary hepatocellular carcinoma incidence. J Natl Cancer Inst 1984;73:1267
29. Levine OS, Vlahov D, Nelson KE. Epidemiology of hepatitis B virus infections among injecting drug users: seroprevalence, risk factors, and viral interactions. Epidemiol Rev 1994;16:418–436
30. Fraumeni JF, Hoover R. Immunosurveillance and cancer: epidemiologic observations. Epidemiology and Cancer Registries in the Pacific Basin (National Cancer Institute Monograph, No. 47). National Cancer Institute, 1977
31. Rabkin CS, Blattner WA. HIV infection and cancers other than non-Hodgkin's lymphoma and Kaposi's sarcoma. In Veral V, Jaffe HW, Weiss RA, Franks LM (eds): Cancer, HIV and AIDS. Cancer Surveys, Vol. 10. The Imperial Cancer Research Fund, Cold Spring Harbor Laboratory Press, 1991
32. de Sanjosé S, Palacio V, Tapur L et al. Prostitution, HIV and cervical neoplasia: a survey in Spain and Colombia. Cancer Epidemiol Biomarkers Prev 2:531–535, 1993
33. Beral V, Peterman TA, Berkelman RL, Jaffe HW. Kaposi's sarcoma among persons with AIDS: a sexually transmitted infection? Lancet 1990;335:123–128
34. McCredie M, Coates MS, Ford JM. Cancer incidence in migrants to New South Wales. Int J Cancer 1990;46:228
35. Grulich AE, Swerdlow AJ, Head J, Marmot MG. Cancer mortality in African and Caribbean migrants to England and Wales. Br J Cancer 1992;66:905–911
36. Steinitz R, Parkin DM, Young JL et al (eds): Cancer incidence in Jewish migrants to Israel, 1961–1981. IARC Scientific Publications No. 98. International Agency for Research on Cancer, Lyon, 1989

37. Bouchardy C, Wanner P, Parkin DM. Cancer mortality among sub-Saharan African migrants in France. Cancer Causes Control 1995;6:539–544
38. Hanley AJG, Choi BCK, Holowaty EJ. Cancer mortality among Chinese migrants: a review. Int J Epidemiol 1995; 24:255–265
39. Muir C, Waterhouse J, Mack T et al (eds): Cancer Incidence in Five Continents, Vol. V. International Agency for Research on Cancer, Lyon, 1987
40. Axelsson G. Hepatocellular cancer in Sweden: incidence 1961–1962 in 1971–1972. Infect Agents Dis 1993;2: 155–160
41. Okuda K, Fujimoto I, Hanai A, Urano Y. Changing incidence of hepatocellular carcinoma in Japan. Cancer Res 1987;47:4967–4972
42. Okuda K. Hepatitis C virus and hepatocellular carcinoma. In Tabor E, Di Bisceglie AM, Purcell RH (eds): Etiology, Pathology, and Treatment of Hepatocellular Carcinoma in North America. Portfolio, The Woodlands, Texas, 1991, pp. 119–126
43. Jin F, Devesa SS, Zheng W et al. Cancer incidence trends in urban Shanghai, 1972–1989. Int J Cancer 1993;53:764–770
44. Lee HS, Han CJ, Kim CY. Predominant etiologic association of hepatitis C virus with hepatocellular carcinoma compared with hepatitis B virus in elderly patients in a hepatitis B-endemic area. Cancer 1993;72:2564–2567
45. Bosch FX, Mũnoz N. Hepatocellular carcinoma in the world: epidemiological questions. In Tabor E, Di Bisceglie AM, Purcell RH (eds): Etiology, Pathology, and Treatment of Hepatocellular Carcinoma. Portfolio, The Woodlands, Texas, 1991
46. Tanaka K, Hirohata T, Fukuda K et al. Risk factors for hepatocellular carcinoma among Japanese women. Cancer Causes Control 1995;6:91–98
47. Schlesselman JJ. Net effect of oral contraceptive use on the risk of cancer in women in the United States. Obstet Gynecol 1995;85:793–801
48. WHO Collaborative Study of Neoplasia and Steroid Contraceptives. Combined oral contraceptives and liver cancer. Int J Cancer 1989;43:254–259
49. Liang TJ, Jeffers LJ, Reddy KR et al. Viral pathogenesis of hepatocellular carcinoma in the United States. Hepatology 1993;18:1326–1333
50. Paterlini P, Gerken G, Nakajima E et al. Polymerase chain reaction to detect hepatitis B virus DNA and RNA sequences in primary liver cancers from patients negative for hepatitis B surface antigen. N Engl J Med 1990;323:80–85
51. Bréchot C, Degos F, Lugassy C et al. Hepatitis B virus DNA in patients with chronic liver disease and negative tests for hepatitis B surface antigen. N Engl J Med 1985;312:270–276
52. Nalpas B. Alcohol and hepatocellular carcinoma. In Bréchot C (ed): Primary Liver Cancer: Etiological and Progression Factors. CRC Press, Boca Raton, 1994
53. Carman WF, Thomas HC. Genetic variation in hepatitis B virus. Gastroenterology 1992;102:711–719
54. Karthigesu VD, Allison LMC, Fortuin M et al. A novel hepatitis B virus variant in the sera of immunized children. J Gen Virol 1994;75:443–448
55. Kuo G, Choo Q-L, Alter HJ et al. An assay for circulating antibodies to a major etiologic virus of human non-A, non-B hepatitis. Science 1989;244:362–364
56. Alter MJ. The detection, transmission, and outcome of hepatitis C virus infection. Infect Agents Dis 1993;2:155–166
57. Hadziyannis S, Tabor E, Kaklamani E et al. A case-control study of hepatitis B and C virus infections in the etiology of hepatocellular carcinoma. Int J Cancer 1995;60:627–631
58. Okamoto H, Kurai K, Okada S et al. Full-length sequence of a hepatitis C virus genome having poor homology to reported isolates: comparative study of four distinct genotypes. Virology 1992;188:331–341
59. Simmonds P, Alberti A, Alter HJ et al. A proposed system for the nomenclature of hepatitis C virus genotypes. Hepatology 1994;19:1321–1324
60. Dusheiko G, Schmilovitz-Weiss H, Brown D et al. Hepatitis C virus genotypes: an investigation of type-specific differences in geographic origin and disease. Hepatology 1994;19: 13–18
61. McOmish F, Yap P, Dow B et al. Geographical distribution of hepatitis C genotypes in blood donors: an international collaborative survey. J Clin Microbiol 1994;32:884–892
62. Austin H. The role of tobacco use and alcohol consumption in the etiology of hepatocellular carcinoma. In Tabor E, Di Bisceglie AM, Purcell RH (eds). Etiology, Pathology, and Treatment of Heptocellular Carcinoma in North America. Portfolio, The Woodlands, Texas, 1991
63. Forman D, Doll R, Peto R. Trends in mortality from carcinoma of the liver and the use of oral contraceptives. Br J Cancer 1983;48:349–354
64. Mant JWF, Vessey MP. Trends in mortality from primary liver cancer in England and Wales 1975–92: influence of oral contraceptives. Br J Cancer 1995; 72:800–803
65. Bosch FX, Muñoz N. Prospects for epidemiological studies on hepatocellular cancer as a model for assessing viral and chemical interactions. In Bartsch H, Hemminki K, O'Neill IK (eds): Methods for Detecting DNA Damaging Agents in Humans: Applications in Cancer Epidemiology and Prevention, IARC Scientific Publications No. 89. International Agency for Research on Cancer, Lyon, 1988
66. Ozturk M, Bressac B, Puisieux A et al. p53 mutation in hepatocellular carcinoma after aflatoxin exposure. Lancet 1991;338:1356–1359
67. Van Rensburg SJ, Cook-Mozaffari P, Van Schalkwyk DJ et al. Hepatocellular carcinoma and dietary aflatoxin in Mozambique and Transkei. Br J Cancer 1985;51:713–726
68. Hsu IC, Metcalf RA, Sun T et al. Mutational hotspot in the p53 gene in human hepatocellular carcinomas. Nature 1991; 350: 427–428
69. Bressac B, Kew M, Wands J, Ozturk M. Selective G to T mutations of p53 gene in hepatocellular carcinoma from southern Africa. Nature 1991;350:429–430
70. Hollstein MC, Wild CP, Bleicher F et al. p53 mutations and aflatoxin B_1 exposure in hepatocellular carcinoma patients from Thailand. Int J Cancer 1993;53:51–55

71. Tabor E. Tumor suppressor genes, growth factor genes, and oncogenes in hepatitis B virus-associated hepatocellular carcinoma. J Med Virol 1994;42:357–365

72. Bannasch P, Imani Khoshkhou N, Hacker HJ et al. Synergistic hepatocarcinogenic effect of hepadnaviral infection and dietary aflatoxin B1 in woodchucks. Cancer Res 1995;55: 3318–3330

73. International Agency for Research on Cancer. Hepatitis Viruses. IARC Monographs of the Evaluation of Carcinogenic Risk to Humans. Vol. 59, IARC, Lyons, 1994

74. Thomas DB. Exogenous steroid hormones and hepatocellular carcinoma. In Tabor E, Di Bisceglie AM, Purcell R (eds): Etiology, Pathology, and Treatment of Hepatocellular Carcinoma. Portfolio, The Woodlands, Texas, 1991, pp. 77–90

3

HEPATITIS B VIRUS AND HEPATOCELLULAR CARCINOMA

PEI-JER CHEN
DING-SHINN CHEN

Hepatocellular carcinoma (HCC) is the most common primary malignancy of the liver[1,2] and the most common cancer in some geographic areas, particularly in the Far East and Africa.[1,2] Intensive epidemiologic studies have supported a correlation between high prevalence of chronic hepatitis B virus (HBV) infection and the high incidence of HCC in these areas. Based on these results, many timely preventive or therapeutic interventions are currently applied to reduce the likelihood of HBV-infected persons developing HCC and to improve patients' survival rate.[3,4]

The close relationship between HBV and HCC has made it one of the most useful and attractive human models to explore the role of viruses in cancer development.[5] The viral genome has been elucidated, and several of the viral genes have been implicated in contributing to carcinogenesis.[6] The majority of HCCs contain integrated HBV genome in the chromosomes, raising the possibility of activation of cellular proto-oncogenes.[7] Despite these interesting observations favoring a direct role of HBV in causing HCC, HBV could also contribute indirectly to hepatocarcinogenesis. Chronic HBV infection provokes a cellular immune response and inflammation, with chronic hepatitis and, often, cirrhosis.[8,9] In patients with cirrhosis, the annual incidence of HCC is 2% to 7%.[10,11]

HBV infection results in pathologic changes in different stages. Evolution from hepatitis, cirrhosis, and HCC is a multistep process in which several critical genetic changes accumulate and in combination eventually transform the hepatocytes.[12] The causal role of HBV in HCC will only be confirmed by a decline in the incidence of HCC after controlling HBV infection by hepatitis B vaccination. Ten years after a universal vaccination program in Taiwan,[13] a reduction of HCC in childen can be observed.

EPIDEMIOLOGIC EVIDENCE FOR THE ASSOCIATION BETWEEN HBV AND HCC

Epidemiologic studies have amassed evidence that strongly supports an association between HBV infection and HCC. The high incidence of HCC parallels the high prevalence of hepatitis B surface antigen (HBsAg) carriers in almost all geographic areas.[1,2] In Southeast Asia, including Taiwan, the incidence of HCC is as high as 10 to 25/100,000 population,[14] accompanied by a high prevalence of HBsAg (10% to 15%).[15] In case control studies, the relative risk of HCC associated with HBsAg ranges from 10 to 20.[16] In cohort studies in which persons with chronic HBV infection are prospectively followed until HCC develops, the relative risk ranges between 7- and 110-fold.[17,18]

Studies in developed countries have confirmed the findings of studies in developing countries. An incidence

TABLE 3-1. Clinical Data and Characteristics of Four Cohort Studies for HCC Occurrence in Populations With Chronic HBV Infection

Characteristics	Japan[19]	Alaska[20]	Canada[21]	Canada[22]
Subjects	513	1400	1069	317
Carrier-years	3745	7815	2340	5235
Mean age	40–55	+	39 ± 12	46 ± 8
HCCs (per 100,000 carrier-years)	240	256	470	0

+ all age group

of about 240 HCC/100,000 HBsAg "carrier-years" was found in Japan,[19] 256 HCCs/100,000 carrier-years in Alaskan Eskimos,[20] and 281 HCCs/100,000 carrier-years in Toronto, Canada.[21] The one exception was a study conducted in Montreal, which reported no cases of HCC among 317 persons chronically infected with HBV who were followed for a mean of 16.2 years.[22] The peak age for HCC in perinatally transmitted HBV is about 59 years,[23,24] much later than the mean age of the Montreal cohort. Perhaps a longer follow-up period would have produced results consistent with the other studies.

EXPERIMENTAL STUDIES

Development of cancer is a multistep process in which several critical genetic changes take place sequentially, resulting in autonomous growth of transformed cells.[25] This model has been well characterized in colorectal cancer[25] and has been proposed and partially supported by experiments in HCC.[12] There are two possible pathways for the involvement of HBV in such a model of HCC development, and they are not mutually exclusive. In the first pathway, the HBV genome may participate directly in causing the genetic changes of carcinogenesis.[26] In the second, persistent HBV infection, but not HBV itself, predisposes hepatocytes to genetic changes resulting from other causes.[26,27]

EVIDENCE FOR A DIRECT ROLE OF HBV IN HCC

Hepatitis B virus has a small genome of 3.2 kb. There are four well-characterized open reading frames.[28] Three encode viral structural proteins: the nucleocapsid core protein, the envelope HBsAg, and the polymerase protein. The functions of these three genes have been clearly defined.[28] The fourth gene encodes the versatile X protein that plays some role in viral infection of animal models[29] and also exerts many diverse effects on cellular functions.[30]

Several other HBV genes may play a role in carcinogenesis. Novel spliced transcripts have been indentified in HBV-infected hepatocytes of HBV-DNA transfected cell lines.[31,32] Although they retain some encoding capacities, these RNAs are not essential for viral replication. In addition, a truncated pre-S2 protein discovered in hepatoma cell lines has been proposed as a second transactivator for cellular gene expression.[33]

Transfection of the entire HBV genome has led to transformation of mouse hepatocytes to mouse cell lines,[34,35] suggesting the presence of a transforming gene. In addition, high levels of expression of X protein in one lineage of transgenic mice created with the HBV gene caused liver cancer[36] without a defined host response and without a background of hepatitis and cirrhosis. These experimental data indicate that under certain circumstances, the X protein itself can transform hepatocytes.

The X gene is a transactivator for some cellular and viral promoters.[30,37] It works not through direct binding to the DNA of target genes, but by interacting with basic RNA polymerase machinery (e.g., the RPB5 subunit[38]) or other cellular factors that modulate transcriptional activities of pol II or III promoters.[39,40] The promoters of several cellular genes, such as c-*myc* and c-*jun*, which are related to cell growth, are activated by the X protein.[41] Some studies show a direct interaction between X protein and the product of the tumor suppressor gene, p53.[42–44] This may prevent p53-mediated cellular apoptosis in a cell culture system.[45] Two groups have shown that X protein activates the *ras*-dependent signaling cascade and leads to both transcriptional activation and proliferation in quiescent cells.[41,46] Interactions between X protein and signaling pathways may represent mechanisms important in hepatocarcinogenesis.

The role of X protein in human HCC is still uncertain. The expression of the X gene is difficult to detect in infected hepatocytes by northern blot,[30] but several groups succeeded in detecting the X protein by immunohistochemical methods.[47,48] In HCC, the X gene transcript can be identified in most HBV-associated HCCs by reverse transcriptase-polymerase chain reaction (RT-PCR) (but not by northern blot analysis), and even in some cases of HBsAg-negative HCC,[49] in which the transcript may be derived from integrated HBV DNA.

Another well-known direct mechanism for HBV involvement is viral genome integration in HCC. HBV replicates via reverse transcription of pregenomic RNA,[28] and the viral genome frequently integrates into the host genome.[7] About 80% of HCCs contain multiple HBV DNA integration in their chromosomes.[50] This re-

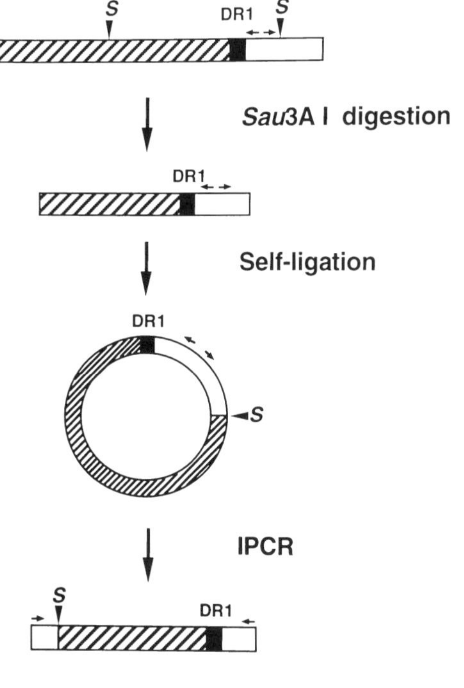

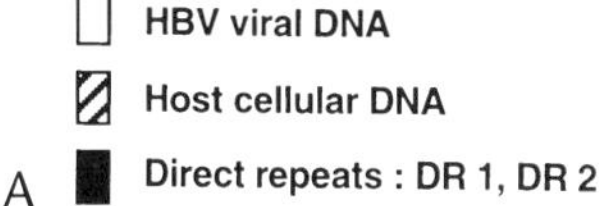

A

FIGURE 3-1. (*A*) Diagram showing the steps for inverse polymerase chain reaction to clone the viral cellular junction fragments from chromosomes of HBsAg-positive HCC. DR1 and 2 designate the two direct repeats in HBV genome, the preferred integration sites in HBV sequences. The small arrows indicate the positions of primers, with their sequences next to viral DR regions. HCC chromosome DNA is digested with restriction enzyme (in this case, Sau3AI) to release the viral-cellular junctional fragment (arrowheads marked with S indicating the Sau3A sites in viral or cellular sequences). Ligation at limiting concentration to be circularized. The circularized fragment was then amplified by primers close to DR regions to yield the product. (*B* & *C*) Representative results for amplification of junctional fragments from two HCCs (37T and 28T). Totally 2.5, 5, 10, or 20 ng (lanes 1 to 4) of circularized HCC DNA was amplified and the products were separated by electrophoresis in agarose gel and visualized by ethidium bromide staining.

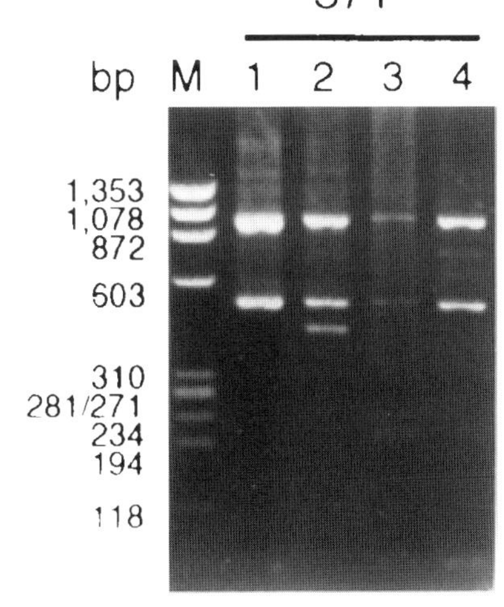

B

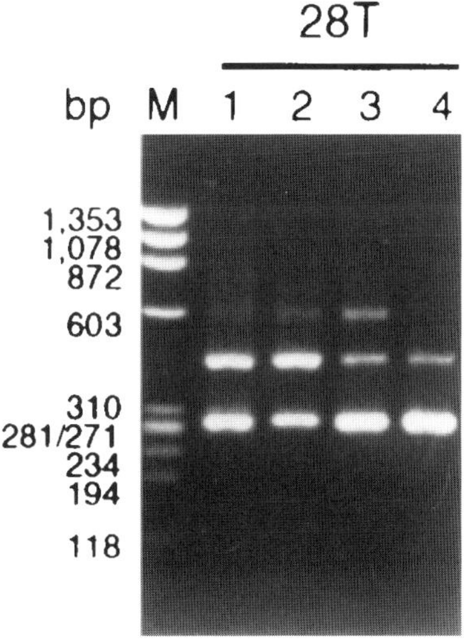

C

sembles insertional mutagenesis in which retroviruses activate proto-oncogene expression, leading to tumor development.[51,52] About 80 to 100 HCC samples have been analyzed for the chromosomal sequences at the HBV integration sites.[53] Rarely, the integration sites are located in the vicinities of growth-regulating genes (e.g., cylcin A gene)[54] or the retinoic acid receptor genes.[55] The majority appear to be integrated at random, suggesting HBV integration does not lead to insertional mutagenesis in most HCCs. Studies in the woodchuck HCC, however, revealed integrations of the woodchuck hepatitis virus near the *myc* gene, *win* and *b3n* loci in 50% to 75% of cases.[56–58]

Since 40% of HBV integration events take place near the viral DR1 or 2 regions of the virus,[59] the regions close to the DR1 or 2 can be used as an anchoring point to amplify the adjacent cellular sequences by inverse PCR[60] (Fig. 3-1A). With appropriate restriction enzymes (e.g., Sau3A) with cleavage sites close to HBV DR1, the HCC DNA is completely digested to free the small viral-cellular junctional fragments. The junctional sequences can be circularized and then amplified with primers of sequences complementary to viral DR1 regions. The immediate cellular flanking sequences can then be analyzed (Fig. 3-1B,C). With more refinement and modification, the method will permit the cloning of most HBV DNA integration sites in HCC. By this approach, some rare but relevant genes might be discovered.

EVIDENCE FOR AN INDIRECT ROLE OF HBV IN HCC

HBV infections in perinatal and early childhood become persistent in 90% of cases. The virus continuously replicates and causes recurrent episodes of hepatitis. The liver responds to persistent inflammation with continuous regeneration and fibrosis that eventually results in cirrhosis (Fig. 3-2).

Clinically, HCC is invariably associated with chronic hepatitis or cirrhosis. About 70% to 90% of HCC develop on a background of cirrhosis.[10] This indirect pathway also gains support from HBV transgenic mice.[27] One lineage of transgenic mice overexpresses the "large" HBsAg, which accumulates in the endoplasmic reticulum. This accumulation may disturb the hepatocyte function to the extent that the cells die spontaneously. After months of inflammation, fibrosis, and a high rate of hepatocyte regeneration, the mice develop cirrhosis and succumb to HCC in high frequency.[61,62]

As cirrhosis is clearly associated with a high risk of HCC, it is imperative to know what lesion in cirrhosis is responsible for the precancerous change. In cirrhosis, the hepatocytes respond with a high rate of regeneration and form a regenerative nodule.[63] Usually in the cirrhotic liver, there are multiple but well-separated regenerative nodules; the latter can be clearly dissected for analysis of clonality. By using molecular clonality markers such as integrated HBV[64] or HPRT polymorphism,[65] a significant proportion (10% to 40%) of the discrete regenerative nodules are shown to be monoclonal in origin. Clinical follow-up study of patients with large regenerative nodules has documented their eventual transition into liver cancer.[66] In some cases, the HCC and its adjacent large hepatic nodules have been resected simultaneously, and both have been shown to retain an identical clonality, supporting a direct evolution from one to the other.[67] These and other findings suggest that the appearance of hepatic regenerative or dysplastic nodules may precede malignant transformation in the development of HCC.[68]

OTHER SYNERGISTIC FACTORS

Although HBV infection plays a major role in HCC development, other factors may promote the process. Epidemiologic correlations have been found between HCC prevalence and urinary aflatoxin excretion,[69–71] although results are controversial.

Other hepatitis viruses, such as HDV and HCV, neither increase the incidence of HCC in HBV-infected patients nor shorten the age of onset of HCC in HBV-infected patients,[23,24] perhaps because dual or multiple virus infections usually result in the dominance of a single virus.[72,73]

Alcohol intake has been associated with increased risk (twofold to fourfold) of HCC development in most case-control studies.[74] Other factors including smoking, genetic polymorphism, and family history also may contribute to HCC development.[75,76] In addition, the remarkable sex difference (male/female ratio about 3 to 8: 1) among HBV-related HCC indicates a possible hormonal influence on hepatocarcinogenesis.

CHILDHOOD HCC IN TAIWAN: A DECLINING TREND 10 YEARS AFTER HBV VACCINATION PROGRAM

One of the earliest universal vaccination programs against HBV was initiated in Taiwan in 1984.[13] The earliest vaccine cohort is now older than 10 years. The prevalence of HBsAg has decreased in this cohort from the previous 10% to 1.3%.[77,78] However, the mean age of HBsAg-positive HCC patients is 55 to 59 years.[23,24] Therefore, three or four decades are needed to determine fully the impact of HBV control on HCC incidence in the Taiwanese population.

Preliminary glimpses of the effect of HBV vaccination on HCC may be found in childhood HCC. Virtually all Taiwanese children who have HCC are HBsAg-positive,[79] as are almost all their mothers.[103] This indicates the critical role of maternal-infant HBV transmission in these HCC patients. These children have a peak age of onset of HCC of about 5 to 9 years (differing from hepatoblastoma, which almost always occurs before 5 years of age[80]). From 1981 to 1991, the annual occurrence of childhood HCC in Taiwan ranged from 4.5 to 7.1 cases/ 1,000,000 children of 6 to 14 years of age. The incidence

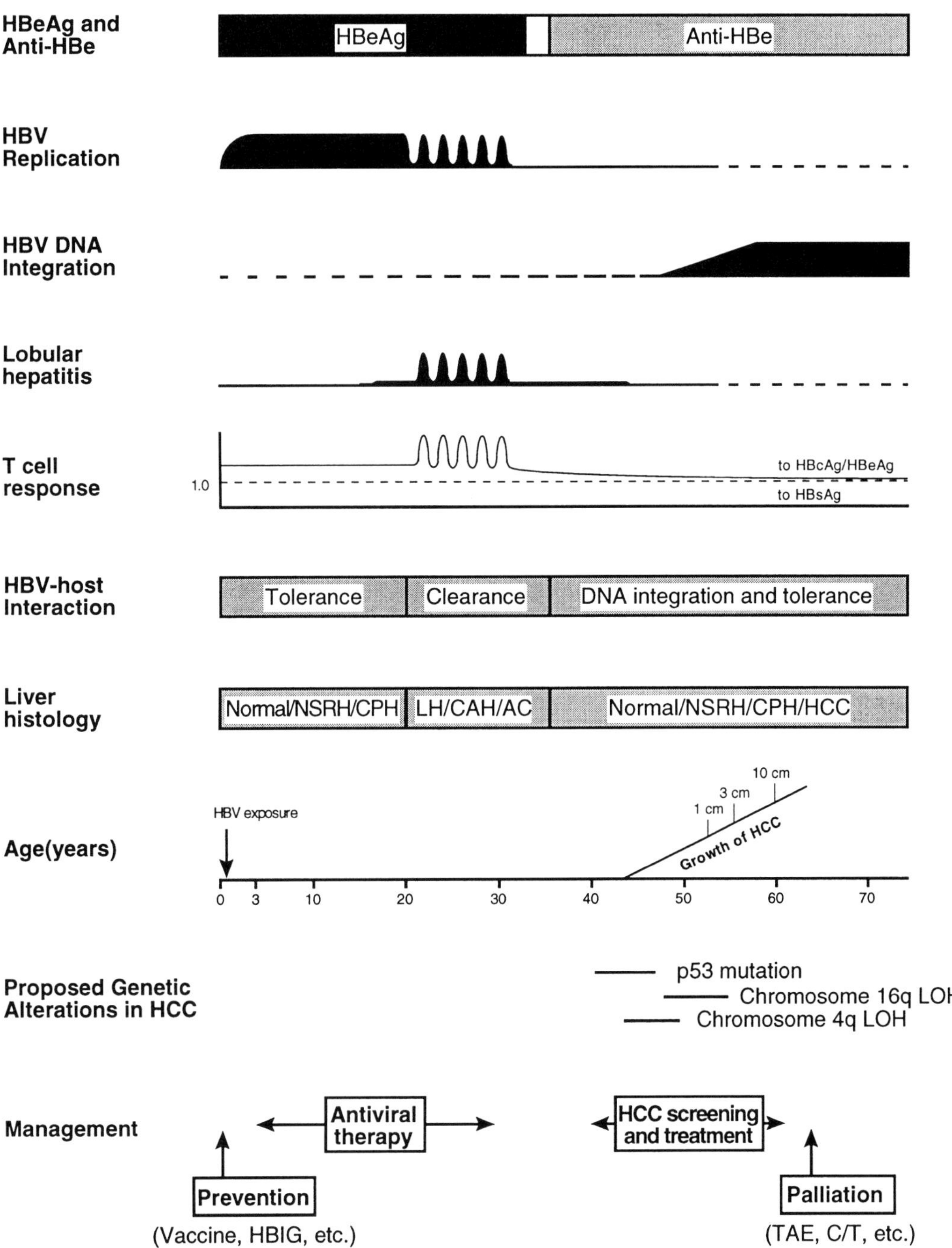

FIGURE 3-2. Natural history of HBV infection in Taiwan and proposed stepwise genetic mutations leading to HCC. HBeAg, hepatitis B e antigen; anti-HBe, antibody against HBeAg; HBcAg, hepatitis B core antigen; NSRH, nonspecific reactive hepatitis; CPH, chronic persistent hepatitis; LH, lobular hepatitis; CAH, chronic active hepatitis; AC, active cirrhosis; LOH, loss of heterozygosity; HBIG, hepatitis B immunoglobulin; TAE, transarterial embolization; C/T, chemotherapy. (Adapted from Chen,[8] with permission.)

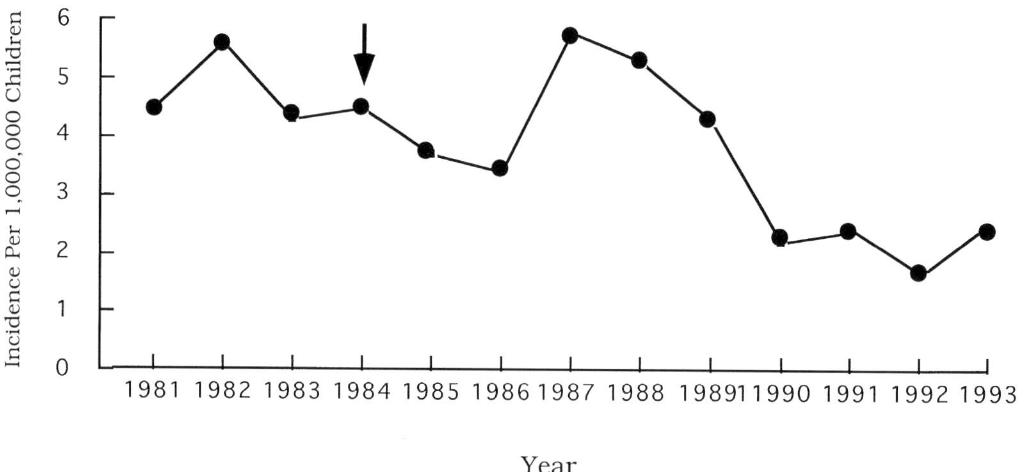

FIGURE 3-3. Liver cancer rates in children 6 to 14 years of age in Taiwan, 1981–1993 (unpublished data). The year, 1984, when mass HBV vaccination was launched, is marked by an arrow.

began to decline to 1.74 and 2.4 cases/1,000,000 children in 1992 and 1993, respectively (Fig. 3-3) (unpublished data). This preliminary observation, if confirmed, will be important evidence to support the causal role of HBV infection in childhood HCC, and it suggests a similar confirmation of the role of HBV in HCC of adults.

PROSPECT

Although most HCCs occur in a background of cirrhosis, a substantial proportion of HCCs develop in chronic hepatitis without cirrhosis. For example, in Japan, about 30% to 40% of HBV-associated HCCs were without cirrhosis[81] (compared to 20% without cirrhosis among all HCCs). The precancerous lesions in such cases are not clear, and the role of HBV in these cases merits further investigation.[82] Limited studies have characterized the HBV DNA integration sites in noncirrhotic HCC, but there seemed to be no preferential sites.[83] The integrated rearranged viral genomes and local genome instability induced by integrations have not yet been explored.

Because cirrhotic patients are at a high risk of developing HCC, they are regularly followed up. Through periodic examinations of α-fetoprotein[84] (AFP) and abdomenal ultrasonography, small HCCs can be identified and patients treated earlier.[3,4] Once the tumor becomes detectable, however, it is usually already about 1 cm in size, representing 10^9 cells in total. In the evolving process of hepatocarcinogenesis, this is quite late. If we could understand the mechanism transforming dysplastic lesions or regenerative nodules to frank HCC,[85] effective prevention procedures could be developed. From this point of view, a recent study suggesting that interferon therapy apparently retarded the occurrence of HCC in patients with HCV-related cirrhosis[86,87] is noteworthy. Whether such a treatment would also be useful to prevent HCC in HBV-related cirrhosis is not known.[87] A better understanding of HCC carcinogenesis also might lead to more effective strategies, as suggested by a promising chemoprevention trial.[88]

The most practical and cost-effective way to prevent HCC is likely to be vaccination against HBV.[77] In Taiwan, universal vaccination reduced chronic HBV infection from 10% to 1.3% in 10 years.[78] A trend of declining incidence of childhood HCC was observed in the latter part of this period (unpublished data), suggesting that the effect of HBV vaccination in controlling HCC has begun to be seen in children.

ACKNOWLEDGMENT

This work was supported by National Science Council and Department of Health, Executive Yuan, Taiwan. The authors are grateful to colleagues in the Department of Internal Medicine and Hepatitis Research Center for their contributions.

REFERENCES

1. Muñoz N, Lincell A. Epidemiology of primary liver cancer. In Correa P, Haenszel H (eds): Epidemiology of Cancer of the Digestive Tract. Martinus Nijhoff, The Hague, 1982; pp. 161–195
2. Simonetti RG, Camma C, Fiorello F et al. Hepatocellular carcinoma. A worldwide problem and the major risk factors. Dig Dis Sci 1991;36:962–972

3. Ohnishi K, Tanabe Y, Ryu M et al. Prognosis of hepatocelluar carcinoma smaller than 5 cm in relation to treatment: study of 100 patients. Hepatology 1987;7:1285–1290
4. Pateron D, Ganne N, Trichet JC et al. Prospective screening for hepatocellular carcinoma in Caucasian patients with cirrhosis. J Hepatol 1994;20:65–71
5. Morris JDH, Eddelstone ALW, Crook T. Viral infection and cancer. Lancet 1995;346:754–758
6. Slagle BL, Lee TH, Butel JS. Hepatitis B virus and hepatocellular carcinoma. Prog Med Virol 1992;39:167–203
7. Bréchot C, Pourcel C, Louis A et al. Presence of integrated hepatitis B virus DNA sequences in cellular DNA in human hepatocellular carcinoma. Nature 1980;286:533–535
8. Chen DS. From hepatitis to hepatoma: lessons from type B viral hepatitis. Science 1993;262:269–270
9. Liaw YF, Tai DY, Chu CM, Chen TJ. The development of cirrhosis in patients with chronic type B hepatitis: a prospective study. Hepatology 1988;8:493–496
10. Okuda K, Nakashima T, Sakamoto K et al. Hepatocellular carcinoma arising in noncirrhotic and highly cirrhotic livers: a comparative study of histopathology and frequency of hepatitis B markers. Cancer 1982;49:450–455
11. Liaw YF, Tai DY, Chu CM et al. Early detection of hepatocelluar carcinoma in patients with chronic type B hepatitis: a prospective study. Gastroenterology 1986;90:263–267
12. Sugimura T. Multistep carcinogenesis: a 1992 prospective. Science 1992;258:603–607
13. Chen DS, Hsu NHM, Sung JL et al. A mass vaccination program in Taiwan against hepatitis B virus infection in infants of hepatitis B surface antigen carrier mothers. JAMA 1987;257:2597–2603
14. Chen DS. Hepatitis B virus infection, its sequelae, and prevention in Taiwan. In Okuda K, Ishak KG (eds): Neoplasms of the Liver. Springer-Verlag, Tokyo, 1987; pp. 71–80
15. Sung JL, Sekine T, Lin TM et al. Hepatitis-associated antigen in hepatocellular carcinoma in Taiwan. J Formos Med Assoc 1972;146:205–210
16. Lu SN, Lin TM, Chen CJ et al. A case-control study of primary hepatocelluar carcinoma in Taiwan. Cancer 1988; 62:2051–2055.
17. Beasley RP, Hwang LY, Lin CC, Chein CS. Hepatocellular carcinoma and hepatitis B virus. A prospective study of 22,707 men in Taiwan. Lancet 1981;2:1129–1133
18. Oshima A, Tsukuma H, Hiyama T et al. Follow-up study of HBsAg-positive blood donors with special reference to effect of drinking and smoking on development of liver cancer. Int J Cancer 1984;34:775–779
19. Sakuma K, Saito N, Kasai M et al. Relative risks of death due to liver disease among Japanese male adults having various statuses for hepatitis B s and e antigen/antibody in serum: a prospective study. Hepatology 1988;8:1642–1646
20. McMahon BJ, Alberts SR, Wainwright RB et al. Hepatitis B-related sequelae: prospective study in 1400 hepatitis B surface antigen-positive Alaska native carriers. Arch Intern Med 1990;150:1051–1054
21. Sherman M, Peltekian KM, Lee C. Screening for hepatocellular carcinoma in chronic carriers of hepatitis B virus: incidence and prevalence of hepatocellular carcinoma in a Northern American urban population. Hepatology 1995;22: 432–438
22. Villeneuve JP, Desrochers M, Infacnte-Rivard C et al. A long-term follow-up of healthy hepatitis B virus surface antigen carriers in Montreal. Gastroenterology 1994;106: 1000–1005
23. Chen DS, Kuo GC, Sung JL et al. Hepatitis C virus infection in an area hyperendemic for hepatitis B and chronic liver diseases: the Taiwan experience. J Infect Dis 1990;162: 817–822
24. Saito I, Miyamura T, Ohbayashi A et al. Hepatitis C virus infection is associated with the development of hepatocellular carcinoma. Proc Natl Acad Sci USA 1990;87:6547–6549
25. Vogelstein B, Fearon ER, Hamilton SR et al. Genetic alterations during colorectal-tumor development. N Engl J Med 1988;319:525–539
26. Okuda K. Hepatocellular carcinoma: recent progress. Hepatology 1992;15:948–963
27. Chisari F. Hepatitis B virus transgenic mice: insights into the virus and the disease. Hepatology 1995;22:1316–1325
28. Ganem D, Varmus HE. The molecular biology of hepatitis B viruses. Annu Rev Biochem 1987;56:651–693
29. Chen HS, Kaneko S, Girones R et al. The woodchuck hepatitis virus X gene is important for establishment of virus infection in woodchucks. J Virol 1993;67:1218–1226
30. Yen TSB. Hepadnaviral X protein: review of recent progress. J Biomed Sci 1996;3:20–30
31. Su TS, Lai CJ, Hunag JL et al. Hepatitis B virus transcript produced by RNA splicing. J Virol 1989;63:4011–4018
32. Chen PJ, Chen CR, Sung JL, Chen DS. Identification of a doubly-spliced viral transcript joining the separated domains for putative protease and reverse transcriptase of hepatitis B virus. J Virol 1989;63:4165–4171
33. Kekule AS, Lauer U, Meyer M et al. The preS2/S region of integrated hepatitis B virus DNA encodes a transcriptional activator. Nature 1990;343:457–460
34. Hohne M, Schaefer S, Seifer M et al. Malignant transformation of immortalized transgenic hepatocytes after transfection with hepatitis B virus DNA. EMBO J 1990;9: 1137–1145
35. Chen SH, Hu CP, Chang C. Hepatitis B virus replication in well differentiated mouse hepatocyte cell lines transformed by plasmid DNA. Cancer Res 1992;52:1329–1335
36. Koike K, Moriya K, Iino S et al. High level expression of hepatitis B virus HBx gene and hepatocarcinogenesis in transgenic mice. Hepatology 1994;19:810–819
37. Spandau DF, Lee CH. Transactivation of viral enhancers by the hepatitis B X protein. J Virol 1988;62:427–432
38. Cheong JH, Yi M, Lin Y, Murakami S. Human RPB5, a subunit shared by eukaryotic RNA polymerases, binds human hepatitis B X protein and may play a role in X transactivation. EMBO J 1995;14:142–150
39. Seto E, Mitchell PJ, Yen TSB. Transactivation by the hepatitis B virus X protein depends on AP-2 and other transcriptional factors. Nature 1990;344:72–74
40. Aufiro B, Schneider RJ. The hepatitis B virus X-gene product

transactivates both RNA polymerase II and III promoters. EMBO J 1990;9:497–504

41. Natoli G, Avantaggiati ML, Chirillo P et al. Induction of the DNA-binding activity of c-jun/c-fos heterodimers by the hepatitis B virus transactivators. Mol Cell Biol 1994;14: 989–998
42. Feitelson MA, Zhu M, Duan LX, London WT. Hepatitis B X antigen and p53 associated in vitro and in liver tissues from patients with primary hepatocellular carcinoma. Oncogene 1993;8:1109–1117
43. Wang XW, Forester K, Yeh H et al. Hepatitis B virus X protein inhibits p53 sequence-specific DNA binding, transcriptional activity and association with transcriptional factor ERCC3. Proc Natl Acad Sci USA 1994;91: 2230–2234
44. Truant R, Antunovic J, Greenblatt J et al. Direct interaction of the hepatitis B virus HBx protein with p53 leads to inhibition by HBx of p53 response element-directed transactivation. J Virol 1995;69:1851–1859
45. Wang XW, Gibson MK, Vermeulen W et al. Abrogation of p53-induced apoptosis by the hepatitis B virus X gene. Cancer Res 1995;55:6012–6016
46. Doria M, Klein N, Lucito R, Schneider J. The hepatitis B virus HBx protein is a dual specificity cytoplasmic activator of Ras and nuclear activator of transcription factors. EMBO J 1995;14:4747–4757
47. Levero M, Jean JO, Balsano C et al. Hepatitis B virus X protein in human cells and anti-HBx antibodies in chronic HBV infection. Virology 1990;174:299–304
48. Haruna Y, Hayashi N, Katayama K et al. Expression of X protein and hepatitis B replication in chronic hepatitis. Hepatology 1991;13:417–421
49. Paterlini P, Poussin K, Kew MC et al. Selective accumulation of the X transcript of hepatitis B virus in patients negative for hepatitis B surface antigen with hepatocellular carcinoma. Hepatology 1995;21:313–321
50. Chen DS, Hoyer BH, Nelson J et al. Detection and properties of hepatitis B viral DNA in liver tissues from patients with hepatocellular carcinoma. Hepatology 1982;2:42s–46s
51. Hayward WS, Neel BG, Astrin S. Activation of a cellular oncogene by promoter insertion in ALV-induced lymphoid leukosis. Nature 1981;290:475–480
52. Neel BG, Hayward WS, Robinson HL et al. Avian leukosis virus-induced tumors have common proviral integration sites and synthesized discrete new RNAs: oncogenesis by promoter insertion. Cell 1981;23:323–334
53. Nagaya T, Nakamura T, Tokino T et al. The mode of hepatitis B virus DNA integration in chromosomes of human hepatocellular carcinoma. Genet Dev 1987;1:773–782
54. Wang J, Chenivesse X, Heigliein B, Bréchot C. Hepatitis B virus integration in a cyclin A gene in a hepatocellular carcinoma. Nature 1990;343:555–557
55. Dejean A, Bougueleret L, Grzeschik KH, Tiollais P. Hepatitis B virus DNA integration in a sequence homologous to v-erb A and steroid hormone receptor in a hepatocellular carcinoma. Nature 1986;322:70–72
56. Hsu TY, Moroy T, Etiemble J et al. Activation of c-*myc* by woodchuck hepatitis virus insertion in hepatocellular carcinoma. Cell 1988;55:627–635
57. Fourel G, Trepo C, Bougueleret L et al. Frequent activation of N-myc genes by hepadnavirus insertion in woodchuck liver tumors. Nature 1990;347:294–280
58. Bruni R, Argentini C, D'Ugo E et al. Recurrence of woodchuck hepatitis virus integration in the *b3n* locus in woodchuck hepatocellular carcinoma. Virology 1995;214: 229–234
59. Shih C, Burke K, Chou MJ et al. Tight clustering of human hepatitis B virus integration sites in hepatoma near a triple-stranded region. J Virol 1987;61:3491–3498
60. Tsuei DJ, Chen PJ, Lai MY et al. Inverse polymerase chain reaction for cloning cellular sequences adjacent to integrated hepatitis B virus DNA in hepatocellular carcinoma. J Virol Methods 1994;49:269–284
61. Chisari FV, Klopchin K, Moriyama T et al. Molecular pathogenesis of hepatocellular carcinoma in hepatitis B virus transgenic mice. Cell 1989;59:1145–1156
62. Moriyama T, Guilhot S, Klopchin K et al. Immunobiology and pathogenesis of hepatocellular injury in hepatitis B virus transgenic mice. Science 1990;248:361–364
63. Wada K, Kondo F, Kondo Y. Large regenerative nodules and dysplastic nodules in cirrhotic livers: a histopathological study. Hepatology 1988;8:1684–1688
64. Chen PJ, Chen DS, Chen CR et al. Clonal origin of recurrent hepatocellular carcinomas. Gastroenterology 1989;96: 527–529
65. Aihara T, Naguchi S, Sasakon Y, Imoaka S. Clonal analysis of regenerative nodules in hepatitis C-induced liver cirrhosis. Gastroenterology 1994;107:1085–1091
66. Arakawa K, Kage M, Sugihara S et al. Emergence of malignant lesions within an adenomatous hyperplastic nodule in a cirrhotic liver: observations in 5 cases. Gastroenterology 1986;91:198–208
67. Tsuda H, Hirohashi S, Shimosato Y et al. Clonal origin of atypical adenomatous hyperplasia of the liver and clonal identity with hepatocellular carcinoma. Gastroenterology 1988;95:1664–1666
68. Takayama T, Makuuchi M, Hirohashi S et al. Malignant transformation of adenomatous hyperplasia to hepatocellular carcinoma. Lancet 1990;336:1150–1153
69. Yeh FS, Yu MC, Mo CC et al. Hepatitis B virus, aflatoxins and hepatocellular carcinoma in southern Guangxi, China. Cancer Res 1989;49:2506–2509
70. Ross RK, Yuan JM, Yu MC et al. Urinary aflatoxin biomarkers and risk of hepatocellular carcinoma. Lancet 1992;339: 943–946
71. Campbell TC, Chen J, Liu J, Parpia B. Nonassociation of aflatoxin with primary liver cancer in a cross-sectional ecological survey in People's Republic of China. Cancer Res 1990;50:6882–6893
72. Liaw YF, Tsai SL, Chang JJ et al. Displacement of hepatitis B virus by hepatitis C virus as the cause of continuing chronic hepatitis. Gastroenterology 1994;106:1048–1053
73. Sheen IS, Liaw YF, Lin DY et al. Role of hepatitis C and delta virus in the termination of chronic hepatitis B surface

antigen carrier state: a multivariate analysis in a longitudinal follow-up study. J Infect Dis 1994;70:358–361

74. Okuda K, Ohnishi K. The role of viral infections in alcoholic liver disease. In Alcoholic Liver Disease: Pathology and Pathogenesis. 2nd Ed. Edward Arnold, London, 1994; pp. 147–159
75. Chen CJ, Liang KY, Chang AS et al. Effects of hepatitis B virus, alcohol drinking, cigarette smoking and familial tendency on hepatocellular carcinoma. Hepatology 1991;13: 398–406
76. Yu MW, Gladek-Yarborough A, Chiamprasert S et al. Cytochrome p4502E1 and glutathione S-transferase M1 polymorphisms and susceptibility to hepatocellular carcinoma. Gastroenterology 1995;109:1266–1273
77. Hsu NHM, Chen DS, Chuang CH et al. Efficacy of a mass hepatitis B vaccination program in Taiwan. JAMA 1988; 260:2231–2235
78. Chen HL, Chang MH, Hsu HY et al. Seroepidemiology of hepatitis B virus infection in children: ten years mass vaccination in Taiwan. JAMA 1996;270:906–908
79. Hsu HC, Wu MZ, Chang MH et al. Childhood hepatocellular carcinoma develops exclusively in hepatitis B surface antigen carriers in three decades in Taiwan: report of 51 cases strongly associated with rapid development of liver cirrhosis. J Hepatol 1987;5:260–267
80. Chang MH, Chen DS, Hsu HC et al. Maternal transmission of hepatitis B virus in childhood hepatocellular carcinoma. Cancer 1989;64:1737–1741
81. Shiratoti Y, Shiina S, Imamura M et al. Characteristic difference of hepatocellular carcinoma between hepatitis B- and C-infection in Japan. Hepatology 1995;22:1027–1033
82. Okuda K. Hepatocellular carcinomas associated with hepatitis B and C virus infections: are they different? Hepatology 1995;22:1883–1885
83. Marchio A, Terris B, Pineau P et al. Analysis of HBV integration sites in liver tumors without accompanying cirrhosis. In Nishioka N, Suzuki H, Mishiro S, Oda T (eds). Viral Hepatitis and Liver Diseases. Springer-Verlag, Tokyo, 1994; pp. 730–733
84. Chen DS, Sung JL. Serum α-fetoprotein in hepatocellular carcinoma. Cancer 1977;40:779–783
85. Ferrell L, Wright T, Lake J et al. Incidence and diagnostic features of macroregenerative nodules vs. small hepatocellular carcinoma in cirrhostic livers. Hepatology 1992;16: 1372–1381
86. Mazzella G, Accogli E, Sottili S et al. Alpha interferon treatment may prevent hepatocellular carcinoma in HCV-related liver cirrhosis. J Hepatol 1996;24:141–147
87. Nishiguchi S, Kuroki T, Nakatani S et al. Randomized trial of effects of interferon alpha on incidence of hepatocellular carcinoma in chronic active hepatitis C with cirrhosis. Lancet 1995;346:1051–1055
88. Muto Y, Moriwaki H, Ninomiya M et al. Prevention of second primary tumors by an acyclic retinoid, polyprenoic acid, in patients with hepatocellular carcinoma. N Engl J Med 1996;334:1561–1567

4

HEPATITIS C VIRUS AND HEPATOCELLULAR CARCINOMA

KUNIO OKUDA

When hepatitis B virus (HBV) was discovered and found to be a cause of chronic hepatitis and cirrhosis, particularly in geographic areas where hepatocellular carcinoma (HCC) is common, it was assumed that this explained the close association between cirrhosis and HCC. In fact, HBV infection was detected in the large majority of HCC patients in countries where HBV infection is endemic.[1]

In many areas of the world, however, it was subsequently found that HBV accounted for only a proportion of patients with chronic hepatitis, and that another type of virus, tentatively called the non-A, non-B hepatitis virus, was the likely cause of the remaining cases.[2,3] It also became clear that some HCC patients had no serologic markers of HBV and no history of alcohol abuse. In 1982, it was first predicted that a non-A, non-B hepatitis virus could account for some of these patients.[4] Epidemiologic surveys in Japan found that the relative proportion of HBV-associated HCC was decreasing[5] and that the incidence of HCC in males had been rising at a remarkable pace since around 1970.[6]

As soon as HCV was discovered[7] and an antibody test was developed,[8] it did not take long to ascertain that patients with HCC who were negative for the hepatitis B surface antigen (HBsAg) often had HCV infection. The prevalence of HCV infection among the general population and among HCC patients is now well established in many countries, and there is no doubt that HCV is associated with HCC. The important question as to how this virus is involved in hepatocarcinogenesis, however, remains to be determined.

EPIDEMIOLOGY OF HCV INFECTION AND HCV-ASSOCIATED HCC

Early reports on the frequency of antibody to HCV (anti-HCV) in the general population and in patients with HCC were based on first-generation tests (detecting the C100–3 antigen), which frequently yielded false-positive results because of hyperglobulinemia[9] and were generally less sensitive and less specific compared with subsequently developed tests. The positivity rate obtained with a more specific and sensitive HCV antibody test in HCC patients not only confirmed results with the first-generation kit but showed a greater association.[10,11] In most geographic areas, anti-HCV is detected in less than 2% of healthy blood donors,[12,13] whereas in patients with HCC, it is detected in greater than 10% and in up to 80% (more than 65% in Japan, Italy, and Spain[14–45]) (Table 4-1). The time trends investigated in countries where HCC incidence is increasing, such as Japan, clearly demonstrate that the increase in HCC incidence is accounted for by the increase in HCV-associated HCC[5]; the incidence of HBV-associated HCC has not changed much (Fig. 4-1).

Temporal changes of HCV prevalence are not yet well known. However, anti-HCV positivity rates in Japan increase with age, with a sharp increase after about age 50 years.[5] Although there is no past record that would assist in elucidating the cause of this antibody distribution in different age groups, infection could have occurred in childhood, perhaps as an effect of the nation-

TABLE 4-1. Prevalence of Anti-HCV Among Patients With Hepatocellular Carcinoma in Selected Countries

Country/Area	Year	% Anti-HCV Positive (no./total)	% Anti-HCV in Controls	Reference
Italy	1989		0.87	14
Milan	1989	65 (86/132)		15
Padua	1989	76 (152/200)		16
Rome	1991	58 (97/78)		17
Naple	1991	72 (63/88)		18
France	1989		0.68	19
Le Kremlin Bicetre	1990	28 (21/74)		20
Paris	1991	58 (32/55)		21
Spain				
Barcelona	1989	75 (72/96)	7.3	22
Pamplona	1992	63 (44/70)		23
U.K.	1990	11 (1/9)	0.18	24
Greece/Athens	1991	39 (72/185)		25
USA	1995		1.4	12
Miami	1990	53 (31/59)		26
Los Angeles	1990	29 (15/51)		27
S. Africa/Johannesburg	1990	29 (110/380)	0.7	28
Mozambique	1990	46 (69/150)		29
Japan	1991		1.15	30
Matsumoto	1991	68 (74/109)		31
Niigata	1990	58 (85/100)		32
Kyushu	1991	68 (62/91)		33
Taiwan				
Taipei	1990	33 (22/66)	0.95	34
Kaohsiung	1991	37 (48/129)		35
Hong Kong	1992	7 (31/414)	0.64	36
China				
Nantong	1993	6 (1/17)		37
South	1993	25 (64/261)		37
North	1991	39 (20/52)		38
Korea/Seoul	1993	28 (28/100)	1.3	39
Thailand	1990	6 (3/47)	2.6	40
Singapore	1991	15 (7/47)	0	41
Indonesia/Jakarta	1991	34 (24/70)		42
India/New Delhi	1992	15 (8/53)		43
Nepal/Kathmandu	1994	10 (6/62)	3.5	44
Saudi Arabia/Riyadh	1992	26 (11/42)	1.5	45

Most of these studies used a first-generation test for anti-/HCV (anti-C100-3), and these figures would have been greater if a second-generation test had been used.

ally mandated mass vaccination program in which the needles were not disposable. Skin wounds are one route of transmission,[12,13] and high seropositivity has been associated with unsanitary medical and paramedical procedures.[46–48] In Japan, blood transfusion-associated non-A, non-B hepatitis was rampant in the 1950s and 1960s.[5] Many of those who had post-transfusion non-A, non-B hepatitis developed HCC after a lapse of at least 20 years.[49] About 40% of HCC patients in Japan have a history of past blood transfusion.[5,31,50] Currently, the prevalence of anti-HCV is near zero below the age of 15 years in Japan.[51]

In some regions of the world, anti-HCV is detected in greater than 50% of blood donors.[52] It remains to be seen whether such high prevalence regions will have an increasing incidence of HCC after a lapse of some years. According to Kiyosawa et al.,[49] it takes on average about 30 years from the time of infection for HCC to develop.

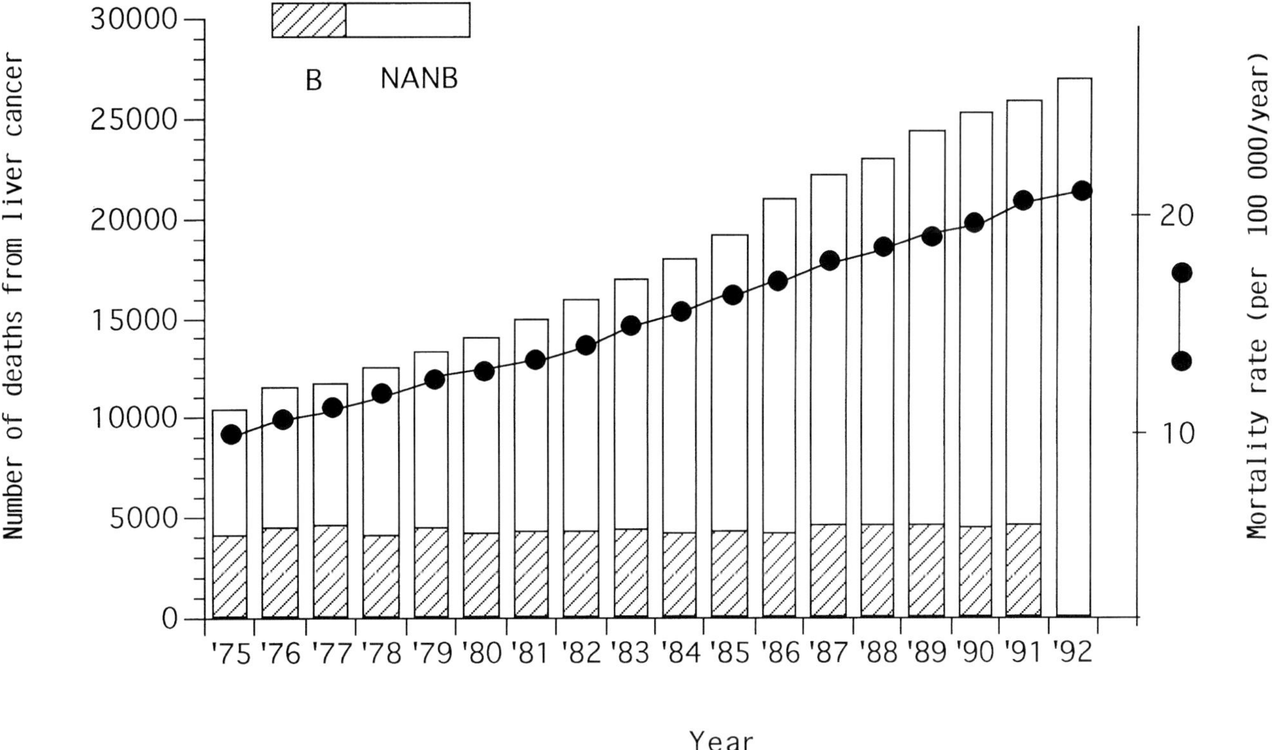

FIGURE 4-1. Time trends in liver cancer mortality in Japan. Relation between HBsAg-positive and -negative (non-A, non-B hepatitis [NANB]) patients based on vital statistics for Japan in 1992 (Statistics & Information Department 1993). The number of deaths of HBsAg-positive patients (shaded) was calculated from HBsAg positivity rates among HCC patients published by the Liver Cancer Study Group of Japan. The number of liver cancer deaths related to HBV is unchanged during the past 18 years, while liver cancer deaths of patients with non-A, non-B hepatitis have more than tripled.

ETIOLOGIC ROLE OF HCV IN HCC

HCV is a plus strand RNA virus and is not reverse transcribed to DNA; hence it is not integrated into the host cell DNA. In contrast, the HBV genome is randomly integrated into hepatocyte DNA, contributing to malignant transformation in an ill-defined manner.[53] Although both viruses cause chronic liver disease and cirrhosis, the etiologic role may differ. The histopathology of HBV-induced chronic liver disease is somewhat different from that induced by HCV. Several clinical and pathologic[54] studies have suggested that inflammation is more active in the liver in HCV-associated HCC when the cancer is found compared with HBV-associated HCC,[35,55] and liver cell proliferation also is active.[56] Generally, cases of HBV-associated HCC occur in younger patients than do cases of HCV-associated HCC.[55] No childhood HCV-associated HCC has yet been reported. In contrast, a report of two pairs of HBsAg-positive brothers developing HCC almost simultaneously in childhood[57] suggests the possibility of germline genetic changes that favor hepatocarcinogenesis in a few cases, although the role of perinatal HBV infection cannot be excluded.

Some of the proteins encoded by the HCV RNA sequences may act like a proto-oncogene product. The nucleotide sequence of HCV is quite variable, and at least six subtypes[58] and quasispecies have been identified. However, Yuwen et al.,[59] analyzing the sequences of HCV RNA in sera of HCC patients from Africa, failed to demonstrate any specific nucleotide sequence in HCC, although the study is preliminary. Rather, certain genotypes tend to produce a more progressive chronic liver disease that is less amenable to interferon treatment and causes HCC more frequently.[60]

COINFECTION OF HBV AND HCV

Some HCC patients have serologic evidence of coinfection with HBV and HCV.[23] Although HCV infection suppresses HBV infection,[61–63] it is generally thought

TABLE 4-2. Relationship of Anti-HCV to HBsAg Status in Hepatocellular Carcinoma

Country	No. Coinfections With HBV and HCV	Anti-HCV Positivity in HBsAg-positive Cases	Anti-HCV Positivity in HBsAg-negative Cases	Reference
Italy	22/132 (17%)	22/41 (54%)	64/91 (70%)	15
Italy	15/167 (9%)	15/53 (28%)	82/114 (72%)	17
Italy	1/78 (1%)	1/8 (13%)	45/70 (64%)	65
France	9/47 (19%)	9/12 (75%)	20/35 (57%)	21
Spain	6/96 (6%)	6/9 (56%)	72/87 (82%)	22
Spain	0/70[a]	0/12 (0%)	44/58 (75%)	23
Greece	61/185 (33%)	61/85 (72%)	41/100 (41%)	25
USA	4/81 (5%)	4/28 (12%)	31/59 (53%)	26
Saudi Arabia	2/42 (5%)	2/16 (13%)	11/26 (42%)	45
Japan	8/100 (8%)	8/42 (19%)	50/58 (86%)	32
Japan	11/180 (6%)	11/75 (16%)	80/105 (76%)	66
Japan	19/253 (8%)	19/87 (22%)	147/166 (89%)	67
Taiwan	7/66 (11%)	7/42 (17%)	15/24 (63%)	34
Taiwan	10/326 (3%)	10/243 (4%)	31/83 (37%)	68
Taiwan	19/129 (15%)	19/81 (24%)	29/48 (60%)	35
China	15/52 (29%)	15/35 (43%)	5/17 (29%)	38
Indonesia	12/70 (17%)	12/41 (29%)	12/29 (41%)	42

[a] When HBV DNA and HCV RNA were studied, 9 of 63 (14%) were positive for both.

that coinfection is more severe than infection with only one of these viruses.[64] The natural history of coinfected persons is not well known.

Anti-HCV is more frequently positive in HBsAg-negative HCC cases in most countries (Table 4-2), suggesting that double infection is not more carcinogenic than single infection. (Most of these studies did not have a control group.) In several exceptional areas such as Greece and China, HBsAg-positive cases were frequently anti-HCV positive; these countries are known for high endemicity of HBV infection. Several studies in which the risk factor was calculated with a control group suggested a synergistic or an additive effect of coinfection.[25,27] According to Chuang et al.,[70] the relative risk for HCC was 13.96 with positive HBsAg, 27.12 with anti-HCV, and was elevated to 40.05 when both were considered simultaneously.

When Colombo et al.[15] analyzed their results of anti-HCV in relation to HBV serology, they noted more frequent detection of both anti-HCV and anti-HBc (54%) in HCC cases than in chronic hepatitis cases (19%). This could be interpreted as showing that past HBV infection could predispose to hepatocarcinogenesis in the presence of ongoing HCV infection. Subsequent studies, however, failed to suggest a synergistic effect (Table 4-3). In fact, the frequency of anti-HCV among anti-HBc-positive HCC cases was lower than that among all HBsAg-negative cases. If past HBV infection were to

TABLE 4-3. Anti-HCV Positivity in Relation to Anti-HBc in HBsAg-Negative HCC Patients

Reference	Anti-HCV Positivity in All HBsAg-Negative Cases	Anti-HCV Positivity in HBsAg-Negative and Anti-HBc Positive Cases
Colombo et al. 1989[15]	70%	54%
Sbolli et al. 1990[65]	64%	22%
Ohkoshi et al. 1990[32]	86%	23%
Saito et al. 1990[69]	69%	59%[a]
Levrero et al. 1991[17]	72%	42%

[a] Anti-HBs-positive patients are also included.

enhance hepatocarcinogenesis, anti-HCV should be detected more frequently.

Several studies have shown that some patients who are serologically negative for HBV may have HBV DNA in serum or tissue[71,72] or an undetectable HBV because of nucleotide sequence changes.[73] Liang et al.[74] studied 91 HCC patients who were negative for HBsAg in the United States. Twenty-six (29%) carried low levels of HBV DNA in serum or liver tissue, 58% had HCV infection, and 15% had evidence of coinfection. Of these 26 HBsAg-negative cases in which HBV DNA was detected, anti-HBc was detected only in six. These results could suggest that HBV infection in the distant past leaves only HBV DNA integrated in liver cell DNA without ongoing viral replication, and that HCC develops after anti-HBc levels become undetectable. Peterlin et al.[75] also found HBV DNA in 11 of 24 HBsAg-negative cases in France, and four of them also had HCV RNA in serum. The issue of the etiologic role of past HBV infection and its additive effect with HCV infection in hepatocarcinogenesis remains to be further eludicated.

PATHOLOGY OF HCV-ASSOCIATED HCC

HCC usually develops in a liver with advanced chronic liver disease and rarely evolves in a normal liver. At autopsy, the liver is cirrhotic in most cases; with frequent early detection as practiced in Japan, the liver is less commonly cirrhotic.

The frequency of the association between cirrhosis and HCC varies somewhat with the critera used for diagnosis of cirrhosis. Pathologic diagnosis is more accurate than clinical, yet the histopathologic diagnosis is not absolute because chronic active hepatitis and cirrhosis frequently coexist in the same liver. Only a few studies have compared the livers with HBV and HCV infection at the time of HCC detection. Shiratori et al.[55] in Tokyo compared 145 HCC cases positive for anti-HCV and negative for HBV seromarkers, 26 cases positive for anti-HCV and HBV antibodies, and 23 cases positive for HBsAg and negative for anti-HCV. There was a significant difference in the severity of liver disease; patients with HBsAg-positive HCC generally had a milder disease, and 65.2% were in the Child A status. The corresponding figure for anti-HCV-positive cases was 37.4%. More than 20% of anti-HCV-positive cases were Child C compared to 8.7% in HBsAg-positive cases. Biopsy histology similarly showed more severe disease in anti-HCV positive cases; 94.1% showed either severe hepatitis (24.8%) or cirrhosis (69.3%). In contrast, 50% of HBsAg-positive cases had only moderately active chronic hepatitis; none had severe chronic hepatitis, and only 50% were cirrhotic. Shimamatsu et al.[54] compared livers with HCV-associated cirrhosis and 21 with HBsAg-positive cirrhosis. They found that the fibrous septa were broader, with smaller regenerative nodules with less regenerative activity in the former; inflammatory reactions were stronger, with prominent lymphoid aggregates in the stroma. The thin stroma with relatively large nodules that had been commonly seen in the past in Japan[76] apparently had been caused by HBV infection.

In other studies, encapsulation with an expanding (and relatively benign) growth pattern was more frequent in non-A, non-B hepatitis-associated HCC, and infiltrating growth was less common.[74] Another study demonstrated that markedly shrunk cirrhotic livers with HCC were more often related to non-A, non-B hepatitis, and the patients were older.[77]

Perhaps HCV-associated HCC emerges more often in an advanced cirrhotic liver in older individuals and grows in a less aggressive fashion.[78]

Cholangiocarcinoma, another but less common primary liver cancer, is not as frequently associated with HCV infection as is HCC.[79] Combined hepatocholangiocarcinoma that sometimes occurs in HCC[80] and behaves very much like HCC, however, is just as commonly associated with HCV infection.[79] This suggests that the cholangiocarcinoma element may be secondary to the HCC element.

HCV RNA IN SERUM AND LIVER TISSUE

The presence of HCV RNA in serum indicates active viral replication. The prevalence of HCV RNA in the sera of patients with HCC in various countries is shown in Table 4-4.[23,81–85] Most studies have demonstrated high HCV RNA positivity rates in HCC patients who have anti-HCV. According to Hagiwara et al.[86] the average HCV RNA titers measured by the method of Becker-

TABLE 4-4. HCV RNA in Serum of Patients With Hepatocellular Carcinoma

	HCV RNA Positivity		
Country	Anti-HCV (+) Cases	Anti-HCV (−) Cases	Reference
Spain	40/42 (96%)	2/28 (7%)	23
France	4/19 (21%)	1/21 (5%)	81
Japan	27/29 (93%)	5/10 (50%)	82
Taiwan	16/21 (76%)	1/10 (10%)	83
South Africa	17/25 (68%)	9/103 (9%)	84
USA	7/10 (70%)	0/21 (0%)	85

Andre and Hahlbrock[87] in asymptomatic blood donors (n = 9) were 5.4 (log_{10} copies/ml), 7.3 in chronic persistent hepatitis (n = 20), 7.9 in chronic active hepatitis (n = 48), 7.8 in cirrhosis (n = 12) and 7.9 in HCC (n = 15). In other words, HCV RNA was present in higher concentration in patients with liver disease than among asymptomatic donors, but among the four disease groups there was no difference. In contrast, an Italian study detected progressively decreasing RNA titers by the branched DNA method from chronic hepatitis to cirrhosis and from cirrhosis to HCC[88] (5700 Keq/ml in chronic hepatitis, 3340 Keq/ml in cirrhosis and 1768 Keq/ml in HCC). It is not clear whether the differences between these studies were due to the method used for quantification or to ethnic and other factors.

If HCV RNA (plus strand) itself is measured in tissue, the detected RNA may be due to the presence of blood; therefore, one has to detect minus strand RNA as a sign of viral replication, as only the plus strand would be expected in blood.[89] A number of studies have shown that both minus and plus strand RNAs are demonstrable in HCC tissue, as well as nontumor liver tissue, in patients with anti-HCV in serum.[90,91] Kurosaki et al.[92] sequenced HCV from HCC and nontumor liver tissues from four cases and found that in one patient, a single species with an identical sequence of the envelope (E2) gene was present in both HCC and nontumorous liver tissues. In the other three patients, there was a mixture of two to five species with different but highly homologous (82% to 99%) E2 genes (quasispecies population). Of ten sequences, four were found in both tissues, two in cancer tissue, and four in noncancer tissue only. Such differences in the constitution of quasispecies population between the two tissues confirm that replication of the virus is occurring in both tissues. Since the tissues failed to show any particular E2 hypervariable region sequence shared by the HCC tissues, a direct contribution of a specific RNA sequence in association with the E2 hypervariable region seems unlikely.

DEVELOPMENT OF HCC IN ASSOCIATION WITH CHRONIC LIVER DISEASE

Kiyosawa et al.[49] analyzed stored sera from patients who developed acute post-transfusion non-A, non-B hepatitis and subsequently chronic liver disease and found that the average interval between acute infection and the diagnosis of cirrhosis was 21.2 ± 9.6 years, and between acute infection and HCC 29.0 ± 13.2 years (Fig. 4-2). In other words, acute HCV infection, if it becomes chronic, can take less than 8 years to progress from cirrhosis to HCC. Other studies in Japan have corroborated Kiyosawa's observations. Kaneko et al.[93] prospectively

FIGURE 4-2. Intervals from post-transfusion hepatitis C to diagnosis of chronic hepatitis, cirrhosis, and HCC in Japan and Los Angeles. (Adapted from Kiyosawa et al.[49] and Tong et al.,[96] with permission.)

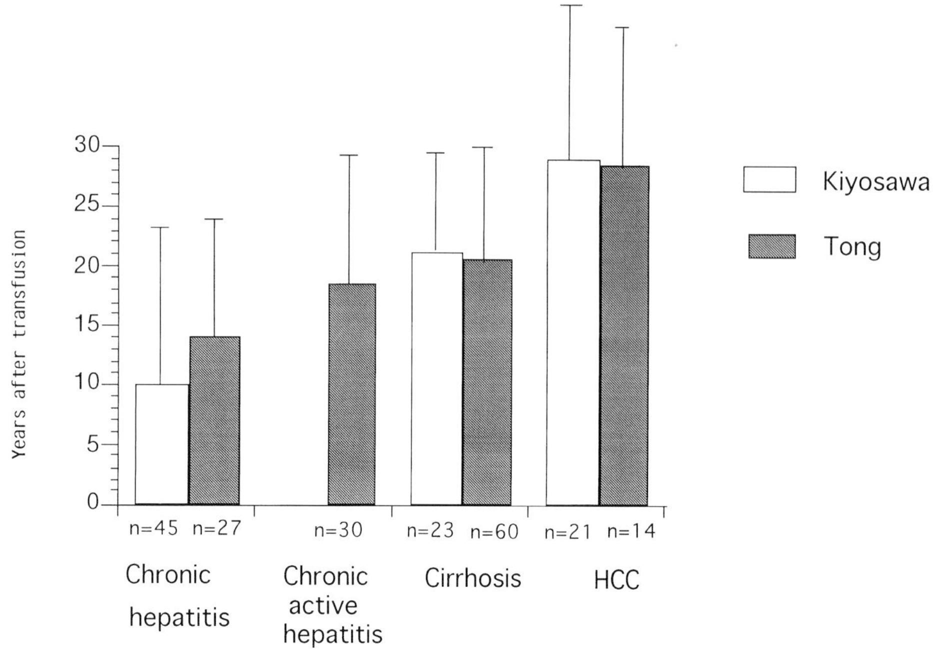

followed up 158 patients with chronic hepatitis C and 70 with C cirrhosis; 14 of the former developed HCC in an average period of 10.1 ± 3.3 years and 44% of the latter did so in 7.3 ± 3.5 years.

Seeff et al.[94] found no increase in mortality from all causes in transfusion-associated non-A, non-B hepatitis compared with control groups after 18 years among 568 patients who had transfusion-associated non-A, non-B hepatitis for an average of 18 years. A small but significant increase in the number of deaths related to liver disease was observed. Further follow-up study at 20 years did not change the overall results.[95] More recently, however, Tong et al.[96] in California followed 131 patients with chronic post-transfusion hepatitis C and found progression of the disease to HCC in a considerable proportion; 60 of the cases developed cirrhosis in an average period of 20.6 ± 10.1 years and 14 HCC in 28.3 ± 11.5 years after blood transfusion (Fig. 4-2). These rates are very similar to those in the Kiyosawa's study in Japan.[49] Nine of the 14 HCC cases in the Tong study were white.

In many studies, the frequency of HCC development among patients with chronic liver disease, particularly cirrhosis, was determined. Ikeda et al.[97] in Tokyo followed 795 consecutive patients with cirrhosis for up to 17 years and analyzed the cumulative rate of HCC development. It was 19.4%, 44.3%, and 58.2% at the end of the fifth, tenth, and fifteenth years, respectively. HCC appeared in 5 years in 14.2% of HBsAg-positive cases and in 21.5% of anti-HCV positive cases; the difference became even greater at the end of 15 years (27.2% vs 75.2%). Using the Cox regression model, it was shown that age, indocyanine green clearance rate, platelet count, α-fetoprotein (AFP) value, alcohol use, and detection of HBsAg were risk factors by univariate analysis. With multivariate analysis, AFP, age, and alcohol use were found to contribute independently to HCC development. Oka et al.[98] showed that 39% of 126 patients with HCC cirrhosis developed HCC in 60 months, equivalent to a 7.8% annual incidence of HCC, the highest rate ever reported. Colombo et al.[99,100] followed 447 Italian patients with well-compensated cirrhosis (62% of viral origin); HCC was found in 7% of these cases at baseline, and another 7% developed HCC during the average follow-up period of 33 months. In this study, the HCC appearance rate was 3.2% per year overall among cirrhotic patients; 28% among those with HCV cirrhosis, and 3% in those with HBV cirrhosis in 5 years. The annual rate of HCC occurrence in patients with cirrhosis has been shown to be more or less similar in Japan, Italy, and France, ranging from 3.0% to 6.5% per year (Table 4-5).[97,99,101–104] Among different etiologic groups, those with HCV cirrhosis had the highest rate of HCC.

ALCOHOL AND HCV-ASSOCIATED HCC

Alcohol may not be a carcinogen or a cocarcinogen, but it may increase conversion of procarcinogen to carcinogen through cytochrome P450 II El, which is inducible by ethanol[105] and may act as a weak promoting agent for induction of hepatocarcinogenesis.[106] Bruix et al.[22] compared 95 patients in Spain with HCC, 106 patients with cirrhosis without HCC, and 177 controls. They found that 76.6% with alcoholic cirrhosis with HCC had anti-HCV and 38.7% with alcoholic cirrhosis without HCC had anti-HCV. Similar results were reported from France by Nalpas et al.[21] Yamauchi et al.[107] studied 63 cases of alcoholic cirrhosis in Japan and 61 with nonalcoholic cirrhosis. The 3-, 5-, and 10-year cumulative rate of HCC occurrence was 13.3%, 41.3%, and 80.7%, respectively, for anti-HCV positive patients with alcoholic cirrhosis. In nonalcoholic HCV cirrhosis, these rates were 7.3%, 23.1%, and 56.5%, respectively. Thus, it appears that hepatocarcinogenesis may be hastened in patients with HCV cirrhosis if they are heavy drinkers. Takada et al.[106] analyzed 369 cases of cirrhosis and found an estimated

TABLE 4-5. Prospective Studies on the Rate of HCC Appearance in Patients With Cirrhosis

		No. of Patients			
Reference	Country	Followed	Developed HCC	Screening Interval (Months)	Annual Rate (%)
Oka et al.[101]	Japan	140	40	3	6.5
Colombo et al.[99]	Italy	447	65	12	3.2
Ikeda et al.[97]	Japan	795	221	1–2	3.9–4.4[a]
Sato et al.[102]	Japan	361	33	3	3.0
Pateron et al.[103]	France	118	14	6	5.8
Cottone et al.[104]	Italy	147	30[b]	6	4.4

[a] For HCV alone, 5%.

[b] 22 of 28, anti-HCV+.

relative risk for HCC development in cirrhotic patients was 8.2 and 8.3 times higher in HBV and HCV carriers, respectively, than in alcoholics without either virus infection.

PORPHYRIA CUTANEA TARDA, HCV, AND HCC

Porphyria cutanea tarda (PCT) is the most common type of porphyria. It is caused by decreased activity of uroporphyrin decarboxylase in the liver, which results in overproduction and accumulation of poorly decarboxylated porphyrin. The disease is thought to be inherited by an autosomal dominant mechanism. The clinical presentation includes photosensitivity, blistering skin lesions, and chronic liver disease. Kordac[108] found HCC in nearly half of necropsied cases of PCT in Czechoslovakia. Solis et al.[109] found HCC in 7.2% of 138 patients with PCT in Spain. Salata et al.[110] found HCC in 13 of 83 patients with unequivocal PCT over an average of 4.8 years in Spain. The age at which cutaneous disease was first noted was 38 years on average, and the mean latent period before HCC detection was 23 years. There is no clear-cut relation of PCT-associated HCC to HBV infection.[111] Earlier histologic studies in the United States have shown that chronic inflammation is commonly seen in the liver of PCT patients.[112] Two recent studies, one from Italy[113] and the other from Spain[114] reported a strong relationship between HCV infection and PCT. Up to 63% of patients with PCT tested positive for anti-HCV.

AUTOIMMUNE LIVER DISEASE, HCV, AND HCC

Primary biliary cirrhosis (PBC) was not known to be associated with HCC until 1984 when Melia et al.[115] reported development of HCC in 5 of 130 cases of PBC in London. In the extensive autopsy registries in Japan, in which more than 30,000 autopsies are recorded annually, not a single case of HCC developed in PBC patients up to 1982. HCC began appearing among PBC patients in 1983, and it has since been seen continually on a yearly basis.[116] In a study in Italy of 160 patients with PBC, anti-HCV was positive in 19.[117] Some Japanese undocumented reports indicated positive anti-HCV in some, but not all patients with PBC developed HCC. Eight cases of HCC that developed on the background of autoimmune hepatitis in England included six with HCV infection.[118] A certain type of autoimmune hepatitis is associated with HCV infection. We need more information about the possible role of HCV infection in autoimmune liver diseases and its relationship to hepatocarcinogenesis.

MANAGEMENT AND PREVENTION OF HCV-ASSOCIATED HCC

Once HCC has emerged in the liver, it is difficult to treat. Although a number of nonsurgical therapeutic modalities have been developed and assessed for efficacy, the results are disappointing.[119] Complete cure is feasible only by surgical removal of tumor. Complete resection is possible and can be successful if HCC is discovered while it is small and if cirrhosis is mild or absent. After resection, if remnant liver is cirrhotic, it will frequently have tumor recurrence after varying time intervals. Early detection before extrahepatic spread and transplantation are the best treatments, but in reality they are only rarely achieved.

Prevention of HCV infection is the primary prevention of HCV-associated HCC. Infection caused by blood transfusion has been nearly eliminated with antibody assays. Treatment of acute hepatitis C with interferon may prevent development of chronic hepatitis, although results vary.[120,121] Treatment of chronic hepatitis C with interferon is of documented efficacy in many cases.[122] In addition, chemoprevention may be possible to prevent emergence of HCC in a liver that has already developed advanced cirrhosis.[98]

SUMMARY

There is sufficient evidence that chronic HCV infection is associated with a risk of developing HCC. The etiologic role of HCV infection in terms of molecular events in hepatocarcinogenesis is not known, but it is clearly different from that of HBV infection. Continuous inflammation, liver cell death, and ongoing viral replication seem to underlie HCV-related hepatocarcinogenesis. It is not yet clear whether the different genotypes of HCV account for the regional differences in the prevalence of HCV-associated HCC. The possible interrelationship of HBV and HCV coinfection needs to be elucidated because of the possible presence of HBV DNA in the liver in the absence of positive serology in some cases. The relative roles of HBV and HCV infections in the epidemiology of HCC are changing throughout the world. HCC is difficult to treat, and major efforts should be directed toward its prevention. Prevention might be achieved by preventing HCV infection, preventing the transition from acute to chronic hepatitis, treating chronic hepatitis C early, and possibly by chemoprevention of HCC in patients with advanced chronic hepatitis C.

REFERENCES

1. Szmuness W. Hepatocellular carcinoma and the hepatitis B virus: evidence for a causal association. Prog Med Virol 1978;24:40–69
2. Dienstag JL. Non-A, non-B hepatitis. I. Recognition, epidemiology, and clinical features. Gastroenterology 1983;85: 439–462
3. Dienstag JL. Non-A, non-B hepatitis. II. Experimental transmission, putative virus agents and markers, and prevention. Gastroenterology 1983;85:743–768
4. Iwama S, Ohnishi K, Nakajima Y et al. A clinical study of hepatocellular carcinoma (HCC) in relation to hepatitis B seromarkers: implication of non-A, non-B hepatitis (NANB). Hepatology 1982;2:117(abstr)
5. Okuda K. Liver Cancer. In Zuckerman AJ, Thomas JC (eds): Viral Hepatitis. Churchill Livingstone, London, 1993, pp. 269–280
6. Okuda K, Fujimoto I, Hanai A, Urano Y. Changing incidence of hepatocellular carcinoma in Japan. Cancer Res 1987;47:4967–4972
7. Choo QL, Kuo G, Wiener LR et al. Isolation of a cDNA clone derived from a blood-borne non-A, non-B viral hepatitis genome. Science 1989;244:359–362
8. Kuo G, Choo QL, Alter HJ et al. An assay for circulating antibodies to a major etiologic virus of human non-A, non-B hepatitis. Science 1989;244:362–364
9. McFarlane IG, Smith HM, Johnson PJ et al. Hepatitis C virus antibodies in chronic active hepatitis: pathogenetic factor or false-positive result? Lancet 1990;335:754–757
10. Colombo M, Rumi MG, Donato MF et al. Hepatitis C antibody in patients with chronic liver disease and hepatocellular carcinoma. Dig Dis Sci 1991;36:1130–1133
11. Manigia A, Vallari D, Di Bisceglie AM. Use of confirmatory tests for hepatitis C virus infection in patients with hepatocellular carcinoma. J Med Virol 1994;43:125–128
12. Alter MJ. Epidemiology of hepatitis C in the West. Semin Liver Dis 1995;15:5–14
13. Mansell CJ, Locarnini SA. Epidemiology of hepatitis C in the East. Semin Liver Dis 1995;15:15–32
14. Sirchia G, Bellobuono A, Giovanetti A, Marconi M. Antibodies to hepatitis C virus in Italian blood donors. Lancet 1989;ii:797
15. Colombo M, Kuo M, Choo QL et al. Prevalence of antibodies to hepatitis C virus in Italian patients with hepatocellular carcinoma. Lancet 1989;ii:1006–1008
16. Simonetti R, Cottonoe M, Craxi A et al. Prevalence of antibodies to hepatitis C virus in hepatocellular carcinoma. Lancet 1989;ii:1338
17. Levrero M, Tagger A, Balsano C et al. Antibodies to hepatitis C virus in patients with hepatocellular carcinoma. J Hepatol 1991;12:60–63
18. Caporaso N, Romano M, Marmo R et al. Hepatitis C infection is an additive risk factor for development of hepatocellular carcinoma in patients with cirrhosis. J Hepatol 1991; 12:367–371
19. Janot C, Courouce AM, Maneiz M. Antibodies to hepatitis C virus in French blood donors. Lancet 1989;ii:796–797
20. Ducreux M, Buffer C, Dussaix E et al. Antibody to hepatitis C virus in hepatocellular carcinoma. Lancet 1990;335:301
21. Nalpas B, Driss F, Pol S et al. Association between HCV and HBV infection in hepatocellular carcinoma and alcoholic liver disease. J Hepatol 1991;12:70–74
22. Bruix J, Barrera JM, Calver X et al. Prevalence of antibodies of hepatitis C virus in Spanish patients with hepatocellular carcinoma and hepatic cirrhosis. Lancet 1989;ii:1004–1006
23. Ruiz J, Sangro B, Cuende JI et al. Hepatitis B and C viral infections in patients with hepatocellular carcinoma. Hepatology 1992;16:637–641
24. Brind AM, Codd AA, Cohen DG et al. Low prevalence of antibody to hepatitis C virus in northeast England. J Med Virol 1990;32:242–248
25. Kaklamani E, Trichopoulos D, Tzonou A et al. Hepatitis B and C viruses and their interaction in the origin of hepatocellular carcinoma. JAMA 1991;265:1974–1976
26. Hasan F, Feffers LJ, Madina M et al. Hepatitis C-associated hepatocellular carcinoma. Hepatology 1990;12:589–591
27. Yu MC, Tong MJ, Coursager P et al. Prevalence of hepatitis B and C viral markers in black and white patients with hepatocellular carcinoma in the United States. J Natl Cancer Inst 1990;82:1038–1041
28. Kew MC, Houghton M, Choo QL, Kuo G. Hepatitis C virus antibodies in southern African blacks with hepatocellular carcinoma. Lancet 1990;335:873–874
29. Dazza M-C, Meneses L-V, Girard P-M et al. Hepatitis C virus antibody and hepatocellular carcinoma. Lancet 1990; 335:1216
30. Nishioka K. Hepatitis C virus infection in Japan. Gastroenterol Jpn 1991;26(suppl 3):152–155
31. Kiyosawa K, Furuta S. Review of hepatitis C in Japan. J Gastroenterol Hepatol 1991;6:383–391
32. Ohkoshi S, Kojima H, Tawaraya H et al. Prevalence of antibody against non-A, non-B hepatitis virus in Japanese patients with hepatocellular carcinoma. Jpn J Cancer Res 1990;81:550–553
33. Tanaka K, Hirohata T, Koga S et al. Hepatitis C and hepatitis B in the etiology of hepatocellular carcinoma in the Japanese population. Cancer Res 1991;2842–2847
34. Chen DS, Kuo GC, Sung L et al. Hepatitis C virus infection in an area hyperendemic for hepatitis B and chronic liver disease: the Taiwan experience. J Infect Dis 1990;162: 817–822
35. Jeng JE, Tsai JF. Hepatitis C virus antibody in hepatocellular carcinoma in Taiwan. J Med Virol 1991;34:74–77
36. Leung NWY, Tam JS, Lai JY et al. Does hepatitis C virus infection contribute to hepatocellular carcinoma in Hong Kong? Cancer 1992;70:4–44
37. Ito S, Yao DF, Nii C et al. Epidemiological characteristics of the incidence of hepatitis C virus (C100-3) antibodies in patients with liver diseases in the Inshore area of the Yangtze river. J Gastroenterol Hepatol 1993;8:232–237
38. Tao QM, Wang Y, Wang H et al. Seroepidemiology of HCV and HBV infections in northern China. Gastroenterol Jpn 1991;26(suppl):156–158
39. Kim BS, Park YM. Prevalence of hepatitis C virus related to

liver diseases in Korea. Gastroenterol Jpn 1993;28(suppl): 17–22

40. Boonmar S, Pojanagaroon B, Watanabe Y et al. Prevalence of hepatitis C virus antibody among healthy blood donors and non-A, non-B hepatitis patients in Thailand. Jpn J Med Sci Biol 1990;43:29–36
41. Oon CJ, Chia SC, Fock KM. Prevalence of hepatitis C in liver diseases and in a random population in Singapore. Proc. 3rd International Symp on Viral Hepatitis and Hepatocellular Carcinoma, Taipei. Gastroenterological Society of the Republic of China, Taipei, 1991, p. 141
42. Sulaiman HA, Noer S, Endardjo S, Hoyaranda E. The prevalence of antibody to hepatitis C virus (anti-HCV) in patients with acute and chronic liver disease in Jakarta, Indonesia. Gastroenterol Jpn 1991;26(suppl 3):179–183
43. Ramesh R, Muhshi A, Panda SK. Prevalence of hepatitis C virus antibodies in chronic liver disease and hepatocellular carcinoma patients in India. J Gastroenterol Hepatol 1991; 7:393–395
44. Shrestha SM, Tsuda F, Okamoto H et al. Hepatitis B virus subtypes and hepatitis C virus genotypes in patients with chronic liver disease in Nepal. Hepatology 1994;19: 805–809
45. Al Karawi MAA, Shariq S, El Shiekh Mohamed AR et al. Hepatitis C virus infection in chronic liver disease and hepatocellular carcinoma in Saudi Arabia. J Gastroenterol Hepatol 1992;7:237–239
46. Suou T, Ikuta Y, Hasegawa M, Kawasaki H. Prevalence of HCV antibodies in Yatsuka town of Simane Prefecture, Japan. Jpn J Gastroenterol 1992;89:113–117
47. Setoguchi Y, Yamamoto K, Ozaki I et al. Prevalence of chronic liver diseases and anti-HCV antibodies in different districts of Saga, Japan. Gastroenterol Jpn 1991;26: 157–161
48. Kiyosawa K, Tanaka E, Sodeyama T et al. Transmission of hepatitis C in an isolated area in Japan: community acquired infection. Gastroenterology 1994;106:1596–1602
49. Kiyosawa K, Sodeyama T, Tanaka E et al. Interelationship of blood transfusion, non-A, non-B hepatitis and hepatocellular carcinoma: analysis by detection of antibody to hepatitis C virus. Hepatology 1990;12:671–675
50. Nishioka K, Watanabe J, Furuta S et al. A high prevalence of antibody to the hepatitis C virus with hepatocellular carcinoma in Japan. Cancer 1991;67:429–433
51. Tanaka E, Sodeyama T, Yoshizawa K et al. Prevalence of hepatitis C virus related C100-3 antibody in school children in Matsumoto area. Acta Hepatol Jpn 1992;32: 205–206
52. Saeed AA, Al-Admawi AM, Rankin D et al. Further observations on the high hepatitis C seroprevalence in Egypt. Proceedings 2nd Conference and Postgraduate Course. African Association for the Study of Liver Disease. Mar. 18–22, Cairo, 1994, Abstract No. 1
53. Okuda K. Hepatocellular carcinoma: recent progress. Hepatology 1992;15:948–963
54. Shimamatsu K, Kage M, Nakashima O, Kojiro M. Pathomorphological study of HCV antibody-positive liver cirrhosis. J Gastroenterol Hepatol 1994;9:624–630
55. Shiratori Y, Shiina S, Imamura M et al. Characteristic difference of hepatocellular carcinoma between hepatitis B- and C-viral infection in Japan. Hepatology 1995;22: 1027–1033
56. Tarao K, Ohkawa S, Shimizu A et al. Significance of hepatocellular proliferation in the development of hepatocellular carcinoma from anti-hepatitis C virus-positive cirrhotic patients. Cancer 1994;73:1149–1154
57. Chang MH, Hsu HC, Lee CY et al. Fraternal hepatocellular carcinoma in young children in two families. Cancer 1984; 53:1807–1910
58. Simmonds P, Alberti A, Alter HJ et al. A proposed system for the nomenclature of hepatitis C viral genotypes. Hepatology 1994;19:1321–1324
59. Yuwen H, Bayley AC, Cairns J, Tabor E. Hepatocellular carcinoma: lack of association with a unique hepatitis C virus necleotide sequence. J Infect Dis 1994;169:706–707
60. Tanaka E, Kiyosawa K, Matsushita T et al. Epidemiology of genotypes of hepatitis C virus in Japanese patients with type C chronic liver diseases. J Gastroenterol Hepatol 1995; 10:538–545
61. Zuckerman AJ. Viral superinfection. Hepatology 1987;7: 184–185
62. Brotman B, Prince AM, Huima T et al. Interference between non-A, non-B and hepatitis B virus infection in chimpanzees. J Med Virol 1983;11:191–205
63. Liaw YF, Tsai SL, Chang JJ et al. Displacement of hepatitis B virus by hepatitis C virus as the cause of continuing chronic hepatitis. Gastroenterology 1994;106:1048–1053
64. Fong TL, Di Bisceglie AM, Waggoner JG et al. The significance of antibody to hepatitis C virus in patients with chronic hepatitis B. Hepatology 1991;14:64–67
65. Sbolli G, Zanotti AR, Tanzi E et al. Serum antibodies to hepatitis C virus in Italian patients with hepatocellular carcinoma. J Med Virol 1990;30:230–232
66. Nishioka K, Watanabe J, Furuta S et al. A high prevalence of antibody to the hepatitis C virus in patients with hepatocellular carcinoma in Japan. Cancer 1991;67:429–433
67. Hamasaki K, Nakata K, Tsutumi T et al. Changes in the prevalence of hepatitis B and C infection in patients with hepatocellular carcinoma in the Nagasaki Prefecture, Japan. J Med Viol 1993;40:146–149
68. Lee SD, Lee FY, Wi JC et al. The prevalence of anti-hepatitis C virus among Chinese patients with hepatocellular carcinoma. Cancer 1992;69:342–345
69. Saito I, Miyamura T, Ohbayashi A et al. Hepatitis C virus infection is associated with the development of hepatocellular carcinoma. Proc Natl Acad Sci USA 1990;87: 6547–6549
70. Chuang WL, Chang WY, Lu SN et al. The role of hepatitis B and C viruses in hepatocellular carcinoma in a hepatitis B endemic area. Cancer 1992;69:2052–2054
71. Brechot C, Degos F, Lugassay C et al. Hepatitis B virus DNA in patients with chronic liver disease and negative tests for hepatitis B surface antigen. N Engl J Med 1985; 312:270–276
72. Blum H, Offensperger WB, Walter E et al. Latent hepatitis B virus infection with full-length viral genome in patients

serologically immune to hepatitis B virus infection. Liver 1988;8:307–316

73. Kremsdorf D, Garreau F, Duclos H et al. Complete nucleotide sequence and viral envelope protein expression of a hepatitis B virus DNA derived from a hepatitis B surface antigen-negative patient. J Hepatol 1993;18:244–250
74. Liang TJ, Jeffers LJ, Reddy KR et al. Viral pathogenesis of hepatocellular carcinoma in the United States. Hepatology 1993;18:1326–1333
75. Peterlin P, Driss F, Nalpas B et al. Persistence of hepatitis B and hepatitis C viral genomes in primary liver cancer from HBsAg-negative patients: a study of a low-endemic area. Hepatology 1993;17:20–29
76. Shikata T. Primary liver carcinoma and liver cirrhosis. In Okuda K, Peters RL (eds): Hepatocellular Carcinoma. Wiley, New York, 1976, pp. 53–71
77. Okuda K, Nakashima T, Sakamoto K et al. Hepatocellular carcinoma arising in noncirrhotic and highly cirrhotic livers: a comparative study of histopathology and frequency of hepatitis B markers. Cancer 1982;49:450–455
78. Okuda K. Hepatocellular carcinomas associated with hepatitis B and C virus infections. Are they any different? Hepatology 1995;22:1883–1885
79. Tomimatsu M, Ishiguro N, Taniai M et al. Hepatitis C virus antibody in patients with primary liver cancer (hepatocellular carcinoma, cholangiocarcinoma, and combined hepatocellular-cholangiocarcinoma) in Japan. Cancer 1993;72: 682–688
80. Okuda K, Kojiro M, Okuda H. Neoplasms of the liver. In Schiff L, Schiff ER (eds): Diseases of the Liver. JB Lippincott, Philadelphia, 1993, pp. 1236–1296
81. Thelu MA, Zarski JP, Dardelet D et al. Low prevalence of hepatitis C virus genome detected by PCR in serum of Caucasian patients with hepatocellular carcinoma. J Hepatol 1992;14:415–416
82. Hagiwara H, Hayashi N, Mita E et al. Detection of hepatitis C virus RNA in chronic non-A, non-B liver disease. Gastroenterology 1992;102:692–694
83. Sheu JC, Huang GT, Shih LN et al. Hepatitis C and B viruses in hepatitis B surface antigen-negative hepatocellular carcinoma. Gastroenterology 1992;103:1322–1327
84. Bukh J, Miller RH, Kew MC, Purcell RH. Hepatitis C virus RNA in southern African blacks with hepatocellular carcinoma. Proc Natl Acad Sci USA 1993;90:1848–1851
85. Magnia A, Vallari D, Di Bisceglie AM. Use of confirmatory tests for hepatitis C viral infection in patients with hepatocellular carcinoma. J Med Virol 1994;43:125–128
86. Hagiwara H, Hayashi N, Mita E et al. Quantitation of hepatitis C virus RNA in serum of asymptomatic blood donors and patients with type C chronic liver disease. Hepatology 1993;17:545–550
87. Becker-Andre M, Hahlbrock K. Absolute mRNA quantification using the polymerase chain reaction (PCR): a novel approach by a PCR aided transcript titration assay (PATTY). Nucleic Acids Res 1989;17:9437–9446
88. Magrin S, Craxi A, Fablano C et al. Hepatitis C viremia in chronic liver disease: relationship to interferon-α or corticosteroid treatment. Hepatology 1994;19:273–279
89. Takehara T, Hayashi N, Mita E et al. Detection of minus strand of hepatitis C virus RNA by reverse transcription and polymerase chain reaction. Implication for hepatitis C virus replication in infected tissue. Hepatology 1992;15: 387–390
90. Gerber MA. Relation of hepatitis C virus to hepatocellular carcinoma. J Hepatol 1993;17(suppl 3): S108–S111
91. Kobayashi S, Hayashi H, Itoh Y et al. Detection of minus-strand hepatitis C virus RNA in tumor tissues of hepatocellular carcinoma. Cancer 1994;73:48–52
92. Kurosaki M, Enomoto N, Sakamoto N et al. Detection and analysis of replicating hepatitis C virus RNA in hepatocellular carcinoma tissues. J Hepatol 1995;22:527–535
93. Kaneko S, Unoura M, Takeuchi M et al. The role of hepatitis C virus in hepatocellular carcinoma in Japan. Intervirology 1994;37:108–113
94. Seeff LB, Tuskell-Bales Z, Wright EC et al. Long-term mortality after transfusion-associated non-A, non-B hepatitis. N Engl J Med 1992;327:1906–1911
95. Seeff LB, NHLBI Study Group. Mortality and morbidity of transfusion-associated type C hepatitis: an NHLBI multicenter study. Hepatology 1995;20:204A(abstract)
96. Tong MJ, El-Farra NS, Reikes AR, Co RL. Clinical outcome after transfusion-associated hepatitis C. N Engl J Med 1995;332:1463–1466
97. Ikeda K, Saitoh S, Koida I et al. A multivariate analysis of risk factors for hepatocellular carcinoma: a prospective observation of 795 patients with viral and alcoholic cirrhosis. Hepatology 1993;18:47–53
98. Oka H, Yamamoto S, Kuroki T et al. Prospective study of chemoprevention of hepatocellular carcinoma with Sho-saiko-to (TJ-9). Cancer 1995;76:743–749
99. Colombo M, de Franchis R, Ninno ED et al. Hepatocellular carcinoma in Italian patients with cirrhosis. N Engl J Med 1991;325:675–680
100. Colombo M. Debate in hepatitis. Should patients with chronic viral hepatitis be screened for hepatocellular carcinoma? Viral Hepatitis Review 1995;1:67–75
101. Oka H, Kurioka N, Kim K et al. Prospective study of early detection of hepatocellular carcinoma in patients with cirrhosis. Hepatology 1990;12:680–687
102. Sato Y, Nakata K, Kato Y et al. Early recognition of hepatocellular carcinoma based on altered profiles of alpha-fetoprotein. N Engl J Med 1993;328:1802–1806
103. Pateron D, Ganne N, Trinchet JC et al. Prospective study of screening for hepatocellular carcinoma in Caucasian patients with cirrhosis. J Hepatol 1994;20:65–71
104. Cottone M, Turri M, Caltagirone M et al. Screening for hepatocellular carcinoma in patients with Child's A cirrhosis: an 8-year prospective study by ultrasound and alphafetoprotein. J Hepatol 1994;21:1029–1034
105. Johanson I, Ekstrom G, Scholte B et al. Ethanol-, fasting- and acetone-inducible cytochrome P-450 in rat liver: regulation and characteristics of enzymes belonging to the IIB and IIE gene subfamilies. Biochemistry 1988;27:1925–1934
106. Takada A, Takase S, Tsutsumi M. Alcohol and hepatic carcinogenesis. In Yirmiya R, Taylor AN (eds): Alcohol,

Immunity, and Cancer. CRC Press, Boca Raton, FL, 1993, pp. 187–209

107. Yamauchi M, Nakahara M, Maezawa Y et al. Prevalence of hepatocellular carcinoma in patients with alcoholic cirrhosis and prior exposure to hepatitis C. Am J Gastroenterol 1993;88:39–43
108. Kordac V. Frequency of occurrence of hepatocellular carcinoma in patients with porphyria cutanea tarda in long-term follow-up. Neoplasm 1972;19:135–139
109. Solis JA, Betancor P, Campos R et al. Association of porphyria cutanea tarda and primary liver cancer. Report of ten cases. J Dermatol 1982;9:131–137
110. Salata H, Cortés JM, Enriques de Salamanca R et al. Porphyria cutanea tarda and hepatocellular carcinoma. Frequency of occurrence and related factors. J Hepatol 1985; 1:477–487
111. Okuda K. Porphyria cutanea tarda and hepatocellular carcinoma: correlations. Hepatology 1986;6:1054–1056
112. Lefkowitch JH, Grossman ME. Hepatic pathology in porphyria cutanea tarda. Liver 1983;3:19–29
113. Fargion S, Piperno A, Capellini MD et al. Hepatitis C virus and porphyria cutanea tarda: evidence of a strong association. Hepatology 1992;16:956–959
114. DeCastro M, Sanchez J, Herrera JF et al. Hepatitis C virus antibodies and liver disease in patients with porphyria cutanea tarda. Hepatology 1993;17:551–557
115. Melia WM, Johnson PJ, Neuberger H et al. Hepatocellular carcinoma in primary biliary cirrhosis: detection by fetoprotein estimation. Gastroenterology 1984;7:660–663
116. Nakanuma Y, Terada T, Doishita K, Miwa A. Hepatocellular carcinoma in primary biliary cirrhosis: an autopsy study. Hepatology 1990;11:1010–1016
117. Bertolini E, Battezzati PM, Zermiani P et al. Hepatitis C virus testing in primary biliary cirrhosis. J Hepatol 1992; 15:207–210
118. Ryder SD, Koskinas J, Rizzi PM et al. Hepatocellular carcinoma complicating autoimmune hepatitis: role of hepatitis C virus. Hepatology 1995;22:718–722
119. Okuda K, Okuda H. Primary liver cell carcinoma. In McIntyre N et al (eds): Oxford Textbook of Clinical Hepatology. Oxford University Press, Oxford, 1991, pp. 1019–1053
120. Omata M, Yokosuka O, Takano S et al. Resolution of acute hepatitis C after therapy with natural beta interferon. Lancet 1991;338:914–915
121. Viladomiu L, Genesca J, Esteban J et al. Interferon alpha in acute post-transfusion hepatitis C: a randomized, controlled trial. Hepatology 1992;15:767–769
122. Fried MW, Hoofnagle JH. Therapy of hepatitis C. Semin Liver Dis 1995;15:82–91

5

AFLATOXIN EXPOSURE AS A RISK FACTOR IN THE ETIOLOGY OF HEPATOCELLULAR CARCINOMA

GERALD N. WOGAN

Abundant epidemiologic and experimental evidence indicates that hepatocellular carcinoma (HCC) is of multifactorial etiology. Infection by hepatitis B is a major risk factor for the disease in Africa and Asia, and hepatitis C virus is of major significance in Japan, Europe, and the United States. Various environmental factors may play etiologic roles in HCC development; roles for consumption of alcoholic beverages, diet, and nutritional status have been suggested. The evidence is stronger for an etiologic role for diets contaminated with aflatoxins than for any other environmental factor.

Aflatoxins, produced by food spoilage molds, have been shown to be carcinogenic when administered to experimental animals. Other known chemical carcinogens include hundreds of compounds representing many chemical classes, including polycyclic aromatic hydrocarbons, aromatic amines, azo compounds, alkylating agents, lactones, N-nitroso compounds, and metals. Many chemicals within these classes have been shown to induce HCC in experimental animals, generally as a result of lifetime feeding of relatively high doses. Often the primary purpose of such experiments has been to elucidate mechanisms of carcinogenesis; however, human populations are rarely, if ever, exposed to significant levels of most of the compounds studied. Other experimental liver carcinogens to which humans are known to be exposed under certain circumstances include fumonisin, sterigmatocystin and other mycotoxins, certain pyrrolizidine alkaloids, cycasin and related glycosides, carcinogenic nitrosamines and nitrosamides formed endogenously (as well as through the interaction of nitrite and nitrosatable substrates in foods and the environment), heterocyclic aromatic amines formed during the cooking of proteinaceous foods, and components of alcoholic beverages such as urethane and ethanol. These substances are not significant etiologic agents for HCC in humans.

AFLATOXIN CARCINOGENESIS IN EXPERIMENTAL ANIMALS

Carcinogenic properties of the aflatoxins, especially aflatoxin B_1 (AFB_1), have been extensively characterized, and much information has been produced relating to mechanisms of action and occurrence as contaminants of foods, as reviewed elsewhere.[1] Feeding of diets naturally contaminated with aflatoxin mixtures or of purified aflatoxin B_1 induced HCC in many species of experimental animals,[1] including fish (rainbow trout, sockeye salmon, and guppy); a bird (duck); rodents (rats, mice, and tree shrew); a carnivore (ferret); and nonhuman primates (Rhesus, cynomolgus, African green monkey, and squirrel monkeys). Although the liver was the primary target organ in most species, tumors of other organs have also been found at different rates in aflatoxin-treated animals. Inasmuch as humans have been shown to metabolize aflatoxin through the same pathways as experimental animals, including activation to AFB_1-8,9-oxide, the ultimate carcinogenic form, it is reasonable to conclude that aflatoxin exposure would represent a carcinogenic hazard for humans.

The amount ("effective dose") of AFB_1 necessary for induction of HCC varies among different animal species. In fish and bird species, effective doses were generally in the range of 10 to 30 ppb in the diet. A particularly wide variation in sensitivity is found among rodent species, with rats responding at levels in the range of 15 to 1000 ppb, and certain strains of mice showing no response at doses up to 150,000 ppb. The tree shrew was intermediate in sensitivity, responding to 2000 ppb. Induction also differs widely among nonhuman primate species[2]; squirrel monkeys developed HCCs when fed a diet containing 2000 ppb AFB_1 for 13 months, but average total doses of 99 to 1225 mg per animal administered orally over periods of 48 to 179 months were required to induce a low prevalence of HCCs (7% to 20%) in Rhesus, African green, and cynomolgus monkeys. In cynomolgus monkeys, tumors in extrahepatic tissues (including adenocarcinomas of the pancreas, adenomas of the biliary and pancreatic ducts, hemangiocarcinoma of the liver, and osteosarcomas) occurred at a much higher rate than liver tumors. These findings indicated that aflatoxin was carcinogenic to extrahepatic tissues in primates. Whether aflatoxin could also be a risk factor for cancers other than HCC in humans has not been studied.

Using data from lifetime feeding studies in rodents and the method of Gold et al.,[3] the effective dose of AFB_1 ("potency" or median toxic dose [TD_{50}] values [expressed as micrograms per kg body weight per day]) was calculated for susceptible and resistant species as follows:[4] Fischer 344 rat, 1.3 (male) and 7.5 (female); Wistar rat, 5.8 (male) and 6.9 (female); Porton rat, 3.1 (male) and 12.5 (female); C3H mouse, >70 (male); C57Bl mouse, >70 (male); Swiss mouse, >5300 (male), Rhesus monkeys treated for an average of 3.3 years, 156; and cynomolgus monkeys treated for 14 years, 848. These values encompass the extremes of observed sensitivity, reflected in the responses of Fischer 344 rats and Swiss mice. The value calculated for Swiss mice is based not on an effective dose, but rather on the highest feeding level, at which no tumors of the liver or other tissues were observed.

ASSOCIATION OF HCC INCIDENCE WITH AFLATOXIN EXPOSURE

In the assessment of AFB_1 as a risk factor for liver cancer in humans, it is of interest to compare the above data from experimental animals with relevant information derived from studies in human populations exposed to the carcinogen through dietary contamination. Extensive epidemiologic studies have established a strong association between HCC and AFB_1 intake.[5] These data provide a basis for calculation of a hypothetical TD_{50} value as an estimate of the potency of AFB_1 as a liver carcinogen for humans. Comparison of AFB_1 intake and HCC incidence data, using the method[3] used in calculation of the above values for experimental animals, produced a TD_{50} value for humans of 132 μg/kg body weight per day.[4] This value was in the same order of magnitude of those calculated for nonhuman primates (156 to 848 mg/kg per day), but substantially lower than those for the most sensitive rodent species (1 to 5 g/kg per day). In making this comparison, however, it is important to acknowledge major uncertainties in the calculated TD_{50}, including the assumption that AFB_1 was ingested at the measured level continuously over a hypothetical life span of 50 years, that there was reliance on crude (i.e., non-age-adjusted) HCC incidence values derived from cancer registry data, and that the impact of hepatitis B virus (HBV) infection was ignored. The calculated TD_{50} value for humans, therefore, must be regarded as only an upper estimate, probably overstating the potency of AFB_1 as a carcinogen in the liver of humans.

In a study of aflatoxin exposure, HBV infection, and HCC incidence in Swaziland, Peers et al.[6] recorded HCC incidence between 1979 and 1983 through a national cancer registry. Prevalence of HBV markers was estimated by analysis of donated blood in the same communities. Aflatoxin intake was estimated by analysis of food samples from households and crop samples collected at representative farms. Across four broad geographic areas, a variation of estimated aflatoxin intake of more than fivefold (from 3.1 to 17.5 g/person per day) was observed. Prevalence of HBsAg was 23%, with little variation (21% to 28%) across subpopulations. HCC incidence varied over a fivefold range and was strongly associated with estimated aflatoxin intake. Analysis of data from ten subregions within the country led the authors to regard aflatoxin exposure as a more important determinant of variation in HCC incidence than HBV infection.

In a similar study of HBV status, aflatoxin exposure, and HCC incidence in males in southern Guangxi, China, by Yeh et al.,[7] the prevalence of HBsAg positivity among 76 people who died of HCC was 91%, in contrast to 23% of all members of the cohort, confirming the importance of HBV as a risk factor for HCC. Within the cohort, there was a 3.5-fold difference in HCC mortality by place of residence. Aflatoxin intakes were calculated on the basis of analysis of food collected in markets, combined with a food consumption questionnaire. Estimated mean aflatoxin intakes of subpopulations varied from 0.3 to 51.8 mg/person per year. When aflatoxin intakes were plotted against corresponding HCC mortality rates in subpopulations, a linear correlation was observed; however, the reported aflatoxin ingestion data represent only approximations of individual intakes, given the manner in which they were obtained.

The collective evidence of aflatoxin carcinogenicity in experimental animals, together with the epidemiologic data summarized above, was considered sufficient to classify aflatoxins as human carcinogens (group 1) by the International Agency for Research on Cancer.[8] This conclusion was significantly influenced by epidemiologic data that were associational in nature and consequently could not provide direct evidence for a causal relationship between aflatoxin exposure and increased risk for HCC in a given individual. Thus, it has been difficult to differentiate and assess the relative contributions of aflatoxin ingestion and HBV infection to HCC incidence in populations exposed to both risk factors concurrently.

MOLECULAR EPIDEMIOLOGY OF AFLATOXIN AS AN ETIOLOGIC AGENT FOR HCC

Incorporation of Biomarkers of Effective Dose into HCC Epidemiology

In the earliest stage of the process of carcinogenesis, exposure to chemical carcinogens leads to their absorption, metabolic activation, and subsequent covalent binding to cellular DNA and proteins. Detection and quantification of these addition products (i.e., DNA and protein adducts), provide biomarkers of exposure and biologically effective dose. Subsequently, replication of carcinogen-damaged DNA results in fixation of mutations that are important in tumor initiation and/or progression. Among various possible biomarkers, the measurement of carcinogen-DNA and carcinogen-protein adducts is of significant interest because they provide molecular, mechanism-based bridges between carcinogen exposures and disease end points.[9,10,11]

Rothman et al.[9] have described a matrix relating biomarker categories to apply them to studies in human populations. Four design categories were included in the matrix: laboratory studies, transitional studies, etiologic studies, and public health applications. In *laboratory studies*, biomarkers are identified and the validity of these markers is established by studies in experimental models. In *transitional studies*, during the gap between development of biomarkers and their application in population-based studies, studies are designed to validate and optimize biomarkers. *Etiologic studies* include case-control studies in which prevalence of exposure or biomarker in cases is compared to that in appropriately matched controls, case-case studies in which tumor characteristics (e.g., anatomic, cellular, chromosomal or molecular) of cases *with* exposure to carcinogen are compared to those of cases *without* exposure, or prospective cohort studies in which specimens from healthy subjects who are followed forward in time are collected and banked. To date, aflatoxins are among a small number of environmental carcinogens that have been extensively studied using this validation scheme, and the studies described here can serve as a useful model for the development, validation, and application of chemical-specific biomarkers in the molecular epidemiology of other cancers in which environmental carcinogens are thought to play etiologic roles.

Laboratory Studies of Aflatoxin-DNA and Albumin Adducts as Biomarkers of Biologically Effective Dose

Aflatoxin-DNA and aflatoxin-protein adducts are direct products of damage to a critical macromolecular target, derived from the ultimate carcinogenic form of AFB_1, the *exo*-aflatoxin B_1-8,9-oxide. Chemical structures of the major aflatoxin macromolecular adducts have been identified.[12,13] While technical limitations preclude routine measurements of aflatoxin-DNA adducts in human tissues, the major DNA adduct species formed in vivo, aflatoxin-N^7-guanine, is rapidly excised and eliminated as the base adduct. Urine is the sole route of excretion of the adduct. Serum albumin is the predominant blood protein to be adducted following aflatoxin ingestion. Because aflatoxin-lysine adducts in albumin are not repaired, adduct levels reflect the 2- to 3-week half-life for circulating albumin. Based on these kinetics, it is assumed that measurements of aflatoxin-N^7-guanine in urine reflect recent exposures, whereas levels of aflatoxin-albumin adducts reflect cumulative, multiple exposures.

Development of biomarker methods to monitor human exposure to aflatoxins required analytic techniques that were sensitive, specific, and applicable to large numbers of samples. An immunoaffinity chromatography/high performance liquid chromatography (HPLC) procedure has been developed to isolate and sensitively measure aflatoxin metabolites, including aflatoxin-N^7-guanine, in biologic samples.[14–16]

Dose-dependent increases in the levels of aflatoxin-N^7-guanine in urine following acute dosing of rats with AFB_1 have been shown.[16,17] Moreover, a striking linear correspondence between amounts of the adduct excreted in urine over the initial 24-hour postdosing period and residual levels of hepatic AFB_1-DNA adducts were observed in both studies. These findings were of crucial importance in establishing that levels of aflatoxin-N^7-guanine excreted in urine were not only accurate measures of exposure and activation, but also provided an accurate measure of DNA damage in liver. Excretion patterns of several other oxidative metabolites of AFB_1

in rat urine were not dose-dependent. The relationship between hepatic and urinary aflatoxin-N^7-guanine reflects the short biologic half-life (8 hours) of aflatoxin-N^7-guanine adducts in liver DNA. Chronic dosing of rats with AFB_1 led to sustained excretion of aflatoxin-N^7-guanine.

Strong concordance between exposure and serum levels of aflatoxin-albumin adducts has also been observed after acute and chronic dosing of rats with AFB_1.[18,19] Because of the longer biologic half-life of the aflatoxin-albumin biomarker in rats (2 to 3 days) and humans (2 to 3 weeks), it is thought to be more useful than urinary markers in chronic exposure settings.

Transitional Studies in Humans in Guangxi Province, PRC and in The Gambia, West Africa

Systematic evaluation of aflatoxin-adduct biomarkers in several human populations has been undertaken. Early studies[20,21] used synchronous fluorescence spectroscopy for analysis of AFB_1-DNA adducts in human urine samples. More than 1000 urine samples collected from residents of Kenya were analyzed, and nearly 13% contained detectable levels of aflatoxin-N^7-guanine. These data provided important evidence that humans had the metabolic capacity to produce and excrete the same aflatoxin-DNA adducts previously detected in experimental animals.

Studies in Guangxi Province, an area in the People's Republic of China with a high incidence of HCC, determined both dietary intake of aflatoxin and levels of urinary aflatoxin biomarkers.[22] The average individual dietary intake of aflatoxins, primarily from contaminated corn, was approximately 275 g and 540 g in males and females, respectively, over the 7-day monitoring period.[9] Total 24-hour urine samples were collected as consecutive 12-hour fractions, beginning on the fourth day of the study. Aflatoxins in the urine samples were measured by radioimmunoassay. Total immunoreactive aflatoxin equivalents in urine did not correspond with aflatoxin intake, indicating that this type of immunoassay did not constitute an appropriate way of determining individual aflatoxin exposure. Therefore, immunoaffinity-HPLC analysis was subsequently performed to determine levels of individual aflatoxin derivatives in urine. Only AFB_1-N^7-guanine and AFM_1 showed dose-dependent relationships between aflatoxin intake and urinary levels, indicating that these two metabolites would be useful biomarkers of exposure. Significantly, these studies also demonstrated that the formation and excretion of AFB-N^7-guanine in urine was similar to that in the F344 rat and human, adding an important element of confirmation to extrapolation from rat to human.

Monitoring levels of aflatoxin-serum albumin adduct in the same study population, a highly significant association between adduct level and intake was observed.[23] About 2% of the ingested AFB_1 was calculated to become covalently bound to serum albumin, similar to that previously observed in rats. When excretion of AFB_1-DNA adducts in urine and levels of aflatoxin serum albumin adducts were compared,[24,25] a statistically significant relationship was seen with a correlation coefficient of 0.73. Thus, both of these markers were useful for human monitoring studies.

A similar study in The Gambia, West Africa,[26,27] involved 10 men and 10 women matched for age, common dietary exposures, and HBsAg status. Aflatoxin intake was measured by analysis of samples of cooked foods collected over a 7-day period. Total 24-hour urine was collected on days 4 through 7 and analyzed for aflatoxin derivatives by the immunoaffinity-HPLC method. Blood samples were collected on days 1 and 8 and analyzed for aflatoxin-albumin adduct levels by immunoassay and by immunoaffinity-HPLC. Mean daily individual aflatoxin intake by all subjects was 1.4 g (range 0 to 29.6 g), and the mean individual total intake over 7 days was 12.0 g (8.2 g by men and 15.7 g by women). Aflatoxin derivatives detected in urine included AFB_1-N^7-guanine, AFB_1 and AFQ_1. Total aflatoxin excretion was significantly correlated with total intake ($p < 0.001$), as was excretion of AFB_1-N^7-guanine ($p < 0.0001$). Serum levels of aflatoxin-albumin adduct were also significantly correlated with total aflatoxin intake ($p < 0.05$). Neither biomarker was affected by HBsAg status.

Etiologic Study of HCC in Male Residents of Shanghai

A study to evaluate the aflatoxin-HCC relationship[28,29] (nested case-control study) was initiated in 1986 in Shanghai to examine the relation between markers for aflatoxin exposure and hepatitis B virus infection and the development of liver cancer in men. Urine samples were collected at the time of entry into the study from 18,244 healthy men between the ages of 45 and 64. Aflatoxin was measured by immunoaffinity chromatography-HPLC analysis. In the subsequent 7 years, 50 of these men developed HCC and were matched for age and residence with 267 control subjects. The relative risk for HCC in subjects who were HBsAg negative and in whom aflatoxin biomarkers were absent was 1.0. There was a significant increase in the relative risk (RR = 3.4) for HCC in those whose urinary aflatoxin biomarkers were positive but who were HBsAg negative. The relative risk for those who were positive for HBsAg, but whose urinary aflatoxin biomarkers were negative, was 7.3. Individuals with both urinary aflatoxin biomarkers and HBsAg in serum had a relative risk for developing HCC of 59.4. Thus, these results showed concordance between the presence of carcinogen-specific biomarkers and cancer risk in humans and an interaction between two major risk factors for HCC, hepatitis B virus, and AFB_1. When individual aflatoxin metabolites were stratified for HCC outcome, the presence of AFB_1-N^7-guanine in urine always resulted in a twofold to threefold elevation in risk of developing HCC.

Genetic Variation in Aflatoxin Detoxifying Enzymes and Susceptibility to HCC

McGlynn et al.[30] have suggested that differences in HCC rates may be attributable to variations among individuals with respect to their ability to detoxify the ultimate carcinogenic derivative AFB_1-8,9-epoxide. Two enzymatic pathways responsible for detoxification have been identified. Epoxide hydrolase catalyzes hydrolysis of the epoxide to AFB_1-diol, and glutathione-S-transferase M1 detoxifies the epoxide by conjugation to glutathione. Lack of or diminution of either of these enzymes might enhance the carcinogenicity of AFB_1 by increasing the availability of AFB_1-epoxide for binding to DNA. A polymorphism for glutathione-S-transferase is found in humans. The null genotype confers an elevated risk because individuals with that genotype have a diminished capacity for conjugation of the aflatoxin epoxide with glutathione. DNA polymorphisms in epoxide hydrolase have also been described, in which the amino acid at position 113, tyrosine in allele 1, is replaced by histidine in allele 2.

Studies were conducted in HCC endemic regions of Ghana and China to test whether high-risk genotypes for either enzyme were associated with elevations serum aflatoxin-albumin adduct levels, with HCC, or with mutations in codon 249 of the p53 gene.[30]

Mutant alleles of both enzymes were associated with the presence of detectable levels of aflatoxin-albumin levels in a cross-sectional study of men in Ghana. Men with detectable levels of adduct (>5 pg/mg albumin) were more likely to have either of the high-risk genotypes than were men without detectable levels of adduct ($p = 0.02$). Similarly, men who were null for glutathione-S-transferase M1 were more likely to have detectable adduct than men with the enzyme ($p = 0.03$). When both genotypes were combined, all of the men with both high-risk genotypes had detectable levels of albumin adducts, compared to only 32% of men with both low-risk genotypes.[30]

Mutant alleles in the two aflatoxin detoxifying enzymes were also overrepresented in male Chinese HCC patients. The frequency of the glutathione-S-transferase M1 null genotype was greater among HCC patients (56%) than among controls (41%), a difference that was statistically significant ($p = 0.047$). The combined presence of HBsAg and either high-risk epoxide hydrolase genotype was associated with an elevation of risk (odds ratio = 77). Mutations in codon 249 of the p53 tumor suppressor genes were observed only in HCC patients with one or both high-risk genotypes.

AFLATOXIN AND MUTATIONS IN THE P53 GENE IN HCC

Data from Studies in Humans

The p53 tumor suppressor gene is the most commonly mutated gene found in a wide variety of human cancers.[31] Mutational spectra of the p53 gene in HCC were initially reported by Hsu et al.[32] and by Bressac et al.,[33] who analyzed tumor DNA of patients from Qidong, PRC, and Mozambique, respectively. Hsu et al.[32] identified a G:C to T:A transversion mutation in the third base of codon 249 of the p53 gene (AGG to AGT, resulting in an arginine to serine substitution in the gene product) in 8 of 16 HCC cases. Bressac et al.[33] identified the same specific mutation in codon 249 of the p53 gene in 3 of 10 HCC cases and another mutation resulting in the same amino acid change at codon 249 in an additional two cases. The high frequency of the G:C to T:A base substitution and the strong localization of the mutation to the third base in codon 249 of the gene were in striking contrast to the more generalized spectra of mutations previously reported for tumors of other tissues. The potential for aflatoxin exposure was comparatively high in both regions, suggesting a possible role for aflatoxin in the induction of the mutations observed.[32,33] Since these initial observations were made, additional studies have revealed that the p53 mutational spectrum in HCC varies significantly by geographic region. Tumors from Qidong County contain an overwhelming preponderance (95%) of G:C to T:A transversions, presumably associated with aflatoxin exposure. In contrast, tumors from Taiwan and Japan have p53 mutation in ≤20% of cases, a few of which were codon 249 mutations. The frequency of the AGG to AGT mutation at codon 249 paralleled the level of aflatoxin exposure,[34] supporting the hypothesis that the carcinogen has a causative role in hepatocarcinogenesis.

Data from Experimental Systems

Aguillar et al.[35] studied mutagenesis of the p53 gene of Hep G2, a human hepatoblastoma cell line. Cells were exposed to AFB_1 in the presence of a rat liver microsome activating system, and mutations were characterized by AFB_1-induced transversion of G:C to T:A in the third position of codon 249. Foster et al.[36] characterized mutations induced in the lacI gene of *Escherichia coli* exposed to AFB_1 activated by rat liver microsomes and found that 89% were G:C to T:A transversions. Other studies have been reported in which the *supF* gene of the pS189 plasmid was the target for mutation by AFB_1. In each instance, G:C to T:A transversion was the predominant mutation induced, following replication of the plasmid in xeroderma pigmentosum cells[37] or human embryonic kidney cells.[38,39] The mutational spectrum induced by AFB_1 has also been characterized in the HPRT gene of cultured human lymphoblasts expressing the CYP1A1 gene[40]; G:C to T:A transversion was the major mutation present at four mutational hotspots.

Molecular Mechanisms of Aflatoxin-DNA Binding and Mutagenesis

The preceding data show that AFB_1 preferentially induces G:C to T:A transversions in the third position of codon 249 in the p53 gene, as well as in other gene sequences. The strong localization of mutations at guanine residues in DNA has been attributed to the fact that the sole covalent DNA adduct formed by metabolically activated AFB_1 is AFB_1-N^7-guanine. This pattern of DNA binding is highly unusual; most bulky carcinogens form a complex spectrum of covalent adducts at nucleophilic sites in DNA. NMR investigations[41–43] of equilibrium binding by AFB_1 to DNA have shown that intercalation of AFB_1 into the DNA helix is a major component of the binding process, and that the aflatoxin moiety intercalates preferentially on the 5′ side of the guanine of AFB_1-8,9-epoxide. The reactive intermediate involved in covalent binding to the N^7 position of guanine residues in DNA has never been detected in biologic materials, but its role as an active intermediate had been inferred from the structures of adducts formed with DNA. Two stereoisomeric forms of AFB_1-8,9-epoxide, *exo-* and *endo-*, were produced by both synthetic and enzymatic activation pathways. The *exo*-epoxide was more efficient, by orders of magnitude, than the *endo*-epoxide, in the formation of biologically active DNA adducts, because steric hindrance prevents efficient intercalation of the *endo-* form of the epoxide. In other studies,[44] an oligonucleotide containing a single AFB_1-N^7-guanine adduct was inserted into the single-stranded genome of bacteriophage M13; replication in SOS-induced *E. coli* yielded a mutation frequency of 4% with a predominant mutation (73%) G to T.

CHEMOPREVENTION FOR REDUCING HCC RISK

Even complete elimination of HBV infection would still leave a residual risk of significant magnitude in regions where aflatoxin contamination of the food supply is common. Elimination of aflatoxin exposures would be a worthwhile long-term objective, but prevention of aflatoxin exposure would be impractical and not economically feasible in many areas of the world. Chemoprotective interventions may provide an alternative approach.

Hepatocarcinogenesis induced by aflatoxin in animals can be prevented using chemopreventive interventions with phenolic antioxidants, 1,2-dithiolethiones, and other agents when they are administered simultaneously with the carcinogen.[45] Oltipraz [4-methyl-5-(2-pyrazinyl)-1,2-dithiole-3-thione] is a particularly effective inhibitor of aflatoxin carcinogenesis in Fisher rats when fed before and throughout carcinogen exposure. Oltipraz effectively reduces urinary excretion of the AFB_1-N^7-guanine adduct and also serum aflatoxin-albumin adducts in this model, in a manner that parallels reductions in DNA adduct formation in liver and inhibition of tumorigenesis. These studies also indicated that measurements of aflatoxin biomarkers reflected the altered risk for disease of the animals receiving chemoprevention.

Oltipraz is currently being evaluated for chemoprevention in Qidong, China.[46] A phase II placebo-controlled chemoprevention trial with oltipraz was conducted in 234 persons during 1995. One of the eligibility criteria was presence of serum aflatoxin-albumin adducts, and levels ranged between 1.3 and 10 pmol/mg albumin.

Elucidation of molecular mechanisms made possible the development and validation of molecular biomarkers of exposure, effective dose, and biologic effect that could be validated independently in experimental models and in human populations exposed to the carcinogen. Essential to the ultimate elucidation of the role of aflatoxin in HCC etiology were the collaborative efforts of epidemiologists and laboratory scientists in application of those biomarkers in well-designed molecular epidemiologic studies capable of producing statistically valid data relating exposure to increased disease risk. Research aimed at elucidation of molecular mechanisms underlying the process of neoplasia and the use of molecular epidemiology in defining the significance of exposure to an environmental carcinogen as an etiologic agent for a major human cancer may permit intervention strategies to reduce the risk of HCC from aflatoxin exposure. The success in this field of research, therefore, may be useful as a template for investigations of other environmentally related cancers.

ACKNOWLEDGMENTS

The author wishes to acknowledge the significant contributions of the many collaborators who participated in studies summarized here. Financial support for work from his laboratory was provided by grants ES00597 and ES05622 from the National Institute for Environmental Health Sciences, NIH.

REFERENCES

1. Busby WF Jr, Wogan GN. Aflatoxins. In Searle CE (ed.): Chemical Carcinogens. 2nd Ed. Vol 12. American Chemical Society, Washington, DC, 1984, pp. 945–1136
2. Adamson RH. Induction of hepatocellular carcinoma in nonhuman primates by chemical carcinogens. Cancer Detect Prev 1989;14:215–220
3. Gold LS, Sawyer CB, Magaw R et al. A carcinogenic potency database of the standardized results of animal bioassays. Environ Health Perspect 1984;58:9–322
4. Wogan GN. Aflatoxins as risk factors for hepatocellular carcinoma in humans. Cancer Res 1992;52:2114s–2118s
5. Bosch FX, Munoz N. Epidemiology of hepatocellular carcinoma. In Bannasch P, Keppler D, Weber G (eds): Liver Cell Carcinoma. Kluwer Academic Publishers, Dordrecht, The Netherlands, 1989, pp. 3–14
6. Peers F, Bosch X, Kaldor J et al. Aflatoxin exposure, hepatitis B virus infection and liver cancer in Swaziland. Int J Cancer 1987;39:545–553
7. Yeh F-S, Yu MC, Mo C-C et al. Hepatitis B virus, aflatoxins, and hepatocellular carcinoma in southern Guangxi, China. Cancer Res 1989;49:2506–2509
8. Some Naturally Occurring Substances: Food Items and Constituents, Heterocyclic Aromatic Amines and Mycotoxins. IARC Monographs on the Evaluation of Carcinogenic Risks to Humans. Lyon: IARC Monographs 1993;56:599
9. Rothman N, Stewart WF, Schulte PA. Incorporating biomarkers into cancer epidemiology: a matrix of biomarker and study design categories. Cancer Epidemiol Biomarkers Prev 1995;4:301–311
10. Wogan GN. Molecular epidemiology in cancer risk assessment and prevention: recent progress and avenues for future research. Environ Health Perspect 1992;98:167–178
11. Hulka B. Epidemiological studies using biological markers: issues for epidemiologists. Cancer Epidemiol Biomarkers Prev 1991;1:13–19
12. Essigmann JM, Croy RG, Nadzan AM et al. Structural identification of the major DNA adduct formed by aflatoxin B_1 in vitro. Proc Natl Acad Sci USA 1977;74:1870–1874
13. Sabbioni G, Skipper P, Buchi G, Tannenbaum SR. Isolation and characterization of the major serum albumin adduct formed by aflatoxin B_1 in vivo in rats. Carcinogenesis 1987; 8:819–824
14. Groopman JD, Trudel LJ, Donahue PR et al. High affinity monoclonal antibodies for aflatoxins and their application to solid phase immunoassays. Proc Natl Acad Sci USA 1984; 81:7728–7731
15. Groopman JD, Donahue K, Zhu J et al. Aflatoxin metabolism in humans: detection of metabolites and nucleic adducts in urine by affinity chromatography. Proc Natl Acad Sci USA 1985;82:6492–6496
16. Groopman JD, Hasler J, Trudel LJ et al. Molecular dosimetry in rat urine of aflatoxin-N^7-guanine and other aflatoxin metabolites by multiple monoclonal antibody affinity chromatography and HPLC. Cancer Res 1992; 52:267–274
17. Bennett RA, Essigmann JM, Wogan GN. Excretion of an aflatoxin-guanine adduct in the urine of aflatoxin B_1-treated rats. Cancer Res 1981;41:650–654
18. Wild CP, Garner RG, Montesano R, Tursi F. Aflatoxin B_1 binding to plasma albumin and liver DNA upon chronic administration to rats. Carcinogenesis 1986;7:853–858
19. Sabbioni G, Skipper P, Buchi G, Tannenbaum SR. Isolation and characterization of the major serum albumin adduct formed by aflatoxin B_1 in vivo in rats. Carcinogenesis 1987; 8:819–824
20. Autrup H, Bradley KA, Shamsuddin AKM et al. Detection of putative adduct with fluorescence characteristics identical to 2,3-dihydro-2-(7′-guanyl)-3-hydroxyaflatoxin B_1 in human urine collected in Murang'a district, Kenya. Carcinogenesis 1983;4:1193–1195
21. Autrup H, Seremet T, Wakhisi J, Wasunna A. Aflatoxin exposure measured by urinary excretion of aflatoxin B_1-guanine adduct and hepatitis B virus infection in areas with different liver cancer incidence in Kenya. Cancer Res 1987; 47:3430–3433
22. Groopman JD, Zhu J, Donahue PR et al. Molecular dosimetry of urinary aflatoxin-DNA adducts in people living in Guangxi Autonomous Region, People's Republic of China. Cancer Res 1992;52:45–52
23. Gan L-S, Skipper PL, Peng X-C et al. Serum albumin adducts in the molecular epidemiology of aflatoxin carcinogenesis: correlation with aflatoxin B_1 intake and urinary excretion of aflatoxin M_1. Carcinogenesis 1988;9:1323–1325
24. Wild CP, Jiang YZ, Sabbioni G et al. Evaluation of methods for quantitation of aflatoxin-albumin adducts and their application to human exposure assessment. Cancer Res 1990; 50:245–251
25. Wild CP, Jiang YZ, Allen SJ et al. Aflatoxin-albumin adducts in human sera from different regions of the world. Carcinogenesis 1990;11:2271–2274
26. Groopman JD, Hall A, Whittle H et al. Molecular dosimetry of aflatoxin-N^7-guanine in human urine obtained in The Gambia, West Africa. Cancer Epidemiol Biomarkers and Prev 1992;1:221–228
27. Wild CP, Hudson G, Sabbioni G et al. Correlation of dietary intake of aflatoxins with the level of albumin bound aflatoxin in peripheral blood in The Gambia, West Africa. Cancer Epidemiol Biomarkers Prev 1992;1:229–234
28. Ross RK, Yuan J-M, Yu MC et al. Urinary aflatoxin biomarkers and risk of hepatocellular carcinoma. Lancet 1992;339: 943–946
29. Qian G-S, Ross RK, Yu MC et al. A follow-up study of urinary markers of aflatoxin exposure and liver cancer risk in Shanghai, People's Republic of China. Cancer Epidemiol Biomarkers Prev 1994;3:3–10
30. McGlynn KA, Rosvold EA, Lustbader ED et al. Susceptibility to hepatocellular carcinoma is associated with genetic variation in the enzymatic detoxification of aflatoxin B_1. Proc Natl Acad Sci USA 1995;92:2384–2387
31. Greenblatt MS, Bennett WP, Hollstein M, Harris CC. Mutations in the p53 tumor suppressor gene: clues to cancer etiology and molecular pathogenesis. Cancer Res 1994;54: 4855–4878
32. Hsu I, Metcalf R, Sun T et al. Mutational hotspot in the

p53 gene in human hepatocellular carcinoma. Nature 1991; 350:427–428

33. Bressac B, Kew M, Wands J, Ozturk M. Selective G to T mutations of p53 in hepatocellular carcinoma from Southern Africa. Nature 1991;350:429–430
34. Aguillar F, Harris CC, Sun T et al. Geographic variation of p53 mutational profile in nonmalignant human liver. Science 1994;264:1317–1319
35. Aguillar F, Perwez Hussain S, Cerutti P. Aflatoxin B_1 induces the transversion of G to T in codon 249 of the p53 tumor suppressor gene in human hepatocytes. Proc Natl Acad Sci USA 1993;90:8586–8590
36. Foster P, Eisenstadt E, Miller J. Base substitution mutations induced by metabolically activated aflatoxin B_1. Proc Natl Acad Sci USA 1983;80:2695–2698
37. Levy D, Groopman JD, Lim S et al. Sequence specificity of aflatoxin-B_1-induced mutations in a plasmid replicated in xeroderma pigmentosum and DNA repair proficient human cells. Cancer Res 1992;52:5668–5673
38. Trotter Y, Waithe WI, Anderson A. Kinds of mutations induced by aflatoxin-B_1 in a shuttle vector replicating in human cells transiently expressing cytochrome P4501A2 cDNA. Mol Carcinog 1992;6:140–147
39. Courtemanche C, Anderson A. Shuttle vector mutagenesis by aflatoxin B_1 in human cells: effects of sequence context on the *supF* muational spectrum. Mutat Res 1994;306:143–151
40. Cariello N, Cui L, Skopek TR. In vitro mutational spectrum of aflatoxin B_1 in the human hypoxanthine guanine phosphoribosyl transferase gene. Cancer Res 1994;54:4436–4441
41. Harris TM. NMR studies of carcinogen reactions with DNA: ethylene dibromide and aflatoxin B_1. J Pharm Biomed Anal 1990;8:195–204
42. Iyer RS, Coles BF, Raney KD et al. DNA adduction by the potent carcinogen aflatoxin B_1. J Am Chem Soc 1994;116: 1604–1609
43. Raney VM, Harris TM, Stone MP. DNA conformation mediates aflatoxin B_1-DNA binding and the formation of guanine N^7 adducts by aflatoxin B_1-8,9-*exo*-epoxide. Chem Res Toxicol 1993;6:64–68
44. Bailey EA, Iyer RS, Stone MP et al. Mutational properties of the primary aflatoxin B_1-DNA adduct. Proc Natl Acad Sci USA 1996;93:1535–1539
45. Kensler TW, Davis EF, Bolton MG. Strategies for chemoprotection against aflatoxin-induced liver cancer. In Eton DL, Groopman JD (eds): The Toxicology of Aflatoxins. Academic Press, San Diego; 1994, pp. 281–306
46. Kensler TW, Groopman JD, Wogan GN. Use of carcinogen-DNA and protein adduct biomarkers for cohort selection and as modifiable endpoints in chemoprevention trials. In Stewart BW, McGregor D, Kleihues P (eds): IARC Monographs on the Principles of Chemoprevention. Vol. 139. IARC Scientific Publication, Lyon, 1996, pp. 237–248

6

MOLECULAR MECHANISMS OF HEPATOCARCINOGENESIS

MICHAEL GEISSLER
ANNETTE GESIEN
JACK R. WANDS

Hepatocellular carcinoma (HCC) is one of the most common and devastating malignant tumors in some parts of the world. Recently, striking advances have occurred in our understanding of hepatocyte growth regulation and how chemical agents and viruses alter these normal growth regulatory pathways during the genesis of liver tumors. The major risk factors for the development of HCC are now well recognized, and both in vivo and in vitro models of neoplastic transformation have established that the pathway to neoplasia has multiple steps as illustrated by the following observations. Aberrant expression of proto-oncogenes or the expression of mutant forms of these genes (i.e., oncogenes) may lead to neoplastic transformation. In addition, induction of programmed cell death or apoptosis and alteration of p53 tumor suppressor gene-dependent cell cycle checkpoint function are involved in hepatic carcinogenesis and tumor promotion. The phenomenon of DNA hypomethylation may represent an epigenetic mechanism involved in hepatocyte transformation. The way in which the possible mechanisms of hepatic oncogenesis operate at the molecular level is still incompletely understood. Transformation of hepatocytes to the malignant phenotype may occur regardless of the etiologic agent (Fig. 6-1) in the context of increased cellular turnover induced by chronic liver injury and regeneration, with genetic mutations being a common phenomenon prior to the development of HCC. For example, hepatitis B virus (HBV)-induced hepatocarcinogenesis has been ascribed to a variety of mechanisms, including (1) the insertional deregulation of cellular growth control genes by the integrated viral DNA sequences commonly found in HCC, (2) the random deregulation of cellular growth control genes by chromosomal aberrations associated with increased hepatocellular turnover, and (3) the mutagenic environment that may exist within the inflamed liver. In addition, there may be transcriptional deregulation of cellular growth control genes by a transactivating protein that is a product of the X gene. Finally, the hepatitis C virus, alcohol, metabolic liver diseases, and certain environmental factors may act predominantly through a pathway of chronic liver injury that eventually leads to cirrhosis. In this regard, the risk of HCC increases several fold in patients with cirrhosis regardless of etiology.

GENETIC BACKGROUND OF HCC

Our knowledge of the genetic basis for HCC risk in humans is limited. Environmental influences are probably more important with respect to hepatocarcinogenesis such as chronic HBV and hepatitis C virus (HCV) infection[1–3] and carcinogen exposure.[4] It is difficult to determine whether a genetic component indeed exists. Clini-

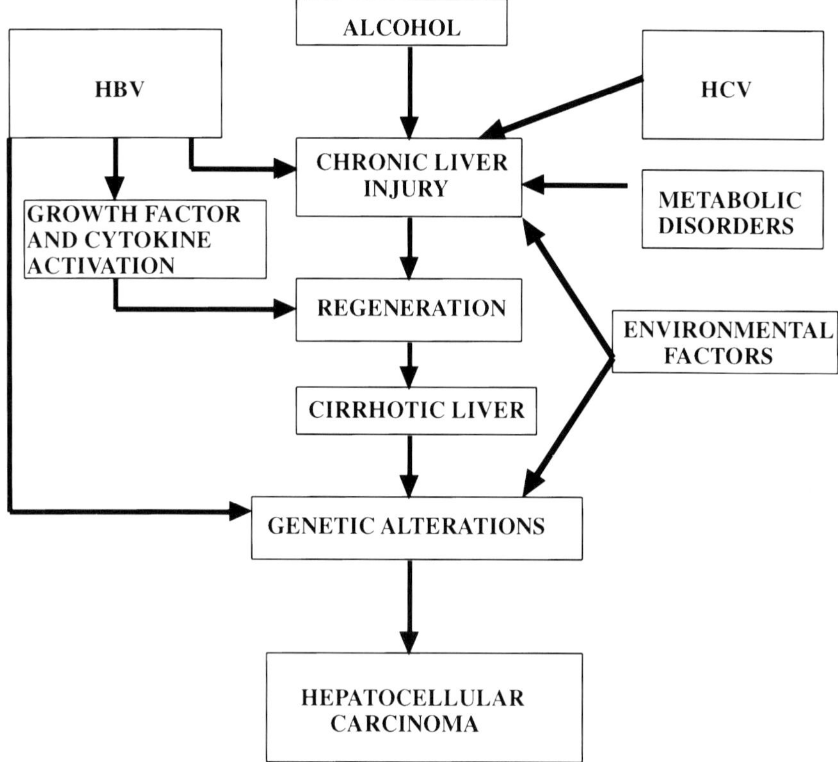

FIGURE 6-1. Etiologic factors involved in the pathogenesis of HCC.

cal studies of several genetic diseases, however, demonstrate the possible participation of genetic factors in the pathogenesis of HCC.

Epidemiology

Several studies have suggested that a high prevalence of HCC may exist in some families, but may be due to environmental risk.[5] However, three studies provide evidence that the risk of HCC development among HBV-infected individuals may be determined by specific susceptibility genes.[6–8] These case control studies of HCC were performed in eastern China and Alaska where a significant risk of developing HCC was observed in parents and siblings of patients with HCC and HBV infection even when chronic HBV infection was taken into account.

Genetic Diseases and Risk of HCC

The importance of cirrhosis in the pathophysiology of HCC is best illustrated by the development of HCC in association with metabolic diseases of the liver (Table 6-1). Several human genetic diseases exist that are associated with the frequent development of hepatocellular adenomas or carcinomas. Chronic liver injury and development of cirrhosis are cardinal features in most of these diseases. Hereditary hemochromatosis is the most common and shows an autosomal recessive pattern of inheritance by linkage analysis using markers on chromosome 6p21.[9] The risk of HCC is extraordinarily high with the cirrhotic form of the disease and approaches the risk of HCC associated with chronic HBV infection.[10,11] Indeed, there are only a few reported cases of HCC occurring in precirrhotic hemochromatosis.[11] The abnormal gene associated with hereditary α_1-antitrypsin deficiency has been mapped to chromosome 14q3,[12] and a variety of mutant alleles has been described.[13,14] Type I tyrosinemia and porphyria cutanea tarda are further examples of metabolic diseases with increased risk of HCC in association with cirrhosis.[15–17] In contrast, type I glycogen storage disease may lead to HCC without chronic liver injury and cirrhosis, suggesting other pathogenetic mechanisms are involved.[18]

Experimental Approaches

Studies of the genetic susceptibility of experimental liver cancer in animals has been approached using comparative studies of inbred animals, linkage analysis to identify cancer susceptibility genes, and assessment of carcinogenic risk in animals that carry specific gene mutations. These studies have led to the identification of several genetic loci that may play a role in the development of

TABLE 6-1. Hepatocellular Carcinoma Associated with Inherited Metabolic Diseases

Disease	Cirrhosis	Associated Conditions	HCC Incidence
Acute intermittent porphyria	—	None	Rare
Porphyria variegata	—	None	Rare
Glyogenosis type I and III	—	Associated or preexisting adenoma	Rare
Hypercitrullinemia	—	None	14%
Hereditary fructose intolerance	—	Steatosis; periportal fibrosis	Very Rare (1 case)
Porphyria cutanea tarda	+ +	Alcoholic liver disease; hemosiderosis; hepatitis C	16–47%
Tyrosinemia	+ +	Large regenerative nodules; liver cell dysplasia	37%
α-1-Antitrypsin deficiency	+ +	Characteristic PAS-positive globules	10–15%
Hemochromatosis	+ + +	Hemosiderosis; iron free foci	40–60%
Wilson's disease	+ +	Copper accumulation; steatosis; Mallory bodies; glycogenated nuclei	Rare

Key: −, no risk for cirrhosis; + +, high risk for cirrhosis; + + +, very high risk for cirrhosis.

these tumors.[19] Further studies at the molecular level will be necessary to prove the association of these altered gene function to the development of HCC.

HEPATIC STEM CELLS AND THEIR ROLE IN HEPATOCARCINOGENESIS

To begin to understand the pathogenesis of HCC, it is of general interest to know which cells become transformed in the liver. Development of experimental HCC probably occurs by multiple molecular mechanisms, which depend in part on both the nature of the carcinogen and the hepatic lesions induced by it. The existence of hepatic stem cells has been controversial.

Stem cells are characterized by the capacity for self-maintenance.[20] In the adult liver, the parenchymal cell population is maintained throughout the life span of the organism. Furthermore, transplantation experiments in a transgenic mouse model have shown that adult hepatocytes have substantial growth potential.[21] The early fetal hepatocytes or hepatoblasts are progenitors of hepatocytes and bile epithelial cells and may be viewed as bipotential precursors. However, adult hepatocytes do not generally retain this bipotential capacity and evidence suggests that transformation of hepatocytes into ductule bile cells may occur.[22] However, such cells were found to be lacking functional characteristics of normal bile duct cells. In contrast, several studies suggest that bile duct epithelium contains a cellular compartment that may differentiate into several cell types.[23–26]

In Vivo Studies

During experimental hepatocarcinogenesis in animal models, distinct cellular alterations have been described and result in the emergence of a morphologically specific cell type called the oval cell. The emergence of such cells generally precedes the development of HCC.[27–37] Similar cells have been observed in the human liver[38,39] and have been implicated in HBV-associated hepatocarcinogenesis.[39] Attention has been directed to the possible function of oval cells as liver progenitor cells, and the findings are consistent with a precursor relationship between oval cells and a hepatocyte lineage.[24,26,31,35] Evidence suggests that oval cells are derived from a progenitor cell compartment represented by the lining cells of the terminal bile ductules (Hering canals) or by periductular cells near the ductules.[23–26,40,41] Oval cells have the capacity to develop into hepatocytes, as well as other cell lineages such as bile duct cells, intestinal epithelial cells, and pancreatic cells[30,31,34,35,42] and therefore may be a precursor cell of hepatic tumors.[24,25,43] It is well established that oval cell proliferation occurs during the early stages of experimental hepatocarcinogenesis, and such cells have the potential to evolve into tumors histologically identified as hepatocellular carcinoma.[28] Oval cells are similar to hepatoblasts in that they have the capacity to develop into different liver parenchymal cell lineages.

The importance of oval cells during early stages of hepatocarcinogenesis is supported by the finding during chemical carcinogenic experiments in rats that oval cells accumulate p53 protein,[44] a molecule central to cell cycle regulation. It has been shown that a variety of carcinogens and toxic agents result in the activation, proliferation, and differentiation of oval cells.[45] These cellular events are often accompanied by increased expression of growth factors such as transforming growth factor-α (TGF-α) and hepatocyte growth factor (HGF). These observations suggest that such agents may be important modulators of oval cell expansion.[46,47] Indeed, two recent studies demonstrated that hepatic ductal cells were continuously entering DNA synthesis after low-dose administration of chemical carcinogens, but the cell number did not increase on continuous administration of the carcinogens because an increased number of cells underwent apoptosis. These findings imply that an equilibrium may exist between the number of cells entering mitosis and the number dying by apoptosis.[48] In this context, the administration of growth factors such as epidermal growth factor (EGF) and HGF appeared to enhance the survival of carcinogen-activated cells by suppressing apoptosis and increasing the number of cells undergoing DNA synthesis.[49–52] C-*myc* expression can induce proliferation of oval cells and is also a potent inducer of apoptosis combined with a deficiency in the availability of growth factors. Down regulation of c-*myc* appears necessary for normal growth arrest and differentiation. Therefore, growth factors along with expression of protooncogenes such as c-*myc* are important regulators of the oval cell with respect to proliferation, differentiation, transformation, and cell death.[28,50,53–55]

In Vitro Studies

No culture system has been developed that conclusively demonstrates differentiation of rat liver epithelium (RLE) cells into hepatocytes or bile epithelial cells, although a recent study demonstrated that oval cell lines underwent a morphologic and functional differentiation along the hepatocyte and bile ductular cell lineages after long-term culture.[56] RLE cells will integrate into the hepatic plates and differentiate morphologically into hepatocytes after intrahepatic transplantation.[57]

Evidence supporting the view that HCC may arise from oval cells is derived in part from tissue culture experiments. Oval cells or RLE cells (cells that share common phenotypic features with oval cells and are regarded as their in vitro counterpart) have been transformed in-vitro. When these transformed cells are injected into nude mice, tumors will be produced displaying a wide range of phenotypes including well-differentiated hepatocellular carcinomas, cholangiomas, hepatoblastomas, and poorly differentiated or anaplastic HCCs.[36,40,58,59] Tumor phenotypes derived from RLE and/or oval cells may depend on the mechanism of transformation and the stage of differentiation of the cells at the time cellular transformation occurs.[60–62]

Therefore, the liver may be composed of two different stem cell compartments, the bipotential hepatocyte and the multipotential nonparenchymal epithelial cell system (Fig. 6-2). Both lineages could provide progenitor cells important for the development of HCC. The hepatocyte is the progenitor cell for liver tumors,[63] and there is evidence that the nonparenchymal (ductular) system is also involved.[63,64] A central issue will be to better understand the involvement of oval cells in the carcinogenic process and to characterize the mechanism(s) that regulate the proliferation of these cells and the factors that govern commitment to a particular cell lineage.

FIGURE 6-2. Pathways of changes and differentiation in hepatic stem cells. (From Thorgeirsson,[23] with permission.)

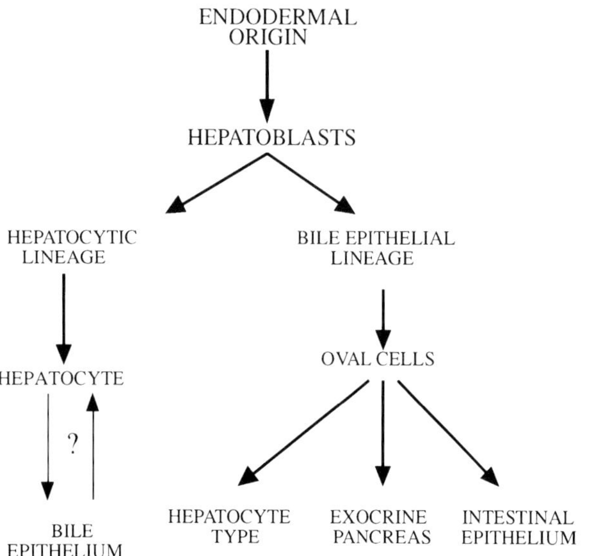

STAGES OF CARCINOGENESIS

Hepatic carcinogenesis is a complex process that histologically progresses from benign precursor lesions to malignant neoplasms and is associated with the accumulation of a series of genetic and epigenetic changes.[65] Three stages—initiation, promotion, and progression,[66]—are identified in a number of different experimental animal model systems.[67] However, studies of age-dependent tumor formation in rats suggest that in fact up to five or six independent steps may be involved in hepatocarcinogenesis.[68]

Approximately 60% of the chemicals determined by the US National Toxicology Program to be carcinogenic in rats and mice give rise principally to liver neoplasms. Most of these compounds function as tumor-promoting agents. Important substances in this regard are contraceptive steroids,[69,70] the antiestrogen compound tamoxifen,[71,72] benzodiazepines,[73] dioxin,[74] peroxisome proliferators,[75] and phenobarbital.[76]

Initiation of cellular transformation involves the formation of abnormal cells containing an irreversible genetic change, occurring either spontaneously or as a result of exposure to chemical or physical agents. Although it has been suggested that initiation events may be reversible since initiated cells are removed from the liver by apoptosis under defined experimental conditions,[77] in general carcinogen-induced DNA damage that leads to an initiating process is generally not reversible.

During the promotion stage, selected cells clonally expand into foci of altered hepatocytes. This promotion step may be reversible[78]; it is greatly influenced by the continuous presence of a promoter agent,[79] and the promoter effect will be observed only after continuous exposure for an extended time.[80,81] Furthermore, dose-response curves of such agents demonstrate an apparent threshold below which promoter effects are not detectable.[82] Evidence suggests that only some of the initiated cells will be clonally expanded into dysplastic hepatic foci under the influence of a promoter.[83,84] These findings suggest that promoters stimulate different subpopulations of initiated cells, which have developed a selective growth advantage due to changes in their genotype. Altered hepatic foci grow progressively and demonstrate increased levels of DNA synthesis when compared with surrounding normal hepatic tissue.[85]

In the progression stage, subsets (1% to 5%) of these foci eventually progress through a process of neoplastic transformation into frank malignancy.[86,87] This process involves additional genetic alterations that include activation of oncogenes and/or inactivation of tumor suppressor genes.[88–94] Initiation and promotion are believed to characterize events under physiologic conditions, and such alterations of the genome may, of course, occur at multiple points in the carcinogenesis process.

Mechanisms of Cell Cycle Regulation

All multicellular organisms have developed control mechanism(s) of cellular proliferation as an essential process for survival. These control events act like molecular switches between the alternative routes, evolving toward cell division, temporary cell-cycle arrest, quiescence, differentiation, or cell death. Under physiologic conditions and even after partial (2/3) hepatectomy, the cell cycle of the hepatocyte is tightly controlled. Several studies have provided insight into the humoral and cellular factors, as well as the patterns of gene expression involved in the hepatocyte cell cycle.[95–97] To pass through the cell cycle requires the successive activation of different cyclin-dependent protein kinases (cdk inhibitors).[98–100] These enzymes are controlled by transient associations with cyclin regulatory subunits, the interaction and binding of inhibitory polypeptides (cdk inhibitors) and the induction of reversible phosphorylation events.[101–103] Such molecular processes act as key regulators[104] of the cell cycle.[105] There are known checkpoints that help prevent genetic damage induced by toxic, mutagenic, or clastogenic agents, generally by providing cells time to repair damaged DNA before proceeding further through the cell cycle.[106–112] There is also evidence that attenuation or loss of the cell cycle checkpoint response and the inability to delay cell cycle progression in response to DNA damage are associated with enhanced sensitivity to toxic agents and genetic instability, contributing to tumor progression.[113–117]

One important restriction checkpoint occurs during the G1 phase of the cell cycle. If this checkpoint is defective, it may lead to deregulated growth with the eventual consequence of malignant transformation. Defects in checkpoint control may be found in tumors,[100] supporting the view that such mutations constitute a common pathway of tumorigenesis. Thus, altered expression of cyclins, cdks, or cdk inhibitors could potentially deregulate the cell cycle program and lead to hepatocellular proliferation in HCC,[118] as well as other tumor types.[119–121]

Tumor-Promoting Agents

ANDROGENS AND ESTROGENS

Males are at a greater risk to develop HCC than females. Furthermore, estrogen receptors increase in tumor cells when HCC develops in males; however, HCCs do not respond to antiestrogenic agents.[122] Villa et al.[123] recently reported that females with HCC displayed "wild type" transcripts of the estrogen receptor in tumors and peritumoral tissues. In contrast, males often displayed variant estrogen receptor transcripts in the tumors, and both normal and abnormal transcripts were found in the peritumoral cirrhotic tissue. As these variant transcripts would predictably give rise to a truncated form of the receptor modified in the hormone binding domain if there was constitutive transcriptional activity, they may favor deregulated proliferation of transformed hepatocytes in the male liver and confer a survival advantage to the neoplastic cells. These findings are supported by several rodent experimental model systems in which males develop HCC with higher frequency and a shorter latency time than females. Androgens appear to play an important role[124,125] in the genesis of these tumors.

In contrast, it is unclear whether secretion of estrogen could explain the sex differences in risk of developing HCC. Animal models suggest a protective role,[126–128] and ovariectomy decreases the promoter effects of chemical carcinogens long term. Synthetic estrogens acted as promoters of hepatocarcinogenesis in rats of both sexes as well as in humans.[129–133] In the resistant hepatocyte model, in which diethylnitrosanine-initiated lesions are promoted with 2-acetylaminofluorene and partial hepatectomy, estrogens did not affect tumor promotion.[134] However, ovariectomy plus testosterone treatment greatly influenced three parameters associated with tumor promotion: acceleration of the dysplastic focus formation, inhibition of proliferation of surrounding hepatocytes, and induction of c-*myc* expression in early hepatic neoplastic lesions. The maintenance of focal cellular proliferation and c-*myc* expression in early tumor nodules derived from males and from testosterone-treated females indicates that sex differentiation may affect growth control.

ORNITHINE DECARBOXYLASE ACTIVITY

Ornithine decarboxylase (ODC) is a rate-limiting enzyme involved in polyamine biosynthesis. ODC appears to play an important role in tumor promotion induced by chemical carcinogens in experimental animal model systems.[135] This enzyme is rapidly degraded in cells and has a half-life of less than 1 hour. Tamori et al.[136] found three-point mutations in ODC cDNAs derived from poorly differentiated human HCC tissue, resulting in formation of truncated but presumably highly stable ODC proteins. Because ODC activity reflects the rate of cell proliferation and is correlated with tumor differentiation in HCC,[137] their findings suggest that stabilization of ODC may be one reason why ODC activity is higher in less differentiated than in more differentiated HCCs. However, only three individual HCCs were examined, and further studies of larger numbers of tumors is necessary before firm conclusions can be reached.

APOLIPROTEIN B mRNA-EDITING PROTEIN

Apoliprotein B mRNA-editing protein deaminates cytidine, creating a new termination codon in the apo-B100 transcript and producing a truncated version termed apo-B48. The cytidine deaminase catalytic subunit of the multiprotein editing complex (APOBEC-1) has been identified, and transgenic mice and rabbits expressing rabbit APOBEC-1[138] have been generated. Unexpectedly, all of the transgenic mice and one rabbit developed liver dysplastic foci, and HCC evolved in many of the transgenic mice. Another hepatic mRNA species encoding for a tyrosine kinase was also found to be edited in the transgenic but not in control mice, suggesting that other mRNAs are affected by the overexpressed enzyme. This phenomenon may lead to aberrant editing of hepatic mRNAs involved in cell growth and regulation, contributing to tumorigenesis.

GROWTH FACTORS

An extensive array of growth factors and their receptors have been identified and may act as positive or negative modulators of cell proliferation and differentiation. The interaction of growth factors with specific membrane receptors triggers a cascade of intracellular signals, resulting in the activation or repression of genes associated with cell growth. Growth factors are generally polypeptides that act directly at short range on cells via autocrine, paracrine, and juxtacrine mechanism(s). Such factors are thereby distinguished from endocrine hormones that act at long range on target tissues after secretion into the blood. The unregulated expression of growth factors or proteins involved in downstream signaling pathways are important contributors to the multistep process of hepatocarcinogenesis.[139,140] Indeed, the products of cellular oncogenes are frequently identified as critical proteins involved in signal transduction pathways mediated by growth factors. Knowledge about the cellular activity of growth factors during hepatic proliferation and transformation is far from complete. Some of the growth factors that may be involved in one or more steps in the development of HCC include insulin, insulin-like growth factor II (IGF), transforming growth factor-α (TGF-α), transforming growth factor-β (TGF-β), epidermal growth factor (EGF), acidic fibroblast growth factor (aFGF) and hepatocyte growth factor (HGF). EGF, HGF, and TGF-α appear to be the most potent growth factors with respect to stimulation of hepatocyte proliferation. Less active in this regard are insulin and aFGF. However, comparative potency on stimulation of hepatocyte proliferation, is based on in vitro studies and may not reflect the actual growth effects obtained under physiologic conditions in vivo.

Insulin-like Growth Factor-2

Insulin-like growth factor-2 (IGF-2) is a polypeptide hormone produced during fetal development and is structurally and functionally related to insulin and insulin-like growth factor-1 (IGF-1).[141] During development, the expression of IGF-2 mRNAs is regulated through the activation of four different promoters (P1-P4) and alternative splicing of 5′ nontranslated leader sequences.[142] Postnatal IGF-2 P1 appears to be activated by liver-enriched activating protein and the CCAAT/enhancer binding protein-α.[143] The biologic activity of IGF-2 is mediated by binding to its receptor and insulin-like growth factor binding proteins (IGFBP). Transcription of the IGFBP-1 gene is stimulated by glucocorticoids, cAMP, and hepatic nuclear factor 3 and inhibited by insulin.[144,145] This gene is highly overexpressed very early in regenerating liver.[146] In situ hybridization studies in woodchuck livers showed that IGF-2, N-*myc*, and IGFBP-4 are up-regulated, whereas IGFBPs 1 and 2 are down-regulated in HCC tumor tissue when compared to normal liver.[147] Further studies are necessary to examine the interference of IGFBPs and IGF-2 at the molecular level during hepatocarcinogenesis. In the liver, IGF-2-mediated signal transduction occurs through binding to either the insulin receptor or the mannose 6 phosphate/insulin-like growth factor-2 receptor (M6P/IGF-2r) since IGF-1 receptors are not present in this tissue.[148] IGF-2 is expressed at high levels in fetal liver; however, the IGF-2 gene transcription rate declines after birth, and very low levels of gene expression are found in the normal adult liver. Re-expression of the fetal pattern of IGF-2 and increased IGF-2 levels of gene expression has been found in chemically induced hepatocarcinogenesis,[149] in transgenic mouse models of hepatocarcinogenesis[150,151] in woodchuck hepatic virus (WHV)-related liver hepatomas,[152–154] and in human HCC.[155–157] IGF-2 appears to reflect tissue-specific gene expression in transformed hepatocytes, and qualitative and quantitative levels of IGF-2 gene expression in HCC depend on the degree of cellular differentiation of the tumors.[158,159] These observations demonstrate that IGF-2 reactivation is a common molecular event in hepatocarcinogenesis regardless of the mammalian species involved and may confer a selective growth advantage on premalignant or transformed hepatocytes by an autocrine mechanism.

Indeed, high levels of IGF-2 mRNA were detected in 45% of HCCs arising from woodchuck livers with persistent WHV infection[154] and IGF-2 was overexpressed in more than 90% of precancerous altered hepatic foci in woodchuck liver.[152] Levels of IGF-2 protein were elevated twofold to threefold in woodchuck serum with chronic active hepatitis, suggesting a role for IGF-2 in the early cellular events before the development of HCC. However, studies derived from transgenic mice indicate that IGF-2 changes occur during the late stages of tumor progression.[160] Furthermore, in situ hybridization studies revealed that IGF-2 expression in woodchuck liver was variably reactivated in altered hepatic foci forming as precursors of HCC,[152,153] a finding that has also been observed in SV40 T antigen-induced tumors.[161]

High levels of IGF-2 RNA have been reported in human HCC and in adjacent uninvolved cirrhotic tissue, sugesting re-expression of fetal transcripts. In contrast, benign liver tumors and cirrhosis expressed the adult form of IGF-2 mRNA.[156] Immunohistochemical staining also has shown that IGF-2 is strongly expressed in HCC and cirrhotic tissues but not in normal liver.[162,163] In a further study, transcripts of fetal IGF-2 were more frequently observed than those of α-fetoprotein (at present the most widely used oncofetal marker of liver cell transformation) in HCCs and surrounding cirrhotic areas. It was suggested that reexpression of fetal IGF-2 mRNA may be an early marker of hepatocyte transformation.[157] Increased levels of high molecular weight forms of IGF-2 produced by HCC have been implicated in the pathogenesis of tumor-associated hypoglycemia.[164]

Results obtained from IGF-1 and IGF-2 transgenic mice suggest that IGF-1, when overexpressed in the liver, may induce hypercellularity and focal dysplasia but does not lead to hepatic malignancy.[165] Although IGF-2 alone is only weakly oncogenic in liver,[166] IGF-2 transgenic animals not only develop HCC but also tumors in other organs that do not express the transgene, indicating that IGF-2 may function in oncogenesis by both autocrine and endocrine mechanisms. Thus, IGF-2 is a weak initiator of the neoplastic process and will promote the growth of tumors in mice. Mating of IGF-2 and TGF-α transgenic mice resulted in a decreased time for development of HCC compared to TGF-α transgenic mice.[147] IGF-2 "knock out" mice that express SV40 T antigen in pancreatic islet cells had significantly reduced tumor growth rates,[161] possibly because lack of IGF-2 gene expression was associated with a fivefold increase in apoptosis. When studies have shown in vitro that IGF-2 expression may block apoptosis,[167] these observations were unrelated to Bcl-2 since Bcl-2 is not normally expressed in liver and was not induced in premalignant hepatic foci of woodchucks with chronic WHV infection.[147]

Transforming Growth Factor-α

Transforming growth factor-α (TGF-α) is a member of a family of structurally related polypeptide growth factors that includes EGF.[168,169] TGF-α and EGF attach to a common cell surface receptor having tyrosine kinase activity.[170] Although TGF-α was originally discovered as a soluble protein in the medium of retrovirally transformed mouse fibroblasts,[171] it has a physiologic role in the growth and development of normal cells and tissues. It acts in an autocrine or paracrine fashion to stimulate directly hepatocyte DNA synthesis.[172] In addition, the membrane-bound forms of TGF-α are also active and can interact with receptors on the surface of adjacent cells, thereby sustaining cell-cell adhesion as well as provide direct stimulation of DNA synthesis.[173] Immunohistochemical studies of HCC cells supported the hypothesis of an autocrine, paracrine, and/or endocrine action of TGF-α and EGF molecules on the growth of HCC.[174] In hepatocyte cultures, TGF-α is more potent than EGF with respect to stimulating DNA synthesis[96,175] and may be a more likely physiologic regulator of liver regeneration than EGF.[95,176] In this regard, increased TGF-α production has been associated with hepatocyte transformation.[177]

TGF-α plays a role in the establishment and maintenance of the malignant phenotype. Increased production of TGF-α and its receptor has been frequently found in human tumors and transformed HCC cell lines in tissue culture.[178] In addition, some cell lines will become transformed following stable transfection with constructs that overexpress TGF-α.[179] Transgenic mice bearing a human TGF-α cDNA under the control of the mouse metallothionein promoter have been shown to develop HCC.[177,180–183] Although the molecular mechanisms by which TGF-α induces hepatic transformation in these animals remain to be elucidated, the long latency period between the expression of the transgene and the development of HCC suggests that TGF-α may serve as a promoting agent. Indeed, one recent study demonstrated that stress promotes the growth of HCC in male TGF-α transgenic mice, emphasizing the fact that multiple factors could be involved in the development of hepatic malignancy.[184]

Hepatocytes derived from TGF-α transgenic animals have been used to establish immortalized cell lines.[185,186] TGF-α overexpression by these cells activates an autocrine growth stimulation loop and permits cells to replicate autonomously in culture. In culture, the TGF-α transgenic hepatocytes behaved similarly to normal hepatocytes supplemented with exogenous EGF and retained a well-differentiated growth pattern. However, when these cells were injected into nude mice, large tumors resembling HCCs arose within 1 month. High level expression of IGF-2 was also observed in these tumors.

In humans with HCC, 65% have elevated TGF-α levels in urine.[187] TGF-α and its receptor (EGFr) have been found to be expressed at high levels in human HCC tissue and not in normal liver.[188,189] Staining for TGF-α in poorly differentiated areas of tumor was less prominent when compared to highly differentiated HCC, which suggests that increased expression of TGF-α and EGFr may be early events of human hepatocarcinogenesis.[189] TGF-α was detected more frequently in individuals whose adjacent nontumorous livers had detectable HBsAg and/or HBcAg. Interestingly, HBsAg was localized within the same hepatocytes as TGF-α in more than half of the cases. Thus, a possible interaction between HBV and TGF-α during hepatocarcinogenesis was indicated by these studies.

Transforming Growth Factor-β

Human transforming growth factor-β (TGF-β) is comprised of three isoforms, TGF-β1, 2, and 3. They are members of a family of structurally and functionally related peptides and include inhibins, activins, and bone morphogenic peptides, many of which regulate cell proliferation and differentiation.[190] TGF-β1 is secreted as a latent, biologically inactive complex.[191] Subsequent proteolytic activation of TGF-β1 by plasmin is facilitated by binding of the latent complex to the M6P/IGF-2 receptor.[192–194] This receptor is ubiquitously expressed in tissues, and following binding there is internalization and subsequent lysosomal degradation of TGF-β or enhancement of extracellular TGF-β activation.[192,195] Once activated, the TGF-β peptide binds to the TGF-β receptor and inhibits hepatocyte proliferation while at the same time stimulating Ito cells to produce more of the latent TGF-β.

TGF-β inhibits epithelial cell proliferation, stimulates cellular differentiation, and augments connective tissue formation. Recently, three TGF-β receptors have been cloned and sequenced.[196–199] Receptors type I and II are members of a new serine/threonine kinase receptor family. Receptor type III lacks an intracellular signaling domain and functions primarily as a binding and presentation molecule for presenting TGF-β to the type I and II receptors.[200,201] During liver regeneration, there is increased expression of all three TGF-β isoforms.[202] In contrast, the TGF-β types I, II, and III receptors are rapidly down-regulated following partial hepatectomy.[203] Type II receptor expression may be responsible for limiting the hepatocyte proliferative response.[204] Inhibition of liver regeneration has been shown after intravenous administration of TGF-β to partially hepatectomized rats.[204] These findings imply that a TGF-β1 sensitive restriction point may exist during the late G1 phase of the cell cycle and results in transient inhibition of DNA synthesis.[191,204]

Under physiologic conditions, TGF-β is believed to counteract the growth-promoting effects of other growth factors such as TGF-α. This negative regulation of proliferation is mediated by the induction of apoptosis in hepatocytes and altered cells in preneoplastic hepatic foci[205–207] TGF-β has been shown to be a potent inhibitor of DNA synthesis in primary hepatocyte cultures[208,209] and HCC cell lines such as HepG2 and Hep3B.[210,211] Thus, TGF-β appears to inhibit the regenerative response. Expression of TGF-β1 may play a role in liver fibrogenesis as well.[212–214]

Increased expression of TGF-β is found in HCC tissue,[178,215,216] and elevated serum levels of TGF-β have been found in patients with HCC.[217] Increased secretion of TGF-β1 by cells that have lost responsiveness to the growth inhibitory activities of TGF-β may facilitate tumor progression by suppression of immune surveillance. Another study, however, demonstrated that TGF-β was not overexpressed in HCC compared to cirrhotic tissue or chronic HBV infected liver.[163] Nonparenchymal mesenchymal Ito cells are the principal source of TGF-β in the liver under most physiologic and pathologic conditions.[208,218] TGF-β1, TGF-β type I, II, and III receptors, as well as M6P/IGF-2 receptor proteins are present at significantly reduced levels in chemically induced HCCs compared to surrounding normal tissue.[219,220] Similarly, human HCCs have a 60% reduction in expression of both the TGF-β type I and II receptors as well as M6P/IGF-2 receptor protein.[221] Furthermore, several groups have demonstrated a loss of heterozygosity at the M6P/IGF-2 receptor locus in 70% of human HCC[222,223] and mutations in the M6P/IGF-2 receptor gene in HCC tissue.[224] Since M6P/IGF-2 receptor expression is increased during liver regeneration,[225] the reduction in HCC is not due to increased cellular proliferation and may be related to transformation TGF-β1 is not expressed by normal hepatocytes and cirrhotic tissue,[226,227] but is stongly expressed in the cytoplasm of altered hepatocytes found in neoplastic nodules.

The TGF-β receptor type II is expressed on the plasma membranes of normal but not transformed hepatocytes. A defect of TGF-β type 2 receptor was observed in a recently established HCC cell line, resulting in partial resistance to the growth inhibitory properties of TGF-β.[228] Thus, when compared to normal hepatocytes, HCC cells not only possess a reduced ability to activate TGF-β (i.e., decreased M6P/IGF-2 receptor) but also a diminished ability to respond to TGF-β (i.e., decreased or nonfunctional TGF-β type I, II, and III receptors). This may explain in part the observation that some patients with HCC have "nonfunctional" elevated TGF-β levels in serum and HCC tissue. Presumably, such transformed hepatocytes would have a growth advantage over normal cells. Chronic exposure to elevated levels of TGF-β may produce a microenvironment that selects transformed hepatocytes resistant to TGF-β.[229] Taken together, the findings suggest that promotion of tumor growth is a process of natural selection of cells resistant to the growth inhibitory environment normally present in the liver with an end result of clonal expansion of cell phenotypes resistant to inhibitory signals.

TUMOR SUPPRESSOR GENES

Mechanisms of Inactivation of Growth Regulatory Genes

Recent investigations have led to the discovery of a class of genes with functional properties opposite to those of the oncogenes or tumor-producing genes. The products of these genes appear to suppress malignant transformation and therefore they have been designated tumor suppressor genes[230,231] (Table 6-2). At the molecular level, mutations, large deletions, alternate splicing, promoter mutations have been found that disrupt the biologic function of these genes in association with the development of human malignancy. Germline mutations of this class of genes may play a role in the rare inherited cancer syndromes. Several investigations have demonstrated allelic chromosomal losses in HCC tissues. In some types of tumors, inactivation of suppressor genes may occur by methylation[232,233] as another mechanism to inactivate such genes. DNA methylation plays a role in the regulation of gene expression. Hypomethylation (i.e., decreased 5-methylcytosine content) may also be required for gene expression to occur. Therefore, hypomethylated genes have an increased potential for expression compared to hypermethylated genes.[234] Alterations in DNA methylation may enhance the expression of oncogenes and/or interfere with the expression of tumor-suppressor genes (Fig. 6-3). Hypomethylation of growth regulatory genes may be a molecular mechanism underlying cell proliferation that contributes to carcinogenesis.[235] Furthermore, it is possible that environmental toxins alter the methylation status of DNA and this event leads to potential mutagenic effects.[236–238]

TABLE 6-2. Loss of Heterozygosity (LOH) in Hepatocellular Carcinoma

Chromosome	Number of Cases with LOH/Informative Cases[a] (%)
1p	9/30 (30%)
	5/6 (83%)
4	15/28 (54%)
5q	11/30 (37%)
8p	39/97 (40%)
10q	9/36 (25%)
11p	12/27 (44%)
13q	27/55 (49%)
16	112/261 (48%)
17p	140/261 (54%)
22q	5/15 (33%)

[a] Only studies with >20% LOH in ≥10 cases have been included in this table.

Retinoblastoma Gene

Involvement of the retinoblastoma (RB) gene in the molecular pathogenesis of HCC has been suggested by a number of studies since chromosomal deletions have been mapped to the RB locus on chromosome 13q.[239–241] Abnormalities of the RB gene have been found in 20% to 25% of HCC including 80% to 86% of HCC with p53 mutations.[242] However, large deletions in the RB gene are a rare event.[243] Kuroki et al.[244] analyzed DNA isolated from 92 HCC for loss of heterozygosity (LOH) at 13 regions on chromosome 13q, using polymorphic microsatellite markers. In 33% of such tumors, LOH was detected, and an additional 22% of the samples were characterized by partial deletions of 13q. Two commonly deleted regions that included the RB and BRCA2 regions were observed.

THE p53 TUMOR SUPPRESSOR GENE AND AFLATOXINS

p53 Protein and HCC

The p53 protein is a multifunctional transcription factor that orchestrates cellular responses to DNA damage and thus conserves genetic stability. Induction of DNA damage activates p53, which in turn induces either cell growth arrest or programmed cell death, depending on the cell type and experimental system. The p53 protein contains a DNA-binding domain in the carboxyterminal region and a transcriptional activation domain within the aminoterminus of the molecule. Thus, p53 controls the G1/S checkpoint in the cell cycle by interacting with cellular genes that are intimately involved in cell cycle regulation.[245] Recent evidence indicates that such alterations of p53 function is found in HCC cell lines.[246–248] Highly specific genetic alterations in the p53 gene were described by two independent groups of investigators in human HCC. There appeared to be a unique association between a specific p53 mutation in HCC derived from two different regions of the world.[90,249] Bressac et al.[338] found 3 G:C to T:A mutations in codon 249 of the p53 gene leading to a substitution of arginine to serine in 10 tumors from southern Africa.[249] Interestingly, the same mutation was also present in two HCC cell lines

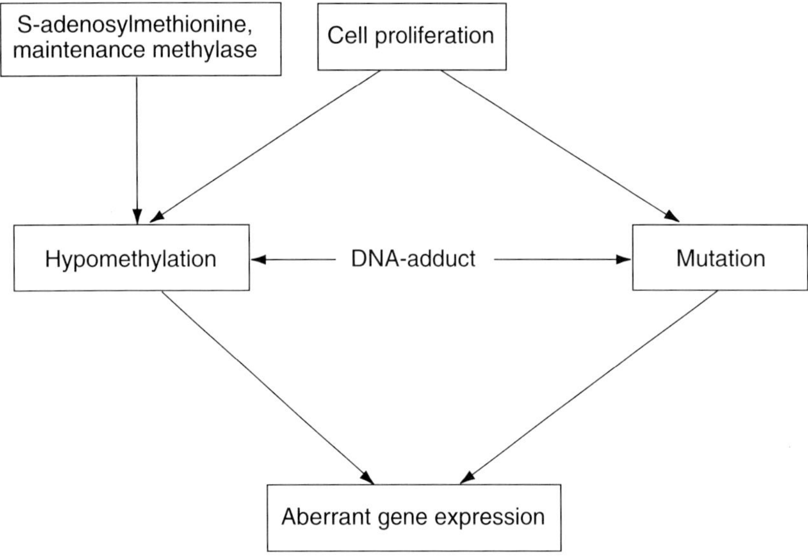

FIGURE 6-3. Effect of methylation on hepatocyte gene expression. (From Counts J, Goodman J. Hypomethylation. In Jirtle RL [ed]: Liver Regeneration and Carcinogenesis. Academic Press, San Diego, 1995, p. 229, with permission.)

derived from African patients but not in cell lines derived from patients residing in other geographic areas. Hsu et al.[90] also described 7 G:C to T:A in codon 249 of the p53 gene and one G:C to C:G substitutions in 16 HCCs derived from the Qidong area of China.[90]

These mutations were consistent with those caused by aflatoxin B1 exposure in experimental animal models. It was suggested that the G:C to T:A mutations were caused by aflatoxin B1 and may contribute to the high incidence of HCC in these areas of the world. This observation was confirmed by additional studies conducted on tumor samples from areas of the world with high endemic exposure to aflatoxin B1 (AFB1)[250–252] (Table 6-3). This mutational event at codon 249 is not entirely specific for aflatoxin exposure[253] and may occur occasionally in tumors derived from other regions of the world. However, the clustering of the codon 249 mutation in HCC derived from high aflatoxin areas of the world represent a molecular clue as to how an environmental toxin contributes to tumor development.

Role of Aflatoxin B1 in Hepatocarcinogenesis

Aflatoxins are produced by the fungi *Aspergillus flavus* and A. *parasiticus*; they contaminate foods such as corn, peanuts, milo, sorgum, and rice in some areas of the world.[254–256] Epidemiologic investigations have revealed a linear relationship between the content of AFB1 in the diet and the risk of HCC.[256,257] The level of aflatoxins found in grains is directly related to the extent to which the food is stored under humid conditions. High aflatoxin areas of the world include certain regions in southern Africa and China. Dietary aflatoxin intake, as expressed in nanograms per kilogram of body weight per day, may vary from 3–5 to 43–53 ng/kg in these regions.[256,258] The risk of HCC is correlated with dietary aflatoxin intake. More important, AFB1 contamination of food and coexisting HBV infection are associated with even higher rates of HCC development within a given population; therefore, the actions of these may be synergistic.[259] The oncogenic role of aflatoxin has clearly been established in experimental animal models in which aflatoxin has reproducibly led to HCC.[260,261]

AFB1 is metabolized by the liver microsomal system to the exo-8, 9-epoxide intermediate. This epoxide binds selectively to guanine residues in cellular DNA to form the N7 guanine adduct[260,261] (Fig. 6-4). The positively charged imidazole ring of this adduct promotes depurination, resulting in the formation of an apurinic (AP) site on the DNA. Alternatively, under slightly basic conditions, the imidazole ring of the N7 guanine adduct opens to form the chemically and biologically stable AFB1 formamidopyrimidine (AFB1-FAPY). The initial N7 adduct, the AFB1-FAPY, and the AP sites, individually or collectively, likely produce the genetic effects of AFB1. The covalent binding of AFB1 to guanine preferentially induces G to T mutations in chromosomal DNA, although several other types of mutations may occur. The primary aflatoxin adduct AFB1-N7-Gua may give rise to a significant proportion of the AFB1-induced mutations.[262] The DNA binding to the AFB1 adduct is followed by an excisional event that removes the AFB1 guanine product from the DNA, and this complex is excreted in the urine of exposed individuals.[257,263–265]

TABLE 6-3. Prevalence of p53 Tumor Suppressor Gene Mutations in Various Geographic Locations

Reference	Geographic Location	AFB1 Exposure	LOH 17p13	Total p53 Mutations	p53 Mutations at Codon 249
Bressac et al., 1991[249]	Southern Africa	high	3/5	5/10	3/10
Hsu et al., 1991[333]	Qidong (China)	high	NA	8/16	8/16
Ozturk et al., 1991[252]	South Africa and southeast coast of China	high	NA	NA	12/72
Patel et al., 1992[270]	Africa and others	high	NA	NA	2/8
Scorsone, 1992[250]	Qidong (China)	high	22/36	NA	21/36
Li et al., 1993[251]	Qidong (China)	high	2/12	9/20	9/20
Ozturk et al., 1991[252]	Various locations	low	NA	NA	0/95
Murakami, 1991[241]	Japan	low	NA	7/43	0/43
Hayward, 1991[279]	Australia	low	NA	NA	0/16
Oda et al., 1992[273]	Japan	low	55/80	49/169	7/169
Patel et al., 1992[270]	UK and others	low	NA	NA	2/64
Challen et al., 1992[272]	UK	low	NA	2/19	0/19
Kress et al., 1992[271]	Germany	low	3/8	2/13	0/13
Hosono et al., 1993[276]	Taiwan	low	3/20	3/29	0/29
Hollstein et al., 1993[277]	Thailand	low	NA	2/15	1/15
Kar et al., 1993[253]	North America	low	NA	NA	0/47
Li et al., 1993	Shanghai (China)	low	6/18	3/18	1/18[a]
Nishda et al., 1993[240]	Japan	low	24/49	17/53	0/53
Nose et al., 1993[274]	Japan	low	5/14	3/20	0/20

Abbreviations: AFB1, aflatoxin B1; LOH, loss of heterozygosity (cases with LOH/informative cases); Arg, arginine; Ser, serine; NA, not available.

[a] This patient had previously resided in Nantong, an area of high AFB1 exposure.

AFB1-guanine adducts have also been detected by immunofluorescent staining in livers of humans and animals exposed to aflatoxin in the diet.[266,267] Susceptibility to HCC may be associated with genetic variation of the enzymes epoxide hydrolase and glutathione S-transferase M1 involved in the detoxification of AFB1.[268]

When one compares the frequency of codon 249 mutations of the p53 gene in HCCs in over 500 specimens analyzed to date, clustering of these specific mutations have been found in only two regions of the world, southern China and South Africa.[90,249–252,338,339] These are two of the highest aflatoxin areas of the world. One recent study describes a mutational hotspot in the p53 gene of HCC derived from Mexico; however, only 21 tumors were examined.[269] Several studies (Table 6-3) of other regions of the world, including North America,[252,253] Europe,[252,270–272] the Middle East,[252] Japan,[241,252,213–275] Taiwan,[276] Thailand,[277] ethnic Chinese in Singapore,[278] and Australia,[279] where aflatoxin levels in food are low or undetectable found no such mutational specificity for codon 249 of exon 7 of the p53 gene. Only one recent study from Taiwan and Japan did not support the hypothesis that codon 249 of the p53 gene is a hot spot for aflatoxin-induced mutagenesis.[280]

The third base of codon 249 of the p53 appears to be preferentially targeted to form adducts with aflatoxin B1.[281,282] In vivo, this specific mutation has not been detected in AFB-induced hyperplastic nodules in rat liver[283] or induction of hepatic tumors in nonhuman primates.[284] These discordant findings could be explained, in part, by species differences in gene structure, drug metabolism, or absence of additional interacting factors.[284] Some more recent investigations in ducks and mice suggested that exposure to aflatoxin alone is not sufficient to induce the unique mutation at codon 249 and implies that other factors may be involved.[285] It is noteworthy that induction of this mutation alone results in a clonal growth advantage for hepatocytes but does not lead to cellular transformation.[286] These findings are consistent with the model of a multistage process of hepatocarcinogenesis. In human studies of HCC with codon 249 mutations, a significant proportion of tumors retain the presence of the "wild type" p53 allele, suggesting that the first step in p53 inactivation was a point mutation in one allele followed by subsequent loss of the "wild type" allele by a deletional event.[250] This hypothesis was supported by the recent observation of codon 249 mutations in the p53 gene in normal liver of aflatoxin-exposed individuals.[287]

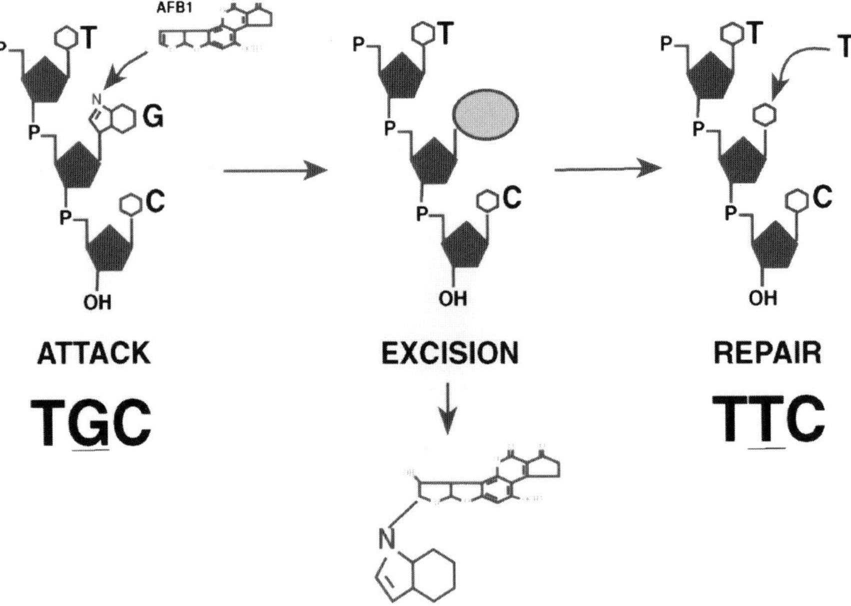

FIGURE 6-4. Aflatoxin B1 binding to guanine residues in DNA leads to an excisional event and subsequent repair by replacement with a thymidine residue. The nucleotide sequence is changed from TGC to T*T*C in this example.

Since the G to T mutation in codon 249 has been primarily identified in patients with chronic HBV infection, it is possible that HBV-induced chronic hepatitis plays an additional role in the frequency of this mutation in high aflatoxin areas of the world. Increased cellular proliferation in the context of chronic inflammation could facilitate fixation of the G:C to T:A transversion in codon 249 and allow selective clonal expansion of the cells containing this mutant p53 gene. Alternatively, loss of G1 checkpoint function by mutated p53 may make hepatocytes more vulnerable to the chromosomal instability induced by long-term HBV infection. This hypothesis is contradicted by the finding that this mutation occurs in non-neoplastic liver of HBV-infected and aflatoxin-exposed individuals in Mozambique, but not in HBV-infected patients and patients not exposed to aflatoxin in North America, suggesting that aflatoxin and not hepatitis per se is the likely cause of this mutation in HCC.[288]

ONCOGENES

Activation of cellular oncogenes, including those of the *ras* family, has been detected in spontaneous and chemically induced preneoplastic lesions of HCC, particularly in rodent models.[289–298] Activated *ras* genes have also been found in preneoplastic lesions of HCC induced by aflatoxin B1 exposure in rats.[299–301] Constitutively elevated and deregulated expression of c-*myc* along with an activated N-*ras* gene has been found in the Hep G2 human hepatoblastoma cell line.[302,303] The expression of the *ras* family of oncogenes, as well as other cellular oncogenes, during experimental hepatocarcinogenesis has been used as evidence that proto-oncogene activation may be an important event in the development of HCC. Although activated forms of cellular oncogenes have been reported in chemically induced rodent liver tumors, a clear sequence of events has not been established. Furthermore, a search for activated oncogenes in human HCCs has not been informative in most instances. Moreover, several recent studies have found little evidence of activated oncogenes in human HCC.[304–309] It is also of interest that no structural or functional changes have been found in a large panel of oncogenes in a transgenic mouse model that develops HCC.[310] Therefore, in contrast to other human tumors, activation of cellular oncogenes is infrequent in human HCC.

HEPATITIS B VIRUS

A fundamental question of whether HBV has a direct role in the initiation of hepatocyte transformation or provides a cellular environment for oncogenesis through nonspecific mechanisms such as liver injury followed by regeneration and the genomic instability associated with increased cellular turnover has not been established.

However, there are several lines of evidence supporting a direct oncogenic role for HBV in hepatocarcinogenesis.

It is now well established that the vast majority of HCCs related to HBV infection contain HBV DNA sequences integrated into the hepatocyte chromosomal DNA. Viral integrations may act as random insertional mutagens and may contribute to secondary chromosomal rearrangements such as inversions, translocations, and deletions. Viral integration sites in early HCC are sometimes near genes involved in the control of cellular proliferation and differentiation. However, many other HCCs have no consistent pattern of integration. In contrast, WHV-DNA integrations insert into or near the *myc* family of nuclear proto-oncogenes and have been found in up to 50% of HCCs. Another line of evidence suggesting a direct oncogenic role for hepadnaviruses in producing HCC are the endogenous *cis*- and *trans*-acting regulatory elements in the viral genome. At least part of the X and truncated pre-S2/S gene sequences are present in many sequenced HBV integration sites.

HBV DNA Integration Sites

Integrated HBV sequences have been documented in established HCC cell lines[311–316] and in greater than 80% of HCC patients with chronic HBV infection.[311,317–325] In many tumors, there are multiple viral integrations (usually three to four but sometimes more than 10). The well-known HCC cell line PLC/PRF/5, for example, carries at least seven HBV integrants.[326–328] In general, hybridization band profiles differ from tumor to tumor, suggesting that integration occurs at various random sites within the cellular DNA. Some integrated HBV genomes appear to provoke secondary chromosomal rearrangements.

The presence of discrete HBV hybridizing bands found in individual tumors suggests clonal expansion of a single transformed hepatocyte. Molecular evidence for a monoclonal origin has been provided by identical Southern blot hybridization patterns of tumor DNA obtained at different locations within the liver.[324,329,330] Occasionally, however, integration sites may vary in different tumor nodules within the same liver,[329,331,333] indicating that some HCCs are multicentric in origin. After surgical removal of a primary HCC, recurrent tumors can be shown to arise from the original residual clone in some cases, and de novo neoplasms in others.[334]

DNA integrations may occur at early stages of some natural HBV infections.[318,335,336] There is also experimental evidence to support this concept. In vitro studies have shown that HBV integrations are evident in cultured primary human fetal hepatocytes as early as 5 days after HBV infection.[337,338] Integrations may be present in chronically infected liver tissue without clinical evidence of cellular transformation, indicating that viral integration precedes the development of HCC.[318,319,339–341] In some studies, discrete hybridization band profiles with chronic liver disease suggest a unique clonal expansion of hepatocytes during liver regeneration.[331,332,342,343] HCC cells and naturally infected hepatocytes may have similar patterns of integration in the same patient.

Molecular Structure of Viral Integrations

The molecular structure of viral integrations has been quite variable, ranging from simple nonrearranged stretches of viral DNA to highly complex rearranged patterns. While the former integration pattern is believed to represent the result of the primary large integration event, the more complex pattern may be a consequence of secondary rearrangements that evolve during either chronic infection or tumor progression. More than 50% of the integrated HBV genomes have at least one viral cellular junction, the so-called cohesive end region that lies between the viral direct repeat 1 and 2 (DR1 and DR2) sequences of the HBV genome,[317,340,344–348] whereas the other end of viral DNA joins cellular DNA at variable positions of the viral genome. It is now understood that DR1 and DR2 represent sites for the initiation of viral minus- and plus-strand DNA synthesis. The sequence within the cohesive end region appears preferred for the recombination between viral and cellular DNA, and thus the viral-viral junctions are commonly found to lie within this region. Integration at this site, together with associated viral deletions and rearrangements, prevents the expression of viral core and polymerase open reading frames, but often leaves the envelope region, the enhancer I element and the 5′ sequences of the viral X gene, intact. In this regard, it has been demonstrated that structurally intact X and/or preS2/S transactivator sequences are found in 81% of integrated viral sequences in HCC tissues and cell lines. In all samples tested, integrated viral DNAs had retained structural functionality as potential transactivators of cellular genes.[349,350]

HBV integrations are commonly associated with microdeletions of about 10 bp in the cellular DNA at the integration site.[345] The frequency of this finding suggests that such microdeletions may arise as a consequence of the general integration mechanism(s). In addition to inducing microdeletions, some integrated HBV genomes appear to be associated with secondary chromosomal rearrangements, including inverted duplications.[347,351–354] Such structures suggest that an initial simple integration event may have occurred followed by gene amplification whereby two copies underwent a recombinational process in a head-to-head orientation; the cohesive end region is commonly found at virus-cell and virus-virus junctions of the integrated HBV DNA.[317,347,348,352,354] Chromosomal translocations have also been found at HBV DNA integration sites, in which the two ends of the HBV DNA are joined

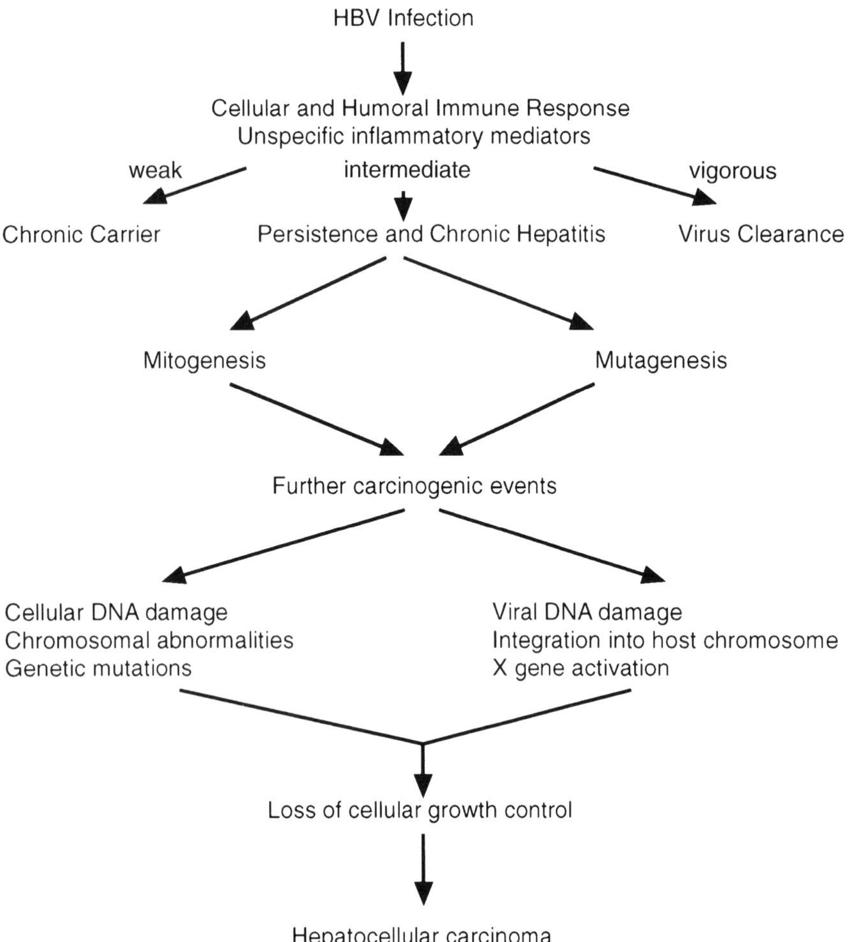

FIGURE 6-5. Proposed roles of HBV in the molecular pathogenesis of HCC. (Adapted from Chisari FV. Hepatitis B virus transgenic mice: insights into the virus and the disease [review]. Hepatology 1995;22:1316–1325, with permission.)

by cellular DNA from different chromosomes. Such associated translocations have been described between chromosomes 17:18,[355] X:17, 5:9,[347] and 17:7.[356] Integration of HBV into hepatocyte DNA may also trigger large chromosome deletions. Rogler et al.[356a] recorded the loss of more than 13.5 kb of cellular DNA on the short arm of chromosome 11 at location 11p13-11p14.[356] It is apparent that large-scale deletions as well as translocations may result in the loss of important cellular genes such as tumor suppressor or other genes involved in the growth process.[357] In rare cases, amplification of a chromosomal region has been found after HBV integration[358] (Fig. 6-5).

Integration and Genomic Instability

In chromosomal DNA studied thus far, HBV DNA integrations appear to have been important in mediating the rearrangement events, suggesting the presence of increased genomic instability.[359] HBV DNA containing the region spanning DR1 has been shown to promote homologous recombination of target DNA even at sites distant from the HBV insertional events.[360] Rearranged regions of the chromosome at some distance from an HBV integration site have also been reported.[361] Many of the integrations are located in fragile sites of the human genome.[362] Although the significance of fragile sites is not well understood, the integration of HBV within these regions may have significance in view of the recent association of fragile sites with unstable DNA sequences and the expansion of triple repeats in several genetic diseases.[363] Spontaneous chromosomal breaks in DNA derived from peripheral blood cells have been found in the same region where rearrangement had been due to HBV integration in an HCC cell line derived from one patient.[364] Chromosome damage and mosaicism of peripheral blood cells during acute and chronic HBV infection have been further documented by others.[365–367] The findings suggest a random mutagenic role for HBV at many different sites within the host genome. In a preliminary study, HBV replicated only in nontumorous cirrhotic liver tissue where genetic instability within the 1p36 region was demonstrated, but not in HCC cells or the Hep40 cell line derived from the HCC where HBV integration in the 1p36 region was observed.[368]

With respect to the importance of regions within the chromosome, it has been proposed that cellular repeat sequences are preferred sites for HBV insertion into human chromosomal DNA.[354,369] In this respect, Alu-type repeats,[348] minisatellite-like repetitive sequences,[369] α-satellite DNA,[354,356] and satellite III sequences[348,370] have been identified at or near HBV integration sites. No clear function has yet been ascribed to the vast majority of such DNA repeat sequences, but it has recently been recognized that they may be involved in the pathogenesis of a number of complex genetic diseases.[371] However, the total number of well-characterized HBV integration sites studied, is still quite small, and an alternative explanation for the apparent preference of HBV insertion into cellular repeat sequence may simply be that it reflects the abundance of these sequences in the human genome.

Viral Integration Within or Near Cellular Genes Governing Growth Regulation

Few examples of HBV integrations within or near known functional cellular genes have been documented. Characterization of a single HBV integration site in a small HCC revealed that HBV inserted into a short genomic DNA sequence sharing striking homology with the genes encoding for nuclear receptors such as the steroid- and c-erb A/thyroid hormone receptors;[372] the overall structure of the gene designated *hap* was similar to that of the DNA-binding hormone receptor genes.[373] The *hap* gene encodes for a second receptor for retinoic acid (RAR-β).[374] It was suggested that read-through transcription occurred from the viral pre-S1 promoter, resulting in overexpression of a truncated RAR-β with altered functions.[375]

In a single small HCC HBV DNA was integrated adjacent to the human cyclin A gene.[118] HBV integration in the cyclin A gene resulted in a strong expression of hybrid HBV-cyclin A transcripts encoding for a stabilized cyclin A, whereas cyclin A- or HBV-specific transcripts were not detected in the nontumorous part of the liver.[376] Constitutive and strong expression of this stabilized cyclin A protein may have led or contributed to increased cell proliferation.

In another HCC, HBV DNA has been found integrated next to a cellular DNA fragment homologous to the tyrosine protein kinase domain of the epidermal growth factor receptor.[377] Insertional activation of the mevalonate kinase (MK) gene in the human hepatoma cell line PLC/PRF/5 has been observed,[378] resulting in overexpression of hybrid transcripts arising from an HBV promoter and resulting in the constitutive overproduction of functionally active mevalonate kinase.

Transactivation Properties of Hepatitis Virus X Protein

Mammalian hepadnaviruses carry in their genome a short open reading frame (ORF) that has been designated as X, since its precise role during the viral life cycle is unknown. The X gene encodes for a 154 amino acid gene product. This gene has an active promoter[379] and was found not to be essential for the viral life cycle in vitro.[380] However, X expression appears to be necessary for the establishment of productive infection in vivo.[381,382] The X protein transactivates transcription of a wide array of promoters that normally regulate transcription of different cellular and viral genes.[383–386] The ability of X to function as a transactivator and the observation that complete and even 3′-truncated functional X ORFs have been described in hepadnavirus DNA integration events in HCC, whereas viral core, envelope, and polymerase encoding genes are often rearranged and not functional in the same integrations,[348,387–392] has led to the suggestion that X may be involved in the development of HBV-associated HCC.

MECHANISM OF TRANSACTIVATION

Several reports have proposed that X may stimulate transcription through a direct interaction at the promoter with components of the transcription machinery, including transcription activator proteins AP-1 and AP-2, cyclic AMP-responsive element binding protein (CREB), and activating transcription factor (ATF-2).[489–491] Furthermore, it X not only interacts with TATA-Box binding protein (TRP)[492] but also increases cellular TBP,[397] binds to the RBP5 subunit of RNA polymerase II, and through these events stimulates transcription.[397,398] The failure of X to directly bind to any defined DNA sequences,[399,400] however, suggests that the transactivation mechanism does not involve a known DNA sequence-specific interaction. Therefore, the biologic role of X may be mediated through an effect on cellular transcription factors,[386,393,401–405] including class III promoters[401] by protein-protein interactions. In this respect, X-mediated stimulation of AP-1- dependent promoters occurs through the activation of various cellular protein kinases including protein kinase C, Raf-1, and Ras.[402,404,406–408] X activates the transcription factor NFkB not only through the Ras/Raf-1-signalling pathway, but also by as yet unidentified Raf-1-independent pathways.[409] Taken together, these studies reveal activation of transcription of many genes by X under experimental conditions that depend in large part on the promoter and the cell system used.

CELLULAR PARTNERS OF X INTERACTIONS

Additional studies suggest that X might act at the cellular level on the proteolytic degradative pathways[391,410] (Huang J., Kwong J., Sun E.C., Liang T.J. Proteasome complex as a potential cellular target of hepatitis B virus X protein. J Vital 1996, 70:5582–91) or on a gene encoding for a DNA repair enzyme,[507] a novel leucine zipper-containing protein called XIP[412] and the p53 protein.[413–416] The results of p53-X interactions, however, have been based on conditions where unnaturally high concentrations of both p53 and X proteins have been used, therefore, the physiologic significance of these observations has been questioned.[417] X protein bound to p53 in vivo blocked entry of p53 into the nucleus in X transgenic mice[418] and thus prevented normal regulation of growth control genes. Such interactions could lead to tumor progression and metastasis in HCC. Further investigations are needed to clarify the role of p53 and X interactions in the pathogenesis of HCC.

Recently, co-expression of TGF-β1 and X were found in dysplastic foci of hepatocytes in X transgenic mice[419]; under these circumstances, X could interact with sequences homologous to a previously defined Egr-1-responsive element[420–422] and could enhance TGF-β1 promoter activity. TGF-β1 was not detectable by immunohistochemical staining in the liver of normal mice and was found exclusively within altered hepatic foci of transgenic mice where X protein was also highly overexpressed. In tumor tissue, both X and TGF-β1 concentrations were elevated. High levels of expression of TGF-β1 mRNA were shown in HCCs but not in control liver, suggesting a regulation of TGF-β1 expression at the transcriptional level. Therefore, an association between X and TGF-β1 expression levels exist under these experimental conditions and illustrate the potential interaction between X and growth factor proteins during tumor development.

X EXPRESSION AND CELLULAR TRANSFORMATION IN VITRO

X has the ability to transform SV40 immortalized mouse hepatocytes in vitro.[423] Transfection of the X gene under the control of the SV40 early promoter into NIH 3T3 cells[424] resulted in X overexpression, and accelerated growth characteristics correlated with these levels of expression. These cells formed tumors following injection into nude mice. These tumors had latency periods up to two and three times longer than tumors induced by *ras* oncogene activation. Transfection of the FMH202 cell line with constructs containing the X gene generated clones with cellular features of malignancy.[425] The duck hepatitis B virus lacks an X ORF, and DHBV replication in primary hepatocyte cultures does not lead to malignant transformation.[426]

TRANSACTIVATING PROPERTIES OF A TRUNCATED HBV ENVELOPE PROTEIN

Another HBV gene product has been reported to possess transcriptional transactivation properties. This envelope protein is the product of a truncated form of the pre-S2/S gene referred to as MHBst (truncated middle hepatitis B surface antigen).[427,428] Transactivating effects comparable to those of X were found with reporter constructs containing SV40, c-*myc* and c-*fos* promoters. Similar effects were also produced with artificially 3′-truncated pre-S2/S sequences. Further mutational analysis defined a range within the S open reading frame (termed "transactivity-on (TAO) region") in which 3′ deletions gave rise to transactivating properties of MHBst.[429] That a structural viral protein gains regulatory functions following truncation is very unusual. Truncated pre-S2/S sequences, however, are frequently found in HBV integration sites in HCC. The potential role of such viral sequences as a transactivator of cellular genes involved in growth control warrants further investigation.

HEPATITIS C VIRUS

HCV Infection and the Development of HCC

The molecular mechanism of HCV-related transformation of hepatocytes remains obscure. There is no evidence that HCV integrates into the cellular DNA. HCV replication may mediate the co-expression of TGF-α and IGF-2 in cirrhotic livers and act as a possible initiating factor for hepatocarcinogenesis.[430] In addition, there is evidence that HCV can be associated with HCC in some patients without the intermediate step of cirrhosis.[431] Recently, it was found that the HCV nonstructural protein 3 (NS3) and the core protein are involved in all transformations.[432,433] Since many HCV nonstructural and structural proteins, however, have not yet been thoroughly investigated at the molecular level, so the mechanisms of this virus in hepatocarcinogenesis remain unclear.

As with HBV, HCV infection offers a paradigm for the role of chronic viral infection in the process of producing chronic liver injury followed by regeneration, cirrhosis, and the subsequent development of HCC[434,435] (Fig. 6-1). After exposure to HCV, a sequence of events takes place over many years with development of chronic hepatitis, cirrhosis and the emergence of HCC up to 30 to 40 years after the onset of chronic infection.[434] When compared with HBV, it appears that HCV- associated HCC emerges more often in the presence of advanced cirrhosis in older individuals.

HCV and Other Associated Diseases in the Pathogenesis of HCC

Little is known about possible interactions between HBV and HCV in patients infected with both viruses with respect to the pathogenesis of HCC. Case control studies have indicated that dual infection with HBV and HCV results in a higher risk for the development of HCC.[436–438] Several studies of HBsAg-negative patients with HCC have shown that some of the patients (with anti-HBc) had both HBV and HCV genomic sequences in tumor and adjacent uninvolved liver tissue.[439–441] The frequency of double infections in HCC patients has been found to be variable.[442] Progression from chronic hepatitis to cirrhosis and HCC may be increased by double infection of HCV and HBV.

HCV infection may also play a role in individuals with autoimmune hepatitis (AIH) and HCC.[443] AIH often progresses to cirrhosis, but the development of HCC is unusual. In summary, the molecular evidence suggests that HCV-associated HCC develops because of the ability of HCV to produce chronic infection, hepatocyte injury, regeneration, and cirrhosis.

ALCOHOL AND HEPATOCELLULAR CARCINOMA

Several mechanisms have been postulated to explain the role of ethanol in promoting the development of HCC.[444–450] These include activation of chemical carcinogens through the induction of the microsomal P-450-dependent biotransformation system,[448] hepatocellular injury induced by ethanol,[451] reduction in the activity of the enzymes involved in the repair of carcinogen-mediated DNA alkylation,[448] suppression of the immune system, and the association of chronic HBV and HCV infection,[452,453] as a consequence of alcohol abuse.[454–458] A recent study in rats suggests that, in addition to the other mentioned mechanisms, an alteration in cellular composition of the liver resulting from oval cell proliferation may be considered as an explanation for the increased incidence of HCC among alcoholics.[459] Fifteen percent of alcoholics with cirrhosis were infected with low level HCV indicating that alcoholics have increased exposure and acquisition of persistent HCV infection for unclear reasons.[460] This virus plays a major role in the pathogenesis of the liver disease in some patients with alcohol abuse and may contribute to some cases of HCV- associated HCC.

ACKNOWLEDGMENTS

The authors gratefully acknowledge Karen Grosso for her help in this work.

REFERENCES

1. Beasley RP. Hepatitis B virus. The major etiology of hepatocellular carcinoma. Cancer 1988;61:1942–1956
2. Beasley RP, Hwang LY, Lin CC, Chien CS. Hepatocellular carcinoma and hepatitis B virus. A prospective study of 22 707 men in Taiwan. Lancet 1981;2:1129–1133
3. Tsukuma H, Hiyama T, Tanaka S et al. Risk factors for hepatocellular carcinoma among patients with chronic liver disease. N Engl J Med 1993;328:1797–1801
4. Qian GS, Ross RK, Yu MC et al. A follow-up study of urinary markers of aflatoxin exposure and liver cancer risk in Shanghai, People's Republic of China. Cancer Epidemiol Biomarkers Prev 1994;3:3–10
5. Fernandez E, La VC, D'Avanzo B et al. Family history and the risk of liver, gallbladder, and pancreatic cancer. Cancer Epidemiol Biomarkers Prev 1994;3:209–212
6. Shen FM, Lee MK, Gong HM et al. Complex segregation analysis of primary hepatocellular carcinoma in Chinese families: interaction of inherited susceptibility and hepatitis B viral infection. Am J Hum Genet 1991;49:88–93
7. Alberts SR, Lanier AP, McMahon BJ et al. Clustering of hepatocellular carcinoma in Alaska Native families. Genet Epidemiol 1991;8:127–139
8. Buetow KH. Genetic studies of human primary hepatocellular carcinoma. Prog Clin Biol Res 1992;376:155–172
9. Gasparini P, Borgato L, Piperno A et al. Linkage analysis of 6p21 polymorphic markers and the hereditary hemochromatosis: localization of the gene centromeric to HLA-F. Hum Mol Genet 1993;2:571–576
10. Bradbear RA, Bain C, Siskind V et al. Cohort study of internal malignancy in genetic hemochromatosis and other chronic nonalcoholic liver diseases. J Natl Cancer Inst 1985;75:81–84
11. Niederau C, Fischer R, Sonnenberg A et al. Survival and causes of death in cirrhotic and in noncirrhotic patients with primary hemochromatosis. N Engl J Med 1985;313:1256–1262
12. Cox DW, Markovic VD, Teshima IE. Genes for immunoglobulin heavy chains and for alpha 1-antitrypsin are localized to specific regions of chromosome 14q. Nature 1982;297:428–430
13. Crystal RG. The alpha 1-antitrypsin gene and its deficiency states. Trends Genet 1989;5:411–417
14. Wu Y, Whitman I, Molmenti E et al. Moore K, Hippenmeyer P, Perlmutter DH. A lag in intracellular degradation of mutant alpha 1-antitrypsin correlates with the liver disease phenotype in homozygous PiZZ alpha 1-antitrypsin deficiency. Proc Natl Acad Sci USA 1994;91:9014–9018
15. Packe GE, Clarke CW. Is porphyria cutanea tarda a risk factor in the development of hepatocellular carcinoma? A case report and review of the literature. Oncology 1985;42:44–47
16. Salata H, Cortes JM, de Salamanca R et al. Porphyria cutanea tarda and hepatocellular carcinoma. Frequency of occurrence and related factors. J Hepatol 1985;1:477–487
17. Van Thiel D, Gartner LM, Thorp FK et al. Resolution of the clinical features of tyrosinemia following orthotopic liver transplantation for hepatoma. J Hepatol 1986;3:42–48
18. Bianchi L. Glycogen storage disease I and hepatocellular tumours. Eur J Pediatr 1993;152:S63–70
19. Drinkwater NR, Lee GH. Genetic susceptibility to liver

cancer. In Jirtle RL (ed): Liver Regeneration and Carcinogenesis. Academic Press, San Diego, 1995, pp. 301–321

20. Lajtha LG. Stem cell concepts. Nouv Rev Fr Hematol 1979; 21:59–65
21. Rhim JA, Sandgren EP, Degen JL et al. Replacement of diseased mouse liver by hepatic cell transplantation. Science 1994;263:1149–1152
22. van Eyken P, Sciot R, Callea F, Desmet VJ. A cytokeratin-immunohistochemical study of focal nodular hyperplasia of the liver: further evidence that ductular metaplasia of hepatocytes contributes to ductular "proliferation." Liver 1989;9:372–377
23. Thorgeirsson SS. Hepatic stem cells. Am J Pathol 1993; 142:1331–1333
24. Sigal SH, Brill S, Fiorino AS, Reid LM. The liver as a stem cell and lineage system. Am J Physiol 1992;239:G139–148
25. Sell S. Is there a liver stem cell? Cancer Res 1990;50: 3811–3815
26. Fausto N. Hepatocyte differentiation and liver progenitor cells. Curr Opin Cell Biol 1990;2:1036–1042
27. Hayner NT, Braun L, Yaswen P et al. Isozyme profiles of oval cells, parenchymal cells, and biliary cells isolated by centrifugal elutriation from normal and preneoplastic livers. Cancer Res 1984;44:332–338
28. Braun L, Mikumo R, Fausto N. Production of hepatocellular carcinoma by oval cells: cell cycle expression of c-myc and p53 at different stages of oval cell transformation. Cancer Res 1989;49:1554–1561
29. Evarts RP, Nagy P, Nakatsukasa H et al. In vivo differentiation of rat liver oval cells into hepatocytes. Cancer Res 1989;49:1541–1547
30. Evarts RP, Nagy P, Marsden E, Thorgeirsson SS. In situ hybridization studies on expression of albumin and alpha-fetoprotein during the early stage of neoplastic transformation in rat liver. Cancer Res 1987;47:5469–5475
31. Evarts RP, Nagy P, Marsden E, Thorgeirsson SS. A precursor-product relationship exists between oval cells and hepatocytes in rat liver. Carcinogenesis 1987;8:1737–1740
32. Sell S, Leffert HL. An evaluation of cellular lineages in the pathogenesis of experimental hepatocellular carcinoma. Hepatology 1982;2:77–86
33. Shinozuka H, Lombardi B, Sell S, Iammarino RM. Early histological and functional alterations of ethionine liver carcinogenesis in rats fed a choline-deficient diet. Cancer Res 1978;38:1092–1098
34. Tatematsu M, Kaku T, Medline A, Farber E. Intestinal metaplasia as a common option of oval cells in relation to cholangiofibrosis in liver of rats exposed to 2-acetylaminofluorene. Lab Invest 1985;52:354–362
35. Lemire JM, Shiojiri N, Fausto N. Oval cell proliferation and the origin of small hepatocytes in liver injury induced by D-galactosamine. Am J Pathol 1991;139:535–552
36. Marceau N. Cell lineages and differentiation programs in epidermal, urothelial and hepatic tissues and their neoplasms. Lab Invest 1990;63:4–20
37. Farber E. Cellular biochemistry of the stepwise development of cancer with chemicals: Cancer Res 1984;44: 5463–5474
38. Gerber MA, Thung SN, Shen S et al. Phenotypic characterization of hepatic proliferation. Antigenic expression by proliferating epithelial cells in fetal liver, massive hepatic necrosis, and nodular transformation of the liver. Am J Pathol 1983;110:70–74
39. Hsia CC, Evarts RP, Nakatsukasa H et al. Occurrence of oval-type cells in hepatitis B virus-associated human hepatocarcinogenesis. Hepatology 1992;16:1327–1333
40. Fausto N. Oval cells and liver carcinogenesis: an analysis of cell lineages in hepatic tumors using oncogene transfection techniques. Prog Clin Biol Res 1990;331:325–334
41. Factor VM, Radaeva SA, Thorgeirsson SS. Origin and fate of oval cells in dipin-induced hepatocarcinogenesis in the mouse. Am J Pathol 1994;145:409–422
42. Germain L, Goyette R, Marceau N. Differential cytokeratin and alpha-fetoprotein expression in morphologically distinct epithelial cells emerging at the early stage of rat hepatocarcinogenesis. Cancer Res 1985;45:673–681
43. Hixson DC, Faris RA, Thompson NL. An antigenic portrait of the liver during carcinogenesis. Pathobiology 1990; 58:65–77
44. Wirnitzer U, Enzmann H, Rosenbruch M, Bomhard EM. Accumulation of p53 protein in chemically induced oval cells during early stages of rodent hepatocarcinogenesis. Carcinogenesis 1995;16:697–701
45. Saeter G, Seglen PO. Cell biology of hepatocarcinogenesis. Crit Rev Oncog 1990;1:437–466
46. Hu Z, Evarts RP, Fujio K et al. Expression of hepatocyte growth factor and c-met genes during hepatic differentiation and liver development in the rat. Am J Pathol 1993; 142:1823–1830
47. Evarts RP, Nakatsukasa H, Marsden ER et al. Expression of transforming growth factor-alpha in regenerating liver and during hepatic differentiation. Mol Carcinog 1992;5: 25–31
48. Bisgaard HC, Nagy P, Santoni RE, Thorgeirsson SS. Proliferation, apoptosis, and induction of hepatic transcription factors are characteristics of the early response of biliary epithelial (oval) cells to chemical carcinogens. Hepatology 1996;23:62–70
49. Nagy P, Bisgaard HC, Santoni RE, Thorgeirsson SS. In vivo infusion of growth factors enhances the mitogenic response of rat hepatic ductal (oval) cells after administration of 2-acetylaminofluorene. Hepatology 1996;23:71–79
50. Harrington EA, Bennett MR, Fanidi A, Evan GI. c-Myc-induced apoptosis in fibroblasts is inhibited by specific cytokines. Embo J 1994;13:3286–3295
51. Fairbairn LJ, Cowling GJ, Reipert BM, Dexter TM. Suppression of apoptosis allows differentiation and development of a multipotent hemopoietic cell line in the absence of added growth factors. Cell 1993;74:823–832
52. Barres BA, Hart IK, Coles HS et al. Cell death and control of cell survival in the oligodendrocyte lineage. Cell 1992; 70:31–46
53. Evan GI, Wyllie AH, Gilbert CS et al. Induction of apoptosis in fibroblasts by c- myc protein. Cell 1992;69: 119–128
54. Hanson KD, Shichiri M, Follansbee MR, Sedivy JM. Effects

of c-myc expression on cell cycle progression. Mol Cell Biol 1994;14:5748–5755

55. Nagy P, Evarts RP, Marsden E et al. Cellular distribution of c-myc transcripts during chemical hepatocarcinogenesis in rats. Cancer Res 1988;48:5522–5527
56. Radaeva S, Steinberg P. Phenotype and differentiation patterns of the oval cell lines OC/CDE 6 and OC/CDE 22 derived from the livers of carcinogen-treated rats. Cancer Res 1995;55:1028–1038
57. Coleman WB, Wennerberg AE, Smith GJ, Grisham JW. Regulation of the differentiation of diploid and some aneuploid rat liver epithelial (stemlike) cells by the hepatic microenvironment. Am J Pathol 1993;142:1373–1382
58. Garfield S, Huber BE, Nagy P et al. Neoplastic transformation and lineage switching of rat liver epithelial cells by retrovirus-associated oncogenes. Mol Carcinog 1988;1: 189–195
59. Tsao MS, Grisham JW. Hepatocarcinomas, cholangiocarcinomas, and hepatoblastomas produced by chemically transformed cultured rat liver epithelial cells. A light- and electron-microscopic analysis. Am J Pathol 1987;127:168–181
60. Bisgaard HC, Parmelee DC, Dunsford HA et al: Keratin 14 protein in cultured nonparenchymal rat hepatic epithelial cells: characterization of keratin 14 and keratin 19 as antigens for the commonly used mouse monoclonal antibody OV-6. Mol Carcinog 1993;7:60–66
61. Bisgaard HC, Ton PT, Nagy P, Thorgeirsson SS. Phenotypic modulation of keratins, vimentin, and alpha-fetoprotein in cultured rat liver epithelial cells after chemical, oncogene, and spontaneous transformation. J Cell Physiol 1994;159:485–494
62. Bisgaard HC, Nagy P, Ton PT et al. Modulation of keratin 14 and alpha-fetoprotein expression during hepatic oval cell proliferation and liver regeneration. J Cell Physiol 1994;159:475–484
63. Farber E. On cells of origin of liver cell cancer. In Sirica AE (ed): The Role of Cell Types in Hepatocarcinogenesis. CRC Press, Boca Raton, Florida. pp. 1992;1–28
64. Sell S, Pierce GB. Maturation arrest of stem cell differentiation is a common pathway for the cellular origin of teratocarcinomas and epithelial cancers. Lab Invest 1994;70: 6–22
65. Boone CW, Kelloff GJ, Steele VE. Natural history of intraepithelial neoplasia in humans with implications for cancer chemoprevention strategy. Cancer Res 1992;52:1651–1659
66. Dragan YP, Pitot HC. The role of the stages of initiation and promotion in phenotypic diversity during hepatocarcinogenesis in the rat. Carcinogenesis 1992;13:739–750
67. Goldsworthy TL, Hanigan MH, Pitot HC. Models of hepatocarcinogenesis in the rat—contrasts and comparisons. Crit Rev Toxicol 1986;17:61–89
68. Okuda K. Hepatocellular carcinoma: recent progress. Hepatology 1992;15:948–963
69. Yager JJ, Yager R. Oral contraceptive steroids as promoters of hepatocarcinogenesis in female Sprague-Dawley rats. Cancer Res 1980;40:3680–3685
70. Baum JK, Bookstein JJ, Holtz F, Klein EW. Possible association between benign hepatomas and oral contraceptives. Lancet 1973;2:926–929
71. Catherino WH, Jordan VC. A risk-benefit assessment of tamoxifen therapy. Drug Saf 1993;8:381–397
72. Williams GM, Iatropoulos MJ, Djordjevic MV, Kaltenberg OP. The triphenylethylene drug tamoxifen is a strong liver carcinogen in the rat. Carcinogenesis 1993;14:315–317
73. Diwan BA, Rice JM, Ward JM. Tumor-promoting activity of benzodiazepine tranquilizers, diazepam and oxazepam, in mouse liver. Carcinogenesis 1986;7:789–794
74. Pitot HC, Goldsworthy TL, Moran S et al. A method to quantitate the relative initiating and promoting potencies of hepatocarcinogenic agents in their dose-response relationships to altered hepatic foci. Carcinogenesis 1987;8: 1491–1499
75. Cattley RC, Popp JA. Differences between the promoting activities of the peroxisome proliferator WY-14,643 and phenobarbital in rat liver. Cancer Res 1989;49:3246–3251
76. Peraino C, Fry RJ, Staffeldt E. Reduction and enhancement by phenobarbital of hepatocarcinogenesis induced in the rat by 2-acetylaminofluorene. Cancer Res 1971;31:1506–1512
77. Grasl KB, Bursch W, Ruttkay NB et al. Food restriction eliminates preneoplastic cells through apoptosis and antagonizes carcinogenesis in rat liver. Proc Natl Acad Sci U S A 1994;91:9995–9999
78. Solt DB, Cayama E, Sarma DS, Farber E. Persistence of resistant putative preneoplastic hepatocytes induced by N-nitrosodiethylamine or N-methyl-N-nitrosourea. Cancer Res 1980;40:1112–1118
79. Hendrich S, Glauert HP, Pitot HC. The phenotypic stability of altered hepatic foci: effects of withdrawal and subsequent readministration of phenobarbital. Carcinogenesis 1986;7:2041–2045
80. Preat V, Lans M, de GJ et al. Influence of the duration and the delay of administration of phenobarbital on its modulating effect on rat hepatocarcinogenesis. Carcinogenesis 1987;8:333–335
81. Laconi E, Denda A, Rao PM et al. Studies on liver tumor promotion in the rat by orotic acid: dose and minimum exposure time required for dietary orotic acid to promote hepatocarcinogenesis. Carcinogenesis 1993;14:1771–1775
82. Pitot HC, Goldsworthy T, Campbell HA, Poland A. Quantitative evaluation of the promotion by 2,3,7,8-tetrachlorodibenzo-p-dioxin of hepatocarcinogenesis from diethylnitrosamine. Cancer Res 1980;40:3616–3620
83. Pereira MA. Rat liver foci bioassay. J Am Coll Toxicol 1983;1:101–106
84. Kaufmann WK, MacKenzie SA, Rahija RJ, Kaufman DG. Quantitative relationship between initiation of hepatocarcinogenesis and induction of altered cell islands. J Cell Biochem 1986;30:1–9
85. Seo MK, Lynch KE, Podolsky DK. Multiplicity of transforming growth factors in human malignant effusions. Cancer Res 1988;48:1792–1797
86. Farber E. Some emerging general principles in the pathogenesis of hepatocellular carcinoma. Cancer Surv 1986;5: 695–718
87. Pitot HC, Dragan Y, Sargent L, Xu YH. Biochemical markers associated with the stages of promotion and progression during hepatocarcinogenesis in the rat. Environ Health Perspect 1991;93:181–189

88. Pitot HC. The molecular biology of carcinogenesis. Cancer 1993;72:962–970

89. Vogelstein B, Kinzler KW. The multistep nature of cancer. Trends Genet 1993;9:138–141

90. Hsu IC, Metcalf RA, Sun T et al. Mutational hotspot in the p53 gene in human hepatocellular carcinomas. Nature 1991;350:427–428

91. Goyette MC, Cho K, Fasching CL et al. Progression of colorectal cancer is associated with multiple tumor suppressor gene defects but inhibition of tumorigenicity is accomplished by correction of any single defect via chromosome transfer. Mol Cell Biol 1992;12:1387–1395

92. Embleton MJ, Butler PC. Reactivity of monoclonal antibodies to oncoproteins with normal rat liver, carcinogen-induced tumours, and premalignant liver lesions. Br J Cancer 1988;57:48–53

93. Cote GJ, Lastra BA, Cook JR et al. Oncogene expression in rat hepatomas and during hepatocarcinogenesis. Cancer Lett 1985;26:121–127

94. Beer DG, Schwarz M, Sawada N, Pitot HC. Expression of H-*ras* and c-*myc* protooncogenes in isolated gamma-glutamyl transpeptidase-positive rat hepatocytes and in hepatocellular carcinomas induced by diethylnitrosamine. Cancer Res 1986;46:2435–2441

95. Michalopoulos GK. Liver regeneration: molecular mechanisms of growth control. FASEB J 1990;4:176–187

96. Fausto N. Growth factors in liver development, regeneration and carcinogenesis. Prog Growth Factor Res 1991;3: 219–234

97. Thompson NL, Mead JE, Braun L et al. Sequential protooncogene expression during rat liver regeneration. Cancer Res 1986;46:3111–3117

98. Nigg EA. Cyclin-dependent protein kinases: key regulators of the eukaryotic cell cycle. Bioessays 1995;17:471–480

99. Reed SI. The role of p34 kinases in the G1 to S-phase transition. Annu Rev Cell Biol 1992;8:529–561

100. Sherr CJ. G1 phase progression: cycling on cue. Cell 1994; 79:551–555

101. Elledge SJ, Harper JW. Cdk inhibitors: on the threshold of checkpoints and development. Curr Opin Cell Biol 1994; 6:847–852

102. Biggs JR, Kraft AS. Inhibitors of cyclin-dependent kinase and cancer. J Mol Med 1995;73:509–514

103. Alexandrow MG, Moses HL. Transforming growth factor beta and cell cycle regulation. Cancer Res 1995;55: 1452–1457

104. Morgan DO. Principles of CDK regulation. Nature 1995; 374:131–134

105. Strauss M, Lukas J, Bartek J. Unrestricted cell cycling and cancer. Nat Med 1995;1:1245–1246

106. Dulic V, Kaufmann WK, Wilson SJ et al. p53-dependent inhibition of cyclin-dependent kinase activities in human fibroblasts during radiation-induced G1 arrest. Cell 1994; 76:1013–1023

107. Kastan MB, Zhan Q, el DW et al. A mammalian cell cycle checkpoint pathway utilizing p53 and GADD45 is defective in ataxia-telangiectasia. Cell 1992;71:587–597

108. Kaufmann WK, Boyer JC, Estabrooks LL, Wilson SJ. Inhibition of replicon initiation in human cells following stabilization of topoisomerase-DNA cleavable complexes. Mol Cell Biol 1991;11:3711–3718

109. Kaufmann WK, Kaufman DG. Cell cycle control, DNA repair and initiation of carcinogenesis. FASEB J 1993;7: 1188–1191

110. Kaufmann WK, Wilson SJ. G1 arrest and cell-cycle-dependent clastogenesis in UV-irradiated human fibroblasts. Mutat Res 1994;314:67–76

111. Murray AW. The genetics of cell cycle checkpoints. Curr Opin Genet Dev 1995;5:5–11

112. Carr AM. Checkpoints take the next step. Science 1996; 271:314–315

113. Yin Y, Tainsky MA, Bischoff FZ et al. Wild-type p53 restores cell cycle control and inhibits gene amplification in cells with mutant p53 alleles. Cell 1992;70:937–948

114. Sanford KK, Price FM, Rhim JS et al. Role of DNA repair in malignant neoplastic transformation of human mammary epithelial cells in culture. Carcinogenesis 1992;13: 1137–1141

115. Paules RS, Levedakou EN, Wilson SJ et al. Defective G2 checkpoint function in cells from individuals with familial cancer syndromes. Cancer Res 1995;55:1763–1773

116. Livingstone LR, White A, Sprouse J et al. Altered cell cycle arrest and gene amplification potential accompany loss of wild-type p53. Cell 1992;70:923–935

117. Kaufmann WK, Levedakou EN, Grady HL et al. Attenuation of G2 checkpoint function precedes human cell immortalization. Cancer Res 1995;55:7–11

118. Wang J, Chenivesse X, Henglein B, Bréchot C. Hepatitis B virus integration in a cyclin A gene in a hepatocellular carcinoma. Nature 1990;343:555–557

119. Buckley MF, Sweeney KJ, Hamilton JA et al. Expression and amplification of cyclin genes in human breast cancer. Oncogene 1993;8:2127–2133

120. Jiang W, Kahn SM, Tomita N et al. Amplification and expression of the human cyclin D gene in esophageal cancer. Cancer Res 1992;52:2980–2983

121. Motokura T, Bloom T, Kim HG et al. A novel cyclin encoded by a bcl1-linked candidate oncogene. Nature 1991; 350:512–515

122. Ng IO, Ng MM, Lai EC, Fan ST. Better survival in female patients with hepatocellular carcinoma. Possible causes from a pathologic approach. Cancer 1995;75:18–22

123. Villa E, Camellini L, Dugani A et al. Variant estrogen receptor messenger RNA species detected in human primary hepatocellular carcinoma. Cancer Res 1995;55:498–500

124. To YC. Physiological and biochemical reviews of sex differences and carcinogenesis with particular reference to the liver. Adv Cancer Res 1973;18:155–209

125. Yamamoto RS, Weisburger EK. The role of hormones on digestive and urinary tract carcinogenesis. Recent Prog Horm Res 1977;33:617–653

126. Cantarow A. Endocrinological aspects of liver disease. Acta Int Cancer 1957;13:740–760

127. Hendrich S, Leveston AO, Pitot HC. Ovariectomy pro-

motes the growth of altered hepatic foci after withdrawal and reintroduction of phenobarbital during hepatocarcinogenesis in rats. Eur J Cancer Prev 1992;1:407–414

128. Katayama S, Ohmori T, Maeura Y et al. Early stages of N-2-fluorenylacetamide-induced hepatocarcinogenesis in male and female rats and effect of gonadectomy on liver neoplastic conversion and neoplastic development. J Natl Cancer Inst 1984;73:141–149

129. Lucier GW, Tritscher A, Goldsworthy T et al. Ovarian hormones enhance 2,3,7,8-tetrachlorodibenzo-p-dioxin-mediated increases, in cell proliferation and preneoplastic foci in a two-stage model for rat hepatocarcinogenesis. Cancer Res 1991;51:1391–1397

130. Wanless IR, Medline A. Role of estrogens as promoters of hepatic neoplasia. Lab Invest 1982;46:313–320

131. Lupulescu A. Estrogen use and cancer risk: a review. Exp Clin Endocrinol 1993;101:204–214

132. Yager JD, Campbell HA, Longnecker DS et al. Enhancement of hepatocarcinogenesis in female rats by ethinyl estradiol and mestranol but not estradiol. Cancer Res 1984; 44:3862–3869

133. Yager JD, Zurlo J, Ni N. Sex hormones and tumor promotion in liver. Proc Soc Exp Biol Med 1991;198:667–674

134. Liao D, Porsch-Hällstrom I, Gustafsson JA, Blanck A. Persistent sex differences in growth control of early rat liver lesions are programmed during promotion in the resistant hepatocyte model. Hepatology 1996;23:835–839

135. Tempero MA, Nishioka K, Knott K, Zetterman RK. Chemoprevention of mouse colon tumors with difluoromethylornithine during and after carcinogen treatment. Cancer Res 1989;49:5793–5797

136. Tamori A, Nishiguchi S, Kuroki T et al. Point mutation of ornithine decarboxylase gene in human hepatocellular carcinoma. Cancer Res 1995;55:3500–3503

137. Tamori A, Nishiguchi S, Kuroki T et al. Relationship of ornithine decarboxylase activity and histological findings in human hepatocellular carcinoma. Hepatology 1994;20: 1179–1186

138. Fishman HA, Orwar O, Scheller RH, Zare RN. Apolipoprotein B mRNA-editing protein induces hepatocellular carcinoma and dysplasia in transgenic animals. Proc Natl Acad Sci U S A 1995;92:8483–8487

139. Aaronson SA. Growth factors and cancer. Science 1991; 254:1146–1153

140. Cross M, Dexter TM. Growth factors in development, transformation, and tumorigenesis. Cell 1991;64:271–280

141. Froesch ER, Schmid C, Schwander J, Zapf J. Actions of insulin-like growth factors. Annu Rev Physiol 1985;47: 443–467

142. Nielsen FC, Christiansen J. Posttranscriptional regulation of insulin-like growth factor II mRNA. Scand J Clin Lab Invest Suppl 1995;220:37–46

143. Liu RT, Suzuki S, Miyamoto T et al. Postnatal liver- specific expression of human insulin-like growth factor-II is highly stimulated by the transcriptional activators liver-enriched activating protein and CCAAT/enhancer binding protein-alpha. Mol Endocrinol 1995;9:424–434

144. O'Brien RM, Noisin EL, Suwanichkul A et al. Hepatic nuclear factor 3- and hormone-regulated expression of the phosphoenolpyruvate carboxykinase and insulin-like growth factor-binding protein 1 genes. Mol Cell Biol 1995; 15:1747–1758

145. Babajko S. Transcriptional regulation of insulin-like growth factor binding protein-1 expression by insulin and cyclic AMP. Growth Regul 1995;5:83–91

146. Mohn KL, Melby AE, Tewari DS et al. The gene encoding rat insulinlike growth factor-binding protein 1 is rapidly and highly induced in regenerating liver. Mol Cell Biol 1991;11:1393–1401

147. Rogler CE, Rogler LE, Yang D et al. Contributions of hepadnavirus research to our understanding of hepatocarcinogenesis. In Jirtle RL (ed): Liver Regeneration and Carcinogenesis. Academic Press, San Diego, 1995, pp. 113–140

148. Cohick WS, Clemmons DR. The insulin-like growth factors. Annu Rev Physiol 1993;55:131–153

149. Ueno T, Takahashi K, Matsuguchi T et al. Reactivation of rat insulin-like growth factor II gene during hepatocarcinogenesis. Carcinogenesis 1988;9:1779–1783

150. Cariani E, Dubois N, Lasserre C et al. Insulin-like growth factor II (IGF-II) mRNA expression during hepatocarcinogenesis in transgenic mice. J Hepatol 1991;13:220–226

151. Schirmacher P, Held WA, Yang D et al. Reactivation of insulin-like growth factor II during hepatocarcinogenesis in transgenic mice suggests a role in malignant growth. Cancer Res 1992;52:2549–2556

152. Yang DY, Rogler CE. Analysis of insulin-like growth factor II (IGF-II) expression in neoplastic nodules and hepatocellular carcinomas of woodchucks utilizing in situ hybridization and immunocytochemistry. Carcinogenesis 1991;12: 1893–1901

153. Yang D, Alt E, Rogler CE. Coordinate expression of N-myc 2 and insulin-like growth factor II in precancerous altered hepatic foci in woodchuck hepatitis virus carriers. Cancer Res 1993;53:2020–2027

154. Fu XX, Su CY, Lee Y et al. Insulinlike growth factor II expression and oval cell proliferation associated with hepatocarcinogenesis in woodchuck hepatitis virus carriers. J Virol 1988;62:3422–3430

155. Bréchot C. Primary Liver Cancer. Etiological and Progression Factors. Paris, CRC Press, 1994

156. Cariani E, Lasserre C, Seurin D et al. Differential expression of insulin-like growth factor II mRNA in human primary liver cancers, benign liver tumors, and liver cirrhosis. Cancer Res 1988;48:6844–6849

157. Cariani E, Lasserre C, Kemeny F et al. Expression of insulin-like growth factor II, alpha-fetoprotein and hepatitis B virus transcripts in human primary liver cancer. Hepatology 1991;13:644–649

158. Hembrough TA, Vasudevan J, Allietta MM et al. Insulin-like growth factor II regulation of gene expression in rat and human hepatomas. J Cell Physiol 1995;162:36–43

159. Lewitt MS, Saunders H, Baxter RC. Interaction of insulin, glucocorticoids, and protein kinase C in the regulation of insulin-like growth factor-binding protein-1 production by H4IIE rat hepatoma cells. J Cell Physiol 1996;166:121–129

160. Sandgren EP. Transgenic models of hepatic growth regula-

tion and hepatocarcinogenesis. In Jirtle RL (ed): Liver Regeneration and Carcinogenesis. Academic Press, San Diego, 1995, pp. 257–306

161. Christofori G, Naik P, Hanahan D. A second signal supplied by insulin-like growth factor II in oncogene-induced tumorigenesis. Nature 1994;369:414–418
162. Seo JH, Park BC. Expression of insulin-like growth factor II in chronic hepatitis B, liver cirrhosis, and hepatocellular carcinoma. Gan To Kagaku Ryoho 1995;3:292–307
163. Park BC, Huh MH, Seo JH. Differential expression of transforming growth factor alpha and insulin-like growth factor II in chronic active hepatitis B, cirrhosis and hepatocellular carcinoma. J Hepatol 1995;22:286–294
164. Shapiro ET, Bell GI, Polonsky KS et al. Tumor hypoglycemia: relationship to high molecular weight insulin-like growth factor-II. J Clin Invest 1990;85:1672–1679
165. Quaife CJ, Mathews LS, Pinkert CA et al. Histopathology associated with elevated levels of growth hormone and insulin-like growth factor I in transgenic mice. Endocrinology 1989;124:40–48
166. Rogler CE, Yang D, Rossetti L et al. Altered body composition and increased frequency of diverse malignancies in insulin-like growth factor-II transgenic mice. J Biol Chem 1994;269:13779–13784
167. Evans G. Integration of cell proliferation and programmed cell death (apoptosis) by c-myc. Cold Spring Harbor Meeting on "Molecular Genetics of Cancer". 1994:Abstract #261
168. Derynck R. Transforming growth factor alpha. Cell 1988; 54:593–595
169. Derynck R. The physiology of transforming growth factor-alpha. Adv Cancer Res 1992;58:27–52
170. Massague J. Epidermal growth factor-like transforming growth factor. II. Interaction with epidermal growth factor receptors in human placenta membranes and A431 cells. J Biol Chem 1983;258:13614–13620
171. de Larco J, Todaro GJ. Growth factors from murine sarcoma virus-transformed cells. Proc Natl Acad Sci U S A 1978; 75:4001–4005
172. Mead JE, Fausto N. Transforming growth factor alpha may be a physiological regulator of liver regeneration by means of an autocrine mechanism. Proc Natl Acad Sci U S A 1989;86:1558–1562
173. Massague J. Transforming growth factor-alpha. A model for membrane-anchored growth factors. J Biol Chem 1990;265: 21393–21396
174. Yamaguchi K, Carr BI, Nalesnik MA. Concomitant and isolated expression of TGF-alpha and EGF-R in human hepatoma cells supports the hypothesis of autocrine, paracrine, and endocrine growth of human hepatoma. J Surg Oncol 1995;58:240–245
175. Webber EM, FitzGerald MJ, Brown PI et al. Transforming growth factor-alpha expression during liver regeneration after partial hepatectomy and toxic injury, and potential interactions between transforming growth factor-alpha and hepatocyte growth factor. Hepatology 1993;18:1422–1431
176. Selden AC, Hodgson HJ. Growth factors and the liver. Gut 1991;32:601–603
177. Lee GH, Merlino G, Fausto N. Development of liver tumors in transforming growth factor alpha transgenic mice. Cancer Res 1992;52:5162–5170
178. Derynck R, Goeddel DV, Ullrich A et al. Synthesis of messenger RNAs for transforming growth factors alpha and beta and the epidermal growth factor receptor by human tumors. Cancer Res 1987;47:707–712
179. Rosenthal A, Lindquist PB, Bringman TS et al. Expression in rat fibroblasts of a human transforming growth factor-alpha cDNA results in transformation. Cell 1986;46: 301–309
180. Jhappan C, Stahle C, Harkins RN et al. TGF alpha overexpression in transgenic mice induces liver neoplasia and abnormal development of the mammary gland and pancreas. Cell 1990;61:1137–1146
181. Sandgren EP, Luetteke NC, Qiu TH, et al. Transforming growth factor alpha dramatically enhances oncogene-induced carcinogenesis in transgenic mouse pancreas and liver. Mol Cell Biol 1993;13:320–330
182. Takagi H, Sharp R, Hammermeister C et al. Molecular and genetic analysis of liver oncogenesis in transforming growth factor alpha transgenic mice. Cancer Res 1992;52: 5171–5177
183. Sandgren EP, Luetteke NC, Palmiter RD et al. Overexpression of TGF alpha in transgenic mice: induction of epithelial hyperplasia, pancreatic metaplasia, and carcinoma of the breast. Cell 1990;61:1121–1135
184. Hilakivi CL, Dickson RB. Stress influence on development of hepatocellular tumors in transgenic mice overexpressing TGF alpha. Acta Oncol 1995;34:907–912
185. Wu JC, Merlino G, Fausto N. Establishment and characterization of differentiated, nontransformed hepatocyte cell lines derived from mice transgenic for transforming growth factor alpha. Proc Natl Acad Sci U S A 1994;91:674–678
186. Wu JC, Merlino G, Cveklova K et al. Autonomous growth in serum-free medium and production of hepatocellular carcinomas by differentiated hepatocyte lines that overexpress transforming growth factor alpha 1. Cancer Res 1994;54: 5964–5973
187. Yeh YC, Tsai JF, Chuang LY et al. Elevation of transforming growth factor alpha and its relationship to the epidermal growth factor and alpha-fetoprotein levels in patients with hepatocellular carcinoma. Cancer Res 1987;47:896–901
188. Hsia CC, Axiotis CA, Di BA, Tabor E. Transforming growth factor-alpha in human hepatocellular carcinoma and coexpression with hepatitis B surface antigen in adjacent liver. Cancer 1992;70:1049–1056
189. Morimitsu Y, Hsia CC, Kojiro M, Tabor E. Nodules of less-differentiated tumor within or adjacent to hepatocellular carcinoma: relative expression of transforming growth factor-alpha and its receptor in the different areas of tumor. Hum Pathol 1995;26:1126–1132
190. Sporn MB, Roberts AB. Transforming growth factor-beta: recent progress and new challenges. J Cell Biol 1992;119: 1017–1021
191. DuBois RN, Hunter EB, Russell WE. Molecular aspects of hepatic regeneration. In Dang CV, Feldman AM (eds): Molecular Basis of Medicine. Mosby-Year Book, 1994

192. Dennis PA, Rifkin DB. Cellular activation of latent transforming growth factor beta requires binding to the cation-independent mannose 6-phosphate/insulin-like growth factor type II receptor. Proc Natl Acad Sci U S A 1991;88:580–584

193. Kovacina KS, Steele PG, Purchio AF et al. Interactions of recombinant and platelet transforming growth factor-beta 1 precursor with the insulin-like growth factor II/mannose 6-phosphate receptor. Biochem Biophys Res Commun 1989;160:393–403

194. Purchio AF, Cooper JA, Brunner AM et al. Identification of mannose 6-phosphate in two asparagine-linked sugar chains of recombinant transforming growth factor-beta 1 precursor. J Biol Chem 1988;263:14211–14215

195. Kojima S, Nara K, Rifkin DB. Requirement for transglutaminase in the activation of latent transforming growth factor-beta in bovine endothelial cells. J Cell Biol 1993;121:439–448

196. Wang XF, Lin HY, Ng EE et al. Expression cloning and characterization of the TGF-beta type III receptor. Cell 1991;67:797–805

197. Lopez CF, Cheifetz S, Doody J et al. Structure and expression of the membrane proteoglycan betaglycan, a component of the TGF-beta receptor system. Cell 1991;67:785–795

198. Lin HY, Wang XF, Ng EE et al. Expression cloning of the TGF-beta type II receptor, a functional transmembrane serine/threonine kinase [published erratum appears in Cell 1992 Sep 18;70:following 1068]. Cell 1992;68:775–785

199. Bassing CH, Yingling JM, Howe DJ et al. A transforming growth factor beta type I receptor that signals to activate gene expression. Science 1994;263:87–89

200. Lopez CF, Wrana JL, Massague J. Betaglycan presents ligand to the TGF beta signaling receptor. Cell 1993;73:1435–1444

201. Segarini PR. TGF-beta receptors: a complicated system of multiple binding proteins. Biochim Biophys Acta 1993;1155:269–275

202. Fausto N, Mead JE. Regulation of liver growth: protooncogenes and transforming growth factors. Lab Invest 1989;60:4–13

203. Chari RS, Price DT, Sue SR et al. Down-regulation of transforming growth factor beta receptor type I, II and III during liver regeneration. Am J Surg 1995;169:126–131

204. Russell WE, Coffey RJ, Ouellette AJ, Moses HL. Type beta transforming growth factor reversibly inhibits the early proliferative response to partial hepatectomy in the rat. Proc Natl Acad Sci U S A 1988;85:5126–5130

205. Bursch W, Oberhammer F, Jirtle RL et al. Transforming growth factor-beta 1 as a signal for induction of cell death by apoptosis. Br J Cancer 1993;67:531–536

206. Ponchel F, Puisieux A, Tabone E et al. Hepatocarcinoma-specific mutant p53–249ser induces mitotic activity but has no effect on transforming growth factor beta 1-mediated apoptosis. Cancer Res 1994;54:2064–2068

207. Benedetti A, Di SA, Svegliati BG, Jezequel AM. Transforming growth factor beta 1 increases the number of apoptotic bodies and decreases intracellular pH in isolated periportal and perivenular rat hepatocytes. Hepatology 1995;22:1488–1498

208. Wollenberg GK, Semple E, Quinn BA, Hayes MA. Inhibition of proliferation of normal, preneoplastic, and neoplastic rat hepatocytes by transforming growth factor-beta. Cancer Res 1987:6595–6599

209. Carr BI, Hayashi I, Branum EL, Moses HL. Inhibition of DNA synthesis in rat hepatocytes by platelet-derived type beta transforming growth factor. Cancer Res 1986;46:2330–2334

210. Inagaki M, Moustakas A, Lin HY et al. Growth inhibition by transforming growth factor beta (TGF-beta) type I is restored in TGF-beta-resistant hepatoma cells after expression of TGF-beta receptor type II cDNA. Proc Natl Acad Sci U S A 1993;90:5359–5363

211. Bigdeli N, Marshall R, Grabow L, Loh W. Tgf-beta inhibits proliferation of the Hep G2 cell line in vitro with concomitant decreases in erythropoietin and alphafetoprotein production. Proc Annu Meet Am Assoc Cancer Res 1992:A436

212. Nakatsukasa H, Nagy P, Evarts RP et al. Cellular distribution of transforming growth factor-beta 1 and procollagen types I, III, and IV transcripts in carbon tetrachloride-induced rat liver fibrosis. J Clin Invest 1990;85:1833–1843

213. Nagy P, Schaff Z, Lapis K. Immunohistochemical detection of transforming growth factor-beta 1 in fibrotic liver disease. Hepatology 1991;14:269–273

214. Castilla A, Prieto J, Fausto N. Transforming growth factors beta 1 and alpha in chronic liver disease: effects of interferon alfa therapy. N Engl J Med 1991;324:933–940

215. Kim SJ, Kehrl JH, Burton J et al. Transactivation of the transforming growth factor beta 1 (TGF-beta 1) gene by human T lymphotropic virus type 1 tax: a potential mechanism for the increased production of TGF-beta 1 in adult T cell leukemia. J Exp Med 1990;172:121–129

216. Unsal H, Yakicier C, Marcais C et al. Genetic heterogeneity of hepatocellular carcinoma. Proc Natl Acad Sci U S A 1994;91:822–826

217. Shirai Y, Kawata S, Ito N et al. Elevated levels of plasma transforming growth factor-beta in patients with hepatocellular carcinoma. Jpn J Cancer Res 1992;83:676–679

218. Nagy P, Evarts RP, McMahon JB, Thorgeirsson SS. Role of TGF-beta in normal differentiation and oncogenesis in rat liver. Mol Carcinog 1989;2:345–354

219. Reisenbichler H, Chari RS, Boyer IJ, Jirtle RL. Transforming growth factor-beta receptors type I, II and III in phenobarbital-promoted rat liver tumors. Carcinogenesis 1994;15:2763–2767

220. Jirtle RL, Hankins GR, Reisenbichler H, Boyer IJ. Regulation of mannose 6-phosphate/insulin-like growth factor-II receptors and transforming growth factor beta during liver tumor promotion with phenobarbital. Carcinogenesis 1994;15:1473–1478

221. Sue SR, Chari RS, Kong FM et al. Transforming growth factor-beta receptors and mannose 6-phosphate/insulin-like growth factor-II receptor expression in human hepatocellular carcinoma. Ann Surg 1995;222:171–178

222. De SA, Hankins GR, Washington MK et al. Frequent loss

of heterozygosity on 6q at the mannose 6-phosphate/insulin-like growth factor II receptor locus in human hepatocellular tumors. Oncogene 1995;10:1725–1729

223. Fujiwara Y, Ohata H, Kuroki T et al. Frequent loss of heterozygosity on 6q at the mannose 6-phosphate/insulin-like growth factor II receptor locus in human hepatocellular tumors. Oncogene 1995;10:1725–1729

224. De SA, Hankins GR, Washington MK et al. M6P/IGF2R gene is mutated in human hepatocellular carcinomas with loss of heterozygosity. Nat Genet 1995;11:447–449

225. Jirtle RL, Carr BI, Scott CD. Modulation of insulin-like growth factor-II/mannose 6-phosphate receptors and transforming growth factor-beta 1 during liver regeneration [published erratum appears in J Biol Chem 1991 Dec 25; 266(36):24860]. J Biol Chem 1991;266:22444–22450

226. Bedossa P, Peltier E, Terris B et al. Transforming growth factor-beta 1 (TGF-beta 1) and TGF-beta 1 receptors in normal, cirrhotic, and neoplastic human livers. Hepatology 1995;21:760–766

227. Hytiroglou P, Theise ND, Schwartz M et al. Transforming growth factor-beta 1 (TGF-beta 1) and TGF-beta 1 receptors in normal, cirrhotic, and neoplastic human livers. Hepatology 1995;21:760–766

228. Bouzahzah B, Nishikawa Y, Simon D, Carr BI. Growth control and gene expression in a new hepatocellular carcinoma cell line, Hep40: inhibitory actions of vitamin K. J Cell Physiol 1995;165:459–467

229. Zhang X, Wang T, Batist G, Tsao MS. Transforming growth factor beta 1 promotes spontaneous transformation of cultured rat liver epithelial cells. Cancer Res 1994;54: 6122–6128

230. Marshall CJ. Tumor suppressor genes. Cell 1991;64: 313–326

231. Weinberg RA. Tumor suppressor genes. Science 1991;254: 1138–1146

232. Merlo A, Herman JG, Mao L et al. 5′ CpG island methylation is associated with transcriptional silencing of the tumor suppressor p16/CDKN2/MTS1 in human cancers. Nat Med 1995;1:686–692

233. Wales MM, Biel MA, el Deiry W et al. p53 activates expression of HIC-1, a new candidate tumour suppressor gene on 17p13.3. Nat Med 1995;1:570–577

234. Vorce RL, Goodman JL. Altered methylation of ras oncogenes in benzidine-induced B6C3F1 mouse liver tumors. Toxicol Appl Pharmacol 1989;100:398–410

235. Goodman JI, Counts JL. Hypomethylation of DNA: a possible nongenotoxic mechanism underlying the role of cell proliferation in carcinogenesis. Environ Health Perspect 1993;5:169–172

236. Ghoshal AK, Farber E. The induction of liver cancer by dietary deficiency of choline and methionine without added carcinogens. Carcinogenesis 1984;5:1367–1370

237. Mikol YB, Hoover KL, Creasia D, Poirier LA. Hepatocarcinogenesis in rats fed methyl-deficient, amino acid-defined diets. Carcinogenesis 1983;4:1619–1629

238. Pogribny IP, Poirier LA, James SJ. Differential sensitivity to loss of cytosine methyl groups within the hepatic p53 gene of folate/methyl deficient rats. Carcinogenesis 1995; 16:2863–2867

239. Walker GJ, Hayward NK, Falvey S, Cooksley WG. Loss of somatic heterozygosity in hepatocellular carcinoma. Cancer Res 1991;51:4367–4370

240. Nishida N, Fukuda Y, Kokuryu H et al. Accumulation of allelic loss on arms of chromosomes 13q, 16q and 17p in the advanced stages of human hepatocellular carcinoma. Int J Cancer 1992;51:862–868

241. Murakami Y, Hayashi K, Hirohashi S, Sekiya T. Aberrations of the tumor suppressor p53 and retinoblastoma genes in human hepatocellular carcinomas. Cancer Res 1991;51: 5520–5525

242. Tabor E. Tumor suppressor genes, growth factor genes, and oncogenes in hepatitis B virus-associated hepatocellular carcinoma. J Med Virol 1994;42:357–365

243. Nagao T, Kondo F, Sato T et al. Expression of the retinoblastoma gene product in human hepatocellular carcinoma. Hum Pathol 1995;26:366–374

244. Kuroki T, Fujiwara Y, Nakamori S et al. Evidence for the presence of two tumour-suppressor genes for hepatocellular carcinoma on chromosome 13q. Br J Cancer 1995;72: 383–385

245. Kern SE, Pietenpol JA, Thiagalingam S et al. Oncogenic forms of p53 inhibit p53-regulated gene expression. Science 1992;256:827–830

246. Bressac B, Galvin KM, Liang TJ et al. Abnormal structure and expression of p53 gene in human hepatocellular carcinoma. Proc Natl Acad Sci U S A 1990;87:1973–1977

247. Hsu IC, Tokiwa T, Bennett W et al. p53 gene mutation and integrated hepatitis B viral DNA sequences in human liver cancer cell lines. Carcinogenesis 1993;14:987–992

248. Livni N, Eid A, Ilan Y et al. p53 expression in patients with cirrhosis with and without hepatocellular carcinoma. Cancer 1995;75:2420–2426

249. Bressac B, Kew M, Wands J, Ozturk M. Selective G to T mutations of p53 gene in hepatocellular carcinoma from southern Africa. Nature 1991;350:429–431

250. Scorsone KA, Zhou YZ, Butel JS, Slagle BL. p53 mutations cluster at codon 249 in hepatitis B virus-positive hepatocellular carcinomas from China. Cancer Res 1992;52: 1635–1638

251. Li D, Cao Y, He L et al. Aberrations of p53 gene in human hepatocellular carcinoma from China. Carcinogenesis 1993;14:169–173

252. Ozturk M. p53 mutation in hepatocellular carcinoma after aflatoxin exposure. Lancet 1991;338:1356–1359

253. Kar S, Jaffe R, Carr BI. Mutation at codon 249 of p53 gene in a human hepatoblastoma. Hepatology 1993;18:566–569

254. Alpert ME, Hutt MS, Wogan GN, Davidson CS. Association between aflatoxin content of food and hepatoma frequency in Uganda. Cancer 1971;28:253–260

255. Peers FG, Linsell CA. Dietary aflatoxins and liver cancer—a population based study in Kenya. Br J Cancer 1973; 27:473–484

256. Van RS, Cook MP, Van SD et al. Hepatocellular carcinoma and dietary aflatoxin in Mozambique and Transkei. Br J Cancer 1985;51:713–726

257. Yeh FS, Yu MC, Mo CC et al. Hepatitis B virus, aflatoxins,

and hepatocellular carcinoma in southern Guangxi, China. Cancer Res 1989;49:2506–2509

258. Groopman JD, Cain LG, Kensler TW. Aflatoxin exposure in human populations: measurements and relationship to cancer. Crit Rev Toxicol 1988;19:113–145

259. Autrup H, Seremet T, Wakhisi J, Wasunna A. Aflatoxin exposure measured by urinary excretion of aflatoxin B1-guanine adduct and hepatitis B virus infection in areas with different liver cancer incidence in Kenya. Cancer Res 1987; 47:3430–3433

260. Groopman JD, Busby WJ, Wogan GN. Nuclear distribution of aflatoxin B1 and its interaction with histones in rat liver in vivo. Cancer Res 1980;40:4343–4351

261. Groopman JD, Donahue PR, Zhu JQ et al. Aflatoxin metabolism in humans: detection of metabolites and nucleic acid adducts in urine by affinity chromatography. Proc Natl Acad Sci U S A 1985;82:6492–6496

262. Baily EA, Iyer RS, Stone MP et al. Mutational properties of the primary aflatoxin B1-DNA adduct. Proc Natl Acad Sci U S A 1996;93:1535–1539

263. Groopman JD, Zhu JQ, Donahue PR et al. Molecular dosimetry of urinary aflatoxin-DNA adducts in people living in Guangxi Autonomous Region, People's Republic of China. Cancer Res 1992;52:45–52

264. Groopman JD, Roebuck BD, Kensler TW. Molecular dosimetry of aflatoxin DNA adducts in humans and experimental rat models. Prog Clin Biol Res 1992;374:139–155

265. Ross RK, Yuan JM, Yu MC et al. Urinary aflatoxin biomarkers and risk of hepatocellular carcinoma. Lancet 1992;339: 943–946

266. Hsieh LL, Hsu SW, Chen DS, Santella RM. Immunological detection of aflatoxin B1-DNA adducts formed in vivo. Cancer Res 1988;48:6328–6331

267. Zhang YJ, Chen CJ, Lee CS et al. Aflatoxin B1-DNA adducts and hepatitis B virus antigens in hepatocellular carcinoma and non-tumorous liver tissue. Carcinogenesis 1991; 12:2247–2252

268. Eriksson P, Kallin B, van Hoof F et al. Susceptibility to hepatocellular carcinoma is associated with genetic variation in the enzymatic detoxification of aflatoxin B1. Proc Natl Acad Sci U S A 1995;92:2384–2387

269. Soini Y, Cheng CS, Bennett WP et al. An aflatoxin-associated, mutational hotspot in the p53 tumor suppressor gene occurs in hepatocellular carcinomas from Mexico. Proc Annu Meet Am Assoc Cancer Res 1995:A971 (abstr) 1995

270. Patel P, Stephenson J, Scheuer PJ, Francis GE. p53 codon 249ser mutations in hepatocellular carcinoma patients with low aflatoxin exposure. Lancet 1992;339:881

271. Kress S, Jahn UR, Buchmann A et al. p53 Mutations in human hepatocellular carcinomas from Germany. Cancer Res 1992;52:3220–3223

272. Challen C, Lunec J, Warren W et al. Analysis of the p53 tumor-suppressor gene in hepatocellular carcinomas from Britain. Hepatology 1992;16:1362–1366

273. Oda T, Tsuda H, Scarpa A et al. p53 gene mutation spectrum in hepatocellular carcinoma. Cancer Res 1992;52: 6358–6364

274. Nose H, Imazeki F, Ohto M, Omata M. p53 gene mutations and 17p allelic deletions in hepatocellular carcinoma from Japan. Cancer 1993;72:355–360

275. Nishida N, Fukuda Y, Kokurya H et al. Role and mutational heterogeneity of the p53 gene in hepatocellular carcinoma. Cancer Res 1993;53:368–372

276. Hosono S, Chou MJ, Lee CS, Shih C. Infrequent mutation of p53 gene in hepatitis B virus positive primary hepatocellular carcinomas. Oncogene 1993;8:491–496

277. Hollstein MC, Wild CP, Bleicher F et al. p53 mutations and aflatoxin B1 exposure in hepatocellular carcinoma patients from Thailand. Int J Cancer 1993;53:51–55

278. Shi CY, Phang TW, Lin Y et al. Codon 249 mutation of the p53 gene is a rare event in hepatocellular carcinomas from ethnic Chinese in Singapore. Br J Cancer 1995;72: 146–149

279. Hayward NK, Walker GJ, Graham W, Cooksley E. Hepatocellular carcinoma mutation. Nature 1991;352:764

280. Hsieh DP, Atkinson DN. Recent aflatoxin exposure and mutation at codon 249 of the human p53 gene: lack of association. Food Addit Contam 1995;12:421–424

281. Puisieux A, Lim S, Groopman J, Ozturk M. Selective targeting of p53 gene mutational hotspots in human cancers by etiologically defined carcinogens. Cancer Res 1991;51: 6185–6189

282. Aguilar F, Hussain SP, Cerutti P. Aflatoxin B1 induces the transversion of G->T in codon 249 of the p53 tumor suppressor gene in human hepatocytes. Proc Natl Acad Sci U S A 1993;90:8586–8590

283. Hulla JE, Chen ZY, Eaton DL. Aflatoxin B1-induced rat hepatic hyperplastic nodules do not exhibit a site-specific mutation within the p53 gene. Cancer Res 1993;53:9–11

284. Fujimoto Y, Hampton LL, Luo LD et al. Low frequency of p53 gene mutation in tumors induced by aflatoxin B1 in nonhuman primates. Cancer Res 1992;52:1044–1046

285. Imazeki F, Yokosuka O, Ohto M, Omata M. Aflatoxin and p53 abnormality in duck hepatocellular carcinoma. J Gastroenterol Hepatol 1995;10:646–649

286. Dumenco L, Oguey D, Wu J et al. Introduction of a murine p53 mutation corresponding to human codon 249 into a murine hepatocyte cell line results in growth advantage, but not in transformation. Hepatology 1995;22:1279–1288

287. Aguilar F, Harris CC, Sun T et al. Geographic variation of p53 mutational profile in nonmalignant human liver. Science 1994;264:1317–1319

288. Kirby G, Batist G, Fotouhi N et al. Allele-specific PCR amplification of p53 codon 249 GCT transversion in liver with hepatitis from aflatoxin B1-exposed and unexposed individuals. Proc Annu Meet Am Assoc Cancer Res 1995: A657(abstr).

289. Ishikawa F, Takaku F, Ochiai M et al. Activated c-raf gene in a rat hepatocellular carcinoma induced by 2-amino-3-methylimidazo[4,5-f]quinoline. Biochem Biophys Res Commun 1985;132:186–192

290. Fox TR, Schumann AM, Watanabe PG, Yano BL et al. Mutational analysis of the H-ras oncogene in spontaneous C57BL/6 and C3H/He mouse liver tumors and tumors induced with genotoxic and nongenotoxic hepatocarcinogens. Cancer Res 1990;50:4014–4019

291. Fox TR, Watanabe PG. Detection of a cellular oncogene in spontaneous liver tumors of B6C3F1 mice. Science 1985; 228:596–597

292. Reynolds SH, Stowers SJ, Patterson RM et al. Activated oncogenes in B6C3F1 mouse liver tumors: implications for risk assessment. Science 1987;237:1309–1316

293. Reynolds SH, Stowers SJ, Maronpot RR et al. Detection and identification of activated oncogenes in spontaneously occurring benign and malignant hepatocellular tumors of the B6C3F1 mouse. Proc Natl Acad Sci U S A 1986;83: 33–37

294. Chandar N, Lombardi B, Locker J. c-myc gene amplification during hepatocarcinogenesis by a choline- devoid diet. Proc Natl Acad Sci U S A 1989;86:2703–2707

295. Suzuki H, Fujita H, Mullauer L et al. Increased expression of c-jun gene during spontaneous hepatocarcinogenesis in LEC rats. Cancer Lett 1990;53:205–212

296. Buchmann A, Bauer HR, Mahr J et al. Mutational activation of the c-Ha-ras gene in liver tumors of different rodent strains: correlation with susceptibility to hepatocarcinogenesis. Proc Natl Acad Sci U S A 1991;88:911–915

297. Dragani TA, Manenti G, Colombo BM et al. Incidence of mutations at codon 61 of the Ha-ras gene in liver tumors of mice genetically susceptible and resistant to hepatocarcinogenesis. Oncogene 1991;6:333–338

298. Pitot HC. Proto-oncogene activation in multistage murine hepatocarcinogenesis. Prog Clin Biol Res 1990;331: 311–324

299. Sinha S, Webber C, Marshall CJ et al. Activation of ras oncogene in aflatoxin-induced rat liver carcinogenesis. Proc Natl Acad Sci U S A 1988;85:3673–3677

300. McMahon G, Davis EF, Huber LJ et al. Characterization of c-Ki-ras and N-ras oncogenes in aflatoxin B1-induced rat liver tumors. Proc Natl Acad Sci U S A 1990;87: 1104–1108

301. Soman NR, Wogan GN. Activation of the c-Ki-ras oncogene in aflatoxin B1-induced hepatocellular carcinoma and adenoma in the rat: detection by denaturing gradient gel electrophoresis. Proc Natl Acad Sci U S A 1993;90: 2045–2049

302. Huber BE, Thorgeirsson SS. Analysis of c-myc expression in a human hepatoma cell line. Cancer Res 1987;47: 3414–3420

303. Richards CA, Short SA, Thorgeirsson SS, Huber BE. Characterization of a transforming N-ras gene in the human hepatoma cell line Hep G2: additional evidence for the importance of c-myc and ras cooperation in hepatocarcinogenesis. Cancer Res 1990;50:1521–1527

304. Lee HS, Rajagopalan MS, Vyas GN. A lack of direct role of hepatitis B virus in the activation of ras and c-myc oncogenes in human hepatocellular carcinogenesis. Hepatology 1988;8:1116–1120

305. Takada S, Koike K. Activated N-ras gene was found in human hepatoma tissue but only in a small fraction of the tumor cells. Oncogene 1989;4:189–193

306. Tsuda H, Hirohashi S, Shimosato Y et al. Low incidence of point mutation of c-Ki-ras and N-ras oncogenes in human hepatocellular carcinoma. Jpn J Cancer Res 1989;80: 196–199

307. Tada M, Omata M, Ohto M. Analysis of ras gene mutations in human hepatic malignant tumors by polymerase chain reaction and direct sequencing. Cancer Res 1990;50: 1121–1124

308 Ogata N, Kamimura T, Asakura H. Point mutation, allelic loss and increased methylation of c-Ha-ras gene in human hepatocellular carcinoma. Hepatology 1991;13:31–37

309. Collier JD, Guo K, Mathew J et al. c-erbB-2 oncogene expression in hepatocellular carcinoma and cholangiocarcinoma. J Hepatol 1992;14:377–380

310. Pasquinelli C, Bhavani K, Chisari FV. Multiple oncogenes and tumor suppressor genes are structurally and functionally intact during hepatocarcinogenesis in hepatitis B virus transgenic mice. Cancer Res 1992;52:2823–2829

311. Bréchot C, Pourcel C, Louise A et al. Presence of integrated hepatitis B virus DNA sequences in cellular DNA of human hepatocellular carcinoma. Nature 1980;286:533–535

312. Chakraborty PR, Ruiz ON, Shouval D, Shafritz DA. Identification of integrated hepatitis B virus DNA and expression of viral RNA in an HBsAg-producing human hepatocellular carcinoma cell line. Nature 1980;286:531–533

313. Edman JC, Gray P, Valenzuela P et al. Integration of hepatitis B virus sequences and their expression in a human hepatoma cell. Nature 1980;286:535–538

314. Marion PL, Salazar FH, Alexander JJ, Robinson WS. State of hepatitis B viral DNA in a human hepatoma cell line. J Virol 1980;33:795–806

315. Chen JY, Harrison TJ, Tsuei DJ et al. Analysis of integrated hepatitis B virus DNA and flanking cellular sequences in the hepatocellular carcinoma cell line HCC36. Intervirology 1994;37:41–46

316. Park JG, Lee JH, Kang MS et al. Characterization of cell lines established from human hepatocellular carcinoma. Int J Cancer 1995;62:276–282

317. Shih C, Burke K, Chou MJ et al. Tight clustering of human hepatitis B virus integration sites in hepatomas near a triple-stranded region. J Virol 1987;61:3491–3498

318. Bréchot C, Hadchouel M, Scotto J et al. State of hepatitis B virus DNA in hepatocytes of patients with hepatitis B surface antigen-positive and -negative liver diseases. Proc Natl Acad Sci U S A 1981;78:3906–3910

319. Koshy R, Maupas P, Muller R, Hofschneider PH. Detection of hepatitis B virus-specific DNA in the genomes of human hepatocellular carcinoma and liver cirrhosis tissues. J Gen Virol 1981;57:95–102

320. Shafritz DA, Kew MC. Identification of integrated hepatitis B virus DNA sequences in human hepatocellular carcinomas. Hepatology 1981;1:1–8

321. Dejean A, Bréchot C, Tiollais P, Wain HS. Characterization of integrated hepatitis B viral DNA cloned from a human hepatoma and the hepatoma-derived cell line PLC/PRF/5. Proc Natl Acad Sci U S A 1983;80:2505–2509

322. Hino O, Kitagawa T, Sugano H. Relationship between serum and histochemical markers for hepatitis B virus and rate of viral integration in hepatocellular carcinomas in Japan. Int J Cancer 1985;35:5–10

323. Miller RH, Lee SC, Liaw YF, Robinson WS. Hepatitis B viral DNA in infected human liver and in hepatocellular carcinoma. J Infect Dis 1985;151:1081–1092

324. Imazeki F, Omata M, Yokosuka O, Okuda K. Integration of hepatitis B virus DNA in hepatocellular carcinoma. Cancer 1986;58:1055–1060

325. Matsubara K, Tokino T. Integration of hepatitis B virus DNA and its implications for hepatocarcinogenesis. Mol Biol Med 1990;7:243–260

326. Koch S, Freytag, von Loringhaven A et al. The genetic organization of integrated hepatitis B virus DNA in the human hepatoma cell line PLC/PRF/5. Nucleic Acids Res 1984;12:6871–6886

327. Shaul Y, Ziemer M, Garcia PD et al. Cloning and analysis of integrated hepatitis virus sequences from a human hepatoma cell line. J Virol 1984;51:776–787

328. Ziemer M, Garcia P, Shaul Y, Rutter WJ. Sequence of hepatitis B virus DNA incorporated into the genome of a human hepatoma cell line. J Virol 1985;53:885–892

329. Esumi M, Aritaka T, Arii M et al. Clonal origin of human hepatoma determined by integration of hepatitis B virus DNA. Cancer Res 1986;46:5767–5771

330. Blum HE, Offensperger WB, Walter E et al. Hepatocellular carcinoma and hepatitis B virus infection: molecular evidence for monoclonal origin and expansion of malignantly transformed hepatocytes. J Cancer Res Clin Oncol 1987; 113:466–472

331. Esumi M, Tanaka Y, Tozuka S, Shikata T. Clonal state of human hepatocellular carcinoma and non-tumorous hepatocytes. Cancer Chemother Pharmacol 1989;23:S1–3

332. Aoki N, Robinson WS. State of hepatitis B viral genomes in cirrhotic and hepatocellular carcinoma nodules. Mol Biol Med 1989;6:395–408

333. Hsu HC, Chiou TJ, Chen JY et al. Clonality and clonal evolution of hepatocellular carcinoma with multiple nodules. Hepatology 1991;13:923–928

334. Chen PJ, Chen DS, Lai MY et al. Clonal origin of recurrent hepatocellular carcinomas. Gastroenterology 1989: 527–529

335. Lugassy C, Bernuau J, Thiers V et al. Sequences of hepatitis B virus DNA in the serum and liver of patients with acute benign and fulminant hepatitis. J Infect Dis 1987;155: 64–71

336. Scotto J, Hadchouel M, Hery C et al. Hepatitis B virus DNA in children's liver diseases: detection by blot hybridisation in liver and serum. Gut 1983;24:618–624

337. Ochiya T, Tsurimoto T, Ueda K et al. An in vitro system for infection with hepatitis B virus that uses primary human fetal hepatocytes. Proc Natl Acad Sci U S A 1989;86: 1875–1879

338. Okubo K, Nakamura T, Tokino T, Matsubara K. Different type of hepatitis B virus (HBV) DNA integrants that may reflect the integration process. Gastroenterol Jpn 1990;2: 23–30

339. Shafritz DA, Shouval D, Sherman HI et al. Integration of hepatitis B virus DNA into the genome of liver cells in chronic liver disease and hepatocellular carcinoma. Studies in percutaneous liver biopsies and post-mortem tissue specimens. N Engl J Med 1981;305:1067–1073

340. Yaginuma K, Kobayashi H, Kobayashi M, Morishima T, et al. Multiple integration site of hepatitis B virus DNA in hepatocellular carcinoma and chronic active hepatitis tissues from children. J Virol 1987;61:1808–1813

341. Takada S, Gotoh Y, Hayashi S et al. Structural rearrangement of integrated hepatitis B virus DNA as well as cellular flanking DNA is present in chronically infected hepatic tissues. J Virol 1990;64:822–828

342. Lai MY, Chen DS, Chen PJ et al. Status of hepatitis B virus DNA in hepatocellular carcinoma: a study based on paired tumor and nontumor liver tissues. J Med Virol 1988;25: 249–258

343. Hadziyannis SJ, Liberman HM, Karvountzis GG, Shafritz DA. Analysis of liver disease, nuclear HBcAg, viral replication, and hepatitis B virus DNA in liver and serum of HBeAg vs. anti-HBe positive carriers of hepatitis B virus. Hepatology 1983;3:656–662

344. Dejean A, Sonigo P, Wain HS, Tiollais P. Specific hepatitis B virus integration in hepatocellular carcinoma DNA through a viral 11-base-pair direct repeat. Proc Natl Acad Sci U S A 1984;81:5350–5354

345. Nakamura T, Tokino T, Nagaya T, Matsubara K. Microdeletion associated with the integration process of hepatitis B virus DNA. Nucleic Acids Res 1988;16:4865–4873

346. Hino O, Ohtake K, Rogler CE. Features of two hepatitis B virus (HBV) DNA integrations suggest mechanisms of HBV integration. J Virol 1989;63:2638–2643

347. Tokino T, Matsubara K. Chromosomal sites for hepatitis B virus integration in human hepatocellular carcinoma. J Virol 1991;65:6761–6764

348. Nagaya T, Nakamura T, Tokino T et al. The mode of hepatitis B virus DNA integration in chromosomes of human hepatocellular carcinoma. Genes Dev 1987;1:773–782

349. Schluter V, Meyer M, Hofschneider PH et al. Integrated hepatitis B virus X and 3′ truncated preS/S sequences derived from human hepatomas encode functionally active transactivators. Oncogene 1994;9:3335–3344

350. Nagasue N, Dhar DK, Makino Y et al. Transactivation of cellular gene expression by hepatitis B viral proteins: a possible molecular mechanism of hepatocarcinogenesis. J Hepatol 1995;23:34–37

351. Zhou YZ, Slagle BL, Donehower LA et al. Structural analysis of a hepatitis B virus genome integrated into chromosome 17p of a human hepatocellular carcinoma. J Virol 1988;62:4224–4231

352. Mizusawa H, Taira M, Yaginuma K et al. Inversely repeating integrated hepatitis B virus DNA and cellular flanking sequences in the human hepatoma-derived cell line huSP. Proc Natl Acad Sci U S A 1985;82:208–212

353. Yaginuma K, Kobayashi M, Yoshida E, Koike K. Hepatitis B virus integration in hepatocellular carcinoma DNA: duplication of cellular flanking sequences at the integration site. Proc Natl Acad Sci U S A 1985;82:4458–4462

354. Ogata N, Tokino T, Kamimura T, Asakura H. A comparison of the molecular structure of integrated hepatitis B virus genomes in hepatocellular carcinoma cells and hepatocytes derived from the same patient. Hepatology 1990;11: 1017–1023

355. Hino O, Shows TB, Rogler CE. Hepatitis B virus integration site in hepatocellular carcinoma at chromosome 17;

18 translocation. Proc Natl Acad Sci U S A 1986;83: 8338–8342
356. Meyer M, Wiedorn KH, Hofschneider PH et al. A chromosome 17:7 translocation is associated with a hepatitis B virus DNA integration in human hepatocellular carcinoma DNA. Hepatology 1992;15:665–671
356a. Rogler CE, Sherman M, Su CY et al. Deletion in chromosome 11p associated with a hepatitis B integration site in hepatocellular carcinoma. Science 1992;230:319–322
357. Solomon E, Borrow J, Goddard AD. Chromosome aberrations and cancer. Science 1991;254:1153–1160
358. Hatada I, Tokino T, Ochiya T, Matsubara K. Co-amplification of integrated hepatitis B virus DNA and transforming gene hst-1 in a hepatocellular carcinoma. Oncogene 1988; 3:537–540
359. Buendia MA. Hepatitis B viruses and hepatocellular carcinoma. Adv Cancer Res 1992;59:167–226
360. Hino O, Tabata S, Hotta Y. Evidence for increased in vitro recombination with insertion of human hepatitis B virus DNA. Proc Natl Acad Sci U S A 1991;88:9248–9252
361. Pasquinelli C, Garreau F, Bougueleret L et al. Rearrangement of a common cellular DNA domain on chromosome 4 in human primary liver tumors. J Virol 1988;62:629–632
362. Simon D, Searls DB, Cao Y et al. Chromosomal site of hepatitis B virus (HBV) integration in a human hepatocellular carcinoma-derived cell line. Cytogenet Cell Genet 1985;39:116–120
363. Richards RI, Sutherland GR. Heritable unstable DNA sequences. Nat Genet 1992;1:7–9
364. Simon D, Knowles BB. Hepatocellular carcinoma cell line and peripheral blood lymphocytes from the same patient contain common chromosomal alterations. Lab Invest 1986;55:657–665
365. Chatterjee B, Ghosh PK. Constitutive heterochromatin polymorphism and chromosome damage in viral hepatitis. Mutat Res 1989;210:49–57
366. Simon D, London WT, Knowles BB. Supernumerary marker chromosomes in peripheral blood cells of hepatitis B virus chronic carriers. Hum Genet 1993;92:457–460
367. Simon D, London T, Hann HW, Knowles BB. Chromosome abnormalities in peripheral blood cells of hepatitis B virus chronic carriers. Cancer Res 1991;51:6176–6179
368. Simon D, Carr BI. Integration of hepatitis B virus and alteration of the 1p36 region found in cancerous tissue of primary hepatocellular carcinoma with viral replication evidenced only in noncancerous, cirrhotic tissue. Hepatology 1995;22:1393–1398
369. Berger I, Shaul Y. Integration of hepatitis B virus: analysis of unoccupied sites. J Virol 1987;61:1180–1186
370. Shaul Y, Garcia PD, Schonberg S, Rutter WJ. Integration of hepatitis B virus DNA in chromosome-specific satellite sequences. J Virol 1986;59:731–734
371. Gusella JF. Elastic DNA elements—boon or blight? N Engl J Med 1993;329:571–572
372. Dejean A, Bougueleret L, Grzeschik KH, Tiollais P. Hepatitis B virus DNA integration in a sequence homologous to v-erb-A and steroid receptor genes in a hepatocellular carcinoma. Nature 1986;322:70–72
373. de The H, Marchio A, Tiollais P, Dejean A. A novel steroid thyroid hormone receptor-related gene inappropriately expressed in human hepatocellular carcinoma. Nature 1987; 330:667–670
374. Brand N, Petkovich M, Krust A et al. Identification of a second human rectinoic acid receptor. Nature 1988;332: 850–853
375. Dejean A, de TH. Hepatitis B virus as an insertional mutagen in a human hepatocellular carcinoma. Mol Biol Med 1990;7:213–222
376. Wang J, Zindy F, Chenivesse X et al. Modification of cyclin A expression by hepatitis B virus DNA integration in a hepatocellular carcinoma. Oncogene 1992;7:1653–1656
377. Zhang XK, Egan JO, Huang D et al. Hepatitis B virus DNA integration and expression of an erb B-like gene in human hepatocellular carcinoma. Biochem Biophys Res Commun 1992;188:344–351
378. Graef E, Caselmann WH, Wells J, Koshy R. Insertional activation of mevalonate kinase by hepatitis B virus DNA in a human hepatoma cell line. Oncogene 1994;9:81–87
379. Treinin M, Laub O. Identification of a promoter element located upstream from the hepatitis B virus X gene. Mol Cell Biol 1987;7:545–548
380. Blum HE, Zhang ZS, Galun E et al. Hepatitis B virus X protein is not central to the viral life cycle in vitro. J Virol 1992;66:1223–1227
381. Chen HS, Kaneko S, Girones R et al. The woodchuck hepatitis virus X gene is important for establishment of virus infection in woodchucks. J Virol 1993;67:1218–1226
382. Zoulim F, Saputelli J, Seeger C. Woodchuck hepatitis virus X protein is required for viral infection in vivo. J Virol 1994;68:2026–2030
383. Twu JS, Schloemer RH. Transcriptional trans-activating function of hepatitis B virus. J Virol 1987;61:3448–3453
384. Spandau DF, Lee CH. Trans-activation of viral enhancers by the hepatitis B virus X protein. J Virol 1988;62:427–434
385. Zahm P, Hofschneider PH, Koshy R. The HBV X-ORF encodes a transactivator: a potential factor in viral hepatocarcinogenesis. Oncogene 1988;3:169–177
386. Colgrove R, Simon G, Ganem D. Transcriptional activation of homologous and heterologous genes by the hepatitis B virus X gene product in cells permissive for viral replication. J Virol 1989;63:4019–4026
387. Ogston CW, Jonak GJ, Rogler CE et al. Cloning and structural analysis of integrated woodchuck hepatitis virus sequences from hepatocellular carcinomas of woodchucks. Cell 1982;29:385–394
388. Tsuei DJ, Hsu TY, Chen JY et al. Analysis of integrated hepatitis B virus DNA and flanking cellular sequences in a childhood hepatocellular carcinoma. J Med Virol 1994; 42:287–293
389. Wollersheim M, Debelka U, Hofschneider PH. A transactivating function encoded in the hepatitis B virus X gene is conserved in the integrated state. Oncogene 1988;3: 545–552
390. Yamamoto S, Nakatake H, Kawamoto S et al. Transactivation of cellular promoters by an integrated hepatitis B virus DNA. Biochem Biophys Res Commun 1993;192:111–118
391. Takada S, Kido H, Fukutomi A et al. Interaction of hepatitis B virus X protein with a serine protease, tryptase TL2 as an inhibitor. Oncogene 1994;9:341–348

392. Balsano C, Avantaggiati ML, Natoli G et al. Full-length and truncated versions of the hepatitis B virus (HBV) X protein (pX) transactivate the c-myc protooncogene at the transcriptional level. Biochem Biophys Res Commun 1991; 176:985–992
393. Seto E, Mitchell PJ, Yen TS. Transactivation by the hepatitis B virus X protein depends on AP-2 and other transcription factors. Nature 1990;344:72–74
394. Unger T, Shaul Y. The X protein of the hepatitis B virus acts as a transcription factor when targeted to its responsive element. EMBO J 1990;9:1889–1895
395. Maguire HF, Hoeffler JP, Siddiqui A. HBV X protein alters the DNA binding specificity of CREB and ATF-2 by protein-protein interactions. Science 1991;252:842–844
396. Qadri I, Maguire HF, Siddiqui A. Hepatitis B virus transactivator protein X interacts with the TATA-binding protein. Proc Natl Acad Sci U S A 1995;92:1003–1007
397. Wang HD, Yuh CH, Dang CV, Johnson DL. The hepatitis B virus X protein increases the cellular level of TATA-binding protein, which mediates transactivation of RNA polymerase III genes. Mol Cell Biol 1995;15:6720–6728
398. Cheong JH, Yi M, Lin Y, Murakami S. Human RPB5, a subunit shared by eukaryotic nuclear RNA polymerases, binds human hepatitis B virus X protein and may play a role in X transactivation. EMBO J 1995;14:143–150
399. Siddiqui A, Gaynor R, Srinivasan A et al. Trans-activation of viral enhancers including long terminal repeat of the human immunodeficiency virus by the hepatitis B virus X protein. Virology 1989;169:479–484
400. Avantaggiati ML, Natoli G, Balsano C et al. The hepatitis B virus (HBV) pX transactivates the c-fos promoter through multiple cis-acting elements. Oncogene 1993;8:1567–1574
401. Aufiero B, Schneider RJ. The hepatitis B virus X-gene product trans-activates both RNA polymerase II and III promoters. EMBO J 1990;9:497–504
402. Cross JC, Wen P, Rutter WJ. Transactivation by hepatitis B virus X protein is promiscuous and dependent on mitogen-activated cellular serine/threonine kinases. Proc Natl Acad Sci U S A 1993;90:8078–8082
403. Lucito R, Schneider RJ. Hepatitis B virus X protein activates transcription factor NF-kappa B without a requirement for protein kinase C. J Virol 1992;66:983–991
404. Kekulé AS, Lauer U, Weiss L et al. Hepatitis B virus transactivator HBx uses a tumour promoter signalling pathway. Nature 1993;361:742–745
405. Natoli G, Avantaggiati ML, Chirillo P et al. Induction of the DNA-binding activity of c-jun/c-fos heterodimers by the hepatitis B virus transactivator pX. Mol Cell Biol 1994; 14:989–998
406. Natoli G, Avantaggiati ML, Chirillo P et al. Ras- and Raf-dependent activation of c-jun transcriptional activity by the hepatitis B virus transactivator pX. Oncogene 1994;9: 2837–2843
407. Doria M, Klein N, Lucito R, Schneider RJ. The hepatitis B virus HBx protien is a dual specificity cytoplasmic activator of Ras and nuclear activator of transcription factors. EMBO J 1995;14:4747–4757
408. Benn J, Schneider RJ. Hepatitis B virus HBx protein activates Ras-GTP complex formation and establishes a Ras, Raf, MAP kinase signaling cascade. Proc Natl Acad Sci U S A 1994;91:10350–10354
409. Chirillo P, Falco M, Puri PL et al. Hepatitis B virus pX activates NF-kappa B-dependent transcription through a Raf-independent pathway. J Virol 1996;70:641–646
410. Huang J, Kwong J, Sun EC, Liang TJ. Proteasome complex as a potential cellular target of hepatitis B virus X protein. J Virol 1996;70:5582–5591
411. Lee T, Elledge S, Butel J. Hepatitis B virus X protein interacts with a probable cellular DNA repair protein. J Virol 1995;69:1107–1114
412. Melegari M, Scaglioni P, Wands JR. Molecular identification and characterization of XIP as a hepatitis B x protein (HBx) interactor that downregulates HBV replication. Hepatology 1996;24:A1125
413. Truant R, Antunovic J, Greenblatt J et al. Direct interaction of the hepatitis B virus HBx protein with p53 leads to inhibition by HBx of p53 response element-directed transactivation. J Virol 1995;69:1851–1859
414. Wang XW, Forrester K, Yeh H et al. Hepatitis B virus X protein inhibits p53 sequence-specific DNA binding, transcriptional activity, and association with transcription factor ERCC3. Proc Natl Acad Sci U S A 1994;91:2230–2234
415. Feitelson MA, Zhu M, Duan LX, London WT. Hepatitis B x antigen and p53 are associated in vitro and in liver tissues from patients with primary hepatocellular carcinoma. Oncogene 1993;8:1109–1117
416. Takada S, Tsuchida N, Kobayashi M, Koike K. Disruption of the function of tumor-suppressor gene p53 by the hepatitis B virus X protein and hepatocarcinogenesis. J Cancer Res Clin Oncol 1995;121:593–601
417. Puisieux A, Ji J, Guillot C et al. p53-mediated cellular response to DNA damage in cells with replicative hepatitis B virus. Proc Natl Acad Sci U S A 1995;92:1342–1346
418. Ueda H, Ullrich SJ, Gangemi JD et al. Functional inactivation but not structural mutation of p53 causes liver cancer. Nat Genet 1995;9:41–47
419. Yoo YD, Ueda H, Park K et al. Regulation of transforming growth factor-beta 1 expression by the hepatitis B virus (HBV) X transactivator. Role in HBV pathogenesis. J Clin Invest 1996;97:388–395
420. Cao XM, Koski RA, Gashler A et al. Identification and characterization of the Egr-1 gene product, a DNA-binding zinc finger protein induced by differentiation and growth signals. Mol Cell Biol 1990;10:1931–1939
421. Milbrandt J. A nerve growth factor-induced gene encodes a possible transcriptional regulatory factor. Science 1987; 238:797–799
422. Sukhatme VP. Early transcriptional events in cell growth: the Egr family. J Am Soc Nephrol 1990;1:859–866
423. Hohne M, Schaefer S, Seifer M et al. Malignant transformation of immortalized transgenic hepatocytes after transfection with hepatitis B virus DNA. EMBO J 1990;9: 1137–1145
424. Shirakata Y, Kawada M, Fujiki Y et al. The X gene of hepatitis B virus induced growth stimulation and tumorigenic transformation of mouse NIH3T3 cells. Jpn J Cancer Res 1989;80:617–621

425. Seifer M, Hohne M, Schaefer S, Gerlich WH. In vitro tumorigenicity of hepatitis B virus DNA and HBx protein. J Hepatol 1991;13:S61–65

426. Tuttleman JS, Pugh JC, Summers JW. In vitro experimental infection of primary duck hepatocyte cultures with duck hepatitis B virus. J Virol 1986;58:17–25

427. Caselmann WH, Meyer M, Kekule AS et al. A trans-activator function is generated by integration of hepatitis B virus preS/S sequences in human hepatocellular carcinoma DNA. Proc Natl Acad Sci U S A 1990;87:2970–2974

428. Kekulé AS, Lauer U, Meyer M et al. The preS2/S region of integrated hepatitis B virus DNA encodes a transcriptional transactivator. Nature 1990;343:457–461

429. Lauer U, Weiss L, Hofschneider PH, Kekulé AS. The hepatitis B virus pre-S/S(t) transactivator is generated by 3′ truncations within a defined region of the S gene. J Virol 1992; 66:5284–5289

430. Tanaka S, Takenaka K, Matsumata T et al. Hepatitis C virus replication is associated with expression of transforming growth factor-alpha and insulin-like growth factor-II in cirrhotic livers. Dig Dis Sci 1996;41:208–215

431. Okino ST, Whitlock JJ. HCV-associated liver cancer without cirrhosis. Lancet 1995;345:413–415

432. Sakamuro D, Furukawa T, Takegami T. Hepatitis C virus nonstructural protein NS3 transforms NIH 3T3 cells. J Virol 1995;69:3893–3896

433. Ray RB, Lagging LM, Meyer K, Ray R. Hepatitis C virus core protein cooperates with ras and transforms primary rat embryo fibroblasts to tumorigenic phenotype. J Virol 1995; 70:4438–4443

434. Kiyosawa K, Sodeyama T, Tanaka E et al. Interrelationship of blood transfusion, non-A, non-B hepatitis and hepatocellular carcinoma: analysis by detection of antibody to hepatitis C virus. Hepatology 1990:671–675

435. Takano S, Yokosuka O, Imazeki F et al. Incidence of hepatocellular carcinoma in chronic hepatitis B and C: a prospective study of 251 patients. Hepatology 1995;21: 650–655

436. Simonetti RG, Camma C, Fiorello F et al. Hepatitis C virus infection as a risk factor for hepatocellular carcinoma in patients with cirrhosis. A case-control study. Ann Intern Med 1992;116:97–102

437. Kaklamani E, Trichopoulos D, Tzonou A et al. Hepatitis B and C viruses and their interaction in the origin of hepatocellular carcinoma. JAMA 1991;265:1974–1976

438. Benvegnu L, Fattovich G, Noventa F et al. Concurrent hepatitis B and C virus infection and risk of hepatocellular carcinoma in cirrhosis. A prospective study. Cancer 1994; 74:2442–2448

439. Paterlini P, Driss F, Nalpas B et al. Persistence of hepatitis B and hepatitis C viral genomes in primary liver cancers from HBsAg-negative patients: a study of a low-endemic area. Hepatology 1993;17:20–29

440. Sheu JC, Huang GT, Shih LN et al. Hepatitis C and B viruses in hepatitis B surface antigen-negative hepatocellular carcinoma. Gastroenterology 1992;103:1322–1327

441. Diamantis ID, McGandy CE, Chen TJ et al. Detection of hepatitis B and C viruses in liver tissue with hepatocellular carcinoma. J Hepatol 1994;20:405–409

442. Shiratori Y, Shiina S, Imamura M et al. Characteristic difference of hepatocellular carcinoma between hepatitis B- and C-viral infection in Japan. Hepatology 1995: 1027–1033

443. Ryder SD, Koskinas J, Rizzi PM et al. Hepatocellular carcinoma complicating autoimmune hepatitis: role of hepatitis C virus. Hepatology 1995;22:718–722

444. Tuyns AJ. Alcohol and cancer. Proc Nutr Soc 1990;49: 145–151

445. Rothman KJ. The proportion of cancer attributable to alcohol consumption. Prev Med 1980;9:174–179

446. Yu MC, Mack T, Hanisch R et al. Hepatitis, alcohol consumption, cigarette smoking, and hepatocellular carcinoma in Los Angeles. Cancer Res 1983;43:6077–6079

447. Prior P. Long-term cancer risk in alcoholism. Alcohol 1988; 23:163–171

448. Lieber CS, Garro A Leo MA MAK KM et al. Alcohol and cancer. Hepatology 1986;6:1005–1019

449. Dourdourekas D, Villa F, Szanto PB, Steigmann F. Hepatocellular carcinoma: relation to alcohol, HB-antigen and alpha-fetoprotein. Am J Gastroenterol 1975;63:307–311

450. Driver HE, Swann PF. Alcohol and human cancer. Anticancer Res 1987;7:309–320

451. Takada A, Nei J, Takase S, Matsuda Y. Effects of ethanol on experimental hepatocarcinogenesis. Hepatology 1986; 6:65–72

452. Břechot C, Nalpas B, Couroućе Am et al. Evidence that hepatitis B virus has a role in liver-cell carcinoma in alcoholic liver disease. N Engl J Med 1982;306:1384–1387

453. Ohnishi K, Iida S, Iwama S et al. The effect of chronic habitual alcohol intake on the development of liver cirrhosis and hepatocellular carcinoma: relation to hepatitis B surface antigen carriage. Cancer 1982;49:672–677

454. Rubin E, Lieber CS. Early fine structural changes in the human liver induced by alcohol. Gastroenterology 1967; 52:1–13

455. Maher JJ. Hepatic fibrosis caused by alcohol. Semin Liver Dis 1990;10:66–74

456. Lane BP, Lieber CS. Ultrastructural alterations in human hepatocytes following ingestion of ethanol with adequate diets. Am J Pathol 1966;49:593–603

457. Baraona E, Leo MA, Borowsky SA, Lieber CS. Alcoholic hepatomegaly: accumulation of protein in the liver. Science 1975;190:794–795

458. Baraona E, Pikkarainen P, Salaspuro M et al. Acute effects of ethanol on hepatic protein synthesis and secretion in the rat. Gastroenterology 1980;79:104–111

459. Smith PG, Tee LB, Yeoh GC. Appearance of oval cells in the liver of rats after long-term exposure to ethanol. Hepatology 1996;23:145–154

460. von Weizsacker F, Maedi E, Brown NV et al. Hepatitis B and C virus infection in HBsAg-negative alcoholics without IV drug abuse or previous blood transfusions. Int Hepatol Commun 1995;4:80–87

7

THE ROLE OF TUMOR SUPPRESSOR GENES IN THE DEVELOPMENT OF HEPATOCELLULAR CARCINOMA

EDWARD TABOR

Hepatocellular carcinoma (HCC), one of the most common human cancers, is closely associated with infections by either the hepatitis B virus (HBV) or the hepatitis C virus (HCV). The mechanisms by which these viruses contribute to the etiology of HCC are only beginning to be understood. Tumor suppressor genes, which normally help prevent cancers from developing, are often unable to function normally in HCC; the possible roles of hepatitis B and C viruses in causing mutations in or interfering with the function of these genes are now being studied.

HBV-infected HCC patients have integrated HBV-DNA in their HCC cells. In general, HBV integrations appear to occur at random[1,2] and do not occur at sites that would be meaningful for carcinogenesis. Integration at sites near genes controlling cell growth has only occasionally been reported.[3,4] The integrated virus may cause multiple genetic changes, or the first in a cascade of successive genetic changes leading to HCC.

In the absence of a consistent integration site, HBV could affect growth-controlling genes at a distant site by transactivation. At least two transactivating proteins of HBV have been identified. The X protein, which has been shown to be able to transactivate retroviral long terminal repeats, can increase the rate of transcription of the oncogenes c-*fos* and c-*myc* by transactivation in vitro.[5] The protein product of a truncated sequence of the preS2/S region of HBV also has been shown to be capable of transactivating the c-*myc* promoter in vitro.[6] The possible role of transactivation by the X protein in hepatocarcinogenesis is supported by reports that mice transgenic for the X gene develop HCC in 90% of males.[7]

In HCC patients infected by HCV, the mechanisms by which HCV could contribute to carcinogenesis remain unclear because HCV is a nonintegrating virus.[8,9] Most HCV-associated cases of HCC have active HCV infections; 70% to 94% of anti-HCV-positive HCC patients have HCV-RNA in their sera.[9,10] HCV-RNA can be detected from most such cases in both HCC and nontumorous liver, or only in the nontumorous liver tissues.[8,11,12] Intact HCV cores can suppress the expression of a variety of cellular genes under experimental conditions;[13] based on these observations, it has been suggested that HCV could interfere with cellular functions by binding to cellular mRNAs.[13]

The inflammation and cirrhosis caused by HCV could function as a "promoter" in the development of HCC. Cirrhosis usually can be found in over 80% of anti-HCV-positive (HBsAg-negative) HCC patients,[14] and HCC develops in 75% of patients with HCV-associated cirrhosis by 15 years after first coming to medical attention for their cirrhosis.[15]

Loss of function of DNA mismatch repair genes also could lead to mutations in tumor suppressor genes. Expansion of a premalignant clone of cells could theoretically select for a p53 mutation. Mismatch repair gene defects, indicated by loss of heterozygosity (LOH) in genomic microsatellites, have been reported in 10/46 (22%) HCCs, as well as in nontumorous liver tissue adjacent to five of the HCCs.[16] In another study, LOH in microsatellites was reported in 30/92 (33%) HCCs.[17] In neither study was the prevalence of HBV or HCV reported.

p53 TUMOR SUPPRESSOR GENE

The p53 tumor suppressor gene is the gene most commonly mutated in human cancers. It is located within a 16-20 kb segment of chromosome 17. The product of this gene, the p53 protein, is a 53 kD phosphorylated 393-amino acid protein that is normally found in the nucleus in its unmutated wild-type form. Wild-type p53 protein regulates cell growth and suppresses tumor formation through two distinct pathways: p53 can initiate the arrest of mitosis at any of several checkpoints, or it can initiate apoptosis (programmed cell death) (Fig. 7-1). These events are mediated by intermediate proteins induced by p53 (Fig. 7-1). Mutations in p53 can interfere with this regulatory control; when HCC and hepatoblastoma cell lines are exposed to genotoxic agents, including UV light, ionizing radiation, and doxyrubicin, cell lines with wild-type p53 have an increase in p53 levels, an increase in p21 (WAF1) expression, and an inhibition of DNA synthesis, whereas cell lines with mutant p53 do not.[18]

FIGURE 7-1. The "gate keeper" functions of p53. The wild-type p53 gene regulates cellular growth, and it functions as a "gate keeper" in controlling the induction of intermediate proteins that induce either cell cycle at rest ("mitotic arrest" at the G_1-S boundary or elsewhere) or apoptosis. The levels of p53 protein are regulated in part by levels of the autocrine mdm2 protein, which binds to p53, and whose levels are reciprocally regulated by p53 protein levels. cdk, cyclin-dependent kinase. (Figure prepared in collaboration with Dr. H. Yuwen.)

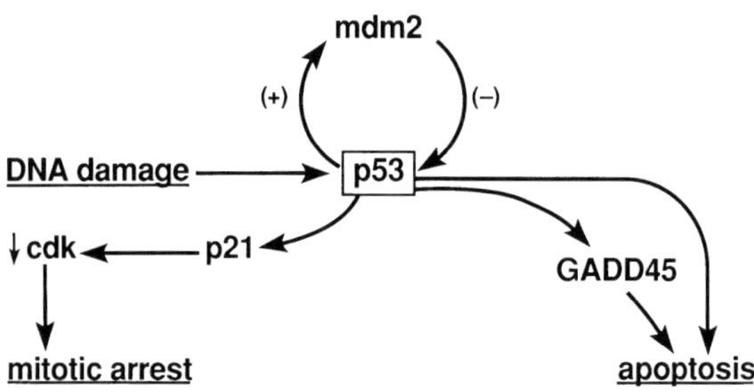

In HCCs, mutations of p53 are common. In some geographic locations, they have a pattern that is unique among human cancers, with 30% to 50% being G to T transversions at codon 249 (Fig. 7-2)[19,20]; in cancers other than HCC, p53 mutations are commonly found at a variety of different codons. These p53 mutations at codon 249 may be caused by ingestion of aflatoxin, because there is a high aflatoxin content of the diet in the geographic regions where these codon 249 mutations occur. Mutations caused by experimental aflatoxin exposure in bacteria[21] and in rats (leading to rat liver tumors)[22] are primarily G to T transversions, and p53 codon 249 mutations have been reported in a human hepatoblastoma cell line after exposure to aflatoxin.[23]

In geographic regions where aflatoxin contamination of the diet is uncommon, p53 mutations are prevalent but occur at sites other than codon 249 (Fig. 7-2). In Japan, 19%[24] and 31%[25] of HCCs had p53 mutations (or 65% when multiple nodules were examined)[26]; codon 249 was the site of none[24,25] or few[26] of the p53 mutations in HCCs from Japan. In Taiwan, 33% of HCCs had p53 mutations,[27] but few of the mutations from Taiwan were at codon 249. Similarly, in a high aflatoxin area of China, 60% of HCCs had p53 mutations (52% G to T transversions at codon 249), whereas in a small sampling from a low aflatoxin area of China, 56% had p53 mutations, none of which were at codon 249.[28] In the United States, 42% of HCCs had p53 mutations, none of which were at codon 249.[29] (Immunohistochemical studies in other United States populations are consistent with these findings.[30])

As with many other human cancers, p53 mutations may be late occurrences in carcinogenesis of the liver in some circumstances. They may occur in association with dedifferentiation to a more aggressive histologic type or the development of metastasis; however, the time when mutations occur could conceivably vary depending on the pathogenesis in different cases. Murakami et al.[24] reported that p53 mutations were found in 4/8 (50%) poorly differentiated HCCs from Japan and in 4/11 (36%) moderately differentiated HCCs, but in none of 24 well-differentiated HCCs. Similar results were reported by Nishida et al.[25] p53 mutations have been detected by single-strand conformation polymorphism (SSCP) in 4/9 (44%) poorly differentiated HCCs, 4/18 (22%) moderately differentiated HCCs, and 0/6 well-differentiated HCCs.[31] (In this study, none of the eight with p53 mutations had HBsAg or anti-HCV.) In patients with multifocal HCC, p53 mutations are usually found only in one of the nodules,[26] which also supports the hypothesis that p53 mutations are a late occurrence. Because the early detection of HCC in Japan is superior to that in most other countries, the prevalence of p53 mutations in studies of HCCs in Japan may be lower than elsewhere, since late mutations in the p53 gene would be underrepresented.

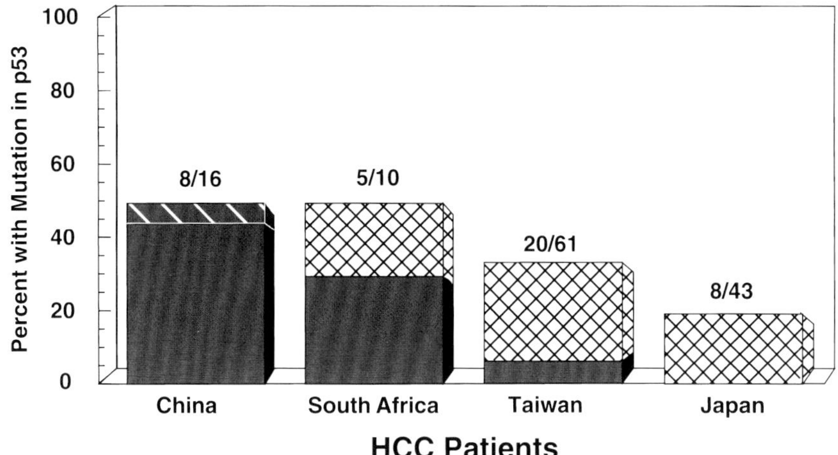

FIGURE 7-2. Percentage of patients with p53 mutations in HCC tissue detected by direct sequencing or single-strand conformation polymorphism (SSCP). Patients are from four countries: China,[19] South Africa,[20] Taiwan,[27] and Japan.[24] ■, mutation at p53 codon 249 (G to T transversion); ▧, mutation at p53 codon 249 (G to C transition, which results in the same amino acid change as a G to T transversion); ▩, mutation at a p53 locus other than codon 249.

The possible occurrence of p53 mutations developing in stepwise progression in conjunction with histologic progression of the tumor is supported by reports of different p53 mutations in different tumor nodules in the same patient. HCC often develops initially as a small well-differentiated tumor, in which a less well-differentiated nodule later arises.[32] One patient has been reported in whom two HCC grade II or III nodules containing two different p53 mutations were surrounded by a grade I nodule containing only wild-type p53.[33] This 58-year-old Japanese patient with more than a 30-year history of chronic hepatitis had anti-HCV, as well as a long history of ethanol use. (Although one of the two mutations was a G to T transversion at codon 249, the mutation was at the second position of the codon rather than the third position, which is the usual site of G to T transversion in HCCs from high-aflatoxin areas.) It remains possible that each mutation was a result of a different carcinogenic influence (in this patient, ethanol and HCV), or that the different mutations reflect a general genetic instability or repair defect. A similar case has been reported of two different p53 mutations identified by SSCP among three HCC nodules of different histologic grades in one patient.[31]

The functions of normal p53 can be inactivated when p53 protein becomes bound by viral or other cellular proteins, in the absence of a p53 mutation. For instance, the transforming proteins (oncoproteins) of three DNA tumor viruses (SV40 T antigen, adenovirus E1B antigen, and human papillomavirus E6 protein) can form stable complexes with wild-type p53 and either prevent its normal function (T antigen, E1B antigen) or induce its degradation (E6 protein). p53 levels in cells are regulated, at least in part, by an autocrine feedback system involving the cellular protein mdm2; under normal conditions, the levels of wild-type p53 and mdm2 inversely regulate each other (Fig. 7-1). When mdm2 is amplified (as a result of pathologic conditions that are not well defined at present), p53 function is interrupted. When the mdm2 protein binds to p53, p53-directed transactivation is inhibited. In studies of human sarcomas, mdm2 is overexpressed in many sarcomas containing wild-type p53 but not in those sarcomas containing mutant p53, suggesting a mechanism of carcinogenesis that is parallel to that involving p53 mutation. Other cellular proteins in the liver have been identified that bind to p53[34] and may play a role in its regulation; abnormal expression of such proteins could contribute to carcinogenesis.

There is evidence that X protein can bind p53 protein, although the biologic role of this remains unclear. X protein can be coimmunoprecipitated with p53 from artificial complexes and from HCC tissues using antibody to either protein.[35] In binding to p53, X protein inhibits p53 transactivation and p53-stimulated transcription in a transient transfection system.[36,37] X protein is itself a transcriptional transactivator. Transgenic mice created with the X gene develop liver tumors in 80% to 90% of cases; when these tumors have evolved to HCC, X and p53 are both detected exclusively in the cytoplasm and are bound to each other.[38] This binding to X could block p53 from entry into the nucleus, and this could be the mechanism for loss of growth control in these cells. (Binding of p53 by X has been shown to block p53-mediated apoptosis, possibly by interfering with up-regulation of the intermediate protein p21 [WAF1][59]). Administration of interferon-α to these mice suppressed X expression in the tumors, eliminated the presence of coimmunoprecipitable bound p53, and permitted the reentry of p53 into the nucleus of almost all cells.[38]

This type of mutation-independent mechanism of p53 inactivation, involving cytoplasmic sequestration of the wild-type protein, has been supported by observations in neuroblastomas[39] and some breast carcinomas.[40] In addition, transforming growth factor β, another negative regulator of cell growth, reduces the level of phosphorylation of p53, thus changing its conformation and causing it to localize in the cytoplasm, where it cannot bind to cellular DNA.[41]

Mutations or deletions in the splice junctions in the introns can also result in transcription of nonfunctional or absent p53 mRNA and the absence of p53 protein in HCCs.[42] Mutations in a splice junction of p53 resulting in aberrant intron retention causing a stop codon insertion has been reported in some human HCCs.[43]

The association of HCC with changes in p53 suggests several possible future approaches to treatment of HCC. Some p53 mutants have a reduced affinity for DNA that can be corrected by altering the carboxyl-terminal end.[44] Restoring wild-type function to mutant p53 may be possible; in vitro, the DNA binding and transcription activation functions of p53 have been restored to colorectal carcinoma cells by microinjection of a monoclonal antibody to p53 (PAb 421).[44] The ability of the p53 protein to bind to DNA is negatively regulated by a 30-amino acid region at the carboxyl-terminal region; deletion of this region, or binding to a part of it by monoclonal antibody to p53 (PAb 421), activates DNA binding. Wild-type p53, transfected using a defective herpes simplex viral vector into a human medulloblastoma cell line containing endogenous mutant p53, produced functionally active wild-type p53 with cell cycle arrest.[45]

Although few studies have formally analyzed p53 in HCV-associated HCC, the association of most HCCs in Japan with HCV infection means that most studies of p53 in Japan reflect the role of HCV. p53 mutations have been found within exons 5 to 10 in 4/15 (27%) HCCs from Japanese patients with serologic evidence of HCV but not HBV infection[46]; the prevalence was reported not to be significantly different from HBV-infected HCC patients in the same study. In another study, 27 HCC patients with detectable HCV-RNA in nontumorous liver or HCC tissue (21 [78%] of whom had anti-HCV) were analyzed for p53 mutations in exons 4, 5, 7, and 8. Either a mutation or LOH at p53 was present in 12/27 (44%) with HCV infection (2 with HBV as well).[47] This was not significantly different from the prevalence they detected in HCC patients with HBV infection alone (5/10; 50%) or those with neither HCV nor HBV (1/8; 13%, not a significant difference).

RB TUMOR SUPPRESSOR GENE

Mutation or deletion of the RB tumor suppressor gene can be found in some HCCs. This gene is located within a 200 kb segment of chromosome 13 that encodes a 110 kD phosphoprotein, pRB, consisting of 928 amino acids. When pRB is underphosphorylated, it localizes in the nucleus, binds tightly to an unidentified "nuclear anchor," and prevents cell growth beyond the G1 phase of the cell cycle. When pRB is phosphorylated, it appears to localize in the cytoplasm, and cell growth can occur. Unrestricted growth occurs when pRB is not functioning. This can occur (1) when the RB gene is deleted or mutated, (2) when proteins produced by certain DNA tumor viruses bind to wild-type pRB (e.g., SV-40 large T antigen, the E7 protein of human papillomavirus, or adenovirus E1A protein), or (3) when pRB is freely phosphorylated because transforming growth factor β1 (TGF-β1), which normally suppresses the enzyme that phosphorylates pRB, is not functioning.[48] Underphosphorylation of pRB may act to restrict cell growth by affecting oncogenes and growth factors. pRB suppresses the transcription of the promoters of the oncogenes c-*myc*[49] and c-*fos*[50] in vitro. It is possible that the release of c-*myc* and c-*fos* from this control plays some role in tumorigenesis associated with pRB dysfunction resulting from any of the mechanisms described previously.

Mutations of the RB gene have been indicated by finding LOH of the RB gene in 25% to 44% of human HCCs,[24,28,51] and undetectable expression of RB by immunohistochemistry in 20% to 29%.[52,53] LOH at the RB gene in HCCs has been reported by others in 13%[31] (65% had anti-HCV and 21% had HBsAg, but none of those with an RB abnormality had either HBsAg or anti-HCV), 10%,[54] and in none.[55] LOH at or near the RB gene was reported in 30 of 92 (33%) HCCs from Japan; this was more common in moderately or poorly differentiated HCCs (26/63; 41%) than in well-differentiated HCCs (2/24; 8%).[17] Sequencing of RB in HCCs has not been reported, presumably because its 27 exons make extensive sequencing difficult.

The identification of HCCs that have deletions or mutations of the RB gene, as well as mutations of the p53 gene, suggests that these could contribute together to carcinogenesis. LOH at the RB gene was detected in six of seven (86%) HCCs with a p53 mutation compared to none of 17 HCCs without a p53 mutation (overall prevalence of changes in both the RB and p53 genes = 6/24 [25%]).[24] All of the seven with abnormalities of p53 (and of RB in six) were poorly or moderately differentiated HCCs. In another study, 8 of 25 (32%) human HCCs had altered expression of pRB (undetectable or detected in less than 1% of nuclei); 4/5 (80%) with undetectable pRB also had apparent p53 mutations as detected by immunohistochemistry.[53] Three of seven (43%) HCC or hepatoblastoma cell lines[56,57] had no detectable pRB by Western immunoblot or immunohistochemistry as well as deletion of p53 or the expression of mutant p53.

By immunohistochemistry, absence of pRB in HCCs has been reported in 4/14 (29%) cases[52]; all four were anti-HCV-positive and HBsAg-negative, as were most of the 14 patients in the study. Three of the four HCCs with undetectable pRB were less than or equal to 2 cm in diameter; three of nine HCCs less than or equal to 2 cm in diameter had absent pRB, and one of five HCCs greater than 2 cm in diameter had absent pRB (not a significant difference).

The intact HCV core protein, which is found only in the cytoplasm, appears to suppress the expression of a variety of cellular genes, including the expression of the RB promoter. It is believed that this suppression occurs at the transcription or translation level.[13]

Homozygous deletions of the $p16^{INK4}$ gene, an inhibitor of cyclin-Cdk complexes (and, hence, of RB protein expression), were found in one of eight (13%) HCC or hepatoblastoma cell lines.[58] RB protein was normally expressed (by immunoprecipitation and Western blot) in five of six cell lines tested[58]; thus, inhibition of RB expression was not associated with a lack of $p16^{INK4}$ expression in these cell lines.

Additional tumor-suppressor genes other than RB have been tentatively identified on chromosome 13 that may be associated with the development of human HCC.[17]

REFERENCES

1. Zhou Y, Butel JS, Li P et al. Integrated state of subgenomic fragments of hepatitis B virus DNA in hepatocellular carcinoma from mainland China. J Natl Cancer Inst 1987;79: 223–231
2. Harrison TJ, Lin Y, Stamps AC et al. Hepatitis B virus-associated hepatocellular carcinoma in African patients. Cancer Detect Prev 1990;14:457–460
3. Dejean A, Bougueleret L, Grzeschik K, Tiollais P. Hepatitis B virus DNA integration in a sequence homologous to *v-erb-A* and steroid receptor genes in a hepatocellular carcinoma. Nature 1986;322:70–72
4. Wang J, Chenivesse X, Henglein B, Bréchot C. Hepatitis B virus integration in a cyclin A gene in a hepatocellular carcinoma. Nature 1990;343:555–557
5. Balsano C, Avantaggiati ML, Natoli G et al. Transactivation of c-fos and c-myc protooncogenes by both full-length and truncated versions of the HBV-X protein. In Hollinger FB, Lemon SM, Margolis H (eds): Viral Hepatitis and Liver Disease. Williams & Wilkins, Baltimore, 1991, pp. 572–576
6. Kekulé AS, Lauer U, Meyer M et al. The *preS2/S* region of integrated hepatitis B virus DNA encodes a transcriptional transactivator. Nature 1990;343:457–461
7. Kim C, Koike K, Saito I et al. HBx gene of hepatitis B virus induced liver cancer in transgenic mice. Nature 1991;351: 317–320
8. Yoneyama T, Takeuchi K, Watanabe Y et al. Detection of hepatitis C virus cDNA sequence by the polymerase chain reaction in hepatocellular carcinoma tissues. Jpn J Med Sci Biol 1990;43:89–94
9. Tabor E, Kobayashi K. Commentary: Hepatitis C virus, a causative infectious agent of non-A, non-B hepatitis: Prevalence and structure—summary of a conference on hepatitis C virus as a cause of hepatocellular carcinoma. J Natl Cancer Inst 1992;84:86–90
10. Park YM, Yoon SK, Chung KW, Kim BS. Detection of HCV RNA using reverse transcription and nested polymerase chain reaction in chronic non-A, non-B liver diseases in Korea. Gastroenterol Jpn 1993;28(suppl 5):12–16
11. Chou W-H, Yoneyama T, Takeuchi K et al. Discrimination of hepatitis C virus in liver tissues from different patients with hepatocellular carcinomas by direct nucleotide sequencing of amplified cDNA of the viral genome. J Clin Microbiol 1991;29:2860–2864
12. Miyamura T, Saito I, Yoneyama T et al. Role of hepatitis C virus in hepatocellular carcinoma. In Hollinger FB, Lemon SM, Margolis H (eds): Viral Hepatitis and Liver Disease. Williams & Wilkins, Baltimore, 1991, pp. 559–562
13. Kim DW, Suzuki R, Harada T et al. *TRANS*-suppression of gene expression by hepatitis C viral core protein. Jpn J Med Sci Biol 1994;47:211–220
14. Hasan F, Jeffers LJ, De Medina M et al. Hepatitis C-associated hepatocellular carcinoma. Hepatology 1990;12: 589–591
15. Ikeda K, Saitoh S, Koida I et al. A multivariate analysis of risk factors for hepatocellular carcinogenesis: a prospective observation of 795 patients with viral and alcoholic cirrhosis. Hepatology 1993;18:47–53
16. Macdonald GA, Greenson JK, Saito K et al. Loss of the DNA mismatch repair genes hMSH2 and/or hMLH1 is an early event in hepatic carcinogenesis. Hepatology 1995;22: 219A (abstr)
17. Kuroki T, Fujiwara Y, Nakamori S et al. Evidence for the presence of two tumour-suppressor genes for hepatocellular carcinoma on chromosome 13q. Br J Cancer 1995;72: 383–385
18. Puisieux A, Jingwei J, Guillot C et al. p53-mediated cellular response to DNA damage in cells with replicative hepatitis B virus. Proc Natl Acad Sci U S A 1995;92:1342–1346
19. Hsu IC, Metcalf RA, Sun T et al. Mutational hotspot in the p53 gene in human hepatocellular carcinomas. Nature 1991; 350:427–428
20. Bressac B, Kew M, Wands J, Ozturk M. Selective G to T mutations of p53 gene in hepatocellular carcinoma from southern Africa. Nature 1991;350:429–431

21. Foster PL, Eisenstadt E, Miller JH. Base substitution mutations induced by metabolically activated aflatoxin B_1. Proc Natl Acad Sci U S A 1983;80:2695–2698

22. McMahon G, Davis EF, Humber LJ et al. Characterization of *c-Ki-ras* and *N-ras* oncogenes in aflatoxin B_1-induced rat liver tumors. Proc Natl Acad Sci U S A 1990;87:1104–1108

23. Aguilar F, Hussain SP, Cerutti P. Aflatoxin B_1 induces the transversion of G-T in codon 249 of the p53 tumor suppressor gene in human hepatocytes. Proc Natl. Acad Sci. U S A 1993;90:8586–8590

24. Murakami Y, Hayashi K, Hirohashi S, Sekiya T. Aberrations of the tumor suppressor p53 and retinoblastoma genes in human hepatocellular carcinoma. Cancer Res 1991;51:5520–5525

25. Nishida N, Fukuda Y, Kokuryu H et al. Role and mutational heterogeneity of the *p53* gene in hepatocellular carcinoma. Cancer Res 1993;53:368–372

26. Oda T, Tsuda H, Scarpa A et al. Mutation pattern of the p53 gene as a diagnostic marker for multiple hepatocellular carcinoma. Cancer Res 1992;52:3674–3678

27. Sheu J, Huang G, Lee P et al. Mutation of p53 gene in hepatocellular carcinoma in Taiwan. Cancer Res 1992;52:6098–6100

28. Fujimoto Y, Hampton LL, Wirth PJ et al. Alterations of tumor suppressor genes and allelic losses in human hepatocellular carcinomas in China. Cancer Res 1994;54:281–285

29. Kazachkov Y, Khaoustov V, Yoffe B et al. p53 Abnormalities in hepatocellular carcinoma from United States patients: analysis of all 11 exons. Carcinogenesis 1996;17:2207–2212.

30. Hsia CC, Kleiner DE, Axiotis CA et al. Mutations of p53 gene in hepatocellular carcinoma: roles of hepatitis B virus and aflatoxin contamination in the diet. J Natl Cancer Inst 1992;84:1638–1641

31. Yumoto Y, Hanafusa T, Hada H et al. Loss of heterozygosity and analysis of mutation of p53 in hepatocellular carcinoma. J Gastroenterol Hepatol 1995;10:179–185

32. Morimitsu Y, Hsia CC, Kojiro M, Tabor E. Nodules of less-differentiated tumor within or adjacent to hepatocellular carcinoma: relative expression of transforming growth factor-α and its receptor in the different areas of tumor. Hum Pathol 1995;26:1126–1132

33. Oda T, Tsuda H, Sakamoto M, Hirohashi S. Different mutations of the *p53* gene in nodule-in-nodule hepatocellular carcinoma as a [sic] evidence for multistage progression. Cancer Lett 1994;83:197–200

34. Yuwen H, Kazachkov Y, Morimitsu Y, Tabor E. Identification of two p53-binding proteins using a recombinant vaccinia virus containing the wild-type human p53 gene. Biochem Biophys Res Comm 1995;213:986–993

35. Feitelson MA, Zhu M, Duan L-X, London WT. Hepatitis B x antigen and p53 are associated in vitro and in liver tissues from patients with primary hepatocellular carcinoma. Oncogene 1993;8:1109–1117

36. Wang XW, Forrester K, Yeh H et al. Hepatitis B virus X protein inhibits p53 sequence-specific DNA binding, transcriptional activity, and association with transcription factor ERCC3. Proc Natl Acad Sci USA 1994;91:2230–2234

37. Truant R, Antunovic J, Greenblatt J et al. Direct interaction of the hepatitis B virus HBx protein with p53 leads to inhibition by HBx of p53 response element-directed transactivation. J Virol 1995;69:1851–1859

38. Ueda H, Ulrich SJ, Gangemi JD et al. Functional inactivation but not structural mutation of p53 causes liver cancer. Nat Genet 1995;9:41–47

39. Moll UM, La Quaglia M, Bénard J, Riou G. Wild-type p53 protein undergoes cytoplasmic sequestration in undifferentiated neuroblastomas but not in differentiated tumors. Proc Natl Acad Sci U S A 1995;92:4407–4411

40. Moll UM, Riou G, Levine AJ. Two distinct mechanisms alter p53 in breast cancer: mutation and nuclear exclusion. Proc Natl Acad Sci U S A 1992;89:7262–7266

41. Raynal S, Jullien P, Lawrence DA. Transforming growth factor-β1 enhances serum-induced dephosphorylation of the p53 protein in cell lines growth-inhibited by this factor. Growth Factors 1994;11:197–203

42. Hsu H-C, Huang A-M, Lai P-L et al. Genetic alterations at the splice junction of p53 gene in human hepatocellular carcinoma. Hepatology 1994;19:122–128

43. Lai M-Y, Chang H-C, Li H-P et al. Splicing mutations of the p53 gene in human hepatocellular carcinoma. Cancer Res 1993;53:1653–1656

44. Abarzúa P, LoSardo JE, Gubler ML, Neri A. Microinjection of monoclonal antibody PAb421 into human SW480 colorectal carcinoma cells restores the transcription activation function to mutant p53. Cancer Res 1995;55:3490–3494

45. Rosenfeld MR, Meneses P, Dalmau J et al. Gene transfer of wild-type p53 results in restoration of tumor-suppressor function in a medulloblastoma cell line. Neurology 1995;45:1533–1539

46. Konishi M, Kikuchi-Yanochita R, Tanaka K et al. Genetic changes and histopathological grades in human hepatocellular carcinomas. Jpn J Cancer Res 1993;84:893–899

47. Teramoto T, Satonaka K, Kitazawa S et al. *p53* gene abnormalities are closely related to hepatoviral infections and occur at a late stage of hepatocarcinogenesis. Cancer Res 1994;54:231–235

48. Laiho M, DeCaprio JA, Ludlow JW et al. Growth inhibition by TGF-β linked to suppression of retinoblastoma protein phosphorylation. Cell 1990;62:175–185

49. Pietenpol JA, Münger K, Howley PM et al. Factor-binding element in the human *c-myc* promoter involved in transcriptional regulation by transforming growth factor β1 and by the retinoblastoma gene product. Proc Natl Acad Sci U S A 1991;88:10227–10231

50. Robbins PD, Horowitz JM, Mulligan RC. Negative regulation of human *c-fos* expression by the retinoblastoma gene product. Nature 1990;346:668–671

51. Zhang X, Xu H-J, Murakami Y et al. Deletions of chromosome 13q, mutations in *retinoblastoma 1*, and retinoblastoma protein state in human hepatocellular carcinoma. Cancer Res 1994;54:4177–4182

52. Kawakita N, Seki S, Sakaguchi H et al. Immunohistochemical analysis of retinoblastoma gene product (pRB) expression in malignant and non-malignant liver diseases. Liver 1994;14:295–301

53. Hsia CC, Di Bisceglie AM, Kleiner DE Jr et al. RB tumor suppressor gene expression in hepatocellular carcinomas from patients infected with the hepatitis B virus. J Med Virol 1994;44:67–73

54. Nakamura T, Iwamura Y, Kaneko M et al. Deletions and rearrangements of the retinoblastoma gene in hepatocellular carcinoma, insulinoma and some neurogenic tumors as found in a study of 121 tumors. Jpn J Clin Oncol 1991;21:325–329

55. T'Ang A, Varley JM, Chakraborty S et al. Structural rearrangements of the retinoblastoma gene in human breast carcinoma. 1988; Science 242:263–266

56. Farshid M, Tabor E. Expression of oncogenes and tumor suppressor genes in human hepatocellular carcinoma and hepatoblastoma cell lines. J Med Virol 1992;38:235–239

57. Farshid M, Hsia CC, Tabor E. Alterations of the RB tumour suppressor gene in hepatocellular carcinoma and hepatoblastoma cell lines in association with abnormal p53 expression. J Viral Hepat 1994;1:45–53

58. Okamoto A, Demetrick DJ, Spillare EA et al. Mutations and altered expression of $p16^{INK4}$ in human cancer. Proc Natl Acad Sci U S A 1994;91:11045–11049

59. Wang XW, Gibson MK, Vermeulen W et al. Abrogation of p53-induced apoptosis by the hepatitis B virus X gene. Cancer Res 1995;55:6012–6016

8

OTHER CAUSES OF HEPATOCELLULAR CARCINOMA

YVES DEUGNIER
BRUNO TURLIN

Besides hepatitis B virus (HBV) and hepatitis C virus (HCV) infections and chemicals, many inherited and acquired conditions are associated with the development of hepatocellular carcinoma (HCC). This chapter reviews current knowledge of these conditions, with emphasis on clarifying, when possible, the respective roles of the condition itself, underlying cirrhosis, and associated environmental and genetic factors in the pathogenesis of such HCCs.

INHERITED DISORDERS

Numerous inherited liver diseases have been associated with HCC, notably hereditary tyrosinemia in childhood, glycogen storage disease in young adults, and genetic hemochromatosis, α-1-antitrypsin deficiency, and porphyria cutanea tarda in adults over age 50 (Table 8-1)

Disorders of Carbohydrate Metabolism

GLYCOGEN STORAGE DISEASE (GSD)

In GSD type I (von Gierke's disease), patients who survive beyond 10 years are prone to develop hepatocellular adenoma(s) (HCA).[1–3] The incidence of such tumors is not precisely known, but it is likely to increase with the longer survival of these patients. Fifty cases of HCA complicating GSD type I had been reported until 1992.[3] HCAs have also been described in GSD type III (Forbes' disease)[3,4] and GSD type VIII.[3] From the 50 cases recorded by Bianchi,[3] 10 (20%) were associated with single or multifocal HCC. Most affected patients were young adult men with a mean age of 27 years (range, 7 to 40 years) who were afflicted with HCA for 2 to 7 years. Usually, the HCCs developed within such preexisting adenomatous lesions as shown by imaging follow-up studies[5] and histologic description of transitional aspects from HCA to HCC in the lesions. Pathologic distinction between benign and malignant tumors may be difficult because GSD-associated HCCs are well-differentiated tumors and atypical lesions ("nodule-in-nodule" pattern and Mallory bodies) are commonly found in GSD-related HCA.[3] Determination of serum α-fetoprotein (AFP) is not very helpful.[6] Interestingly, underlying cirrhosis is never present. This suggests a role of abnormal glycogen storage in initiating and/or promoting liver growth and malignancy, possibly through glucagon/insulin imbalance.[3] Regular ultrasound screening for HCA and then for HCC is suitable in GSD type I patients.[7] When performed early, liver transplantation potentially may cure both the metabolic disease and the tumor.[4]

HEREDITARY FRUCTOSE INTOLERANCE

One case of HCC has been reported in a 49-year-old man without cirrhosis who had suspected hereditary fructose intolerance.[8]

The authors are indebted to Michael Kluk for reviewing the manuscript and to Rémi Trinquart for his excellent technical assistance.

TABLE 8-1. Main Inherited and Acquired Conditions Associated With HCC in Adults[a]

Absence of Underlying Cirrhosis
Inherited conditions
Glycogen storage disease
Paucity of intrahepatic bile ducts
Acquired Conditions
Oral contraceptives
Anabolic-androgenic steroids
Presence of Associated Cirrhosis
Inherited conditions
Genetic hemochromatosis
α-1-Antitrypsin deficiency
Porphyrias (especially porphyria cutanea tarda)
Membranous obstruction of inferior vena cava
Acquired Conditions
HBV and HCV infections
Aflatoxin, chemicals, and tobacco
Alcohol
Chronic autoimmune hepatitis
Primary biliary cirrhosis
Primary sclerosing cholangitis

[a] Listed according to the presence or absence of underlying cirrhosis. (For conditions shown in *italics*, some cases may occur in noncirrhotic patients.)

Disorders of Protein Metabolism

α-1-ANTITRYPSIN DEFICIENCY (A1ATD)

- *Homozygous (PiZZ) A1ATD*. HCC has been reported in case series and numerous individual case reports in homozygous A1ATD adult patients (see Poley[9] for review). Eriksson et al.[10] found 17 cases (6%) of homozygous A1ATD among 297 autopsied cases of HCC and demonstrated that male A1ATD homozygotes were at high risk for both cirrhosis (odds ratio = 7.8; CI = 2.4 to 24.7) and HCC (odds ratio = 20; CI = 3.5 to 114), compared with the general population. Interestingly, 9 of these 17 patients (53%) did not have cirrhosis, but only had mild inflammation of the liver, fibrosis or both. Whether the Z allele is directly involved in liver carcinogenesis remains unknown.
- *Heterozygous (PiMZ) A1ATD*. Early studies have reported conflicting data on the prevalence of heterozygous A1ATD among patients with HCC (see Poley[9] for review). Recent data do not support a significant role of the heterozygous state in the development of HCC. On one hand, Rabinovitz et al.[11] found that the prevalence of heterozygous A1ATD in 59 HCC patients was not increased compared with that in the general population (6.8% vs 8.5%). On the other hand, the prevalence of HCC in patients with heterozygous A1ATD patients with cirrhosis was comparable to that in patients with cirrhosis of other etiologies.[12] Moreover, most patients (67%) with both heterozygous A1ATD-associated cirrhosis and HCC had positive serum HBV and/or HCV markers.[12] Thus, PiMZ genotype is unlikely to be a risk factor for HCC.[12] Finally, a few cases of HCC complicating noncirrhotic heterozygous A1ATD have been described. Most were fibrolamellar carcinomas.[11,13] Whether there is a relationship between this rare neoplasm and the PiMZ phenotype remains unknown.
- *Other A1ATD phenotypes*. There is no evidence of an increased risk for HCC in PiSZ A1ATD.[9]

HEREDITARY TYROSINEMIA

The prevalence of HCC in tyrosinemia patients over 2 years of age is high, ranging from 18% in a recent international survey (including 108 patients with tyrosinemia type I[14]) to 35% in a previous study of Weinberg et al.[15] Early liver transplantation may explain the lower frequency of HCC in the recent series. HCC was equally distributed between boys and girls aged 2 to 12 years.[14] Serum AFP levels were usually high, even in the absence of HCC. As reported by Ishak and Sharp,[16] HCC complicating tyrosinemia arises in a cirrhotic liver with fatty change, cholestasis, pseudoacinar transformation of the hepatic plates, and pericellular and periportal fibrosis. Regenerative nodules are often difficult to distinguish from multifocal HCC. Large and small liver cell dysplasia is frequently present in the nontumorous liver.[17] Chromosome breakage[18] and DNA ploidy abnormalities[19] have been described in patients with tyrosinemia type I complicated with HCC. Accumulation of the intermediates of tyrosine metabolism, which act as natural alkylating agents and cause genetic instability, has been proposed as a mechanism of development of HCC.[18] Because of the high risk of liver malignancy in tyrosinemia type I patients who are over the age of 2 years, liver transplantation is recommended early in the course of the disease.[17,20]

HYPERCITRULLINEMIA

Hypercitrullinemia is a urea cycle disorder related to argininosuccinate synthetase deficiency. As reported by Nakayama et al.,[21] HCC occurs in 14% of adult-onset cases. There is no underlying cirrhosis. In vivo and in vitro studies suggest that citrulline may act as a carcinogenic factor.[21]

Disorders of Porphyrin Metabolism

PORPHYRIA CUTANEA TARDA (PCT)

Numerous cases of HCC complicating PCT have been reported (see Lim and Mascaro[22] for review). The prevalence of HCC in PCT patients ranges from 39% to 47% in autopsy series[23] and from 7% to 16% in case-control[24] and follow-up[23,25] studies. Almost all HCCs occurred in men older than 50 years with preexisting cirrhosis and a long-standing history of symptomatic PCT. The role of additional risk factors such as HBV infection, HCV infection,[26] iron overload, and chronic alcoholism is likely but not proven. Whether porphyrins are carcinogenic per se[27] remains controversial. Rarely, PCT evolves as a paraneoplastic syndrome associated with HCC. In such cases, symptoms of PCT are not detected much more than 1 year before the diagnosis of HCC and can resolve after surgical removal of the tumor.[22]

Variegate porphyria[28–30] and acute intermittent porphyria[27,28,31,32] have been occasionally complicated by HCC.

Chronic Cholestatic Syndromes

PAUCITY (OR HYPOPLASIA) OF INTRAHEPATIC BILE DUCTS

Nine cases of Alagille's syndrome (or arteriohepatic dysplasia) have been reported to be complicated by HCC.[33,34] Among these nine patients, four were children and five were adults (three males and two females) aged 25 to 48 years. In the adult cases, HCC developed in either a normal[33–35] or a fibrotic but noncirrhotic liver.[36,37] Some data suggest that arteriohepatic dysplasia may result from a contiguous gene-deletion syndrome with deletion of multiple gene loci.[38] It is tempting to hypothesize that HCC complicating noncirrhotic arteriohepatic dysplasia might be related to genetic abnormalities, especially the deletion of a tumor suppressor gene locus.[39]

Biliary atresia and congenital hepatic fibrosis have been reported to be rarely complicated by HCC.[40]

In Byler syndrome (progressive familial intrahepatic cholestasis), an autosomal recessive disease, HCC can develop before 3 years of age when cirrhosis is also present.[41]

Metal Storage Diseases

WILSON'S DISEASE AND THE ROLE OF COPPER

As recently reviewed by Cheng et al.,[42] only 11 cases of HCC in Wilson's disease have been reported. Patients were 14 to 72 years (six were older than 40 years). Eight were male. All presented with underlying cirrhosis. No relationship was found between the duration of penicillamine therapy (range from 1 week to 33 years) and the development of HCC. On the basis of the low incidence of HCC in patients with the liver damage of Wilson's disease and on the basis of experimental studies in rats,[43,44] it has been proposed that copper may have a protective effect against cancer. However, this was not confirmed by studies in mice[45] and in a mutant copper-overloaded rat strain with hereditary hepatitis and hepatoma.[46]

HEMOCHROMATOSIS AND THE ROLE OF IRON

Risk for HCC in Hemochromatosis

Studies have confirmed the high incidence of primary liver cancer, mainly HCC, in patients with genetic hemochromatosis.[47–52] Primary liver cancer accounts for 30%[50] to 36.4%[49] of deaths in early series and up to 45%[52] of deaths in recent studies. The relative risk for the development of primary liver cancer in hemochromatosis patients with cirrhosis has been calculated as greater than 200.[49,50]

Presentation of HCC Complicating Hemochromatosis

The main clinical, biologic, and pathologic features of HCC complicating hemochromatosis are similar to those of other HCCs.[53] Magnetic resonance imaging may be useful to detect early HCCs arising in iron-overloaded hemochromatosis livers of patients with hemochromatosis[54] (Fig. 8-1). Iron-free foci (IFF)[55,56] (defined as clear-cut sublobular nodules of hepatocytes free of iron or with significantly less iron than the surrounding parenchyma) (Figs. 8-2 and 8-3) were found in 7.6% of 185 patients with uncomplicated hemochromatosis[56] and in 83% of hemochromatosis patients with HCC.[53] Evidence from experimental[57] and clinical[56] data (Table 8-2), points to the possible involvement of IFF as an early step toward HCC.

FIGURE 8-1. Detection of hepatocellular carcinoma by magnetic resonance imaging in a patient with genetic hemochromatosis. The tumor is devoid of iron and then appears as a normal or hyperintense image when compared to the hypointense surrounding iron-overloaded parenchyma.

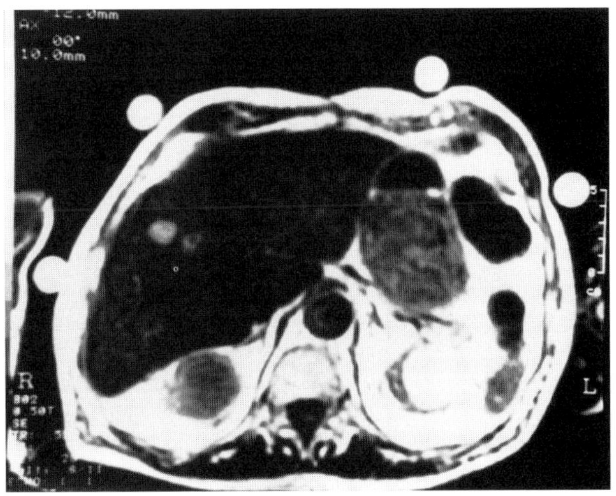

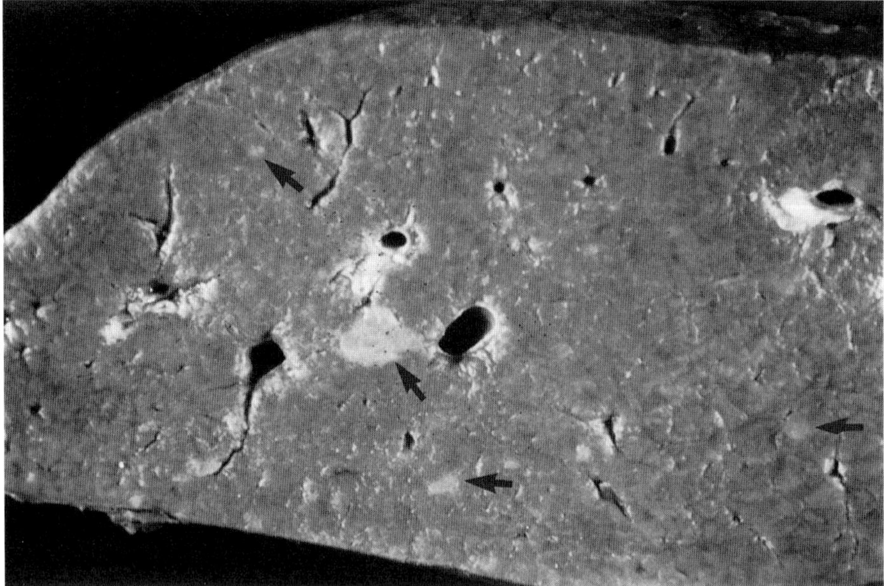

FIGURE 8-2. Numerous macroscopic pale nodules corresponding to iron-free-foci (arrows) in a noncirrhotic hemochromatosis liver in a 65-year-old man with hemochromatosis and hepatocellular carcinoma.

FIGURE 8-3. Histologic aspect of an iron-free-focus (IFF) in genetic hemochromatosis. Hepatocytes are free of iron compared to the iron-overloaded surrounding parenchyma. Rare iron deposits are seen in sinusoidal cells within IFF. (Perls' stain, ×150.)

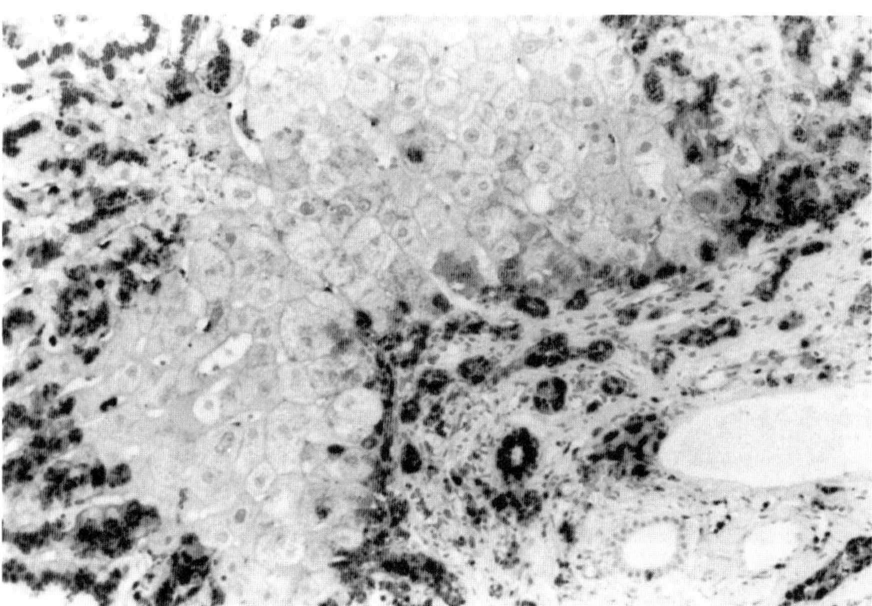

TABLE 8-2. Demonstration of the Preneoplastic Significance of Iron-free-foci (IFF) in Genetic Hemochromatosis: Comparison Between Hemochromatosis Patients With IFF and Hemochromatosis Controls Without IFF

	IFF-Positive Patients	IFF-Negative Controls
Age (years-mean ± SD)	51 ± 8	51 ± 8
Liver iron concentration (N < 36 μmol/g)	435 ± 174	409 ± 153
Removed iron (g)	15 ± 5	18 ± 9
Cirrhosis (%)	67%	63%
Duration of follow-up (years-mean ± SD)	7 ± 6	8 ± 6
HCC at the end of follow-up (%)	50%	8%

Controls were matched by sex, age, amount of liver iron excess, and stage of fibrosis. The two groups were identical except for the incidence of HCC at the end of follow-up period (X^2 test, $p = 0.001$). Data from Deugnier et al.[56]

Roles of Iron, Cirrhosis and Noniron Related Factors

HCC develops in some highly iron-overloaded hemochromatosis patients with cirrhosis.[50,53,58] At least six cases of HCC, however, that developed in noncirrhotic (but fibrotic) hemochromatosis livers (Fig. 8-4) have been reported (see Deugnier et al.[53] for review), suggesting that cirrhosis is not an absolute prerequisite. Thus, iron could be a (co)carcinogenic factor. This is supported by the demonstration of an increased risk for various types of cancer in patients with elevated body iron stores[59–62] and of a relationship between hepatic parenchymal iron excess and HCC development in nonhemochromatosis patients.[63,64] In hemochromatosis patients with cirrhosis, however, the risk for HCC persists long after iron depletion. Indeed, although there is some evidence of a promoting effect of iron on tumor cell growth in vivo[65,66] and in vitro,[67,68] a direct carcinogenic effect of iron has not been documented in rats,[69] and dietary iron overload mimicking noncirrhotic human hemochromatosis was not shown to either initiate or promote the formation of preneoplastic lesions in the rat liver.[70] In hemochromatosis patients, risk factors for HCC are the same as in other HCC patients: male sex, age greater than 50 years, cirrhosis, chronic alcoholism,[53,58] tobacco smoking,[53] and HBV infection.[58] Exposure to parenteral blood products was also a significant risk factor for HCC development in 53 hemochromatosis patients,[53] suggesting a pos-

FIGURE 8-4. Hepatocellular carcinoma from a noncirrhotic hemochromatosis patient. Note the dark color of the nontumorous liver and the regular aspect of liver capsule.

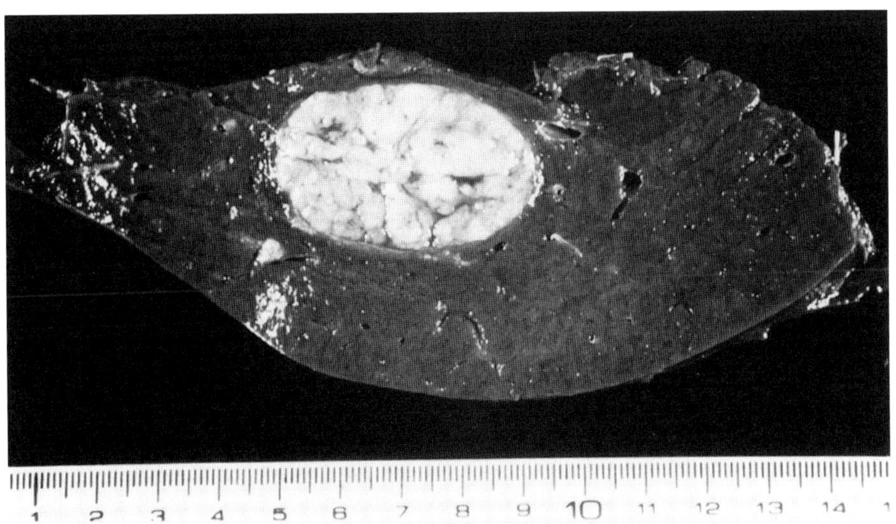

sibility of HCV infection as a risk factor, but was not shown to increase HCC risk in 152 Italian hemochromatosis patients.[58]

Cirrhotic hemochromatosis patients older than 50 years are at risk to develop HCC whether or not iron overload has been removed. Such patients should be screened for early HCC, especially when IFF are found on their initial liver biopsy, or when chronic alcoholism or hepatitis virus infection is present.[53,58]

Hepatic Vascular Anomalies

MEMBRANOUS OBSTRUCTION OF THE INFERIOR VENA CAVA (MOVC)

Simson[71] first pointed out a relationship between MOVC and the development of HCC in a South African black population. More recently, a large epidemiologic survey in Japan[72] reported 10 cases of HCC in 157 patients with the Budd-Chiari syndrome (BCS) (6.4%). BCS was related to MOVC in 93% of patients. The HCC patients (five men and five women) were aged 18 to 65 years. Eight were cirrhotic. The mean duration between the onset of BCS and the diagnosis of HCC was 6.8 ± 6.5 years (range, 1 to 18 years). Only one patient was hepatitis B surface antigen (HBsAg) positive. Anti-HCV testing was not done. This large study confirmed previous results of smaller series from the United States[73] and from South Africa,[74] which indicated a prevalence of 25% (2/8 cases) and 40% (6/14 cases), respectively, of HCC in MOVC patients. As proposed by Kew et al.,[74] environmental factors could be involved in the development of HCC in MOVC. Despite being a risk factor for HCC, however, MOVC is not an important cause of HCC because its prevalence in HCC patients is <1% in Japan[72] and 3.7% in South Africa.[74]

OTHER VASCULAR DISEASES

Cases of HCC have been occasionally reported in hereditary hemorrhagic telangiectasia (Osler-Rendu-Weber disease)[75] and in ataxia-telangiectasia.[76]

Extrahepatic Inherited Conditions

Several cases of HCC have been reported in familial polyposis of the colon.[77–79] Occasional cases have been described in neurofibromatosis, Soto's syndrome, and situs inversus.[40]

ACQUIRED DISEASES

Alcohol and exogenous sex hormones as risk factors for the development of HCC are reviewed. Attention will be also focused on the occurrence of HCC in some dysimmune chronic liver diseases (Table 8-1).

Alcohol

There is some epidemiologic evidence of a relationship between alcohol consumption and HCC. Whether this association is due to cirrhosis remains unclear.

EPIDEMIOLOGIC STUDIES

In Chronic Alcoholism

Finnish,[80] Danish,[81] Japanese,[82–84] Chinese,[85] and Swedish[86] large-scale follow-up studies of alcohol abuse and HCC consistently demonstrated that alcoholism carried a relative risk of 2 for HCC, with a significant dose-response relationship. Few case-control studies[87–89] have not found any significant positive association between alcohol consumption and HCC; most[90–97] indicated about a twofold increase of HCC risk related to alcohol use, at least in heavy drinkers. In general, there was no evidence of a confounding effect of either associated HBV infection or current cigarette smoking. However, these studies, present several limitations:

1. Misclassifications may have occurred because of the difficulty in assessing drinking patterns and because of misdiagnosis of liver tumors metastatic from alcohol-related extrahepatic cancers.
2. Other risk factors such as age, sex, cirrhosis, tobacco use, HBV infection, parenteral exposure to blood products, and long-term oral contraceptive use have never been considered together.
3. HBV infection might be underdiagnosed in alcoholics because of unusual serologic patterns of HBV infection in these patients (see Nalpas et al.[98] for review).
4. The possible role of HCV infection has not been evaluated (the prevalence of anti-HCV antibodies is higher in alcoholics than in the general population [see Nalpas et al.[98] for review]).

In Alcoholic Cirrhosis

The incidence of HCC in alcoholic cirrhosis has been reported either similar to or slightly lower than in nonalcoholic cirrhosis patients (see Mandelli et al.[99] for review) with an overall lifetime risk (culled from many studies) around 15%. Once cirrhosis is present, cessation of drinking does not prevent HCC.[100] This may suggest that, in alcoholic cirrhosis, the risk of HCC is closely related to cirrhosis.

In Nonalcoholic Cirrhosis

Ikeda et al.[101] found that the total alcohol amount ingested before the diagnosis of cirrhosis was an independent risk factor for HCC in anti-HCV positive patients with alcoholic cirrhosis. Likewise, one case-control report[53] and one follow-up study[58] of hemochromatosis patients found that alcohol abuse was associated with a higher risk for HCC development. However, these findings were not confirmed by other studies.[84,86,102] Indeed,

Hirayama[84] did not find any effect of daily alcohol intake on the risk of HCC in cirrhotic patients, and Adami et al.[86] found that alcoholism with cirrhosis did not increase the risk of HCC more than cirrhosis alone. Tsukuma et al.[102] reported that, among patients with cirrhosis, HCC risk was increased in former heavy drinkers but was insignificant in current heavy drinkers. Thus, epidemiologic data pertaining to alcohol consumption and HCC indicate an independent, moderate, positive relationship, especially in heavy drinkers. Whether the risk is due to cirrhosis, environmental factors, or to a direct carcinogenic effect of ethanol remains unclear.

It is unlikely that ethanol initiates liver carcinogenesis (see Naccarato and Farinati[103] for review). On the other hand, a promoting effect of alcohol is plausible but not proven. Ethanol has been shown experimentally to activate environmental carcinogens by inducing cytochrome P450, to interfere with DNA repair, and to promote hepatocellular regeneration (see Naccarato and Farinati[103]).

Steroid Hormones

EXOGENOUS HORMONES

Oral Contraceptives (OC)

In the 1970s and early 1980s, case reports of HCC diagnosed in young noncirrhotic women focused attention on a possible relationship between the use of OC and HCC. Since then, case-control studies in North American,[93,104–106] British,[107,108] and Italian[109,110] women have consistently shown that the use of combined OC in areas not endemic for HBV infection results in an increase of the relative risk for HCC from 1.5 to 14.5 (mean = 3.2; 95% CI = 1.7–5.9) as calculated by Thomas[111] from five of these studies.[104,105,107–109] HCC relative risk was strongly related to the duration of OC use, ranging from 7.2 to 20.1 in long-term users (5 years) (mean = 10.3; 95%; CI = 4.5–23.6).[111] Case-control studies conducted in countries endemic for HBV infection[112,113] failed to find any increase of HCC risk, even in long-term OC users. It is likely that, in these countries, the risk related to OC is masked by the risk from HBV infection.

Presentation of OC-related HCCs differs from that of other HCCs.[114] Patients are usually younger and do not have a history of chronic liver disease. Most are symptomatic at the time of diagnosis. The most frequent symptoms are abdominal pain, hepatomegaly, and nausea or vomiting. In 25% of patients, the presenting sign is an acute abdomen secondary to intratumoral or intraperitoneal bleeding. Serum AFP levels are usually normal or only moderately elevated. The HCC has a macroscopic and histopathologic appearance similar to that of other HCCs, except for the absence of associated cirrhosis (Fig. 8-5) and the more frequent finding of peliosis in both the tumor and the surrounding liver (Fig. 8-6). The distinction between carcinoma and adenoma is sometimes difficult in these patients, especially in well-differentiated HCCs or in ruptured tumors. Diagnosis may be more difficult in case of HCCs arising in a preexisting HCA (see Thung and Gerber[115] for review). These HCCs may be estrogen-dependent. Indeed, regression of these HCCs has been reported after cessation of OC use.

FIGURE 8-5. Hepatocellular carcinoma in a 23-year-old woman who had been using oral contraceptives for 7 years. This large tumor developed in a noncirrhotic liver. Hemorrhagic foci are seen at the lower part of the tumor.

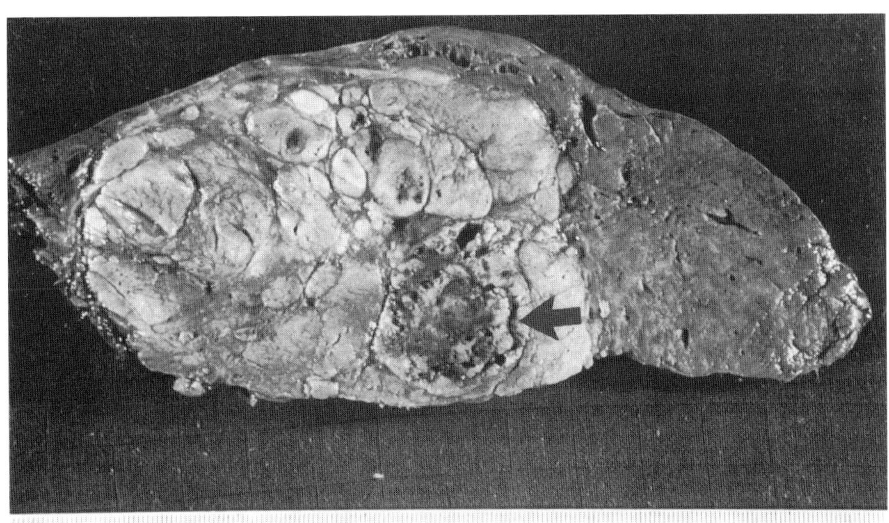

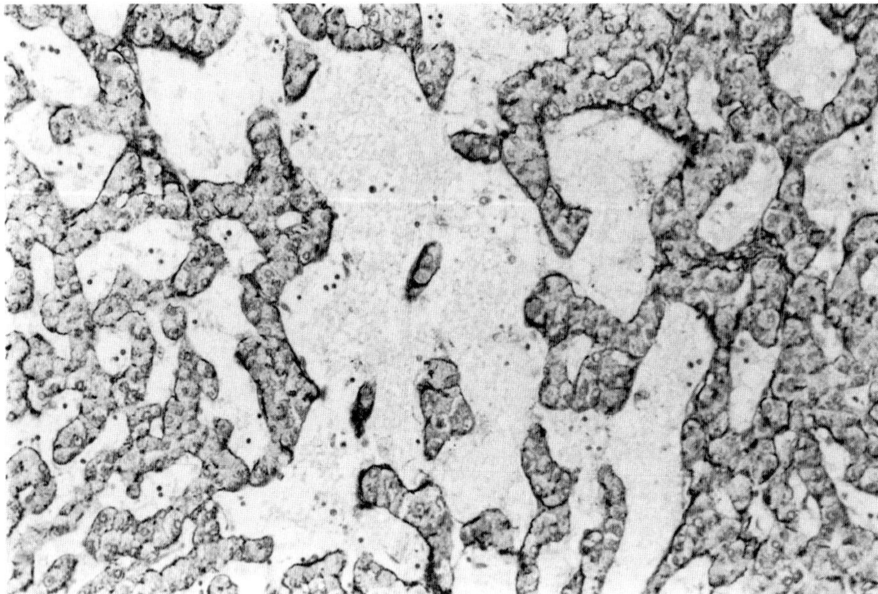

FIGURE 8-6. Peliosis in the nontumorous liver parenchyma of a young woman with hepatocellular carcinoma related to long-term oral contraceptive use. Atrophic plates of hepatocytes are distorted by blood-filling spaces. (Gordon-Sweet stain, ×100.)

Whether these particular tumors were true HCCs or atypical hepatocellular adenomas is unclear. The fibrolamellar variant of HCC has not been found to be significantly related to the use of OC.[116] Estrogens may enhance the vascularity and growth of hepatocytic tumors. This would explain the increased risk of hemorrhage and rupture in OC-related HCCs.[114] Experimental data suggest that estrogens are more likely to promote than to initiate liver cell tumors, but their effects vary widely according to study protocols, gender, strains, and species (see Farrel[117] for review). Estrogen receptors have been demonstrated in the mammalian liver[118]; low concentrations were also detected in 14% to 40% of human HCCs.[119–122] However, studies suggesting that estrogens could stimulate hepatocellular proliferation by stimulating specific receptors[123,124] have not been confirmed by recent studies.[125] This may explain the absence of a significant antitumoral effect of tamoxifen, an estrogen receptor-blocker, in HCC patients.[126]

Progesterone

Injectable progesterone contraceptives have not been found to increase the relative risk of liver cancer in two studies conducted in areas endemic for HBV infection.[112,113]

Hormone Replacement Therapy

Hormone replacement therapy as a risk factor of HCC has not been studied. Although there is evidence of increasing rates of liver cancer over time in some countries, it has not been studied in those where estrogens and/or progestins are used at menopause.[111]

Anabolic-Androgenic Steroid Therapy (AAS)

Several small series and individual case reports suggest anabolic-androgenic steroids may contribute to the development of HCC. However, no case-control study has been reported because of the rarity of such tumors.

The main features of AAS-associated HCCs have been reviewed.[117,127–129] Most patients (81%) were males aged 6 to 68 years.[129] All but two had been treated by 17-alkylated AASs for Fanconi's anemia (27%), aplastic anemia, hypogonadism, improvement of athlete performance, or conditioning in female transsexuals.[129] Abdominal pain and discomfort, weight loss, and fatigue were the most frequent opening symptoms.[127,128] Jaundice was present in 25% of cases at presentation.[127,128] In some patients, HCC was revealed by intratumoral or intraperitoneal hemorrhage.[127,128] In most cases, serum AFP level was normal.[129] Extrahepatic metastasis was rare (four cases), and death was related to liver disease in six patients only.[129] Tumor regression after cessation of AAS therapy was reported in three cases of non-Fanconi's anemia.[129] These findings suggest overdiagnosis of malignancy in AAS-associated hepatocellular tumors.[117,130] Most cases diagnosed as HCC have been well-differentiated tumors occurring in noncirrhotic livers with occasional peliosis hepatis, and cholestasis,[127] which may be difficult to distinguish from adenoma with

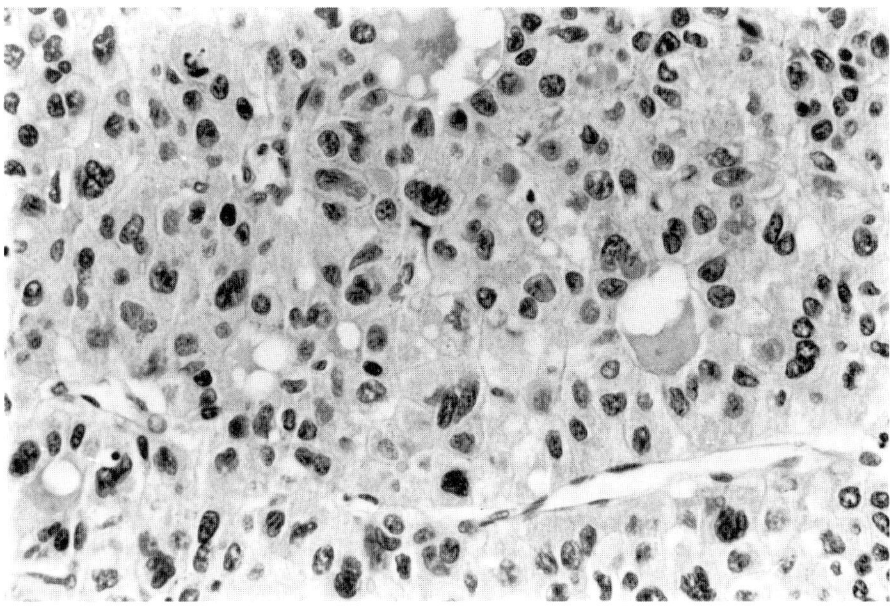

FIGURE 8-7. Liver tumor diagnosed as hepatocellular carcinoma in a 3-year-old girl treated with steroids for Fanconi's anemia. Tumor cells are shown with bizarre large nuclei, often multiple nuclei, and are arranged as thick plates with some acinar figures. (H&E, ×150.)

areas of dysplasia (Fig. 8-7).[131] A few cases of poorly differentiated tumors attributed to AAS use have been described.[134,135] It is possible that these tumors were not related to AASs because they developed in cirrhotic livers in patients with Fanconi's anemia[117,129] with increased risk of viral hepatitis because of repeated transfusions.[133] These patients are also susceptible to malignancy even in the absence of AAS therapy.[134,135]

There is little experimental evidence that AASs are able to initiate liver carcinogenesis in animals,[136] but they act as promotors both in rats with chemically induced tumors[137] and in vitro.[138] Mechanisms by which AASs can promote tumor growth in humans remain poorly understood. Androgen receptors[121,122,139,140] and androgen receptor mRNA[139] have been found in HCC tissues, usually at higher concentrations than in the surrounding liver.[122] It is likely that AASs could modulate cell growth through these receptors. AASs could also act indirectly by modifying the metabolism of exogenous carcinogens through their cholestatic effect or by induction of liver enzymes.[141,142]

ENDOGENOUS HORMONES

HCC is more frequent in males than in females (ratio 3:1 to 8:1). A higher prevalence of cirrhosis and of environmental risk factors in men may account for this difference, as suggested by a recent study.[102] However, based on epidemiologic, biologic, and experimental observations, however, modulation of human hepatocarcinogenesis by estrogens or androgens is plausible.

Epidemiologic Studies

Epidemiologic studies of the effect of gender on hepatocarcinogenesis are difficult to interpret because of inadequate information on associated confounding risk factors, especially HBV and HCV infections. An association between parity and HCC has been reported.[143–145] The relative risk was 1.6 for women with one pregnancy, 3.5[144] with four or more pregnancies, and 3.8 with seven or more pregnancies.[143] Other studies[146,147] failed to find such an association, perhaps because of differences in the prevalence of HBV and HCV infections.[145,147] Lau et al.[148] recorded 29 cases of HCC in pregnant women, 43% (10/23) of whom presented with underlying cirrhosis, mostly related to HBV infection.

Biological Data

Nagasue et al.[149] showed that, in male cirrhotics, the estrone testosterone ratio was higher in patients with HCC than in patients without HCC. Similar findings were reported by Farinati et al.[150] but only in alcohol cirrhosis.

Experimental Data

Studies in rats and mice have shown that chemical hepatocarcinogenesis depends on gender and the hormonal status of the animals.[117]

Autoimmune Diseases

CHRONIC AUTOIMMUNE HEPATITIS (CAIH)

The risk of HCC in CAIH is low, even in patients with long-standing cirrhosis. In a 10-year follow-up study of 124 patients with corticosteroid-treated severe CAIH, Wang and Czaja[151] found only three cases (2%) of HCC. Ryder et al.[152] reported eight cases (3.7%) of HCC in a 9-year follow-up study of 217 patients with treated CAIH. Interestingly, six of these eight HCC cases had evidence of HCV infection (anti-HCV), serum HCV-RNA, or liver HCV-RNA; five had been infected by HCV after the onset of CAIH, usually by blood transfusion. The mean duration between HCV infection and the development of HCC was 7 years. Thus, an unsuspected HCV infection might be involved in cases of HCC complicating CAIH.[152] When associated HCV infection is found, screening for HCC development should be prompt.

PRIMARY BILIARY CIRRHOSIS (PBC)

All studies[153–157] but one[158] have found an excess risk of HCC in PBC. In three large studies,[155–157] HCC was reported in 4.1% to 4.6% of patients with PBC; the cases all occurred in patients over 50 years old with cirrhosis. In two other studies[153,154] with a 5-year follow-up, HCC was found in 2.2% of patients. Loof et al.[158] found that, despite an increase in overall risk for cancer, HCCs were not increased in PBC.

PRIMARY SCLEROSING CHOLANGITIS (PSC)

Five well-documented cases of HCC complicating PSC have been reported (see Votte-Lambert et al.[159] for review). Patients were 26 to 62 years of age; all but one were males. Ulcerative colitis was present in four cases. At least three patients had cirrhosis. Data on HCV infection were not available.[159]

SUMMARY

Almost any chronic liver disease, regardless of its cause, may be complicated by HCC. Most cases of HCC arise in a cirrhotic liver. Therefore, cirrhosis is considered as a major preneoplastic state, but it is not an absolute prerequisite to the development of HCC, as shown by the occurrence of HCCs both in noncirrhotic chronic liver diseases and in otherwise apparently normal livers. In addition, HCC is far from being an inevitable complication of cirrhosis, even long-standing cirrhosis. Thus, hepatocarcinogenesis in humans appears to be a multifactorial process.

REFERENCES

1. Coire C, Quizilbash A, Castelli M. Hepatic adenomata in type Ia glycogen storage disease. Arch Pathol Lab Med 1987;111:166–169
2. Poe R, Snover D. Adenomas in glycogen storage disease: two cases with unusual histological features. Am J Surg Pathol 1988;12:477–483
3. Bianchi L. Glycogen storage disease I and hepatocellular tumours. Eur J Pediatr 1993; 152(suppl 1):S63–S70
4. Leese T, Farges O, Bismuth H. Liver cell adenomas. Ann Surg 1988; 208:558–564
5. Grosmann H, Ram P, Coleman R et al. Hepatic ultrasonography in type I glycogen storage disease (von Gierke disease). Detection of hepatic adenoma and carcinoma. Radiology 1981;141:753–756
6. Limmer J, Fleig W, Leupold D et al. Hepatocellular carcinoma in type I glycogen storage disease. Hepatology 1988; 8:531–537
7. Conti J, Kemeny N. Type Ia glycogenosis associated with hepatocellular carcinoma. Cancer 1992;69:1320–1322
8. See G, Marchal G, Odièvre M. Hépatocarcinome chez un adulte suspect d'une intolérance héréditaire au fructose. Ann Pediatr 1984;31:49–51
9. Poley JR. Malignant liver disease in alpha 1-antitrypsin deficiency. Acta Paediatr Suppl 1994;393:27–32
10. Eriksson S, Carlson J, Velez R. Risk of cirrhosis and primary liver cancer in alpha-1-antitrypsin deficiency. N Engl J Med 1986;314:736–739
11. Rabinovitz M, Gavaler J, Kelly R et al. Lack of increase in heterozygous alpha1-antitrypsin deficiency among patients with hepatocellular and bile duct carcinoma. Hepatology 1992;15:407–410
12. Propst T, Propst A, Dietze O et al. Prevalence of hepatocellular carcinoma in alpha-1-antitrypsin deficiency. J Hepatol 1994;21:1006–1011
13. Govindarajan S, Ashcavai M, Peters R. Alpha-1-antitrypsin phenotypes in hepatocellular carcinoma. Hepatology 1981;1:628–631
14. van Spronsen F, Thomasse Y, Smit GPA, et al. Hereditary tyrosinemia type 1: a new clinical classification with difference in prognosis on dietary treatment. Hepatology 1994; 20:1187–1191
15. Weinberg A, Mize C, Worthen H. The occurrence of hepatoma in the chronic form of hereditary tyrosinemia. J Pediatr 1976;88:434–438
16. Ishak K, Sharp H. Metabolic errors and liver disease. In MacSween R, Anthony P, Scheuer P (eds): Pathology of the Liver. Churchill Livingstone, Edinburgh, 1994, pp. 123–218
17. Manowski Z, Silver M, Roberts E et al. Liver cell dysplasia and early liver transplantation in hereditary tyrosinemia. Mod Pathol 1990;3:694–701
18. Gilbert-Barness E, Barness L, Meisner L. Chromosomal instability in hereditary tyrosinemia type I. Pediatr Pathol 1990;10:243–252
19. Zerbini C, Weinberg D, Hollister K, Perez-Atayde A. DNA

ploidy abnormalities in the liver of children with hereditary tyrosinemia type I. Correlation with histopathologic features. Am J Pathol 1992; 140:1111–1119

20. Dehner L, Snover D, Sharp H et al. Hereditary tyrosinemia type 1 (chronic form). Hum Pathol 1989;20:149–158
21. Nakayama M, Okamoto Y, Morita T et al. Promoting effect of citrulline in hepatocarcinogenesis: possible mechanism in hypercitrullinemia. Hepatology 1990;11:819–823
22. Lim HW, Mascaro JM. The porphyrias and hepatocellular carcinoma. Dermatol Clin 1995;13:135–142
23. Siersema PD, ten Kate FJ, Mulder PG, Wilson JH. Hepatocellular carcinoma in porphyria cutanea tarda: frequency and factors related to its occurrence. Liver 1992;12:56–61
24. Solis J, Betancor P, Campos R et al. Association of porphyria cutanea tarda and primary liver cancer: report of ten cases. J Dermatol 1982;9:131–137
25. Salata H, Cortés J, Enriquez de Salamanca R et al. Porphyria cutanea tarda and hepatocellular carcinoma. Frequency of occurrence and related factors. J Hepatol 1985;1:477–487
26. DeCastro M, Sanchez J, Herrera J et al. Hepatitis C virus antibodies and liver disease in patients with porphyria cutanea tarda. Hepatology 1993;17:551–557
27. Bengtsson N, Hardell L. Porphyrias, porphyrins and hepatocellular carcinoma. Br J Cancer 1986;54:115–117
28. Kauppinen R, Mustajoki P. Acute hepatic porphyria and hepatocellular carcinoma. Br J Cancer 1988;57:117–120
29. Tidman MJ, Higghins EM, Elder G, MacDonald DM. Variegate porphyria associated with hepatocellular carcinoma. Br J Dermatol 1989;121:503–505
30. Germanaud J, Luthier F, Causse X et al. A case of association between hepatocellular carcinoma and porphyria variegata. Scand J Gastroenterol 1994;29:671–672
31. Lithner F, Wetterberg L. Hepatocellular carcinoma in acute intermittent porphyria. Acta Med Scand 1984;215: 271–274
32. Hardell L, Bengtsson N, Johnson U et al. Aetiological aspects of primary liver cancer with special regard to alcohol, organic solvents and acute intermittent porphyria: an epidemiological investigation. Br J Cancer 1984;50:389–397
33. Bach N, Kahn H, Thung SN et al. Hepatocellular carcinoma in a long-term survivor of intrahepatic biliary duct hypoplasia. Am J Gastroenterol 1991;86:1527–1530
34. Keeffe E, Pinson C, Ragsdale J, Zonana J. Hepatocellular carcinoma in arteriohepatic dysplasia. Am J Gastoenterol 1993;88:1446–1448
35. Adams P. Hepatocellular carcinoma associated with arteriohepatic dysplasia. Dig Dis Sci 1986;31:438–442
36. Rabinovitz M, Imperial J, Shade R. Hepatocellular carcinoma in Alagille's syndrome: a family study. J Pediatr Gastroenterol Nutr 1989;8:26–30
37. Le Bail B, Bioulac-Sage P, Arnoux R et al. Late occurrence of a hepatocellular carcinoma in a patient with incomplete Alagille syndrome. Gastroenterology 1990;99:1514–1516
38. Schnittger S, Hofers C, Heidemann P. Molecular and cytogenetic analysis of an interstitial 20p deletion associated with syndromic intrahepatic ductular hypoplasia (Alagille syndrome). Hum Genet 1989; 83:239–244
39. Knudson AJ. Genes that predispose to cancer. Mutat Res 1991;247:185–190
40. Weinberg A, Finegold M. Primary hepatic tumors in childhood. Hum Pathol 1983;14:512–537
41. Quillin SP, Brink JA. Hepatoma complicating Byler disease. Am J Roentgenol 1992;159:432–433
42. Cheng WS, Govindarajan S, Redeker AG. Hepatocellular carcinoma in a case of Wilson's disease. Liver 1992;12: 42–45
43. Kamamoto Y, Makiura S, Sugihara S. The inhibitory effect of copper on diethonine carcinogenesis in rats. Cancer Res 1973;33:1129–1135
44. Yamane Y, Sakai K, Umeda T. Suppressive effect of cupric acetate on DNA alkylation, DNA synthesis and tumorigenesis in the liver of dimethylnitrosamine-treated rats. Jpn J Cancer Res (Gann) 1984;75:1062–1069
45. Tariq MA, Preiss IL. Fluctuations in Fe, Cu, Zn, Br, As, Se, and Rb concentrations in C57L/J mice bearing BW7756 murine hepatoma using radioisotope-induced X-ray fluorescence. Biol Trace Elem Res 1994;42:97–114
46. Powell CJ. Copper-overload causes cancer? The LEC rat: a model for human hepatitis, liver cancer, and much more. Hum Exp Toxicol 1994;13:910–912
47. MacSween R, Scott A. Hepatic cirrhosis: a clinico-pathological review of 520 cases. J Clin Pathol 1973;26:936–942
48. Bomford A, Williams R. Long term results of venesection therapy in idiopathic haemochromatosis. Q Med J 1976; 45:611–623
49. Bradbear R, Bain C, Siskind V et al. Cohort study of internal malignancy in genetic hemochromatosis and other chronic non-alcoholic liver disease. J Nat Cancer Inst 1985; 75:81–84
50. Niederau C, Fischer R, Sonnenberg A et al. Survival and causes of death in cirrhotic and noncirrhotic patients with primary hemochromatosis. N Engl J Med 1985;313: 1256–1262
51. Tiniakos G, Williams R. Cirrhotic process, liver cell carcinoma and extrahepatic malignant tumors in idiopathic haemochromatosis: study of 71 patients treated with venesection therapy. Appl Pathol 1988;6:128–138
52. Fargion S, Mandelli C, Piperno A et al. Survival and prognostic factors in 212 Italian patients with genetic hemochromatosis. Hepatology 1992;15:655–659
53. Deugnier Y, Guyader D, Crantock L et al. Primary liver cancer in genetic hemochromatosis: a clinical, pathological and pathogenetic study of 54 cases. Gastroenterology 1993; 104:228–234
54. Gandon Y, Guyader D, Heautot JF et al. Hemochromatosis: diagnosis and quantification of liver iron with gradient-echo MR imaging. Radiology 1994;193:533–538
55. Deugnier Y, Loréal O, Turlin B et al. Liver pathology in genetic hemochromatosis: a review of 135 homozygous cases, and their bioclinical correlations. Gastroenterology 1992;102:2050–2059
56. Deugnier YM, Charalambous P, Le Quilleuc D et al. Preneoplastic significance of hepatic iron-free foci in genetic hemochromatosis: a study of 185 patients. Hepatology 1993;18:1363–1369

57. Hirota N, Williams G. The sensitivity and heterogeneity of histochemical markers for altered foci involved in liver carcinogenesis. Am J Pathol 1979;95:317–328

58. Fargion S, Fracanzani A, Piperno A et al. Prognostic factors for hepatocellular carcinoma in genetic hemochromatosis. Hepatology 1994;20:1426–1431

59. Stevens R, Jones Y, Micozzi M, Taylor P. Body iron stores and the risk of cancer. N Engl J Med 1988;319:1047–1052

60. Stevens R, Graubard B, Micozzi M et al. Moderate elevation of body iron level and increased risk of cancer occurrence and death. Int J Cancer 1994;56:364–369

61. van Asperen I, Feskens E, Bowles C, Kromhout D. Body iron stores and mortality due to cancer and ischaemic heart disease: a 17-year follow-up study of elderly men and women. Int J Epidemiol 1995;24:665–670

62. Nelson R, Davis F, Persky V, Becker E. Risk of neoplastic and other diseases among people with heterozygosity for hereditary hemochromatosis. Cancer 1995;76:875–879

63. Turlin B, Juguet F, Moirand R et al. Increased liver iron stores in patients with hepatocellular carcinoma developed on a noncirrhotic liver. Hepatology 1995;22:446–450

64. Gangaidzo I, Gordeuk V. Hepatocellular carcinoma and African iron overload. Gut 1995;37:727–730

65. Thompson H, Kennedy K, Witt M, Juzefyk J. Effect of dietary iron deficiency or excess on the induction of mammary carcinogenesis by 1-methyl-1-nitrosurea. Carcinogenesis 1991;12:111–114

66. Hann HW, Stahlhut MW, Rubin R, Maddrey WC. Antitumor effect of deferoxamine on human hepatocellular carcinoma growing in athymic nude mice. Cancer 1992;70: 2051–2056

67. Bergeron R, Streiff R, Elliot G. Influence of iron on in vivo proliferation and lethality of L1210 cells. J Nutr 1985;115: 369–374

68. Hann H, Stahlhut M, Hann C. Effect of iron and deferoxamine on cell growth and in vitro ferritin synthesis in human hepatoma cell lines. Hepatology 1990;11:566–569

69. Park C, Bacon B, Brittenham E, Tavill A. Pathology of dietary carbonyl iron overload. Lab Invest 1987;57: 555–563

70. Stäl P, Hultcrantz R, Moller L, Ericksson L. The effects of dietary iron on initiation and promotion in chemical hepatocarcinogenesis. Hepatology 1995;21:521–528

71. Simson I. Membranous obstruction of the inferior vena cava and hepatocellular carcinoma in South Africa. Gastroenterology 1982;82:171–178

72. Okuda H, Yamagata H, Obata H et al. Epidemiological and clinical features of Budd-Chiari syndrome in Japan. J Hepatol 1995;22:1–9

73. Rector WJ, Xu Y, Goldstein L et al. Membranous obstruction of the inferior vena cava in the United States. Medicine 1985;64:134–143

74. Kew M, McKnight A, Hodkinson J et al. The role of membranous obstruction of the inferior vena cava in the etiology of hepatocellular carcinoma in southern African blacks. Hepatology 1989; 9:121–125

75. Jameson C. Primary hepatocellular carcinoma in hereditary haemorrhagic telangiectasia. Histopathology 1989;15: 550–552

76. Weinstein S, Scottalini A, Loo S et al. Ataxiatelangiectasia with hepatocellular carcinoma in a 15 year old girl and studies of her kindred. Arch Pathol Lab Med 1985;109: 1000–1004

77. Weinberger J, Cohen Z, Berk T. Polyposis coli preceded by hepatocellular carcinoma. Dis Colon Rectum 1981;24: 296–300

78. Zeze F, Ohsato K, Mitani H et al. Hepatocellular carcinoma associated with familial polyposis of the colon. Dis Colon Rectum 1983;26:465–468

79. Laferla G, Kaye S, Crean G. Hepatocellular carcinoma and gastric carcinoma associated with familial polyposis coli. J Surg Oncol 1988; 38:19–21

80. Hakulinen T, Lehtimäki L, Lehtonen M, Teppo L. Cancer mortality among two male cohorts with increased alcohol consumption. J Natl Cancer Inst 1974;52:1711–1714

81. Jensen O. Cancer morbidity and causes of death among Danish brewery workers. Int J Cancer 1979;23:454–463

82. Kono S, Ikeda M, Tokudome S et al. Cigarette smoking, alcohol and cancer mortality: a cohort study of male Japanese physicians. Jpn J Cancer Res (Gann) 1987;78: 1323–1328

83. Shibata A, Hirohatu T, Toshima H, Tashiro H. The role of drinking and cigarette smoking in the excess deaths from liver cancer. Jpn J Cancer Res (Gann) 1986;77:287–295

84. Hirayama T. A large-scale cohort study on risk factors for primary liver cancer, with special reference to the role of cigarette smoking. Cancer Chemothep Pharmacol 1989;23 (suppl):S114–S117

85. Chen C, Yu M, Wang C et al. Multiple risk factors of hepatocellular carcinoma: a cohort study of 13737 male adults in Taiwan. J Gastroenterol Hepatol 1993;8:S83–S87

86. Adami H, Hsing A, McLaughlin J. Alcoholism and liver cirrhosis in the etiology of primary liver cancer. Int J Cancer 1992;51:898–902

87. Lam K, Yu M, Leung J, Henderson B. Hepatitis B virus and cigarette smoking: risk factors for hepatocellular carcinoma in Hong Kong. Cancer Res 1982;42:5246–5248

88. Trichopoulos D, Day N, Kaklamani E et al. Tobacco smoking, hepatitis B virus and ethanol consumption in the etiology of hepatocellular carcinoma. Int J Cancer 1987;39: 45–49

89. Arico S, Corrao G, Torchio P et al. A strong negative association between alcohol consumption and the risk of hepatocellular carcinoma in cirrhotic patients. A case-control study. Eur J Epidemiol 1994;10:251–257

90. Oshima A, Tsukuma H, Hirayama T et al. Follow-up study of HBsAg-positive blood donors with special reference to effect of drinking and smoking on development of liver cancer. Int J Cancer 1984;34:775–779

91. Austin H, Delzell E, Grufferman S et al. A case-control study of hepatocellular carcinoma and the hepatitis B virus, cigarette smoking, and alcohol consumption. Cancer Res 1986;46:962–966

92. Tanaka K, Hirohata T, Fukuda K et al. Risk factors for

hepatocellular carcinoma among Japanese women. Cancer Causes Control 1995;6:91–98

93. Yu M, Tong M, Govindarajan S, Henderson B. Nonviral risk factors for hepatocellular carcinoma in a low-risk population, the non-Asians of Los Angeles County, California. J Natl Cancer Inst 1991;83:1820–1826
94. La Vecchia C, Negri E, Decarli A et al. Risk factors for hepatocellular carcinoma in Northern Italy. Int J Cancer 1988;42:872–876
95. Tsukuma H, Himaya T, Oshima A et al. A case-control study of hepatocellular carcinoma in Osaka. Jpn Int J Cancer 1990;45:231–236
96. Tanaka K, Hirohata T, Takeshita S et al. Hepatitis B virus, cigarette smoking and alcohol consumption in the development of hepatocellular carcinoma: a case-control study in Fukuoka. Jpn Int J Cancer 1992;51:509–514
97. Mohamed A, Kew M, Groeneveld H. Alcohol consumption as a risk factor for hepatocellular carcinoma in urban southern African Blacks. Int J Cancer 1992;51:537–541
98. Nalpas B, Feitelson M, Bréchot C, Rubin E. Alcohol, hepatotropic viruses, and hepatocellular carcinoma. Alcohol Clin Exp Res 1995;19:1089–1095
99. Mandelli C, Fraquelli M, Fargion S et al. Comparable frequency of hepatocellular carcinoma in cirrhosis of different aetiology. Eur J Gastroenterol Hepatol 1994;6:1129–1134
100. Lee F. Cirrhosis and hepatoma in alcoholics. Gut 1966;7: 77–85
101. Ikeda K, Saitoh S, Koida I et al. A multivariate analysis of risk factors for hepatocellular carcinogenesis: a prospective observation of 795 patients with viral and alcoholic cirrhosis. Hepatology 1993;18:47–53
102. Tsukuma H, Hiyama T, Tanaka S et al. Risk factors for hepatocellular carcinoma among patients with chronic liver disease. N Engl J Med 1993;328:1797–1801
103. Naccarato R, Farinati F. Hepatocellular carcinoma, alcohol, and cirrhosis: facts and hypotheses. Dig Dis Sci 1991; 36:1137–1142
104. Henderson B, Preston-Martin S, Edmondson H et al. Hepatocellular carcinoma and oral contraceptives. Br J Cancer 1983;48:437–440
105. Palmer J, Rosenberg L, Kaufman D et al. Oral contraceptives and liver cancer. Am J Epidemiol 1989;130:878–882
106. Hsing A, Hoover R, McLaughlin J et al. Oral contraceptives and primary liver cancer among young women. Cancer Causes Control 1992;3:43–48
107. Neuberger J, Forman D, Doll R, Williams R. Oral contraceptives and hepatocellular carcinoma. Br Med J 1986;292: 1355–1357
108. Forman D, Vincent T, Doll R. Cancer of the liver and the use of oral contraceptives. Br Med J 1986;292:1357–1361
109. La Vecchia C, Negri E, Parazzini F. Oral contraceptives and primary liver cancer. Br J Cancer 1989;59:460–461
110. Tavani A, Negri E, Parazzini F et al. Female hormone utilisation and risk of hepatocellular carcinoma. Br J Cancer 1993;67:635–637
111. Thomas D. Exogenous steroid hormones and hepatocellular Carcinoma. In Tabor E, Di Bisceglie A, Purcell R (eds): Etiology, Pathology, and Treatment of Hepatocellular Carcinoma in North America. Portfolio, The Woodlands, Texas, 1991, pp.67–89
112. WHO Collaborative Study of Neoplasia and Steroid Contraceptives. Combined oral contraceptives and oral cancer. Int J Cancer 1989;43:254–259
113. Kew M, Song E, Mohammed A, Hodkinson J. Contraceptive steroids as a risk factor for hepatocellular carcinoma: a case-control study in South African black women. Hepatology 1990;11:298–302
114. Hromas R, Srigley J, Murray J. Clinical and pathological comparison of young adult women with hepatocellular carcinoma with and without exposure to oral contraceptives. Am J Gastroenterol 1985;80:479–485
115. Thung S, Gerber M. Development of malignancy in benign tumors of the liver. In Tabor E, Di Bisceglie A, Purcell R (eds): Etiology, Pathology, and Treatment of Hepatocellular Carcinoma in North America. Portfolio, The Woodlands, Texas, 1991, pp. 209–215
116. Goodman Z, Ishak K. Hepatocellular carcinoma in women: probable lack of etiologic association with oral contraceptive steroids. Hepatology 1982;2:440–444
117. Farrel G. Hepatic tumors. In Farrel G (ed): Drug-induced Liver Disease. Churchill Livingstone, Edinburgh, 1994, pp. 489–510
118. Eagon P, Porter L, Francavilla A et al. Estrogen and androgen receptors in liver: their role in liver disease and regeneration. Semin Liver Dis 1985;5:59–69
119. Ohnishi S, Murakami T, Moriyama T et al. Androgen and estrogen receptors in hepatocellular carcinoma and in the surrounding liver tissue. Hepatology 1986;6:440–443
120. Nagasue N, Ito A, Yukaya H, Ogawa Y. Estrogen receptors in hepatocellular carcinoma. Cancer 1986;57:87–91
121. Nagasue N, Kohno H, Chang Y et al. Androgen and estrogen receptors in hepatocellular carcinoma and the surrounding liver in women. Cancer 1989;63:112–116
122. Boix L, Bruix J, Castells A et al. Sex hormone receptors in hepatocellular carcinoma. Is there a rationale for hormonal treatment? J Hepatol 1993;17:187–191
123. Fisher B, Ganduz N, Saffer E, Zheng S. Relation of estrogen and its receptor to rat liver growth and regeneration. Cancer Res 1984;44:2410–2415
124. Francavilla A, Di Leo A, Eagon P et al. Regenerating rat liver: correlations between estrogen receptor localization and deoxyribonucleic acid synthesis. Gastroenterology 1984;86:552–557
125. Liddle C, Farrel G. The role of estrogen receptor in liver regeneration in the male rat. J Gastroenterol Hepatol 1993; 8:524–529
126. Castells A, Bruix J, Bru C et al. Treatment of hepatocellular carcinoma with tamoxifen: a double-blind placebo-controlled trial in 120 patients. Gastroenterology 1995;109: 917–922
127. Ishak K. Hepatic neoplasms associated with contraceptive and anabolic steroids. Recent Results Cancer Res 1979;66: 73–128
128. Ishak K, Zimmerman H. Hepatotoxic effects of the anabolic/androgenic steroids. Semin Liv Dis 1987;7:230–236

129. Soe K, Soe M, Gluud C. Liver pathology associated with the use of anabolic-androgenic steroids. Liver 1992;12:73–79

130. Anthony P. Hepatoma associated with androgenic steroids? Lancet 1975;1:685–686

131. Anthony P, Bannash P. Tumours and tumour-like lesions of the liver and biliary tract. In MacSween R, Anthony P, Scheuer P et al (eds): Pathology of the Liver. Churchill Livingstone, Edinburgh, 1994; pp. 635–711

132. Johnson F, Feagler J, Lerner K et al. Association of androgenic-anabolic steroid therapy with development of hepatocellular carcinoma. Lancet 1972;2:1273–1276

133. Gleeson D, Newbould M, Taylor P et al. Androgen associated hepatocellular carcinoma with an aggressive course. Gut 1991;32:1084–1086

134. Sarna G, Tomasulo P, Lotz M et al. Multiple neoplasms in two siblings with a variant form of Fanconi's anemia. Cancer 1975;36:1029–1033

135. Cattan D, Vésin P, Wautier J et al. Liver tumours and steroid hormones. Lancet 1974;1:878

136. Higashi S, Tomita T, Mizumoto R, Nakakuki K. Development of hepatoma in rats following oral administration of synthetic estrogen and progesterone. Jpn J Cancer Res (Gann) 1980;40:3680–3685

137. Reuber M. Effects of age and testosterone on the induction of hyperplastic nodules, carcinomas and cirrhosis of the liver in rats ingesting N-2-fluenyldiacetamide. Eur J Cancer 1976;12:137–141

138. Erdstein J, Wisebord S, Miskin S, Miskin S. Effect of several sex steroid hormones on the growth rate of three Morris hepatoma tumor lines. Hepatology 1989;9:621–624

139. Nakagama H, Gunji T, Ohnishi S. Expression of androgen receptor mRNA in human hepatocellular carcinomas and hepatoma cell lines. Hepatology 1991;14:99–102

140. Nagasue N, Kohno H, Yamanoi A et al. Progesterone receptor in hepatocellular carcinoma: correlation with androgen and estrogen receptors. Cancer 1991;67:2501–2505

141. Paradinas F, Bull T, Westaby D, Murray-Lyon I. Hyperplasia and prolapse of hepatocytes into hepatic veins during long-term methyltestosterone therapy: possible relationships of these changes to the development of peliosis hepatis and liver tumours. Histopathology 1977;1:225–246

142. Taylor W, Snowball S, Lesna M. The effects of long-term administration of methyltestosterone on the development of liver lesions in BALB/c mice. J Pathol 1984;143:211–218

143. Stanford JL, Thomas DB. Reproductive factors in the etiology of hepatocellular carcinoma. The WHO Collaborative Study of Neoplasia and Steroid Contraceptives. Cancer Causes Control 1992;3:37–42

144. La Vecchia C, Negri E, Franceschi S, d'Avanzo B. Reproductive factors and the risk of hepatocellular carcinoma in women. Int J Cancer 1992;52:351–354

145. Tzonou A, Zavitsanos X, Hsieh C, Trichopoulos D. Liveborn children and risk of hepatocellular carcinoma. Cancer Causes Control 1992;3:171–174

146. Hsing A, McLaughlin J, Hrubec Z et al. Parity and primary liver cancer among young women. J Natl Cancer Inst 1990; 84:1118–1119

147. Lambe M, Trichopoulos D, Hsieh CC et al. Parity and hepatocellular carcinoma: a population-based study in Sweden. Int J Cancer 1993;55:745–747

148. Lau W, Leung W, Ho S et al. Hepatocellular carcinoma during pregnancy and its comparison with other pregnancy-associated malignancies. Cancer 1995;75:2669–2676

149. Nagasue N, Ogawa Y, Yukaka H et al. Serum levels of estrogens and testosterone in cirrhotic men with and without hepatocellular carcinoma. Gastroenterology 1985;88: 768–772

150. Farinati F, De Maria N, Marafin C et al. Hepatocellular carcinoma in alcoholic cirrhosis: is sex hormone imbalance a pathogenetic factor? Eur J Gastroenterol Hepatol 1995; 7:145–150

151. Wang K, Czaja A. Hepatocellular carcinoma in corticosteroid-treated severe autoimmune chronic active hepatitis. Hepatology 1988; 8:1679–1683

152. Ryder S, Koskinas J, Rizzi P et al. Hepatocellular carcinoma complicating autoimmune hepatitis: role of hepatitis C virus. Hepatology 1995;22:718–722

153. Farinati F, Floreani A, De Maria N et al. Hepatocellular carcinoma in primary biliary cirrhosis. J Hepatol 1994;21: 315–316

154. Floreani A, Biagini M, Chiaramonte M et al. Incidence of hepatic and extra-hepatic malignancies in primary biliary cirrhosis (PBC). Ital J Gastroenterol 1993;25:473–476

155. Krasner N, Johnson P, Portmann B et al. Hepatocellular carcinoma in primary biliary cirrhosis: report of four cases. Gut 1979;20:255–258

156. Melia W, Johnson P, Neuberger J et al. Hepatocellular carcinoma in primary biliary cirrhosis: detection by alpha-fetoprotein estimation. Gastroenterology 1984;87:660–663

157. Nakanuma Y, Terada T, Doishita K, Miwa A. Hepatocellular carcinoma in primary biliary cirrhosis: an autopsy study. Hepatology 1990;11:1010–1016

158. Loof L, Adami H, Sparen P et al. Cancer risk in primary biliary cirrhosis: a population-based study from Sweden. Hepatology 1994;20:101–104

159. Votte-Lambert A, Samuel D, Reynes M et al. Hepatocellular carcinoma complicating primary sclerosing cholangitis. Gastroenterol Clin Biol 1993;17:604–605

SECTION III
PATHOLOGY OF HEPATOCELLULAR CARCINOMA AND EXPERIMENTAL SYSTEMS

9

PATHOLOGY TECHNIQUES AND GRADING SYSTEMS IN THE DIAGNOSIS OF HCC

ZSUZSA SCHAFF
PETER NAGY

Over the last 10 years, significant progress in the diagnosis and management of hepatocellular carcinoma (HCC) has been achieved with visually guided methods of laparoscopy, laparotomy, imaging techniques such as ultrasonography, and computed tomography and with the extensive use of immunohistochemistry, flow cytometry, and molecular biology.[1–4] The more advanced pathologic methods help to establish the diagnosis in an earlier stage of the tumor development and to clarify the type of the cancer. They can add predictive information for the prognosis of the patient.[4] Despite these improvements, however, the diagnosis of HCC is still problematic in the early stages.[4] This chapter describes the basic and more sophisticated pathology techniques in the diagnosis of HCC. It also addresses the different morphologic classifications and grading systems of HCC currently used and accepted by the scientific community.

PATHOLOGY TECHNIQUES

Tissue Sampling

BIOPSY

Despite progress using noninvasive procedures in the diagnosis of liver diseases, biopsy is still one of the most important tools to establish the diagnosis, to provide prognosis, and to monitor therapy.[5–7] The selection of the best method of biopsy to obtain sufficient tissue for diagnosis of a focal liver lesion including HCC is highly important. The best results can be achieved if the focal lesion is first visualized either directly, by laparoscopy, or indirectly by ultrasonography or computed tomography.[5,7,8] Core or fine needle aspiration on palpable liver masses can be performed without image guidance.[9]

Methods for biopsy include percutaneous,[10] surgical,[5] transjugular,[11–15] laparoscopic,[16,17] or fine needle aspiration.[9,18–22] The choice of method depends on the size and localization of the focal lesion,[5] presence of ascites, portal hypertension, coagulation disorders, and massive obesity.[11–15]

FINE NEEDLE ASPIRATION CYTOLOGY

Cytology[9,18,19,21,23,24] can be used successfully in detection of malignancies, for differentiation of primary and secondary liver tumors[9] and even in the staging.[25] Sampling of lesions that are otherwise unreachable by punch biopsy is sometimes possible by fine needle aspiration.[5] The cytologic characteristics of HCC, based on examining the individual cells, have been described.[26,27] These features include the resemblance of the tumor cells to normal polygonal hepatocytes with central nucleus, eosinophilic and granular cytoplasm, prominent nu-

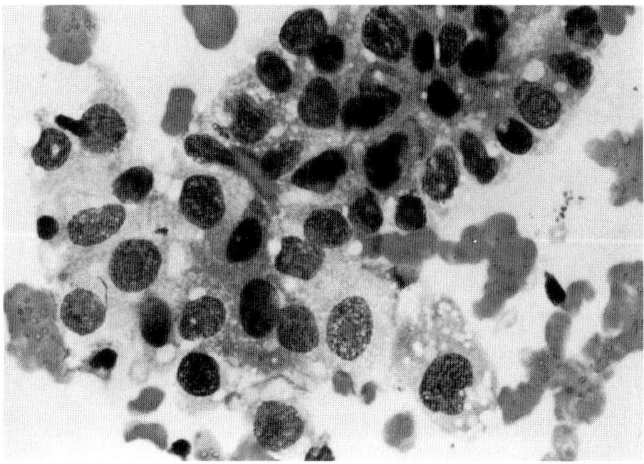

FIGURE 9-1. Fine needle aspiration cytology of HCC. The tumor cells resemble hepatocytes and have large nuclei, prominent nucleoli, and a wide cytoplasm (H&E, ×630).

cleoli, intranuclear pseudoinclusions, giant and multinucleated cells, different forms of cytoplasmic vacuoles, and inclusions such as hyalin globules, Mallory hyalin, and signs of bile secretion[26–28] (Figs. 9-1, 9-2A). Good correlation has been reported between cellular features and cytology and histology[28] (Fig. 9-2). It has been suggested that tumor cells separated or surrounded by sinusoidal endothelial cells, "capping" cell groups, or located around central capillary cores might form characteristic cytologic patterns, which could be classified according to the WHO histologic classification[25,29] as trabecular, pseudoglandular, and compact. The diagnosis and classification of HCC by fine needle aspirate cytology should not be based only on cellular features that might not be characteristic in certain cases and may vary from case to case, but also on their pattern in association with the sinusoidal stroma.[9] Some groups advocate the examination of cell blocks in addition to smears in fine needle aspiration biopsy of focal liver lesions.[23,30–34]

Several fixatives and stains are available for smears taken from HCCs.[9,35] Some authors prefer hematoxylin and eosin (H&E) to Papanicolaou or Giemsa stains for HCC.[9] The air-dried rehydration technique[9,35] has been found particularly satisfactory for HCC because the tumor cells stand out conspicuously against the background.[9]

Another advantage of fine needle aspiration in HCC is the lower risk of complications compared to conventional needle biopsy, especially hemorrhage,[9] which might be particularly dangerous when the HCC is situated near the liver surface.[6] Immunohistochemistry, electron microscopy,[23,33,34,36] flow cytometry, DNA content analysis,[37] and biologic assays[38] can be applied to specimens obtained by fine needle aspiration.

COMPLICATIONS OF LIVER BIOPSY

Liver needle biopsy, particularly fine needle aspiration, is considered a safe procedure, with an overall low mortality rate between 0.01% and 0.1%.[5–7] Bleeding is the most frequent complication of liver biopsy,[5,39] especially in focal liver lesions with a high vascular content or in tumors of vascular origin.[5–7,12,39–42] Bile leakage is less common than hemorrhage, and it is usually associated with biliary obstruction.[7,43,44] Few cases of bacteremia and septicemia[7,45–47] have been reported after liver biopsy. Subcutaneous tumor implantation in the biopsy track rarely occurs.[48]

FIXATION, PROCESSING, AND STAINING

Before performing the liver biopsy, the clinician should know what kind of examination is required to gain the most information from the sample. It is especially important in the diagnosis of focal liver lesions when HCC is suspected. For routine purposes, 10% buffered neutral formalin, maintained for at least 2 to 3 hours, is the best fixative.[3,5] Formalin fixation is usually appropriate for immunohistochemical detection of the majority of antigens as well. Occasionally, however, specific improved preservation methods such as AMeX[49] and rapid freezing of the liver in liquid nitrogen or in a mixture of isopen-

FIGURE 9-2. *(A)* Fine needle aspiration cytology and *(B)* histology of a moderately differentiated HCC. Cytoplasmic inclusions can be seen in both specimens (H&E, ×630).

A

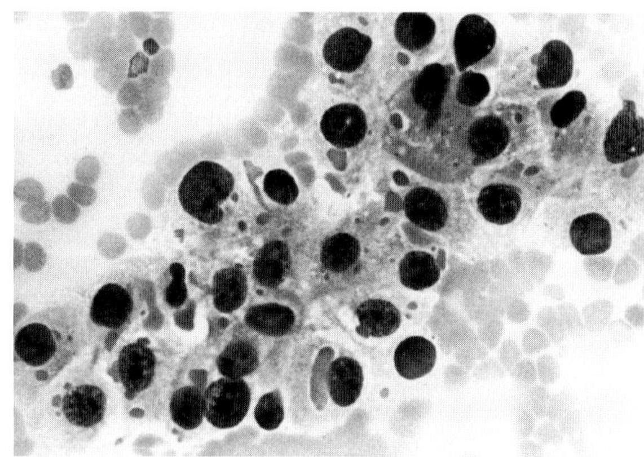

B

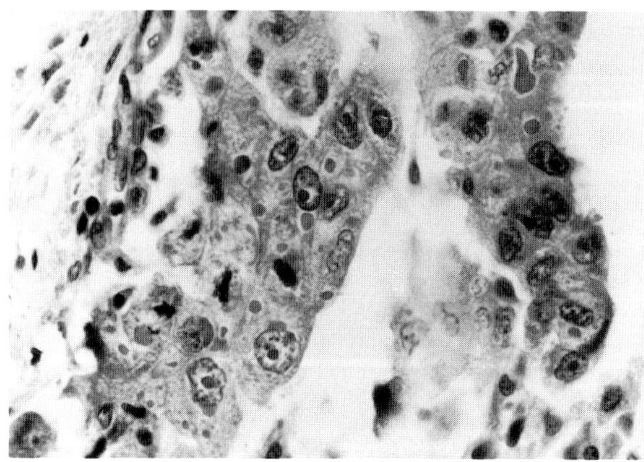

tane and dry ice might be necessary[3,5] for special immunohistochemistry, enzyme histochemistry, and molecular biologic studies.[3,5] The best fixative for electron microscopy is 2.5% to 3% buffered glutaraldehyde.[3,50]

After routine processing and embedding in paraffin, several sections 3 to 5 μm thick should be cut and stained.[51] H&E and several special stains should be used routinely. The periodic acid-Schiff (PAS) reaction is useful in the diagnosis of HCC by detecting glycogen and to differentiate the tumor cells from the surrounding hepatocytes. PAS reaction after diastase digestion (dPAS) detects α-1-antitrypsin globules, fibrinogen, and epithelial mucin, which is useful in the differentiation of mucin-negative HCC from cholangiocellular carcinoma (CCC) or from certain metastatic tumors. Large intranuclear pseudoinclusions occurring in several forms of HCC can be visualized after the dPAS reaction. Stains for connective tissue (e.g., Masson's trichrome) or reticulin stains (e.g., Gomori) outline the differences in the architecture of the tumorous and nontumorous liver and help establish the presence of cirrhosis in the surrounding liver. Shikata's orcein stain, Victoria blue or aldehyde fuchson stains can detect elastic tissue and identify hepatitis B surface antigen (HBsAg).[52] Copper-associated protein can be detected by orcein staining.[53] Iron stains (e.g., Mallory stain or Prussian blue) are important for detection of hemosiderin in the surrounding liver and help show the bile pigment, which might be undetected in H&E staining.[3] The demonstration of nucleolar organizer regions (NOR) might be useful in the differentiation of HCC from benign lesions and to follow the multistep development of nodular lesions in the liver.[54] The proteins associated with the NOR can be silver-stained (Ag-NOR proteins) and can be characterized by argyrophilia.[55–58]

ENZYME HISTOCHEMISTRY

The multistep process of hepatocarcinogenesis has been studied extensively in animals using enzyme histochemistry in the recognition and characterization of early lesions. Enzyme histochemistry requires fresh tissue, snap frozen in liquid nitrogen, and has been used mainly for research purposes.

Changes in the activity of key enzymes such as glucose-6-phosphatase (G6Pase), γ-glutamyl transpeptidase (GGT), membrane-bound adenosine triphosphatase (ATPase), β-glucuronidase, serine hydratase, and acid phosphatase also can be observed in human hepatic tumors.[59–62]

Enzymes characteristic of mature hepatocytes, especially G6Pase and canalicular ATPase, are usually decreased during tumor development, while those characteristic of fetal cell types (for example GGT) reappear.

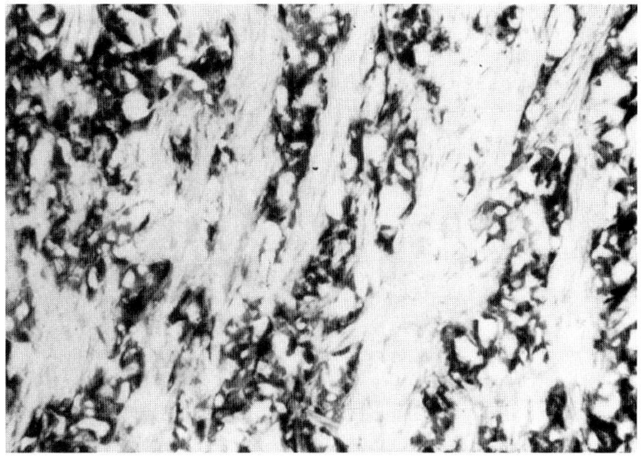

FIGURE 9-3. Strong GGT histochemical reaction in a fibrolamellar HCC. The connective tissue is negative with this stain. (×160.)

However, the enzyme pattern in human liver tumors does not always follow this scheme.[61]

HCCs show an increase in GGT activity (Fig. 9-3), whereas the activities of G6Pase (Fig. 9-4) and ATPase (Fig. 9-5) are lost in the majority of cases, but not all.[59,63] HCCs have in general more variations in enzyme activity than benign liver lesions and nontumorous hepatic alterations such as cirrhosis or chronic hepatitis.[61,64] The pattern of the phenotypic enzyme activity changes in human liver tumors, especially in HCCs, are not as characteristic as in experimental hepatocarcinogenesis models and cannot be used in the differential diagnosis of lesions in human focal liver lesions. Increased activity of GGT and loss of ATPase were observed in most cases of focal nodular hyperplasia.[59] Hepatocellular adenomas presented ATPase and G6Pase activity but not GGT.[59,62]

IMMUNOHISTOCHEMISTRY

Several stains can be used to prove the epithelial origin of the tumor and/or to detect proliferative activity. This can be useful in the differential diagnosis of HCC.

Cytokeratins

Cytokeratins (CK) and epithelial membrane antigen (EMA) are considered useful markers of epithelial origin.[65–69] Adult hepatocytes express CK8 and CK18, while biliary epithelial cells also express CK7 and CK19.[70,71] It was previously thought that HCC, cholangiocellular carcinoma (CCC), and metastatic tumors could be distinguished based on CK expression.[65,67] However, 50% of HCC cases express bile duct type CK (CK7, CK19), in addition to CK8 and CK18.[68] This may perhaps indicate that the CK pattern is not preserved during hepatocarcinogenesis, that HCCs sometimes ex-

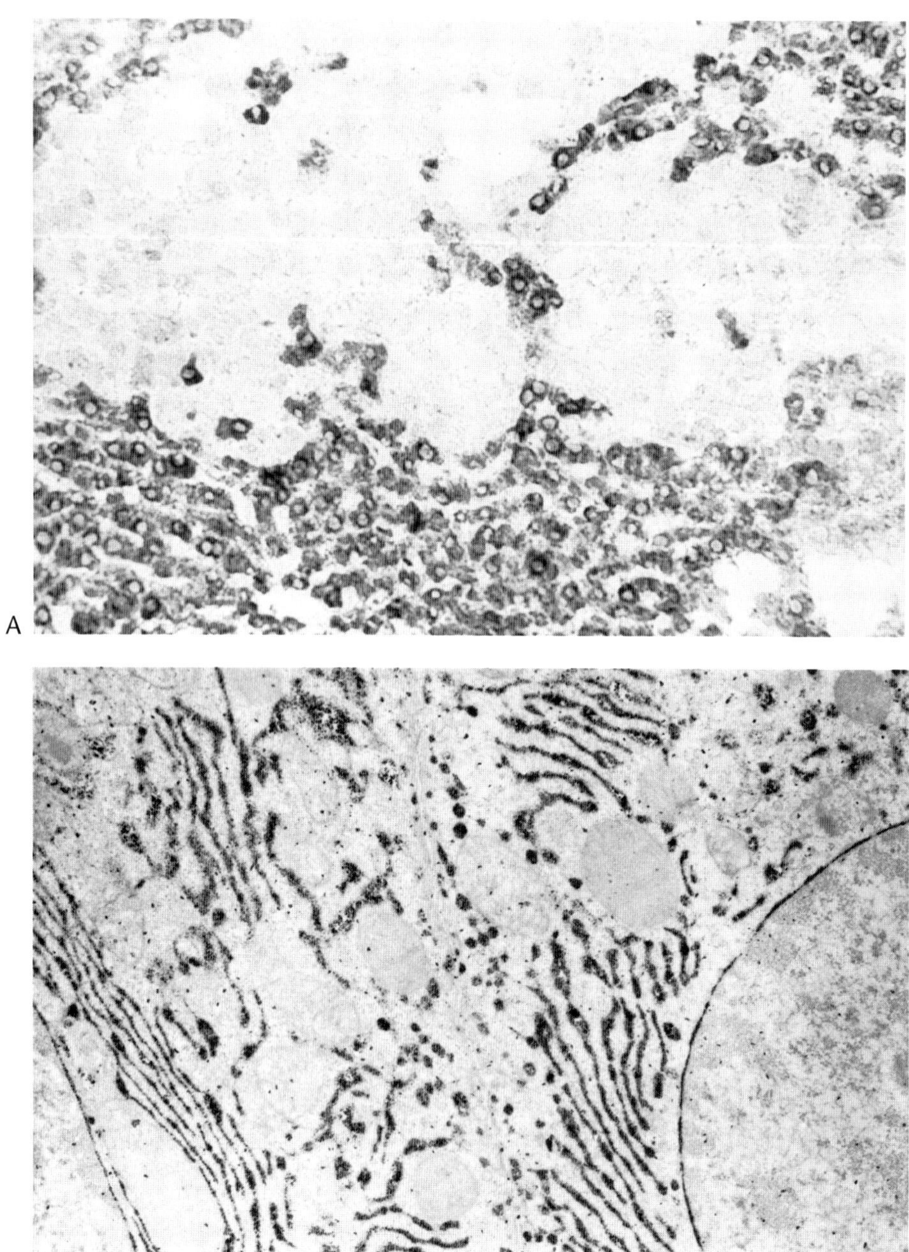

FIGURE 9-4. Strong G6Pase histochemical reaction (black area) in the liver surrounding the HCC cells, which are negative *(A)*. A positive G6Pase reaction in a hepatocyte by electron microscopy *(B)* (Original magnification: Fig. A ×160; Fig. B ×10000.)

press an aberrant differentiation,[72] or that dedifferentiation can occur as part of hepatocarcinogenesis.

Several monoclonal antibodies to cytokeratins with different specificities have been used. CAM 5.2, a monoclonal antikeratin antibody recognizes CK8, CK18, and CK19[73] and reacts with most HCCs.[65] AE1 recognizes CK10, CK14, CK15, CK16, and CK19 and reacts with bile duct epithelium but not with hepatocytes. Some authors have found no reaction of AE1 with HCCs,[65] and others found it reacted with 52% to 70% of HCCs.[33,74] AE3 recognizes all basic keratins, but it does not react with hepatocytes[75]; it reacts with none[76] to 30% of HCCs.[33] Sarcomatoid elements can be identified in both HCCs and CCCs; CK8 has been suggested as an excellent marker in the differential diagnosis of sarcomatoid cancers and metastatic or primary sarcomas of the liver.[77]

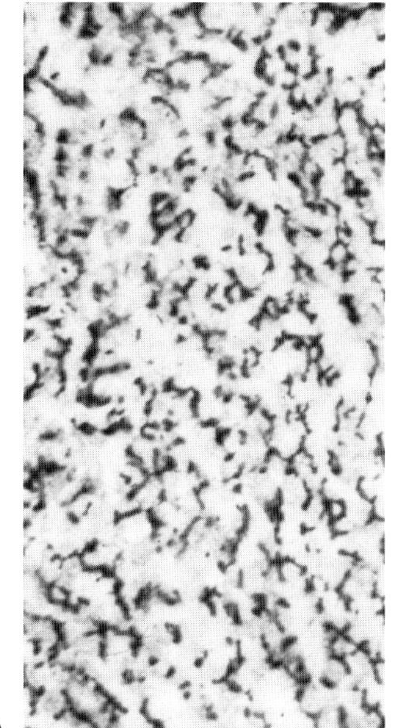

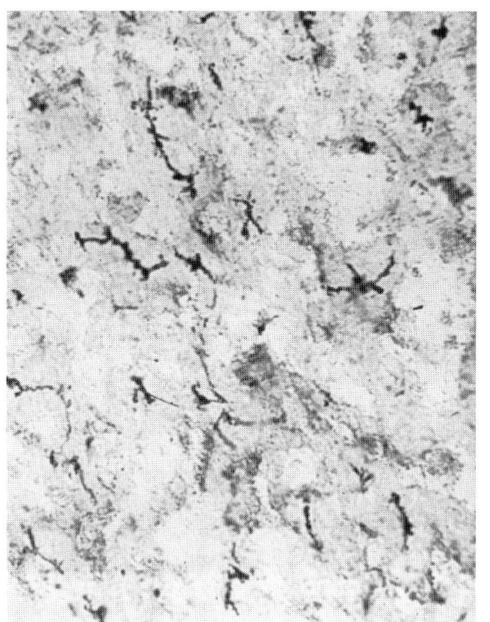

FIGURE 9-5. *(A)* ATPase histochemical reaction outlines the bile canaliculi in the normal liver, but *(B)* it is partly lost in a well-differentiated HCC. (Fig. A ×100; Fig. B ×400.)

Thus, the expression of "bile duct type" CKs in HCCs suggests that the CK profile may not be a reliable way to distinguish HCCs from cholangiocellular carcinoma or from liver metastases.[2,72]

Several other antibodies to epithelial antigens, including Leu-M1, B72.3, HMFG-2, BCA-225, and Ber-EP4, have been used in the differentiation of primary and metastatic liver tumors.[33] BCA-225 was the only monoclonal antibody in which there was a significant difference between HCC and metastatic adenocarcinomas.[33] Cholangiocellular carcinomas had a staining profile similar to that of metastatic carcinoma.[33]

Carcinoembryonic Antigen

Many studies suggested the usefulness of carcinoembryonic antigen (CEA) in distinguishing HCCs from metastatic carcinomas in the liver, especially those from the gastrointestinal tract.[76,78–83] The detection rate of CEA with a monoclonal antibody in HCCs is low[66,78,79,81,82] compared to CCCs and metastatic tumors of endodermal origin, in which it is positive in the majority of cases. A polyclonal-antibody to CEA (pCEA), however, outlined a bile canalicular staining pattern in 71% of HCCs, but it was absent in all metastatic carcinomas and cholangiocarcinomas.[33] Reaction with pCEA is also useful in hepatic fine needle aspiration specimens; a canalicular staining pattern is an indication of benign or malignant hepatocytes.[84,85] The staining of bile canaliculi with pCEA antibody results from cross-reactivity with biliary

FIGURE 9-6. Immunohistochemical detection of *(A)* TGF-α and *(B)* HBsAg in cirrhotic tissue surrounding HCC nodule. (×400.)

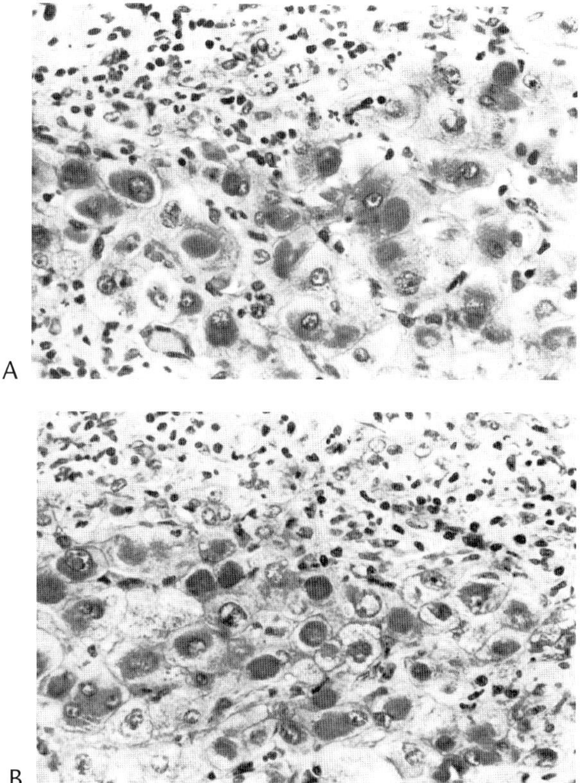

glycoprotein I, which is normally expressed in the glycocalix on the bile canalicular and bile ductal cells.[80] Poorly differentiated HCCs tend to be negative or exhibit a lower percentage of bile canalicular staining for CEA, in contrast to moderately or well-differentiated HCCs.[33]

α-Fetoprotein and α-1-Antitrypsin

Antibodies to α-fetoprotein (AFP) and α-1-antitrypsin (AAT) although commonly used, lack specifity for HCC.[78–81] The expression of AFP in HCC is usually weak in contrast to hepatoblastomas and the normal fetal liver.[2] However, poorly differentiated HCCs may not be positive for bile canalicular-CEA stain but express AFP, which suggests that AFP is still a worthwhile diagnostic stain.[33]

Growth Factors, Adhesion Molecules, and Integrins

Expression of several growth factors, adhesion molecules, and integrins have been studied in primary and metastatic liver tumors and cirrhosis.[86–92] Transforming

FIGURE 9-7. *(A & B)* In situ hybridization with a radioactive TGF-α probe in the same area as in Fig. 9-6 (Autoradiography, no counterstain; Fig. A ×160; Fig. B ×250.)

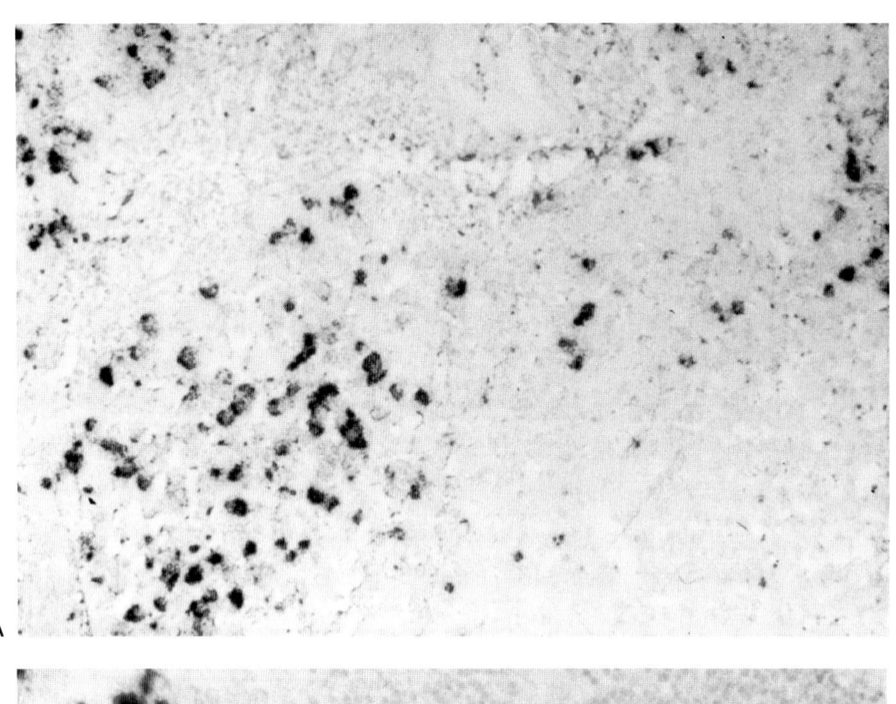

A

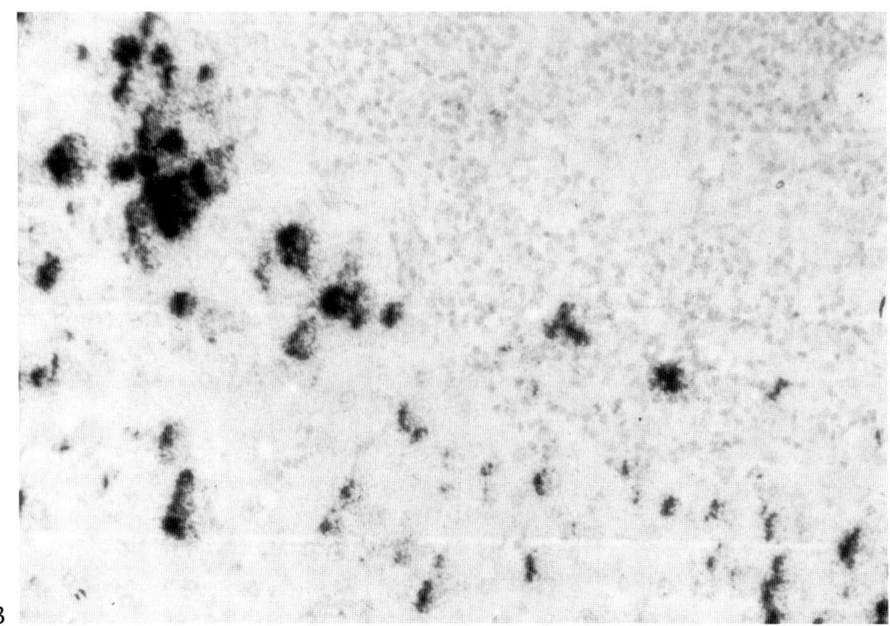

B

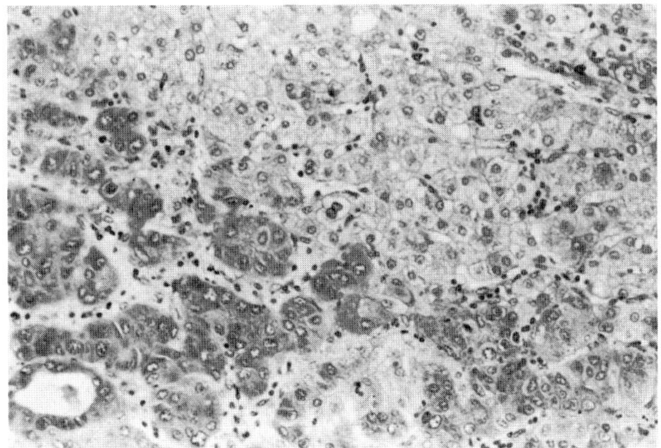

FIGURE 9-8. Strong diffuse cytoplasmic TGF-α immunoreaction in a differentiated, HCC, in contrast to the surrounding liver, which is negative. (H&E ×250.)

growth factor-α (TGF-α) was increased in a majority of HCCs, FNHs, and cirrhotic livers[86,87,89] (Figs. 9-6 to 9-8). Hepatitis B virus (HBV) up-regulated the expression of TGF-α[86–88] and HBsAg expression co-localized with increased TGF-α by immunohistochemistry (Fig. 9-6). The increased expression of TGF-α can be proved by in situ hybridization as well (Fig. 9-7). The TGF-α-positive HCC cells are clearly separated from the negative surrounding hepatocytes (Fig. 9-8).

Up-regulation of the CD44 adhesion molecule in poorly differentiated HCCs and down-regulation in metastatic tumors were found.[90] Integrins were down-regulated in poorly differentiated HCCs, and a relatively high activity of integrins α-2, α-3 and β-1 in metastatic tumors was observed.[90] Detection of the VLA-α1 and VLA-β4 integrin subunits, which highlight the cellular phenotypes of HCC and CCC, respectively, might be helpful in the differential diagnosis between the two tumors.[91] The differences in integrin receptor expression by HCC and CCC might be responsible for the altered adhesive properties of the tumor cells.[91] Various endothelium-associated antigens were detected in the sinusoids in HCC to a different extent than in normal and cirrhotic livers.[92] Most specific endothelial markers, such as lectin UEA1 and anti-CD-34, stained large numbers of sinusoids in all of the HCCs investigated.[92] BMA120 and antibodies against von Willebrand factor and CD-31 stained a smaller number of sinusoids and with lower intensity, and they failed to stain the sinusoids in some of the tumors.[90] Staining with anti-CD34 in cirrhotic livers was very weak; this antibody may be useful for distinguishing well-differentiated HCC from nonneoplastic liver tissue.[90]

Oncogenes and Other Markers

Bcl-2 protein, which has a role in prolongating of cell survival by blocking apoptosis, is expressed by bile ductules and small duct epithelium, but not by hepatocytes or large bile duct epithelium.[93] All HCCs studied were bcl-2-negative, in contrast to the high percentage of positive cases among CCCs.[93]

Several markers can be used for evaluation of cell proliferation, including the detection of proliferating cell nuclear antigen (PCNA),[94–98] Ki-67 staining,[99] and DNA-flow cytometry. PCNA is a nuclear protein synthetized in G1/S phase and is related to cell proliferative activity.[94] A significant correlation between the PCNA proliferation index in HCC detected by immunohistochemistry and tumor invasion, histologic grade of HCC, and prognosis has been found.[100–106] Hepatocellular adenoma and HCC have been distinguished by detecting Ki-67 positive cells in the tissue.[107,108] Ras p21 overexpression[109,110] and c-*myc* overexpression[109,111] have been detected in a large proportion of HCCs. p53 gene mutations have been observed in many HCCs in association with HBV-infection and aflatoxin exposure.[112–115] However, positive staining for p53, indicating the overexpression or mutation and prolonged half-life of p53 protein, also was detected in the nuclei of tumor cells of HCCs in geographic areas in which aflatoxin contamination of the diet was low[116] (Fig. 9-9). Altered expression of the retinoblastoma (RB) gene was detected by immunohistochemistry in high percentage of HCC cases.[117,118]

SPECIAL MICROSCOPY TECHNIQUES

Fluorescence and Confocal Laser Scanning Microscopy

Immunolocalization of certain antigens requires the use of frozen sections after short periods of fixation only.[119] Immunofluorescence techniques applied with higher magnification can be achieved using the laser-scanning confocal microscope.[119–121] Newly formed bile canaliculi accompanied by an accumulation of the membrane skel-

FIGURE 9-9. Intensive nuclear immunstaining for p53 in HCC. (No counterstain, ×160.)

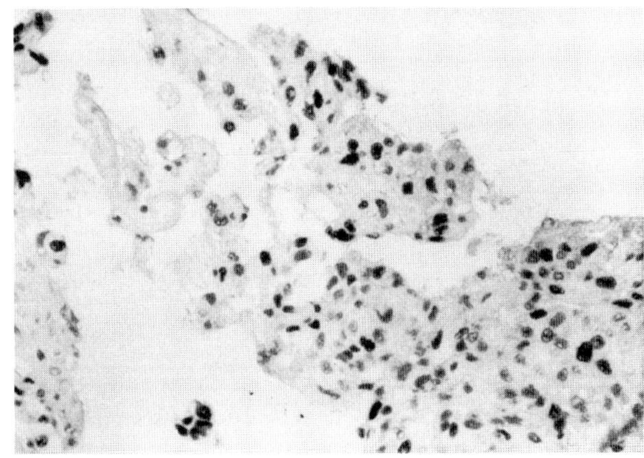

etal protein can be observed by confocal microscopy.[119,120,122]

Polarization microscopy is rarely applied in the examination of liver tumors. It might be useful, however, in studying the portal macrophages, Kupffer cells, and amyloid after congo-red stain, to visualize different foreign, birefringent materials.[3]

Phase contrast microscopy is applied more in association with in vitro experimental studies than in the analysis of human liver tumors in tissue sections. However, Thorotrast particles, for example, can be detected with this method in hemangioendothelioma.[3]

Electron Microscopy

Transmission EM is a useful method to differentiate liver tumors.[123–125] The hepatic origin of the tumor sometimes can be proved by ultrastructural features, such as the presence of bile canaliculi (Fig. 9-10), bile pigment (Fig. 9-10A), sinusoid formation, intranuclear pseudoinclusions (Fig. 9-11), and fingerprint-like organization of the endoplasmic reticulum (Fig. 9-12).[126] The degree of differentiation of the HCC can be followed by EM.[123,124] In well-differentiated HCCs, the trabecular arrangement of the polygonal tumor cells, resembling hepatocytes, bile canaliculi with microvilli and intact tight junctions, bile plugs (Fig. 9-10), and the formation of Disse space-like channels (Fig. 9-13A) can be seen.[123,124] In poorly differentiated HCCs, the prominent, large nucleoli (Fig. 9-11), nuclear membrane invaginations, nuclear pseudoinclusions containing material of cytoplasmic origin (Fig. 9-11), and glycogen rosettes (Fig. 9-13A) help establish the diagnosis.[123]

Different inclusions detected by light microscopy can be analysed by EM. Enlarged giant mitochondria,

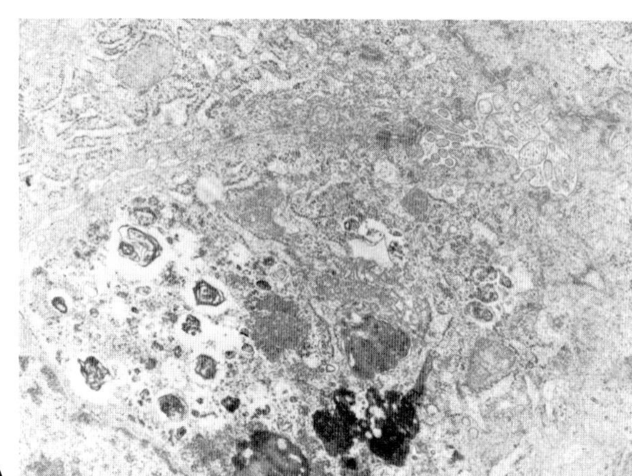

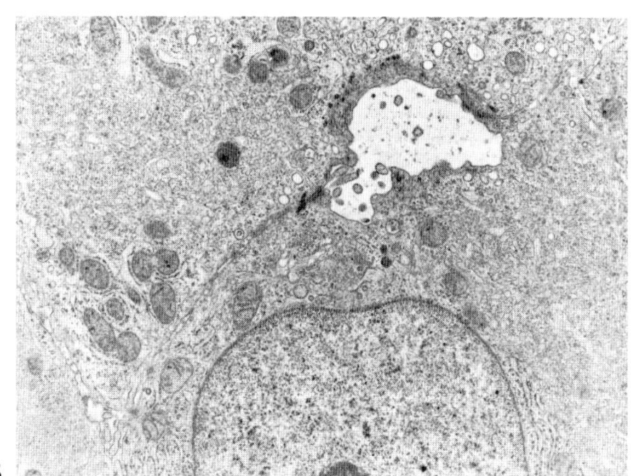

FIGURE 9-10. *(A)* Bile pigment and *(B)* bile canaliculus in a well-differentiated HCC by electron microscopy (Double contrast, original magnification: Fig. A, ×5000; Fig. B, ×3000.)

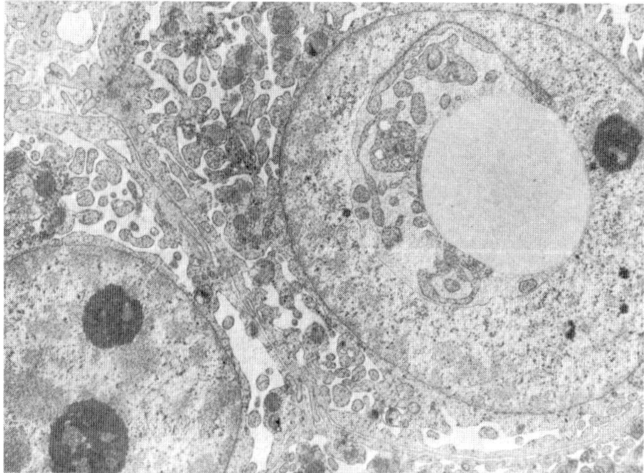

FIGURE 9-11. Intranuclear pseudoinclusions in HCC and papillary endoplasmic reticulum by electron microscopy. (Double contrast, ×3000.)

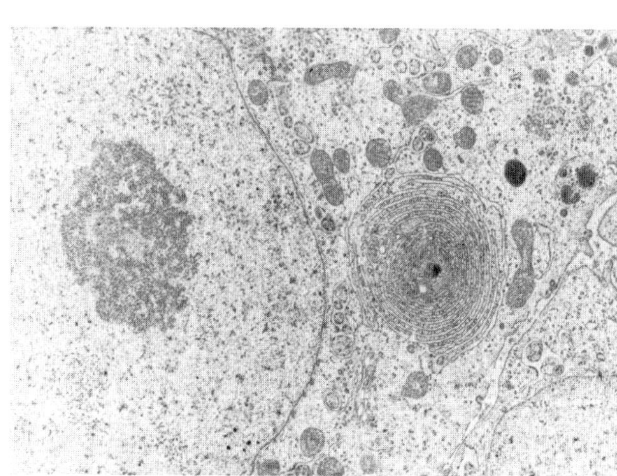

FIGURE 9-12. Fingerprint-like organization of the endoplasmic reticulum in HCC by electron microscopy. (Double contrast, ×3300.)

A
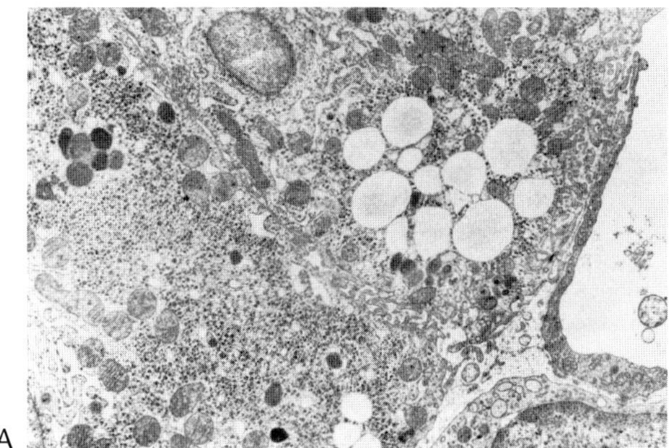

B
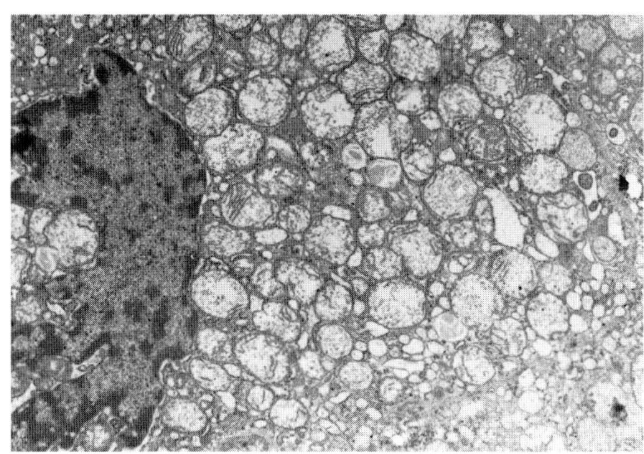

FIGURE 9-13. The cytoplasm is filled with glycogen granules and lipid droplets in clear cell HCC *(A)* and with mitochondria in fibrolamellar HCC *(B)*. (Double contrast, ×3000.)

Mallory bodies, extended endoplasmic reticulum cisternae containing electron dense α-1-antitrypsin, lipid inclusions (Figs. 9-11, 9-13A), cytoplasmic fibrillar inclusions, autophagic vacuoles, and focal cytoplasmic necrosis are common.[123,124]

Special types of HCCs have distinctive ultrastructural features. Clear cell carcinomas contain large fields of glycogen rosettes and a few lipid droplets[124] (Fig. 9-13A). The cells of fibrolamellar carcinoma are packed with organelles, particularly with mitochondria (Fig. 9-13B).[124,127]

Scanning electron microscopy (SEM) has provided considerable knowledge regarding the three-dimensional structure of the liver[123,124]; however, its diagnostic use is limited in liver tumors. The combination of SEM with x-ray analysis may have diagnostic utility in the identification of particulate materials such as Thorotrast, silica, gold, or copper, although it is rarely used in the study of liver tumors.

MORPHOMETRY

Various cytohistologic parameters can be useful for HCCs, particularly in the diagnosis of well-differentiated HCCs. Measurement of cell density (number of cells/mm^2), cell, nuclear and nucleolar size, nucleocytoplasmic ratio, and the index of anisokaryosis help identify preneoplastic foci and nodules, hepatomas, and dysplastic cells.[37,128–138] A morphometric analysis often can differentiate cirrhosis and adenomatous hyperplasia from small and/or highly differentiated HCC[130,131,133]; hepatic nodules presenting a nuclear density greater than two times that of controls can be identified as HCCs.[133] Microtrabecular HCC should be considered when a nodule has a nuclear density exceeding 1.3 times that of the extranodular tissue.[133] Karyometric analysis of liver cell dysplasia and HCC may[135] or may not[137] support the notion of dysplasia being precancerous.

DNA ploidy can be measured by image cytometry of Feulgen-stained sections.[129] The DNA content in small and well-differentiated HCCs was evaluated by densitometry on smears obtained by ultrasound-guided fine needle aspiration biopsy.[37] A progressive increase in aneuploidy was observed in repeated fine needle aspiration biopsies with the increasing size of the nodules.[37] These methods indicated that aneuploidy in adenomatous hyperplasia is an indicator of malignant potential.[136]

These techniques may be particularly useful in cases of early HCC, where diagnosis might be a problem.[134]

Flow Cytometry

Flow cytometry for analysis of cellular DNA from fresh or paraffin-embedded tissues can be useful for establishing a correlation between DNA content, S-phase fraction, and the grade of malignancy or prognosis.[139–147] An elevated fraction of diploid cells and reduction in the polyploid population have been found in human and experimental animal HCCs with an inverse correlation with grading and proliferation rates.[142] Ploidy reductions also were observed in chronic hepatitis and cirrhosis,[142] euploidy also can be found in some HCCs.[144]

Molecular Biology

Molecular biology has an increasing diagnostic application in pathology.[148–154] Analysis of DNA and RNA by Southern and northern blotting, by in situ hybridization (Fig. 9-7), polymerase chain reaction (PCR) and in situ PCR on fresh, frozen, or paraffin-embedded archive material[148,149,151,155] has been widely used in the study of human HCC, including studies to detect sequences of hepatitis B virus (HBV)[156–159] and hepatitis C virus (HCV),[152,160] to detect p53 mutations,[117,158,161–163] changes in RB expression,[117,163–165] and changes in expression of several oncogenes.[117,164,166,167] Overexpression of integrin α-6 may predict a poorer outcome in HCCs.[168] RT-PCR analysis detected sequences of fibronectin isoforms in malignant but not in nonmalignant hepatic tissue.[169] The identification of albumin mRNA by in situ hybridization has also been suggested as a good marker for HCC.[170]

MORPHOLOGIC CHARACTERISTICS AND GRADING OF HCC

Gross Anatomy

Several classifications of HCC have been prepared based on gross anatomy of the tumor. Eggel[171] distinguished nodular, massive, and diffuse types of HCC based on autopsy studies.[1,2,7,172,173] All three forms of HCC could occur with cirrhosis or an otherwise normal liver.[172] The nodular form of HCC consists of large nodules, sharply delineated from the surrounding liver. The massive type of HCC occupies a large area, almost an entire lobule of the liver, and infiltrates the neighboring hepatic tissue with small satellite nodules. In the diffuse type, multiple tumor nodules infiltrate the entire liver. Peters[174] subclassified HCCs into diffuse, multicentric, inductive, expanding, megalonodular, and sclerosing types. A pedunculated[175] and an encapsulated type[176] were recognized as less common growth patterns of HCC. A new classification[176] based on growth patterns of HCC in relation to the surrounding liver parenchyma and blood vessels was suggested[176]: infiltrative (spreading), expanding (solitary), multinodular (multiple), and mixed forms.

More recently, another more detailed classification system for HCC was published based on collaborative study of autopsy material obtained from Japan, the United States and South Africa.[173,177] The expanding (subclassified into cirrhotomimetic, pseudoadenomatous and sclerosing types), spreading (with cirrhotomimetic and infiltrative types), multifocal, and intermediate variants were distinguished.[173,177] The gross appearance of the growth patterns differs in the three geographic areas, possibly correlated with etiologic factors.[173]

HISTOLOGY OF HCC

Histologic Pattern of HCC

Based on the structural organization of tumor cells, the World Health Organization (WHO) proposed the following histologic classification of HCC,[29] which has been accepted and widely used.[1,2,6]

- Trabecular type (sinusoidal): tumor cells are arranged in cords of variable cell thickness separated by sinusoids. Fibrosis is absent or minimal (Fig. 9-14)
- Pseudoglandular type (acinar): tumor cells form glandlike structures. Canaliculi with or without bile are common. Glandlike spaces may derive from central degeneration and are filled with cellular debris, exudate, and macrophages (Fig. 9-15)
- Compact type: solid mass of cells, sinusoids are inconspicuous (Figs. 9-16, 9-17)
- Scirrhous type: significant fibrous stroma separating cords of tumor cells (Fig. 9-17).

FIGURE 9-14. Grade I trabecular HCC. The tumor contains vascular channels and the cells are arranged in cords (trabecules). (H&E, ×160.)

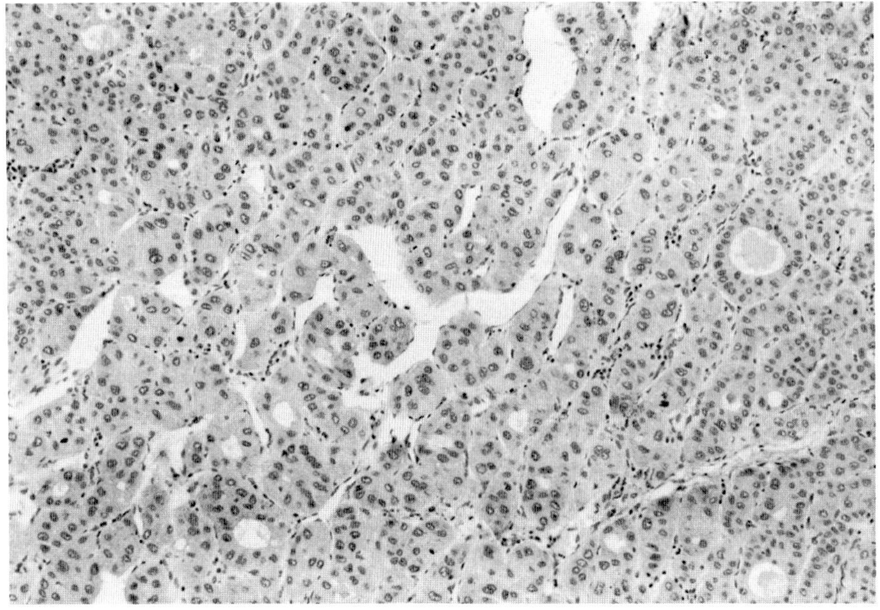

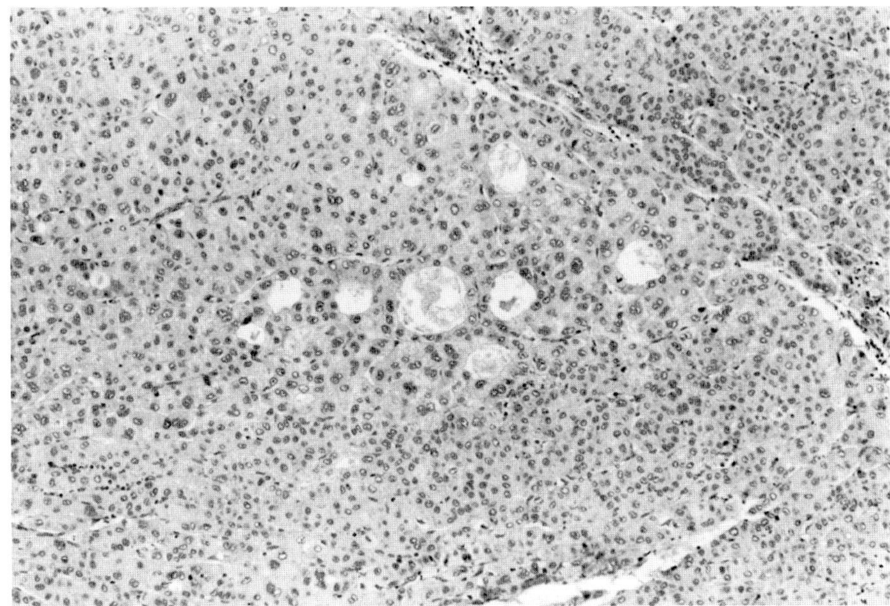

FIGURE 9-15. Grade II HCC. Trabecular and pseudoglandular pattern can be seen. (H&E, ×160.)

At the edges of the tumor and surrounding liver border, the histologic growth patterns have been classified as replacing or sinusoidal patterns.[179]

In the replacing pattern, the tumor cells grow as if they were replacing the hepatocytes in the liver cell trabecules (Fig. 9-18). This can be demonstrated by silver impregnation stains.

In the sinusoidal growth pattern, the tumor cells grow in the sinusoids. Cords of atrophic hepatocytes can be seen at the borders of the tumor infiltration.

FIGURE 9-16. Grade III HCC. Solid mass of cells, occasional trabecule formation, and nuclear polymorphism. (H&E, ×160.)

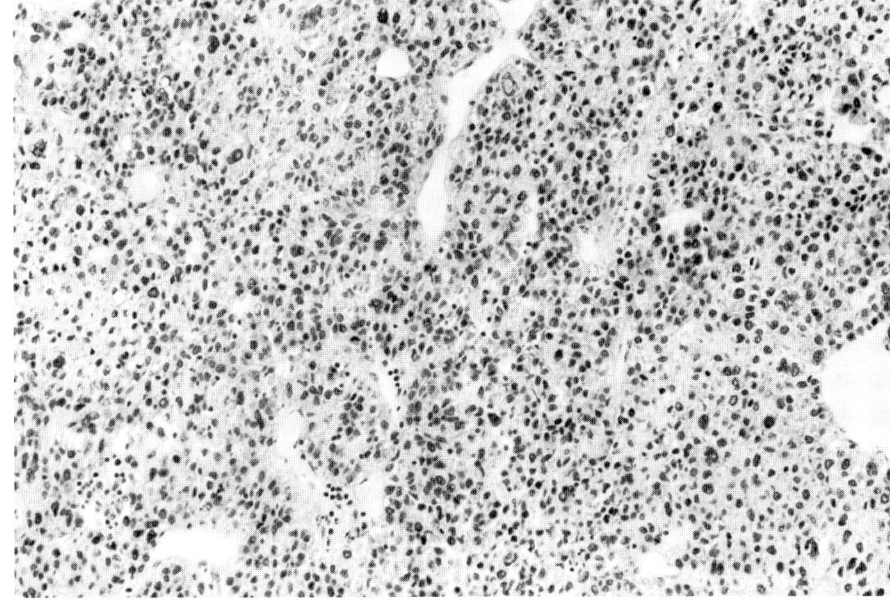

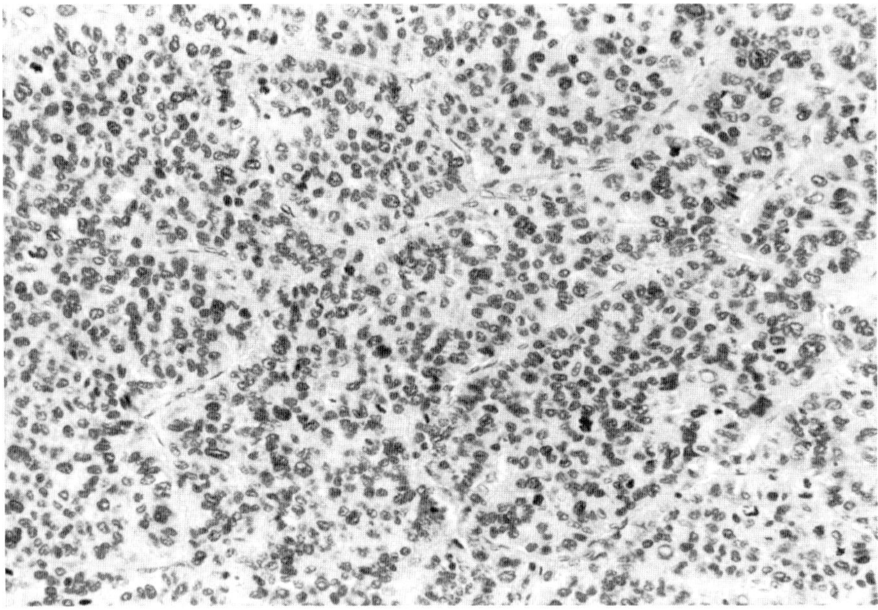

FIGURE 9-17. Grade IV HCC. Compact type, no trabecule formation (H&E, ×160).

Cytologic Variations

The cells of "typical" HCC share certain features with hepatocytes[1,2,6,29,172,173] (Fig. 9-19). Variations from these include the following:

- Hepatic: The most common cytologic variation. The tumor cells are polygonal with large eosinophilic cytoplasm rich in organelles[50] (Fig. 9-20).
- Pleomorphic: Wide differences in cell size and shape. Bizarre giant cells are common (Fig. 9-21).
- Clear cell: Result from the presence of glycogen and fat (Figs. 9-13A, 9-22). This type might be confused with renal cell carcinoma. Clear cells can be predominant but usually occupy only part of the HCC and have been suggested to be associated with better prognosis,[180–183] although this has not been confirmed by others.[184,185]
- Oncocyte-like cells: Characterized by eosinophilic cytoplasm caused by the large number of mitochondria; these occur mainly in the fibrolamellar variant of HCC (Figs. 9-13B, 9-23).
- Spindle cells, small cells, rhabdoid cells, etc. occur occasionally (Fig. 9-24).

Inclusions of several types located in the nuclei and cytoplasm of tumor cells are common findings. The more significant and common ones are the nuclear pseudoinclusions (Figs. 9-11, 9-19), Mallory hyalin, globular hyalin bodies, pale bodies, ground-glass inclusions, and pigment granules.[1,2,29,50]

Degree of Differentiation and Grading of HCC

The basic criteria of grading HCC include cytoplasmic eosinophilia, nuclear chromatism, nuclear cytoplasmic ratio, cohesiveness of the tumor cells, bile secretion, and histologic structure.[173] Edmondson and Steiner[172] divided HCC into four grades from I to IV. Many HCCs, however, contain more than one grade of tumor, usually in areas separated from each other by fine fibrous septa.[1,173]

Grade I HCC is the best preserved highly differentiated form, closely resembling the normal liver (Fig. 9-14). These hepatocyte-like tumor cells are arranged in trabecules as in normal liver. Grade I HCCs constitute only 3.3% of liver tumors,[186] but they can also be found in association with areas of grade II HCC.[172]

Grade II HCC still shows a marked resemblance of tumor cells to hepatocytes (Figs. 9-15, 9-18). The cytoplasm is still eosinophilic, but the nuclei are usually larger and the nucleoli are more prominent. Glandular-like patterns are seen, often filled with bile or proteinaceous material.

Grade III HCC lacks the trabecular or glandular pattern (Fig. 9-16); more single cells or solid groups of tumor cells are isolated from the cords, occasionally intravascular. Tumorous syncytial giant cells and bizarre hyperchromatic nuclei are numerous (Fig. 9-16). The nuclear/cytoplasmic ratio is increased and the cytoplasm is less acidophilic.

Grade IV HCC has large, hyperchromatic nuclei that often occupy almost the entire cell (Fig. 9-17). The

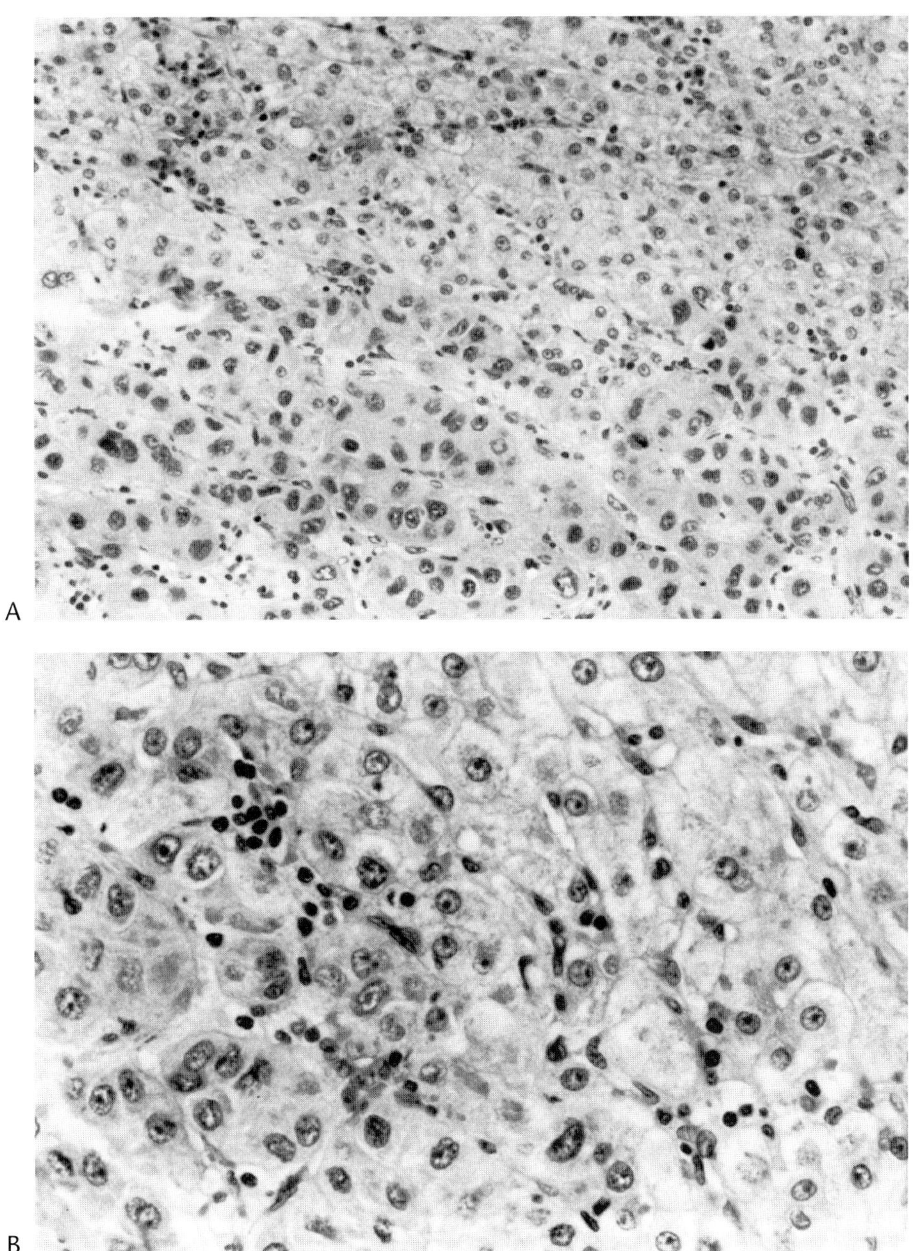

FIGURE 9-18. *(A & B)* "Replacing" pattern of cell growth in HCC. The tumor cells, which have basophilic (darker) cytoplasm and nuclear atypia, grow in trabecules similar to the surrounding hepatocytes. (H&E; Fig. A, ×200; Fig. B, ×400.)

cytoplasm tends to be basophilic. Trabecules or acini are seldom seen. The growth is medullary in character (Fig. 9-17); the cells are loosely coherent. Spindle cells rather than giant cells are common.

Sugihara et al.[187] classified the HCC differentiation into three categories using a slightly different system.

Well-differentiated HCC consist of a trabecular pattern with 2- to 3-cell thick cords. This corresponds to Grade I carcinoma according to Edmondson and Steiner.[172] However, this category also includes tumor areas of intermediate features between Grade I and II (Figs. 9-14, 9-15).

Moderately differentiated HCC have a "typical" trabecular pattern.

Poorly differentiated HCC were divided into three subclasses: (1) trabecular (associated with numerous giant cells) (Fig 9-21), (2) solid (Fig. 9-17), and (3) sarcomatous appearance (Fig. 9-24).

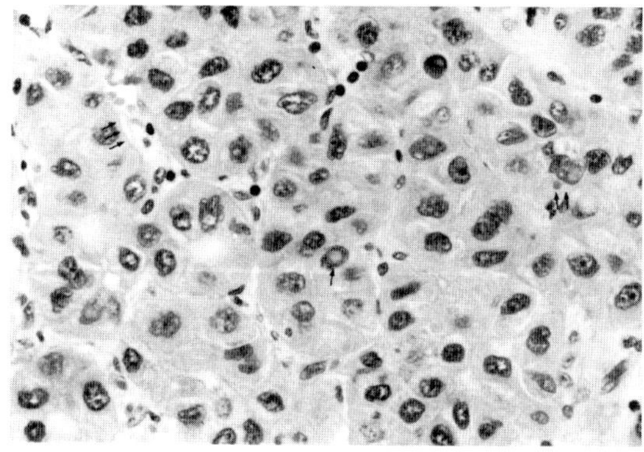

FIGURE 9-19. Nuclear pseudoinclusions (♠), intracytoplasmic bile pigment (♠♠), sinusoid-like spaces (♠♠♠) in a well-differentiated HCC. (H&E, ×400.)

Special Types of HCC

There are distinct subtypes of HCC in which the histology and natural history of the tumor are unique: fibrolamellar carcinoma (Fig. 9-23), clear cell liver-cell carcinoma (Fig. 9-22), pedunculated liver-cell carcinoma, and small or minute carcinoma.

Correlation of Histologic Grading with Other Markers and Biologic Characteristics

The size of an HCC correlates with the degree of differentiation; HCCs smaller than 20 mm in diameter were well-differentiated; tumors larger than 30 mm were moderately differentiated.[189] In comparing the degree of differentiation of HCC less than 20 mm in the biopsy and autopsy specimens of the same patient, it was found that the tumors originally diagnosed as well differentiated at biopsy were moderately differentiated at autopsy[187]; moderately differentiated tumors at biopsy were poorly differentiated at autopsy. Among the tumors larger than 3 cm at biopsy, the histologic type remained unchanged.[187] Data suggest that currently available treatment has no effect on the grade of tumor; among 200 advanced HCCs after treatment, no well-differentiated tumors were found.[187]

Correlation has been found between magnetic resonance (MR) images and histopathologic findings.[190] Hyperintensity on spin echo (SE) T1-weighted images and isointensity on SE T2W significantly correlated with grade I tumors.[188] No MR feature demonstrated significant correlation with grade II or grade III tumors.[188] In another MR study, it was found that on T2-weighted images, grade II HCCs had significantly greater tumor/phantom signal intensity value than grade I HCCs.[189] The nuclear/cytoplasmic ratio was found to be an important factor relating the signal intensity to the histologic grade of HCCs on T2-weighted images.[189]

Based on the study of glucose metabolism with fluorodeoxyglycose in HCC by PET scan technique, the kinetic rate constants and uptake values were significantly higher in poorly differentiated HCCs than in those of more differentiated HCCs.[190]

Proliferation markers, including DNA-content measured by flow cytometry or cytophotometry, have been

FIGURE 9-20. "Hepatic" (liverlike) cytologic variation of HCC. The tumor cells (star) highly resemble hepatocytes (asterisk). (H&E, ×200.)

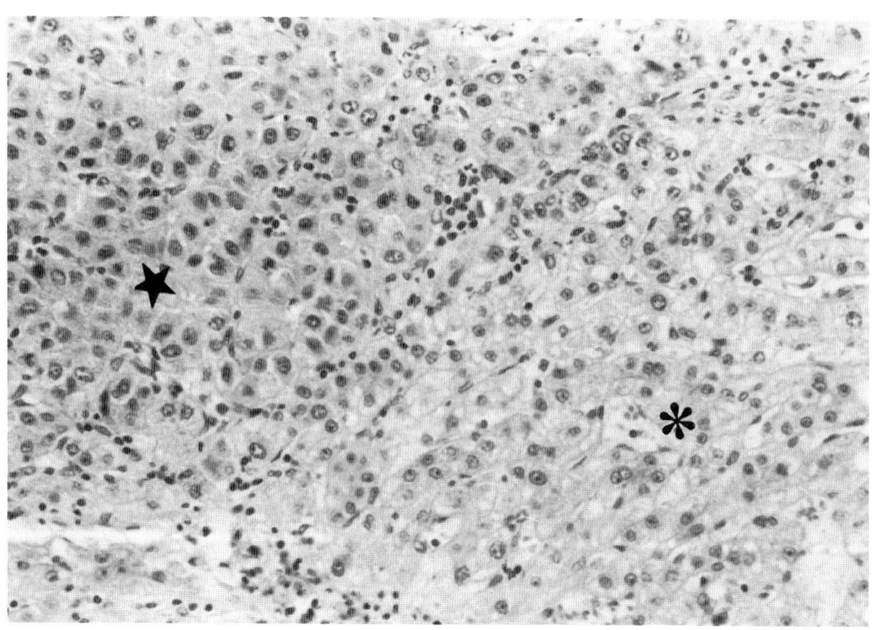

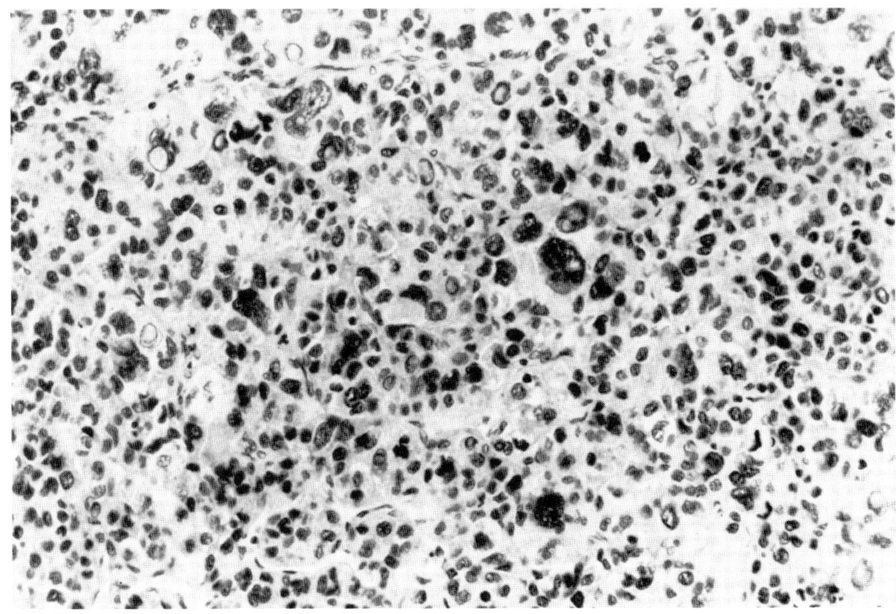

FIGURE 9-21. Pleomorphic variation of HCC. (H&E, ×200.)

correlated in several studies with the degree of differentiation.[149] After an increase in tumor size, the number of nondiploid cases increased.[146] In other studies, the ploidy level showed no correlation with the histopathologic grading.[144,145] The DNA pattern showed no significant correlation with survival rates of 60 patients with HCC who underwent hepatic resection.[146]

PCNA is detected by immunohistochemistry in a higher percentage in poorly differentiated, faster growing HCCs.[98] p53 overexpression corresponded well with PCNA positivity; there was no correlation between c-*myc* overexpression[98] and histologic grading. In a study of 68 intratumoral nodular lesions within 34 HCCs composed of two distinct subpopulations,[191] p53 mutations

FIGURE 9-22. Clear cell variation of HCC. (H&E, ×200.)

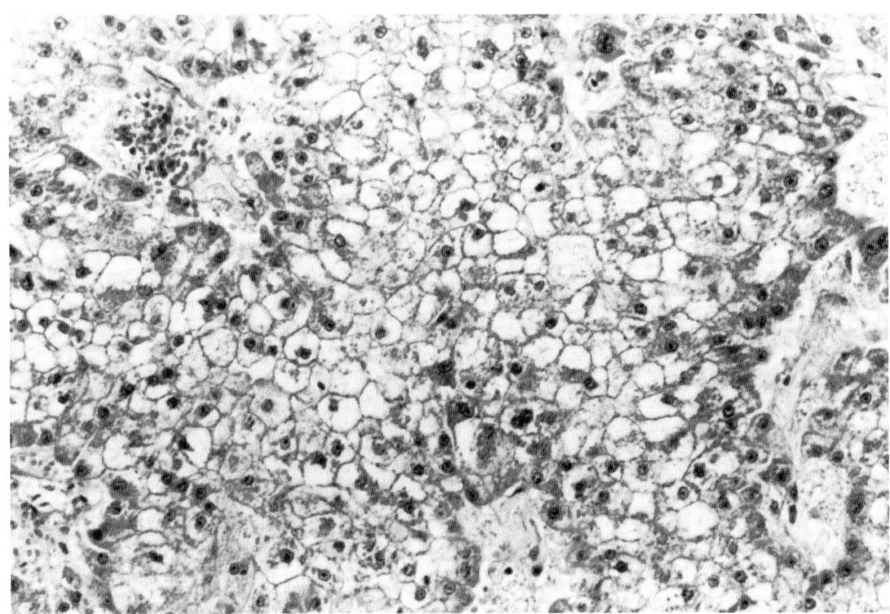

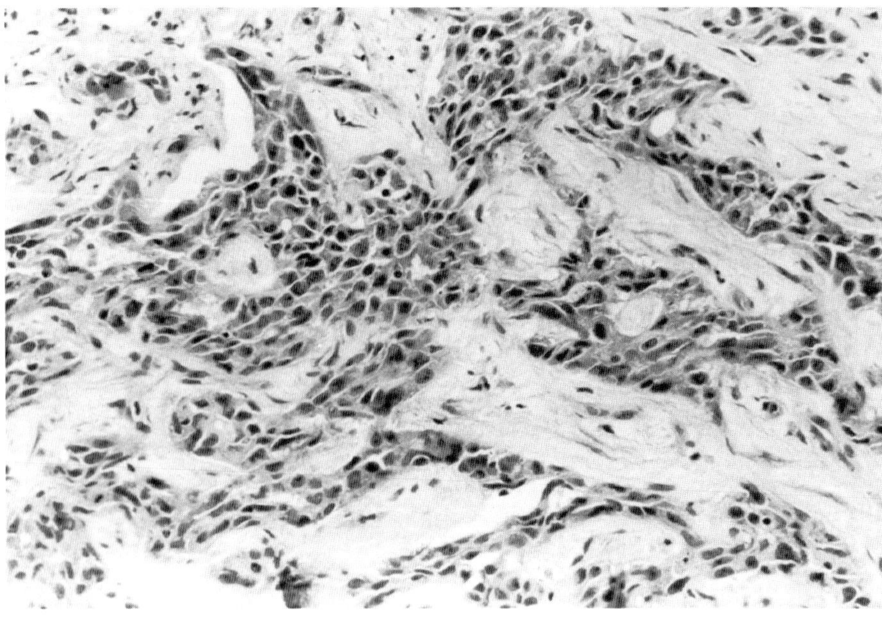

FIGURE 9-23. Oncocyte-like cells in fibrolamellar HCC. (H&E, ×200.)

were found in none of eight grade I lesions and 5 of 29 grade II lesions (17%). Abnormalities of both p53 and of RB have been noted in poorly or moderately differentiated HCCs.[164]

The intensity of immunoreactivity of TGF-α and epidermal growth factor have been reported to be related to the grading of the HCC, with less intense stainings observed in the less differentiated tumor areas.[88] A relationship was detected between positive AFP immunoreaction and poorly differentiated HCC.[192]

Noncirrhotic livers can be divided into two groups: those showing a tendency to increasing grade of dedifferentiation as the degree of fibrosis increases and those showing an inverse correlation between the extent of fibrosis and differentiation.[193] HCCs arising in cirrhotic livers tend to be more differentiated than those in non-

FIGURE 9-24. Sarcomatoid-like cells in HCC. (H&E, ×200.)

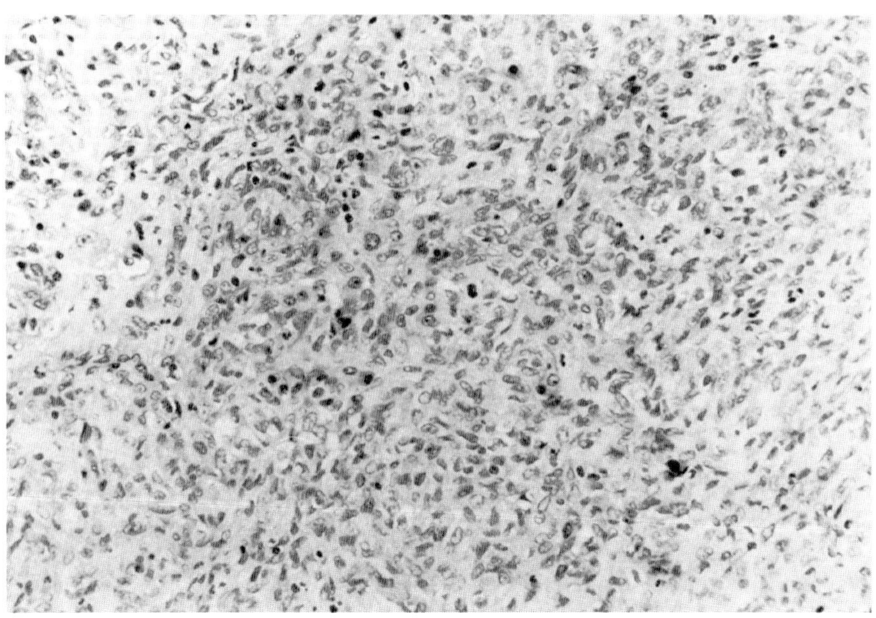

cirrhotic livers.[193] A relationship between the histologic grade of HCC and its metastatizing capacity was demonstrated at autopsy in a study of 100 consecutive cases of HCC associated with cirrhosis.[194]

TNM Classification of HCC

The importance of prognostic factors in cancers, including HCC, has been widely recognized and analyzed in several studies.[195] T(umor) N(odes) M(etastasis) classification is generally the most important indicator for prognosis of patients with cancer.[196–198] Cirrhosis does not affect the TNM classification.[197] In the TNM classification of HCC [196–198] the clinical (cTNM) and pathologic (pTNM) categories correspond to each other.[204] The TNM classification consists of primary tumor size (T), regional lymph nodes (N), and distant metastases (M).

The primary tumor size (T) is classified as follows[196]:

Tx: Primary tumor cannot be assessed

T0: no evidence of primary tumor

T1: Solitary, < 2 cm, without vascular invasion

T2: Solitary, < 2 cm, with vascular invasion

Multiple, one lobe, < 2 cm, without vascular invasion

Solitary, > 2 cm, without vascular invasion

T3: Solitary, > 2 cm, with vascular invasion

Multiple, one lobe, < 2 cm, with vascular invasion

Multiple, one lobe, > 2 cm, with or without vascular invasion

T4: Multiple, > one lobe

Invasion of major branch of portal or hepatic veins.

For the purposes of this classification, a plane projecting between the bed of the gall bladder and the inferior vena cava defines two "lobes" of the liver.[196,197]

The regional lymph nodes (N), the hilar nodes located in the hepatoduodenal ligament,[205] are classified as follows:

Nx: regional lymph nodes cannot be assessed

N0: no regional lymph node metastasis

N1: regional lymph node metastasis

Distant metastases can be absent (M0) or present (M1).[196]

The TNM classification for HCC has been proved to have significant prognostic value in both multivariate[199,200] and univariate analysis[201,202] as for other tumors.[203] After surgical treatment of the tumor, the outcome is influenced by the completeness of tumor removal, which is described by the residual tumor (R) classification as R0, no residual tumor; R1, microscopic residual tumor; and R2, macroscopic residual tumor.[204] The TNM and pTNM consider the extent of the tumor before treatment; the R classification describes the tumor after surgical treatment.[195] There are correlations between TNM and R classification because R0 resection is less frequently possible in higher tumor stages.[195]

REFERENCES

1. Schaff Z, Lapis K, Henson DE. Liver. Pathology of incipient neoplasia. In Henson DE, Albores-Saavedra J (eds): Major Problems in Pathology, 2nd Ed. WB Saunders, Philadelphia, 1993, pp. 151–166
2. Anthony PP, Bannasch P. Tumours and tumour-like lesions of the liver and biliary tract. In MacSween RNM, Anthony PP, Scheuer PJ et al. (eds): Pathology of the Liver. Churchill Livingstone, Edinburgh, 1994, pp. 635–667
3. Ishak KG. Hepatic histopathology. In Schiff L, Schiff ER (eds): Diseases of the Liver. JB Lippincott, Philadelphia, 1993, pp. 145–188
4. The Liver Cancer Study Group of Japan. Predictive factors for long term prognosis after partial hepatectomy for patients with hepatocellular carcinoma in Japan. Cancer 1994;74:2772–2780
5. Thung SN, Schaffner F. Liver biopsy. In MacSween RNM, Anthony PP, Scheuer PJ et al (eds): Pathology of the Liver. Churchill Livingstone, Edinburgh, 1994, pp. 787–795
6. Okuda K, Kojiro M, Okuda H. Neoplasms of the liver. In Schiff L, Schiff ER, (eds): Diseases of the Liver. Lippincott-Raven, Philadelphia, 1993, pp. 1236–1295
7. Schiff ER, Schiff L. Needle biopsy of the liver. In Schiff L, Schiff ER (eds): Diseases of the Liver. Lippincott-Raven, Philadelphia, 1993, pp. 216–225
8. Hansen SW, Jensen F, Pedersen NT et al (eds): Detection of liver metastases in small cell lung cancer: a comparison of peritoneoscopy with liver biopsy and ultrasonography with fine needle aspiration. J Clin Oncol 1987;5:255–259
9. Kung ITM, Chan SK, Fung KH. Fine-needle aspiration in hepatocellular carcinoma. Combined cytologic and histologic approach. Cancer 1991;67:673–680
10. Luning M, Schroeder K, Wolff H, Kranz Hoppe E. Percutaneous biopsy of the liver. Cardiovasc Intervent Radiol 1991; 14:40–42
11. Lebrec D, Goldfarb G, Degott C et al. Transvenous liver biopsy. An experience based on 1000 hepatic tissue samplings with this procedure. Gastroenterology 1992;83: 338–340
12. McAfee JM, Keeffe EB, Lee RG, Rösch J. Transjugular liver biopsy. Hepatology 1992; 14:726–732
13. Coor P, Beningfield SJ, Davey N. Transjugular liver biopsy: a review of 200 biopsies. Clin Radiol 1992;45:238–239
14. Lipchik EO, Cohen EB, Mewissen MW. Transvenous liver

biopsy in critically ill patients: adequacy of tissue samples. Radiology 1991;181:497–499

15. Bull HJM, Gilmore IT, Bradley RD et al. Experience with transjugular liver biopsy. Gut 1983;24:1057–1060
16. Jeffers L, Spiegelman G, Reddy R et al. Laparoscopically directed fine needle aspiration for the diagnosis of hepatocellular carcinoma: a safe and accurate technique. Gastrointest Endosc 1988;34:235–237
17. Fornari F, Rapaccini GL, Cavanna L et al. Diagnosis of hepatic lesions: ultrasonically guided fine needle biopsy or laparoscopy? Gastrointest Endosc 1988;34:231–234
18. Bocking A. Cytological vs histological evaluation of percutaneous biopsies. Cardiovasc Intervent Radiol 1991;14: 5–12
19. Wee A, Nilsson B, Tan LK, Yap I. Fine-needle aspiration biopsy of hepatocellular carcinoma. Diagnostic dilemma at the ends of the spectrum. Acta Cytol 1994;38:347–354
20. Bru C, Maroto A, Bruix J et al. Diagnostic accuracy of fine needle aspiration biopsy in patients with hepatocellular carcinoma. Dig Dis Sci 1989;34:1763–1769
21. Pitman MB, Szyfelbein WM. Significance of endothelium in the fine-needle aspiration biopsy diagnosis of hepatocellular carcinoma. Diagn Cytopathol 1995;12:208–214
22. Wakely PE, Silverman JF, Geisinger KR, Frable WJ. Fine needle biopsy aspiration cytology of hepatoblastoma. Mod Pathol 1990;3:688–693
23. Guindi M, Yazdi HM, Gilliatt MA. Fine needle aspiration biopsy of hepatocellular carcinoma. Value of immunocytochemical and ultrastructural studies. Acta Cytol 1994;38: 385–391
24. Tao LC, Ho CS, McLoughlin MJ et al (eds): Cytologic diagnosis of hepatocellular carcinoma by fine-needle aspiration biopsy. Cancer 1984;53:547–552
25. Dusenbery D, Dodd GD, Carr Bl. Percutaneous fine-needle aspiration of portal vein thrombi as a staging technique for hepatocellular carcinoma. Cancer 1995;75:2057–2062
26. Ali MA, Akhtar M, Mattingly RC. Morphologic spectrum of hepatocellular carcinoma in fine needle aspiration biopsies. Acta Cytol 1986;30:294–302
27. Bottles K, Cohen MB, Holly EA et al. A step-wise logistic regression analysis of hepatocellular carcinoma. Cancer 1988;62:558–563
28. Noguchi S, Yamamoto R, Tatsuta M et al. Cell features and patterns in fine-needle aspirates of hepatocellular carcinoma. Cancer 1986;58:321–328
29. Gibson JB, Sobin LH. Histological typing of tumours of the liver, biliary tract and pancreas. International Histological Classification of Tumours. No. 20. WHO, Geneva, 1978
30. Cochand-Priolett B, Chagnon S, Ferrand J et al. Comparison of cytologic examination of smears and histologic examination of tissue cores obtained by fine needle aspiration biopsy of the liver. Acta Cytol 1987;31:476–480
31. Bognel C, Rougier P, Leclere J et al. Fine needle aspiration of the liver and pancreas with ultrasound guidance. Acta Cytol 1988;32:22–25
32. Pinto MM, Avila NA, Heller CI, Criscoulo EM. Fine needle aspiration of the liver. Acta Cytolo 1988;32:15–21
33. Ma CK, Zarbo RJ, Frierson HF Jr, Lee MW. Comparative immunohistochemical study of primary and metastatic carcinomas of the liver. Am J Clin Pathol 1993;99:551–557
34. Papotti M, Pacchioni D, Negro F et al. Albumin gene expression in liver tumors: diagnostic interest in fine needle aspiration biopsies. Mod Pathol 1994;7: 271–275
35. Chan JKC, Kung ITM. Rehydration of air-dried smears with normal saline. Am J Clin Pathol 1988;89:30–34
36. Bedrossian CW, Davile RM, Merenda G. Immunocytochemical evaluation of liver fine needle aspirations. Arch Pathol Lab Med 1989;113:1225–1230
37. Zeppa P, Vetrani A, Palombini L et al. Evolution of DNA content in small and well-differentiated hepatocarcinoma. Anal Quant Cytol Histol 1993;15:12–22
38. Fukushima H. Subrenal capsule assay using liver cancer specimens obtained by fine needle biopsy. Kurume Med J 1991;38:181–186
39. Cohen MB, A-Kader HH, Lambers D, Heubi JE. Complications of percutaneous liver biopsy in children. Gastroenterology 1992;102:629–632
40. Karpas CM, Parvon EE. Fatal haemorrhage following needle biopsy of hepatic hemangioendothelioma. NY State J Med 1971;71:770–772
41. Kato M, Sugawara F, Okada A et al. Hemangioma of the liver. Am J Surg 1975;129:698–704
42. McGill DR, Rabola I, Zurmeister AR, Ott BJ. A 21 year experience with major haemorrhage after percutaneous liver biopsy. Gastroenterology 1990;99:1396–1400
43. Kelly ML, Mosenthal WT, Milne J. Bile leaking following Menghini needle liver biopsy. JAMA 1971;216:333
44. Conn HO. Liver biopsy in extrahepatic biliary obstruction and in other "contraindicated" disorders. Gastroenterology 1975;68:817–821
45. McCloskey RV, Gold M, Weser E. Bacteremia after liver biopsy. Arch Intern Med 1973;132: 213–215
46. Vincente MVF, Ranz HFM, del Arbol RLK, Bouza EP. Septicaemia as a complication of liver biopsy. Am J Gastroenterol 1981;76:145–147
47. Domingo M, Grau J, Vasquez A et al. Septic shock and bacteremia associated with laparoscopic guided liver biopsy: report on two cases. Endoscopy 1989;21:240–241
48. Goletti O, Chiarugi M, Buccianti P, Macchiarini P. Subcutaneous implantation of liver metastasis after fine needle biopsy. Eur J Surg Oncol 1992;18:636–637
49. Sato Y, Mukai K, Watanabe S et al. The AMeX Method. A simplified technique of tissue processing and paraffin embedding with improved preservation of antigens for immunostaining. Am J Pathol 1986;125:431–435
50. Schaff Z, Lapis K, Sáffrány L. The ultrastructure of primary hepatocellular cancer in man. Virchows Arch A Pathol Anat 1971;352:340–358
51. Luna IG. Manual of histologic staining methods of the Armed Forces Institute of Pathology. 3rd Ed. Mc-Graw-Hill, New York, 1968
52. Shikata T, Uzawa T, Yoshiwara N et al. Staining methods of Australia antigen in paraffin section: detection of cytoplasmic inclusions bodies. Jpn J Exp Med 1974;44:25–36

53. Sipponen P. Orcein positive hepatocellular material in long-standing biliary diseases.I. Histochemical characteristics. Scand J Gastroenterol 1976;11:545–552

54. Aoki K, Sakamoto M, Hirohashi S. Nucleolar organizer regions in small nodular lesions representing early stages of human hepatocarcinogenesis. Cancer 1994;73:289–293

55. Derenzini M, Pession A, Treré D. Quantity of nucleolar silver-stained proteins is related to proliferating activity in cancer cells. Lab Invest 1990;63:137–140

56. Crocker J, McGovern J. Nucleolar organizer regions in normal, cirrhotic and carcinomatous livers. J Clin Pathol 1988; 41:1044–1048

57. Nonomura A, Mizukami Y, Matsubara F, Nakanuma Y. Identification of nucleolar organizer regions in non-neoplastic and neoplastic hepatocytes by the silver-staining techniques. Liver 1990;10:229–238

58. Terasaki S, Terada T, Nakanuma Y et al. Argyrophilic nucleolar organizer regions and alpha-fetoprotein in adenomatous hyperplasia in human cirrhotic livers. Am J Clin Pathol 1991;95:850–857

59. Schaff Z, Lapis K, Henson DE. Liver. In Henson DE, Albores-Saavedra J (eds): Pathology of Incipient Neoplasia. WB Saunders, Philadelphia, 1986, pp. 167–202

60. Schaff Z, Lapis K. Liver cancer and viruses. In Roberfroid MB, Préat V (eds): Experimental Hepatocarcinogenesis. Plenum Press, New York, 1988, pp. 63–76

61. Lapis K, Jeney A, Schaff Z et al. Enzyme pattern changes in preneoplastic and neoplastic lesions of the liver. In Okolicsányi L, Csomós G, Crepaldi G: (eds): Assessment and Management of Hepatobiliary Disease. Springer, Berlin, 1987, pp. 171–186

62. Gerber MA, Thung SN. Enzyme patterns in human hepatocellular carcinoma. Am J Pathol 1980;98:395–400

63. Uchida T, Miyata H, Shikata T. Human hepatocellular carcinoma and putative precancerous disorders. Their enzyme histochemical study. Arch Pathol Lab Med 1981;105: 180–186

64. Taketa K, Shimamura J, Ueda M et al. Profiles of carbohydrate-metabolizing enzymes in human hepatocellular carcinomas and preneoplastic livers. Cancer Res 1988;48: 467–474

65. Johnson DE, Herndier BG, Medeiros LJ et al. The diagnostic utility of the keratin profiles of hepatocellular carcinoma and cholangiocarcinoma. Am J Surg Pathol 1988;12: 187–197

66. Desmet VJ, van Eyken P, Sciot R. Cytokeratins for probing cell lineage relationships in developing liver. Hepatology 1990;12:1249–1251

67. Fischer HP, Altmannsberger M, Weber K, Osborn M. Keratin polypeptides in malignant epithelial liver tumors: differential diagnostic and histogenetic aspects. Am J Pathol 1987;127:530–537

68. van Eyken P, Sciot R, Paterson A et al. Cytokeratin expression in hepatocellular carcinoma: an immunohistochemical study. Hum Pathol 1988;19:562–568

69. Balaton AJ, Nehama-Sibony M, Gotheil C et al. Distinction between hepatocellular carcinoma, cholangiocarcinoma, and metastatic carcinoma based on immunohistochemical staining for carcinoembryonic antigen and for cytokeratin 19 on paraffin sections. J Pathol 1988;156: 305–310

70. Moll R, Franke WW, Schiller DL. The catalog of human cytokeratins: patterns of expression in normal epithelia, tumors and cultured cells. Cell 1982;31:11–24

71. Denk H, Krepler R, Lackinger E et al. Biochemical and immunocytochemical analysis of the intermediate filament cytoskeleton in human hepatocellular carcinomas and in hepatic neoplastic nodules of mice. Lab Invest 1982;46: 584–596

72. Van Eyken P, Desmet VJ. Cytokeratins and the liver. Liver 1993;13:113–122

73. Leader M, Patel J, Makin C, Henry K. An analysis of the sensitivity and specificity of the cytokeratin marker CAM 5.2 for epithelial tumours: results of a study of 203 sarcomas, 50 carcinomas and malignant melanomas. Histopathology 1986;10:1315–1324

74. Battifora H. Diagnostic uses of antibodies to keratins: a review and immunohistochemical comparison of seven monoclonal and three polyclonal antibodies. In Fenoglio CM, Wolff M, (eds): Progress in Surgical Pathology. Vol. 8. Masson, New York, 1988, pp. 1–15

75. Tseng SC, Jarvinen MJ, Nelson WG et al. Correlation of specific keratins with different types of epithelial differentiation: monoclonal antibody studies. Cell 1982;30: 361–372

76. Christensen WN, Boitnott JK, Kuhajda FP. Immunoperoxidase staining as a diagnostic aid for hepatocellular carcinoma. Mod Pathol 1989;2:8–12

77. Haratake J, Horie A. An immunohistochemical study of sarcomatoid liver carcinomas. Cancer 1991;68:93–97

78. Ganjei P, Nadji M, Albores-Saavedra J, Moralkes AR. Histologic markers in primary and metastatic tumors of the liver. Cancer 1988;62:1994–1998

79. Ferrandez-Izquierdo A, Llombart-Bosh A. Immunohistochemical characterization of 130 cases of primary hepatic carcinomas. Pathol Res Pract 1987;182:783–791

80. Koelma IA, Nap M, Huitema S et al. Hepatocellular carcinoma, adenoma, and focal nodular hyperplasia: comparative histopathologic study with immunohistochemical parameters. Arch Pathol Lab Med 1986;110:1035–1040

81. Brumm C, Schulze C, Charles K et al. The significance of alpha-fetoprotein and other tumour markers in differential immunocytochemistry of primary liver tumors. Histopathology 1989;14:503–513

82. Thung SN, Gerber MA, Sarno E, Popper H. Distribution of five antigens in hepatocellular carcinoma. Lab Invest 1979;41:101–105

83. Hurlimann J, Gardiol D. Immunohistochemistry in the differential diagnosis of liver carcinomas. Am J Surg Pathol 1991;15:280–288

84. Rishi M, Kovatich A, Ehya H. Utility of polyclonal and monoclonal antibodies against carcinoembryonic antigen in hepatic fine-needle aspirates. Diagn Cytopathol 1994; 11:358–361

85. Rebello Pinto M, Koelma IA, Kumar D. Fine needle aspiration of focal liver lesions. Cytopathology 1994;5:359–568

86. Hsia CC, Axiotis CA, Di Bisceglie A, Tabor E. Transforming growth factor-alpha in human hepatocellular carcinoma and coexpression with hepatitis B surface antigen in adjacent liver. Cancer 1992;70:1049–1056

87. Schaff Z, Hsia CC, Sárosi I, Tabor E. Overexpression of transforming growth factor-α in hepatocellular carcinoma and focal nodular hyperplasia from European patients. Hum Pathol 1994;25:644–651

88. Morimitsu Y, Hsia CC, Kojiro M, Tabor E. Nodules of less-differentiated tumor within or adjacent to hepatocellular carcinoma: Relative expression of transforming growth factor-α and its receptor in the different areas of tumor. Hum Pathol 1995;26:1126–1132

89. Tabor E, Farshid M, Di Bisceglie A, Hsia CC. Increased expression of transforming growth factor α after transfection of a human hepatoblastoma cell line with the hepatitis B virus. J Med Virol 1991;37:271–273

90. Jaskiewicz K, Chasen MR. Differential expression of transforming growth factor alpha, adhesion molecules and integrins in primary, metastatic liver tumors and in liver cirrhosis. Anticancer Res 1995;15:559–562

91. Volpes R, van den Oord J, Desmet VJ. Integrins as differential cell lineage markers of primary liver tumors. Am J Pathol 1993;142:1483–1492

92. Ruck P, Xiao JC, Kaiserling E. Immunoreactivity of sinusoids in hepatocellular carcinoma. An immunohistochemical study using lectin UEA-1 and antibodies against endothelial markers, including CD34. Arch Pathol Lab Med 1995;119:173–178

93. Charlotte F, L'Herminé A, Martin N et al. Immunohistochemical detection of bcl-2 protein in normal and pathological human liver. Am J Pathol 1994;144:460–465

94. Ng IOL, Lai ECS, Fan ST et al. Prognostic significance of proliferating cell nuclear antigen expression in hepatocellular carcinoma. Cancer 1994;73:2268–2274

95. Hall PA, Levison DA, Woods AL et al. Proliferating cell nuclear antigen (PCNA) immunolocalization in paraffin sections: an index of cell proliferation with evidence of deregulated expression in some neoplasms. J Pathol 1990; 162:285–294

96. Bravo R, MacDonald-Bravo H. Existence of two populations of cyclin/proliferating cell nuclear antigen during the cell cycle: association with DNA replication sites. J Cell Biol 1987;105:1549–1554

97. Mathews MB, Bernstein RM, Fransa BR Jr, Garriels JI. Identity of the proliferating cell nuclear antigen and cyclin. Nature 1984;309:374–376

98. Saegusa M, Takano Y, Kishimoto H et al. Comparative analysis of p53 and c-myc expression and cell proliferation in human hepatocellular carcinomas: an enhanced immunohistochemical approach. J Cancer Res Clin Oncol 1993; 119:737–744

99. van Dierendock JH, Wijsman JH, Keijzer et al. Cell-cycle-related staining patterns of anti-proliferating cell nuclear antigen monoclonal antibodies: comparison with BrdUrd labelling and Ki-67 staining. Am J Pathol 1991;138: 1165–1172

100. Kawakita N, Seki S, Yanai A et al. Immunocytochemical identification of proliferative hepatocytes using monoclonal antibody to proliferating cell nuclear antigen (PCNA/cyclin). Am J Clin Pathol 1992;97(suppl 1): S14–S20

101. Ojanguren JJ. Proliferating cell nuclear antigen expression in normal, regenerative and neoplastic liver. Hum Pathol 1993;24:905–908

102. Taniai M, Tomimatsu M, Okuda H et al. Immunohistochemical detection of proliferating cell nuclear antigen in hepatocellular carcinoma: relationship to histological grade. J Gastroenterol Hepatol 1993;8:420–425

103. Saiki I, Une Y, Uchino J. DNA ploidy pattern, p53 immunohistochemical overexpression and PCNA labelling index in "single nodular" human hepatocellular carcinomas from the viewpoint of biological malignant potential. Gan To Kagaku Ryoho 1995;22(suppl 2):103–109

104. Adachi E, Hashimoto H, Tsuneyoshi M. Proliferating cell nuclear antigen in hepatocellular carcinoma and small cell liver dysplasia. Cancer 1993;72:2902–2909

105. Nishimori H, Tsukishiro T, Nambu S et al. Analysis of proliferating cell nuclear antigen-positive cells in hepatocellular carcinoma: comparisons with clinical findings. J Gastroenterol Hepatol 1994;9:425–432

106. Nakajima T, Kagawa K, Ueda K et al. Evaluation of hepatic proliferative activity in chronic liver diseases and hepatocellular carcinomas by proliferating cell nuclear antigen (PCNA) immunohistochemical staining of methanol-fixed tissues. J Gastroenterol 1994;29:450–454

107. Grigioni WF, D'Errico A, Bacci F et al. Primary liver neoplasms: evaluation of proliferative index using MoAb Ki67. J Pathol 1989;158:23–30

108. Than KW, Okayasu I, Akashi T. Histopathological and immunohistochemical analysis of adenomatosus hyperplasia and hepatocellular carcinoma: cellularity, thickness of cell cord and Ki-67 proliferative activity. Bull Tokyo Med Dent Univ 1995;42:67–81

109. Tiniakos D, Spandidos DA, Kakkanas A et al. Expression of *ras* and *myc* oncogenes in human hepatocellular carcinoma and non-neoplastic liver tissue. Anticancer Res 1989; 9:715–722

110. Nonomura A, Ohta G, Hayashi M et al. Immunohistochemical detection of ras oncogene p21 product in liver cirrhosis and hepatocellular carcinoma. Am J Gastroenterol 1987;82:512–518

111. Lee H, Rajagopalan MS, Vyas GN. A lack of direct role of hepatitis B virus in the activation of ras and c-myc oncogenes in human hepatocellular carcinogenesis. Hepatology 1988;8:1116–1120

112. Ozturk M, Bressac B, Puisieux PL et al. p53 mutation in hepatocellular carcinoma after aflatoxin exposure. Lancet 1991;338:1356–1359

113. Hsia CC, Kleiner DE, Axiotis CA et al. Mutations of p53 gene in hepatocellular carcinoma: roles of hepatitis B virus and aflatoxin contamination in the diet. J Natl Cancer Inst 1992;84:1638–1641

114. Livni N, Eid A, Ilan Y et al. p53 expression in patients with cirrhosis with and without hepatocellular carcinoma. Cancer 1995;75:2420–2426

115. Wee A, The M, Raju GC. p53 expression in hepatocellular carcinoma in a population in Singapore with endemic hepatitis B virus infection. J Clin Pathol 1995;48:236–238
116. Schaff Z, Sárosi L, Hsia CC et al. p53 in malignant and benign liver lesions. Eur J Cancer 1995;31A:1847–1850
117. Farshid M, Tabor E. Expression of oncogenes and tumor suppressor genes in human hepatocellular carcinoma and hepatoblastoma cell lines. J Med Virol 1992;38:235–239
118. Seki S, Kawakita N, Yanai A et al. Expression of the retinoblastoma gene product in human hepatocellular carcinoma. Hum Pathol 1995;26:366–374
119. Vassy J, Rigaut JP, Briane D, Kraemer M. Confocal microscopy immunofluorescence localization of desmin and other intermediate filament proteins in fetal rat livers. Hepatology 1993;17:293–300
120. Vassy J, Rigaut JP, Hill AM, Foucrier J. Analysis by confocal scanning laser microscopy imaging of the spatial distribution of intermediate filaments in foetal and adult rat liver cells. J Microsc 1990;157:91–104
121. Laurent M, Johannin G, Gilbert N et al. Power and limits of laser scanning confocal microscopy. Biol Cell 1994;80: 229–240
122. Sormunen R, Eskelinen S, Lehto VP. Bile canaliculus formation in cultured HEPG2 cells. Lab Invest 1993;68: 652–662
123. Schaff Z, Lapis K. Fine structure of hepatocytes during the etiology of several common pathologies. J Electron Microsc Tech 1990;14:179–207
124. Phillips MJ, Poucell S, Patterson J, Valencia P. The Liver. An Atlas and Text of Ultrastructural Pathology. Raven Press, New York, 1987
125. Tanikawa K. Ultrastructural Aspects of the Liver and its Disorders. Igaku-Shoin, Tokyo, 1979
126. Henderson DW, Papadimitrious JM. Ultrastructural Appearance of Tumors. A Diagnostic Atlas. Churchill Livingstone, New York, 1982
127. Lapis K, Schaff Z, Kopper L et al. Das fibrolamelläre Leberkarzinom. Zentralbl Allg Pathol 1990;136:135–149
128. Okada S, Ishii H, Nose H et al. Intratumoral DNA heterogeneity of small hepatocellular carcinoma. Cancer 1995; 75:444–450
129. Rubin EM, DeRose PB, Cohen C. Comparative image cytometric DNA ploidy of liver cell dysplasia and hepatocellular carcinoma. Mod Pathol 1994;7:677–680
130. Le Bail B, Belleannée G, Bernard PH et al. Adenomatous hyperplasia in cirrhotic livers: histological evaluation, cellular density and proliferative activity of 35 macronodular lesions in the cirrhotic explants of 10 adult French patients. Hum Pathol 1995;26:897–906
131. Kondo F, Wada K, Kondo Y. Morphometric analysis of hepatocellular carcinoma. Virchows Arch 1988;413: 425–430
132. Kondo F, Wada K, Nagato Y et al. Biopsy diagnosis of well-differentiated hepatocellular carcinoma based on new morphologhic criteria. Hepatology 1989;9:751–755
133. Nagato Y, Kondo F, Kondo Y et al. Histological and morphometrical indicators for a biopsy diagnosis of well-differentiated hepatocellular carcinoma. Hepatology 1991;14: 473–478
134. Ferrel LD, Crawford JM, Dhillon AP et al. Proposal for standardized criteria for the diagnosis of benign, borderline and malignant hepatocellular lesions arising in chronic advanced liver disease. Am J Surg Pathol 1993;17:1113–1123
135. Henmi A, Uchida T, Shikata T. Karyometric analysis of liver cell dysplasia and hepatocellular carcinoma: evidence against precancerous nature of liver cell dysplasia. Cancer 1985;55:2594–2599
136. Orsatti G, Theise ND, Thung SN, Paronetto F. DNA image cytometric analysis of macroregenerative nodules (adenomatous hyperplasia) of the liver: evidence in support of their preneoplastic nature. Hepatology 1993;17:621–627
137. Roncalli M, Borzio M, Tombesi MV et al. A morphometric study of liver cell dysplasia. Hum Pathol 1988;19:471–474
138. Ueda K, Terada T, Nakanuma Y, Matsui O. Vascular supply in adenomatous hyperplasia of the liver and hepatocellular carcinoma: a morphometric study. Hum Pathol 1992;23: 619–626
139. Hedley DW, Friedlander MI, Taylor IW et al. Method for analysis of cellular DNA content of paraffin-embedded pathological material using flow cytometry. J Histochem Cytochem 1983;31:1333–1335
140. Cope C, Rowe D, Delbridge L et al. Comparison of image analysis and flow cytometric determination of cellular DNA content. J Clin Pathol 1991;44:147–151
141. Koss LG, Czerniak B, Herz F, Wersto RP. Flow cytometric measurements of DNA and other cell components in human tumors: a critical appraisal. Hum Pathol 1989;20: 528–548
142. Anti M, Marra G, Rapaccini GL et al. DNA ploidy pattern in human chronic liver diseases and hepatic nodular lesions. Cancer 1994;73:281–288
143. Chiu JH, Kao HL, Wu LH et al. Prediction of relapse or survival after resection in human hepatomas by DNA flow cytometry. J Clin Invest 1992;89:539–545
144. Kopper L, Lapis K, Schaff Z et al. Flow cytometric analysis of DNA content in focal nodular hyperplasia and hepatocellular carcinoma. Neoplasma 1991;38:257–263
145. Fujimoto J, Okamoto E, Yamanaka N et al. Flow cytometric DNA analysis of hepatocellular carcinoma. Cancer 1991; 67:939–944
146. Ezaki T, Kanematsu T, Okamura T et al. DNA analysis of hepatocellular carcinoma and clinicopathologic implications. Cancer 1988;61:106–109
147. Schmidt D, Wischmeyer P, Leuschner I et al. DNA analysis in hepatoblastoma by flow and image cytometry. Cancer 1993;72:2914–2919
148. Coates PJ. Paraffin section molecular biology: review of current techniques. J Histotechnol 1991;14:263–268
149. Arends MJ, Bird CC. Recombinant DNA technology and its diagnostic applications. Histopathology 1992;21: 303–313
150. Stanta G, Schneider C. RNA extracted from paraffin-embedded human tissues is amenable to analysis by PCR amplification. Biotechniques 1991;11:304–308
151. Coates PJ, d'Ardenne AJ, Khan G et al. Simplified proce-

dures for applying the polymerase chain reaction to routinely fixed paraffin wax sections. J Clin Pathol 1991;44: 115–118
152. Gerber MA, Shieh YS, Shim KS et al. Detection of replicative hepatitis C virus sequences in hepatocellular carcinoma. Am J Pathol 1992;141:1271–1277
153. Komminoth P, Long AA. In-situ polymerase chain reaction. Virchows Arch 1993;64:67–73
154. Chen RH, Fuggle SV. In situ cDNA polymerase chain reaction: a novel technique for detection mRNA expression. Am J Pathol 1993;143:1527–1534
155. Goodrow TL, Prahalada SR, Storer RD et al. Polymerase chain reactions/sequencing analysis of ras mutations in paraffin-embedded tissues as compared with 3T3 transfection and polymerase chain reaction/sequencing of frozen tumor deoxyribonucleic acids. Lab Invest 1992;66:504–511
156. Diamantis ID, McGandy CE, Chen TJ et al. Hepatitis B X-gene expression in hepatocellular carcinoma. J Hepatol 1992;15:400–403
157. Manzin A, Menzo S, Bagnarelli P et al. Sequence analysis of the hepatitis B virus pre-C region in hepatocellular carcinoma (HCC) and nontumoral liver tissues from HCC patients. Virology 1992;188:890–895
158. Goldblum JR, Bartos RE, Carr KA, Frank TS. Hepatitis B and alterations of the p53 tumor suppressor gene in hepatocellular carcinoma. Am J Surg Pathol 1993;17:1244–1251
159. Paterlini P, Poussin K, Kew M et al. Selective accumulation of the X transcript of hepatitis B virus in patients negative for hepatitis B surface antigen with hepatocellular carcinoma. Hepatology 1995;21:313–321
160. Takeda S, Shibata M, Morishima T et al. Hepatitis C virus infection in hepatocellular carcinoma: detection of plus-strand and minus-strand viral RNA. Cancer 1992;70: 2255–2259
161. Shieh YS, Nguyen C, Vocal MV, Chu HW. Tumor-suppressor p53 gene in hepatitis C and B virus-associated human hepatocellular carcinoma. Int J Cancer 1993;54: 558–562
162. Tanaka S, Toh Y, Adachi E et al. Tumor progression in hepatocellular carcinoma may be mediated by p53 mutation. Cancer Res 1993;53:2884–2887
163. Murakami Y, Hayashi K, Hirohashi S, Sekiya T. Aberrations of the tumor suppressor p53 and retinoblastoma genes in human hepatocellular carcinomas. Cancer Res 1991;51: 5520–5525
164. Hsia CC, Di Bisceglie AM, Kleiner DE et al. RB tumor suppressor gene expression in hepatocellular carcinomas from patients infected with the hepatitis B virus. J Med Virol 1994;44:67–73
165. Ogata N, Kamimura T, Asakura H. Point mutation, allelic loss and increased methylation of c-Ha-Ras gene in human hepatocellular carcinoma. Hepatology 1991;13:31–37
166. Tabor E. Tumor suppressor genes, growth factor genes, and oncogens in hepatitis B virus-associated hepatocellular carcinoma. J Med Virol 1994;42:357–365
167. Stork P, Loda M, Bosari S et al. Detection of K-ras mutations in pancreatic and hepatic neoplasms by non-isotopic mismatched polymerase chain reaction. Oncogene 1991;6: 857–862
168. Begum NA, Mori M, Matsumata T et al. Differential display and integrin alpha 6 messenger RNA overexpression in hepatocellular carcinoma. Hepatology 1995;22:1447–1455
169. Tavian D, De Petro G, Colombi et al. RT-PCR detection of fibronectin EDA+ and EDB+ mRNA isoforms: molecular markers for hepatocellular carcinoma. Int J Cancer 1994; 56:820–825
170. Murray GI, Paterson PJ, Melvin WT. In situ hybridization of albumin mRNA in normal liver and hepatocellular carcinoma with a digoxigenin labelled oligonucleotide probe. J Clin Pathol 1992;45:21–24
171. Eggel H. Ueber das primäre Carcinom der Leber. Beitr Pathol Anat 1901;30:506–604
172. Edmondson HA, Steiner PE. Primary carcinoma of the liver. Cancer 1954;7:462–503
173. Tumors of the liver and intrahepatic bile ducts. In Craig JR, Peters R, Edmondson HA (eds): Atlas of Tumor Pathology (Second series Fascicle 26). Armed Forces Institute of Pathology Washington, 1989
174. Peters RI. Pathology of hepatocellular carcinoma. In Okuda K, Peters RL (eds): Hepatocellular Carcinoma. John Wiley, New York, 1976, pp. 107–169
175. Horie Y, Katoh S, Yoshida H et al. Pedunculated hepatocellular carcinoma. Report of three cases and review of literature. Cancer 1983;51:746–751
176. Nakashima T, Okuda K, Kojiro M et al. Pathology of hepatocellular carcinoma in Japan. Cancer 1983;51:863–877
177. Okuda KL, Peters RL, Simson IW. Gross anatomic features of hepatocellular carcinoma from three disparate geographical areas. Cancer 1984;54:2165–2173
178. Okuda K, Nakashima T, Obata H, Kubo Y. Clinicopathological studies of minute hepatocellular carcinoma. Gastroenterology 1977;73:109–115
179. Nakashima T, Kojiro M, Kawano Y et al. Histologic growth pattern of hepatocellular carcinoma: relationship to orcein (hepatitis B surface antigen)-positive cells in cancer tissue. Hum Pathol 1982;13:563–568
180. Edmondson HA. Tumors of the Liver and Intrahepatic Bile Ducts. Armed Forces Institute of Pathology, Washington DC, 1958
181. Lai CL, Wu PC, Lam KC, Toda D. Histologic prognostic indicators in hepatocellular carcinoma. Cancer 1980;44: 1677–1683
182. Buchannan TF, Huvos AG. Clear-cell carcinoma of the liver: a clinicopathologic study of 13 patients. Am J Clin Pathol 1974;61:529–539
183. Kishi K, Shikata T, Hirohashi S et al. Hepatocellular carcinoma: a clinical and pathologic analysis of 57 hepatectomy cases. Cancer 1983;51:542–548
184. Hsu HC, Sheu JC, Lin YH et al. Prognostic histologic features of resected small hepatocellular carcinoma (HCC) in Taiwan: a comparison with resected large HCC. Cancer 1985;56:672–680
185. El-Domeiri AA, Huvos AG, Goldsmith HS et al. Primary malignant tumor of the liver. Cancer 1971;27:7–11
186. Okuda K and the Liver Cancer Study Group of Japan. Primary liver cancers in Japan. Cancer 1980;45:2663–2669

187. Sugihara S, Nakashima O, Kojiro M et al. The morphologic transition in hepatocellular carcinoma: a comparison of the individual histologic features disclosed by ultrasound-guided fine-needle biopsy with those of autopsy. Cancer 1992;70:1488–1492

188. Bartolozzi C, Lencioni R, Caramella D et al. The magnetic resonance and histological correlations in hepatocellular carcinoma. Radiol Med (Torino) 1994;87:90–95

189. Inoue E, Kuroda C, Narumi Y et al. Magnetic resonance imaging-histologic correlation of small hepatocellular carcinomas and adenomatous hyperplasias. Invest Radiol 1993;28:691–697

190. Torizuka T, Tamaki N, Inokuma T et al. In vivo assessment of glucose metabolism in hepatocellular carcinoma with FDG-PET. J Nucl Med 1995;36:1811–1817

191. Tanaka S, Toh Y, Adachi E et al. Tumor progression in hepatocellular carcinoma may be mediated by p53 mutation. Cancer Res 1993;53:2884–2887

192. Brumm C, Schulze C, Charels K et al. The significance of alpha-fetoprotein and other tumour markers in differential immunocytochemistry of primary liver tumours. Histopathology 1989;14:503–513

193. Okuda K, Nakashima T, Sakamoto K et al. Hepatocellular carcinoma arising in noncirrhotic and highly cirrhotic livers: a comparative study of histopathology and frequency of hepatitis B markers. Cancer 1982;49:450–455

194. Kenmochi K, Sughihara S, Kojiro M. Relationship of histologic grade of hepatocellular carcinoma (HCC) to tumor size, and demonstration of tumor cells of multiple different grades in single small HCC. Liver 1987;7:18–26

195. Wittekind C. Hepatocellular carcinoma. In Hermanek P, Gospodarowicz MK, Henson DE et al. (eds): Prognostic Factors in Cancer. Springer, Heidelberg, 1995, pp. 88–93

196. Hermanek P, Sobin LH (eds): UICC TNM Classification of Malignant Tumors. 4th Ed. 2nd Rev. Springer, Berlin, 1992

197. Spiessl B, Beahrs OH, Hermanek P et al. TNM Atlas, 4th Ed. Springer, Berlin, 1989

198. Hermanek P, Sobin LH. UICC TNM classification of malignant tumours, 4th Ed. Springer, Berlin, 1987

199. Iwatsuki S, Starzl TE, Sheahan DG et al. Hepatic resection versus transplantation for hepatocellular carcinoma. Ann Surg 1991;214:221–229

200. Ringe B, Pichlmayr R, Wittekind C, Tusch G. Surgical treatment of hepatocellular carcinoma: experience with liver resection and transplantation in 198 patients. World J Surg 1991;15:270–285

201. Tang Z-Y, Yu Y-Q, Zhou X-D et al. Surgery of small hepatocellular carcinoma: analysis of 144 cases. Cancer 1989;64: 536–541

202. Zhao G, Su S, Borek D et al. Long survival and prognostic factors in hepatocellular carcinoma. J Surg Oncol 1990;45: 257–260

203. Hermanek P, Hutter RVP, Sobin LH. Prognostic grouping: the next step in tumor classification. J Cancer Res Clin Oncol 1990;116:513–516

204. Hermanek P, Wittekind C. Residual tumor (R) classification and prognosis. Semin Surg Oncol 1994;10:12–20

10

PATHOLOGY OF EARLY HEPATOCELLULAR CARCINOMA AND PRENEOPLASTIC LESIONS IN THE LIVER

YOICHIRO KONDO

The pathologic features of hepatocellular carcinoma (HCC) have been described by Edmondson and Steiner,[1] Edmondson,[2] Peters,[3] and Craig et al.[4] Recent advances in diagnostic imaging techniques have facilitated early detection of small space-occupying lesions in the liver, including small HCCs in the early developing stage. It was soon realized that these small HCC nodules presented a well-differentiated histologic appearance and could not be reasonably categorized based on previously established criteria. Accordingly, the Liver Cancer Study Group of Japan proposed a new standard for the histologic diagnosis of early HCC and possible premalignant changes.[5] Except for representative cases, however, evaluation of atypical changes seen in early HCC or premalignant lesions is still lacking consensus among investigators, indicating further need for elaboration of the criteria.

The best way to understand the morphologic basis of early HCC is by histologic examination of a small tumor nodule that is composed of well-differentiated HCC; in such a nodule, a wide variety of cellular and structural changes can be observed, ranging from almost normal to overt atypia. Several possible candidates have been suggested as precursor lesions of early HCC. Both completely benign changes and malignant changes are present in these putative precursor lesions.

For the differential diagnosis of early HCC, it is also important to know the reactive and/or proliferative changes of hepatocytes that can be seen in various disease conditions. In fact, certain dysplastic changes resembling those seen in early HCC do arise in regenerating livers, benign tumors, or tumorlike conditions. This chapter describes morphologic findings in early HCCs and related hepatocellular proliferative changes, together with brief comments regarding a differential diagnosis of these lesions.

EARLY HEPATOCELLULAR CARCINOMA

Early HCC has been defined as a small HCC not greater than 2 cm in diameter that is histologically well differentiated and is arranged in a thin trabecular fashion, compatible with Edmondson grade I HCC.[5] The carcinoma cells closely simulate normal hepatocytes, but differ in the presence of several noticeable changes described later. In discussing the pathology of early HCC, it should first be realized that there is a significant range of over-

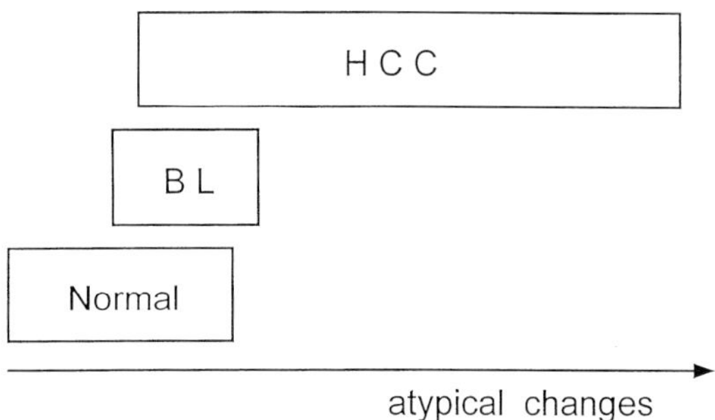

FIGURE 10-1. Schematic presentation of ranges of atypical changes in hepatocellular carcinoma (HCC) and normal hepatocytes with partial overlapping. Borderline lesions (BL) including premalignant changes can be found in an intermediate zone.

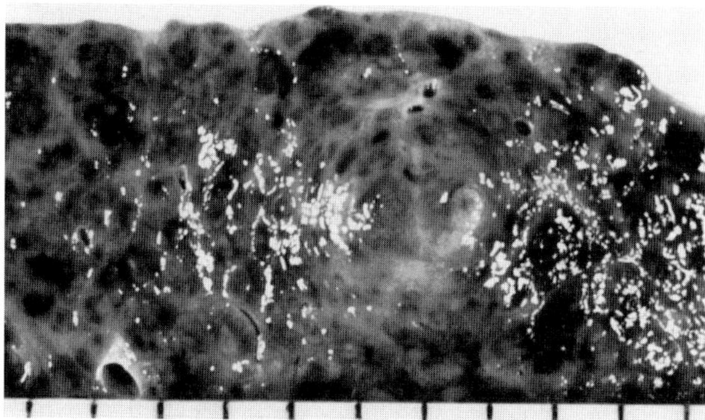

FIGURE 10-2. A bulging nodule of early hepatocellular carcinoma with an ill-defined border (about 1 cm in diameter).

lapping histologic manifestations between early HCC and benign reactive hepatocellular changes, schematically shown in Fig. 10-1. The discrimination of early HCC from these benign changes is often impossible when judged by a single parameter (e.g., nuclear atypism). Atypical changes seen in early HCCs are usually diagnosed by assessments of both the gross anatomic and histologic findings. The great majority of early HCC cases may be misjudged if overt atypical changes are used as the sole criterion for their identification.

Gross Appearance

Based on tumor shape and histologic growth patterns, Kanai et al.[6] classified small HCCs into single nodular type, single nodular type with extranodular outgrowth, contiguous multinodular type, and poorly demarcated type. Early HCCs would develop into any one of these types according to differences in histologic growth patterns. Early HCC nodules, however, are usually more vaguely demarcated due to a unique pattern of early invasive growth[7] (Fig. 10-2). When examined grossly, they bulge from the cut surface and have a grayish-white or yellowish appearance, reflecting fatty change of tumor cells.[7]

Histology

The degree of differentiation of early HCC has been referred to as "extremely well," "very well," or "highly" differentiated to emphasize the similarity of the HCC to normal hepatocytes. In low magnification, the tumors are often poorly demarcated and contain remnants of portal tracts and the septa of cirrhosis (Fig. 10-3).

TUMOR HEPATOCYTES

Tumor hepatocytes are arranged in thin cords or trabeculae that are, by definition, two or three cells thick.[5] When the three-cell thick trabeculae predominate, the

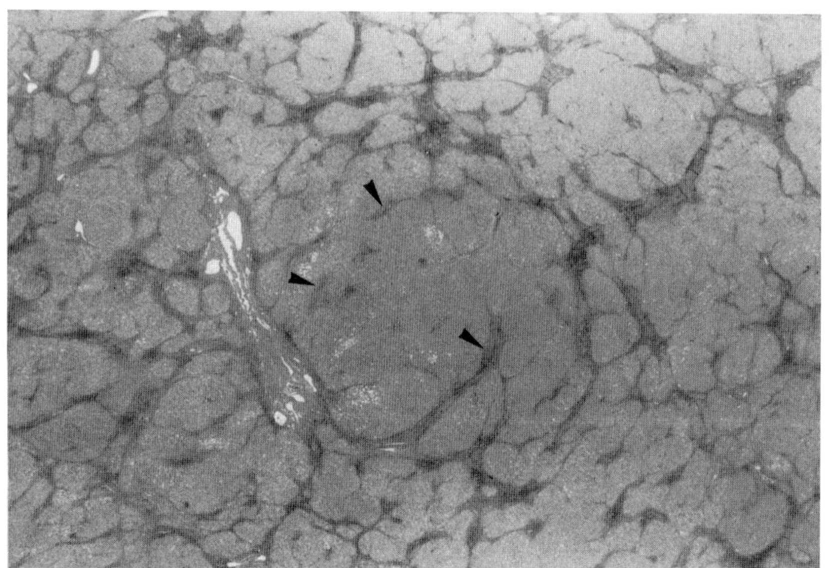

FIGURE 10-3. A minute nodule of early hepatocellular carcinoma (about 0.6 cm in diameter) showing increased staining. Tumor margin is obscure and portal tracts (arrowheads), as well as remnants of cirrhotic septa, are recognizable within the nodule. (H&E.).

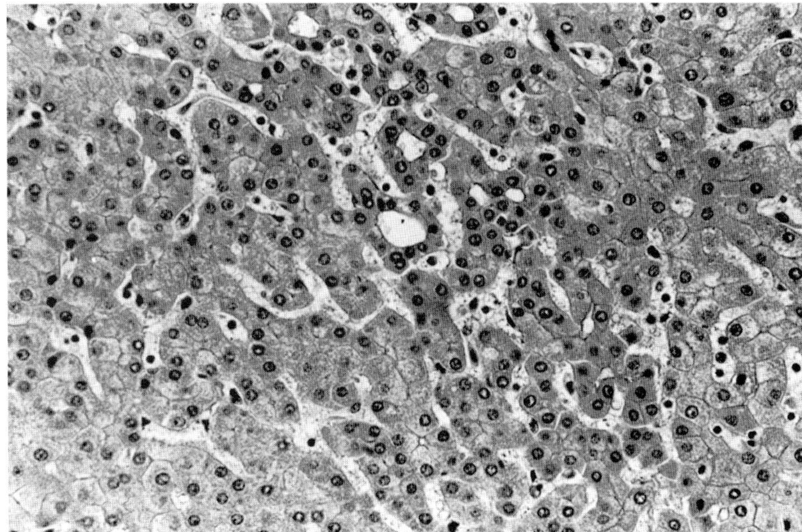

FIGURE 10-4. Well-differentiated hepatocellular carcinoma of the trabecular type. Tumor cells present no atypical changes except for focal nuclear crowding and acinar formation. (H&E.)

feature is consistent with that seen in advanced HCC and apparently conflicts with the definition of "extremely well-differentiated." According to our definition, early HCC nodules are composed of thin cell cords that are less than 3 cells thick (Figs. 10-4 and 10-5). Therefore, we have proposed the descriptive term *normotrabecular type* to denote the representative cell arrangements seen in early HCC.[8–10] Notably, in the normotrabecular type of HCC, the cell cords are clearly encircled by reticulin fibers (Fig. 10-5) and thus separated from the sinusoidal blood spaces. This normal-appearing cord structure is often distorted by microacinar formation resulting from mild dilation of the bile canaliculi (Figs. 10-4 and 10-5). The change is focally observed and differs somewhat from typical pseudoglandular formation in advanced HCC.

The normotrabecular pattern is also distorted in association with an increased nuclear density, which is usually accompanied by a gradual loss of the reticulin framework. Basement membrane components (e.g., fibronectin, laminin, and type IV collagen), can still be demonstrated by immunohistochemistry.[11] The normotrabecular type of HCC, on the other hand, may have structural alteration due to interstitial invasion characterized by formation of tumor cell cords that have become more slender or fragmented.

NUCLEAR DENSITY

Increased nuclear density (nuclear crowding) in hepatic cords is a notable finding of early HCC and has been recommended by many investigators as the most reliable diagnostic indicator. Nonetheless, mitotic figures are very rare and have no diagnostic importance. In thin tumor cell trabeculae of early HCC, the nuclei of tumor cells are significantly uniform, and their mean size is almost identical to that of hepatocytes in normal or cirrhotic livers, whereas mean cell size is apparently reduced.[10,12] This is mainly responsible for the increased

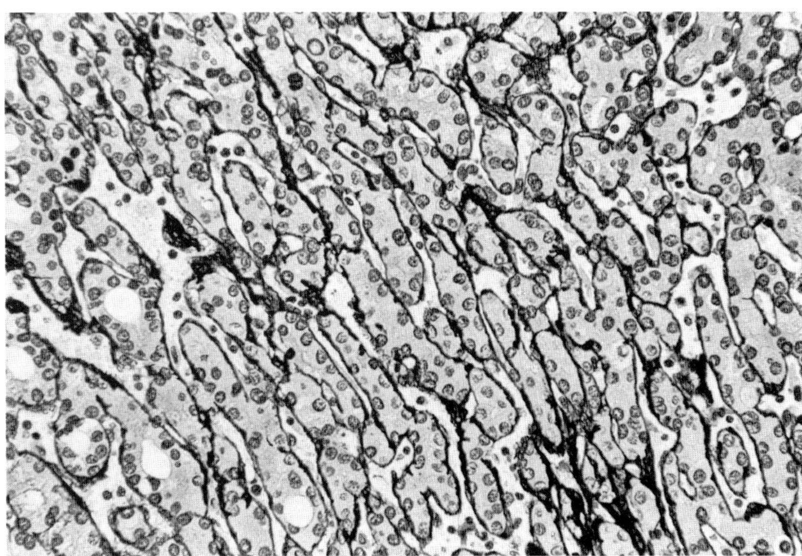

FIGURE 10-5. Thin tumor cell cords completely surrounded by reticulin fibers. Despite a marked increase in nuclear density, the cords are basically two cells thick. Acinar formation is also seen. (Reticulin fiber stain.)

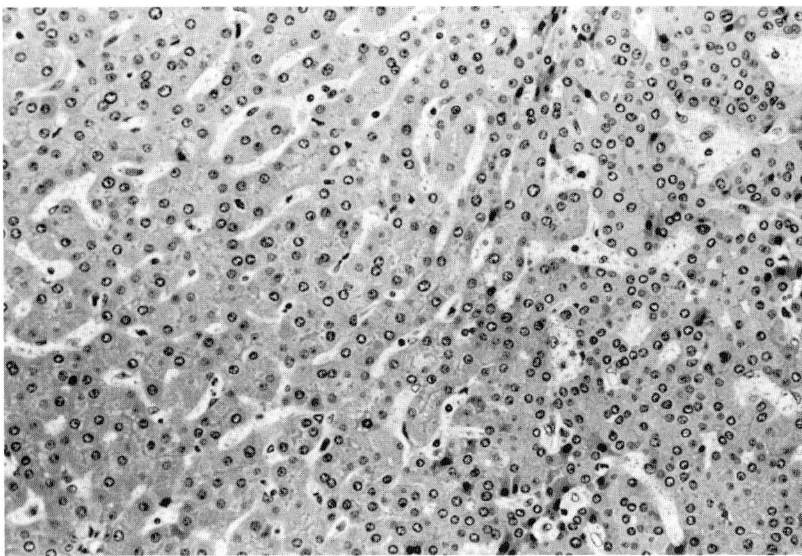

FIGURE 10-6. Transitional change from well to moderately differentiated hepatocellular carcinoma. Gradual increase of nuclear density and irregular thickening of cell cords are seen. (H&E.)

nuclear density and elevation of the nuclear cytoplasmic (N:C) ratio. The high N:C ratio becomes more prominent in the thick trabeculae seen in larger HCC nodules. As for the crucial diagnostic value of nuclear density, there is general consensus that the hepatic nodules composed of cell cords with a nuclear density larger than two times that of controls could be classified as HCC.[10,12] Actually, however, such a high value of nuclear density may not be a prerequisite to the diagnosis of well-differentiated HCC because of the concurrent presence of other atypical changes. The increased nuclear density usually results in progressive thickening of trabecular structure (Fig. 10-6), which can be recognized as a distinctive atypical change. In liver cell atrophy, the nuclear density would enter into the range of that seen in HCCs due to the marked reduction in cell size.[10]

Cell cords included in early HCC nodules are not uniform but rather vary in grade of nuclear density, and there may be areas with only a mild increase in nuclear density (Fig. 10-4). The heterogeneity of the nuclear density could be explained by postulating different functional activities and/or proliferative phases of tumor cell populations within the same nodule.

CELL ATYPIA

In well-differentiated HCC, cell atypia may be very mild or virtually absent. Following active proliferation of tumor cells, nuclear abnormalities appear.[8,13] While the cell nuclei mostly remain round and uniform, they sometimes become oval, uneven, or slightly lobulated. Simultaneously, an increase in coarse chromatin can be observed, giving rise to a hyperchromatic nuclear appearance (Fig. 10-7). Thickening of the nuclear membrane is another manifestation of nuclear atypia. Nucleolar enlargement may be seen but less than in advanced HCC. Progression of the nuclear atypia is usually related

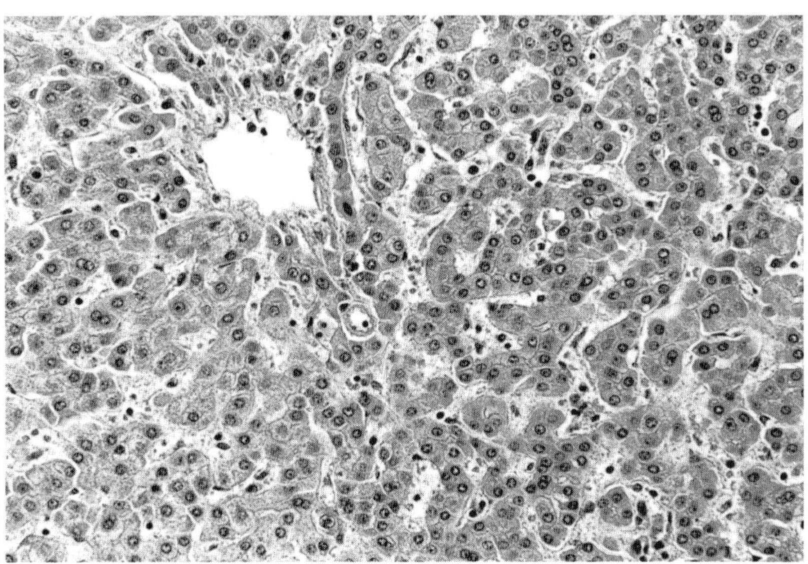

FIGURE 10-7. Appearance of atypical nuclear changes. Marked increase in nuclear chromatin and/or thickening of nuclear membrane can be seen. A small portal vein branch and an arteriole, remnants of portal triad, are embedded within tumor parenchyma. (H&E.)

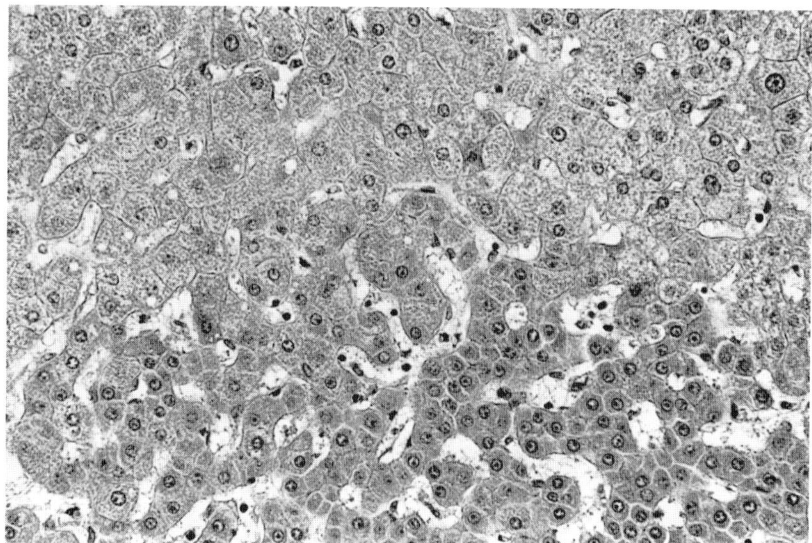

FIGURE 10-8. "Replacing" growth of well-differentiated HCC. Tumor cell cords (lower portion) are fused with benign hepatic cords (upper portion).

to the gradual thickening of tumor cell trabeculae (Fig. 10-7).

Cytoplasmic changes often can also be seen. In general, there is increased basophilic or eosinophilic cytoplasmic staining in routine heatoxylin-eosin staining, which may be of diagnostic use.[8,9] For unknown reasons, tumor cells have a remarkable tendency to undergo fatty change or clear cell alteration, especially in smaller nodules.[7] Consequently, a small nodule in the liver with prominent fatty change should be carefully examined to detect early HCC.[7] Intracytoplasmic accumulation of Mallory bodies (alcoholic hyaline) may also be a common finding.[14]

GROWTH PATTERNS

"Replacing" Growth

Nakashima et al.[15] classified the invasive growth of advanced HCCs at tumor-nontumor boundaries into "sinusoidal," "replacing," and "encapsulated" patterns.[15] In the "replacing" type, tumor cells grow into the cord of normal liver cells and seem to replace but not destroy them (Fig. 10-8). The reticulin framework of the tumor is continuous with that of the liver cell cord.[16] Both malignant and benign hepatocytes are directly attached to each other, but ultrastructurally, no junctional complexes could be demonstrated.[16] This "replacing" growth pattern has generally been regarded as a representative invasive pattern of early HCC. If tumor cells are much less differentiated, the tumor-nontumor boundary can be clearly recognized. In early HCC, the boundary is often recognizable as an obscure zone, rather than a clear line, due to the subtle blend of normal hepatocytes and well-differentiated tumor cells (Fig. 10-8). This histologic finding accounts for the ill-defined margin of early HCC nodules on gross examination.

The invasive outgrowth of early HCC may be more accelerated and become random in noncirrhotic livers, because of the absence of intervening fibrous septa.[17]

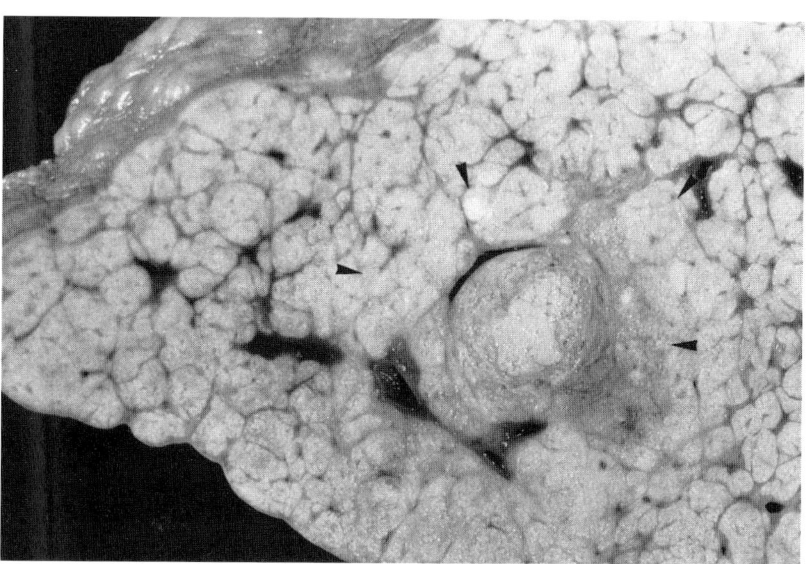

FIGURE 10-9. Nodule-in-nodule lesion consisting of a central mass and an ill-defined peripheral area (arrowheads) of invasive tumor growth.

Determination of the tumor margin in such a case is difficult even for experts.

Nodule-in-nodule Lesions

Arakawa et al.[18] described adenomatous hyperplastic nodules containing small malignant areas. They speculated that these nodule-in-nodule lesions represent an early stage of hepatocarcinogenesis and that an adenomatous hyperplastic nodule occurring in a cirrhotic liver is preneoplastic. Since this original report, the nodule-in-nodule lesion has been widely recognized as a developmental step of early HCC. In a representative case, the lesion can be grossly identified (Fig. 10-9) and histologically separated into two distinctive elements consisting of a core of overt HCC (Fig. 10-10A) and a surrounding area of proliferating hepatocytes of equivocal nature (Fig. 10-10B). The overt HCC tends to be progressive[19,20]

Interstitial Invasion

Interstitial invasion of tumor cells in advanced HCC can be easily recognized due to the prominent cellular as well as structural atypia. In contrast, in early HCC, tumor

FIGURE 10-10. Nodule-in-nodule lesion. (H&E.) (A) Moderately differentiated hepatocellular carcinoma seen in a central portion. (B) Well-differentiated hepatocellular carcinoma of the trabecular type widely distributed around peripheral zone. Insidious invasion into the septal connective tissue is seen.

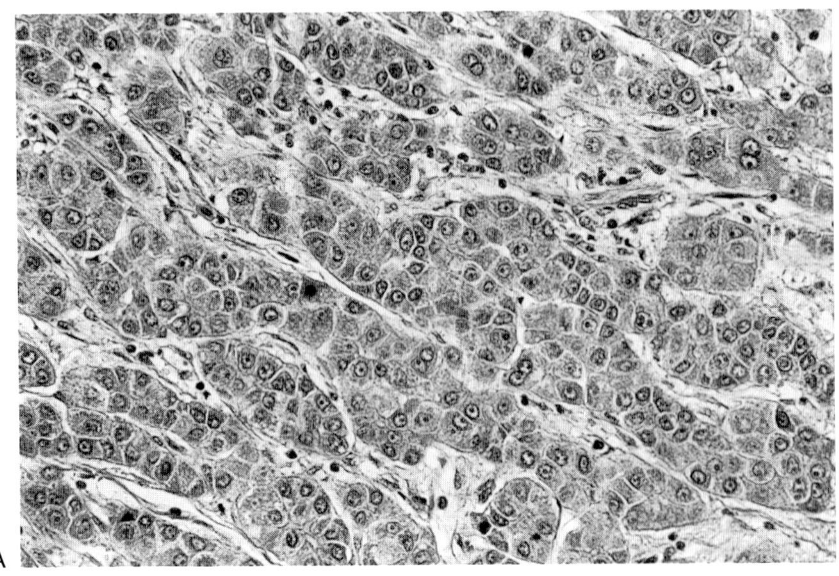

A

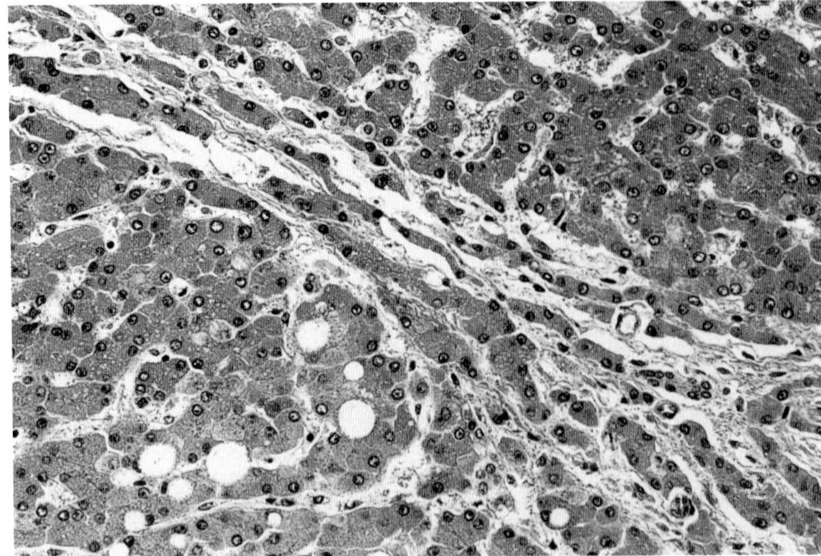

B

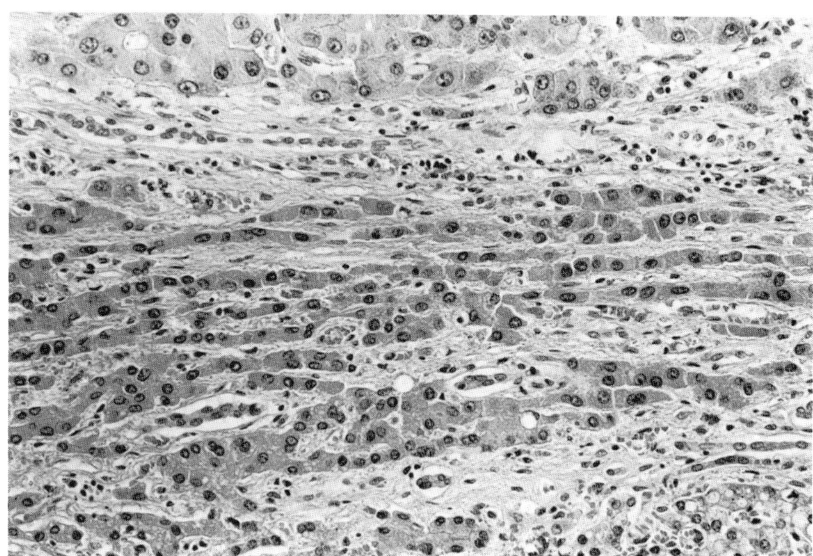

FIGURE 10-11. Interstitial invasion of well-differentiated HCC characterized by formation of streaks of slender cell cords along septal collagen fibers. (H&E.)

cells are so well differentiated that their invasion may be inconspicuous and may be either overlooked or mistaken for a fibrosing process in otherwise normal hepatocytes. For an exact diagnosis, therefore, precise knowledge about the unique pattern of interstitial invasion of well-differentiated HCC is first required.

Well-differentiated tumor cells that have entered into the septa of cirrhosis may produce short slender cell cords, which are often of single-cell thickness (Fig. 10-11). These slender cell cords are often longitudinally arranged along collagen fibers, thereby producing a characteristic streak pattern[8,21] (Fig. 10-11). The invading tumor cells resemble dissociated normal hepatocytes enclosed within septal connective tissue. However, they have no reticulin framework and are directly attached to coarse collagenous fibers (Fig. 10-12A). In contrast, nontumorous hepatocytes are clearly encircled by reticulin fibers (Fig. 10-12B), even in hepatocytes undergoing piecemeal necrosis. In addition, hepatocytes isolated within the interstitium may undergo progressive atrophy or pseudo-bile duct formation. The formation of the bare cell cords, lacking a reticulin framework, is considered to be a transient adaptation of tumor cells for promoting their migration through dense collagen fibers. The malignant nature of the slender cell cords is demonstrated by their close association with more atypical cell groups producing thick cell trabeculae with occasional vascular involvement (Fig. 10-13).

In early HCC nodules, the continued existence of portal areas has been emphasized.[6] The number of portal areas contained in small HCC nodules has been reported as less than 50% of those in cirrhotic livers; the number progressively decreases with enlargement of tumor size.[17] Portal areas included in early HCC nodules may be encompassed by tumor cells, resulting in variable diminution of fibrous elements. In places, individual components of portal triads are separated by tumor cells and then completely embedded in the tumor parenchyma (Fig. 10-7). These features are frequently, if not specifically, observed in early HCC.

Portal areas are also infiltrated by dissociated tumor cells that are irregularly dispersed within the portal connective tissue.[21] The change partly resembles piecemeal necrosis in chronic active hepatitis, but the relationship between the parenchymal cells and interstitium is completely reversed; hence the term *reversed piecemeal necrosis* can be applied to describe this type of interstitial invasion in well-differentiated HCC (Fig. 10-14). Reversed piecemeal necrosis is sometimes very inconspicuous, but when detected, it can be a crucial indicator of malignancy.[22]

Vascular Invasion

It has been stated that vascular invasion and intrahepatic metastases are rare in early HCCs,[20] but they can be encountered if a detailed histologic examination is performed.[8,23] In early HCCs, tumor cells invading the interstitium may resemble normal hepatocytes and involve small vascular branches (Fig. 10-13). These benign-appearing tumor cells may also invade the walls of much larger veins (Fig. 10-15).

Proliferative Cell Activity

The growth rate of small HCCs varies from case to case as demonstrated by clinical follow-up studies and by the doubling time of the tumor, which may range from several months to a few years.[24,25] Recently, many methods have been introduced for assessing the proliferative activity of HCCs, including silver staining for nuclear organizer regions (AgNOR)[17,26,27] or inmunostaining for proliferating cell nuclear antigen (PCNA),[28] Ki67,[29] MIB-I,[30] (Fig. 10-16) and DNA polymerase-α,[31] and in situ hybridization for histone H3 mRNA.[32] The evalu-

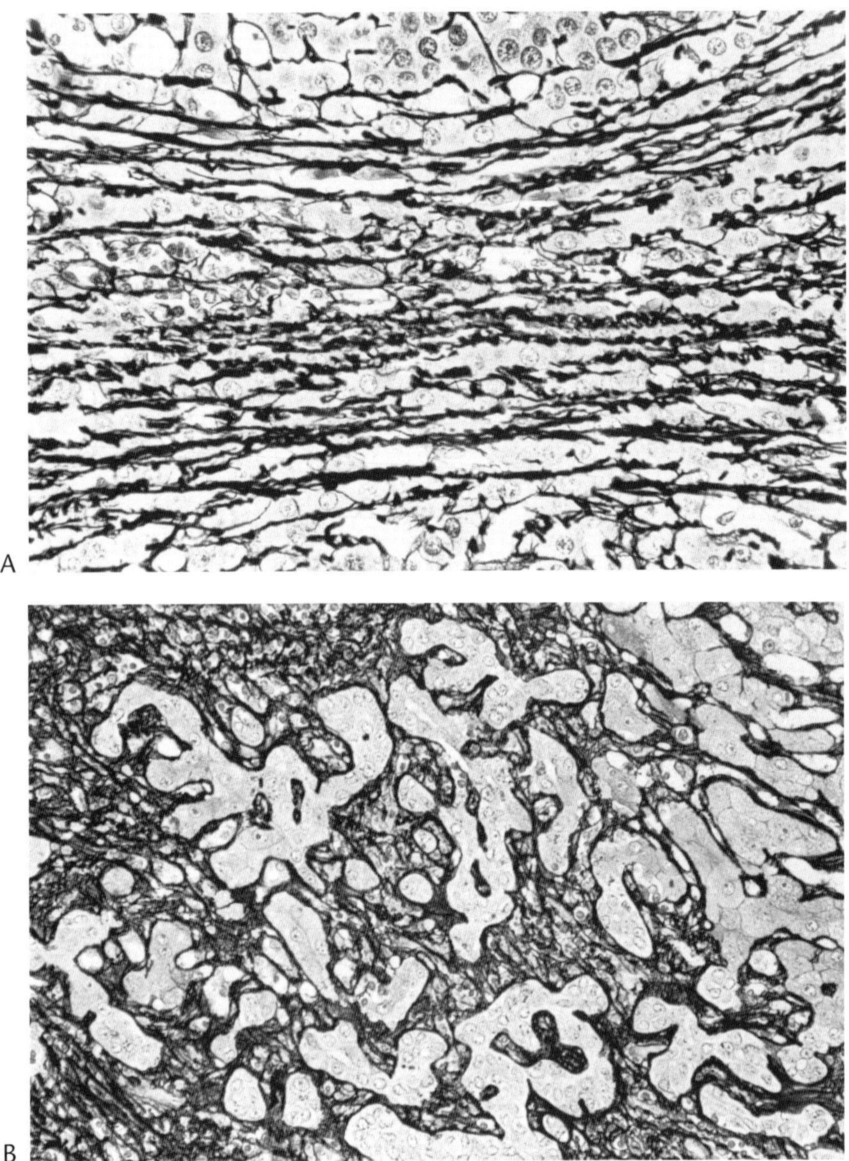

FIGURE 10-12. Reticulin fiber stain revealing association of malignant and benign hepatocytes with interstitial collagen fibers. (A) Invading tumor cells in direct contact with coarse collagen fibers. (B) In cirrhosis, hepatic cell cords are twisted but clearly circumscribed by a thick reticulin framework.

ation of proliferative activity is made by counting the number of positively stained cells and is expressed as a labeling index. The labeling index of early HCC reported by various investigators has been quite diverse, owing to the methods used. When correlated with the Edmondson grade of differentation, however, the results are fairly uniform. The labeling index in well-differentiated HCCs is significantly lower than that of less differentiated HCCs, but higher than that of control liver tissues. When examining a nodule-in-nodule lesion, proliferative cell activities in a core portion were shown to be higher than those of a surrounding area composed of well-differentiated HCC.[26] Tumor cells that have already invaded interstitial connective tissues may be rather suppressed in their proliferative activities.[17]

In many malignant neoplasms, oncogene mutations and expressions of growth factors and/or corresponding receptors have been studied extensively and found to be correlated with tumor cell proliferation. In HCCs, information concerning the correlation is still fragmentary or controversial. For example, intense expression of transforming growth factor-α and its receptor was observed in well-differentiated HCCs but not in less-differentiated HCCs.[33] Conversely, aberrant p53 expression

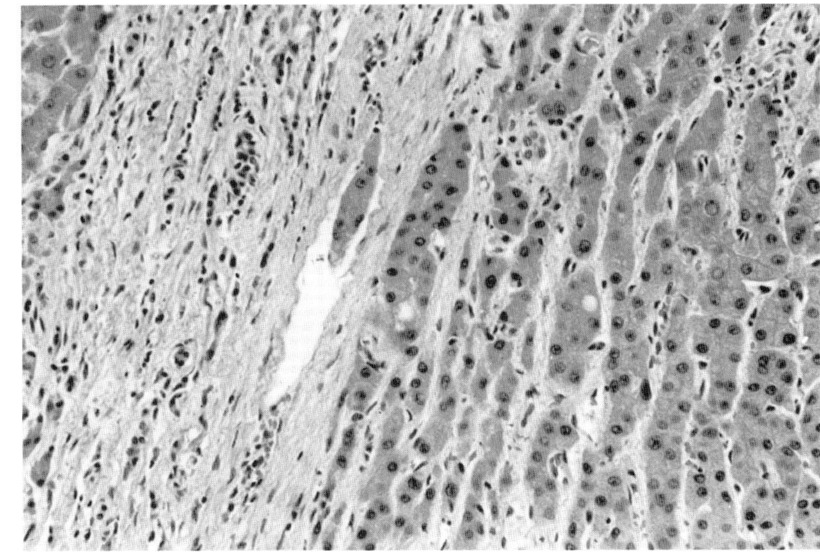

FIGURE 10-13. Tumor cell cords of variable thickness formed in septal connective tissue. Note hyperchromatic atypical nuclei. Vascular invasion is also seen. (H&E.)

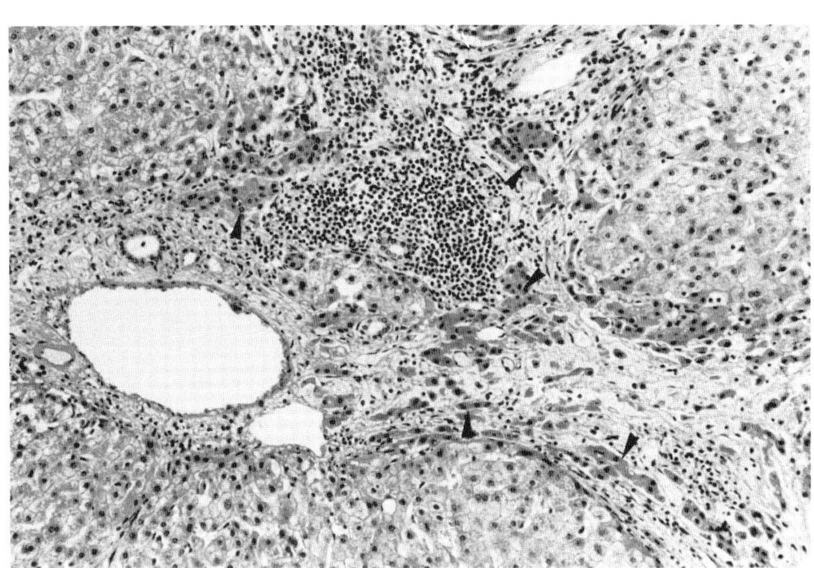

FIGURE 10-14. A portal tract within a tumor infiltrated by tumor cells with increased cytoplasmic stainability (arrowheads). (H&E.)

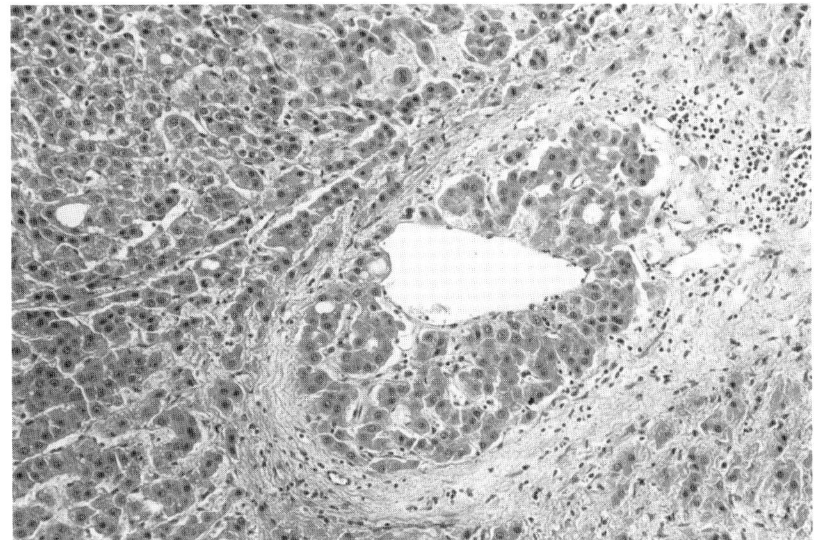

FIGURE 10-15. Tumor cells accumulated beneath the endothelial cells of a vein, a unique feature of the vascular involvement seen in well-differentiated HCC.

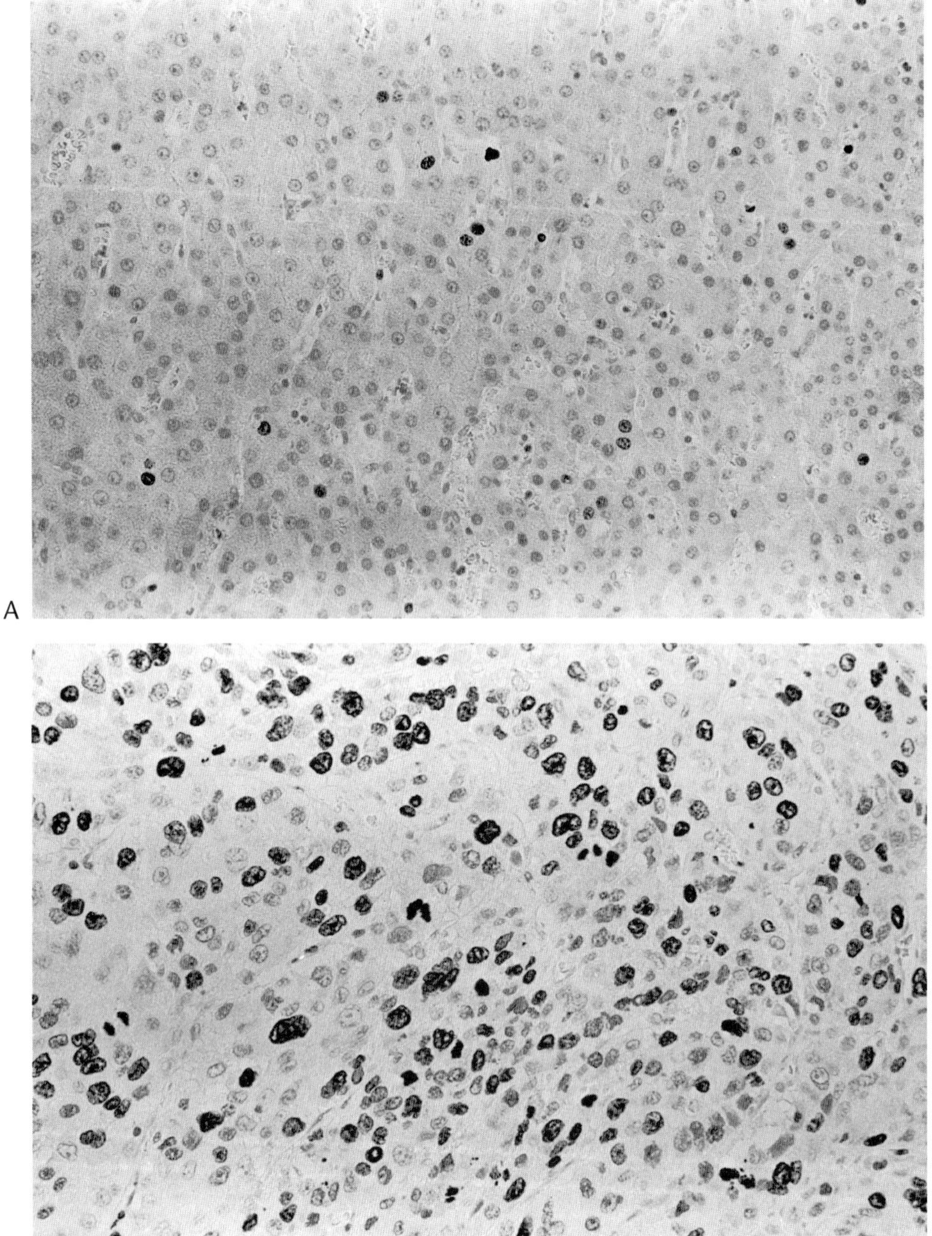

FIGURE 10-16. Immunostaining for MIB-1 in well-differentiated (A) and poorly differentiated (B) HCC. Proliferative activity is demonstrated by dark stained nuclei. A remarkable difference in the labeling index is seen between the two tissues. (Courtesy Dr. T. Nagao.)

is detected mainly in less-differentiated HCC cases and is correlated with greater proliferative cell activity.[30,34]

Multifocal Carcinoma

In advanced HCCs, a primary lesion is often accompanied by formation of a large tumor embolus within the portal vein system; smaller tumor nodules scattered in the liver usually are explained as being metastatic. When there are multifocal small tumor nodules of similar size and appearance in cirrhotic livers, however, it can be difficult to decide whether they are attributable to multicentric primary tumors or intrahepatic metastasis from a single primary nodule. The categorization of multifocal HCC has been based on comparative gross and histologic examinations of each nodule, referring to the presence or absence of vascular involvement. In general, portal type metastatic HCC nodules are found within a small branch of the portal vein and, to a certain extent, the vascular architecture is preserved.[35] In the less common lobular type of metastasis, metastatic foci are produced within the parenchyma as a consequence of intrasinusoidal seeding of carcinoma cells. In a few instances, such an intralobular focus has a well-differentiated trabecular growth pattern that must be discriminated from a primary lesion of early HCC.[36]

The nature of tumor nodules can be determined by evaluating the integration pattern of the hepatitis B virus (HBV), which is identical among tumor cells that are derived from the same cell clone. By using this marker, Esumi et al.[37] accurately identified metastatic foci within the liver, lymph nodes, and various remote organs. Hsu et al.[38] conducted a similar study; in a few multifocal HCC cases, they identified three or four different integration patterns of the HBV genome. To devise a more convenient procedure that could be used even in the absence of HBV, Oda et al.[39] evaluated the mutation pattern of p53 in HCCs to identify multifocal cases.[39] The diagnostic usefulness of p53 mutations is

FIGURE 10-17. Biopsy samples. (H&E.) (A) Early HCC of the normotrabecular type showing small thin cell cords crowded with hyperchromatic nuclei. Indefinite acinar formation is also seen (arrowhead). (B) Control specimen obtained from extranodular tissue.

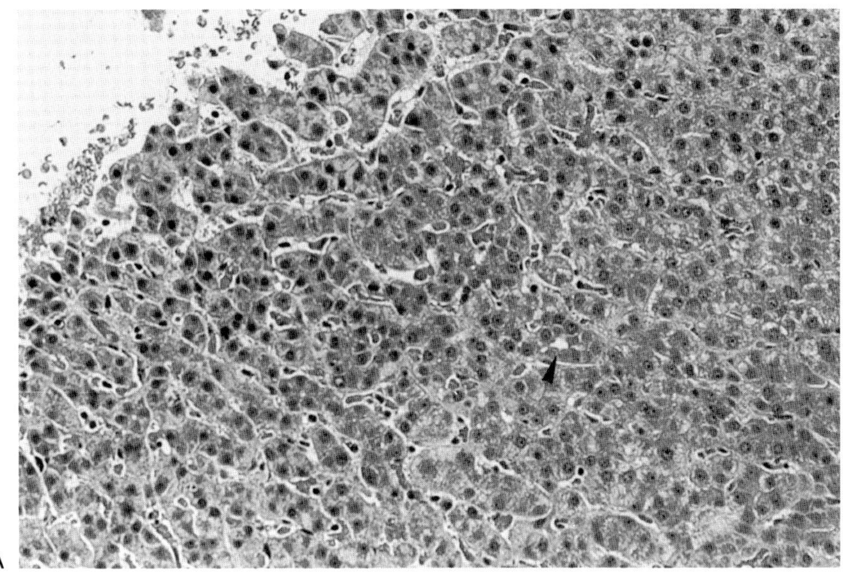

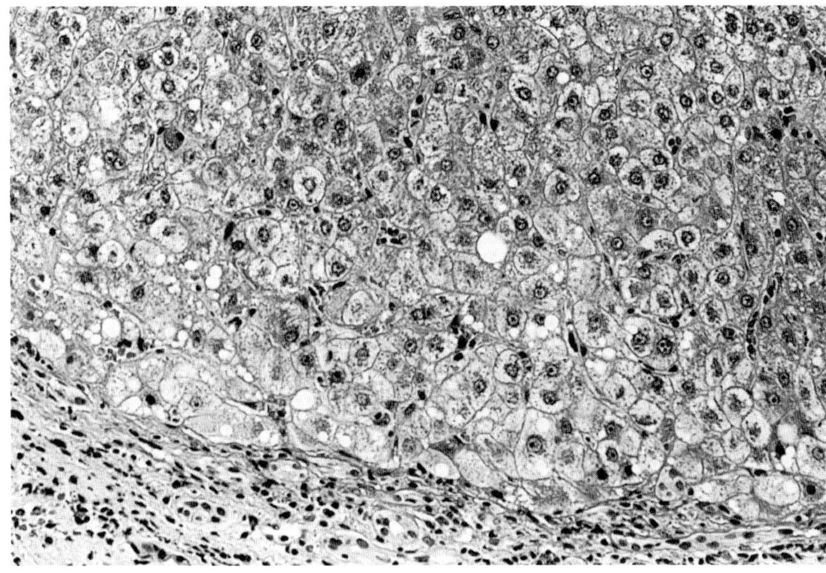

limited, because the mutation is a relatively late event in cancer and hence may not be detected in early HCC.

Biopsy Diagnosis

In Japan and other Asian countries where HBV and HCV infections are followed, a large number of patients with chronic liver disease undergo biopsy examination of small hepatic masses. Histologic findings seen in a biopsied nodule are best evaluated in comparison with those of control extranodular tissue from the same liver[12,40] (Fig. 10-17).

Well-differentiated HCC can be diagnosed in this way, but not in all cases, because only a limited portion of a nodule is available for the histologic examination. Furthermore, interstitial tumor invasion, a reliable indicator of malignancy, is rarely observed in biopsy specimens. An increase in nuclear density has been particularly useful[12,40]; a nuclear density greater than two times that of controls can be classified as overt HCC.[12] It has also been suggested from statistical analysis that the possibility of well-differentiated HCC should be considered when a nodule has a nuclear density exceeding 1.3 times that of the extranodular tissue. In biopsy specimens, however, the value is quite variable from case to case as well as from area to area.

When the possibility of well-differentiated HCC cannot be excluded, the lesion should be classified as "borderline" to avoid a risk of underdiagnosis. Although a few follow-up studies have been carried out on biopsied hepatic nodules,[25,41] there is no comprehensive survey for the ultimate fate of these borderline lesions. Furthermore, several benign nodular lesions known to arise from the normal liver sometimes display changes similar to those seen in well-differentiated HCCs, and biopsy diagnosis of these lesions should be made with care.

PUTATIVE PREMALIGNANT CHANGES

Liver Cell Dysplasia

Many attempts have been made to detect possible precursors morphologically related to HCC. To describe some of these, the term *liver cell dysplasia* was proposed by Anthony et al.[42] to refer to cellular enlargement, a combination of cellular enlargement, nuclear pleomorphism, and multinucleation of hepatocytes occurring in groups or whole cirrhotic nodules (Fig. 10-18). Because of its close association with HBV infection, cirrhosis, and HCC, it was suggested that liver cell dysplasia could be a precancerous lesion. A recent study has confirmed that the incidence of HCC is statistically more frequent in patients with liver cell dysplasia than in those without.[43] Despite these results, many investigators have concluded that there is no direct connection between liver cell dysplasia and HCC. In fact, liver cell dysplasia is too widely distributed to be regarded as a real precarcinomatous change. In addition, the remarkable nuclear pleomorphism seen in liver cell dysplasia is very different from the appearance of nuclei in early HCC.

Watanabe et al.[44] described clusters of atypical cells in chronic liver disease that were smaller than normal hepatocytes and had relatively large nuclei. They called these cells "small dysplastic cells." It has been suggested that these are more likely candidates for precursor cells than are the cells of liver cell dysplasia. This suggestion appears attractive, but these small dysplastic hepatocytes have not been described in detail, nor have the morphologic steps leading to early HCC been proposed.

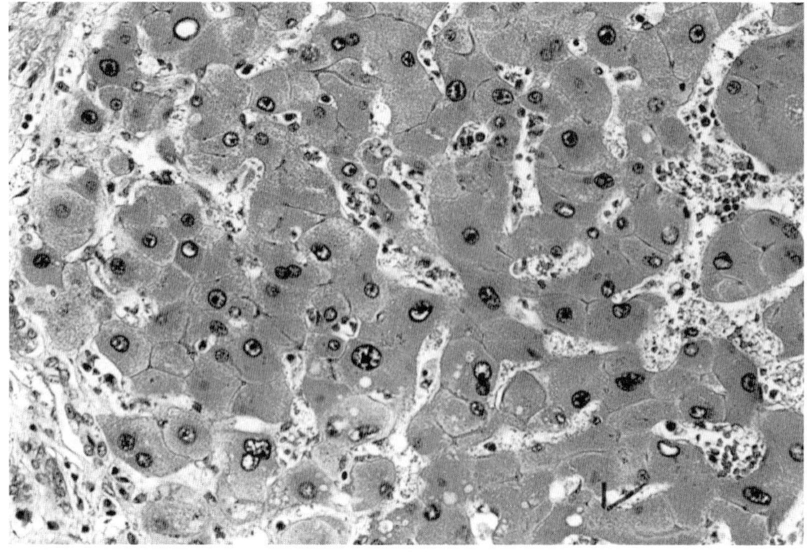

FIGURE 10-18. Liver cell dysplasia showing prominent nuclear enlargement and pleomorphism. (H&E.)

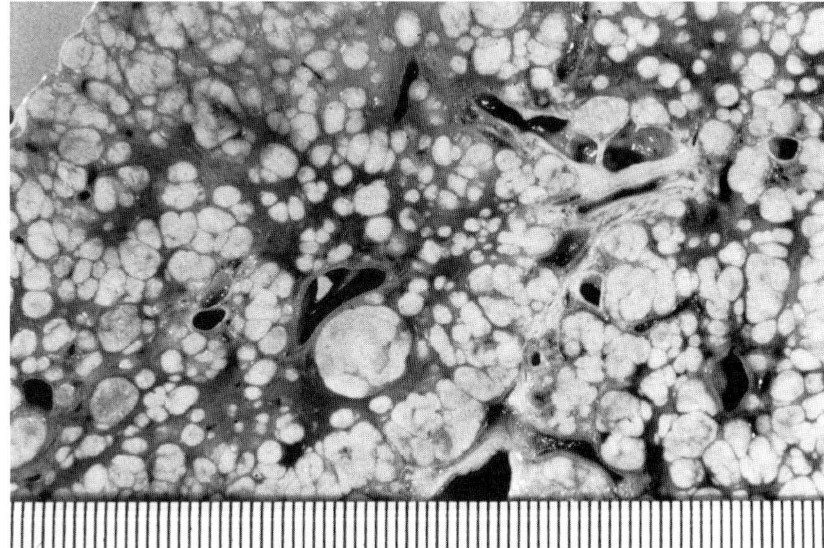

FIGURE 10-19. A discrete round nodule (about 1 cm in diameter) arising in a cirrhotic liver. Its nature cannot be determined from its gross anatomic features.

Another putative premalignant lesion, "paraplasia," described by Edmondson,[2,3] consists of cells with altered growth that form nodules distinct from simple regeneration. The hepatocytes in these nodules proliferate and expand, often compressing the adjacent hepatocytes. Paraplastic hepatocytes seem to be composed of diverse cell populations ranging from actively regenerating hepatocytes to well-differentiated HCC cells.

Preformed Nodule

Aside from small HCCs, cirrhotic livers occasionally contain discrete nodules (1 to 2 cm in diameter) apparently larger than regenerative nodules (Fig. 10-19). These nodules have been classified by an international working party to standardize the terminology and histologic manifestations.[45]

LARGE REGENERATIVE NODULE

Large regenerative nodules have also been referred to as adenomatous hyperplasia or macroregenerative nodules type I.[46] Histologically, fragmentary strands of connective tissues are scattered within the nodule, a remnant of the preexisting septa of cirrhosis. The portal areas are scattered and have variable degrees of structural distortion. Large regenerative nodules have no significant histologic differences from extranodular sites. A typical large regenerative nodule presents a completely benign appearance without any suggestion of a potentiality for malignant transformation. The proliferative cell activities so far examined have been almost identical or even suppressed when compared with those of hepatocytes in simple regenerative nodules.

Although the ultimate fate of these large regenerative nodules has still not fully been determined, it has been confirmed that they do regress and eventually vanish into the parenchyma of cirrhotic livers.[41] At present, therefore, it appears that many of the large regenerative nodules are not preneoplastic lesions.

The morphogenesis of large regenerative nodules is unknown, but two processes may be considered. First, it has been strongly suggested that local disturbance of the blood supply induces active hepatocyte proliferation and results in the nodular formation.[47,48] Second, large regenerative nodules may develop as a consequence of hepatic regeneration of several lobular units after local necrosis.

HYPERPLASTIC CHANGE

There are nodules that differ from simple large regenerative nodules by the presence of variable regenerative or hyperplastic changes (Figs. 10-20 and 10-21). Regenerating hepatocytes may be discernible as a sheet of or as clusters of small basophilic hepatocytes. A mild increase in nuclear density is common in the regenerating area (Fig. 10-21); mitotic figures are rare. Microacinar formation, a diagnostic hallmark of well-differentiated HCC, is rarely seen. Portal areas are generally replaced by regenerating hepatocytes and are reduced in number and size. This feature may partially mimic "reversed piecemeal necrosis" characteristic of interstitial invasion of well-differentiated HCC. Consequently, an isolated bile duct or small artery is occasionally found embedded in the parenchyma. It is not unlikely that these are misinterpreted as premalignant. The "atypical hepatocyte groups," however, have a homogeneous cytologic appearance and are present not only within a discrete larger nodule but are also scattered in neighboring hepatic parenchyma (Fig. 10-20).

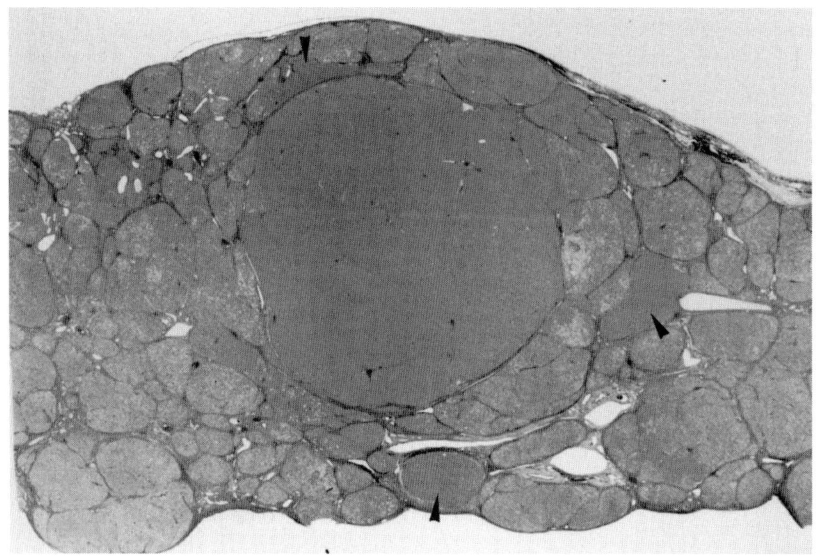

FIGURE 10-20. A possible example of multifocal occurrence of hyperplastic change. Hyperplastic hepatocytes have histologically increased cytoplasmic basophilia that can be seen in a central larger nodule as well as neighboring some pseudolobules (arrowheads). (H&E.)

PREMALIGNANT NODULE

In contrast to large regenerative nodules, premalignant nodules contain apparent atypical changes, but these are still insufficient for a diagnosis of HCC. Furuya et al.[46] classified minute hepatic nodules into macroregenerative nodules type I (consistent with large regenerative nodules) and type II (proliferative focus of hepatocytes with mild cellular and structural atypia). In addition, the type II nodules occasionally contain an area of HCC. Unfortunately, the essential features of the "mild atypia" are still unclear, and there is no substantial information relating to evolution of the macroregenerative nodules to early HCC.

Similarly, Wada et al.[49] classified two types of nodules arising in cirrhotic livers: large regenerative nodules and dysplastic nodules. The dysplastic nodules showed increased cytoplasmic basophilia, nuclear crowding, microacinar formation (Fig. 10-22), and other atypical changes, findings that also are common in early HCC. Invasive outgrowth was occasionally seen in these dysplastic nodules. These dysplastic nodules thus appear to be malignant and a possible stepwise process of hepatocarcinogenesis via large regenerative nodule and dysplastic nodule to early HCC is suggested.

A similar concept of sequential steps for the development of HCC has also been introduced, consisting of adenomatous hyperplasia, atypical adenomatous hyperplasia, to early HCC.[7,13,18,20,25,26,28,50–53] Sakamoto et al.[20] were able to select from small hepatic nodules many early HCCs with a very well-differentiated appearance, consistent with Edmondson grade I HCC. These early HCCs each contained a focal area identical to adenomatous hyperplasia, reminiscent of a possible precursor lesion. In several other nodules, areas of overt HCC (Edmondson grade II HCC) were found on a background of

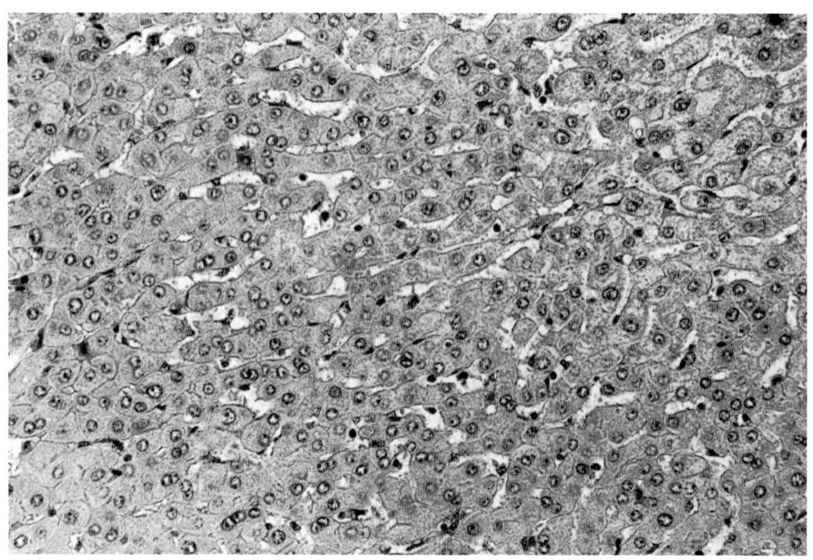

FIGURE 10-21. A portion of a regenerative, hyperplastic nodule produced around a tumor that had undergone transarterial embolization. A considerable increase in the nuclear density and an irregular cord structure are seen, simulating well-differentiated hepatocellular carcinoma. (H&E.)

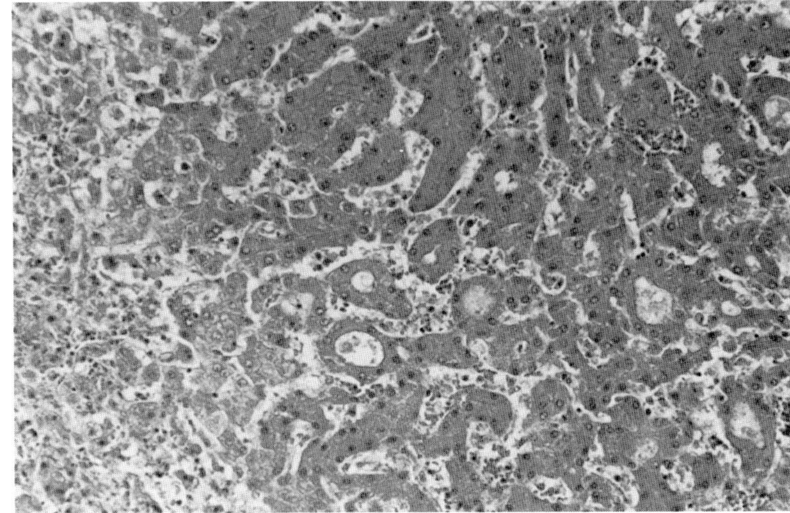

FIGURE 10-22. A portion of a well-circumscribed nodule with gross anatomic appearance similar to that of a large regenerative nodule. Histologically, however, acinar formation, a dysplastic change, is evident adjacent to a necrotic area. (H&E.)

grade I HCC. They speculated that such a nodule-in-nodule lesion might indicate progression of early HCC to more malignant and advanced HCC. The development of HCC from adenomatous hyperplasia has been more directly demonstrated by the observation that histologically proven nodules of adenomatous hyperplasia eventually showed rapid volume growth comparable with HCC.[25] The sequential steps from atypical adenomatous hyperplasia to early HCC were confirmed by morphometric analysis,[13] immunohistochemistry for cell proliferative activity,[28,54] and clinicopathologic investigations.[51]

In summary, it can be realized by reviewing the previous reports that the characterization of premalignant nodules is still a matter of controversy. For instance, some investigators believe that it is difficult to distinguish atypical adenomatous hyperplasia from extremely well-differentiated HCC. It is also uncertain whether atypical adenomatous hyperplasia is benign or malignant. Moreover, an overt cancerous area is often detected within a nodule of atypical adenomatous hyperplasia. The margin of such a nodule is ill defined, as it is in early HCC. The putative premalignant lesions thus seem to have been rather arbitrarily categorized in the previous studies. Because no consistent nomenclature or diagnostic criteria have been put forward to describe premalignant lesions, Ferrell et al.[54] designated the nodules with atypical features not diagnostic of HCC as "borderline lesions."

NODULAR LESIONS ARISING FROM NORMAL LIVERS

Many tumors or tumorlike lesions arise from an otherwise normal liver. Of these, three benign lesions may be important to distinguish them from early HCC, comprising hepatocellular adenoma, focal nodular hyperplasia, and nodular regenerative hyperplasia. Each of these lesions is a distinctive lesion with virtually no potentiality of malignant transformation.

Hepatocellular Adenoma

Hepatocellular adenoma usually has a huge solitary hepatic mass. Several etiologic factors have been implicated,[55] including oral contraceptives, anabolic steroids, and metabolic disorders.[4] The majority of adenoma cases are probably related to the use of oral contraceptives, so that the incidence is extremely low in some countries. Interestingly, patient withdrawal from estrogenic compounds or anabolic steroids leads to regression of large hepatocellular adenoma nodules.

Hepatocellular adenomas are well demarcated, and the cut surface is often characterized by peliotic change or intense hemorrhage. Hepatocytes in an adenoma nodule are arranged in cords or sheets mimicking the normal hepatic architecture. They often become swollen and clear (Fig. 10-23) because of excess intracytoplasmic accumulation of fat or glycogen or because of hydropic changes. Atypical changes are mild and nuclear crowding is rarely encountered; occasional acinar formation is seen. Bile ducts are absent, and thin-walled vessels are seen randomly scattered within a tumor. Hepatocellular adenomas with these classic changes are easily defined.

In contrast, anabolic steroid-associated hepatocellular adenomas frequently display obvious atypical changes that resemble HCCs, including nodule-in-nodule growth patterns and acinar formation.[4] For a differential diagnosis, the adenomas have a low nucleus:cytoplasm ratio, whereas HCCs have high ratios.[4]

Focal Nodular Hyperplasia

Focal nodular hyperplasia is an uncommon nodular hepatic lesion that preferentially occurs in younger women. In view of its close association with vascular changes, it

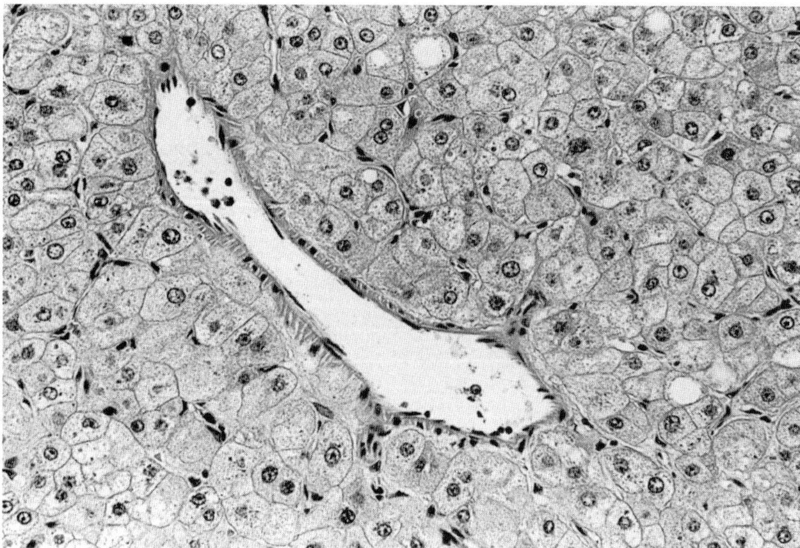

FIGURE 10-23. Liver cell adenoma composed of a sheet of swollen, relatively clear hepatocytes. No atypical changes are recognizable. A thin-walled artery is seen unaccompanied by a vein. (H&E.)

is likely that focal vascular abnormalities with greater blood flow result in unusual proliferation of hepatocytes in an involved area.[48] The nodule has a central scar and radiating thin septal connective tissue that divide the parenchyma into lobular compartments.[56] As a result, the area resembles cirrhosis. The interstitial tissue is infiltrated by many mononuclear cells and variable amounts of neutrophils. Characteristically, a number of bile ductules are seen, perhaps a result of metaplastic transformation of hepatocytes.

In a representative nodule of focal nodular hyperplasia with the preceding features, there is no problem of differential diagnosis. In a developing small nodule, however, the typical central scar may be absent and atypical changes are observed, probably related to the active proliferation of hepatocytes. The cell cords are thickened and distorted, with mild nuclear crowding and scattered acinar formation (Fig. 10-24). The changes resemble those seen in early HCC, thus making differential diagnosis difficult unless other hallmarks of focal nodular hyperplasia are demonstrated.

Nodular Regenerative Hyperplasia

Unlike the focal lesions of hepatocellular adenoma and focal nodular hyperplasia, nodular regenerative hyperplasia is a diffuse hepatic disease. The basic pathologic change is the formation of minute nodules of hyperplastic hepatocytes involving the whole liver.[57] The size of these micronodules is almost the same as that of normal hepatic lobules. In addition, scattered larger nodules also may be encountered. The gross appearance resembles cirrhosis, but individual nodular units are not circumscribed by fibrous septa. Instead, they are surrounded by compressed, atrophic hepatic cords. Nodular regenerative hyperplasia tends to develop in association with certain

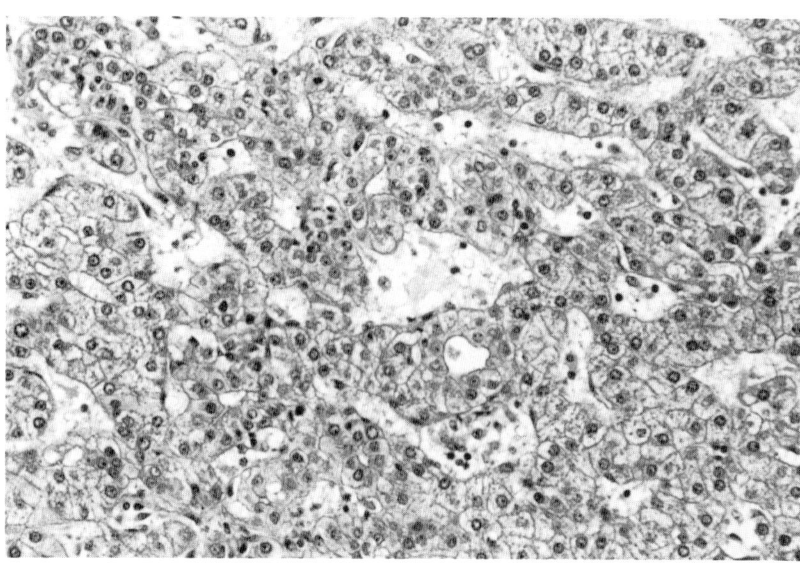

FIGURE 10-24. A small nodule of focal regenerative hyperplasia showing atypical changes, such as irregular trabecular structure with acinar formation. This nodule had once been misinterpreted as well-differentiated HCC. (H&E.)

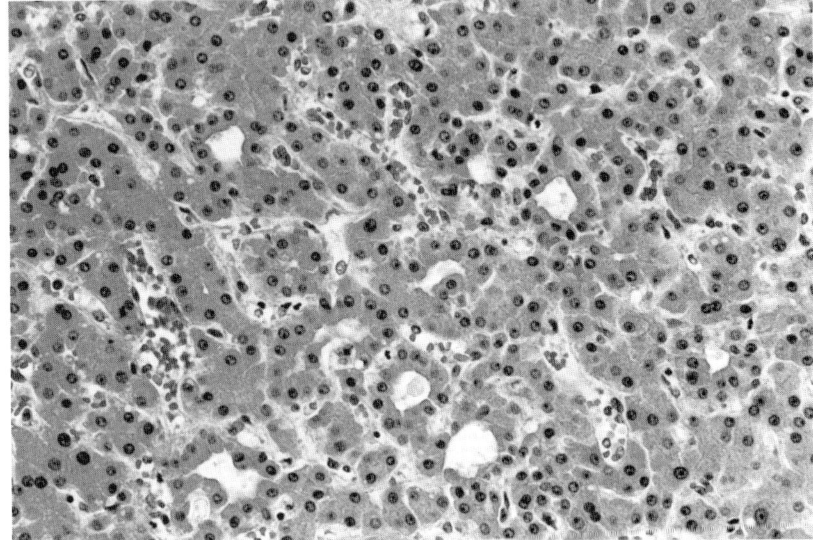

FIGURE 10-25. Nodular regenerative hyperplasia. Focal nuclear crowding, hyperchromatic nuclei, and frequent acinar formation are seen. From this picture alone, well-differentiated hepatocellular carcinoma may be strongly suspected. (H&E.)

diseases such as rheumatoid diseases, dysgammaglobulinemia, or hematologic disorders. Portal hypertension is the most serious complication of nodular regenerative hyperplasia. Circulatory abnormalities of the hepatic vascular system have been implicated in the pathogenesis.[47]

Nodular foci are composed of hyperplastic hepatocytes arranged in cords, which are more or less distorted and hypernucleated. Acinar or pseudoglandular formation is common (Fig. 10-25). The hypertrophic cell cords gradually merge into peripheral attenuated cell cords. Except for acinar formation, the atypical changes are not so prominent, and the exact diagnosis is possible when diffuse distribution of the unique nodular change is confirmed.

REFERENCES

1. Edmondson HA, Steiner PE. Primary carcinoma of the liver. A study of 100 cases among 48,900 necropsies. Cancer 1945; 7:462–563
2. Edmondson HA. Tumor of the liver and intrahepatic bile ducts. In Atlas of Tumor Pathology, Section VII. Armed Forces Institute of Pathology, Washington, DC, 1958
3. Peters RL. Pathology of hepatocellular carcinoma. In Okuda K, Paters RL (eds): Hepatocellular Carcinoma. Wiley, New York, 1976, p.107
4. Craig JR, Peters RL, Edmondson HA. Tumors of the Liver and Intrahepatic Bile Ducts. Second series, Fasicle 26. Armed Forces Institute of Pathology, Washington DC, 1989
5. Liver Cancer Study Group of Japan. The General Rule for the Clinical and Pathological Study of Primary Liver Cancer, 3rd Ed. Kanahara, Tokyo, 1992
6. Kanai T, Hirohashi S, Upton MP et al. Pathology of small hepatocellular carcinoma: a proposal for new gross classification. Cancer 1987;60:810–819
7. Kojiro M, Sugihara S, Nakashima O. Pathomorphologic characteristics of early hepatocellular carcinoma. Gann Monogr Cancer Res 1991;38:29–37
8. Kondo Y, Kondo F, Wada K, Okabayashi A. Pathologic features of small hepatocellular carcinoma. Acta Pathol Jpn 1986;36:1149–1161
9. Kondo F, Hirooka N, Wada K, Kondo Y. Morphogical clues for the diagnosis of small hepatocellular carcinomas. Virchows Arch Pathol Anat 1987;411:15–21
10. Kondo F, Wada K, Kondo Y. Morphometric analysis of hepatocellular carcinoma. Virchows Arch Pathol Anat 1988;413: 425–430
11. Donato MF, Colombo M, Matarazzo M, Paronetto F. Distribution of basement membrane components in human hepatocellular carcinoma. Cancer 1989;63:272–279
12. Nagato Y, Kondo F, Kondo Y et al. Histological and morphometrical indicators for a biopsy diagnosis of well-differentiated hepatocellular carcinoma. Hepatology 1991;14: 473–478
13. Terada T, Ueda K, Nakanuma Y. Histopathological and morphometric analysis of atypical adenomatous hyperplasia of human cirrhotic livers. Virchows Arch Pathol Anat 1993; 422:381–388
14. Nakanuma Y, Ohta. Is Mallory body formation a preneoplastic change? A study of 181 cases of liver bearing hepatocellular carcinoma and 82 cases of cirrhosis. Cancer 1985;55: 2400–2404
15. Nakashima T, Kojiro M, Kawano Y et al. Histologic growth pattern of hepatocellular carcinoma. Relationship to orcein (hepatitis B surface antigen)-positive cells in cancer tissue. Hum Pathol 1982;13:563–568
16. Sugihara S, Kojiro M, Nakashima T. Ultrastructural study of hepatocellular carcinoma with replacing pattern. Acta Pathol Jpn 1985;35:549–559
17. Tomizawa M, Kondo F, Kondo Y. Growth patterns and interstitial invasion of small hepatocellular carcinoma. Pathol Int 1995;45:352–358

18. Arakawa M, Kage M, Sugihara S et al. Emergence of malignant lesions within an adenomatous hyperplastic nodule in a cirrhotic liver: observations in five cases. Gastroenterology 1986;91:192–208
19. Kenmochi K, Sugihara S, Kojiro M. Relationship of histologic grade of hepatocellular carcinoma (HCC) to tumor size, and demonstration of tumor cells of multiple different grades in single small HCC. Liver 1987;7:18–26
20. Sakamoto M, Hirohashi S, Shimosato Y. Early stages of multistep hepatocarcinogenesis: adenomatous hyperplasia and early hepatocellular carcinoma. Hum Pathol 1991;22:172–178
21. Kondo F, Kondo Y, Nagato Y et al. Interstitial tumor cell invasion in small hepatocellular carcinoma. Evaluation in microsopic and low magnification views. J Gastroenterol Hepatol 1994;9:604–612
22. Nakano M, Saito A, Takasaki K et al. A histopathologic study of early hepatocellular carcinoma. Portal tract invasion and progression to advanced hepatocellular carcinoma. Acta Hepatol Jpn 1990;31:754–762
23. Wakasa K, Sakurai M, Okamura J, Kuroda C. Pathological study of small hepatocellular carcinoma: frequency of their invasion. Virchows Arch Pathol Anat 1985;407:259–270
24. Ebara M, Ohto M, Shinagawa T et al. Natural history of minute hepatocellular carcinoma smaller than three centimeters complicating cirrhosis. A study in 22 patients. Gastroenterology 1986;90:289–298
25. Takayama T, Makuuchi M, Hirohashi S et al. Malignant transformation of adenomatous hyperplasia to hepatocellular carcinoma. Lancet 1990;336:1150–1153
26. Aoki K, Sakamoto M, Hirohashi S. Nuclear organizer regions in small nodular lesions representing early stages of human hepatocarcinogenesis. Cancer 1994;73:289–293
27. Nagao T, Ishida Y, Yamazaki K, Kond Y. Nuclear organizer regions in hepatocellular carcinoma related to the cell cycle, cell proliferation and histologic grade. Pathol Res Pract 1995;191:967–972
28. Terada T, Nakanuma Y. Cell proliferative activity in adenomatous hyperplasia of the liver and small hepatocellular carcinoma. An immunohistochemical study demonstrating proliferating cell nuclear antigen. Cancer 1992;70:591–598
29. Grigioni WF, D'Errico A, Bacci F et al. Primary liver neoplasms: evaluation of proliferative index using MoAb Ki67. J Pathol 1989;158:23–29
30. Nagao T, Kondo F, Sato T et al. Immunohistochemical detection of abberant p53 expression in hepatocellular carcinoma. Correlation with cell proliferation activity indices, including mitotic index and MIB-1 immunostaining. Hum Pathol 1995;26:326–333
31. Seki S, Sakaguchi H, Kawakita N et al. Identification and fine structure of proliferating hepatocytes in malignant and nonmalignant liver diseases by use of a monoclonal antibody against DNA polymerase alpha. Hum Pathol 1990;21:1020–1030
32. Nagao T, Ishida Y, Kondo Y. Determination of S-phase cells by in situ hybridization for histone H3 mRNA in hepatocellular carcinoma. Correlation with histologic grade and other cell proliferative markers. Mod Pathol 1996;9:99–104
33. Morimitsu T, Hsia CC, Kojiro M, Tabor E. Nodules of less-differentiated tumor within or adjacent to hepatocellular carcinoma: relative expression of transforming growth factor and its receptor in the different areas of tumor. Hum Pathol 1995;26:1126–1132
34. D'Errico A, Grigioni WF, Fiorentino M et al. Overexpression of p53 protein and Ki67 proliferative index in hepatocellular carcinoma. An immunohistochemical study on 109 Italian patients. Pathol Int 1994;44:682–687
35. Kondo Y, Wada K. Intrahepatic metastasis of hepatocellular carcinoma. A histopathologic study. Hum Pathol 1991;22:125–130
36. Komatsu T, Kondo Y, Yamamoto Y, Isono K. Hepatocellular carcinoma presenting well differentiated, normotrabecular patterns in peripheral or metastatic loci. Analysis of 103 resected cases. Acta Pathol Jpn 1990;40:887–893
37. Esumi M, Arifata T, Arii M et al. Clonal origin of human hepatoma determined by integration of hepatitis B virus DNA. Cancer Res 1986;46:5767–5771
38. Hsu HC, Chiou TJ, Chen JY et al. Clonality and clonal evolution of hepatocellular carcinoma with multiple nodules. Hepatology 1991;13:923–928
39. Oda T, Tsuda H, Scarpa A et al. Mutation pattern of the p53 gene as a diagnostic marker for multiple hepatocellular carcinoma. Cancer Res 1992;52:3674–3678
40. Kondo F, Wada K, Nagato Y et al. Biopsy diagnosis of well-differentiated hepatocellular carcinoma based on new morphologic criteria. Hepatology 1989;9:751–755
41. Kondo F, Ebara M, Sugiura N et al. Histological features and clinical course of large regenerative nodules. Evaluation of their precancerous potentiality. Hepatology 1990;12:592–598
42. Anthony PP, Vogel CL, Barker LF. Liver cell dysplasia: a premalignant condition. J Clin Pathol 1973;26:217–223
43. Borzio M, Bruno S, Roncalli M et al. Liver cell dysplasia is a major risk factor for hepatocellular carcinoma in cirrhosis: a prospective study. Gastroenterology 1995;108:812–817
44. Watanabe S, Okita K, Harada T et al. Morphologic studies of the liver cell dysplasia. Cancer 1983;51:2197–2205
45. International Working Party. Terminology of nodular hepatocellular lesions. Hepatology 1995;22:983–993
46. Furuya K, Nakamura M, Yamamoto Y et al. Macroregenerative nodule of the liver: a clinicopathologic study of 345 autopsy cases of chronic liver disease. Cancer 1988;61:99–105
47. Wanless IR, Godwin TA, Allen F, Feder A. Nodular regenerative hyperplasia of the liver in hematologic disorders: a possible response to obliterative portal venopathy. A morphometric study of nine cases with an hypothesis on the pathogenesis. Medicine 1980;59:367–379
48. Wanless IR, Mawdsley C, Adams R. On the pathogenesis of focal nodular hyperplasia of the liver. Hepatology 1985;5:1192–1200
49. Wada K, Kondo F, Kondo Y. Large regenerative nodules and dysplastic nodules in cirrhotic livers: a histopathologic study. Hepatology 1988;8:1684–1688
50. Terada T, Terasaki S, Nakanuma Y. A clinicopathologic study of adenomatous hyperplasia of the liver in 209 consecu-

tive cirrhotic livers examined by autopsy. Cancer 1993;72: 1551–1556

51. Grigioni WF, D'Errico A, Bacci F et al. Small liver masses in cirrhotic patients: a pathological clue for the morphogenesis of human hepatocellular carcinoma. Acta Pathol Jpn 1989;39:520–527
52. Tsuda H, Hirohashi S, Shimosato Y et al. Clonal origin of atypical adenomatous hyperplasia of the liver and clonal identity with hepatocellular carcinoma. Gastroenterology 1988;95:1664–1666
53. Eguchi A, Nakashima O, Okudaira S et al. Adenomatous hyperplasia in the vicinity of small hepatocellular carcinoma. Hepatology 1992;15:843–848
54. Ferrell L, Crawford JM, Dhillon AP et al. Proposal for standardized criteria for the diagnosis of benign, borderline and malignant hepatocellular lesions arising in chronic advanced liver disease. Am J Surg Pathol 1993;17:1113–1123
55. Anthony PP. Tumours and tumour-like lesions of the liver and biliary tract. In MacSween NM, Anthony PP, Scheuer PJ et al (eds): Pathology of the Liver. 3rd Ed. Churchill Livingstone, Edinburgh, 1994, p. 635
56. Knowles DM, Wolff M. Focal nodular hyperplasia of the liver. A clinicopathologic study and review of the literature. Hum Pathol 1976;7:533–545
57. Stromeyer FW, Ishak KG. Nodular transformation (nodular "regenerative" hyperplasia) of the liver. A clinicopathologic study of 30 cases. Hum Pathol 1981;12:60–71

COLOR PLATES

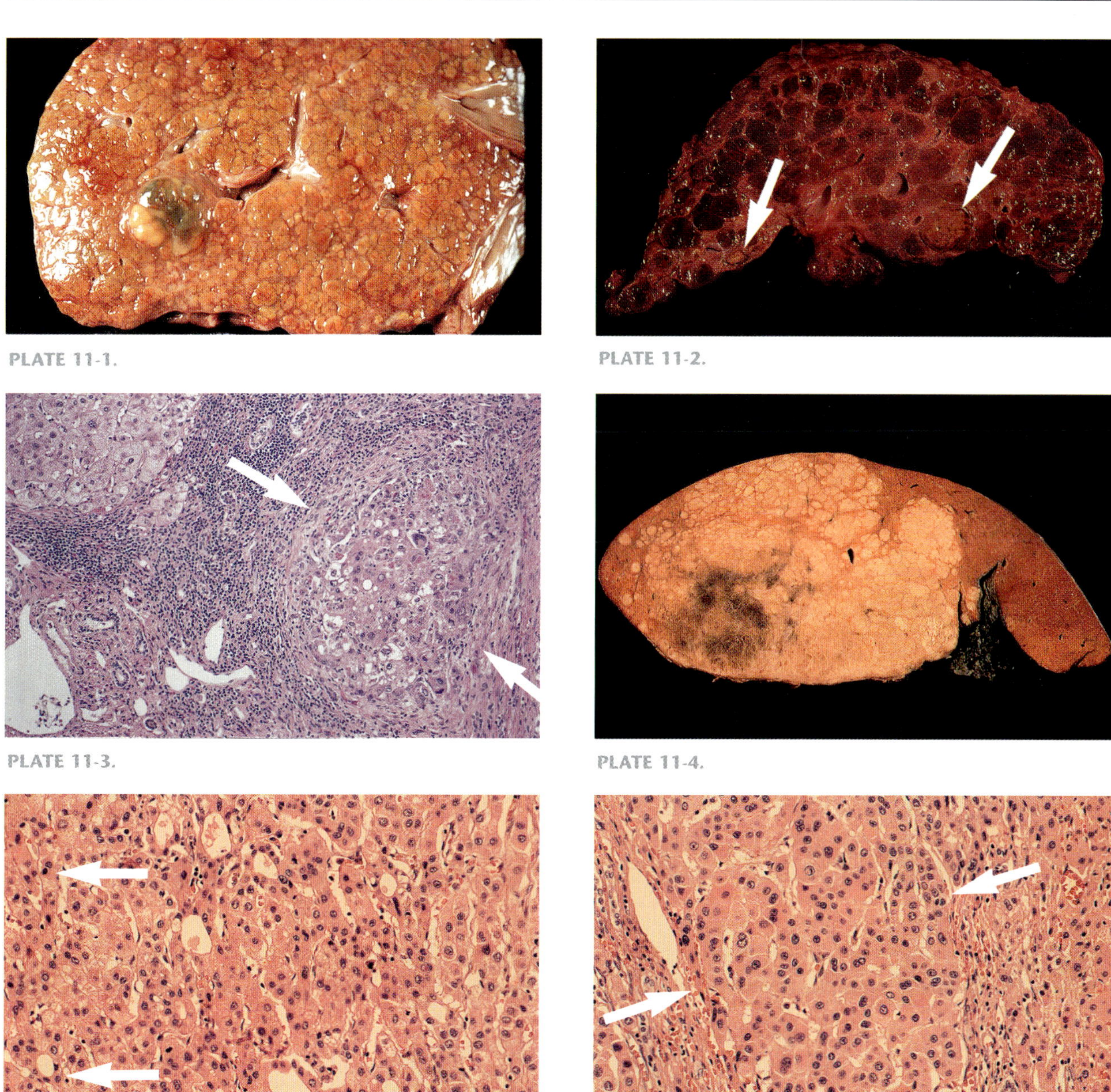

PLATE 11-1.

PLATE 11-2.

PLATE 11-3.

PLATE 11-4.

PLATE 11-5.

PLATE 11-6.

PLATE 11-1. Bile-producing hepatocellular carcinoma arising in a micronodular cirrhosis secondary to alcoholic liver disease.

PLATE 11-2. Macronodular cirrhosis with numerous macroregenerative nodules with multicentric hepatocellular carcinoma in a patient with chronic hepatitis B (arrows).

PLATE 11-3. Chronic hepatitis C and cirrhosis with multiple small hepatocellular carcinomas (arrows). (H&E, ×100.)

PLATE 11-4. A large hepatocellular carcinoma in a dark brown liver with hemochromatosis.

PLATE 11-5. Hepatocellular carcinoma arising in a macroregenerative nodule. The periphery of the tumor consists of hyperplastic hepatocytes (arrows). (H&E, ×250.)

PLATE 11-6. Well-differentiated hepatocellular carcinoma arising not in a macroregenerative nodule, but from and replacing a small cirrhotic nodule (arrows). (H&E, ×250.)

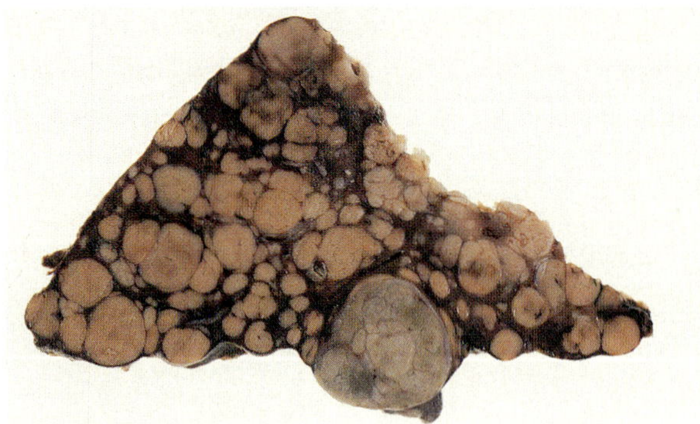

PLATE 12-1.

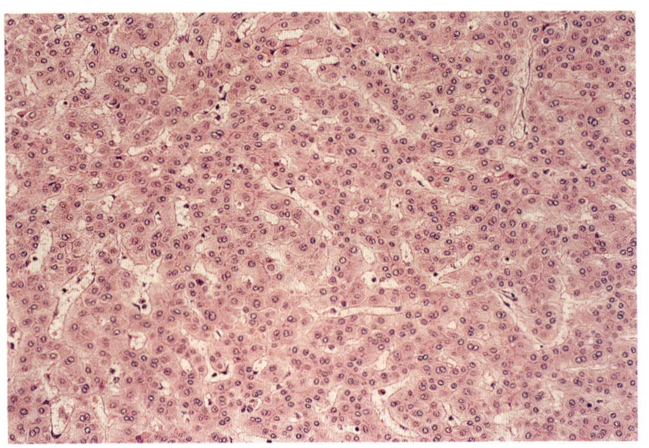

PLATE 12-2A.

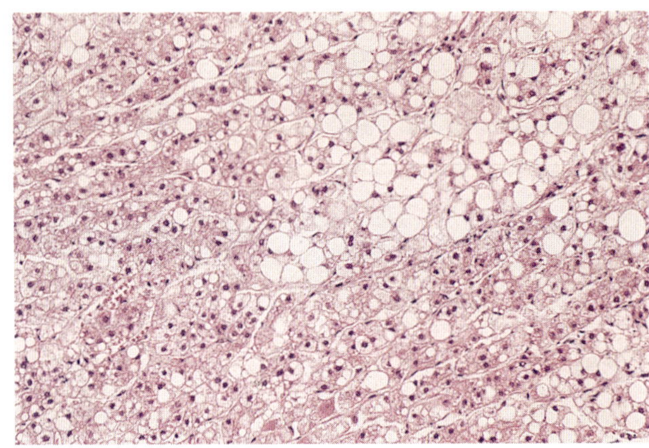

PLATE 12-2B.

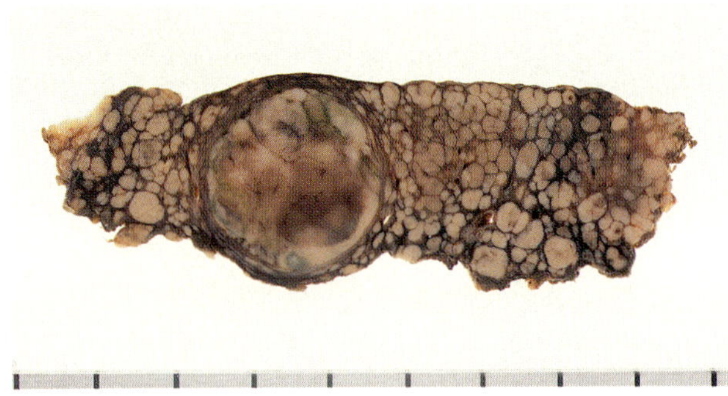

PLATE 12-3A.

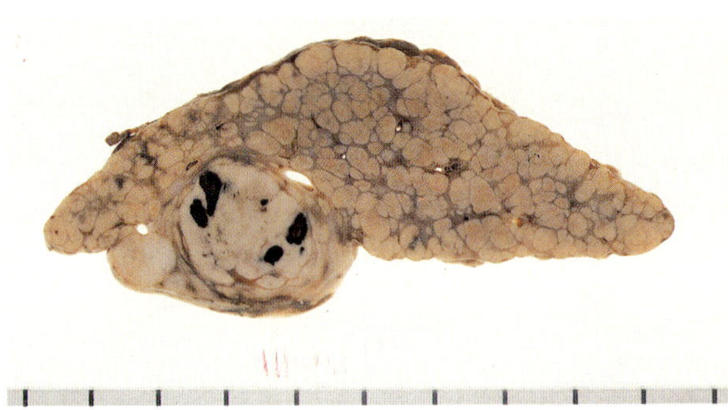

PLATE 12-3B.

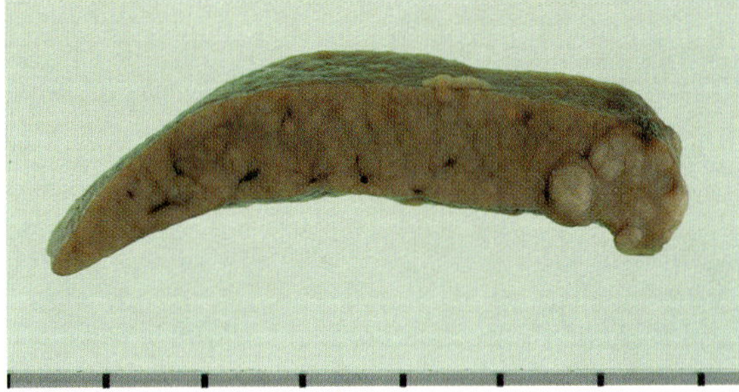

PLATE 12-3C.

PLATE 12-1. Small hepatocellular carcinoma of a distinct nodular type. The tumor presents thin fibrous capsule and septa. Hepatitis C virus-associated cirrhosis is present.

PLATE 12-2. Typical histologic features of well-differentiated hepatocellular carcinoma (HCC). *(A)* HCC with little atypia shows irregular thin trabecular pattern. *(B)* Diffuse fatty change in HCC tissue.

PLATE 12-3. Modified gross classification by Liver Cancer Study Group of Japan. *(A)* Single nodular type. A well-encapsulated cancer nodule without perinodular tumor growth. *(B)* Nodular pattern with a perinodular tumor growth. *(C)* Multinodular confluent type.

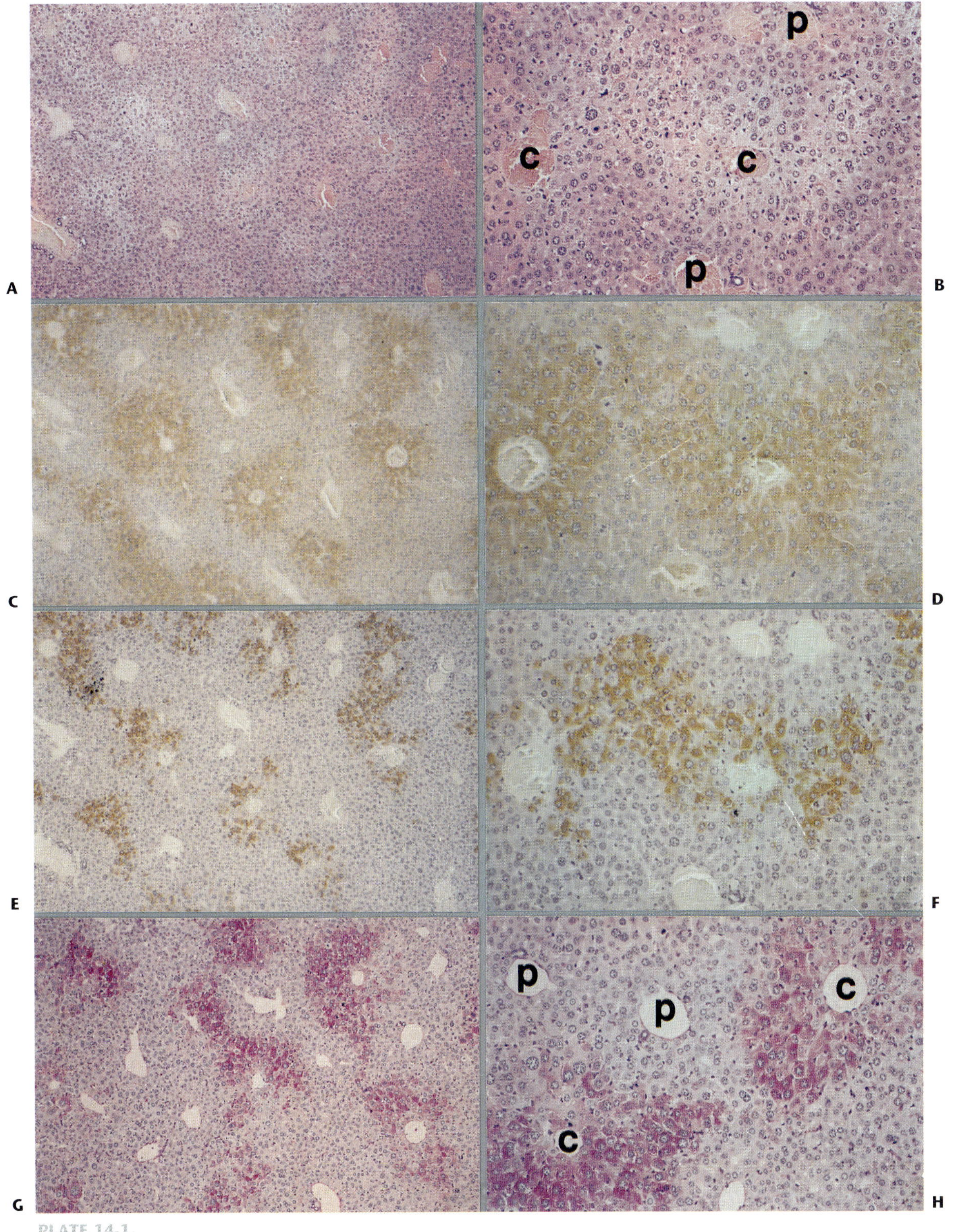

PLATE 14-1.

PLATE 14-1. Early focal lesions of altered hepatocytes in the livers of HBx transgenic mice. Sections of liver from a male mouse sacrificed at 2 months of age and stained with hematoxylin and eosin (H&E) *(A, B)*, rabbit anti-HBx *(C, D)*, rabbit anti-TGFβ1 *(E, F)*, or periodic acid-Schiff *(G, H)*. Both low (Plates A, C, E, G) and high (Plates B, D, F, H) magnification views are shown. The immunostained sections were visualized by the avidin-biotin complex method. The H&E, anti-HBx, and anti-TGFβ1 sections are serial cuts. The central veins (c) and portal veins (p) are indicated.

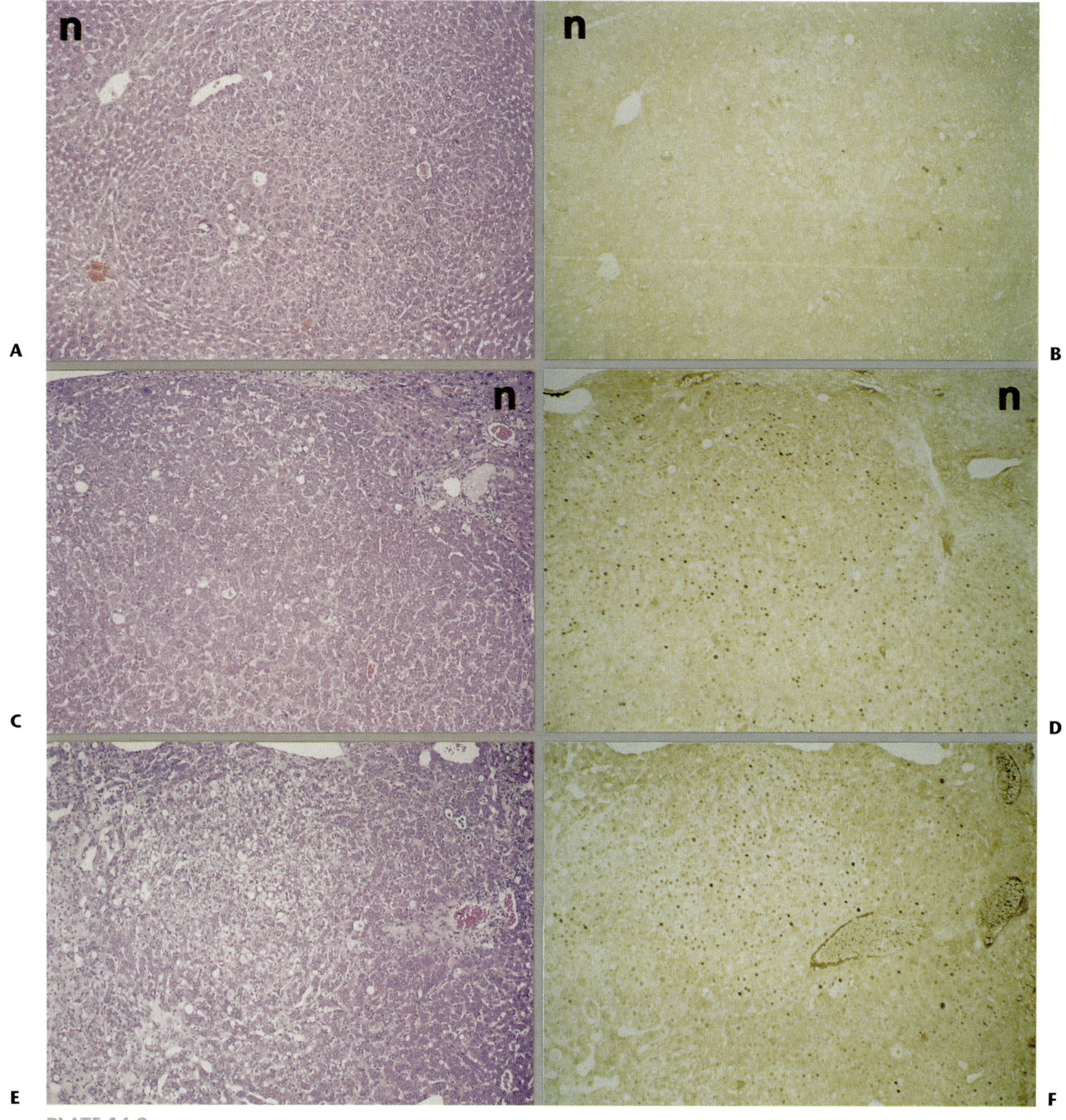

PLATE 14-2. Tumor nodules in the liver of HBx transgenic mice. Sections of tumor lesions from three independent transgenic mice were stained with either hematoxylin and eosin *(A, C, E)* or anti-PCNA *(B, D, F)*. The adjacent normal region of the liver (n) is indicated.

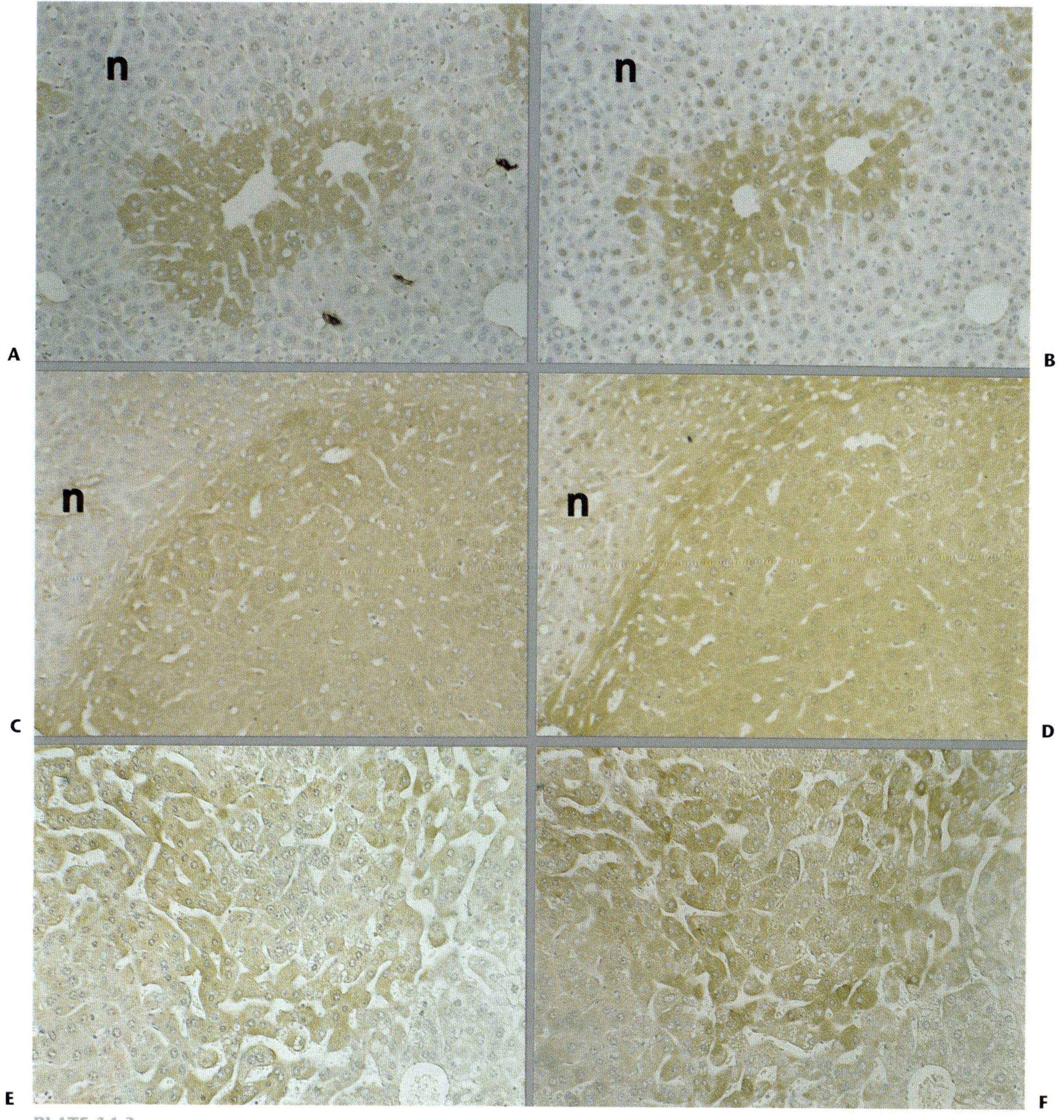

PLATE 14-3.

PLATE 14-3. Immunostaining of p53 in the liver of HBx transgenic mice. Serial sections of an altered focus *(A, B)*, an adenoma *(C, D)*, and a hepatocellular carcinoma *(E, F)* from different transgenic mice were immunostained with either rabbit anti-HBx *(Plates A, C, E)* or rabbit anti-p53 *(Plates B, D, F)*. The immunostained sections were visualized by the avidin-biotin complex method. The adjacent normal region of the liver (n) is indicated.

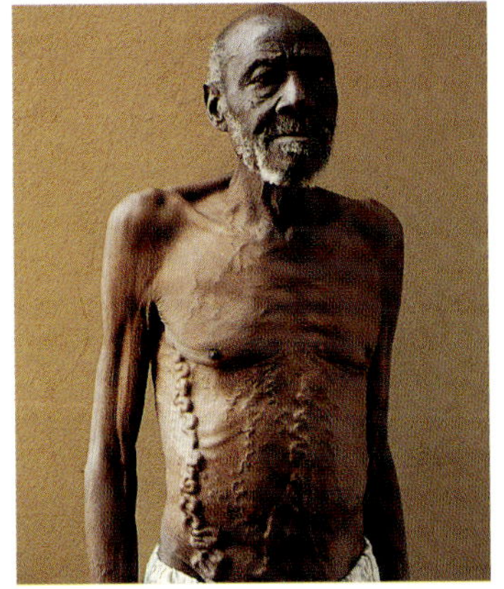

PLATE 20-1.

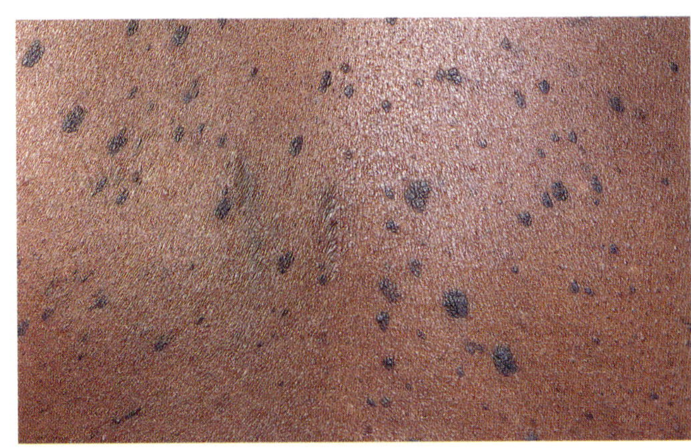

PLATE 20-2.

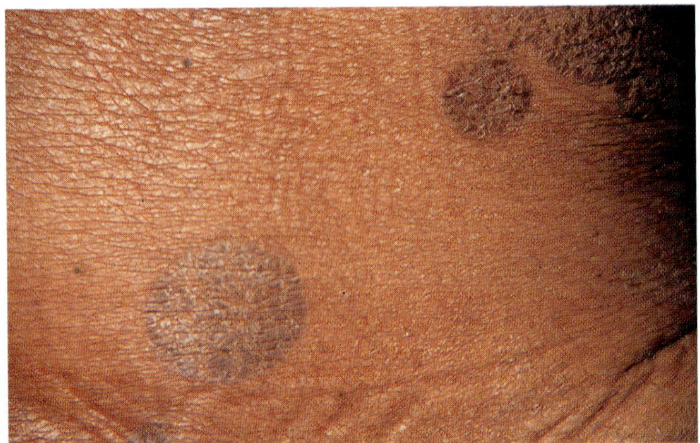

PLATE 20-3.

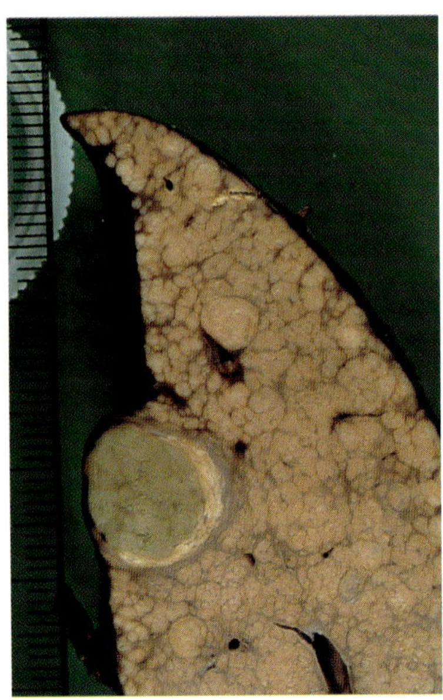

PLATE 21-1.

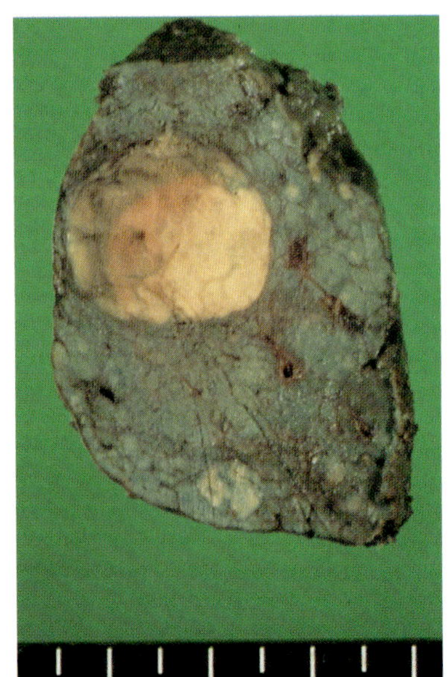

PLATE 21-2.

PLATE 20-1. Markedly dilated and tortuous collateral veins in a patient with membranous obstruction of the inferior vena cava.

PLATE 20-2. Leser-Trélat sign.

PLATE 20-3. Pityriasis rotunda.

PLATE 21-1. Resected specimen from a patient with hypoechoic hepatocellular carcinoma.

PLATE 21-2. Resected specimen from a patient with hyperechoic hepatocellular carcinoma. Fatty change can be seen within the nodule.

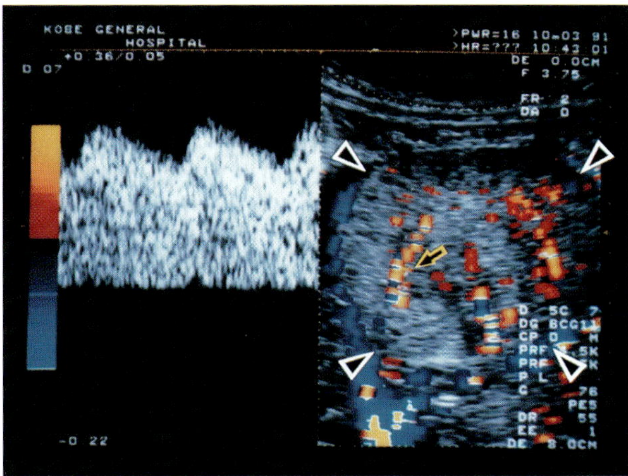

PLATE 21-3.

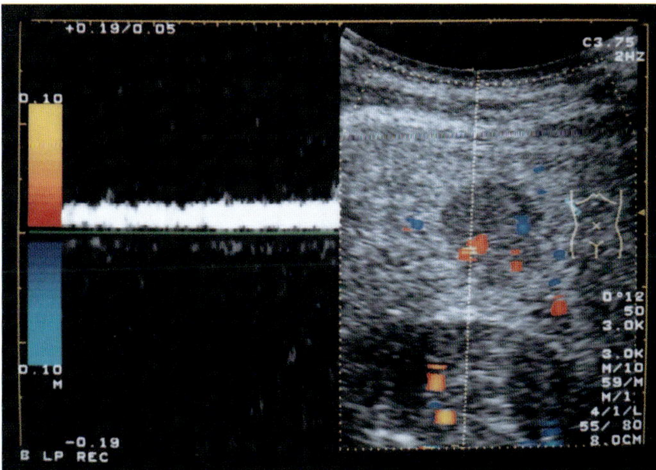

PLATE 21-4.

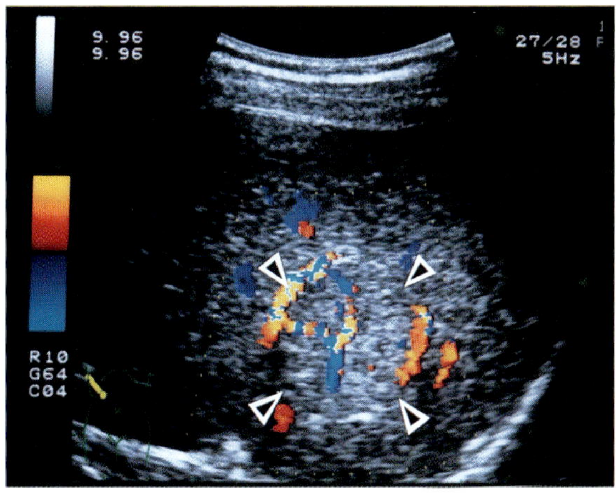

PLATE 21-5.

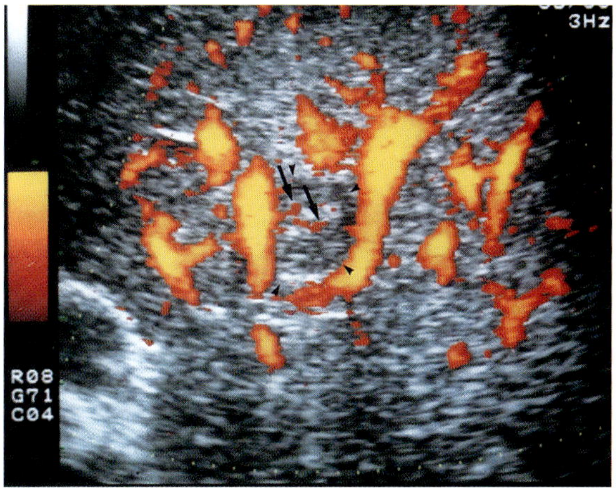

PLATE 21-6.

PLATE 21-3. Color Doppler appearance of typical hepatocellular carcinoma (arrowheads). Intratumoral pulsatile signal (arrow) is clearly demonstrated.

PLATE 21-4. Color Doppler appearance of typical adenomatous hyperplasia. Afferent continuous waveform signal not associated with pulsatile signal can be demonstrated.

PLATE 21-5. Color Doppler findings of focal nodular hyperplasia. Centrifugal flow pattern is clearly demonstrated.

PLATE 21-6. Apparent color flow signals (arrows) are demonstrated by power Doppler imaging within the nodule (arrowhead) of a 1-cm-diameter hepatocellular carcinoma.

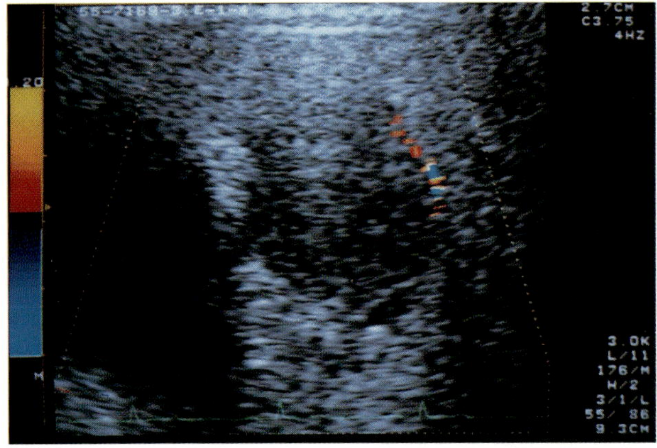

PLATE 21-7A.

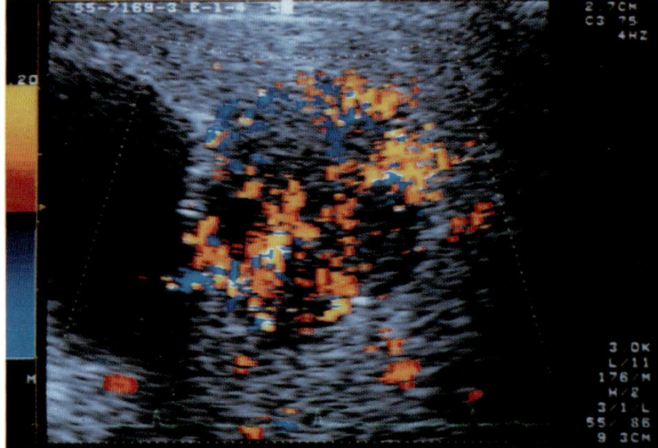

PLATE 21-7B.

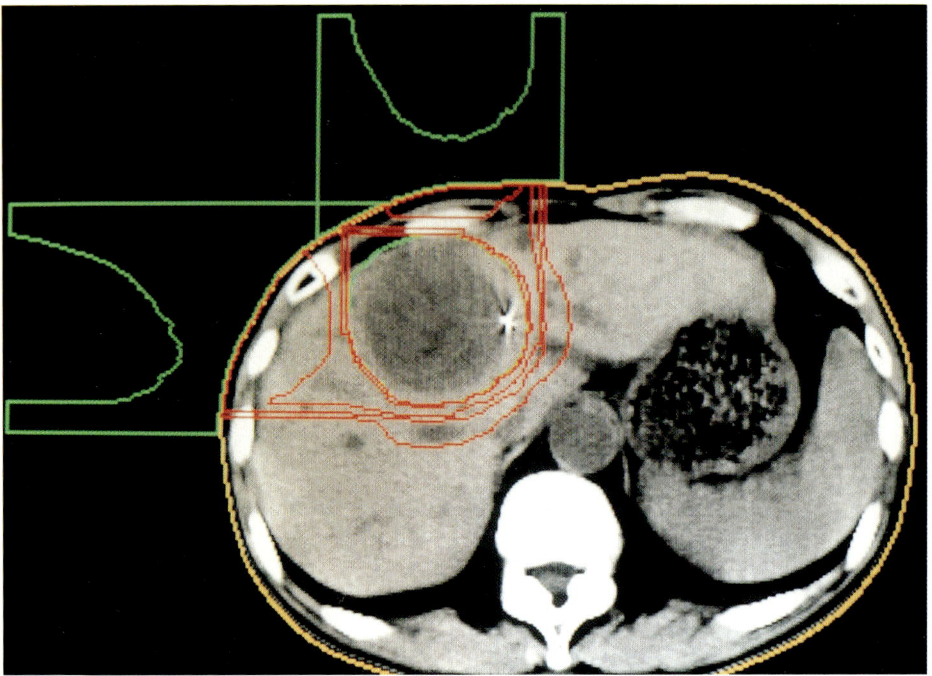

PLATE 34-1.

PLATE 21-7. *(A)* Color signal is not demonstrated within a 5-cm-diameter hepatocellular carcinoma (HCC) by plain color Doppler. *(B)* Abundant color flow signal can be seen upon enhanced color Doppler study with intravenous injection of the contrast medium Levovist, suggesting HCC.

PLATE 34-1. Dose contour of proton beam in a patient with hepatocellular carcinoma who was irradiated with proton beam. Iso-dose curves of proton beams show that radiation dose deposited in the normal tissue of the liver surrounding the tumor is minimal.

11

CIRRHOSIS AND HEPATOCELLULAR CARCINOMA

SWAN N. THUNG
MICHAEL A. GERBER

Hepatocellular carcinoma (HCC) is one of the most common fatal malignant neoplasms in the world. The etiology of HCC appears to be multifactorial, and several events seem to be necessary for malignant transformation to occur. The striking geographic differences in the incidence of HCC suggest that environmental factors frequently contribute to its development. One common factor in about three-fourths of HCC, however, is the association with cirrhosis. In fact, cirrhosis has been considered a preneoplastic condition. The incidence of HCC varies depending on the etiology and type of associated cirrhosis.

CIRRHOSIS OF DIFFERENT ETIOLOGIES AND TYPES

About 75% of all HCCs worldwide are associated with cirrhosis, in addition one of three other factors: hepatitis B virus (HBV) infection,[1–3] hepatitis C virus (HCV) infection,[3,4] or alcoholism.[5–7] (Figs. 11-1 through 11-3 and Plates 11-1 through 11-3). Any other form of chronic liver disease that leads to cirrhosis may also be complicated by HCC. These include inherited metabolic diseases such as genetic hemochromatosis,[8,9] (Fig. 11-4 and Plate 11-4) α_1-antitrypsin deficiency,[10,11] Wilson's disease,[12–14] and autoimmune liver diseases such as primary biliary cirrhosis[15–18] and autoimmune hepatitis.[19–21] Cirrhosis, therefore, may be a premalignant condition, regardless of the etiology.[22–24]

Of the various types of cirrhosis, macronodular or the mixed macronodular and micronodular cirrhosis are most frequently associated with HCC, and micronodular cirrhosis is complicated by HCC less often. Active proliferation, as evidenced by the presence of large or macroregenerative nodules (MRN) and small liver cell dysplasia in a cirrhotic liver, has been considered an important step in the process of malignant transformation.[25–32]

CIRRHOSIS AS A PRENEOPLASTIC CONDITION

Cirrhosis is the end result of chronic hepatocellular necrosis, inflammation, and fibrosis and is defined morphologically as a diffuse process with septal fibrosis and regenerative nodules.[33] The strong correlation between cirrhosis and HCC suggests that they may be due to a common cause or that the development of cirrhosis involves the same steps or mechanisms as hepatocarcinogenesis. Malignant transformation itself involves the processes of initiation, promotion, and progression, steps that are provided by cirrhotic livers.

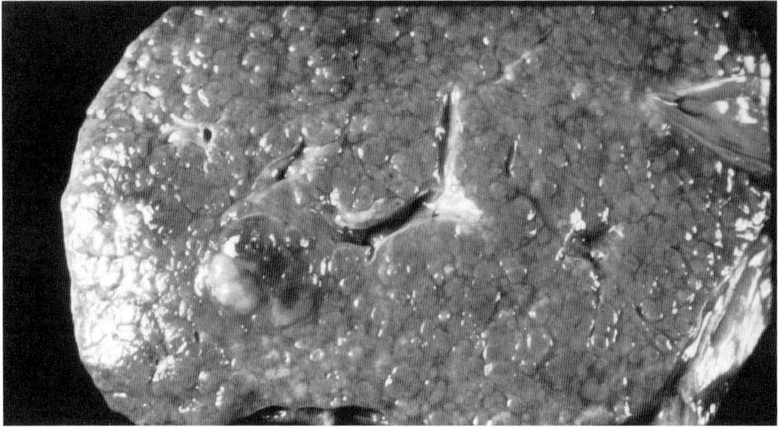

FIGURE 11-1. Bile-producing hepatocellular carcinoma arising in a micronodular cirrhosis secondary to alcoholic liver disease. (See also Plate 11-1.)

INITIATION AND SOMATIC MUTATIONS

A somatic mutation represents the earliest irreversible step during initiation and most likely occurs when hepatocytes are damaged and undergo mitoses.[34,35] A variety of carcinogens may act directly as initiators. The integration of hepatitis B virus (HBV) into the host genome is one example (besides the possible role of this virus in tumor promotion and progression).[36–38] Single-site and multiple-site integrations have been observed in HBV infection,[39] with or without major rearrangements of cellular DNA.[40] The integration pattern of HBV DNA in the tumorous and nontumorous liver tissues of the same patient may be either the same or different.

Different sites of integration have been reported. In some cases, the HBV genome may be integrated within a gene that regulates cell growth (e.g., the cyclin A gene),[41] within the retinoic acid receptor gene, which regulates cell differentiation,[42] or in chromosome 17,

FIGURE 11-2. Macronodular cirrhosis with numerous macroregenerative nodules and multicentric hepatocellular carcinoma (arrows) in a patient with chronic hepatitis B. (See also Plate 11-2.)

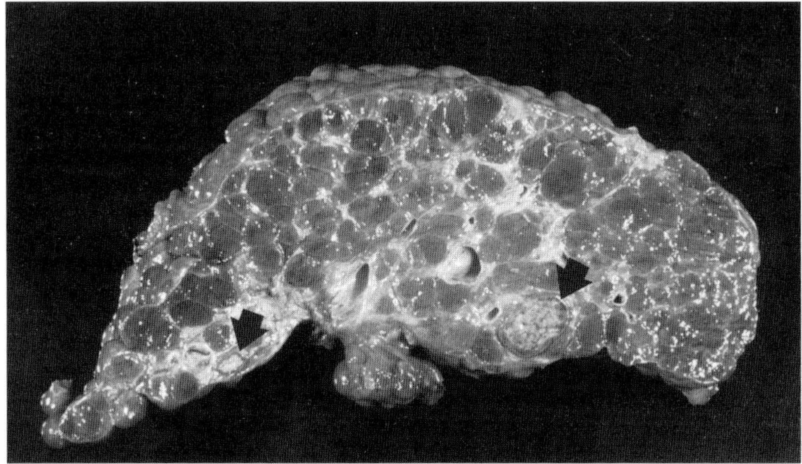

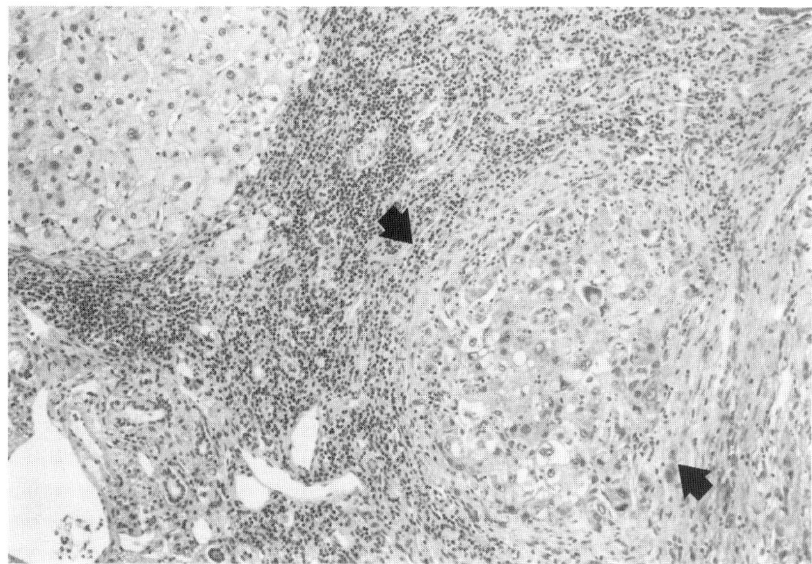

FIGURE 11-3. Chronic hepatitis C and cirrhosis with multiple small hepatocellular carcinomas (one of which is delineated by arrows). (H&E, ×100.) (See also Plate 11-3.)

which could lead to alterations of the p53 tumor suppressor gene.[43,44]

The efficiency of initiation is related to cellular replicative DNA synthesis and cell division,[45,46] which follows liver injury. Repetitive mitoses favor carcinogenesis. In the HBV transgenic mouse, which overproduces the HBV large envelope protein, HCC develops following liver cell injury, inflammation, and regenerative hyperplasia. This places large numbers of hepatocytes at risk for the development of transforming mutations[47] and may represent a general mechanism of hepatocarcinogenesis in any necroinflammatory liver disease. Nitric oxide derived from macrophages in liver injury, which may play a role in the elimination of injured hepatocytes by inducing apoptosis via DNA fragmentation, can cause other types of DNA damage such as DNA strand breaks

FIGURE 11-4. A large hepatocellular carcinoma in a dark brown liver with hemochromatosis. (See also Plate 11-4.)

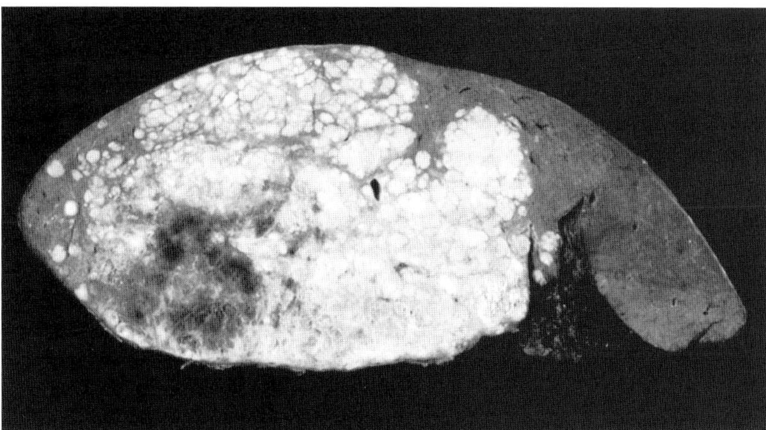

and oxidative base alterations, which may lead to carcinogenesis.[48]

REGENERATION OF HEPATOCYTES

Hepatocytes in the normal adult liver rarely divide, but they do so following parenchymal injury and loss. Regeneration of hepatocytes is a promoting factor for hepatocarcinogenesis. HCC develops more frequently in cirrhosis of the macronodular type than in micronodular cirrhosis[22–24] (Figs. 11-5 and 11-6 and Plates 11-5 and 11-6), and even more so when macroregenerative nodules (MRNs) are present. MRNs are defined as large hepatic nodules that are distinct in color, texture, or the degree to which they bulge from the surrounding cirrhotic liver parenchyma; they are at least 8 mm in diameter.[26,29,49] They can be found in a wide variety of chronic liver diseases including viral hepatitis, autoimmune hepatitis, primary biliary cirrhosis, primary sclerosing cholangitis, primary hemochromatosis, α_1-antitrypsin deficiency and alcoholic liver injury.[29,30,49,50] It has been suggested that MRNs, particularly atypical MRNs or type II MRNs, develop as a result of extensive regeneration in a cirrhotic liver[51] and that these highly proliferative nodules are more susceptible to carcinogenic events.[50–54] The development of HCC in a cirrhotic liver with lesions indicative of proliferation (such as nodule-in-nodule lesions and the small cell dysplasia often seen in MRNs type II) underlines the importance of hepatocyte proliferation.[55] This is also supported by hepatocarcinogenesis in HBV transgenic mice, in which the development of HCC strongly correlates with the degree of the necroinflammatory process and the level of hepatocellular proliferation following hepatocellular injury.[52]

ONCOGENES

Proto-oncogenes or cellular oncogenes are cellular genes that are involved in cell proliferation.[57] Specific transcriptional patterns of proto-oncogene expression during physiologic cellular growth and differentiation have been demonstrated for a variety of cell types in developing and adult tissues.[58] The products of a number of oncogenes have been identified as nuclear proteins, tyrosine kinases, growth factors, or their receptors.[57–59]

Sequential induction of the c-*ets*,[60] c-*fos*,[61,62] and c-*jun*[63] genes is initiated within minutes in regenerating rat livers after partial hepatectomy, followed by c-*myc*[62,64,65] and then by c-Ki-*ras* and c-Ha-*ras*.[61,66,67] The expression of cellular oncogenes such as c-K-*ras* and c-*fos* during liver regeneration in human liver diseases, including cirrhosis, has been documented.[68]

A series of changes in these genes that control hepatocyte growth or interference with the protein products of these genes, may play an important role in the etiology

FIGURE 11-5. Hepatocellular carcinoma arising in a macroregenerative nodule. The periphery of the tumor consists of hyperplastic hepatocytes (arrows). (H&E, ×250.) (See also Plate 11-5.)

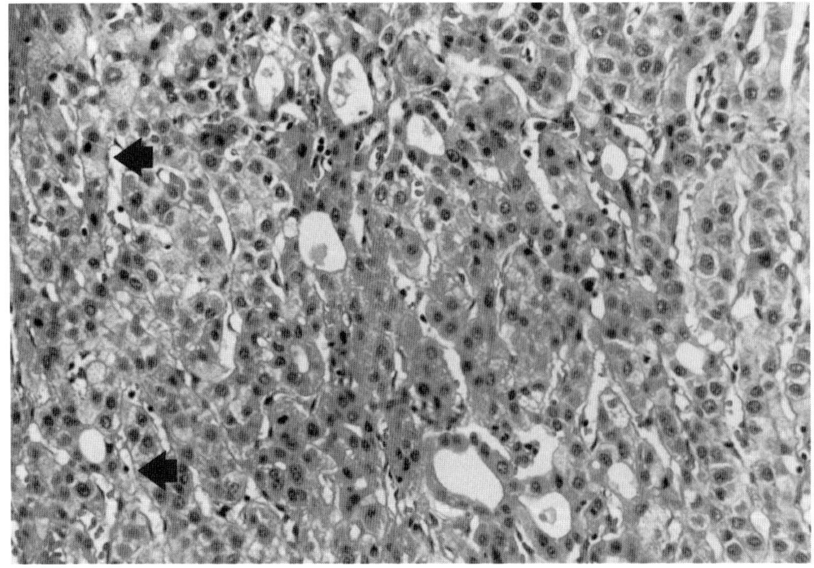

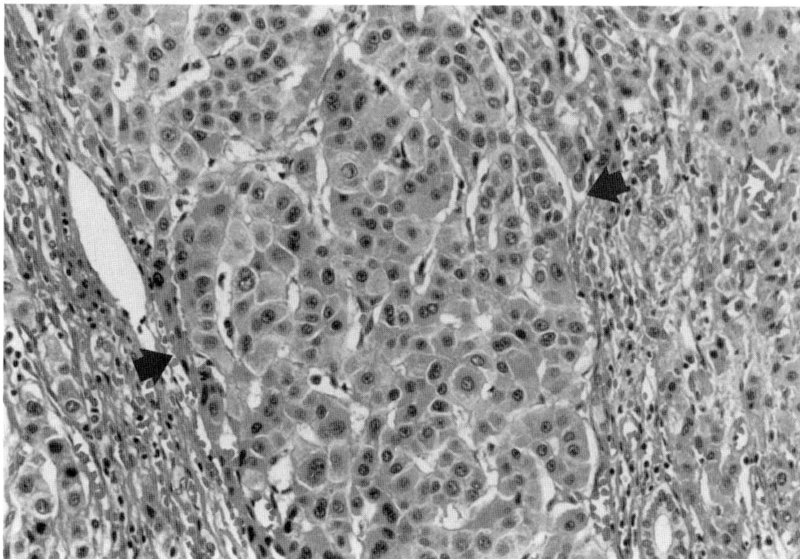

FIGURE 11-6. Well-differentiated hepatocellular carcinoma arising not in a macroregenerative nodule, but from and replacing a small cirrhotic nodule (arrows). (H&E, ×250.) (See also Plate 11-6.)

of HCC.[69,70] Rearrangement and/or amplification of N-*ras* and c-*myc* genes,[71] as well as others, including N-*myc*, H-*ras*, *abl*, *fos*, *src*, c-erb B-2 and *raf*, have been observed in HCCs,[72,73] but not in non-neoplastic liver disease.[68] Overexpression of c-*myc* is a common finding in most studies of human HCCs,[72,74,76] possibly due to trans-activation of the c-*myc* promoter by mutant p53 protein[77] or by the protein product of either the HBV X gene or of a truncated HBV pre S2/S sequence.[78,79] Mutations or amplication of c-*myc*, however, are uncommon in HCC.[80,81] Transfection of rat liver epithelial cells ("oval cells") in culture with activated c-Ha-*ras* produced HCCs when injected subcutaneously into nude mice.[82]

TUMOR SUPPRESSOR GENES

Alterations of tumor suppressor genes have been associated with a variety of human cancers. The products of the p53 and RB genes act as tumor suppressors[83,84]; mutations or inactivation of these may facilitate cell immortalization and transformation.[84,85] Their mutations, which often require inactivation of both alleles of the genes, have been reported to be late events in human hepatocarcinogenesis and, therefore, may play an important role in tumor progression.[86] In HBV transgenic mice, however, the development of HCCs is not accompanied by structural or functional alterations of the p53 and RB genes.[87]

p53

The p53 tumor suppressor gene is located on chromosome 17 and is often mutated or inactivated in human HCC.[76] The product of this gene, the p53 protein in its "wild-type" form, is found in the nucleus and appears to suppress tumor formation.[83,88] The incidence of mutations of the p53 gene in HCC shows a striking geographic variation.[87,88] Point mutations at codon 249[89–92] are found especially in HCCs of patients from southern Africa and Southeast Asia, but generally not in other parts of the world, such as North America, Europe, the Middle East, and Japan.[90–93] It has been suggested that a mutation at codon 249 identifies an endemic form of HCC strongly associated with dietary aflatoxin B1 intake and possibly with HBV infection.[90,92–94] Mutation at codon 249 involving G to T transversion has also been reported in a hepatoblastoma from a child without known exposure to aflatoxin B1 or hepatitis B or C viruses.[95] Mutational hot spots in the p53 gene other than at codon 249 have also been described in HCCs (e.g., at codon 166 in exon 5 and at codon 286 in exon 8).[96] There seems to be a difference in the pattern of p53 mutational changes depending on whether HCC is associated with HBV or hepatitis C virus (HCV) infection.[97] In addition, inactivation of the functions of p53 gene or its product can occur when transforming proteins of DNA tumor viruses (SV40 T antigen, adenovirus E1B antigen, and HPV E6 protein) form complexes with the wild-type p53 protein.[98,102] Structural abnormalities of the p53 gene were observed more frequently in advanced HCCs, suggesting a role in tumor progression,[86,97] rather than in tumor initiation.

RB GENE

Mutation or deletion of the RB tumor suppressor gene has been reported in various types of tumors including HCC.[100,101] The gene is located on chromosome 13 and encodes for a 110 kd phosphoprotein (pRB). When pRB is underphosphorylated, it suppresses cell proliferation, but when pRB is phosphorylated, cell growth can occur.[76] Unrestricted cellular growth resulting in tumorigenesis may occur when the restraint provided by pRB is no longer available. This may follow (1) RB gene deletion or mutation; (2) binding of proteins of DNA tumor viruses (e.g., the large T antigen of SV 40,[102] the adenovirus E1A protein,[103] and the human papillomavirus type 16 E7 antigen)[104,105]; and (3) when transforming growth factor-β1 (TGF-β1), which normally suppresses the enzyme that phosphorylates the RB protein, is not functioning.[106] An additive effect of p53 and RB gene mutations or deletions in carcinogenesis has been suggested. In human HCC cell lines, RB gene aberrations are rare, and p53 abnormalities are more frequently found.[107]

GROWTH FACTORS

Normal cell growth is regulated by proto-oncogene products and growth factors, which act in concert.[108] Growth factors activate gene expression programs that involve proto-oncogenes and proto-oncogene receptors.[109] Growth factor genes are often activated in HCCs, usually without mutations. Some of these genes can be activated by removal of the restraining influences of normally functioning tumor suppressor genes. The inappropriate or prolonged expression of growth factor genes may lead to uncontrolled growth and result in tumor formation. Growth factors such as hepatocyte growth factor (HGF), epidermal growth factor (EGF), and transforming growth factor α (TGF-α) play important functions in triggering and initiating the early events required for liver regeneration.[110,111] Their overexpression[112,113] and that of others such as fibroblast growth factor (FGF),[114] and insulin-like growth factor II (IGF-II)[115,116] have been described in HCCs. The detection of greater quantities of TGF-α in the more differentiated portions of HCCs suggests that its increased expression may be an early event in human hepatocarcinogenesis.[117] Expression of TGF-α has also been described in focal nodular hyperplasia[118] and in chronic hepatitis B and C.[119]

REFERENCES

1. Hadengue A, N'Dri N, Benhamou J-P. Relative risk of hepatocellular carcinoma in HBsAg positive vs. alcoholic cirrhosis. A cross-sectional study. Liver 1990;10:147–151
2. Beasley RP, Hwang LY, Lin CC, Chien CS. Hepatocellular carcinoma and hepatitis B virus: a prospective study of 22,707 men in Taiwan. Lancet 1981;2:1129–1133
3. Ikeda K, Saitoh S, Koida I et al. A multivariate analysis of risk factors for hepatocellular carcinogenesis: a prospective observation of 795 patients with viral and alcoholic cirrhosis. Hepatology 1993;18:47–53
4. Thung SN, Hytiroglou P, Fiel I, Theise ND. Preneoplastic lesions in chronic hepatitis C. In Kobayashi K, Purcell RH, Shimotohno K, Tabor E, (eds). Hepatitis C Virus and Its Involvement in the Development of Hepatocellular Carcinoma. Princeton Scientific Publishing Co, Princeton, 1996, pp. 1–8
5. Hardell L, Bengtsson NO, Jonsson U et al. Aetiological aspects on primary liver cancer with special regard to alcohol, organic solvents and acute intermittent porphyria—an epidemiological investigation. Br J Cancer 1984;50: 389–397
6. De Bac C, Stroffolini T, Gaeta GB et al. Pathogenic factors in cirrhosis with and without hepatocellular carcinoma: a multi-center Italian study. Hepatology 1994;20:1225–1230
7. Tsukuma H, Hiyama T, Tanaka S et al. Risk factors for hepatocellular carcinoma among patients with chronic liver disease. N Engl J Med 1993;328:1797–1801
8. Bradbear RA, Halliday JW, Bassett ML et al. Hepatocellular carcinoma in hemochromatosis. In Okuda K, Ishak KG (eds). Neoplasms of the Liver. Springer-Verlag, Tokyo, 1987, pp. 189–197
9. Fargion S, Fracanzani AL, Piperno A et al. Prognostic factors for hepatocellular carcinoma in genetic hemochromatosis. Hepatology 1994;20:1426–1431
10. Berg NO, Erickson S. Liver disease in adults with 1-antitrypsin deficiency. N Engl J Med 1972;287:1264–1267
11. Reid CL, Wiener GJ, Cox DW et al: Diffuse hepatocellular dysplasia and carcinoma associated with the Malton variant of 1-antitrypsin. Gastroenterology 1987;93:181–187
12. Wilkinson ML, Portmann B, Williams R. Wilson's disease and hepatocellular carcinoma: possible protective role of copper. Gut 1983;24:767–771
13. Polio J, Enriquez RE, Chow A et al. Hepatocellular carcinoma in Wilson's disease. Case report and review of the literature. J Clin Gastroenterol 1989;11:220–226
14. Cheng WSC, Govindarajan S, Redeker AG. Hepatocellular carcinoma in a case of Wilson's disease. Liver 1992;12: 42–45
15. Nakanuma Y, Terada T, Doishita K et al. Hepatocellular carcinoma in primary biliary cirrhosis: an autopsy study. Hepatology 1990;11:1010–1016
16. Gluskin LE, Guariglia P, Payne JA et al. Hepatocellular carcinoma in a patient with precirrhotic primary biliary cirrhosis. J Clin Gastroenterol 1985;7:441–444
17. Melia WM, Johnson PJ, Neuberger H et al. Hepatocellular

carcinoma in primary biliary cirrhosis: detection by α-fetoprotein estimation. Gastroenterology 1984;87:660–663

18. Min AD, Schluger LK, Thung SN et al. Hepatocellular carcinoma in patients with end-stage primary biliary cirrhosis undergoing liver transplantation. Hepatology 1994;20: 152A
19. Wang KK, Czaja AJ. Hepatocellular carcinoma in corticosteroid treated severe autoimmune chronic active hepatitis. Hepatology 1988;8:1679–1683
20. Burroughs AK, Bassendine MF, Thomas HC, Sherlock S. Primary liver cancer in autoimmune chronic liver disease. Br Med J 1981;1:273
21. Thung SN, Bach N, Jordon D, Schaffner F. Hepatocellular carcinoma associated with autoimmune chronic active hepatitis. Mt Sinai J Med 1990;57:165–168
22. Okuda K, Liver Cancer Study Group of Japan. Primary liver cancers. Cancer 1980;45:2663–2669
23. Anthony PP. Primary carcinoma of the liver: a study of 282 cases in Ugandan Africans. J Pathol Bacteriol 1973;110: 37–49
24. Kew MC, Popper H. Relationship between hepatocellular carcinoma and cirrhosis. Semin Liver Dis 1984;4:136–146
25. Kondo F, Ebara M, Sugiura N et al. Histological features and clinical course of large regenerative nodules: evaluation of their pre-cancerous potentiality. Hepatology 1990;12: 592–598
26. Furuya K, Nakamura M, Yamamoto Y et al. Macroregenerative nodule of the liver: a clinicopathologic study of 345 autopsy cases of chronic liver disease. Cancer 1988;61: 99–105
27. Takayama T, Makuuchi M, Hirohashi S et al. Malignant transformation of adenomatous hyperplasia to hepatocellular carcinoma. Lancet 1990;336:1150–1153
28. Eguchi A, Nakashima O, Okudaira S et al. Adenomatous hyperplasia in the vicinity of small hepatocellular carcinoma. Hepatology 1992;15:843–848
29. Ferrell L, Wright T, Lake J et al. Incidence and diagnostic features of macroregenerative nodules vs. small hepatocellular carcinoma in cirrhotic livers. Hepatology 1992;16: 1372–1381
30. Hytiroglou P, Theise ND, Schwartz M et al. Macroregenerative nodules in a series of adult cirrhotic liver explants: issues of classification and nomenclature. Hepatology 1995; 21:703–708
31. Ohno Y, Shiga J, Machinami R. A histopathological analysis of five cases of adenomatous hyperplasia containing minute hepatocellular carcinoma. Acta Pathol Jpn 1990;40: 267–278
32. Nakanuma Y, Terada T, Ueda K et al. Adenomatous hyperplasia of the liver as a pre-cancerous lesion. Liver 1993;13: 1–9
33. Anthony PP, Ishak KG, Nayak NC et al. The morphology of cirrhosis, definition, nomenclature and classification. Bull WHO 1977;55:521–531
34. Goldfarb S, Pugh TD. The origin and significance of hyperplastic hepatocellular islands and nodules in hepatic carcinogenesis. J Am Coll Toxicol 1982;1:119–144
35. Pitot HC, Dragan YP. Facts and theories concerning the mechanisms of carcinogenesis. FASEB J 1991;5:2280–2286
36. Popper H, Thung SN, McMahon BJ et al. Evolution of hepatocellular carcinoma associated with chronic hepatitis B virus infection in Alaskan Eskimos. Arch Pathol Lab Med 1988;112:498–504
37. Haruna Y, Hayashi N, Kamada T et al. Expression of hepatitis C virus in hepatocellular carcinoma. Cancer 1994;73: 2253–2258
38. Popper H, Gerber MA, Thung SN. The relation of hepatocellular carcinoma to infection with hepatitis B and related viruses in man and animals. Hepatology 1982;2(suppl):1–9
39. Chang MH, Chen P-J, Chen J-Y et al. Hepatitis B virus integration in hepatitis B virus-related hepatocellular carcinoma in childhood. Hepatology 1991;13:316–320
40. Hino O, Shows TB, Rogler CE. Hepatitis B virus integration site in hepatocellular carcinoma at chromosome 17; 18 translocation. Proc Natl Acad Sci U S A 1986;83: 8338–8342
41. Wang J, Chinevesse X, Henglein B, Bréchot C. Hepatitis B virus integration in a cyclin A gene in a hepatocellular carcinoma. Nature 1990;343:555–557
42. Dejean A, Bougueleret L, Grzeschik K, Tiollais P. Hepatitis B virus DNA integration in a sequence homologous to v-erb-A and steroid receptor genes in a hepatocellular carcinoma 1986;322:70–72
43. Tokino T, Fukushige S, Nakamura T et al. Chromosomal translocation and inverted duplication associated with integrated hepatitis B virus in hepatocellular carcinoma. J Virol 1987;61:3848–3854
44. Zhou Y, Slagle BL, Donehower LA et al. Structural analysis of a hepatitis B virus genome integrated into chromosome 17p of a human hepatocellular carcinoma. J Virol 1988;62: 4224–4231
45. Ishikawa T, Takayama S, Kitagawa T. Correlation between time of partial hepatectomy after a single treatment with diethylnitrosamine and induction of adenosine triphosphatase-deficient islands in rat liver. Cancer Res 1980;40: 4261–4264
46. Warwick GP. Effect of the cell cycle on carcinogenesis. Fed Proc 1971;30:1760–1765
47. Dunsford HA, Sell S, Chisari FV. Hepatocarcinogenesis due to chronic liver cell injury in hepatitis B virus transgenic mice. Cancer Res 1990;50:3400–3407
48. Watanabe N, Kurose I, Higuchi H et al. Macrophage-derived mitotic oxide promotes fragmentation, single strand break and oxidative damage of DNA in rat hepatocytes. Gastroenterology 1996;110:A1358
49. Theise ND, Schwartz M, Miller C et al. Macroregenerative nodules and hepatocellular carcinoma in forty-four sequential adult liver explants with cirrhosis. Hepatology 1992; 16:949–955
50. LeBail B, Belleannee G, Bernard P-H et al. Adenomatous hyperplasia in cirrhotic livers: histological evaluation, cellular density, and proliferative activity of 35 lesions in the cirrhotic explants of 10 adult French patients. Hum Pathol 1995;26:897–906
51. Sakamoto M, Hirohashi S, Shimosato Y. Early stages of

multistep hepatocarcinogenesis: adenomatous hyperplasia and early hepatocellular carcinoma. Hum Pathol 1991;22: 172–178

52. Terasaki S, Terada T, Nakanuma Y et al. Argyrophilic nucleolar organizer regions and α-fetoprotein in adenomatous hyperplasia in human cirrhotic livers. Am J Clin Pathol 1991;95:850–857
53. Grigioni W, D'Errico A, Bacci F et al: Primary liver neoplasms: evaluation of proliferative index using MoAb Ki 67. J Pathol 1989;158:23–29
54. Terada T, Nakanuma Y. Cell proliferative activity of adenomatous hyperplasia in the liver and small hepatocellular carcinoma. An immunohistochemical study demonstrating proliferating cell nuclear antigen. Cancer 1992;70:591–598
55. Theise ND. Macroregenerative (dysplastic) nodules and hepatocarcinogenesis: theoretical and clinical considerations. Semin Liv Dis 1995;15:360–371
56. Huang S-N, Chisari FV. Strong, sustained hepatocellular proliferation precedes hepatocarcinogenesis in hepatitis B surface antigen transgenic mice. Hepatology 1995;21: 620–626
57. Bishop JM. Cellular oncogenes and retroviruses. Annu Rev Biochem 1983;52:301–305
58. Klein G, Klein E. Evolution of tumors and the impact of molecular oncology. Nature 1985;315:190–195
59. Weinberg RA. The action of oncogenes in the cytoplasm and nucleus. Science 1985;230:770–783
60. Bhat NK, Fisher RJ, Fujiwara S et al. Temporal and tissue-specific expression of mouse ets genes. Proc Natl Acad Sci U S A 1987;84:3161–3165
61. Kerr LD, Holt JT, Matrisian LM. Growth factors regulate transin gene expression by c-fos-dependent and c-fos independent pathways. Science 1988;242:1424–1427
62. Thompson NL, Mead JE, Braun L et al. Sequential proto-oncogene expression during rat liver regeneration. Cancer Res 1986;46:3111–3117
63. Alcorn JA, Feitelberg SP, Brenner DA. Transient induction of c-jun during hepatic regeneration. Hepatology 1990; 11:909–915
64. Makino R, Hayashi K, Sugimura T. C-myc transcript is induced in rat liver at a very early stage of regeneration or by cycloheximide treatment. Nature 1984;310:697–698
65. Sobczak J, Tournier MF, Lotti AM, Duguet M. Gene expression in regenerating liver in relation to cell proliferation and stress. Eur J Biochem 1989;180:49–53
66. Sasaki Y, Hayashi N, Morita Y et al. Cellular analysis of c-Ha-ras gene expression in rat liver after CCl^4 administration. Hepatology 1989;10:494–500
67. Goyette M, Petropoulos CJ, Shank PR, Fausto N. Expression of a cellular oncogene during liver regeneration. Science 1983;219:510–512
68. Haritani H, Esumi M, Uchida T, Shikata T. Oncogene expression in the liver tissue of patients with non-neoplastic liver disease. Cancer 1991;67:2594–2598
69. Tatosyan AG, Galetzki SA, Kisseljava NP et al. Oncogene expression in human tumors. Int J Cancer 1985;35: 731–736
70. Slamon DJ, deKernion JB, Verma IM, Cline MJ. Expression of cellular oncogenes in human malignancies. Science 1984;224:256–262
71. Gu JR, Hu L-F, Cheng Y-C, Wan D-F. Oncogenes in human primary hepatic cancer. J Cell Phys Suppl 1986;4: 13–20
72. Farshid M, Tabor E. Expression of oncogenes and tumor suppressor genes in human hepatocellular carcinoma and hepatoblastoma cell lines. J Med Virol 1992;38:235–239
73. Voravud N, Foster CS, Gilbertson JA et al. Oncogene expression in cholangiocarcinoma and in normal hepatic development. Human Pathol 1989;20:1163–1168
74. Zhang X, Huang D, Qiu D, Chiu J. The expression of c-myc and C-N-ras in human cirrhotic livers, hepatocellular carcinomas and liver tissue surrounding the tumors. Oncogene 1990;5:909–914
75. Saito H, Morizane T, Watanabe T et al. Protooncogene expression in three human hepatoma cell lines, HCC-M, HCC-T and PLC/PRF/5. Keio J Med 1991;40:139–145
76. Tabor E. Tumor suppressor genes, growth factor genes, and oncogenes in hepatitis B virus-associated hepatocellular carcinoma. J Med Virol 1994;42:357–365
77. Moses HL. Transforming growth factors and cancer. New insights. Proc Am Assoc Cancer Res 1992;33:560
78. Balsano C, Avantaggiati ML, Natoli G et al. Transactivation of c-fos and c-myc protooncogenes by both full-length and truncated versions of the HBV-X protein. In Hollinger FB, Lemon SM, Margolis H (eds): Viral Hepatitis and Liver Disease. Williams and Wilkins, Baltimore, 1991, pp. 572–576
79. Koshy R, Meyer M, Kekulé AS et al. Altered functions of hepatitis B virus proteins as a consequence of viral DNA integration may lead to hepatocyte transformation. In Hollinger FB, Lemon SM, Margolis H (eds): Viral Hepatitis and Liver Disease. Williams and Wilkins, Baltimore, 1991, pp. 566–572
80. Fukuda K, Ogasawara S, Maruiwa M et al. Structural alterations in c-myc and c-Ha-ras protooncogenes in human hepatocellular carcinoma. Kurume Med J 1988;35:77–87
81. Gu J. Oncogenes in human and duck primary hepatic cancer. In Robinson W, Koike K, Will H (eds): Hepadna Viruses. Liss, New York, 1987, pp. 303–316
82. Goyette M, Faris R, Braun L et al. Expression of hepatocyte and oval cell antigens in hepatocellular carcinomas produced by oncogene-transfected liver epithelial cells. Cancer Res 1990;50:4809–4817
83. Finlay CA, Hinds PW, Levine AJ. The p53 protooncogene can act as a suppressor of transformation. Cell 1989;57: 1083–1093
84. Huang HJS, Yee JK, Shew JY et al. Suppression of the neoplastic phenotype by replacement of the RB gene in human cancer cells. Science 1988;242:1563–1566
85. Hinds P, Finlay C, Levine AJ. Mutation is required to activate the p53 gene for cooperation with the ras oncogene and transformation. J Virol 1989;63:739–746
86. Murakami Y, Hayashi K, Hirohashi S, Sekiya T. Aberrations of the tumor suppressor p53 and retinoblastoma genes in human hepatocellular carcinoma. Cancer Res 1991;51: 5520–5525

87. Pasqiunelli C, Bhavani K, Chisari FV. Multiple oncogenes and tumor suppressor genes are structurally and functionally intact during hepatocarcinogenesis in hepatitis B virus transgenic mice. Cancer Res 1992;52:2823–2829

88. Puisieux A, Ponchel F, Ozturk M. p53 as a growth suppressor gene in HBV related hepatocellular carcinoma cells. Oncogene 1993;8:487–490

89. Hollstein M, Sidransky D, Vogelstein B, Harris CC. p53 mutations in human cancers. Science 1991;253:49–53

90. Ozturk M, Bressac B, Puisieux A et al. p53 mutations in hepatocellular carcinoma after aflatoxin exposure. Lancet 1991;338:1356–1359

91. Bressac B, Kew M, Wands J, Ozturk M. Selective G to T mutations of p53 gene in hepatocellular carcinoma from southern Africa. Nature 1991;350:429–431

92. Hsu IC, Metcalf RA, Sun T et al. Mutational hotspot in p53 gene in human hepatocellular carcinomas. Nature 1991;350:427–428

93. Choi SW, Hytiroglou P, Geller SA et al. p53 antigen expression in primary malignant epithelial tumors of the liver. An immunohistochemical study. Liver 1993;13: 172–176

94. Hsia CC, Kleiner DE Jr, Axiotis CA et al. Mutations of p53 gene in hepatocellular carcinoma: roles of hepatitis B virus and aflatoxin contamination in the diet. J Natl Cancer Inst 1992;84:1638–1641

95. Kar S, Jaffe R, Carr BI. Mutation at codon 249 of p53 gene in a human hepatoblastoma. Hepatology 1993;18:566–569

96. Diamantis ID, McGandy C, Chen T-J et al. A new mutational hotspot in the p53 gene in human hepatocellular carcinoma. J Hepatol 1994;20:553–556

97. Teramoto T, Satonaka K, Kitazawa S et al. p53 gene abnormalities are closely related to hepatoviral infections and occur at a late stage of hepatocarcinogenesis. Cancer Res 1994;54:231–235

98. Scheffner M, Werness BA, Huibregtse JM et al. The E6 oncoprotein encoded by the human papillomavirus type 16 and 18 promotes degradation of p53. Cell 1990;63: 1129–1136

99. Tabor E, Kobayashi K. Current issues in hepatocellular carcinoma: hepatitis B virus, hepatitis C virus, and the p53 tumor suppressor gene. In Nishioka K, Suzuki H, Mishiro S, Oda T, (eds): Viral Hepatitis and Liver Disease. Springer-Verlag, Tokyo, 1994, pp. 669–671

100. Hsia CC, Di Bisceglie AM, Kleiner DE Jr et al. RB tumor suppressor gene expression in hepatocellular carcinomas from patients infected with the hepatitis B virus. J Med Virol 1994;44:67–73

101. Farshid M, Tabor E. Localizing mutations in the RB tumor suppressor gene in human hepatocellular carcinoma cell lines by single strand conformation polymorphism. Hepatology 1993;18:183A

102. DeCaprio JA, Ludlow JW, Figge J et al. SV40 large tumor antigen forms a specific complex with the product of the retinoblastoma susceptibility gene. Cell 1988;54:275–283

103. Whyte P, Buchkovich KJ, Horowitz JM et al. Association between an oncogene and an anti-oncogene: the adenovirus E1A proteins bind to the retinoblastoma gene product. Nature 1986;334:124–128

104. Dyson N, Howley PM, Munger K, Harlow E. The human papilloma virus-16 E7 oncoprotein is able to bind to the retinoblastoma gene product. Science 1989;243:934–937

105. Green BL, Squire JH, Goddard A et al. Mechanism of oncogenesis in retinoblastoma. Lab Invest 1990;62:394–408

106. Laiho M, DeCaprio JA, Ludlow JW et al. Growth inhibition by TGF-α linked to suppression of retinoblastoma protein phosphorylation. Cell 1990;62:175–185

107. Puisieux A, Galvin K, Troalen F et al. Retinoblastoma and p53 tumor suppressor genes in human hepatoma cell lines. FASEB J 1993;7:1407–1413

108. Fausto N. Proto-oncogenes and growth factors associated with normal and abnormal liver growth. Dig Dis Sci 1991; 36:653–658

109. Bishop JM. The molecular genetics of cancer. Science 1987; 235:305–311

110. Weir E, Chen Q, DeFrances MC et al. Rapid induction of mRNAs for liver regeneration factor and insulin-like growth factor binding protein-1 in primary cultures of rat hepatocytes by hepatocyte growth factor and epidermal growth factor. Hepatology 1994;20:955–960

111. Matsumoto K, Nakamura T. Hepatocyte growth factor. Molecular structure and implications for a central role in liver regeneration. J Gastroenterol Hepatol 1991;6:509–519

112. Chuang L-Y, Tsai J-H, Yeh Y-C et al. Epidermal growth factor-related transforming growth factors in the urine of patients with hepatocellular carcinoma. Hepatology 1991; 13:1112–1116

113. Hsia CC, Thorgeirsson SS, Tabor E. Expression of hepatitis B surface and core antigens and transforming growth factor-α in "oval cells" of the liver in patients with hepatocellular carcinoma. J Med Virol 1994;43:216–221

114. Motoo Y, Sawabu N, Nakanuma Y. Expression of epidermal growth factor and fibroblast growth factor in human hepatocellular carcinoma: an immunohistochemical study. Liver 1991;11:272–277

115. Lamas E, LeBail B, Housset C et al. Localization of insulin-like growth factor-II and hepatitis B virus mRNAs and proteins in human hepatocellular carcinomas. Lab Invest 1991; 64:98–101

116. Su Q, Liu Y-F, Zhang J-F et al. Expression of insulin-like growth factor II in hepatitis B, cirrhosis and hepatocellular carcinoma: its relationship with hepatitis B virus antigen expression. Hepatology 1994;20:788–799

117. Morimitsu Y, Hsia CC, Kojiro M, Tabor E. Nodules of less-differentiated tumor within or adjacent to hepatocellular carcinoma: relative expression of transforming growth factor-α and its receptor in the different areas of tumor. Hum Pathol 1995;26:1126–1132

118. Schaff Z, Hsia CC, Sarosi I, Tabor E. Overexpression of transforming growth factor-α in hepatocellular carcinoma and focal nodular hyperplasia from European patients. Hum Pathol 1994;25:644–651

119. Morimitsu Y, Kleiner DE, Conjeevaram HS et al. Expression of transforming growth factor-α in the liver before and after interferon alpha therapy for chronic hepatitis B. Hepatology 1995;22:1021–1026

12

PATHOLOGY OF HEPATOCELLULAR CARCINOMA

MASAMICHI KOJIRO

Remarkable advances in diagnostic imaging and other diagnostic modalities have made possible the early diagnosis of hepatocellular carcinoma (HCC). Much new clinical and pathologic information about small HCCs has become known; however, many HCCs are still detected in advanced stages.

HEPATOCELLULAR CARCINOMA AND HEPATITIS VIRUS-RELATED CIRRHOSIS

Approximately 80% of HCC are associated with cirrhosis, mostly posthepatitic cirrhosis, worldwide. In most Asian countries, this is hepatitis B virus (HBV)-related,[1] or hepatitis C virus (HCV)-related cirrhosis. HCC is now more closely related to HCV than to HBV in some areas, including Japan.[2–6] Recently, it also has been noted that the morphology of HBV-related cirrhosis (type B cirrhosis) is significantly different from HCV-related cirrhosis (type C cirrhosis).[7]

Morphologic Characteristics of Liver Cirrhosis Associated with Hepatocellular Carcinoma

The striking morphologic differences between type B cirrhosis and type C cirrhosis are the different sizes of the regenerative nodules, different degrees of fibrosis, and different degrees of active inflammation. In type C cirrhosis, the regenerative nodules are significantly smaller and fibrous septa extend broadly and irregularly from the portal area. Active inflammation with piecemeal necrosis is frequently observed in type C cirrhosis (Fig. 12-1). In type B cirrhosis, the regenerative nodules are larger than those of type C cirrhosis, the fibrous septa are relatively thin and regular in shape, and active inflammation is infrequently seen (Fig. 12-2). Histometrical analysis of the HCC-associated liver shows that the size of regenerative nodules in type B cirrhosis is approximately three times greater than those in type C cirrhosis, and the area of fibrosis in type C cirrhosis is three times larger than that in type B cirrhosis. There are some differences in autopsy cases compared with the surgical cases in the size of the regenerative nodules because of terminal events in the course of the disease (Fig. 12-3).

These differences may be related to the severity and duration of active inflammation in the portal and periportal areas. Type C cirrhosis shows stronger inflammatory reactions than type B cirrhosis, associated with piecemeal necrosis along the fibrous septa. The reason for such marked inflammatory reactions in the portal areas in type C cirrhosis is not known, but it may be related to continuous replication of HCV in the hepatocytes. Such active inflammation in type C cirrhosis might reflect viral replication and the host's immune reaction. Replication of HBV has been reported to decrease along with progression of the disease, while the number of virus copies in serum is low but gradually in-

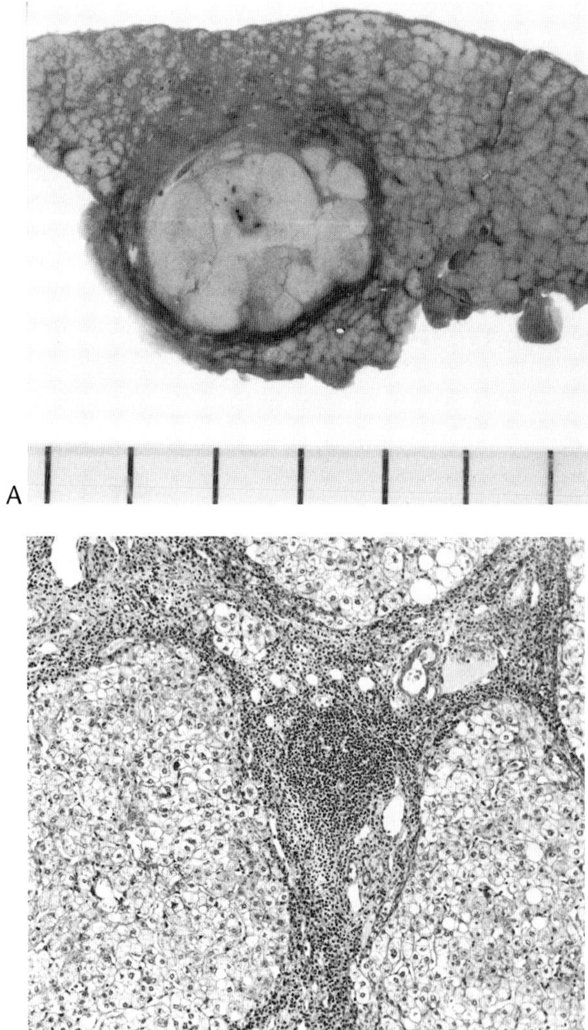

FIGURE 12-1. Anti-HCV antibody-positive (type C) cirrhosis with HCC. (*A*) Gross features are characterized by small and irregularly shaped regenerative nodules. (*B*) Active inflammation with piecemeal necrosis is prominent in the fibrous septa.

creases in hepatitis C patients. In addition, regenerative activity in the parenchyma differs between type B and C cirrhosis. In general, type C cirrhosis is accompanied by weak regenerative activity compared to type B cirrhosis. In the latter, marked regenerative features are commonly found, such as a "paving stone" arrangement of hepatocytes. Persistent active inflammation from chronic hepatitis may lead to smaller and indistinct regenerative nodules in type C cirrhosis. Meanwhile, subsided inflammation and marked liver cell regeneration may form the larger regenerative nodules seen in type B cirrhosis.

Chronological Changes in the Morphology of Cirrhosis Associated with Hepatocellular Carcinoma

In Japan, the incidence of HCC has been increasing since the 1970s as a result of a remarkable increase of non-HBV-related cases, mostly HCV-related cases.[8] Among 67 cases of cirrhosis associated with HCC from 1970 to 1975, 26 (38.8%) were macronodular, which is characterized by large regenerative nodules 5 to 10 mm in diameter and relatively thin, fibrous septa; 35 (52.2%) were mixed type, consisting of a mixture of small and large regenerative nodules, with small regenerative nodules predominant; six were micronodular cirrhosis. Hepatitis B surface antigen (HBsAg) was detected in 57.1% of the macronodular type and 22.2% of the mixed type. In comparison, among 44 of HCC cases from 1989 to 1994, macronodular cirrhosis was found in only six (13.6%), and four (66.7%) of these were HBsAg-positive. Thirty-seven cases (84.1%) from 1989 to 1994 were associated with the mixed macronodular and micronodular cirrhosis; 15 (93.8%) of 16 mixed type cirrhoses examined were positive for antibody to HCV (anti-HCV) and only 1 (5.3%) of 19 mixed type cirrhoses examined was HBsAg-positive. One was micronodular type, with small regenerative nodules about 2 to 3 mm in diameter despite no history of heavy alcohol abuse. These findings are believed to reflect the remarkable change in the proportion of HBV- and HCV-associated cases among patients with chronic HCC in the last two to three decades.

Comparison of HCC with Type B and Type C Cirrhosis

A clinicopathologic study of surgically resected HCCs has shown some significant differences among HCCs associated with type B cirrhosis and those associated with type C cirrhosis.[9–11] In a comparison of 35 resected HCCs associated with type B cirrhosis and 100 resected cases with type C cirrhosis, the mean age of patients with HCCs with type B cirrhosis was 50.6 + 9.9 (SD) years and 64.3 + 7.3 (SD) years ($p < 0.001$) with type C cirrhosis. The mean value of indocyanine green retention rate at 15 minutes (ICG R15) was 30% in HCCs with type C cirrhosis and 16% in the cases with type B cirrhosis. The higher ICG R15 indicates that liver function was worse in HCCs with type C cirrhosis.

Tumor size ranged from 1.5 to 11.5 cm, with a mean of 4.5 ± 2.7 (SD) cm in HCCs associated with type B cirrhosis, and 0.7 to 15.1 cm with a mean of 3.1 ± 1.9 (SD) cm in cases with type C cirrhosis. The frequency of tumors less than 3.0 cm in diameter was 65% in HCCs with type C cirrhosis and 28% in type B cirrhosis ($p < 0.0002$). However, there were no significant differences in histologic features of the tumors in the two groups.

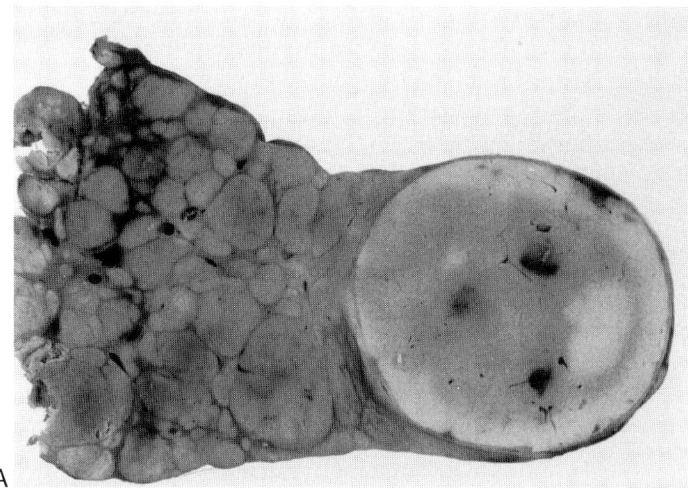

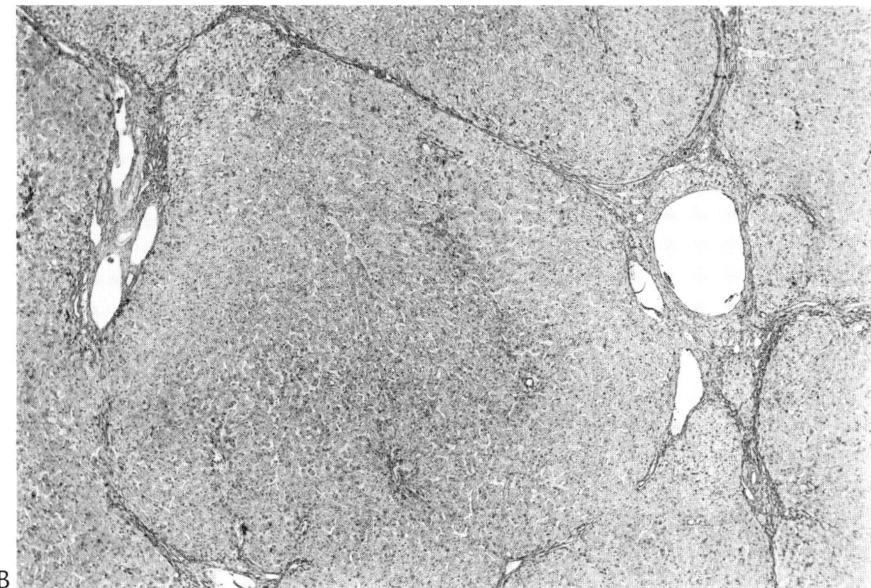

FIGURE 12-2. HBsAg-positive (HBV) cirrhosis with HCC. (*A*) Regenerative nodules are large and regular in shape compared with those of HCV-associated cirrhosis. (*B*) The large regenerative nodules are surrounded by thin, fibrous septa with little inflammation.

There are some possible explanations for the differences in patient age and tumor size between HCCs with type C cirrhosis and those with type B cirrhosis. The age differences may be explained by the sources of virus transmission. Although perinatal and mother-to-infant infections are common sources in HBV carriers, HCV is mainly transmitted by blood transfusion, dialysis, and intravenous drug abuse, situations generally occurring many years after birth. With regard to the difference in tumor size, patients with type C cirrhosis may be more likely to have an imaging examination because of worse liver function. Accordingly, HCC would be detected in an earlier stage. Furthermore, it may be difficult to detect minute tumors in type B cirrhosis because the large regenerative nodules might conceal a small tumor.

DEVELOPMENTAL PROCESS OF HCC FROM EARLY TO ADVANCED STAGES

The remarkable advances in various diagnostic imaging techniques and the introduction and popularization of ultrasound-guided fine needle biopsy have led to the

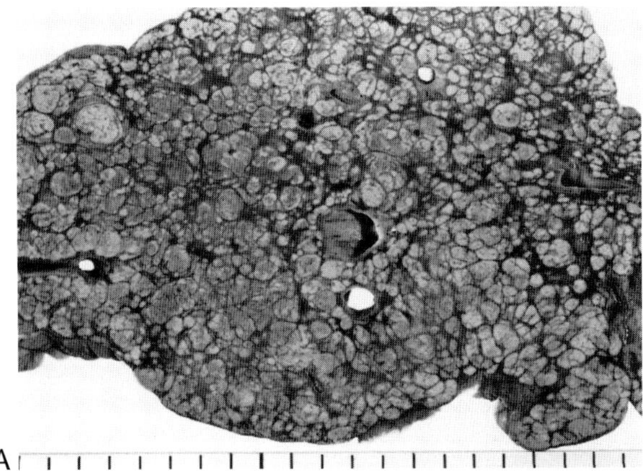

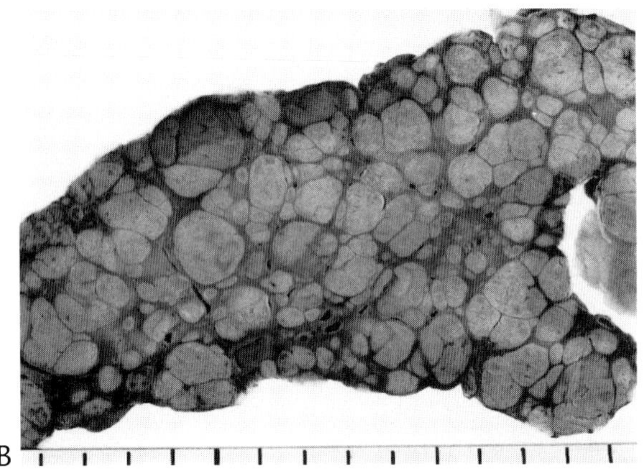

FIGURE 12-3. Autopsy findings of cirrhosis. (*A*) HCV-associated cirrhosis presents the features of the mixed macronodular and micronodular cirrhosis, but micronodular is predominant. (*B*) HBV-associated cirrhosis has a typical form of macronodular cirrhosis.

early detection and resection of more small HCCs.[12,13] Accordingly, new information about the pathomorphologic characteristics and developmental process of early HCC has been obtained through the histologic examinations of resected HCC tissues in various sizes and of biopsy specimens from minute tumors.[14–16] The most valuable information is that the majority of HCCs first appear as well-differentiated cancer and proliferate with gradual dedifferentiation. In addition, a certain proportion of HCCs associated with cirrhosis develop from hyperplastic nodular lesions, such as adenomatous hyperplasia.[17–19]

Morphologic Characteristics of Early HCC

GROSS FEATURES

Small HCCs less than 2 cm in diameter can be categorized as either a distinct nodular type or an indistinct nodular type. Many resected small HCCs are the distinct nodular type, in which there is a distinct nodule, often with a fibrous capsule and/or fibrous septa (Fig. 12-4 and Plate 12-1). The indistinct nodular type is about 1 to 1.5 cm in diameter. Although most tumors in this indistinct nodules category can be clearly detected either as a hypoechoic or hyperechoic nodular lesion in ultrasound, in gross observation of surgically resected specimens the nodule is usually obscure or difficult to distinguish from the surrounding cirrhotic liver (Fig. 12-5). These findings are considered to be the characteristics of the smallest clinically detectable HCC.

Histologically, small HCCs of the indistinct nodular type are composed of uniformly proliferated well-differentiated cancerous tissue; many portal tracts can be seen, as well as fibrous septa of regenerative nodules, in varying degrees within the cancerous tissue (Fig. 12-6). At the tumor-nontumor boundary, well-differentiated HCC cells proliferate along the adjacent liver cell cord, and there is no capsule formation at the boundary. When the diameter of the indistinct nodular small HCC reaches about 1.0 to 1.5 cm, a fibrous capsule is formed on the tumor boundary, and fibrous septa are formed within the nodule. The fibrous capsule and septa can be seen in more than 70% of HCC nodules that are 2 cm in diameter and a rate that is equivalent to that seen in advanced HCC. These findings suggest that early HCC may change its characteristics when it reaches 1 to 2 cm in diameter, at which time it may develop some of the qualities of advanced cancer.

HISTOLOGIC FEATURES

The most important histologic characteristic of early HCC less than 1 to 1.5 cm in diameter is that the majority of the tumors consist solely of well-differentiated can-

FIGURE 12-4. Small HCC of a distinct nodular type. The tumor presents with a thin, fibrous capsule and septa. HCV-associated cirrhosis is present. (See also Plate 12-1.)

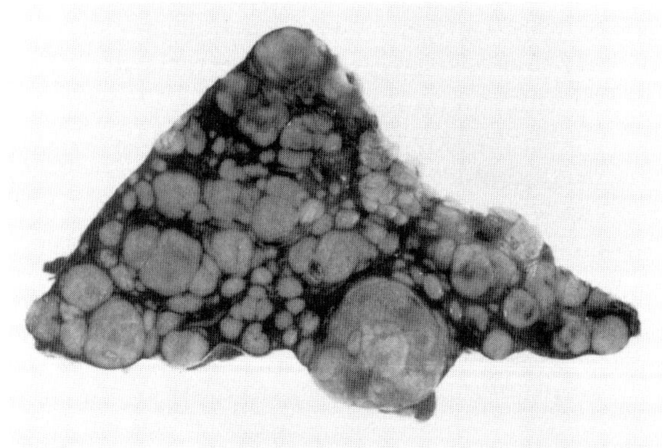

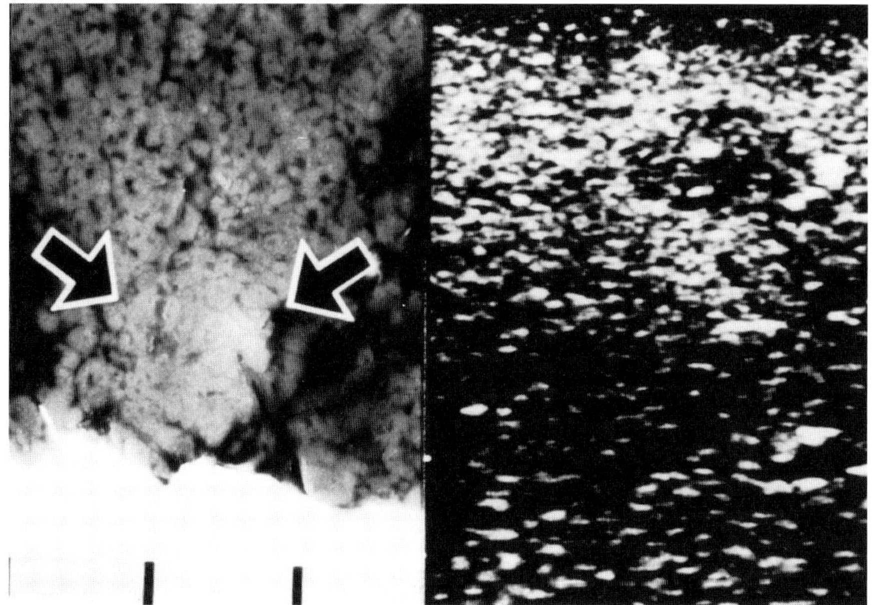

FIGURE 12-5. Small HCC with indistinct margins. The hypoechoic nodule was detected by ultrasonography during the follow-up study of the cirrhotic patient (anti-HCV-positive) and well-differentiated HCC was confirmed by biopsy. In the surgical specimen, the boundary of the cancerous lesion with a diameter of 1 cm (arrows) is unclear.

FIGURE 12-6. Small HCC with indistinct margins in HCV-associated cirrhosis. (*A*) Vaguely nodular HCC, 1.2 cm in diameter. (*B*) Uniform proliferation of well-differentiated cancerous tissue containing portal tracts within the lesion.

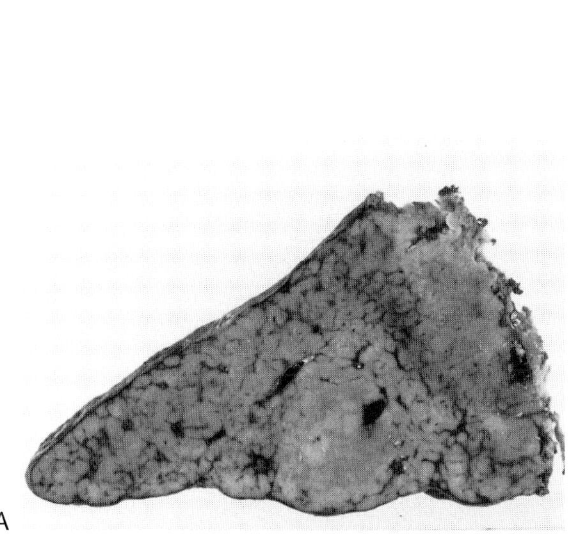

A

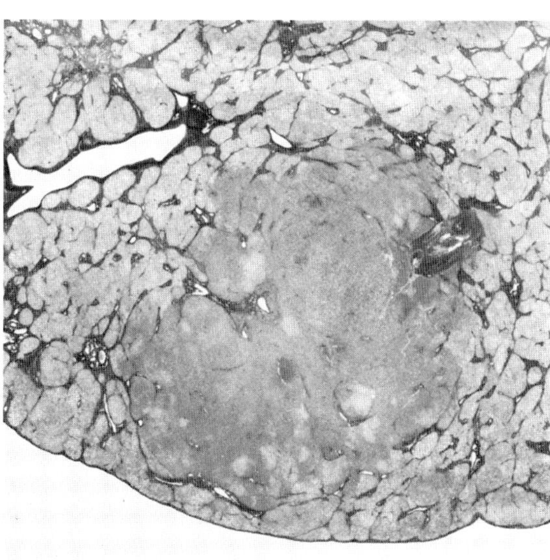

B

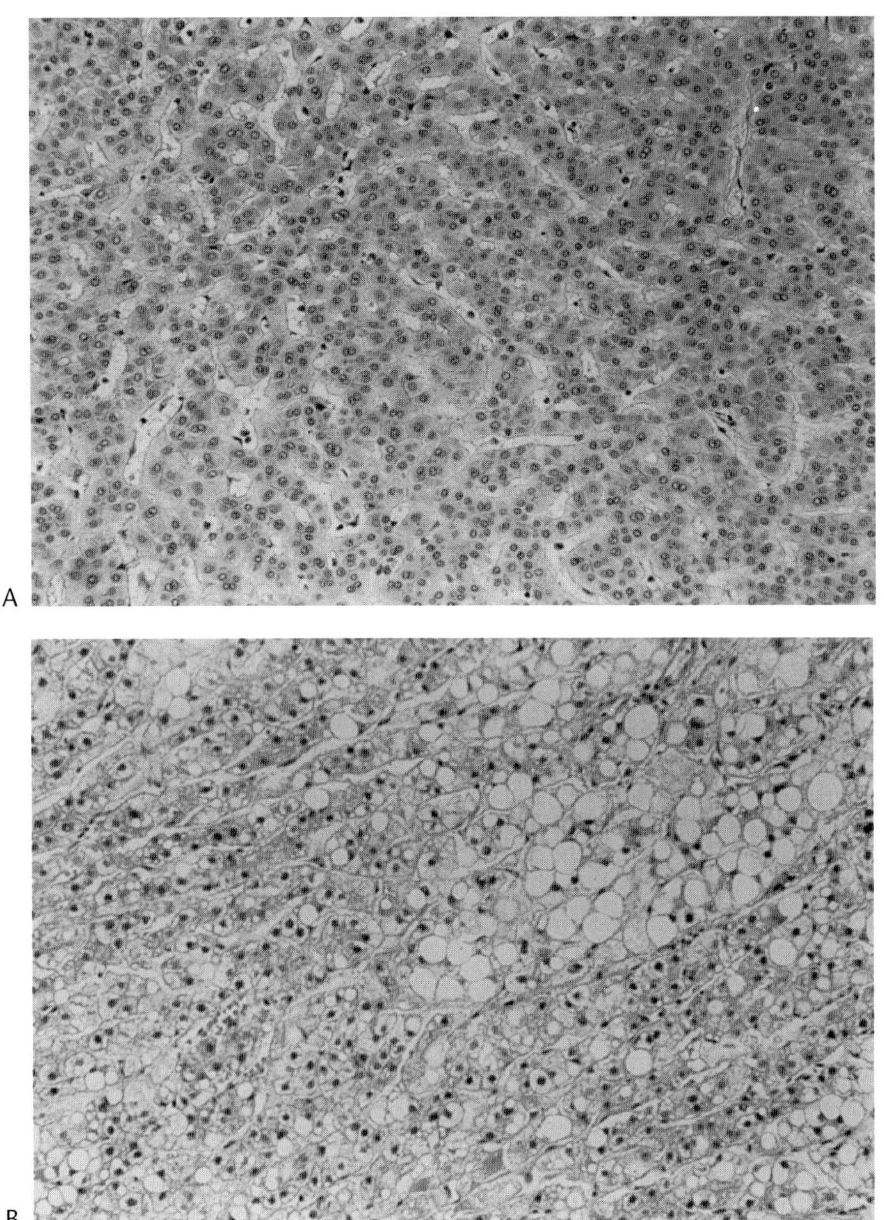

FIGURE 12-7. Typical histologic features of well-differentiated HCC. (*A*) HCC with little atypia show irregular, thin, trabecular pattern. (*B*) Diffuse fatty change in HCC tissue. (See also Plate 12-2.)

cerous tissues, with little cellular and structural atypia[14–16] (Fig. 12-7 and Plate 12-3). Such an early HCC lesion has the following five characteristics in varying degrees: (1) increased cell density associated with the increase of nucleus:cytoplasm ratio, (2) increased eosinophilic staining affinity, (3) irregular thin trabecular pattern, (4) acinar and/or pseudoglandular pattern, and (5) fatty changes and/or clear cell changes of cancer cells. Fatty changes are observed in approximately 40% of HCCs less than 2 cm diameter, which makes the other characteristic changes (e.g., increased cell density and appearance of irregular thin trabecular pattern) indistinguishable, and consequently makes histologic diagnosis, especially biopsy diagnosis, difficult.

TUMOR DEDIFFERENTIATION AND PROLIFERATION

Well-differentiated HCC proliferates along with its dedifferentiation. This can result in histologic variations within a single nodule. Cancer nodules with less than 1 cm of diameter consist of uniform distribution of well-differentiated cancerous tissues, whereas approximately 40% of cancer nodules 1.1 to 3 cm in diameter consist of more than two cancerous tissues of varying differentiation levels. In such an HCC nodule, moderately or poorly differentiated tissues are always found inside the lesion, and well-differentiated tissues outside. The well-differentiated area diminishes in size as the tumor size increases.[20]

The most typical case with dedifferentiation morphologically shows a nodule-in-nodule appearance in which moderately or poorly differentiated cancerous tissues proliferate in an expansive fashion within a well-differentiated cancer nodule (Fig. 12-8). Generally, when moderately differentiated cancer tissues without fatty changes are present within a well-differentiated cancerous nodule with fatty changes, the moderately differentiated cancerous tissues are surmised to be a newer development in clinical observations using ultrasonography. In observation of a hyperechoic small cancerous nodule, either a hypoechoic or isoechoic area appears

FIGURE 12-8. Nodule-in-nodule appearance in HCC. (*A*) Well-differentiated HCC nodule contains a moderately differentiated cancer nodule. (*B*) Moderately differentiated tumor is proliferating in an expansive fashion. *(Figure continues.)*

A

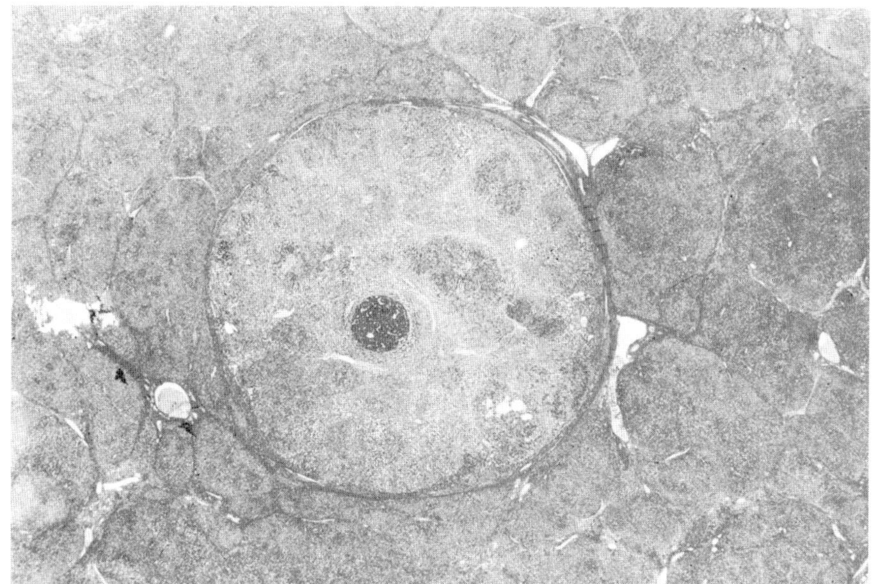

B

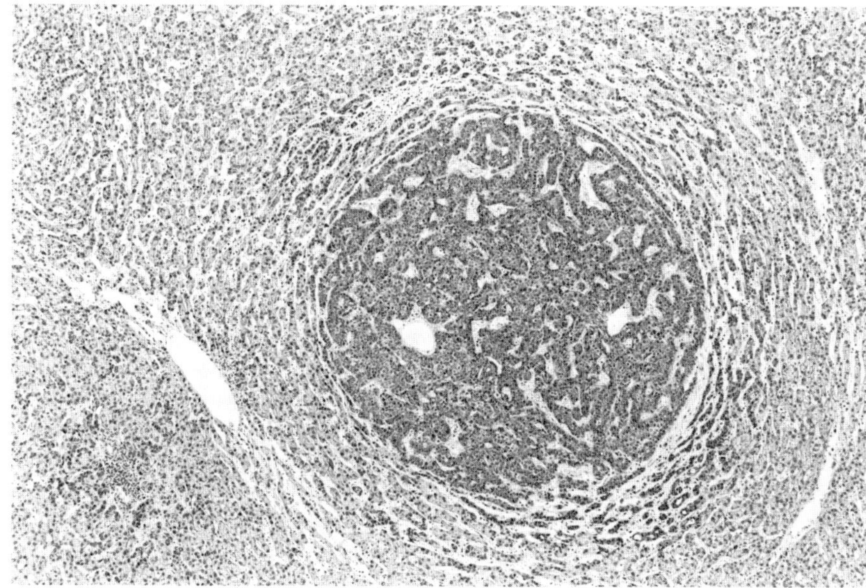

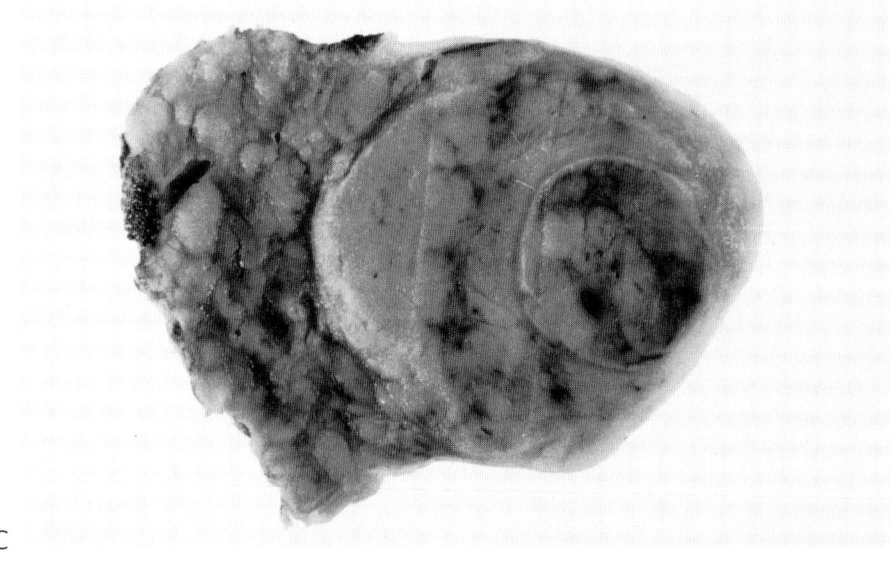

C

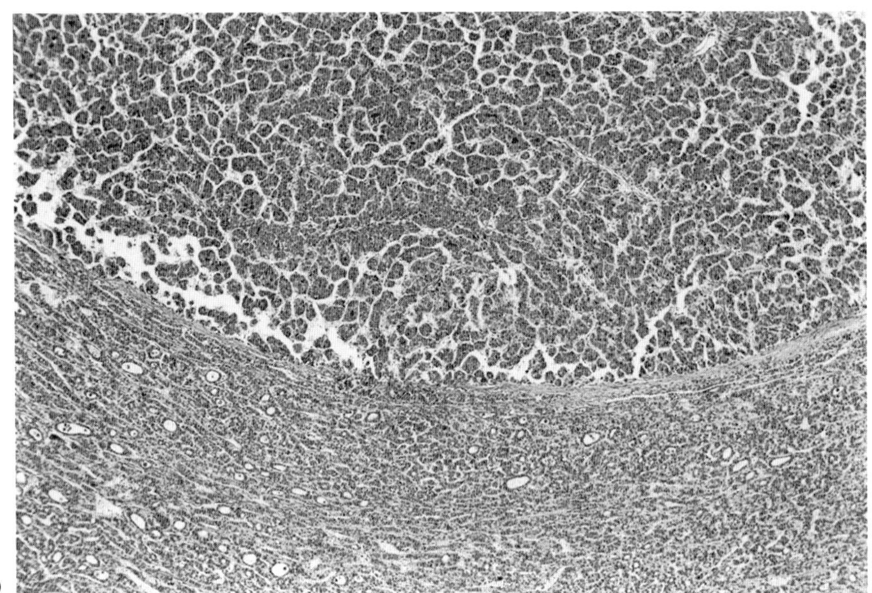

D

FIGURE 12-8 *(Continued). (C)* HCC 2.2 cm in diameter presents a typical nodule-in-nodule appearance. *(D)* The inner tumor consists of moderately differentiated cancerous tissue and is proliferating in an expasive fashion oppressing surrounding well-differentiated cancerous tissue.

within the hyperechoic nodule, gradually increases its area while the hyperechoic area becomes smaller, and then the nodule starts to grow. This suggests that progress of dedifferentiation of the tumor is closely related to the tumor proliferation.

CLONAL DEDIFFERENTIATION OF HCC CELLS IN A SINGLE TUMOR NODULE

A well-differentiated HCC cell line (HAK-1A) and a poorly differentiated HCC cell line (HAK-1B) have been established from a surgically obtained HCC nodule, which measured 2.7×2.2 cm and presented a nodule-in-nodule appearance with a clear boundary between well-differentiated and moderately/poorly differentiated cancer tissues[21] (Fig. 12-9). These two cell lines show morphologically and biologically different characteristics: the doubling time of HAK-1A is approximately three times longer than that of HAK-1B; the DNA ploidy pattern is diploid in HAK-1A but aneuploid in HAK-1B; and HAK-1B is easily transplantable to nude mice but HAK-1A is not, because of its weak proliferative activity. In these two cell lines, however, there are

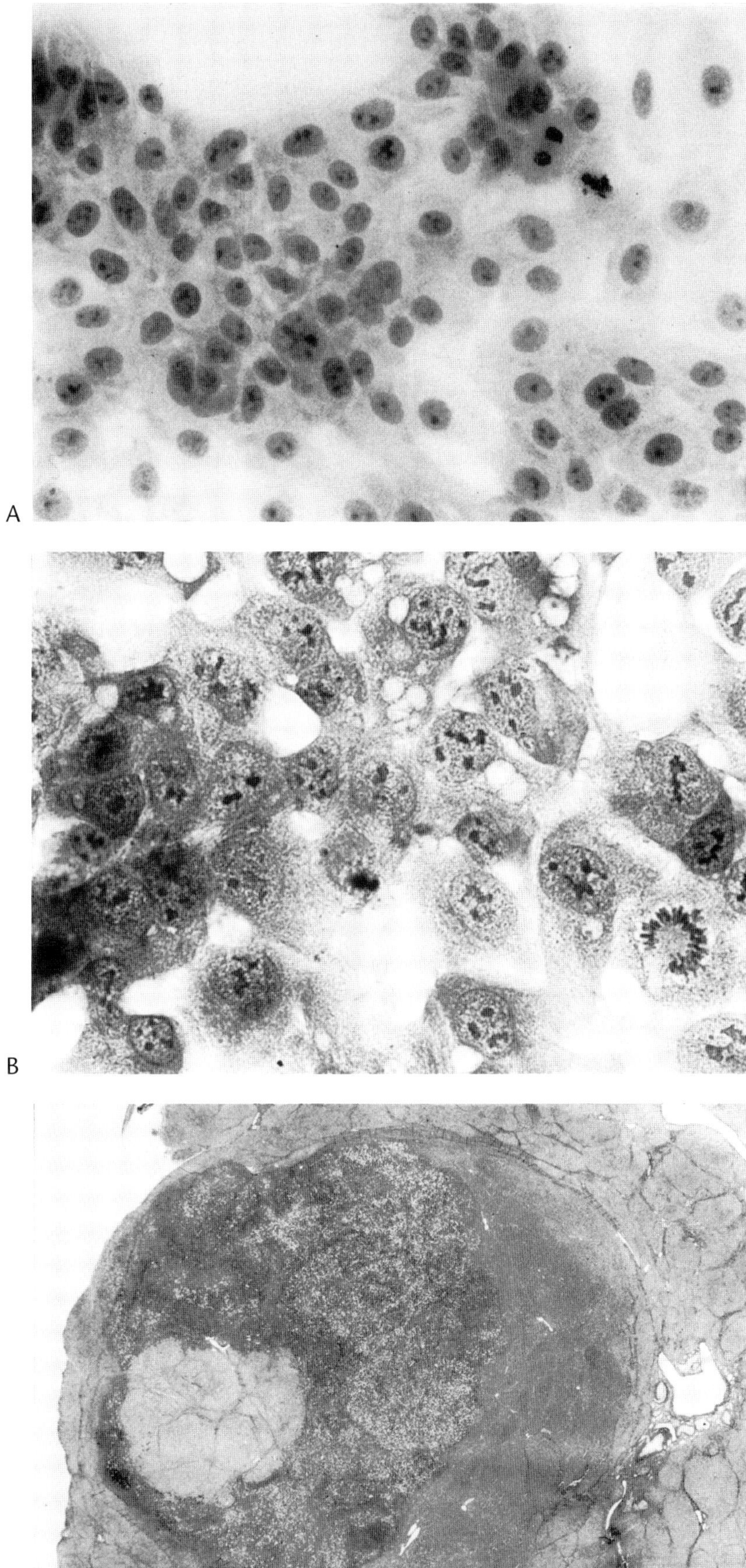

FIGURE 12-9. Two distinct HCC cell lines established from a cancer nodule with a nodule-in-nodule appearance. (*A*) Well-differentiated cancer cell line (HAK-1A) has abundant eosinophilic cytoplasm and round to ovoid nuclei with little atypia.(*B*) Poorly differentiated cancer cell line (HAK-1B) has significantly larger and highly atypic cells compared with HAK-1A. (*C*) The original tumor with a three-layered nodule-in-nodule appearance, in which poorly differentiated cancerous tissue is located in the most inner nodule and well-differentiated cancerous tissues are in the outer layers.

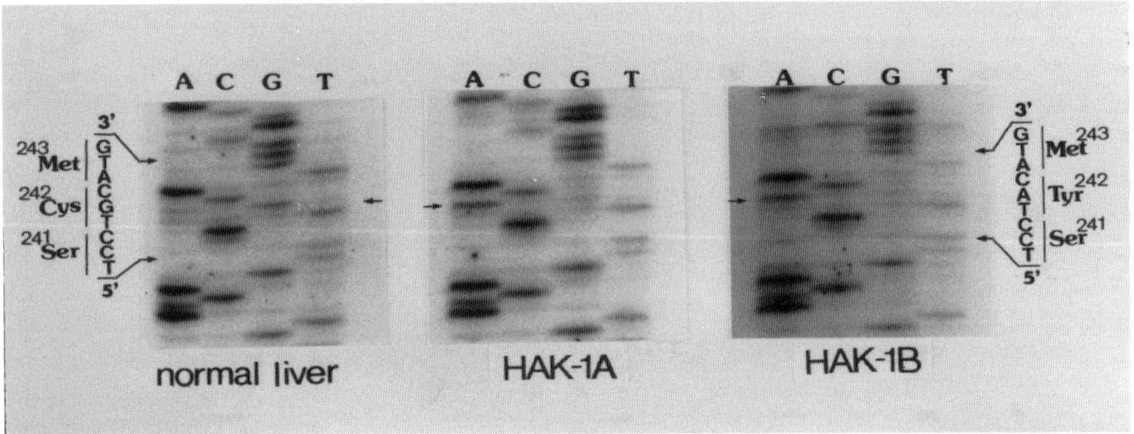

FIGURE 12-10. Nucleotide sequence analysis of exon 7 of the p53 gene showing an identical mutation of p53 at codon 242 (arrows) in well-differentiated cancer cells (HAK-1A) and poorly differentiated cancer cells (HAK-1B).

identical genetic abnormalities on chromosomes 2 and 17, and nucleotide sequence analysis of exon 7 of the p53 gene shows an identical point mutation of p53 at codon 242 (Fig. 12-10). These findings strongly suggest that the two cell lines have the same clonal origin, and that HAK-1B, which is poorly differentiated, might have developed from dedifferentiation of the cells from which HAK-1A was derived, which is well differentiated. Therefore, in HCC nodules consisting of cancerous tissues of different histologic grades, it is conceivable that less-differentiated cancer cells developed via dedifferentiation of the well-differentiated cells.[22–25]

The following developmental process can be postulated. Human HCC could develop as a well-differentiated cancer in a hyperplastic nodular lesion, such as adenomatous hyperplasia (AH), or it could arise de novo. When the tumor grows to about 1 to 1.5 cm in diameter, dedifferentiation of the well-differentiated cancer cells occurs; moderately and/or poorly differentiated cancerous tissues proliferate within the well-differentiated nodule and replace the well-differentiated tissues. They start to grow expansively and develop into an advanced HCC.

MORPHOLOGY OF ADVANCED HCC

Gross Features

The gross features of advanced HCC vary depending on the size of the tumor and the presence or absence of cirrhosis. The majority of advanced HCCs are expansive and/or infiltrative tumors with varying numbers and sizes of intrahepatic metastases. Many HCCs associated with cirrhosis are well-demarcated encapsulated tumors, but those without cirrhosis tend to show "massive" form. It has been reported that the gross appearance of HCC varies in different geographic areas. Okuda et al.[26] compared the gross features of HCC in the United States, South Africa, and Japan and found that the most striking difference among these three countries was the high incidence of encapsulated HCC in Japan in contrast to the other countries. However, there were no specific differences in the morphology of HCCs between Spain and Japan other than the predominance of mixed macronodular and micronodular cirrhosis among Japanese cases and micronodular cirrhosis among Spanish cases.[27]

Gross Classification of HCC

The classic gross classification proposed by Eggel[28] in 1901 has been widely used up to the present time, in which HCC was classified into massive, nodular and diffuse types (Fig. 12-11). The massive type consists of a large single tumor occupying almost the entire lobe. The nodular type is composed of a single nodular tumor or varying numbers of nodular tumors of different sizes. The diffuse type is characterized by distribution of numerous small tumor nodules throughout the liver. However, it is difficult to classify surgically resected HCCs, which are relatively small, using Eggel's classification, which is based on autopsy cases with larger tumors. In the past few decades, a few new classification systems have been proposed, but none has been widely accepted.[26,29,30]

Recently, The Liver Cancer Study Group of Japan proposed the subclassification of nodular HCCs into sin-

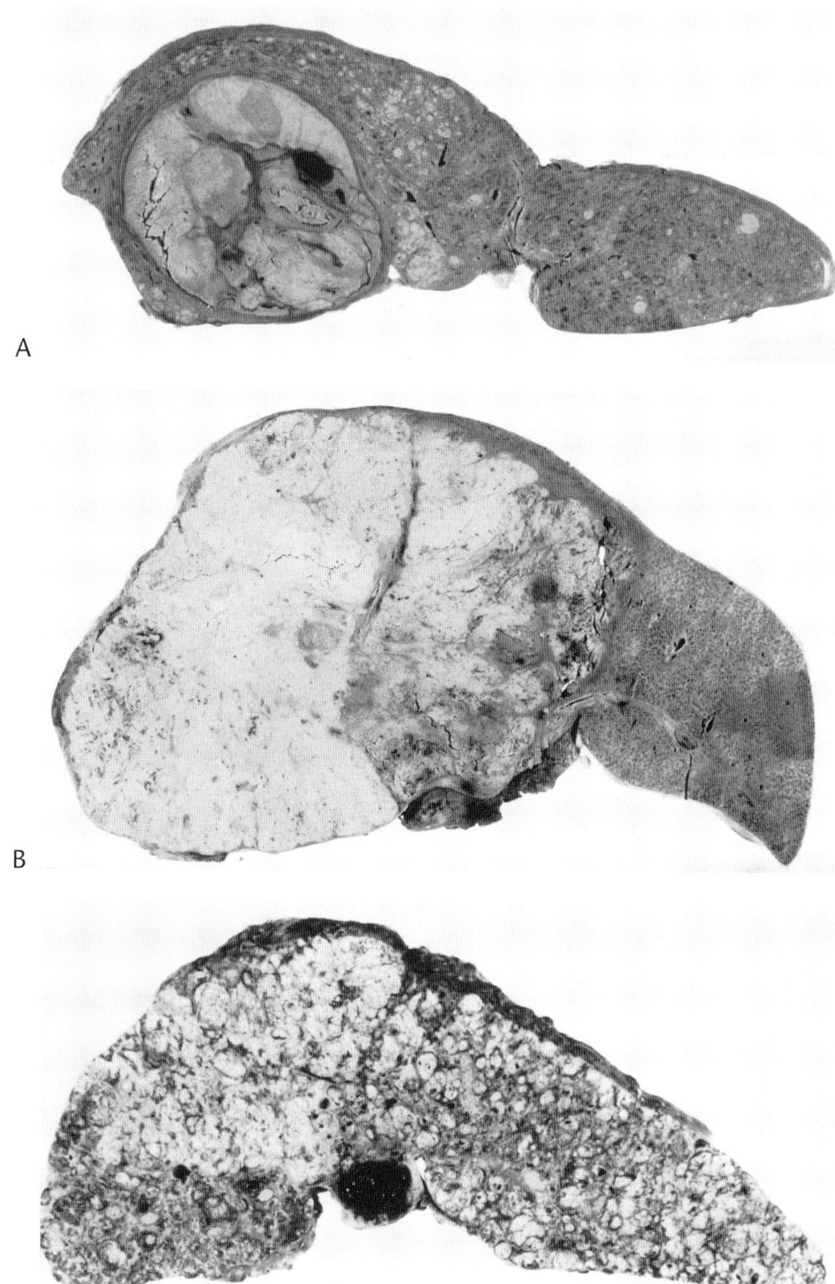

FIGURE 12-11. Eggel's gross classification of hepatocellular carcinoma. (*A*) Nodular type. Tumor is encapsulated and is divided by fibrous septa. (*B*) Massive type. The massive tumor occupies the entire right lobe of noncirrhotic liver.(C) Diffuse type. Numerous small cancer nodules, 5 to 10 mm in diameter, distributed throughout the cirrhotic liver.

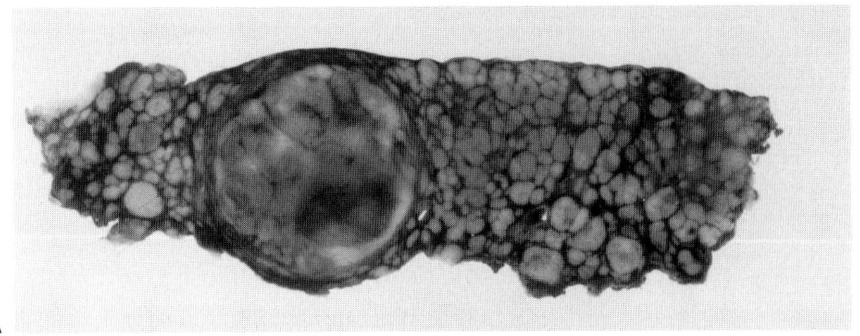

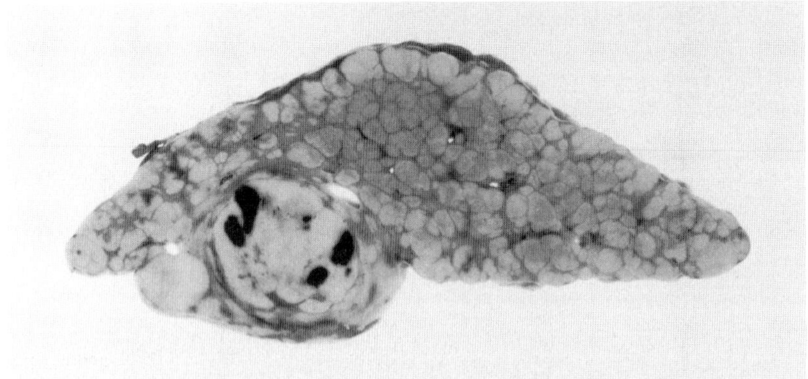

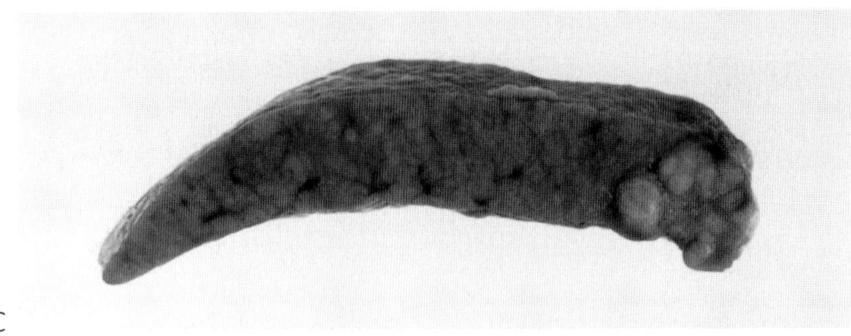

FIGURE 12-12. Modified gross classification by Liver Cancer Study Group of Japan. (*A*) Single nodular type. A well-encapsulated cancer nodule without perinodular tumor growth. (*B*) Nodular type with a perinodular tumor growth. (*C*) Multinodular confluent type. (See also Plate 12-3.)

gle nodular type, single nodular type with perinodular tumor growth, and confluent multinodular type (Fig. 12-12 and Plate 12-3). This subclassification system has been widely accepted in Japan.[31]

Histologic Features of HCC

HCC is generally composed of the tumor parenchyma, consisting of cancer cells and stroma, the latter comprising sinusoid-like blood spaces lined by a single layer of endothelial cells, and represents a trabecular pattern of varying thickness.

HISTOLOGIC CLASSIFICATION

Classification by Histologic Grade

According to histologic grade, HCC is classified into well-differentiated, moderately differentiated, poorly differentiated, and undifferentiated types.

Well-differentiated HCC: This carcinoma is characterized by the increased cell density with an irregular thin trabecular pattern with frequent areas of pseudoglandular patterns and fatty change. The HCC cells lack distinct cellular and nuclear atypia. Well-differentiated carcinoma is common among HCCs $<$ 2 cm in diameter, but it is rare in advanced tumors. This carcinoma corresponds to grade 1 carcinoma of the Edmondson-Steiner classification (Fig. 12-13A).[32]

Moderately differentiated HCC: This carcinoma is characterized by a classic trabecular pattern in which tumor cells are arranged in layers that are several cells thick. A pseudoglandular pattern is frequently observed. Cancer cells have abundant eosinophilic cytoplasm and round nuclei with distinct nucleoli. The nucleus: cytoplasm ratio is almost equal to that of the nontumorous hepatocyte. This carcinoma corresponds to grade II to III carcinoma of the Edmondson-Steiner classification

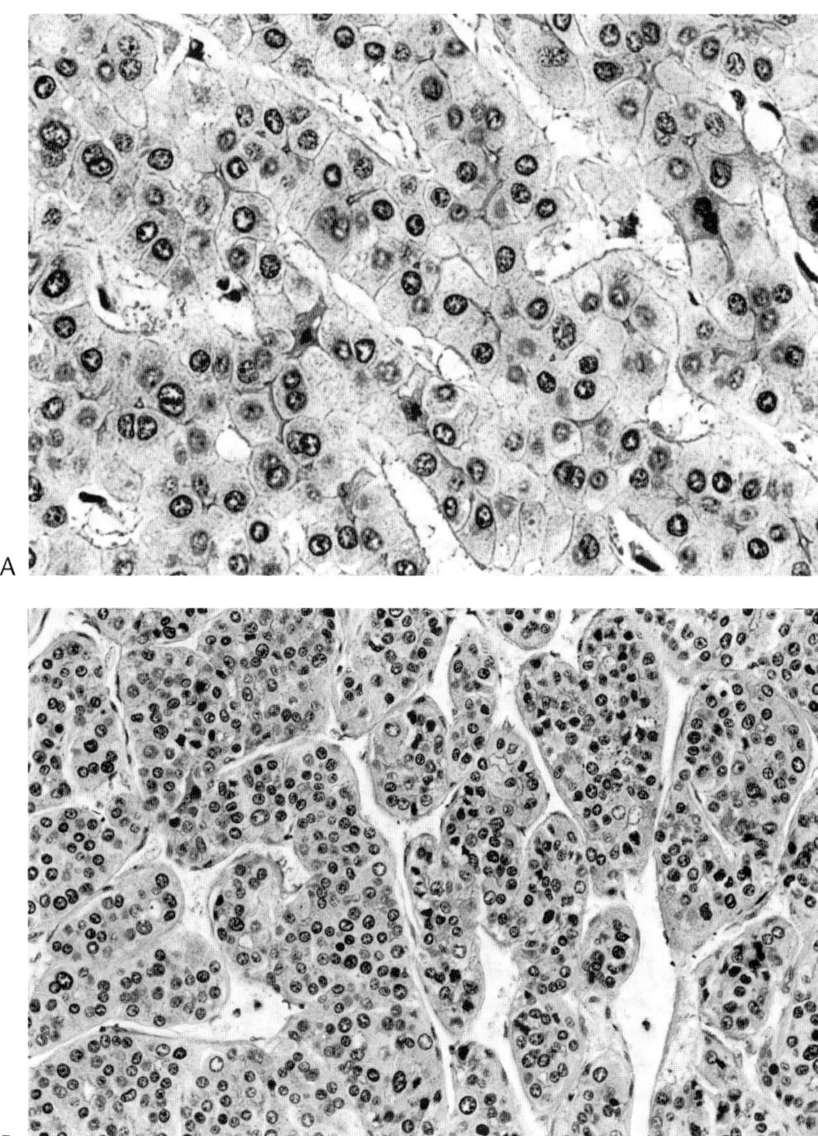

FIGURE 12-13. Histologic classification of HCC. (*A*) Well-differentiated type. Cancer cells with abundant eosinophilic cytoplasm show little atypia and are arranged in an irregular, thin, trabecular pattern. (*B*) Moderately differentiated type. Cancer cells are proliferating in a classical trabecular pattern. *(Figure continues.)*

and is most common among advanced HCCs (Fig. 12-13B).

Poorly differentiated HCC: Cancer cells of poorly differentiated HCCs show a compact (solid) growth pattern without showing a trabecular pattern. A slitlike blood vessel is sporadically observed in the tumor. Cancer cells show an increased nucleus:cytoplasm ratio and frequently show pleomorphism, including mononucleated and/or multinucleated giant cells. This carcinoma corresponds to grade III to IV carcinoma of the Edmondson-Steiner classification (Fig. 12-13C).

Undifferentiated carcinoma: Cancer cells in undifferentiated HCC have scant cytoplasm with short spindle-shaped and/or round nuclei. They proliferate in a solid or medullary pattern. It is often difficult to diagnose this carcinoma only by histologic findings. This carcinoma corresponds to grade IV carcinoma of the Edmondson-Steiner classification (Fig. 12-13D).

WHO Classification

HISTOLOGIC CLASSIFICATION

The histologic classification proposed by WHO has been accepted worldwide.[33] In this system, HCC is classified into five subtypes according to the histologic pattern: trabecular (platelike), pseudoglandular (acinar), compact, scirrhous, and fibrolamellar carcinoma.

The trabecular and pseudoglandular patterns are the most common in well- to moderately differentiated HCCs (Figs. 12-13A, B; 12-14A). The compact pattern

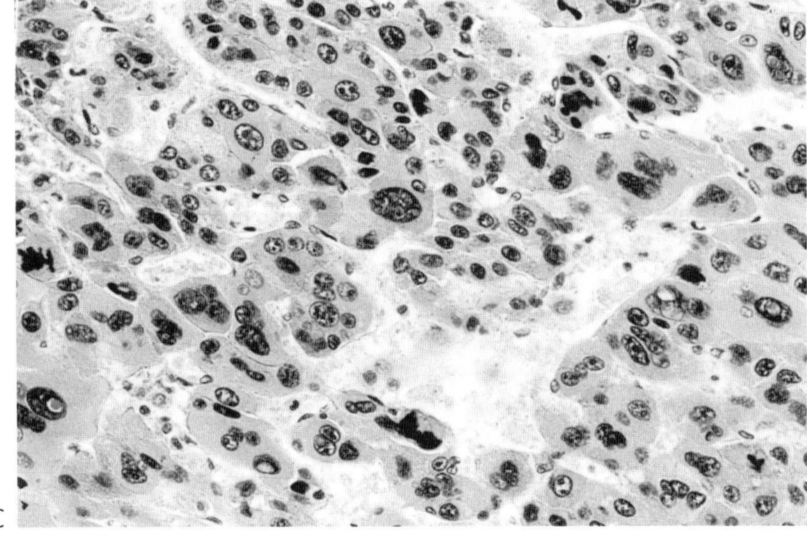

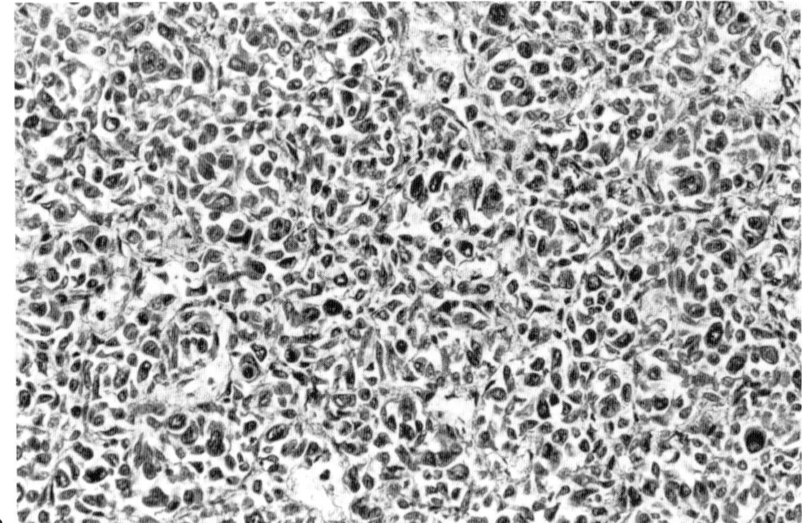

FIGURE 12-13 *(Continued).* (C) Poorly differentiated type. Pleomorphic cancer cells including mononuclear and multinuclear giant cells are proliferating in a vague trabecular pattern. (*D*) Undifferentiated carcinoma. Highly atypical cancer cells with scant cytoplasm are proliferating in a solid pattern; it is difficult to differentiate this tumor from sarcoma only by histologic findings.

is generally observed in poorly differentiated HCCs. The scirrhous pattern is characterized by abundant fibrous stroma separating cords of tumor cells, and it is often seen following radiation, chemotherapy, or infarction. However, varying degrees of the scirrhous pattern are also found in HCCs without any known etiologic factors (Fig. 12-14B). In our institute, scirrhous HCC accounts for approximately 3.8% of surgical cases without preoperative anticancer therapies. HCC with a scirrhous appearance must be distinguished from cholangiocarcinoma and from metastatic carcinoma. Fibrolamellar carcinomas are usually not associated with cirrhosis and occur most frequently in adolescents or young adults; it has a more favorable prognosis than that of other HCCs. Although fibrolamellar carcinoma is often encountered in Western countries, it is rare in Asian countries. Among 760 consecutive autopsy cases and 450 surgical cases of HCC in our institution, none were fibrolamellar carcinoma.

CYTOLOGIC VARIANTS

Cytologic variants of HCC are seen, including pleomorphic, clear cell, oncocyte-like, and spindle cell (pseudosarcomatous or sarcomatoid) variants.

The pleomorphic variant is characterized by bizarre pleomorphic cells. It is common in poorly differentiated HCCs (Fig. 13C).[29]

The clear cell variant of HCC is characterized by tumor cells with a clear cytoplasm, which is due to the presence of abundant glycogen (Fig. 12-15A, B). This variant is sometimes difficult to distinguish from some metastatic carcinomas such as renal cell carcinoma of clear cell type, adrenal carcinoma, and clear cell adenocarcinoma of the ovary. It has been reported that HCC of the clear cell variant has a favorable prognosis compared with that of other variants,[34] but no significant difference in prognosis was seen in our study of 20 cases of clear cell HCC among 215 consecutively resected HCCs.[35] Occasionally, sarcomatoid HCCs, consisting of

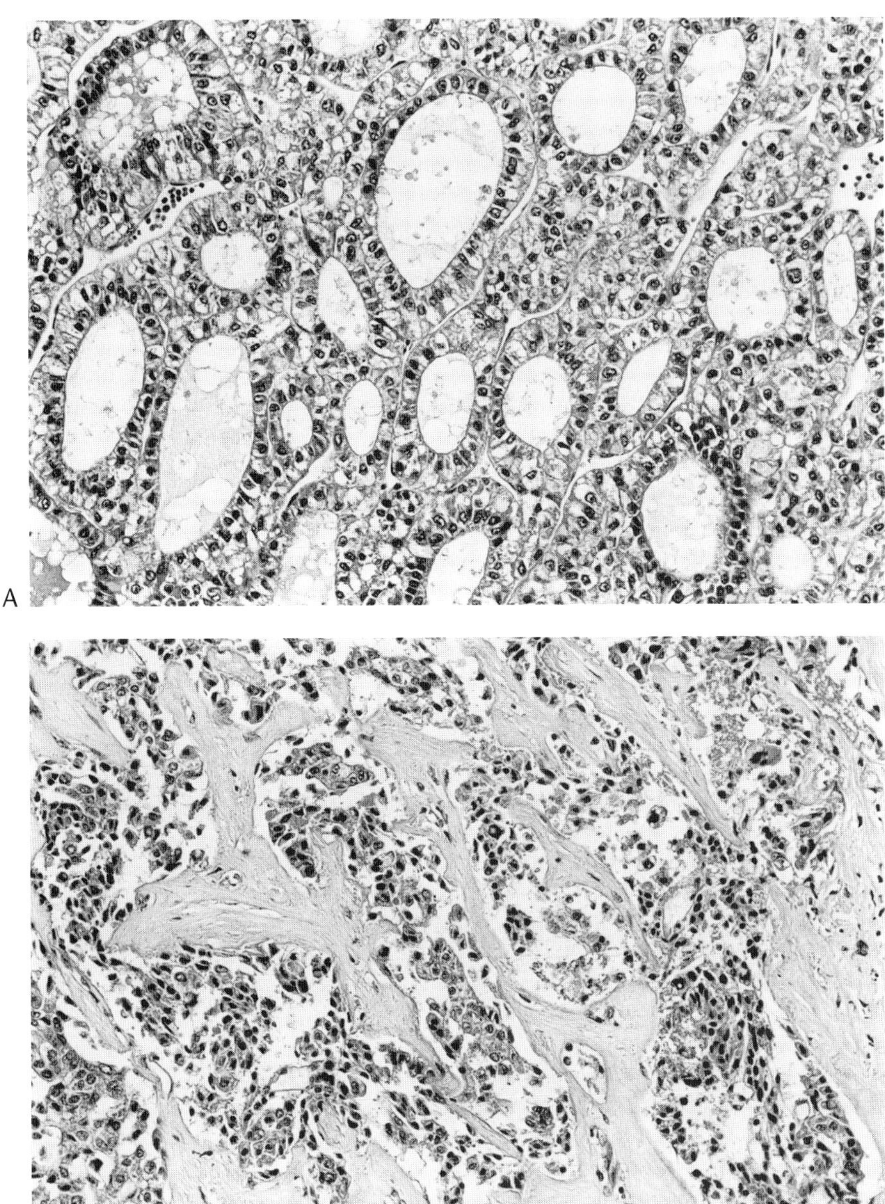

FIGURE 12-14. Structural variations in HCC. (*A*) Pseudoglandular type. Trabecular pattern is obscure due to marked glandular pattern and varying sized glandlike structures that contain proteinaceous fluid. (*B*) Scirrhous type. Blood spaces are replaced by hyalinized connective tissue.

spindle-shaped or pleomorphic anaplastic tumor cells, are found in part or most of the tumor with or without a transitional feature between trabecular HCC and the sarcomatoid area (Fig. 12-15C).[36,37] This may be a sarcomatoid variant rather than the combination of true sarcoma and HCC. Among more than 62 surgically resected HCCs less than 2 cm in diameter in our institution, none had a sarcomatoid appearance, whereas about 4% of advanced HCCs had a sarcomatoid appearance. Thus, the sarcomatoid cytologic variant of HCC may be caused by phenotypic changes of cancer cells that occur during the course of the disease. Anticancer therapy may contribute to the phenotypic change in HCC cells; sarcomatoid HCC is significantly more prevalent among HCC cases treated with transcatheter arterial chemoembolization therapy compared with nontreated cases.[38]

INTRACYTOPLASMIC INCLUSIONS IN HCC

Mallory bodies are seen not only in alcoholic hepatitis, but also frequently in HCC (Fig. 12-16A). They are ir-

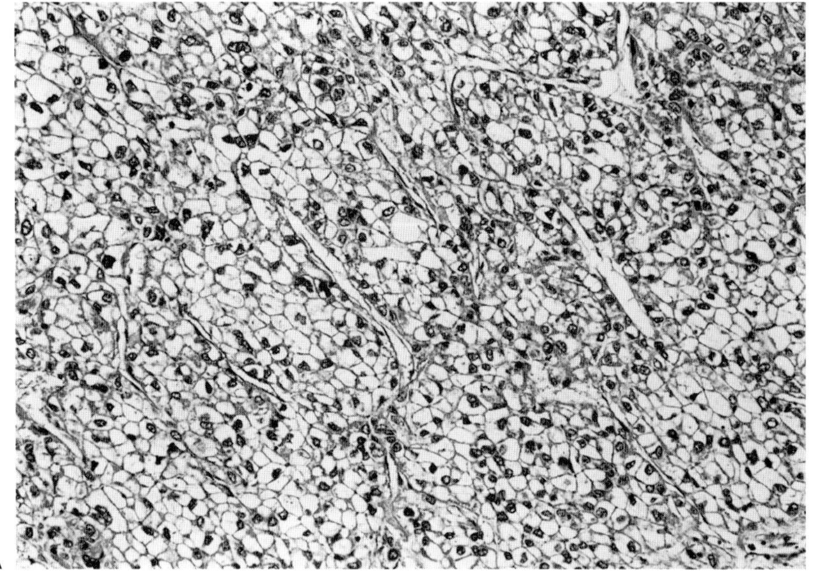
A

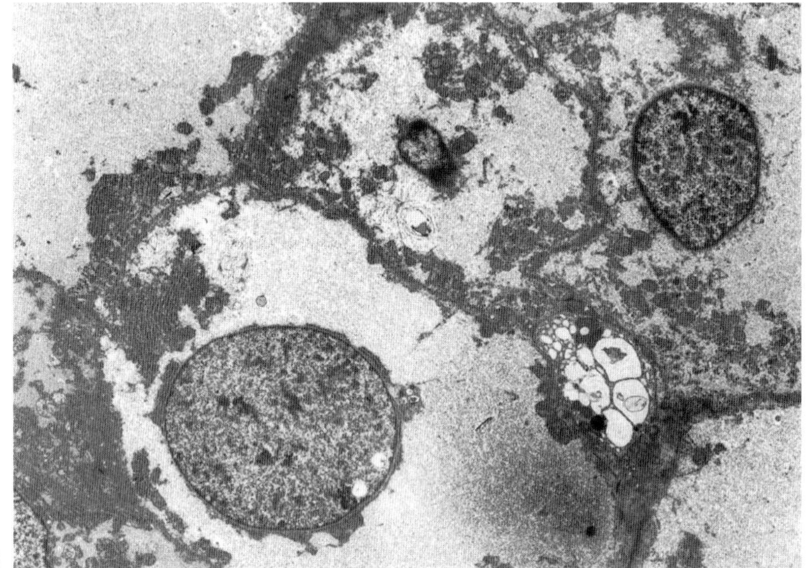
B

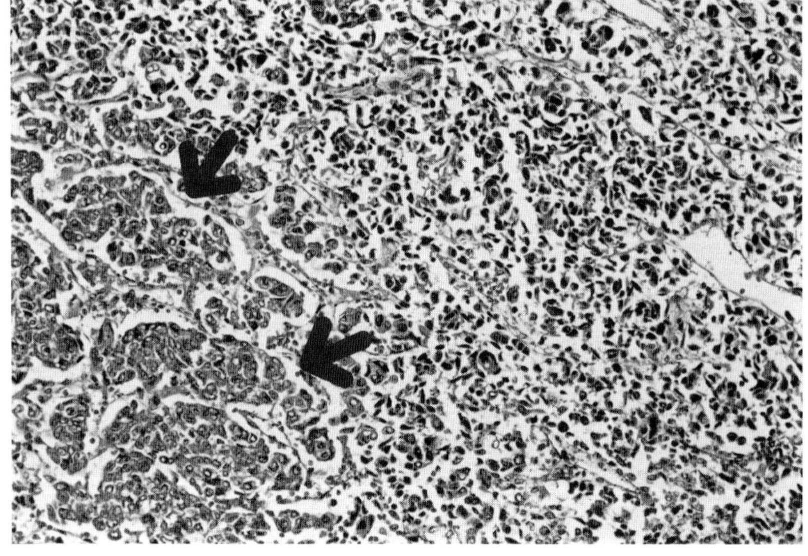
C

FIGURE 12-15. Cytologic variation in HCC. (*A,B*) Clear cell HCC. The cytoplasm of the HCC cells is watery and clear and is filled with numerous glycogen particles ultrastructurally. (*C*) Sarcomatoid HCC. Anaplastic tumor cells and vaguely trabecular carcinoma nests (arrows) are admixed with transitional features.

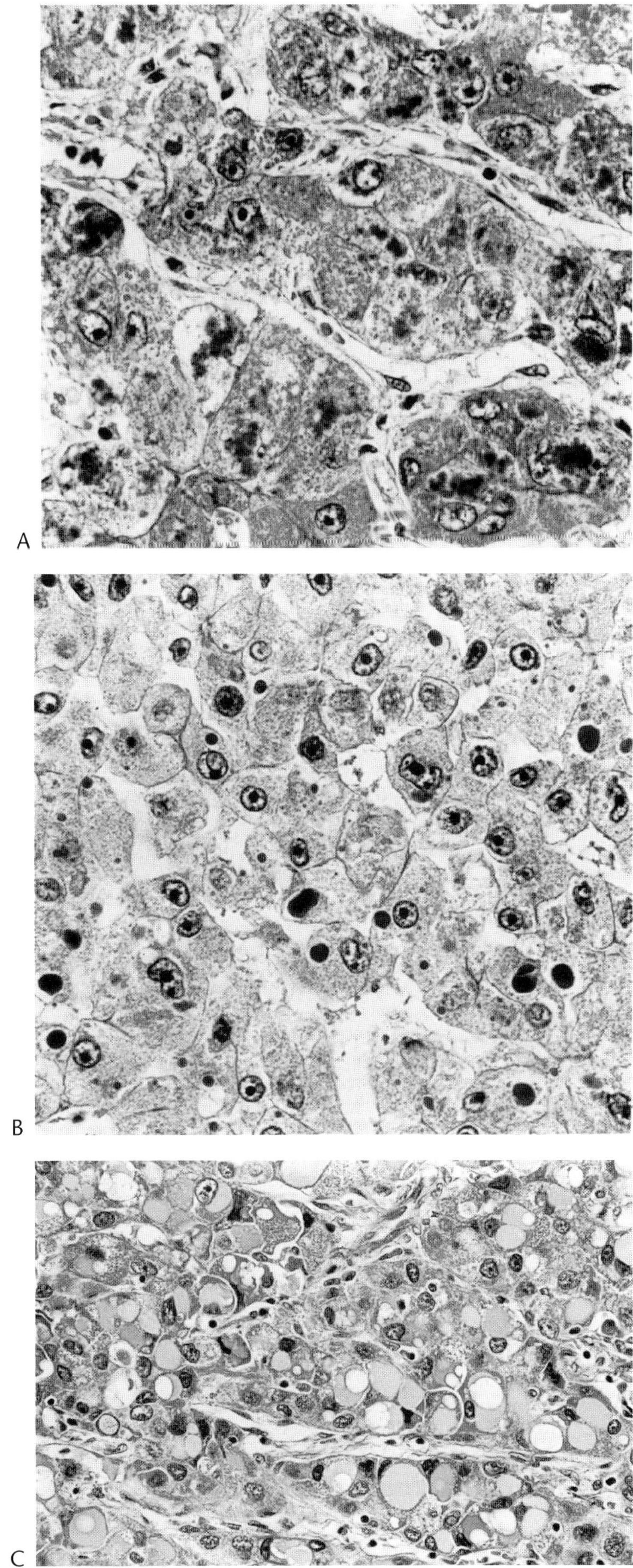

FIGURE 12-16. Hyaline inclusions in HCC. (*A*) Reticular hyalin (Mallory bodies). (*B*) Globular hyalin. (C) Pale bodies.

regular in shape and acidophilic, and they are not stained by periodic acid Schiff (PAS). Ultrastructurally, they are composed of an accumulation of intermediate filaments.[39]

GLOBULAR HYALINS

Globular hyalins are brightly stained with eosin and round to ovoid in shape (Fig. 12-16B). Most globular hyalins are diastase-resistant PAS positive.

Pale bodies are round to ovoid in shape and lightly eosinophilic (Fig. 12-16C). They stain positively with antifibrinogen antibody, and they are observed ultrastructurally as an accumulation of fibrils (fibrinogen) in the endoplasmic reticula, with cystic dilatation.[40,41] Pale bodies are frequently found in fibrolamellar carcinomas and in about 4% of HCCs.

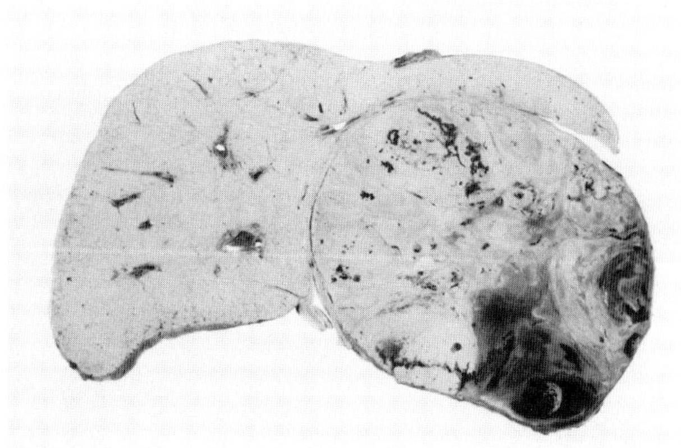

FIGURE 12-17. Pedunculated hepatocellular carcinoma. Massive tumor is proliferating extrahepatically with fibrous peduncle.

Extrahepatic Metastasis in HCC

Extrahepatic metastasis occurs at a relatively late stage. The incidence of extrahepatic metastasis in HCC range from 50% to 70% in Western countries.[42,43] Among 660 consecutive autopsy cases of HCC in Japan (in our institute), extrahepatic metastases were found in 503 cases (76.2%). The incidence of extrahepatic metastases tends to be slightly higher in HCC without cirrhosis than in HCC with cirrhosis. Peters[44] reported extrahepatic metastases in 67.0% and 46.2% among HCCs without and with cirrhosis, respectively. Our own study in Japan found an incidence 74.2% and 58.4%, respectively. Extrahepatic metastases are more common when HCC cells are proliferating along the sinusoids in an infiltrative fashion.

Hematogeneous metastases are much more common than lymphatic ones in HCC, occurring in 50.8% and 25.5% of cases, respectively, in our series. Hematogeneous metastasis was seen in lungs (47.6%), adrenal glands (8.3%), bone (5.6%), gastrointestinal tract (4.7%), gall bladder (3.5%), and pancreas (3.0%) in our series.

Lymphatic metastasis is found in 25.5% of 660 consecutive autopsy cases of HCC[45] and is frequent in the hepatic hilar lymph nodes (58.3%), peripancreatic lymph nodes (54.2%), perigastric nodes (45.8%), periaortic nodes (33.3%), and superficial lymph nodes (e.g. cervical nodes 10%).

Unusual Tumor Growth in HCC

HCC often shows unusual tumor growth, such as pedunculated tumor growth, intrabile duct tumor growth, and intra-atrial tumor growth through the inferior vena cava. The pathologic characteristics of such unusual growth patterns must be understood to make an accurate imaging diagnosis.

PEDUNCULATED HCC

Massive extrahepatic tumor growth with little tumor invasion into the liver is occasionally found in HCC. Most of these pedunculated HCCs are found in the subcapsular portion of the liver and grow extrahepatically with or without a pedicle (Fig. 12-17).

INTRA-BILE DUCT TUMOR GROWTH IN HCC

Tumor invasion into the hepatic duct and/or common bile duct accounts for about 6% of advanced HCCs seen at autopsy.[46] In most cases with tumor invasion into the hepatic duct and/or common bile duct, progressive obstructive jaundice is one of the major clinical signs (Fig. 12-18). Lin[47] referred to cases that present difficult problems in diagnosis as "icteric hepatoma." Patients with HCC growing into the bile duct have a significantly shorter survival after the time of diagnosis than patients with the usual HCC. However, the survival period has been extended in some cases by earlier diagnosis. Massive hemorrhage in the bile duct (hemobilia) resulting from intrabile duct tumor growth is occasionally observed.

INTRA-ATRIAL TUMOR GROWTH IN HCC

It is rather common to find tumor growth in the right atrium in some malignant neoplasms such as HCC, renal cell carcinoma, pulmonary carcinoma, and pancreatic carcinoma. Edmondson and Steiner[32] observed tumor extension into the right atrium in only 1 of 100 autopsy cases of primary liver cancer. Among 439 autopsy cases of HCC in the past two decades in our institute, tumor extended into the inferior vena cava in 48 (10.9%) cases and into the right atrium in 18 (4.8%) cases (Fig. 12-19). The tumor traversed the tricuspid valves and entered the ventricle in 5 of the 18 cases, and direct tumor invasion

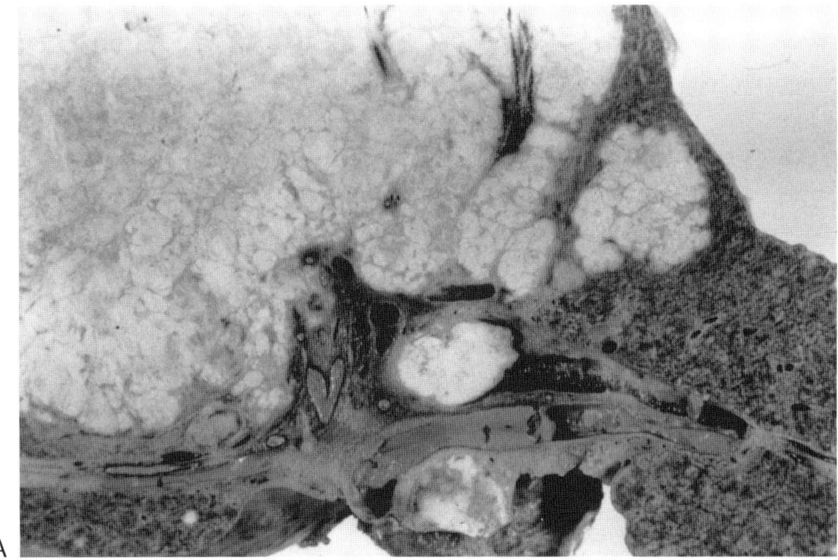

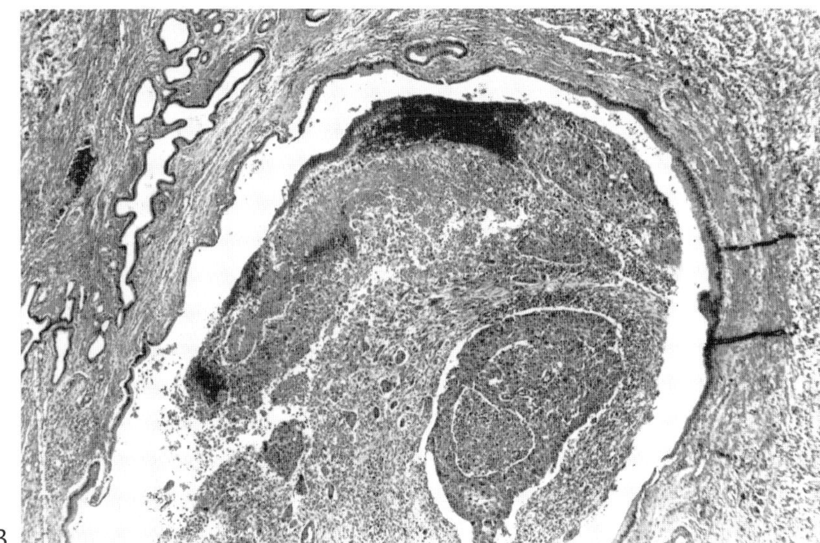

FIGURE 12-18. Hepatocllular carcinoma with intra-bile duct tumor growth. (*A*) The patient presented progressive obstructive jaudice shortly before death, and autopsy disclosed tumor growth into the bifurcation of the hepatic duct. (*B*) Tumor casts extend into the bile duct branches.

into the myocardium was found in two cases. The reason for the discrepancy in the incidence of HCC cases with intra-atrial tumor growth between the experience of Edmondson and Steiner and ours can be explained by the increase in survival time in the past decade. The average survival time after diagnosis of HCC was only 3 months until 1970, but was more than 1 year in the decade from 1985 to 1995.

It is uncommon to see serious clinical signs due to intra-atrial tumor growth. Only a few patients present with diuretic-resistant lower extremity edema and/or marked venous dilatation of the abdominal wall. Patients with intra-atrial tumor growth rarely have sudden cardiac arrest or severe dyspnea due to obstruction of tricuspid valves by ball-shaped tumor thrombus in the right atrium. We have had only one case among 18 autopsy cases of HCC with right atrial tumor growth.[48]

COMBINED HEPATOCELLULAR AND CHOLANGIOCARCINOMA

According to the WHO classification, combined hepatocellular and cholangiocarcinoma (combined HCC-CCC) is defined as a tumor containing unequivocal elements of HCC and cholangiocarcinoma (CCC) that are intimately admixed[33] (Fig. 12-20A,B). The reported frequency of combined HCC-CCC in autopsy cases varies from 2.5% to 14.2%.[49–52]

Clinicopathologic Features

Our 23 surgically resected cases of combined HCC-CCC accounted for 6.3% of surgical cases of primary liver cancer.[53] The mean patient age was 64.0 years, the same as that of patients with HCCs, and the male:female ratio

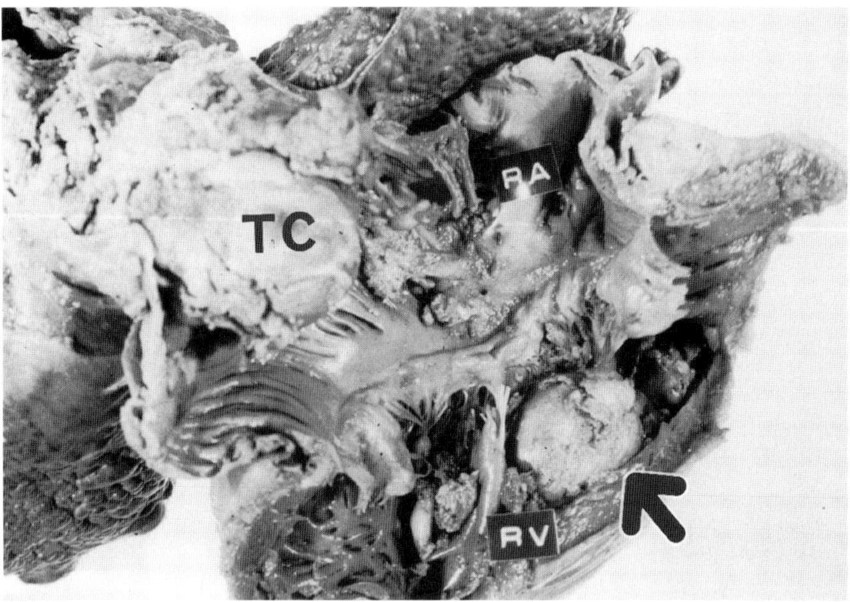

FIGURE 12-19. Tumor growth into the right atrium (RA) and ventricle (RV). Tumor cast (TC) is extending from the hepatic vein to the right atrium, and a ball-shaped tumor cast is also found in the right ventricle (arrow). The tumor growth into the right atrium was noted 8 months before patient death without significant symptoms.

was 1.9:1, which is closer to the ratio of CCC. Serum α-fetoprotein is detected in 70% of the cases, but its levels are relatively low (< 1,000 ng/ml) in most cases. Carcinoembryonic antigen (CEA) is detected in 18%, and its levels are also low (> 4.1 ng/ml). Low levels of these tumor markers appear to be one of the characteristics of combined HCC-CCC. Among combined HCC-CCC cases, 17% to 20% were positive for hepatitis B surface antigen, and 70% for antibody to hepatitis C virus. These results are almost the same as those for HCC patients in Japan. HCC-CCC was not diagnosed before hepatectomy in many of the 23 patients, even though they had had ultrasound-guided tumor biopsy because it is difficult to obtain both the HCC and the CCC components at biopsy.

Combined HCC-CCC can be divided macroscopically into a separated type, with HCC and CCC clearly separated (17%); an HCC predominant type, which resembles HCC (49%); and a CCC predominant type (34%). Cirrhosis was found associated in 9 of 23 cases (40%) (50% in the separated type, 55% in the HCC predominant type, 13% in the CCC predominant type).

Both HCC and CCC components can be clearly distinguished in 17% of cases, corresponding macroscopically to a separated type. In others, HCC and CCC are contiguous with transitional features (66%), macroscopically corresponding to either the HCC predominant type or the CCC predominant. Cancerous tissues that can be interpreted as either HCC or CCC are considered an intermediate form of HCC and CCC (17%).

Although the histogenesis of combined HCC-CCC is still obscure, the following three possible mechanisms are possible: (1) It could be a double cancer; (2) HCC could differentiate to CCC in part; or (3) the cancer could arise in an intermediate (transitional) cell that differentiates to both HCC and CCC. A cell line has been established[54] from an HCC that transformed to adenocarcinoma after culturing. The presence of intermediate cells has been questioned in human liver; however, combined HCC-CCC with intermediate features of HCC and CCC could be interpreted as having originated from intermediate cells.

To reveal CCC components, the demonstration of mucin production by mucicarmin stain has been widely used. Furthermore, the immunohistochemical demonstration of cytokeratins 7 and 19, which are considered to be specific to bile duct epithelial cells, is more useful in demonstrating the CCC components than the HCC components (Fig. 12-20C). In the 23 combined HCC-CCC cases, cytokeratins 7 and 19 were positive in all CCC components of the HCC predominant type and in all the CCC predominant type, as well as in three of the four intermediate-type cases.

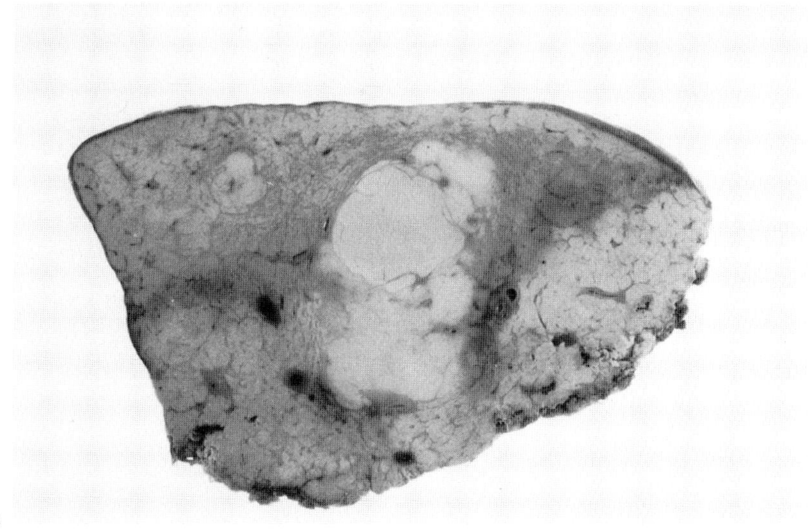

A

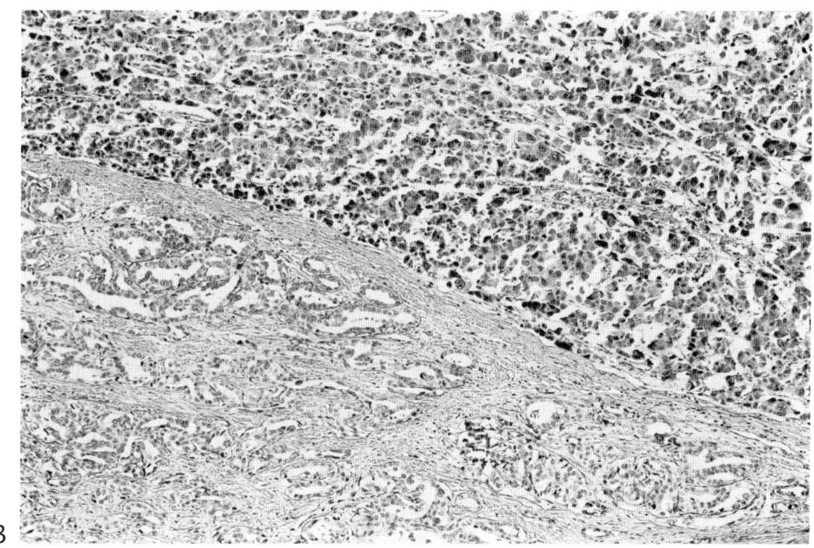

B

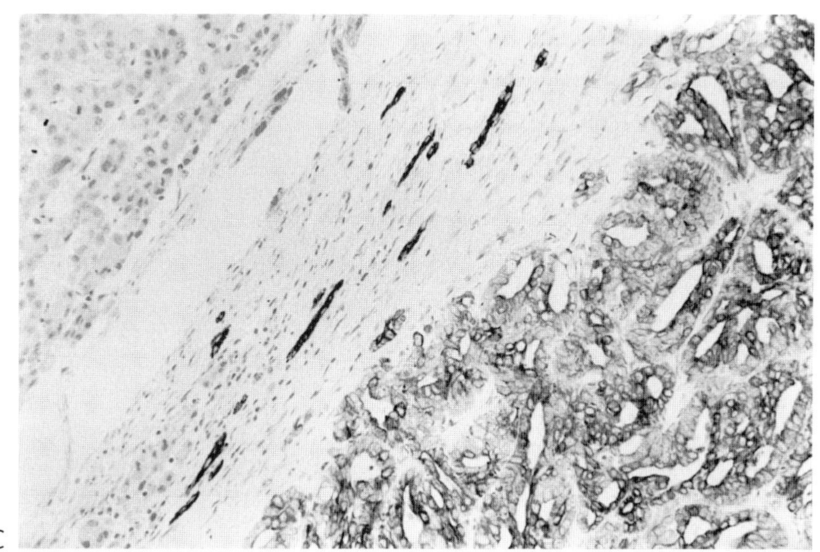

C

FIGURE 12-20. Combined hepatocellular and cholangiocarcinoma (surgical case). (*A*) The nodular tumor consists of HCC; infiltrative tumor around the nodular tumor consists of cholangiocarcinoma. HCV-associated cirrhosis was present. (*B*) Histologically, the HCC and cholangiocarcinoma are clearly separated. (*C*) Positive reaction to cytokeratin 7 in cholangiocarcinoma component. Cytokeratin 7 is markedly positive in cholangiocarcinoma component (lower right), but negative in hepatocellular components (upper left). It also is strongly positive in noncancerous ductules along the boundary (avidin-biotin complex method).

REFERENCES

1. Munoz N, Bosch X. Epidemiology of hepatocellular carcinoma. In Okuda K, Ishak KG (eds): Neoplasms of the Liver, Springer-Verlag, Tokyo, 1987, pp. 3–19
2. Kiyosawa K, Sodeyama T, Tanaka E et al. Interrelationship of blood transfusion, non-A, non-B hepatitis and hepatocellular carcinoma: analysis by detection of antibody to hepatitis C. Hepatology 1990;12:671–675
3. Colombo M, Kuo G, Choo QL et al. Prevalence of hepatitis C virus in Italian patients with hepatocellular carcinoma. Lancet 1989;2:1006–1008
4. Levrero M, Tagger A, Balsano C et al. Antibodies to hepatitis C virus in patients with hepatocellular carcinoma. J Hepatol 1991;12:60–63
5. Bruix J, Barrera JM, Calvet X et al. Prevalence to antibodies to hepatic C virus in Spanish patients with hepatocellular carcinoma and hepatic cirrhosis. Lancet 1989;2:1004–1006
6. Saito I, Miysamura T, Ohbayashi A et al. Hepatitis C virus infection is associated with the development of hepatocellular carcinoma. Proc Natl Acad Sci U S A 1990;87: 6547–6549
7. Shimamatsu K, Kage M, Nakashima O, Kojiro M: Pathomorphological study of HCV antibody positive liver cirrhosis. J Gastroenterol Hepatol 1994;9:624–630
8. Okuda K, Fujimoto I, Hanai A, Urano Y. Changing incidence of hepatocellular carcinoma in Japan. Cancer Res 1987;47:4967–4972
9. Shiratori Y, Shiina S, Imamura M et al. Characteristic difference of hepatocellular carcinoma between hepatitis B- and C-viral infection in Japan. Hepatology 1995;22:1027–1033
10. Takenaka K, Yamamoto K, Taketomi A et al. A comparison of of the surgical results in patients with hepatitis B versus hepatitis C-related hepatocellular carcinoma. Hepatology 1995;22:20–24
11. Takazawa T, Nakashima O, Sueda J et al. Clinicopathologic comparison of hepatitis B virus-related and hepatitis C virus-related hepatocellular carcinoma (submitted).
12. Okuda K: Hepatocellular carcinoma: recent progress. Hepatology 1992;15:948–963
13. Ohto M, Karasawa E, Tsuchiya Y et al. Ultrasonically guided percutaneous contrast medium ingestion and aspiration biopsy using a real time transducer. Radiology 1980;136: 171–176
14. Kondo Y, Niwa Y, Akikusa B et al. A histopathologic study of early hepatocellular carcinoma. Cancer 1983;52:687–692
15. Nakashima O, Sugihara S, Kage M. Pathomorphologic characteristics of small hepatocellular carcinoma: a special reference to small hepatocellular carcinoma with indistinct margins. Hepatology 1995;22:101–105
16. Kojiro M, Sugihara S, Nakashima O. Pathomorphologic characteristics of early hepatocellular carcinoma. In Okuda K, Tobe T, Kitagawa T (eds): Early Detection and Treatment of Liver Cancer. Japan Scientific Societies Press, Tokyo, 1991, pp. 29–33
17. Takayama T, Makuuchi M, Hirohashi S et al. Malignant transformation of adenomatous hyperplasia to hepatocellular carcinoma. Lancet 1990;336:1150–1153
18. Sakamoto M, Hirohashi S, Shimosato Y. Early stage of multistep hepatocarcinogenesis: adenomatous hyperplasia and early hepatocellular carcinoma. Hum Pathol 1991;22: 172–178
19. Arakawa M, Kage M, Sugihara S et al. Emergence of malignant lesions within an adenomatous hyperplastic nodule in a cirrhotic liver. Observations in five cases. Gastroenterology 1986;91:198–208
20. Kenmochi K, Sugihara S, Kojiro M. Relationship of histologic grade of hepatocellular carcinoma (HCC) to tumor size, and demonstration of tumor cells of multiple different grades in a single small HCC. Liver 1987;7:18–26
21. Yano H, Iemura A, Fukuda K et al. Establishment of two distinct human hepatocellular carcinoma cell lines from a single nodule showing clonal dedifferentiation of cancer cells. Hepatology 1993;18:320–327
22. Rim KS, Sakamoto M, Watanabe H et al. Pathology and DNA cytophotometry of small hepatocellular carcinoma with a nodule-in-nodule appearance: evidence for stepwise progression of hepatocellular carcinoma. Jpn J Clin Oncol 1992;23:26–33
23. Sakamoto M, Ino Y, Fujii T, Hirohashi S. Phenotype changes in tumor vessels associated with the progression of hepatocellular carcinoma. Jpn J Clin Oncol 1993;23:98–104
24. Okada S, Ishii H, Nose H et al. Intratumoral DNA heterogeneity of small hepatocellular carcinoma. Cancer 1995;75: 444–450
25. Tsuda H, Zhang W, Shimosato Y et al. Allele loss on chromosome 16 associated with progression of human hepatocellular carcinoma. Proc Natl Acad Sci U S A 1990;87: 6791–6794
26. Okuda K, Peters RL, Simson IW. Gross anatomic features of hepatocellular carcinoma from three disparate geographic areas. Proposal of new classification. Cancer 1984;54: 2165–2163
27. Kojiro M, Nakashima O, Kiyomatsu K et al. Comparative study of HCC between Japan and Spain. In Sung JL, Chen DS (eds): Viral Hepatitis and Hepatocellular Carcinoma. Excerpta Medica, Amsterdam, 1990, pp. 545–548
28. Eggel H. Uber das primare Carcinom der Leber. Beitr Pathol Anat 1901;30:506
29. Nakashima T, Kojiro M. Hepatocellular Carcinoma. Tokyo, Springer, 1987, p. 56
30. Kanai T, Hirohashi S, Upton MP et al. Pathology of small hepatocellular carcinoma. A proposal for a new gross classification. Cancer 1987;60:810–819
31. Liver Cancer Study Group of Japan. The General Rules for the Clinical and Pathological Study of Primary Liver Cancer. 3rd Ed. Kanehara Shuppan Tokyo, 1992, p. 14 (in Japanese)
32. Edmondson H, Steiner PE: Primary carcinoma of the liver: a study of 100 cases among 48,900 necropsies. Cancer 1954; 7:462–503
33. Ishak KG, Anthony PP, Sobin LH. Histological Typing of Tumours of the Liver, 2nd Ed. WHO International Histological Classification of Tumours. Springer-Verlag, Berlin, 1994, p. 20
34. Lai CL, Wu PC, Lam KC, Lok ASF. Histologic prognostic indicators in hepatocellular carcinoma. Cancer 1979;44: 1677–1683

35. Yang SH, Watanabe J, Nakashima O, Kojiro M. Clinicopathologic study on clear cell hepatocellular carcinoma. Pathol Intern 1996;46:503–509
36. Kakizoe S, Kojiro M, Nakashima T. Hepatocellular carcinoma with sarcomatous change: clinicopathologic and immunohistochemical studies of 14 autopsy cases. Cancer 1987; 59:310–316
37. Maeda T, Adachi E, Kajiyama K et al. Spindle cell hepatocellular carcinoma. A clinicopathologic and immunohistochemical analysis of 15 cases. Cancer 1995;77:51–57
38. Kojiro M, Sugihara S, Kakizoe S et al. Hepatocellular carcinoma with sarcomatous change: a special reference to the relationship with anticancer therapy. Cancer Chemother Pharmacol 1989;23 (suppl):4–8
39. Nakanuma Y, Ohta G. Is Mallory body formation a preneoplastic change? A study of 181 cases of liver bearing hepatocellular carcinoma and 82 cases of cirrhosis. Cancer 1984; 55:2400–2404
40. Stromeyer FW, Ishak KG, Gerber MA, Mathew T. Ground-glass cells in hepatocellular carcinoma. Am J Clin Pathol 1980;74:254–258
41. Nakashima O, Sugihara S, Eguchi A et al. Pathomorphologic study of pale bodies in hepatocellular carcinoma. Acta Pathol Jpn 1992;42:414–417
42. MacDonald RA. Primary carcinoma of the liver. Arch Intern Med 1957;99:266–279
43. MacSween RNM. A clinicopathological review of 100 cases of primary malignant tumors of the liver. J Clin Pathol 1974; 27:669–682
44. Peters RL. Pathology of hepatocellular carcinoma. In Okuda K, Peters RL (eds): Hepatocellular Carcinoma. Wiley, New York, 1976, pp. 107–168
45. Watanabe J, Nakashima O, Kojiro M. Clinicopathologic study on lymph node metastasis of hepatocellular carcinoma: a retrospective study of 660 consecutive autopsy cases. Jpn J Clin Oncol 1994;24:37–41
46. Kojiro M, Kawabata K, Kawano Y et al. Hepatocellular carcinoma presenting as intrabile duct tumor growth: a clinicopathologic study of 24 cases. Cancer 1982;49:2144–2124
47. Lin TY: Tumor of the liver, part 1, primary malignant tumors. In Bockus HL, Berk JE, Haubrich WS et al (eds): Gastroenterology. 3rd Ed. WB Saunders, Philadelphia, 1972, pp. 22
48. Kojiro M, Nakahara H, Sugihara S et al. Hepatocellular carcinoma with intraatrial tumor growth: a clinicopathologic study of 18 autopsy cases. Arch Pathol Lab Med 1984;108: 989–992
49. Allen RA, Lisa JL. Combined liver cell and bile duct carcinoma. Am J Pathol 1949;25:647–655
50. Edmondson HA, Peters RL. Neoplasms of the liver. In Schiff L, Schiff ER (eds): Diseases of the Liver. 5th Ed. JB Lippincott, Philadelphia, 1982, pp. 1101
51. Goodman ZD, Isha KG, Langlos JM et al. Combined hepatocellular-cholangioma. A histological and immunohistological study. Cancer 1985;55:124–135
52. Nakahara H. Clinicopathological study of combined hepatocellular and cholangiocarcinoma. Acta Hepatol Jpn 1986; 27:1431–1438
53. Taguchi J, Nakashima O, Tanaka M et al. A clinicopathological study on combined hepatocellular and cholangiocarcinoma. J Gastroenterol Hepatol 1996;11:758–764
54. Yano H, Kojiro M, Nakashima T. A new human hepatocellular carcinoma cell line (KYN-1) with a transformation to adenocarcinoma. In Vitro 1986;22:637–646

13

ANIMAL HEPADNAVIRUSES AS A MODEL OF CARCINOGENESIS

PASCAL PINEAU
PIERRE TIOLLAIS

AN OVERVIEW OF THE HEPADNAVIRIDAE FAMILY

The Hepadnaviridae family shares unique features that allow classification in a specific virus group: (1) common DNA size and genetic organization, (2) similar polypeptides and antigenic composition, (3) a unique mechanism of replication, and (4) analogous virion size and structure.[1] Their hosts belong to different groups of vertebrates. In addition to the human pathogen hepatitis B virus (HBV), which is the prototypic member of the family[2] (Fig. 13-1), two other well-documented mammalian hepadnaviruses infect rodents of the Sciuridae family (Fig. 13-1). These are the woodchuck hepatitis virus (WHV), which infects the woodchuck (*Marmota monax*)[3]; and the ground squirrel hepatitis virus (GSHV), which infects the Californian ground squirrel (*Spermophilus beecheyi*)[4]; the Canadian ground squirrel (*S. richardsonii*),[5] and the eastern grey squirrel (*S. carolinensis*).[6] Recently, the Arctic Squirrel Hepatitis Virus (ASHV), which infects Alaskan squirrels (*S. parriyi kenicotti*), was discovered (Buendia MA, personal communication, 1996). The identical genetic organization of mammalian hepadnaviruses allows gathering them in the *Orthohepadnavirus* genus. The genome of the avian hepadnaviruses lacks the fourth open reading frame coding for the X gene, and thus these viruses constitute the separate *Avihepadnavirus* genus.[7] Avian hepadnaviruses are represented by the duck hepatitis B virus (DHBV), which infects domestic ducks (*Anas domesticus*)[8] (Fig. 13-1), and the heron hepatitis B virus (HHBV), which infects the gray heron (*Ardea cinerea*).[9] Data yet to be confirmed suggest that many novel hepadnaviruses may infect various other hosts.[10]

NATURAL HISTORY AND HISTOPATHOLOGIC FEATURES OF LIVER TUMORS IN ANIMALS INFECTED BY HEPADNAVIRUSES

Woodchucks

The WHV chronic carriers have a high rate of developing hepatocellular carcinoma (HCC).[11] As shown by experimental infections beginning early in life (similar to the situation in humans) more than 50% of infected animals develop chronic hepatitis.[12] The lifetime risk for developing a primary liver tumor approaches 100% among chronic carriers, suggesting that WHV acts as a complete carcinogen (Table 13-1). It has been reported that prior WHV infection with seroconversion to anti-WHs also is associated with a risk (5% to 17%) of developing HCC.[13–15] The tumor is generally detected before age 4 years, corresponding to one-third of the woodchuck's life span.[16] Based on the duration of chronic infection before the development of HCC and on the proportion (~ 15%) of chronic carriers of WHV developing HCC,[17] WHV is a more efficient tumorigenic agent than

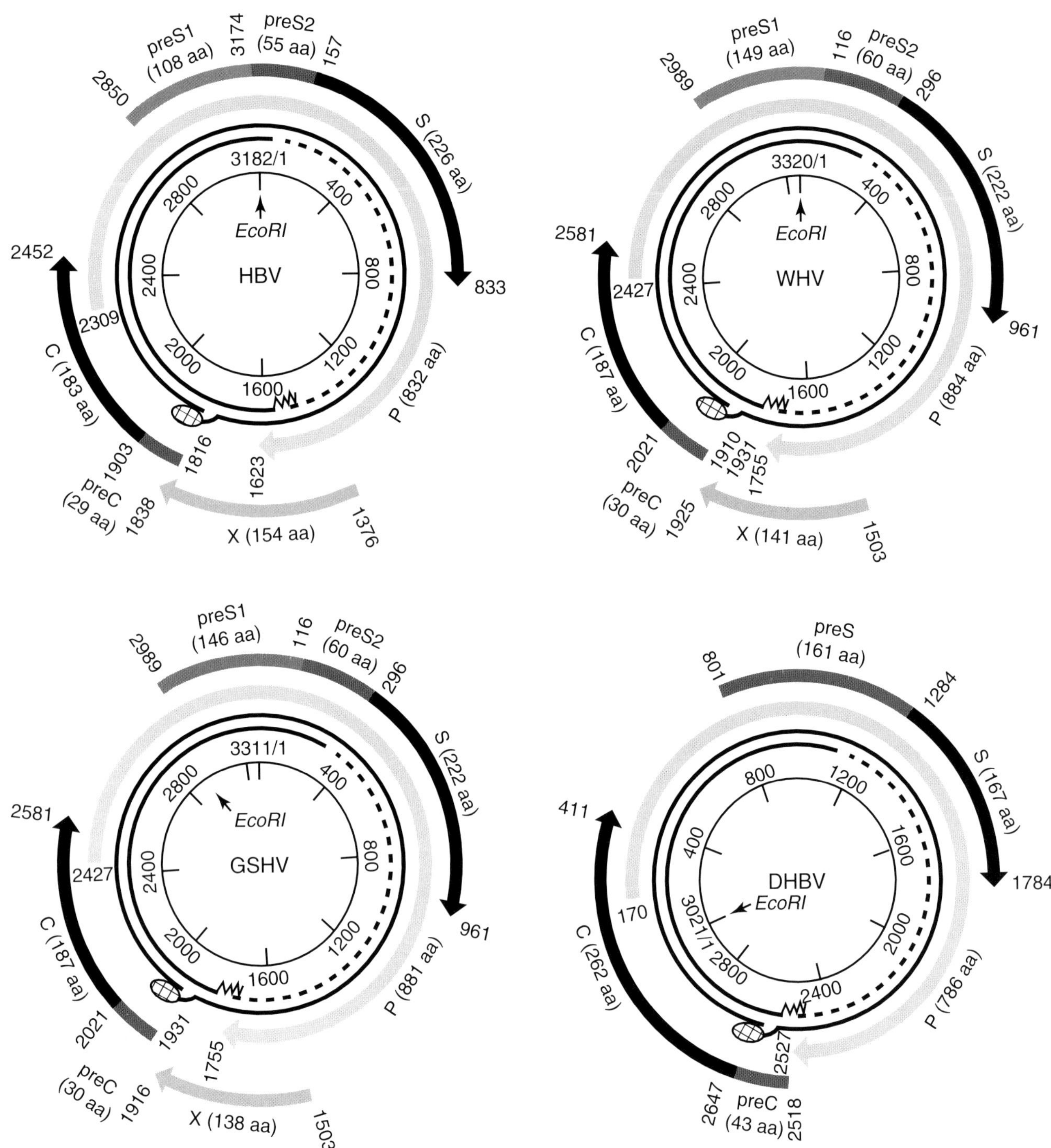

FIGURE 13-1. Structure and genetic organization in the Hepadnavirus family. A short jagged line indicates the oligoribonucleotide priming DNA(+) strand synthesis. The P-gene-derived protein covalently linked to the 5′ end of the DNA(−) strand is indicated by a hatched oval. The arrows symbolize the open reading frames (ORF) encoded on the DNA minus strand. The numbering at each extremity of the ORF indicates their positions in the genome according to the EcoRI site.

TABLE 13-1. Comparison of Oncogenic Potentials Among the Principal Hepadnaviruses

	HBV	WHV	GSHV	DHBV
Histopathologic features of chronically infected livers	Chronic active hepatitis, cirrhosis ++	Mild hepatitis, no cirrhosis	Mild hepatitis, no cirrhosis	Chronic hepatitis, infrequent cirrhosis
HCC incidence	15%	90%	45%	Low (circumscribed to Qidong region of China)
Latence (age of onset)	20–30 years (2nd part of life span)	2–4 years (1st part of life span)	5–6 years (2nd part of life span)	3–5 years or more (half life span)
Clonal pattern of viral DNA integration (% of tumors)	+ (70–80%)	+ (80–90%)	+ (20–25%)	Sporadic
Myc gene alterations	Overexpression of c-*myc* (>90%)	Insertional mutagenesis (85%) and overexpression of N-*myc2* and c-*myc*	Amplification (40%) or overexpression of c-*myc*	?
p53 status	High rates of codon 249 mutations in Mozambique and Qidong (China)	No mutation described	One mutation published (codon 176)	No mutation described
Co-carcinogens	AFB1, sex steroids? others?, HCV	—	?	+ (AFB1)

Abbreviations: HBV, hepatitis B virus; WHV, woodchuck hepatitis virus; GSHV, ground squirrel hepatitis virus; DHBV, duck hepatitis B virus; HCC, hepatocellular carcinoma.

HBV. Chemical carcinogenesis experiments have shown that rodent hepatocytes are exquisitely susceptible to transformation, in contrast to the absence of effect of most rodent carcinogens on humans.[18] Thus, the relative intrinsic oncogenic potential of HBV and WHV appears difficult to assess in the absence of a common host. In addition, data provided by experimental infection highlight the determinant influence of the genetic background of the individual host in these models. In the woodchuck model, the similar rates of HCC among naturally and experimentally infected animals probably rule out any potential cocarcinogenic effect of environmental factors.[19,20] One of the most original features of woodchuck hepatocarcinogenesis is the absence of a male predominance, such as that observed in humans with HCC and for chemical hepatocarcinogenesis in mice and rats.[20,21]

Most woodchucks infected with WHV have a mild to moderate chronic active hepatitis associated with an inflammatory cell infiltration in portal tracts, a few necrotic foci, and early fibrosis.[10,20] Sequential histologic investigations of infected livers show a gradual deterioration with age. In contrast to humans with HBV,[22] cirrhosis is never observed in WHV-infected woodchucks.[23] Ductular proliferation associated with cystic cholangiomas has also been reported in WHV-infected woodchucks[23,26] as in ducks infected with DHBV.[24,25] Apoptosis is often seen along with the cytolysis in livers of WHV chronic carriers.[26]

Preneoplastic changes in infected woodchucks include foci of altered hepatocytes (clear cell or basophilic) similar to those observed during chemical hepatocarcinogenesis.[23,26,27] Aneuploidy can be seen in 50% of WHV-infected woodchucks with chronic active hepatitis, reaching 63% in basophilic foci. Woodchuck HCCs are aneuploid in 90% of cases. Interestingly, different ploidy peaks can be found in different areas of the tumor, indicating heterogeneity within a single tumor,[23] as seen with heterogeneity of c-*myc* expression.[28] In woodchucks, HCCs are generally well differentiated and trabecular[16,20,23] and are sometimes multifocal.[29,30]

Squirrels

In California, ground squirrels infected with GSHV, HCC development is less frequent (~ 46%) and occurs at least 18 to 24 months later in the squirrel's life span than in woodchucks.[31,32] GSHV-infected ground squirrels characteristically develop only minor liver inflammation[24,33] (Table 13-1). It has been reported that many hepatic malignancies in squirrels arise with no serologic evidence of GSHV infection,[32,34] raising the possibility of a different noninfectious etiology of HCC in these rodents.[35] Cholangiocellular carcinomas (CCC) are sometimes encountered concomitantly with HCC in both infected and uninfected squirrels.[34]

It appears that viral determinants may control the

oncogenic potential of the different hepadnaviruses. Newborn woodchucks infected with WHV develop HCC more rapidly than woodchucks experimentally infected with GSHV, even if the virus replication rate and liver hispathologic changes are the same.[36] A few HCCs have also been detected in two of the three other squirrel species that are commonly infected with GSHV, *S. richardsonii* and *S. parriyi kenicotti*.[36]

Ducks

In contrast to the situation observed in mammals infected with hepadnaviruses, the association of DHBV infection and HCC is uncommon and limited to domestic brown ducks in the Qidong region of China where the virus is congenitally present in the flocks.[25,37,38] A recent study of duck liver disease in the Qidong region reveals that 70% of the HCCs are positive for DHBV DNA.[25]

The development of HCC may be a late event in ducks.[37] However, a recent study by Duflot et al,[25] described HCC as occurring mainly in the first half of the duck's life span (Table 13-1).

Duck HCCs are a well-differentiated trabecular type in more than 80% of cases.[25] The histopathology of the nontumorous liver reveals a portal infiltration and an infrequent evolution toward cirrhosis.[25,37,39] Overall, changes in DHBV-infected livers seem to be milder than in HBV-infected humans.[25,40] Some variations in the histology of DHBV-infected livers may reflect differences in the susceptibility of ducks or in the course of natural and experimental infections.[33,37]

One of the key features of duck liver histopathology is a high prevalence of ductular proliferation and the presence of viral antigens in bile duct cells.[24,25,37] Biliary cell proliferation is usually associated with aflatoxin B1 (AFB1) exposure or helminth infestation,[41] which may play etiologic roles in some HCCs.[25,37,39] In fact, cholangiocellular carcinomas, which may be caused by helminth infections, represent a substantial proportion of neoplasias identified in naturally infected Qidong ducks or AFB1-dosed Pekin ducks.[25,33] The hypothesis suggesting the presence of a specific causative environmental factor in the Qidong region is supported by the fact that neoplastic pathology is never observed early in the life of naturally or experimentally DHBV-infected ducks outside of China.[25]

MOLECULAR ASPECTS

Structural and Functional Characteristics of Hepadnaviral DNA in Animal Hepatocellular Carcinomas

WHV

As with HCC and HBV in humans, the majority (80% to 90%) of HCCs arising in WHV-infected woodchucks contain an integrated viral sequence[42] (Table 13-1). As with HBV, the integration process of WHV is a relatively early event, taking place in the chronic hepatitis phase.[13,43] In animals with serologic evidence of recovery, Southern blot analysis has revealed the presence of integrated WHV in low levels (0.1 to 0.3 copies per cell).[13] Contrasting with the situation observed in humans, high levels of WHV replication are found in the liver.[13] An early extinction of viral gene expression occurs in the preneoplastic stage.[44]

WHV integrants share general features with their HBV counterparts: different sites of integration in the host genome[45–47] and frequent complex rearrangements of viral and cellular sequences at the integration site, including deletions or inverted duplication.[43,48–52] So far, no replication-competent integrants have been cloned. Abnormal WHV RNAs could be detected in 30% of HCC samples in studies by Wei et al. in our laboratory.[59] In woodchucks, the virus seems to act as an insertional mutagen,[30,50,53] a situation infrequently encountered in humans.[54,55]

It was believed initially that rearrangements such as deletions in the cohesive region or inverted duplications occur only after integration.[56,57] The recent cloning of mutant WHV genomes in serum of woodchucks raises the hypothesis that such mutant forms appear before integration or alternatively. One may imagine that a functional virus concurrently present in the cell allows packaging and liberation of a minor proportion (4% of circulating virions) of the mutant virus (expressed from the integrants) into the circulation. A novel polymerase chain reaction (PCR)-based method, "fixed-flanking primer PCR" (FFP-PCR), suitable for the molecular characterization of integrated WHV or other hepadnavirus has been described[58]

The X gene product of HBV has the capacity to enhance the activity of cellular genes through transcription factors or by interfering with various cellular transduction pathways.[60,61] As a result of integration, the X open reading frame is frequently disrupted in its 3′ region in humans and woodchucks, but it has been demonstrated that truncated X proteins of HBV frequently retain their transactivating capacity.[62] The analysis of cDNAs from two woodchuck HCCs revealed hybrid virus-cell transcripts containing carboxy-truncated sequences of the X gene. The co-transcribed cellular sequences were providing signals for transcription termination. One of these transcripts exhibited a transactivating capacity in transient transfection assays.[59] These observations support the hypothesis that the WHV X gene participates in tumorigenesis in woodchucks.[51,59]

GSHV

GSHV DNA is integrated only in a minority of Beecheyi ground squirrel (*S. beecheyi*) HCCs (20% to 25%)[31,34] (Table 13-1). To date, only two GSHV integrations have been cloned. Their analysis revealed that GSHV integrants shared common features with other hepadnaviruses. Transy, in our laboratory, found the viral sequences to be composed of defective or rearranged genomes. The recombination breakpoints were located close to the direct repeat DR1. As with HBV, no cellular coding sequence was found in the vicinity of the integrated viral sequences.[63] Southern-blot analysis of HCC DNA from Richardson ground squirrels (*S. richardsonii*) revealed high molecular weight DNA fragments hybridizing with a GSHV probe in 3 of 10 cases.[64] In contrast, examination of molecular events occurring in woodchucks experimentally infected with GSHV revealed the presence of viral integrants in all tumor samples tested.[35] Taken together, these observations suggest that host factors exist that determine the capacity of hepadnaviruses to integrate.

DHBV

The absence of the X open reading frame in the genome of avian hepadnaviruses (Fig. 13-1) may provide a partial explanation for the different carcinogenic potentials of mammalian and avian Hepadnaviridae. In a recent study of a large series of duck HCCs, DHBV DNA was found in 68% of the tumors.[25] Few DHBV genome integrations in duck HCCs[65] have been extensively characterized.[38] In fact, a clonal pattern of DHBV DNA integrations is detectable only in a minority of the tumors[41,34,38,40] (Table 13-1). DHBV integrants are similar to HBV integrants,[52] so DHBV is probably a relevant model for the integration process of HBV and its consequences. The cloning of three DHBV integrants revealed several common features with HBV integrants: (1) no integrated full length genome, (2) inversely duplicated structures encompassing viral and flanking cellular DNA, and (3) virus-cell junctions frequently located in the vicinity of direct repeat sequences, DR1 and DR2.[38,66] One of the integrants was amplified several times, along with the adjacent cellular sequences.[38] The recent molecular dissection of the DHBV integration process in the LMH chicken hepatoma cell line revealed that the integration substrate may be a double-stranded linear genome contained in a fraction of DHBV virions; the double-stranded DNA and the cellular target site undergo a multistep enzymatic modification leading to integration.[66]

The Role of *myc* Genes in Hepadnavirus-induced Liver Carcinogenesis of Rodents

In a great proportion of woodchuck HCCs, the WHV acts as an insertional mutagen in *myc* family genes. The *myc* genes are proto-oncogenes present in all vertebrates species that act as regulators of gene expression. Overexpression of c-*myc* has been associated with a broad range of human cancers.[67] Both c-*myc* and N-*myc* constitute frequent targets of retroviral insertion in murine T-cell lymphomas.[68–70]

c-*myc* GENE IN THE WOODCHUCK MODEL

In a few cases of woodchuck HCC, c-*myc* is constitutionally overexpressed. C-*myc* overexpression was triggered by chromosomal rearrangements upstream or within the first exon of the c-*myc* gene. WHV DNA, however, was not integrated near the c-*myc* coding regions, possibly excluding a direct role of WHV in c-*myc* activation. In one instance, the c-*myc* gene was fused at the 5′ end of a transcriptionally functional liver-specific locus, *hcr*, and chimaeric transcripts resulted from this fusion.[71] The *hcr* locus was highly expressed in hepatocytes but not in other cell types. The function is still unknown of this potential 37-amino acid-encoding open frame reading.[72] Thus, in some woodchuck HCC, the chromosomal aberrations appear to be similar to those found in Burkitt's lymphomas.[28]

In three cases, WHV integration was located in the vicinity (5′ or 3′) of the c-*myc* coding domain acting through an enhancer insertion mechanism, as described previously for retroviral proviruses. In two cases, chimaeric WHV-*myc* transcripts were detected at high levels.[30,50] Recently two other cases have been characterized (Fourel G: personal communication, 1996) (Fig. 13-2). The insertional mutagenesis of c-*myc* seems to be involved in 10% of WHV-associated HCCs.[73]

N-*myc* GENES IN THE WOODCHUCK MODEL

The most frequent site of WHV integration is by far the N-*myc2* locus, found in 55% of 56 woodchuck HCC samples studied in our laboratory by G. Fourel in the group of M. Buendia[30,53] (Fig. 13-2). WHV integrants were clustered in a 3kb region upstream of N-*myc2* or in the 3′ untranslated sequence of N-*myc2*.[30] The N-*myc1* locus represents only a minor target of integration for WHV (detected in that locus in only one tumor).[53] The N-*myc2* gene is a functional retrotransposon specific to the Sciuridae family. Physiologic expression of N-*myc2* is detectable at low levels in brain tissue only.[74] The N-*myc2* gene is overexpressed without rearrangement in most woodchuck HCCs, in which expression levels can be one hundred times higher than in normal brain tissue.[53,74]

Alternatively, hybrid transcripts of N-*myc2*-WHV can be produced.[30,53] In woodchuck HCCs, WHV integrants are able to enhance N-*myc2* expression in apparently any orientation, suggesting an enhancer insertion mechanism of activation.[30,42,46]

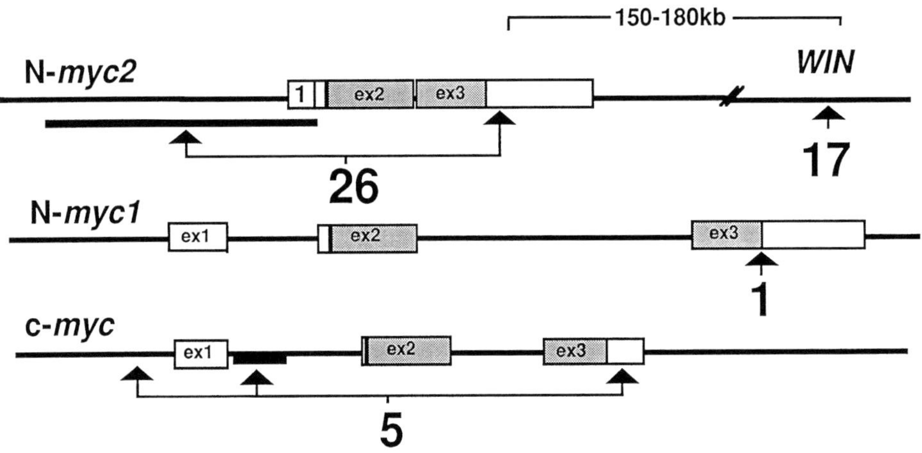

FIGURE 13-2. Mapping of the WHV integration sites in the different *myc* genes in 56 woodchuck hepatocellular carcinomas. Exons are represented by boxes, and the coding regions are shaded. Arrows and horizontal bars represent the principal clusters of integration. The number of integrations corresponding to each locus is mentioned below the arrows (with the authorization of Genevieve Fourel and Marie-Annick Buendia).

The recent analysis of four woodchuck HCCs displaying no rearrangement in the N-*myc2* locus, but harboring a strong overexpression of that gene, revealed that WHV was integrated in a 20-kb region named *win* at a distance of 150 to 180 kb from N-*myc2*.[46] To date, WHV DNA has been found integrated in the *win* locus in 17 of 56 woodchuck HCCs (Fourel G: personal communication, 1996) (Fig. 13-2). It has been proposed that, in these tumors, the WHV enhancer may act at a long distance to activate N-*myc2* expression.[46] Taken together, it appears that WHV DNA is integrated either in one of the *myc* loci or in the *win* locus in more than 85% of cases.

N-*myc2* activation results in an enhanced mitogenic activity of cells accompanied by an increased propensity to undergo apoptosis. However, cultured hepatocytes transfected with an N-*myc2* expression vector were not able to grow in soft agar and then were not fully malignant.[75] The commitment to apoptosis may be counteracted by overexpression of the insulin-like growth factor II (IGF II), as observed in foci of altered hepatocytes in vivo and in cells expressing N-*myc2* in vitro.[44,75]

myc GENES IN THE SQUIRREL MODEL

GSHV DNA integration does not result in insertional activation of *myc* genes.[34] Extensive analysis of a few GSHV integration sites does not provide evidence of insertional mutagenesis.[63] However, c-*myc* amplification can be detected in ground squirrel HCC in 40% of cases, with an increased level of c-*myc* messenger RNA[34] (Table 13-1).

Investigating the oncogenic potential of WHV and GSHV in one host, the newborn woodchuck, Hansen et al.[35] noticed striking differences in the mechanisms of *myc* activation. In GSHV-induced tumors, c-*myc* amplification and overexpression were common. Rearrangement of the N-*myc* locus occurred in only one case (6%). In WHV-induced tumors, N-*myc* gene rearrangements and overexpression were the preferential event.

Thus, molecular analysis of hepadnavirus-associated oncogenesis in rodents provides strong evidence that members of the *myc* family genes, although activated by different pathways, are critical factors in carcinogenesis. Although insertional activation of a *myc* proto-oncogene has never been observed in a human HCC, a few cases with *myc* amplification and an almost constant overexpression have been described.[76]

Cocarcinogenic Factors in Hepadnavirus-infected Animals

Human HCC is considered to have a multifactorial etiology. Contamination of the diet by mycotoxins may contribute to the etiology of HCCs, as suggested by hepatocarcinogenicity of these compounds in various animal species[77,78] (Table 13-1).

Recent experiments on WHV-infected woodchucks showed that aflatoxin B1 (AFB1) administration results in a significantly earlier appearance and a higher incidence of HCC. In uninfected woodchucks receiving AFB1 alone, no hepatic neoplasms were detected; however, more pronounced inflammation and simultaneous fibrotic changes were noted in livers of AFB1-treated animals. These data provide evidence of a synergistic hepatocarcinogenic effect of hepadnaviral infection and AFB1 in woodchucks. The phenotypes of preneoplastic lesions were essentially similar in the different groups of animals, which suggested these different oncogenic agents might trigger analogous molecular and cellular mechanisms leading to cell transformation.[26]

Domestic ducks are considered to be extremely sensitive to toxic and carcinogenic effects of AFB1.[24] To determine the respective contribution to hepatocarcinogenesis of hepadnavirus infection and AFB1 exposure, Pekin ducks have been used as a model.[24,33,37,40] The results have been controversial. Some authors consider that the two risk factors may act synergistically on tumor development, and others could not detect any cooperation between DHBV and AFB1.[37,40] AFB1 appears to be a more potent carcinogenic agent than DHBV, which is not able to produce HCC alone in controlled experimental conditions[24,33] (Table 13-1).

Biochemical studies showed that in vitro production of the AFB1 main metabolite, aflatoxin B1-8,9 epoxide, by hepatic microsomes, is more efficient in ducks than in F344 rats. In addition, AFB1-DNA adducts reached higher levels in ducks than in F344 rats. This process and the subsequent DNA repair reaction were not altered by concomitant DHBV infection.[24] Major differences in the design of cocarcinogenesis studies, including differences in conditions of duckling infection, duration, dose and route of administration of AFB1, and length of follow-up make global conclusions difficult.

p53 Gene in Animal Models

In contrast to p53 in human HCC,[79,80] examination of the p53 tumor suppressor gene in 16 duck HCCs did not reveal any mutations in codon 249 (Table 13-1). The duck HCCs, whether positive or negative for DHBV, were from the Qidong region of China, where codon 249 mutations have been commonly identified in humans. Differences in the sequences of the human and avian p53 genes could partially explain the absence of mutation.[81] Similarly, analysis of the p53 gene (exons 4–9) in 18 HCCs from GSHV-infected ground squirrels and 11 HCCs from WHV-infected woodchucks revealed a lower rate of p53 mutation in either than in human HCCs. In an HCC from an AFB1-treated squirrel only one mutation was found, located in codon 176; no major rearrangement of the p53 gene was detected in any sample[82] (Table 13-1). Rarity of p53 mutations correlated with the presence of X gene in human HCCs, perhaps because of viral interference with p53 function,[83] and may be similar to the situation in hepadnavirus-infected Sciuridae.

Mutations in p53 gene are rarely observed in chemically induced liver tumors from other rodents.[84] However, two studies in rats have reported high rates of mutation after AFB1 and tamoxifen treatments, suggesting that specific environmental contaminants may target p53.[85,86]

Other Molecular Factors in WHV-associated HCCs and Their Progression

ONCOGENES AND GROWTH FACTORS

As in human HCCs,[87] the expression of insulin-like growth factor II (IGF II), a fetal growth factor, is frequently activated in woodchuck HCCs.[27] However, its level of expression differs from one tumor to another and even within the same sample.[88,89] Careful examination of altered hepatic foci considered to be preneoplastic lesions has revealed IGF II overexpression in nearly all lesions.[44] In addition, IGF II was reported to have a strong anti-apoptotic effect on N-*myc2*-expressing rodent hepatic cells in culture.[75] IGF II has been implicated in the progression of various tumors, including HCC.[90–92] Taken together, these data suggest that IGF II overexpression may be involved in progression toward malignancy.[44] The recent designation of the mannose 6-phosphate/insulin-like growth factor II receptor gene (IGF2R) as a tumor suppressor gene in human HCC substantiates the hypothesis of a critical implication of the IGFII/IGF2R pathway in hepatocarcinogenesis.[93,94]

Other cellular oncogenes including *ras*, *src*, *raf*, and *erb*-A did not have enhanced levels of transcription in woodchuck HCCs.[28] Expression of immediate-early genes of the *fos-jun* family have been found to be frequently activated in woodchuck HCCs.[95]

METABOLIC PHENOTYPE

Using a cDNA substractive library isolated from WHV-infected woodchuck HCC, the two genes most significantly stimulated encoded two acute-phase reactant serum proteins, hemopexin and α-1 acid glycoprotein. The significance of this observation remains to be elucidated.[96]

Other metabolic aberrations have been identified in WHV-induced hepatocarcinogenesis. These alterations detected by cytochemistry involve enzymes of carbohydrate metabolism. Glucose-6-phosphate dehydrogenase or malate dehydrogenase is frequently activated, and reduction in the activity of glycogen phosphorylase can be observed. (In humans, excessive storage of glycogen is frequently encountered in liver tumors.[97]) It has been suggested that these changes may represent a general biologic response of the liver to oncogenic agents, but their role in malignant transformation is still unclear.[98] The strong impact of metabolic stimuli such as insulin/glucagon balance on WHV transcriptional regulatory elements located upstream of c-*myc* has been reported recently. In a transgenic mouse model with HCC developing in 100% of mice and containing a WHV-*myc* integration, the activity of a viral enhancer was apparently controlled by glucose uptake.[99]

NITRATES, NITRIC OXIDE, AND N-NITROSO COMPOUND PRODUCTION

Nitrate exposure and the subsequent formation of N-nitroso compounds is considered as a potential risk factor in human cancer because of their mutagenic action on cellular DNA.[100,101] It has recently been observed that chronic WHV infection sharply enhanced in vivo and in vitro excretion of nitrate and N-dimethylnitrosamine (NDMA) in woodchucks.[102,103] In addition, the measurements of the urinary recovery of nitrate suggested that its catabolism was quantitatively similar in humans and woodchucks.[102] Similarly, SV40 large T antigen-immortalized woodchuck hepatocytes produced nitric oxide after oxydation of L-arginine.[104,105]

It has been hypothesized that immunostimulation of inflammatory cells such as Kupffer cells may have a tumor-promoting effect on liver through an enhanced production of nitroso compounds. The endogenous formation of NDMA, a potent carcinogen in animals, may be the result of the L-arginine oxidation process.[102] WHV surface antigen particles present in the cell culture medium of primary woodchuck hepatocytes is sufficient concentration to increase nitric oxide (NO) free radical synthesis. Thus, WHV-induced hepatocarcinogenicity may in part result from long-term exposure of liver cells to NO free radicals.[106]

Similar experiments on human hepatocytes revealed that lipopolysaccharides and cytokines cause cells to produce NO through amino acid oxidation catalyzed by nitric oxide synthase.[107] In humans, increased nitrosation potential has been detected during cirrhosis and trematode infestation of the liver.[41] In contrast, the ability of WHV-infected cells to activate other genotoxic substances such as cigarette smoke components seems to be rather limited.[108]

The animal hepadnaviruses have provided valuable models in hepatocarcinogenesis. The extensive similarity in viral genetic material and the integrated forms of human and animals viruses will probably allow complete elucidation of the integration process. The study of woodchuck HCC permitted some major breakthroughs in the understanding of viral oncogenesis. However, it should be pointed out that the molecular phenotype of malignant cells and notably effector genes in rodent tumors are quite different from those observed in human beings.

ACKNOWLEDGMENTS

We are grateful to Marie-Annick Buendia for helpful discussion and critical reading of the manuscript.

P.P. was supported by grants from the Fondation pour la Recherche Médicale and the Institut Electricité-Santé.

REFERENCES

1. Robinson WS. Hepadnaviridae and their replication. In Fields BN, Knipe DM (eds): Virology. Vol. 2. 2nd Ed. Raven Press, New York, 1990, pp. 2137–2169
2. Tiollais P, Pourcel C, Dejean A. The hepatitis B virus. Nature 1985;317:489–495
3. Summers J, Smolec JM, Snyder R. A virus similar to human hepatitis B virus associated with hepatitis and hepatoma in woodchucks. Proc Natl Acad Sci U S A 1978;75: 4533–4537
4. Marion PL, Oshiro L, Regnery DC et al. A virus in Beechey ground squirrels that is related to hepatitis B virus of man. Proc Natl Acad Sci U S A 1980;77:2941–2945
5. Minuk GY, Shaffer EA, Hoar DI, Kelly J. Ground squirrel hepatitis virus (GSHV) infection and hepatocellular carcinoma in the Canadian Richardson ground squirrel (*Spermophilus richardsonii*). Liver 1986;6:350–356
6. Feitelson MA, Millman I, Halbherr T et al. A newly identified hepatitis B type virus in tree squirrels. Proc Natl Acad Sci U S A 1986;83:2233–2237
7. Rothnie HM, Chapdelaine Y, Hohn T. Pararetroviruses and retroviruses: a comparative review of viral structure and gene expression strategies. Adv Virus Res 1994;44:1–67
8. Mason WS, Seal G, Summers J. Virus of Pekin ducks with structural and biological relatedness to human hepatitis B virus. Virology 1980;36:829–836
9. Sprengel R, Kaleta EF, Will H. Isolation and characterization of a hepatitis B virus endemic in herons. J Virol 1988; 62:3832–3839
10. Sherker AH, Marion PL. Hepadnaviruses and hepatocellular carcinoma. Annu Rev microbiol 1991;45:475–508
11. Snyder RL, Tyler G, Summers J. Chronic hepatitis and hepatocellular carcinoma associated with woodchuck hepatitis virus. Am J Pathol 1982;107:422–425
12. Mast EE, Alter MJ. Epidemiology of viral hepatitis: an overview. Semin Virol 1993;4:273–283
13. Korba BE, Wells F, Baldwin B et al. Hepatocellular carcinoma in woodchuck hepatitis virus-infected woodchucks: presence of viral DNA in tumor tissue from chronic carriers and animals serologically recovered from acute infections. Hepatology 1989;9:461–470
14. Gerin JL, Cote PJ, Korba BE et al. Hepatitis B virus and liver cancer: the woodchuck as an experimental model of hepadnavirus-induced liver cancer. In Hollinger FB, Lemon SM, Margolis HS (eds): Viral Hepatitis and Liver Disease. Williams & Wilkins, Houston, 1990, pp. 556–559
15. Paterlini P, Gerken G, Nakajima E et al. Polymerase chain reaction to detect hepatitis B virus DNA and RNA sequences in primary liver cancers from patients negative for hepatitis B surface antigen. N Engl J Med 1990;323:80–85
16. Popper H, Roth L, Purcell RH et al. Hepatocarcinogenicity of the woodchuck hepatitis virus. Proc Natl Acad Sci U S A 1987;84:866–870
17. Hollinger FB. Hepatitis B virus. In Fields BN, Knipe DM (eds): Virology. Lippincott-Raven, New York, 1990; pp. 2171–2236

18. Anthony PP, Bannasch P. Tumours and tumour-like lesions of the liver and biliary tract. In MacSween RNM, Anthony PP, Scheuer PJ et al (eds): Pathology of the Liver. Churchill Livingstone, Edinburgh, 1994, pp. 629–711
19. Gerin JL, Cote PJ, Korba BE, Tennant BC. Hepadnavirus-induced liver cancer in woodchucks. Cancer Detect Prev 1989;14:227–229
20. Tennant BC, Gerin JL. The woodchuck model of hepatitis B virus infection. In I.M. A, Boyer JL, Fausto N et al (eds): The Liver: Biology and Pathobiology. Raven Press, New York, 1994, pp. 1455–1466
21. Yu M-W, Chen C-J. Elevated serum testosterone levels and risk of hepatocellular carcinoma. Cancer Res 1993;53: 790–794
22. Okuda K, Okuda H. Carcinome primitif du foie. In Benhamou J-P, Bircher J, MacIntyre N et al (eds): Hepatologie Clinique. Medecine/Sciences Flammarion, Paris, 1993, pp. 1019–1053
23. Mi L-J, Patil J, Hornbuckle WE et al. DNA ploidy analysis of hepatic preneoplastic and neoplastic lesions in woodchucks experimentally infected with woodchuck hepatitis virus. Hepatology 1994;20:21–29
24. Seawright AA, Snowden RT, Olubuyide O et al. A comparison of the effects of aflatoxin B1 on the livers of rats and duck hepatitis B virus-infected and noninfected ducks. Hepatology 1993;18:188–193
25. Duflot A, Mehrotra R, Yu S-Z et al. Spectrum of liver disease and duck hepatitis B virus infection in a large series of Chinese ducks with hepatocellular carcinoma. Hepatology 1995;21:1483–1491
26. Bannasch P, Khoshkhou NI, Hacker HJ et al. Synergistic hepatocarcinogenic effect of hepadnaviral infection and dietary aflatoxin B1 in woodchucks. Cancer Res 1995;55: 3318–3330
27. Rogler CE, Hino O, Su CY. Molecular aspects of persistent woodchuck hepatitis virus and hepatitis B virus infection and hepatocellular carcinoma. Hepatology 1987;7: 74S–78S
28. Möröy T, Marchio A, Etiemble J et al. Rearrangement and enhanced expression of c-*myc* in hepatocellular carcinoma of hepatitis virus infected woodchucks. Nature 1986;324: 276–279
29. Shimoda A, Kaneko S, Uchijima M et al. Clonal origin of mammalian hepatitis B virus-related hepatocellular carcinoma. J Med Virol 1990;30:282–286
30. Wei Y, Fourel G, Ponzetto A et al. Hepadnavirus integration: mechanisms of activation of the N-*myc2* retrotransposon in woodchuck liver tumors. J Virol 1992;66:5265–5276
31. Marion PL, VanDavelaar MJ, Knight SS et al. Hepatocellular carcinoma in ground squirrels persistently infected with ground squirrel hepatitis virus. Proc Natl Acad Sci U S A 1986;83:4543–4546
32. Marion PL. Ground squirrel hepatitis virus. In McLachlan A (ed): Molecular Biology of the Hepatitis B Virus. CRC Press, Boca Raton, 1991, pp. 39–51
33. Cullen J, Marion PL, Sherman GJ et al. Hepatic neoplasms in aflatoxin B1-treated congenital duck hepatitis B virus-infected and virus-free Pekin ducks. Cancer Res 1990;50: 4072–4080
34. Transy C, Fourel G, Robinson WS et al. Frequent amplification of c-*myc* in ground squirrel liver tumors associated with past or ongoing infection with a hepadnavirus. Proc Natl Acad Sci U S A 1992;89:3874–3878
35. Hansen LJ, Tennant BC, Seeger C, Ganem D. Differential activation of myc gene family members in hepatic carcinogenesis by closely related hepatitis B viruses. Mol Cell Biol 1993;13:659–667
36. Seeger C, Baldwin B, Hornbuckle WE et al. Woodchuck hepatitis virus is a more efficient oncogenic agent than ground squirrel hepatitis virus in a common host. J Virol 1991;65:1673–1679
37. Uchida T, Suzuki K, Esumi M et al. Influence of aflatoxin B1 intoxication on duck livers with DHBV infection. Cancer Res 1988;48:1559–1565
38. Imazeki F, Yaginuma K, Omata M et al. Integrated structures of duck hepatitis B virus DNA in hepatocellular carcinoma. J Virol 1988;63:861–865
39. Cova L, Mehrotra R, Wild CP et al. Duck hepatitis B virus infection, aflatoxin B1 and liver cancer in domestic Chinese ducks. Br J Cancer 1994;69:104–109
40. Cova L, Wild CP, Mehrotra R et al. Contribution of aflatoxin B1 and hepatitis B infection in the induction of liver tumors in ducks. Cancer Res 1990;50:2156–2163
41. Srivatanakul P, Ohshima H, Khlat M et al. *O. viverrini* infestation and endogenous nitrosamines as risk factors for cholangiocarcinoma in Thailand. Int J Cancer 1991;48:821
42. Buendia MA. Mammalian hepatitis B viruses and primary liver cancer. Semin Cancer Biol 1992;3
43. Rogler CE, Summers J. Cloning and structural analysis of integrated woodchuck hepatitis virus sequences from a chronically infected liver. J Virol 1984;50:832–837
44. Yang D, Alt E, Rogler CE. Coordinate expression of N-*myc2* and insulin-like growth factor II in pre-cancerous altered hepatic foci in woodchuck hepatitis virus carriers. Cancer Res 1993;53:2020–2027
45. Mizuno Y, Murakami S, Matsushita F et al. Chromosomal assignment of woodchuck hepatitis virus (WHV) DNA integrations sites in a woodchuck hepatocellular carcinoma-derived cell line (WH257GE10). Int J Cancer 1989;43: 652–657
46. Fourel G, Couturier J, Wei Y et al. Evidence for long-range oncogene activation by hepadnavirus insertion. EMBO J 1994;13:2526–2534
47. Tokino T, Matsubara K. Chromosomal sites for hepatitis B virus integration in human hepatocellular carcinoma. J Virol 1991;65:6761–6764
48. Ogston CW, Jonak GJ, Rogler CE et al. Cloning and structural analysis of integrated woodchuck hepatitis virus sequences from hepatocellular carcinomas of woodchucks. Cell 1982;29:385–394
49. Kaneko S, Oshima T, Kodama K et al. Stable integration of woodchuck hepatitis virus DNA in transplanted tumors and established tissue culture cells derived from a woodchuck primary hepatocellular carcinoma. Cancer Res 1986; 46:3608–3613
50. Hsu TY, Möröy T, Etiemble J et al. Activation of c-*myc* by woodchuck hepatitis virus insertion in hepatocellular carcinoma. Cell 1988;55:627–635

51. Yamazoe M, Nakai S, Ogasawara N, Yoshikawa H. Integration of woodchuck hepatitis virus (WHV) DNA at two chromosomal sites (V_k and *gag*-like) in a hepatocellular carcinoma. Gene 1991;100:139–146
52. Schröder CH, Zentgraf H. Hepatitis B virus related hepatocellular carcinoma: chronicity of infection—the opening of different pathways of malignant transformation? Biochim Biophys Acta 1990;1032:137–156
53. Fourel G, Trépo C, Bougueleret L et al. Frequent activation of N-*myc* genes by hepadnavirus insertion in woodchuck liver tumours. Nature 1990;347:294–298
54. Dejean A, Bougueleret L, Grzeschik KH, Tiollais P. Hepatitis B virus DNA integration in a sequence homologous to v-*erbA* and steroid receptor genes in a hepatocellular carcinoma. Nature 1986;322:70–72
55. Wang J, Chenivesse X, Henglein B, Bréchot C. Hepatitis B virus integration in a cyclin A gene in a human hepatocellular carcinoma. Nature 1990;343:555–557
56. Kew MC, Miller RH, Chen H-S et al. Mutant woodchuck hepatitis virus genomes from virions resemble rearranged hepadnaviral integrants in hepatocellular carcinoma. Proc Natl Acad Sci U S A 1993;90:10211–10215
57. Kew MC. Do mutant woodchuck hepatitis viruses play a role in hepatocellular carcinoma? Res Virol 1993;144: 293–296
58. Bruni R, Argentini C, D'Ugo E et al. A PCR-based strategy for rapid mapping of hepadnavirus integrated sequences in hepatocellular carcinoma. J Virol Methods 1995;52: 347–360
59. Wei Y, Etiemble J, Fourel G et al. Hepadnavirus integration generates virus-cell cotranscripts carrying 3′ truncated X genes in human and woodchuck liver tumors. J Med Virol 1995;45:82–90
60. Cross JC, Wen P, Rutter WJ. Transactivation by hepatitis B virus X protein is promiscuous and dependent on mitogen-activated cellular serine/threonine kinases. Proc Natl Acad Sci U S A 1993;90:8078–8082
61. Kekulé AS, Lauer U, Weiss L et al. Hepatitis B virus transactivator HBx uses a tumour promoter signalling pathway. Nature 1993;361:742–745
62. Rakotomahanina CK, Hilger C, Fink T et al. Biological activities of a putative truncated hepatitis B virus X gene product fused to a polylysin stretch. Oncogene 1994;9: 2613–2621
63. Transy C, Renard CA, Buendia MA. Analysis of integrated ground squirrel hepatitis virus and flanking host DNA in two hepatocellular carcinomas. J Virol 1994;68:5291–5295
64. Tennant BC, Mrosovsky N, McLean K et al. Hepatocellular carcinoma in Richardson's ground squirrels (*Spermophilus richardsonii*): evidence for association with hepatitis B-like virus infection. Hepatology 1991;13:1215–1222
65. Yokosuka O, Omata M, Zhou S et al. Duck hepatitis B virus DNA in liver and serum of Chinese ducks: integration of viral DNA in a hepatocellular carcinoma. Proc Natl Acad Sci U S A 1985;82:5180–5184
66. Gong SS, Jensen AD, Wang H, Rogler CE. Duck hepatitis B virus integrations in LMH chicken hepatoma cells: identification and characterization of new episomally derived integrations. J Virol 1995;69:8102–8108
67. DePinho RA, Schreiber-Agus N, Alt FW. Myc family oncogenes in the development of normal and neoplastic cells. Adv Cancer Res 1991;57:1–45
68. Corcoran LM, Adams JM, Dunn AR, Cory S. Murine T-lymphomas in which the cellular *myc* oncogene has been activated by retrovirus insertion. Cell 1984;37:113–122
69. Selten G, Cuypers HT, Zijlstra M et al. Involvement of c-*myc* in MuL V-induced T cell lymphomas in mice: frequency and mechanisms of activation. EMBO J 1984;3: 3215–3222
70. Van Lohuizen M, Breuer M, Berns A. N-*myc* is frequently activated by proviral insertion in MuL V-induced T-cell lymphomas. EMBO J 1989;8:133–136
71. Etiemble J, Möröy T, Jacquemin E et al. Fused transcripts of c-*myc* and a new cellular locus, *hcr*, in a primary liver tumor. Oncogene 1989;4:51–57
72. Möröy T, Etiemble J, Bougueleret L et al. Structure and expression of *hcr*, a locus rearranged with c-*myc* in a woodchuck hepatocellular carcinoma. Oncogene 1989;4:59–65
73. Buendia MA, Pineau P. The complex role of hepatitis B virus in human carcinogenesis. In Barbanti-Brodano G (ed): DNA Tumor Viruses: Oncogenic Mechanisms. Plenum Press, New York, 1995, pp. 171–193
74. Fourel G, Transy C, Tennant BC, Buendia MA. Expression of the woodchuck N-*myc2* retroposon in brain and in liver tumors is driven by a cryptic N-*myc* promoter. Mol Cell Biol 1992;12:5336–5344
75. Ueda K, Ganem D. Apoptosis is induced by N-*myc* expression in hepatocytes, a frequent event in hepadnavirus oncogenesis, and is blocked by insulin-like growth factor II. J Virol 1996;70:1375–1383
76. Tabor E. Tumor suppressor genes, growth factor genes, and oncogenes in hepatitis B virus-associated hepatocellular carcinoma. J Med Virol 1994;42:357–365
77. Wogan GN. Aflatoxins as risk factors for hepatocellular carcinoma in humans. Cancer Res 1992;52:2114–2118
78. Buendia MA. Hepatitis B viruses and hepatocellular carcinoma. Adv Cancer Res 1992;59:167–226
79. Hsu IC, Metcalf RA, Sun T et al. Mutational hotspot in the p53 gene in human hepatocellular carcinomas. Nature 1991;350:427–428
80. Bressac B, Kew M, Wands J, Ozturk M. Selective G to T mutations of p53 gene in hepatocellular carcinoma from southern Africa. Nature 1991;350:429–431
81. Duflot A, Hollstein M, Mehrotra R et al. Absence of p53 mutation at codon 249 in duck hepatocellular carcinomas from the high incidence area of Qidong (China). Carcinogenesis 1994;15:1353–1357
82. Rivkina MB, Cullen JM, Robinson WS, Marion PL. State of the p53 gene in hepatocellular carcinomas in ground squirrels and woodchucks with past and ongoing infection with hepadnaviruses. Cancer Res. 1994;54:5430–5437
83. Unsal H, Yakicier C, Marçais C et al. Genetic heterogeneity of hepatocellular carcinoma. Proc Natl Acad Sci U S A 1994;91:822–826
84. Stanley LA. Molecular aspects of chemical carcinogenesis: the roles of oncogenes and tumour suppressor genes. Toxicology 1995;96:173–194

85. Lilleberg SL, Cabonce MA, Raju NR et al. Alterations in the structural gene and the expression of p53 in rat liver tumors induced by aflatoxin B1. Mol Carcinog 1992;6: 159–172

86. Vancutsem PM, Lazarus P, Williams GM. Frequent and specific mutations of the rat p53 gene in hepatocarcinomas induced by tamoxifen. Cancer Res. 1994;54:3864–3867

87. Cariani E, Lasserre C, Seurin D et al. Differential expression of insulin-like growth factor II mRNA in human primary liver cancers, benign liver tumors, and liver cirrhosis. Cancer Res 1988;48:6844–6849

88. Fu XX, Su CY, Lee Y et al. Insulin like growth factor II expression and oval cell proliferation associated with hepatocarcinogenesis in woodchuck hepatitis virus carriers. J Virol 1988;62:3422–3430

89. Yang DY, Rogler CE. Analysis of insulin-like growth factor II (IGF-II) expression in neoplastic nodules and hepatocellular carcinomas of woodchucks utilizing in situ hybridization and immunocytochemistry. Carcinogenesis 1991;12: 1893–1901

90. Steller MA, Delgado C, Zou Z. Insulin-like growth factor II mediates epidermal growth factor-induced mitogenesis in cervical cancer cells. Proc Natl Acad Sci U S A 1995; 92:4533–4537

91. Christofori G, Naik P, Hanahan D. A second signal supplied by insulin-like growth factor II in oncogene-induced tumorigenesis. Nature 1994;369:414–418

92. Ito T, Sasaki Y, Wands JR. Overexpression of human insulin receptor substrate 1 induces cellular transformation with activation of mitogen-activated protein kinases. Mol Cell Biol 1996;13:943–951

93. DeSouza AT, Hankins GR, Washington MK et al. Frequent loss of heterozygosity on 6q at the mannose-6-phosphate/insulin-like growth factor II receptor locus in human hepatocellular tumors. Oncogene 1995;10:1725–1729

94. DeSouza A, Hankins GR, Washington MK et al. *M6P/IGF2R* gene is mutated in human hepatocellular carcinoma with loss of heterozygosity. Nat Genet 1995;11:447–449

95. Hsu TY, Fourel G, Etiemble J et al. Integration of hepatitis virus DNA near c-*myc* in woodchuck hepatocellular carcinoma. Gastroenterol Jpn 1990;25:43–48

96. Darabi A, Gross S, Watabe M et al. Differential gene expression in experimental hepatocellular carcinoma induced by woodchuck hepatitis B virus. Cancer Lett 1995; 95:153–159

97. Ishak KG. Pathology of hepatic malignancy. In Terblanche J (ed): Hepatobiliary Malignancy: Its Multidisciplinary Management. Edward Arnold, London, 1994; 3 pp. 3–26

98. Toshkov I, Hacker HJ, Roggendorf M, Bannasch P. Phenotypic patterns of preneoplastic and neoplastic hepatic lesions in woodchuck infected with woodchucks hepatitis virus. J Cancer Res Clin Oncol 1990;116:581–590

99. Etiemble J, Degott C, Renard CA et al. Liver-specific expression and high oncogenic efficiency of a c-*myc* transgene activated by woodchuck hepatitis virus insertion. Oncogene 1994;9:727–737

100. Bartsch H, Montesano R. Relevance of nitrosamines to human cancer. Carcinogenesis 1984;5:1381–1393

101. Pitot HC, Dragan YP. Chemical induction of hepatic neoplasia. In Arias IM, Boyer JL, Fausto N et al (eds): The Liver: Biology and Pathobiology. Raven Press, New York, 1994

102. Liu RH, Baldwin B, Tennant BC, Hotchkiss JH. Elevated formation of nitrate and *N*-nitrosodimethylamine in woodchucks (*Marmota monax*) associated with chronic woodchuck hepatitis virus infection. Cancer Res 1991;51: 3925–3929

103. Liu RH, Jacob JR, Tennant BC, Hotchkiss JH. Nitrite and nitrosamine synthesis by hepatocytes isolated from normal woodchucks (*Marmota monax*) and woodchucks chronically infected with woodchuck hepatitis virus. Cancer Res 1992; 52:4139–4143

104. Liu RH, Jacob JR, Hotchkiss JH, Tennant BC. Synthesis of nitric oxide and nitrosamine by immortalized woodchuck hepatocytes. Carcinogenesis 1993;14:1609–1613

105. Jacob JR, Liu RH, Roneker CA et al. Characterization and immortalization of woodchuck hepatocytes isolated from normal and hepadnavirus-infected woodchucks (*Marmota monax*). Exp Cell Res 1994;212:42–48

106. Liu RH, Jacob JR, Hotchkiss JH et al. Woodchuck hepatitis virus surface antigen induces nitric oxide synthesis in hepatocytes: possible role in hepatocarcinogenesis. Carcinogenesis 1994;15:2875–2877

107. Nussler A, DiSilvio M, Billiar TR et al. Stimulation of the nitric oxide synthase pathway in human hepatocytes by cytokines and endotoxin. J Exp Med 1992;176:261–264

108. DeFlora S, Izzotti A, D'Agostini F et al. Metabolic activation of a cigarette smoke condensate by woodchuck liver, as related to sex, pregnancy, hepatitis virus infection and primary hepatocellular carcinoma. Mutat Res 1994;324: 153–158

14

A TRANSGENIC MOUSE MODEL OF HBV-RELATED HEPATOCELLULAR CARCINOMA

HIROYUKI UEDA
SHOWGO OHKOSHI
CHANG-MIN KIM
GILBERT JAY

Hepatitis B virus (HBV) infection is a public health problem of global importance.[1] It has been estimated that 5% of the world population are persistently infected by this virus. In southeast Asia and central Africa, where more than 10% of the population are HBV carriers, chronic active hepatitis and cirrhosis are major causes of mortality. Moreover, epidemiologic studies have clearly shown the importance of HBV in hepatocellular carcinoma (HCC), one of the most common cancers in the world.[2] Among individuals who are chronically infected by HBV, 50% will develop HCC.

The HBV genome is unusual in several ways.[1,3] When obtained from the virion, it is composed of two open DNA strands, a full-length minus strand of about 3,200 nucleotides, and an incomplete plus strand that is variable in length. The positions of the 5′ ends of the two strands are fixed, and their base-pairing ensures the circular structure of the intact viral genome (Fig. 14-1). When inside the cell, the HBV genome can exist in two states: free DNA is detected during the acute and some chronic stages of infection, and integrated DNA sequences are found during chronic infection and in HCC. In the process of viral replication, an RNA copy of the HBV genome is made as a replication intermediate and a reverse transcriptase is subsequently involved in the synthesis of virion DNA.[4] Although HBV is hepatotropic, HBV DNA has also been detected in other tissues.[5,6]

Consequences of viral infection are unpredictable and range from inapparent forms to acute hepatitis and severe chronic liver disease. The study of HBV has been difficult because of the lack of a cell culture system that will allow virus propagation. Much of what we know about the replication and expression of HBV comes from the study of other closely related hepadnaviruses, such as the woodchuck hepatitis virus (WHV)[7] and the Beechey ground squirrel hepatitis virus (GSHV).[8]

The HBV genome contains four translational open reading frames (ORFs) and the products of these four ORFs, designated S, C, P, and X, have been identified.[1,3] The S region has three in-phase translation initiation codons and encodes the 409 amino acid "large" protein, the 281 amino acid "middle" protein, and the 226 amino acid "major" hepatitis B surface antigen (HBsAg) protein, which form the viral envelope (Fig. 14-1). The C region encodes the 193 amino acid hepatitis B core anti-

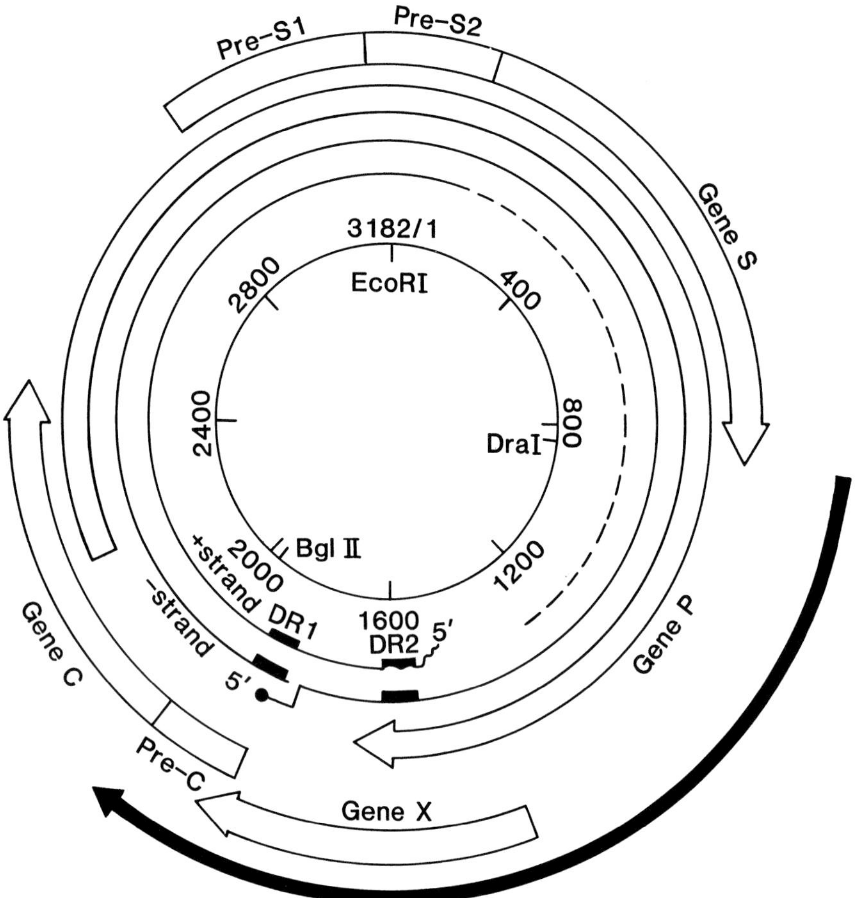

FIGURE 14-1. Schematic representation of the genomic organization of the human HBV. The thin lines represent the two DNA strands of the viral genome. The broad arrows represent the four ORFs. The filled arrow indicates the segment of DNA that was used to generate the X gene transgenic mice in the studies described in this chapter.

gen (HBcAg), which forms the viral capsid. The P region encodes the 832 amino acid DNA polymerase that possesses reverse transcriptase activity. The X region encodes a polypeptide (HBxAg), 145 to 154 amino acids depending on the subtype of the virus, that can transactivate viral gene expression.

All four ORFs are expressed from the minus strand of the genome.[3] Three distinct transcriptional promoters and a single polyadenylation site have been identified. Two major poly(A)$^+$ RNAs have been detected in the infected liver.[9,10] A 2.1-kb transcript initiating at position 3,155 encodes the major HBsAg, and a 3.5 kb transcript from approximately position 1,818 is the messenger RNA for HBcAg and probably for the DNA polymerase. A minor 0.65-kb transcript with multiple start sites located between positions 1,250 and 1,350 encodes HBxAg.[11,12] All three transcripts terminate at the unique poly(A) site at position 1,934.[13,14] Transcription initiation at the various promoter regions is apparently controlled by two transcriptional enhancers, one located between positions 1,011 and 1,076[15–17] and the other between positions 1,513 and 1,593.[18,19] These HBV enhancers confer liver specificity to each of the viral promoters.[20,21]

There is increasing evidence that HBV can contribute to the causation of HCC. This association is suggested by three lines of evidence: epidemiologic observations, animal models, and molecular biologic analysis. Between 85% and 90% of HCC cases worldwide occur in individuals who are chronically infected with HBV. The relative risk of developing HCC for individuals who are positive for HBsAg is 217 compared with those who are negative, and the lifetime risk of HCC in males with chronic HBV infection is high.[22,23] In studies with the related WHV, the risk is even greater; every experimentally infected woodchuck that became positive for the

WHV surface antigen for more than 1 year developed HCC.[24,25] In humans, HBV DNA sequences are invariably found integrated in the host genome in HCC.[26–29] The number of integration sites varies from 1 to 12, and the HBV sequences can be either complete genomes or rearranged subgenomic fragments.[30]

The underlying molecular mechanism for the etiology of HCC remains unclear, but several possible mechanisms have been suggested.[22,31] It has been suggested that the continuous liver necrosis and regeneration that accompany chronic hepatitis have allowed selection of a second genetic event that is responsible for the malignancy. Consistent with the possibility is the observation that the risk of HCC is considerably greater in HBsAg-positive persons with cirrhosis than among HBsAg-positive persons without cirrhosis.[2] Another theory is that the malignancy arises as a consequence of the random integration of viral regulatory sequences and fortuitous activation of an adjacent cellular oncogene, as has been shown with other viral systems, since HBV carries liver-specific transcriptional enhancers[18–21] and HBV DNA was always found inserted into the genome of tumor cells.[26–29] Different cellular genes may be activated by the HBV transcriptional enhancers that will result in uncontrolled cell proliferation and neoplasia.[32] For that reason and until large numbers of flanking host sequences have been analyzed, it will be difficult to rule out this possibility. Since most but not all cancer-causing viruses carry a transforming gene, it has also been suggested that HBV might have a gene whose product could function to alter the growth properties of the host cell.

Given the high incidence of HCC worldwide (from 0.5 to 1.0 million new cases occur every year in China alone), a concerted effort to define the mechanism of etiology of this malignancy is needed. While in vitro approaches, such as the use of tissue culture, have been rewarding in other systems, they have not proven very useful for HCC. This deficiency has called for the use of in vivo approaches that offer a more accurate view of the whole picture.

TRANSGENIC MICE

A transgenic mouse model of a human disease may often provide the first unequivocal proof that a particular gene is responsible for causing the pathologic changes that occur with that disease. They also can provide a system to dissect carefully the successive events that lead to the disease state and can provide a custom-designed whole animal system to test potential therapies. Most important, new concepts relating to gene expression and gene function in a disease often emerge from transgenic studies.

The most widely and successfully used method for generating transgenic mice is by direct microinjection of DNA into the pronuclei of fertilized eggs.[33] The actual procedure can be divided into three phases:

1. Generation and recovery of single-cell embryos. On day −3 (with respect to the day of microinjection), sexually immature female mice are injected intraperitoneally with pregnant mare's serum, which mimics follicle-stimulating hormone in inducing large numbers of preimplantation embryos. On day −1, the mice are injected with human chorionic gonadotropin, which mimics luteinizing hormone in inducing the rupture of mature follicles, and the animals are placed with reproductively active males. The following morning, they are inspected for the presence of a vaginal plug, which would be indicative of successful mating. Successfully mated females are sacrificed, the ovaries are dissected, and eggs are removed. The fertilized eggs are placed into microdrops of culture medium under a layer of mineral oil.
2. Microinjection of pronuclei. This procedure is performed on an inverted microscope with two micromanipulators. The left micromanipulator is used to control the holding pipette. Each egg to be injected is positioned so that the male pronucleus is clearly visible. The right micromanipulator controls the injection pipette carrying a DNA solution. To carry out pronuclear injection, the pipette is pushed through the zona pellucida and vitelline membrane and into the male pronucleus. About 200 molecules of DNA are delivered by activating the microinjector.
3. Embryo transfer. Pseudopregnant "foster mother" mice are generated by mating randomly cycling, sexually mature females to vasectomized males. Pseudopregnant females are anesthetized, and a small incision is made lateral to the spinal chord at a level just below the ribs. The ovary is pulled out through the body wall, and the ovarian bursa is opened. The ostium, located between the ovary and the oviduct, is visualized, and the microinjected embryos are delivered with an implantation pipette through the ostium into the oviduct. The incision is closed with a single suture, and the procedure is repeated for the other ovary.

The use of transgenic mice to study viral gene function and pathogenesis has been well documented.[34–42] An advantage of the transgenic model is that the incorporation of viral sequences into every cell of the mouse bypasses the initial steps of viral infection. This effectively circumvents any species barrier that may be imposed by host-specific receptors and avoids problems that may be associated with the route of viral administration. However, the presence of the viral transgene(s) in every cell may allow expression in cell types that would not normally be susceptible to viral infection. This situation may result in pathologic changes in the transgenic mice that are not clinically relevant to humans. However, it may sometimes be an advantage that the transgenic mice may show pathologies that are rare in infected humans, that perhaps may occur because certain cell types are difficult to infect naturally and may only be seen in a minority of cases.

The suggestion of a direct involvement of viral gene products in the development of HCC is particularly attractive in view of the finding that HBV encodes a viral transactivator,[43–45] the X protein, which at least in cell culture can function as a transcriptional control element to upregulate the expression of other viral genes.[46,47] Since viral transactivators act through the host biosynthetic machinery, they are likely to perturb the expression of cellular genes and the differentiated functions of the infected cell. We have previously shown that transactivator genes from different human viruses, such as the human immunodeficiency virus,[38] human T-lymphotropic virus,[36,37] human adenovirus,[41] and human JC and BK papovaviruses,[34,35,39] when introduced into the germline of mice, induced specific malignancies that are similar to those that develop in humans infected by the same viruses. Given the importance of a clear understanding of the consequences of HBV infection, we undertook to determine whether the expression of the X gene alone would suffice to induce HCC in transgenic mice and to define its underlying mechanism of action.[42,48]

The X transgenic mice were derived by microinjection of a 1.15-kb DNA fragment of HBV subtype *adr*, which spans nucleotide positions 707 to 1,856 in the viral genome,[49] into single-cell embryos derived from outbred CD1 mice. This segment of DNA contains not only the entire coding region of the X gene (map positions 1,246 to 1,710),[49] but also the transcriptional enhancers (map positions 1,011 to 1,076 and 1,513 to 1,593),[15–19] the principal RNA start sites (map positions 1,184, 1,203, and 1,214),[50] and the polyadenylation site (map 1,788).[49] Multiple transgenic mice, each with at least one intact copy of the transgene stably integrated into the host genome, were identified, and three of them were randomly selected to be bred into permanent lines.[42]

EXPRESSION OF THE X GENE

Despite the presence of the X gene in every cell in the transgenic mouse, its expression is restricted to only certain adult tissues. Analysis of total mRNA extracted from various tissues reveals the presence of the 0.7-kb X transcript in the liver and, to a lesser extent, the kidney. Similar tissue topism was seen for each of the independent transgenic lines. Selective expression in liver and kidney is consistent with the detection of HBV DNA sequences in these tissues of infected individuals[5,6] and suggests that the hepatotropic property of this virus is determined, at least in part, at the level of viral gene expression. The HBV transcriptional promoter and enhancer within the transgene are probably responsible, possibly by interacting with tissue-specific transcription factors required for viral gene expression.

Histologic examination of hematoxylin and eosin (H&E) stained liver sections from the transgenic mice reveals multifocal areas of poorly stained hepatocytes (Fig. 14-2A; see also Plate 14-1) that are not detected in sections from nontransgenic littermates. These altered foci are found in all hepatic lobes of every mouse, beginning when the mice are about 4 weeks of age and become increasingly apparent with age. A high-magnification view of a typical altered focus reveals that it is made up of hepatocytes with poorly stained granular cytoplasm and nuclei that are highly variable in size (Fig. 14-2B). While dysplastic in appearance, these hepatocytes show no morphologic evidence of increased proliferation.

Increased cytoplasmic vacuolation in hepatocytes from these mice prompted us to investigate whether these hepatocytes contain an increased level of glycogen, a characteristic of preneoplastic cells in experimental chemical carcinogenesis.[51] Indeed, periodic acid-Schiff staining reveals selective staining of cells of the altered foci (Fig. 14-2G, H), indicating an abundance of glycogen storage.

Since these changes are detected in the transgenic mice and not in the nontransgenic littermates, they must be attributed to the X gene. Immunohistochemical staining of serial sections from one of the transgenic mouse livers using a rabbit antibody directed against the X protein for one section and H&E for the other show perfect overlap between the altered foci (Fig. 14-2A, B) and anti-X immunoreactivity (Fig. 14-2C, D). This finding could suggest that expression of the HBx protein in hepatocytes was directly responsible for the observed morphologic and biochemical changes in the livers of these mice.

Expression of the X gene in the transgenic mice is not only tissue restricted but also differentiation specific. Periportal hepatocytes are less well-differentiated and retain the capacity to proliferate, while perivenous hepatocytes become terminally differentiated and lose their capacity to divide; X expression is restricted to hepatocytes around the central vein and is never detected in cells around the portal triad (Fig. 14-2B, D). This observation suggests that host factors required for HBV gene expression are selectively present in hepatocytes with a low replicative potential and a more differentiated profile. This may explain why HBV does not replicate in hepatocytes growing in culture. Dividing liver cells cannot support viral gene expression and, hence, would not permit productive virus infection.

DEVELOPMENT OF HCC

As the transgenic mice reach 8 to 10 months of age, independent tumor nodules become evident in the liver on the background of altered foci (Fig. 14-3A; see also

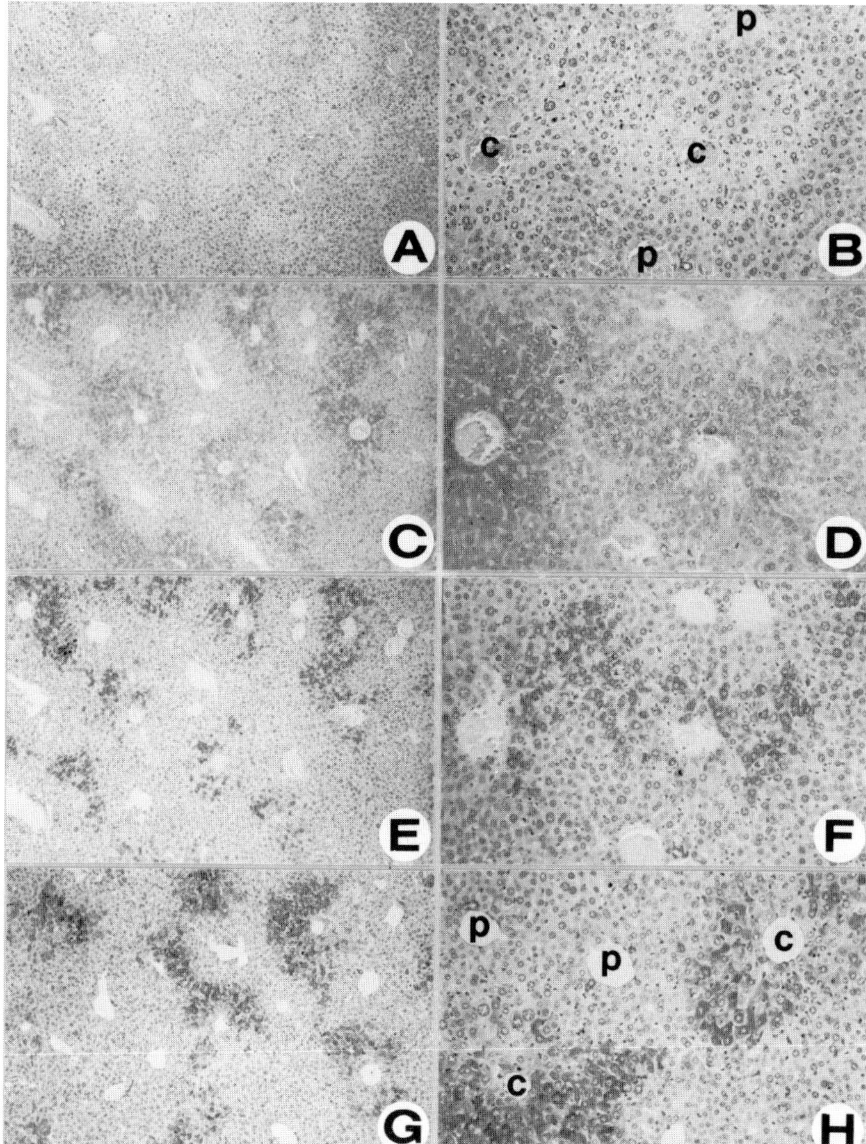

FIGURE 14-2. Early focal lesions of altered hepatocytes in the livers of the X gene transgenic mice. Sections of liver from a male mouse sacrificed at 2 months of age and stained with either H&E *(A, B)*, rabbit antibody to the X protein (anti-HBx) *(C, D)*, rabbit anti-TGF-β1 *(E, F)*, or periodic acid-Schiff *(G, H)*. Both low (A, C, E, G) and high (B, D, F, H) magnification views are shown. The immunostained sections were visualized by the avidin-biotin complex method. The H&E, anti-HBx, and anti-TGF-β1 sections are serial cuts. The central veins (c) and portal veins (p) are indicated. (See also Plate 14-1.)

Plate 14-2). These nodules are frequently made up of basophilic cells that proliferate and compress the neighboring normal parenchyma; they have the characteristics of adenomas. Like cells in the altered foci, those that make up the nodules also accumulate relatively high levels of the X protein (Fig. 14-4C) and contain large amounts of glycogen. Unlike in the altered foci, however, α-fetoprotein is detected in the tumors. Serum alanine aminotransferase concentration in transgenic mice bearing tumors is consistently within the normal range, indicating that there is no extensive liver cell damage present.

Most of the transgenic mice develop HCCs during their lifespan. Male mice develop tumors with a higher penetrance and at an earlier age. The number of tumor nodules per animal varies from mouse to mouse. This is

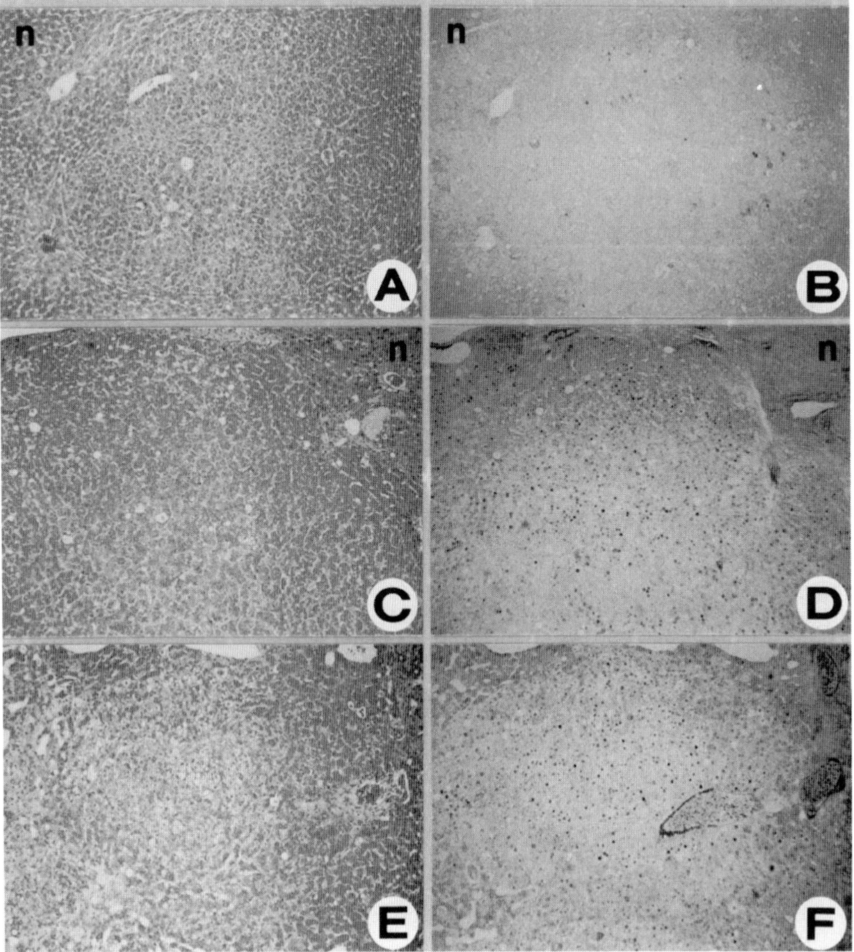

FIGURE 14-3. Tumor nodules in the liver of X gene transgenic mice. Sections of tumor lesions from three independent transgenic mice were stained with either H&E *(A, C, E)* or anti-PCNA *(B, D, F)*. The adjacent normal region of the liver (n) is indicated. (See also Plate 14-2.)

consistent with the epidemiologic observation that there are more men than women with chronic HBV infection developing HCC. The possible roles of male or female hormones could be tested easily in this transgenic model.

The early tumor lesions have no mitotic figures by H&E staining (Fig. 14-3A). Immunostaining of serial sections with an antibody directed against the proliferating cell nuclear antigen (PCNA), an essential DNA replication protein, reveals only an occasional immunoreactive cell within the tumor nodule (Fig. 14-3B). This finding suggests that the early tumors are slow-growing benign lesions. However, the relative number of PCNA-positive cells increases markedly as the tumor nodules become larger (Fig. 14-3C, D), and the morphology of the tumor cells changes markedly. Within nodules made up of basophilic tumor cells, isolated clusters of clear cells with extensive cytoplasmic vacuolation are seen (Fig. 14-3E). These clear cells appear to arise from among the basophilic cells and are highly PCNA-positive (Fig. 14-3F). Within larger tumors, there is frequently a mix of basophilic and clear cell types, each with high anti-PCNA immunoreactivity. This may suggest a continuous evolution of tumor cells with an increasingly elevated index. As in humans, the histopathology of individual tumors may vary, as may the level of accumulation of the X protein (Fig. 14-4E; see also Plate 14-3).

The high rate of tumor development in each of the transgenic mice suggests that expression of the X gene might lead to neoplastic changes in the liver. Indeed, it has been increasingly observed that HCC arises in some patients who have cleared HBsAg and HBV from serum, in whom the HBV genome, either in full or in part, has been integrated into the host cell chromosome.[52] What appears to be a common characteristic of HBV-related HCC is the presence of the X gene sequences[53] and the X antigen[54] in the tumor cells.

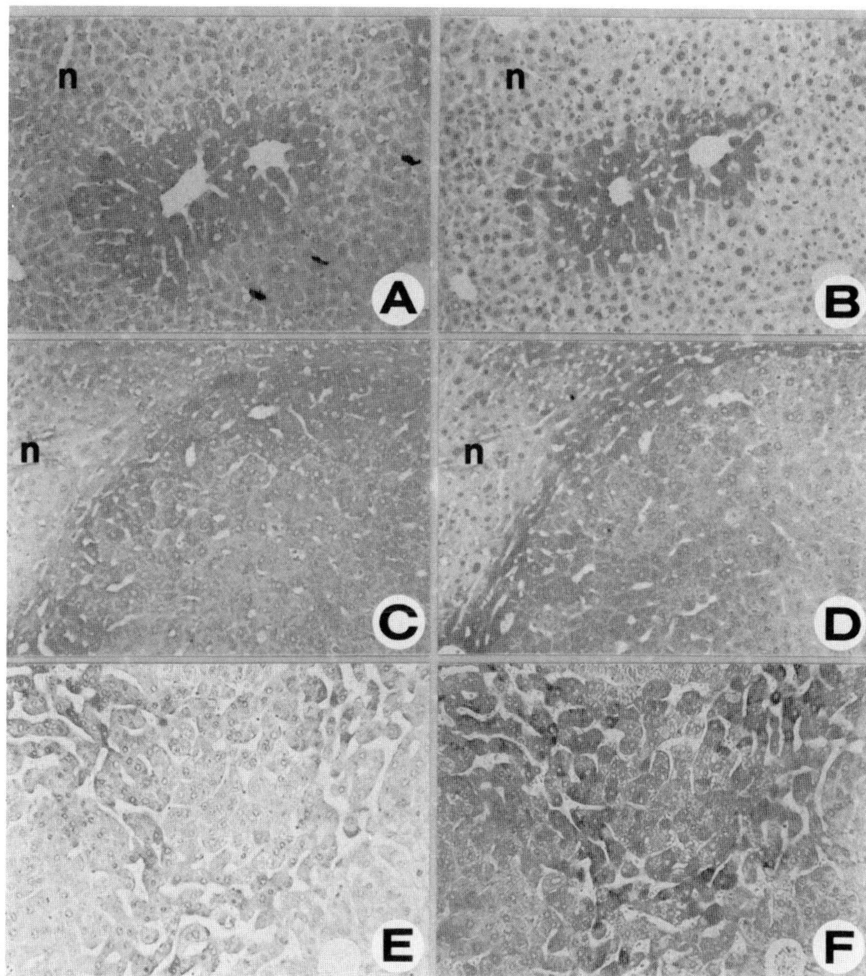

FIGURE 14-4. Immunostaining of p53 in the liver of X gene transgenic mice. Serial sections of an altered focus *(A, B)*, an adenoma *(C, D)*, and a hepatocellular carcinoma *(E, F)* from different transgenic mice were immunostained with either rabbit antibody to X protein (A, C, E) or rabbit anti-p53 (B,D,F). The immunostained were visualized by the avidin-biotin complex method. The adjacent normal region of the liver (n) is indicated. (See also Plate 14-3.)

TRANSCRIPTIONAL ACTIVATION OF TRANSFORMING GROWTH FACTOR-β1

Not every hepatocyte that expresses the transgene develops into a tumor cell. This suggests that X protein is necessary but not sufficient to induce neoplastic change. The long latency necessary for tumors to develop further suggests that additional event(s) are required but rare. There is now increasing evidence that epigenetic alterations involving changes in gene expression and gene function are important in the process of carcinogenesis. Not only does the hepatocyte have to be able to support the expression of the X gene above a threshold level, it must also have in place the functional target(s) for the X protein to act and ensure the effects of the X protein are coupled to the additional events necessary for the tumor to develop. Even after the cell has become a tumor, the resulting tumor cells continue to undergo adaptive changes that presumably would render them autonomous. Identification of the underlying epigenetic changes is crucial if we are to understand how HBV induces HCC.

Transforming growth factor-β (TGF-β1) has been shown to inhibit hepatocyte proliferation during liver regeneration,[55,56] to stimulate the production of extracellular matrix proteins by hepatocytes during cirrhosis,[57,58] and to play a role in the development of HCC.[59] To determine whether TGF-β1 may be a target of X, we looked for a correlation between expression of the two proteins in HCCs from transgenic mice.[60] Immunohistochemical staining using a rabbit antibody directed against TGF-β1 was positive in transgenic livers but not in control livers. TGF-β1 is found selectively in hepatocytes that form the altered foci. Analysis of serial liver sections stained either with antibody to X protein (Fig. 14-2C) or anti-TGF-β1 (Fig. 14-2E) shows overlapping immunoreactivity, suggesting that expression of HBx might lead to the overexpression of TGF-β1. Whereas every cell within an altered focus expresses X, only a subset of them also expresses TGF-β1 (cf. Fig. 14-3D, F). Because of the large number of cells expressing TGF-β1, this argues for an epigenetic rather than genetic mechanism underlying the activation process.

By deletional analysis of the TGF-β1 promoter region in transfected HepG2 cells, X transactivation was shown to be mediated through cis-acting elements that form the binding sites for the Egr-1 transcription factor.[60] Additionally, using a GAL4–Egr-1 fusion protein we showed that X can mediate transactivation through Egr-1, and using a GST–Egr-1 fusion protein provided evidence for direct physical binding between X and Egr-1. Together, these findings suggest that the binding of X to the Egr-1 transcription factor in HBV-infected hepatocytes allows complex formation at specific cites within the TGF-β1 promoter region and concomitant activation of TGF-β1 expression. One can speculate that activation of TGF-β1 by X places a cell in a state that is compatible with transformation.

FUNCTIONAL INACTIVATION OF p53

There is increasing evidence for the involvement of tumor suppressor genes in the neoplastic transformation of cells. These genes have a normal function of inducing growth arrest in appropriate differentiated cells; loss of that function will result in uncontrolled growth. Mutations of the p53 tumor suppressor gene have been found in as many as half of all human malignancies.[61]

Immunohistochemical staining of an altered focus (of the type described above) with a rabbit antibody against p53 protein reveals an alteration in the subcellular distribution of p53.[48] p53 in cells in normal hepatocytes of the transgenic mice is found exclusively within the nucleus, but in hepatocytes within the altered foci there is also abundant cytoplasmic p53 (Fig. 14-4B). If the nuclear localization of p53 reflects its essential role in that compartment of the cell, partial redistribution to the cytoplasm may have deleterious consequences for the cell. Within an adenoma with sustained cytoplasmic accumulation of X (Fig. 14-4C), p53 molecules were entirely absent from the nucleus of the tumor cells (Fig. 14-4D). It is possible that altered hepatocytes from benign tumor cells, such as those of an adenoma, are distinguished by the extent of cytoplasmic sequestration of p53; as long as some of the p53 enters the nucleus of hepatocytes in the altered foci, the cells can still undergo growth arrest.

The correlation between the extent of cytoplasmic accumulation of the X protein in the altered foci (Fig. 14-4A) and the degree of cytoplasmic sequestration of the p53 protein is further illustrated by an analysis of a carcinoma lesion (Fig. 14-4E, F). This correlation suggests that the two proteins maybe physically associated with one another. Incubation of a tumor cell extract with antibodies to one protein, followed by immunoblot analysis of the resulting immune complex with antibodies to the second protein, shows abundant reactivity.[48] With this approach, it is possible to demonstrate that all of the p53 molecules are bound to the X molecules and that the latter are in excess within the tumor cells. The physical binding of p53 to X could explain the cytoplasmic sequestration of the tumor suppressor protein and the loss of growth arrest resulting in HCCs.

What determines the extent of complex formation between the two proteins and, hence, the progression from altered foci to tumors remains obscure. Since both X[62] and p53[63] have been shown to undergo post-translational modification, one might suspect that these changes could facilitate the interaction between them. If that is the case, this event may be the rate-limiting step that ultimately dictates the long latency and incomplete penetrance of tumor development.

MUTATION OF p53 IS A LATE EVENT

Consistent with our suggestion that functional inactivation of p53 by X leads to malignant transformation of hepatocytes in the transgenic mouse, we do not find by single-strand conformational polymorphism (SSCP) analysis[64] any point mutation in the p53 gene in tumor nodules dissected from paraffin block. We suspect that, over time, this functional inactivation of p53 will provide positive selection among the proliferating tumor cells for structural mutations of the p53 gene. Such cells will then have a growth advantage over those without the mutation. Indeed, p53 mutations can be detected by SSCP analysis in minor cell populations when larger HCCs from these transgenic mice are analyzed. We suspect that since the tumors in these transgenic mice are polyclonal in nature, resulting from multiple independent events, the mice succumb to the tumor before "selected" tumor cells with actual mutations of p53 have a chance to expand and take over.

These findings in transgenic mice agree with clinical observations made regarding the involvement of p53 mutations in human HCCs. First, only 30% to 50% of HBV-related HCCs have detectable mutations in the p53 gene,[53, 65–71] suggesting that such genetic alterations are not a prerequisite for the development of HCCs. Second, mutations are selectively detected in those HCCs that are most aggressive,[72–75] suggesting that mutations are likely to be a late event in tumor progression. Third, different regions from the same HCC can have different p53 mutations,[73] suggesting that separate independent events arise from the same parent tumor. These observations are in agreement with our suggestion that functional inactivation of p53 is the basis for the initial tumor development and that in turn provides the necessary selective pressure for subsequent mutations that will give rise to cells with more malignant characteristics

SYNERGY BETWEEN X AND AFLATOXIN B_1

The etiology of most forms of human cancers is multifactorial in nature, involving both genetics and the environment.[76] Each step in the process may be influenced by one or more specific cofactors. In the case of HCC, dietary exposure to aflatoxin B_1 (AFB_1) has not only been linked to the development of liver cancer in epidemiologic studies, but also suggested to act synergistically with HBV.[77,78] AFB_1 is a mutagen that induces G to T transversions.[79] Our studies are consistent with the suggestion that p53 mutation is likely to be a late event in the development of HBV-related HCC in the absence of AFB_1.

To understand the possible synergism between HBV and AFB_1, we examined whether AFB_1 could shorten the latency for the development of liver tumors in the X transgenic mice and, if so, whether p53 mutations can be detected in these tumors.[80] While low-dose AFB_1 can indeed induce earlier detection of tumors in the transgenic mice, the existence of synergistic p53 mutations was not confirmed in these tumors.[80] This suggests that AFB_1 acts in the transgenic model in a manner other than by causing p53 gene mutation. These findings do not, however, exclude the possibility that AFB_1 can act at a later stage.

CONCLUSIONS

Transgenic technology is a valuable approach for the dissection of complex disease mechanisms. As with any animal model, potential artifacts may be inherent in the experimental system. Information derived from the analysis of transgenic animals can be confirmed by comparing them to patients with the relevant disease. A clear understanding of a disease at the molecular level would no doubt facilitate the development of treatments.

REFERENCES

1. Tiollais P, Pourcel C, Dejean A. The hepatitis B virus. Nature 1985;317:489–495
2. Beasley RB, Hwang L-Y. In Vyas GN (ed): Viral Hepatitis and Liver Disease. Grune & Stratton, New York, 1984, p. 209–224
3. Tiollais P, Charnay P, Vyas GN. Biology of hepatitis B virus. Science 1981;213:406–411
4. Seeger C, Ganem D, Varmus HE. Biochemical and genetic evidence for the hepatits B virus replication strategy. Science 1986;232:477–484
5. Siddiqui A. Hepatitis B virus DNA in Kaposi sarcoma. Proc Natl Acad Sci USA 1983;80:4861–4864
6. Dejean A, Lugassy C, Zafrani S et al. Detection of hepatitis B virus DNA in pancreas, kidney and skin of two human carriers of the virus. J Gen Virol 1984;65:651–655
7. Summers J, Smolec J, Snyder R. A virus similar to human hepatitis B virus associated with hepatitis and hepatoma in woodchucks. Proc Natl Acad Sci USA 1978;75:4533–4537
8. Marion PL, Oshiro LS, Regnery DC et al. A virus in Beechey ground squirrels that is related to hepatitis B virus of humans. Proc Natl Acad Sci USA 1980;77:2941–2945
9. Pourcel G, Louise A, Gervais M et al. Transcription of the hepatitis B surface antigen gene in mouse cells transformed with cloned viral DNA. J Virol 1982;42:100–105.
10. Gough, N. Core and E antigen synthesis in rodent cells transformed with hepatitis B virus DNA is associated with greater than genome length viral messenger RNAs. J Mol Biol 1983; 165:683–699
11. Siddiqui A, Jameel S, Mapoles J. Expression of the hepatitis B virus X gene in mammalian cells. Proc Natl Acad Sci USA 1987;84:2513–2517
12. Kaneko S, Miller RH. X-region-specific transcript in mammalian hepatitis B virus-infected liver. J Virol 1988;62: 3979–3984
13. Cattaneo R, Will H, Hernandez N, Schaller H. Signals regulating hepatitis B surface antigen transcription. Nature 1983; 305:336–338
14. Cattaneo R, Will H, Schaller H. Hepatitis B virus transcription in the infected liver. EMBO J 1984;3:2191–2196
15. Shaul Y, Rutter WJ, Laub O. A human hepatitis B viral enhancer element. EMBO J 1985;4:427–430
16. Elfassi E. Broad specificity of the hepatitis B enhancer function. Virology 1987;160:259–262
17. Vannice JL, Levinson AD. Properties of the human hepatitis B virus enhancer: position effects and cell-type nonspecificity. J Virol 1988;62:1305–1313
18. Wang Y, Chen P, Wu X et al. A new enhancer element ENII identified in the X gene of hepatitis B virus. J Virol 1990;64:3977–3981
19. Yuh C-H, Ting L-P. The genome of hepatitis B virus contains a second enhancer: cooperation of two elements within this enhancer is required for its function. J Virol 1990;64: 4281–4287
20. Antonucci TK, Rutter WJ. Hepatitis B virus (HBV) pro-

moters are regulated by the HBV enhancer in a tissue-specific manner. J Virol 1989;63:579–583

21. Honigwachs J, Faktor O, Dikstein R et al. Liver-specific expression of hepatitis B virus is determined by the combined action of the core gene promoter and the enhancer. J Virol 1989;63:919–924
22. Beasley RP, Hwang L-Y, Lin C-C, Chien C-S. Hepatocellular carcinoma and hepatitis B virus. Lancet 1981;II: 1129–1133
23. Beasley RP, Lin C-C, Chien C–S et al. Geographic distribution of HBsAg carriers in China. Hepatology 1982;2: 553–556
24. Summers J. Three recently described animal virus models for human hepatitis B virus. Hepatology 1981;1:179–183
25. Popper H, Roth L, Purcell RH et al. Hepatocarcinogenicity of the woodchuck hepatitis virus. Proc Natl Acad Sci USA 1987;84:866–870
26. Marion PL, Salazar FH, Alexander JJ, Robinson WS. State of hepatitis B viral DNA in a human hepatoma cell line. J Virol 1980;35:795–806
27. Chakraborty PR, Ruiz-Opazo N, Shouval D, Shafritz DA. Identification of integrated hepatitis B virus DNA and expression of viral RNA in an HBsAg-producing human hepatocellular carcinoma cell line. Nature 1980;286:531–533
28. Bréchot C, Pourcel C, Louis A et al. Presence of integrated hepatitis B virus DNA sequences in cellular DNA of human hepatocellular carcinoma. Nature 1980;286:533–535
29. Edman JC, Gray P, Valenzuela P et al. Integration of hepatitis B virus sequences and their expression in a human hepatoma cell. Nature 1980;286:535–538
30. Nagaya T, Nakamura T, Tokino T et al. The mode of hepatitis B virus DNA integration in chromosomes of human hepatocellular carcinoma. Genes Dev 1987;1:773–782
31. Szmuness W. Hepatocellular carcinoma and the hepatitis B virus: evidence for a causal association. Prog Med Virol 1978; 24:40–69
32. Peters G. In Reddy EP, Skalka AM, Curran T (eds): Oncogene Handbook. Elsevier, New York, 1988, p. 487–559
33. Brinster RL, Chen HY, Trumbauer ME et al. Factors affecting the efficiency of introducing foreign DNA into mice by microinjecting eggs. Proc Natl Acad Sci USA 1985;82: 4438–4442
34. Small JA, Scangos G, Cork L et al. The early region of human papovavirus JC induces dysmyelination in transgenic mice. Cell 1986;46:13–18
35. Small JA, Khoury G, Jay G et al. Early regions of JC virus and BK virus induce distinct and tissue-specific tumors in transgenic mice. Proc Natl Acad Sci USA 1986;83: 8288–8292
36. Nerenberg M, Hinrichs SH, Reynolds RK et al. The *tat* gene of human T-lymphotropic virus type I induces mesenchymal tumors in transgenic mice. Science 1987;237:1324–1329
37. Hinrichs SH, Nerenberg M, Reynolds RK et al. A transgenic mouse model for human neurofibromatosis. Science 1987; 237:1340–1343
38. Vogel J, Hinrichs SH, Reynolds RK et al. The HIV *tat* gene induces dermal lesions resembling Kaposi's sarcoma in transgenic mice. Nature 1988;335:606–611
39. Reynolds RK, Hoekzema GS, Vogel J et al. Multiple endocrine neoplasia induced by the promiscuous expression of a viral oncogene. Proc Natl Acad Sci USA 1988;85: 3135–3139
40. Green JE, Hinrichs SH, Vogel J, Jay G. Exocrinopathy resembling Sjögren's syndrome in HTLV-I *tax* transgenic mice. Nature 1989;341:72–74
41. Koike K, Hinrichs SH, Isselbacher KJ, Jay G. Transgenic mouse model for human gastric carcinoma. Proc Natl Acad Sci USA 1989;86:5615–5619
42. Kim C-M, Koike K, Saito I et al. The HBx gene of hepatitis B virus induces liver cancer. Nature 1991;351:317–320
43. Twu J-S, Schloemer RH. Transcriptional *trans*-activating function of hepatitis B virus. J Virol 1987;61:3448–3453
44. Spandau DF, Lee CH. *trans*-Activation of viral enhancers by the hepatitis B virus X protein. J Virol 1988;62:427–434
45. Seto E, Zhou D-X, Peterlin BM, Yen TSB. Trans-activation by the hepatitis B virus X protein shows cell-type specificity. Virology 1989;173:764–766
46. Two JS, Robinson WS. Hepatitis B virus X gene can transactivate heterologous viral sequence. Proc Natl Acad Sci USA 1989;86:2046–2050
47. Siddiqui A, Gaynor R, Srinivasan A et al. Trans-activation of viral enhancers including long terminal repeat of the human immunodeficiency virus by the hepatitis B virus X protein. Virology 1989;169:479–494
48. Ueda H, Ullrich SJ, Gangemi JD et al. Functional inactivation but not structural mutation of p53 causes liver cancer. Nature Genet 1995;9:41–47
49. Fujiyama A, Miyanohara A, Nozaki C et al. Cloning and structural analyses of hepatitis B virus DNAs, subtype adr. Nucleic Acids Res 1983;11:4601–4610
50. Treinin M, Laub O. Identification of a promoter element upstream from the hepatitis B virus X gene. Mol Cell Biol 1987;7:545–548
51. Klimek F, Mayer D, Bannasch P. Biochemical microanalysis of glycogen content and glucose-6-phosphate dehydrogenase activity in focal lesions of the rat liver induced by *N*-nitrosomorpholine. Carcinogenesis 1984;5:265–268
52. Chen DS. From hepatitis to hepatoma: lessons from type B viral hepatitis. Science 1993;262:369–370
53. Unsal H, Yakicier C, Marcais C et al. Genetic heterogeneity of hepatocellular carcinoma. Proc Natl Acad Sci USA 1994; 91:822–826
54. Feitelson MA, Clayton MM. X antigen polypeptides in the sera of hepatitis B virus-infected patients. Virology 1990; 177:367–371
55. Braun L, Mead JE, Panzica M et al. Transforming growth factor mRNA increases during liver regenerations: a possible paracrine mechanism of growth regulation. Proc Natl Acad Sci USA 1988;86:1539–1543
56. Fausto N, Mead JE. Regulation of liver growth: protooncogenes and transforming growth factors. Lab Invest 1989;60: 4–13
57. Czaja MF, Weiner FR, Flanders KC et al. In vitro and in vivo association of transforming growth factor-β1 with hepatic fibrosis. J Cell Biol 1989;108:2477–2482

58. Nakatsukasa H, Nagy P, Evarts RP et al. Cellular distribution of transforming growth factor-β1 and procollagen types I, III, and IV transcripts in carbon tetrachloride-induced rat liver fibrosis. J Clin Invest 1990;85:1833–1843

59. Ito N, Kawata S, Tamura S et al. Elevated levels of transforming growth factor-β messenger RNA and its polypeptide in human hepatocellular carcinoma. Cancer Res 1991;51: 4080–4083

60. Yoo YD, Ueda H, Park K et al. Regulation of transforming growth factor-β1 expression by the hepatitis B virus (HBV) X transactivator: role in pathogenesis. J Clin Invest 1996; 97:1–8

61. Harris CC, Hollstein M. Clinical implications of the p53 tumor-suppressor gene. N Engl J Med 1993;329:1318–1327

62. Schek N, Bartenschlager R, Kuhn C, Schaller H. Phosphorylation and rapid turnover of hepatitis B virus X-protein expressed in Hep G2 cells from a recombinant vaccinia virus. Oncogene 1991;6:1735–1744

63. Ullrich SJ, Anderson CW, Mercer WE, Appella E. The p53 tumor suppressor protein, a modulator of cell proliferation. J Biol Chem 1992;267:15259–15262

64. Orita M, Suzuki Y, Sekiya T, Hayashi K. Rapid and sensitive detection of point mutations and DNA polymorphisms using the polymerase chain reaction. Genomics 1989;5:874–879

65. Hsu IC, Metcalf RA, Sun T et al. Mutational hotspot in the p53 gene in human hepatocellular carcinomas. Nature 1991; 350:427–428

66. Bressac B, Kew MC, Wand JR, Ozturk M. Selective G to T mutations of p53 gene in hepatocellular carcinoma from southern Africa. Nature 1991;350:429–431

67. Hosono S, Lee C-S, Chou M-J et al. Molecular analysis of the p53 alleles in primary hepatocellular carcinomas and cell lines. Oncogene 1991;6:237–243

68. Buetow KH, Sheffield VC, Zhu M et al. Low frequency of p53 mutations observed in a diverse collection of primary hepatocellular carcinomas. Proc Natl Acad Sci USA 1992; 89:9622–9626

69. Sheu JC, Huang GT, Lee PH et al. Mutation of p53 gene in hepatocellular carcinoma in Taiwan. Cancer Res 1992; 52:6098–6100

71. Nishida N, Fukuda Y, Kokuryu H et al. Role and mutational heterogeneity of the p53 gene in hepatocellular carcinoma. Cancer Res 1993;53:368–372

72. Hsu H-C, Tseng H-J, Lai P-L et al. Expression of p53 gene in 184 unifocal hepatocellular carcinomas: association with tumor growth and invasiveness. Cancer Res 1993;53: 4691–4694

73. Tanaka S, Toh Y, Adachi E et al. Tumor progression in hepatocellular carcinoma may be mediated by p53 mutation. Cancer Res 1993;53:2884–2887

74. Oda T, Tsuda H, Scarpa A et al. p53 gene mutation spectrum in hepatocellular carcinoma. Cancer Res 1992;52: 6358–6364

75. Teramoto T, Satonaka K, Kitazawa S et al. p53 gene abnormalities are closely related to hepatoviral infections and occur at a late stage of hepatocarcinogenesis. Cancer Res 1994;54:231–235

76. Harris CC, Sun T-T. Multifactorial etiology of human liver cancer. Carcinogenesis 1984;5:697–701

77. Yeh F-S, Yu MC, Mo C-C et al. Hepatitis B virus, aflatoxins, and hepatocellular carcinoma in southern Guangxi, China. Cancer Res 1989;49:2506–2509

78. Ross R, Yuan J-M, Yu M et al. Urinary aflatoxin biomarkers and risk of hepatocellular carcinoma. Lancet 1992;339: 943–946

79. Aguila F, Hussain SP, Cerutti P. Aflatoxin B_1 induces the transversion of G-T in codon 249 of the p53 tumor suppressor gene in human hepatocytes. Proc Natl Acad Sci USA 1993;90:8586–8590

80. Ueda H, Ohkoshi S, Harris CC, Jay G. Synergism between the *HBx* gene and aflatoxin B_1 in the development of murine liver cancer. Int J Oncol 1995;7:735–740

15

EXPERIMENTAL CHEMICAL HEPATOCARCINOGENESIS

PETER BANNASCH
HEIDE ZERBAN

Hepatocarcinogenesis induced by chemicals in laboratory animals has been used as a model system for human hepatocarcinogenesis and neoplastic development in general for more than half a century. M.B. Schmidt[1] was the first to describe the experimental induction of a hepatocellular neoplasm in a mouse that had received scarlet red per os in an unsuccessful attempt to stain fat in vivo. It was, however, Sasaki and Yoshida[2] who produced a high incidence of hepatocellular carcinomas (HCC) by the systematic feeding of rats with the carcinogenic component of scarlet red, the azo dye *o*-aminoazotoluene, that established chemical hepatocarcinogenesis as a main tool in cancer research. A large number of additional chemical hepatocarcinogens belonging to various chemical classes have been identified.[3–7] In animal experiments, the rodent liver has been shown to represent a favored target tissue for chemical carcinogens.[8] Although rodents continue to remain the preferred animal species for studying chemical hepatocarcinogenesis, a broad spectrum of other species including primates are also susceptible to the chemical induction of hepatic neoplasia.[9–12]

In addition to the link between chemical structure and biologic effects, the metabolism of chemical hepatocarcinogens[3–6] and dose-response relationships[13,14] have been studied in great detail. These areas are important for extrapolation from the results of carcinogenesis bioassays in laboratory animals to humans, but observations on the pathogenesis of experimental liver tumors are of particular interest.[15,16] Nearly all types of primary liver tumors known from human pathology can be produced by chemicals in laboratory animals, especially in rats.[9,17,18] The malignant variants of these neoplasms have been classified as HCCs, cholangiocellular carcinomas, angiosarcomas, and perisinusoidal (Ito) cell sarcomas (Fig. 15-1). Sequential cellular and molecular changes preceding these neoplasms have been observed and analyzed in several experimental models of chemical hepatocarcinogenesis.[12,19] This holds particularly true for preneoplastic foci of altered hepatocytes (FAH), which emerge weeks or months before hepatocellular adenomas and HCCs appear.[16,20,21] The consistent development of FAH early during experimental hepatocarcinogenesis suggested their utilization for carcinogenicity testing[22] and prompted several laboratories to introduce medium-term carcinogenesis bioassays based on the detection of FAH.[23–26] FAH have also been discovered in humans bearing hepatocellular neoplasms and/or suffering from liver cirrhosis.[27,28] Further analysis of FAH and their progression to hepatocellular adenomas and HCCs in experimental animal models and humans offers one of the most promising approaches to the elucidation of the molecular mechanisms of neoplastic conversion of the hepatocyte.[16]

CHEMICAL HEPATOCARCINOGENS

A large number of compounds representing many classes of chemicals have been shown to induce liver neoplasms in laboratory animals.[3–7] Representatives of the ever-

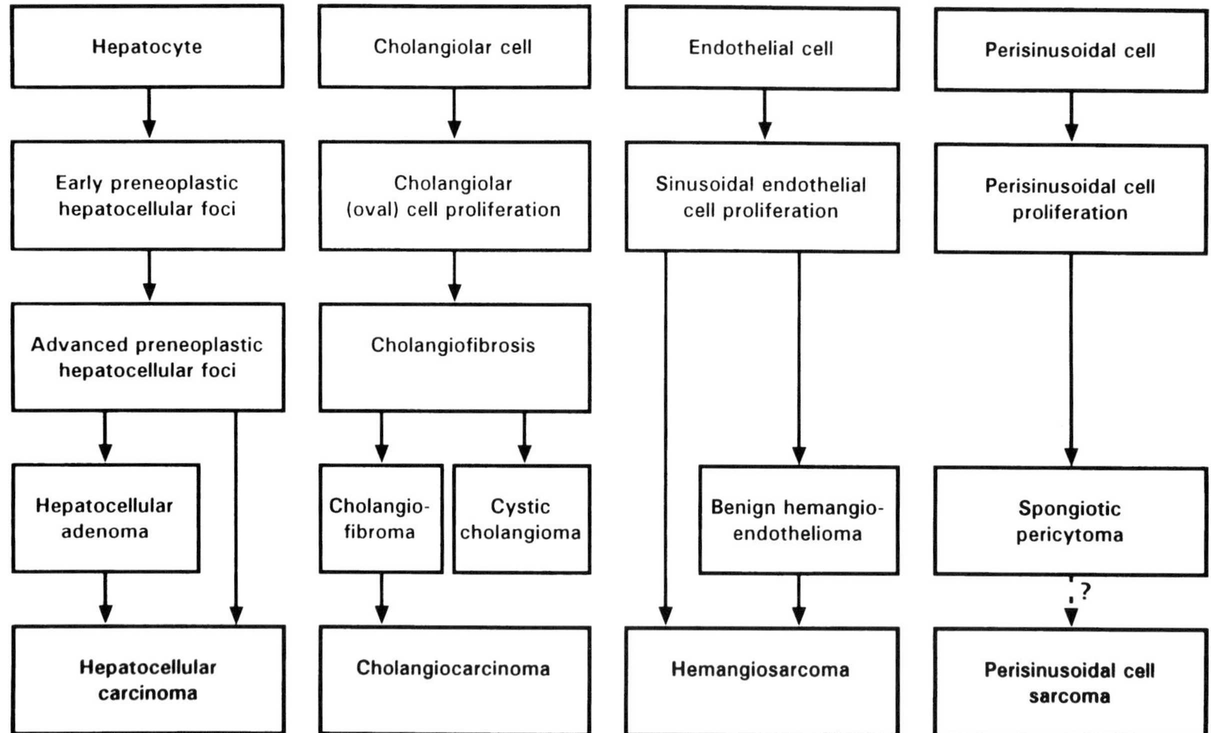

Figure 15-1. Schematic diagram of sequential preneoplastic and neoplastic lesions arising from the four main target cells of chemical hepatocarcinogens in rodent liver. (From Bannasch,[16] with permission.)

growing catalogue of hepatocarcinogenic chemicals are listed in Table 15-1, including the recently discovered tamoxifen.[29–31] The immense number of hepatocarcinogens identified in laboratory animals sharply contrasts with the few compounds for which epidemiologic studies provide sufficient evidence for a similar effect in humans. However, this discrepancy should not detract from the finding of several striking interspecies similarities in the hepatocarcinogenic effects of chemicals. This applies particularly to the aflatoxin B_1 (AFB_1) and vinyl chloride, whose hepatocarcinogenic effects were first detected in rodents, and which were later found to affect not only the same target tissue but also the same target cells in rodents and humans. In both groups, AFB_1 is preferentially involved in the development of hepatocellular carcinomas,[32] whereas vinyl chloride mainly induces liver angiosarcomas derived from the sinusoidal endothelial cells.[17] Another example of analogous carcinogenic effects is the increased incidence of hepatocellular neoplasms, predominantly adenomas and peliosis hepatis in rats treated with different steroids (e.g., ethinyl estradiol, norethisterone) and the increased risk of the development of hepatocellular adenomas in women using combined oral contraceptives.[33] Similar lesions may also develop in men and women treated with androgenic anabolic steroids. These observations suggest that all chemicals that induce liver neoplasms in laboratory animals should be seriously considered as risk factors for humans, even though convincing epidemiologic data may not be available at present. It is true, however, that the extrapolation of data from animals to humans is complicated by many factors such as the dose and duration of administration of the chemical; the age, sex, and genetic background of the animal; and the intrinsic or compound-related cell proliferation.[34]

In some situations, chemicals that are clearly carcinogenic in humans have not been shown to be so in rodents. Epidemiologic observations indicate that chronic exposure to arsenic and arsenic compounds may induce neoplasms, especially angiosarcomas, in the human liver.[35] Although arsenic has not been established unequivocally as a carcinogen in rodents, some evidence for hepatocarcinogenic activity in rats has been presented.[35] The well-established hepatocarcinogenic effect of chronic abuse of alcoholic beverages in humans[36] lacks an experimental counterpart. Ethanol has never been demonstrated to induce liver neoplasms in experimental animals but may modulate hepatocarcinogenesis elicited by various oncogenic agents, including chemicals and hepatitis viruses.[37,38]

TABLE 15-1. Representative Hepatocarcinogens in Laboratory Animals and Humans

Laboratory Animals	Humans
Natural products	
Aflatoxins	Aflatoxins
Sterigmatocystin	
Luteoskyrin	
Cyclochlorotine (Yellow rice toxin)	
Pyrrolizidine alkaloids	
Cycasin	
Safrole (Isafrole, dihydrosafrole)	
Tannic acid and tannins	
Coumarin	
Griseofulvin	
Hormones and drugs	
Ethinyl estradiol	
Norethisterone	
Dehydroepiandrosterone	
Tamoxifen	
Clofibrate	
Nafenopin	Oral contraceptives, combined [androgenic (anabolic) steroids][a]
Azathioprin	Azathioprine
Phenobarbital	
Oxazepam	
Aromatic amines	
o-Aminoazotoluene	
4-Dimethylaminoazobenzene	
2-Acetylaminofluorene	
Nitrosamines	
Dimethylnitrosamine	
Diethylnitrosamine	
N-Nitrosomorpholine	
N-Nitrosopiperidine	
Halogenated aliphatic compounds	
Carbon tetrachloride	
Chloroform	
Trichlorethylene	
Vinyl chloride	Vinyl chloride
Organochlorine pesticides	
Aramite	
2,2-Bis(*p*-chlorophenyl)-1,1,1-trichloroethane (DDT)	
Aldrin	
Dieldrin	
Polychlorinated biphenyls	
3,3′,4,4′-Tetrachlorobiphenyl	[Polychlorinated biphenyls]
Peroxisome proliferators (other than drugs)	
Di(2-ethylhexyl)phthalate	
Wy-14,643	
Miscellaneous	
Ethionine	
Thioacetamide	
2,3,7,8-Tetrachlorodibenzo-*p*-dioxin (TCDD)	
[Arsenic]	Arsenic
	Alcoholic beverages

[a] Brackets indicate suspected hepatocarcinogen.

THE METABOLISM OF CHEMICAL HEPATOCARCINOGENS AND THEIR INTERACTION WITH CELLULAR MACROMOLECULES

The majority of chemical hepatocarcinogens are not carcinogenic per se but require metabolic activation.[3–6,39,40] The biotransformation of inactive chemicals (procarcinogens) to active metabolites (ultimate carcinogens) frequently passes through intermediates (proximate carcinogens) and is carried out by enzymes of the intracellular mixed function oxygenase system, particularly cytochrome P450 species, which are located in the endoplasmic reticulum and require NADPH and oxygen. These enzymes can catalyze several chemical reactions, including aromatic ring hydroxylation, aliphatic hydroxylation, oxidative demethylation, and *N*-hydroxylation, on various organic compounds. For example, 2-acetylaminofluorene is metabolized not only by ring hydroxylation but also by hydroxylation of the nitrogen of the acetylamino group of the molecule as a first step in becoming reactive.[41] In contrast, AFB_1[42] and vinyl chloride[43] are activated through epoxidation. The processes of procarcinogen activation, which are particularly well developed and versatile in the liver, are functionally closely connected with inactivation steps, resulting in more soluble, secretable derivatives. The final fate of chemical hepatocarcinogens depends largely on the balance between these two processes. The ultimate carcinogens act as electrophiles that may exert biologic effects through spontaneous covalent binding to cellular macromolecules such as proteins, RNA, and DNA.[39] Damage to nuclear DNA is considered the most important early event in hepatocarcinogenesis, but alterations in mitochondrial DNA, in RNA, and in soluble or structural proteins have also been described.[44,45] Electrophilic intermediates of many chemical carcinogens give rise to a variety of DNA adducts, involving binding to various sites in the four bases of DNA as well as to the phosphate backbone.[46,47] The formation and possible persistence of DNA adducts are influenced by many factors, including distribution, metabolic activation and detoxification of the chemical carcinogen, and the proliferation and repair capacities of the target cell. Some of these DNA adducts, particularly those that are only slowly repaired (e.g., O^4-methylguanine[48] or O^4-ethylthymidine[49]) are promutagenic and, therefore, may lead to mutations in the target tissue upon replication.[6,50] It has been emphasized recently, however, that the quantitative and qualitative patterns of mutagenesis for a specific adduct are potentially quite variable and changeable, depending on diverse factors including the DNA sequence context.[51] Castro et al.[52] reported that the intensity of CCl_4 hepatocarcinogenicity in three different species (C3H mice, Syrian golden hamsters, and Sprague-Dawley rats) did not correlate with the covalent binding of CCl_4 reactive metabolites to total DNA but rather to binding to histone and nonhistone nuclear proteins. Amino acids such as methionine may also be targets of the ultimate forms of chemical hepatocarcinogens.[44]

In addition to chemicals that react directly with DNA and have, hence, been classified as "DNA reactive" or "genotoxic," a rapidly increasing number of "nongenotoxic" compounds have been identified that apparently do not interact directly with DNA but, nevertheless, produce liver neoplasms in rodents, suggesting alternative mechanisms of action.[53,54] Mutagenicity and carcinogenicity are not closely correlated in hepatocarcinogenesis.[55] Nongenotoxic hepatocarcinogens may act as weak carcinogens or strong carcinogens in rodent liver; they comprise compounds such as phenobarbital, methapyrilene, chloroform, and a diverse group of chemicals including drugs (e.g., clofibrate, ciprofibrate, tamoxifen), hormones (e.g., dehydroepiandrosterone), phthalate esters, plasticizers, and herbicides, all of which have the ability to increase the number of peroxisomes in hepatocytes (peroxisome proliferators). It has been proposed that oxidative DNA damage due to a marked increase in free radical-generating enzymes of peroxisomal β-oxidation via H_2O_2 might initiate carcinogenesis by these compounds.[56] However, recent studies failed to demonstrate any significant genotoxic effect of peroxisome proliferators, even under conditions that enhance the production of oxygen free radicals,[57] and modification of DNA by active oxygen radicals does not necessarily lead to initiation of carcinogenesis.[58] In addition, investigations on the morphogenesis of hepatocellular neoplasms induced by the peroxisomal proliferator dehydroepiandrosterone have shown that the preneoplastic foci preceding the appearance of these neoplasms do not develop from the perivenular zones, in which the most pronounced peroxisomal proliferation occurs, but from periportal areas, in which the prevailing cellular alteration is a proliferation of mitochondria.[59]

The regulation of gene expression and cellular differentiation is associated with changes in DNA methylation that have also been proposed as being essential for hepatic carcinogenesis.[60] Prolonged feeding of diets that are deficient in sources of transferable methyl groups, such as choline and methionine, has been shown to induce a high incidence of HCC without added carcinogens.[61–64] Due to the requirement for choline and methionine in the formation of *S*-adenosylmethionine, diets deficient in these methyl donors may lead to hypomethylation of DNA in particular genes, which can be considered to gain an increased potential for expression compared to their hypermethylated counterpart.[60] In fact, hypomethylation and increased expression of several proto-oncogenes (c-Ha-*ras*, c-Ki-*ras*, c-*myc*, c-*fos*) not only were found after prolonged feeding but also were detected within 1 to 4 weeks after starting the methyl-deficient diets.[65–67] However, the nongenotoxic hepatocarcinogen methapyrilene has been reported to lead to an increase in deoxycytidine methylation.[68]

Using ^{32}P-postlabeling for the analysis of DNA alterations, nonpolar covalent DNA modifications were detected in rat liver, so-called I-compounds (which resembled persistent DNA adducts produced by 2-acetylaminofluorene) under a variety of conditions, including aging, regeneration, and treatment with various chemicals.[69–71] The concentration of these I-compounds increased with aging,[69] but no changes or a reduced accumulation were found in liver DNA of rats administered 2,3,7,8-tetrachlorodibenzo-*p*-dioxin[70] or phenobarbital,[72] and of rats fed a choline-deficient diet.[73] The treatment of rats with several different hepatocarcinogenic estrogens resulted in an increase in non-I-compound DNA adducts in the liver.[74] A qualitatively identical major adduct pattern was observed in several tissues and species after administration of various chemical carcinogens, with the patterns being species and tissue dependent rather than carcinogen dependent, suggesting that they are more closely related to genetically determined, normal metabolic activities than to exposure to environmental carcinogens.[75] Generally, the genetic background of the host has a profound impact on the risk for the development of liver cancer as discussed in detail by Drinkwater and Lee.[76]

DOSE-RESPONSE RELATIONSHIPS IN CHEMICAL HEPATOCARCINOGENESIS

The development of liver neoplasms induced by chemicals is a complex multistage process (Fig. 15-1) that is influenced by many factors, especially the dose and the duration of carcinogenic treatment.[13,14,77] In addition to preneoplastic and neoplastic lesions, nonspecific changes and regenerative responses show characteristic dose-response relationships. Thus, perivenular cytotoxic changes resulting in cell death increase with dose but are rapidly reversible and may be replaced by parenchymal regeneration after withdrawal of the compound.[77,78] However, once fibrotic or cirrhotic changes develop as a consequence of parenchymal necrosis, these alterations may persist and may accompany hepatocarcinogenesis. In contrast, after administration of low doses of hepatocarcinogens that do not lead to appreciable parenchymal necrosis, the evolution of hepatocellular neoplasms is not complicated by any fibrosis or cirrhosis.[79] The proliferation of oval cells has also been shown to be dose dependent; these are rare or absent after low-dose treatment, but often replace pronounced parenchymal necrosis produced by high doses and have at least the potential to give rise to preneoplastic cholangiofibrosis and cholangiocellular neoplasms after long lag periods.[80]

The dose-response relationships for production of malignant liver neoplasms, mainly HCCs, by chemicals have been studied in great detail in rodents. Early investigations with 4-dimethylaminoazobenzene in rats (Druckrey[13,81]) indicated that the primary carcinogenic effects of all individual doses, even the smallest, persist and remain irreversible over the entire lifespan of the rats, accumulating until tumor formation. Accordingly, the carcinogenic action was considered as a function of all consecutive doses and called the *summation action*. Discontinuation of treatment with the same compound at total dose levels of 200, 300, 500, 700, and 1,000 mg per rat, respectively, in so-called stop experiments revealed that the carcinogenic action is not only irreversible but progresses with time although the causal agent is no longer present. In similar studies with the more potent hepatocarcinogen, diethylnitrosamine, in BDII rats[82] medium total doses [D_{50}] and the medium induction time [t_{50}] were calculated up to the appearance of malignant liver tumors in 50% of the treated rats for each of nine dosage groups (Table 15-2). It is evident that the total dose needed to produce carcinomas with small daily doses over a long period is not greater but significantly smaller than that with higher doses (Table 15-2), indicating an accelerated process without a threshold dose for this carcinogen.[14,82] In principle, the less potent hepatocarcinogens dimethylnitrosamine, *N*-nitrosopyrrolidine, and *N*-nitrosopiperidine gave similar dose-response curves for the induction of liver neoplasms, including hepatocellular, cholangiocellular, and vascular tumors. However, the development of liver neoplasms in the lower dose ranges would not have been predicted by simple extrapolation to lower doses.[14] This observation emphasizes the importance of experimental determinations of the effects of low doses to assess potential human exposure instead of theoretical conclusions from the effects of high doses.

In studies using preneoplastic FAH as end points in rats, a close statistical correlation between the dose and time of carcinogen treatment and the number and size of FAH was found in all cases.[83–92] A quantitative relationship between the early induction of defined volumes of FAH and the appearance of liver neoplasms at later time points was found.[88–90] There was also a linear dose-response relationship for the induction of FAH by doses of diethanolnitrosamine ranging from 0.2 to 25 mg/kg body weight per day at dose levels that were too low to result in manifestation of neoplasms during the lifespan of the animal species used (Fig. 15-2).[88,89] Thus, in accordance with the results of the investigations on the dose-response relationship of the induction of hepatocellular neoplasms in rats,[13] there was no indication of a threshold below which the carcinogen had no effect.[88,89]

More recently, however, several authors reported nonlinearity for the induction of preneoplastic FAH by low exposures of rats to diethylnitrosamine,[91] 2-acetyl-

TABLE 15-2. Diethylnitrosamine Carcinogenesis: Medium Total Dose and Induction Time Dependent on Daily Dosage[a]

Daily Dosage (d)	No. with Carcinomas/ No. of Survivors (No. of Animals)	Total Dose (D_{50})	Induction Time (t_{50}) (Days)	Standard Deviation (s) (%)
14.2	5/5	1000	68	8
9.6	25/25	963	101	1
4.8	25/25	660	137	3
2.4	34/34	460	192	4.7
1.2	36/36	285	238	6.5
0.6	49/49	213	355	7.1
0.3	67/67	137	457	8.9
0.15	27/30	91	609	6.3
0.075	5/7	64	840	—

[a] In milligrams per kilogram body weight, BD II rats.

(From Druckrey et al.,[82] with permission.)

Figure 15-2. Dose-time relationship of preneoplastic cell areas compared with that of liver tumors. An area density of 1% for glucose-6-phosphate dehydrogenase (G6PDH) and of 0.05% for γ-glutamyltransferase (GGT), respectively, was taken as the constant parameter of foci of altered hepatocytes. The incidence of 50% lethality from liver tumors served as the parameter for tumor development. The time taken to achieve these effects is plotted against the corresponding dose of *N*-nitrosodiethanolamine (NDELA). The parallelism of the three lines indicates an identical dose-time response dependence of G6PDH- and GGT-positive areas and of tumor development. (From Zerban et al.,[89] with permission.)

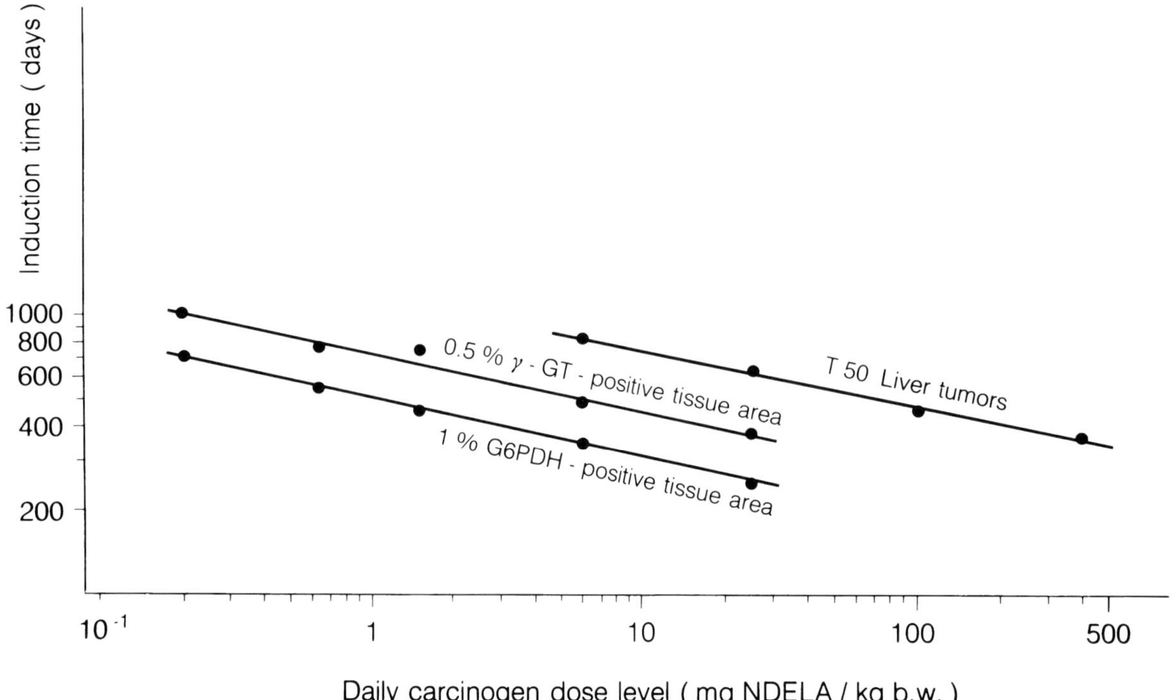

aminofluorene,[93] and N-nitrosomorpholine.[92] When N-nitrosomorpholine was given in the drinking water at dose levels ranging from 0.006 to 60 mg/L, a steep increase in the number of FAH and the parenchymal portion occupied by FAH was observed in the dose range from 6 to 60 mg N-nitrosomorpholine/L whereas a dose-dependent increase in FAH was less pronounced or not detectable at the lower dose levels. These findings are in line with observations on the incidence of liver neoplasms after treatment of rats with a wide dose range of N-nitrosomorpholine.[94] The dose-response curve for the induction of liver neoplasms showed a steeper slope in the higher dose range compared with a rather flat slope after lower doses.

These observations on the dose dependence of the development of FAH and hepatocellular neoplasms suggest that some effects of the chemicals contribute to carcinogenesis over the whole dose range, whereas other effects exert a carcinogenic influence only at higher dose levels.[92] Quantitative stereologic studies on the cellular phenotype of FAH revealed that not only the number and size but also the cellular composition of these lesions strongly depend on the dose and duration of the carcinogenic treatment and the time point of the carcinogenic process investigated (see below).[95–99]

INTERACTION BETWEEN DIFFERENT CHEMICALS IN HEPATOCARCINOGENESIS

Hepatocarcinogenesis induced by chemicals may be enhanced or inhibited by the additional administration of other chemicals through modulation of processes such as biotransformation, adduct formation, expression of phenotypic cellular changes, and neoplastic growth.[7,100,101] The synergistic effect of two or more carcinogens, syncarcinogenesis,[102,103] occurs only when the carcinogens involved have the same target tissue.[104] The carcinogens can be administered concurrently or sequentially,[100] and syncarcinogenesis is considered to result from the summation of the irreversible primary lesions caused by each compound.[104] In rodent liver, syncarcinogenic effects were demonstrated for the combined[105–109] or sequential[110–112] exposure to various hepatocarcinogens. However, the concurrent or sequential administration of two carcinogens may also result in the reduction of carcinogenicity, for example, when the induction of drug metabolizing enzymes by one of the carcinogens favors the detoxification rather than the activation of the other carcinogen.[100]

For many chemicals that are not regarded as "complete" carcinogens but rather as "cocarcinogens" or "promoters," it has been shown that their administration to rodents previously exposed to "initiating" hepatocarcinogens "promotes" the production of hepatocellular neoplasms.[6,7,100,113–115] Peraino and colleagues[113] were the first to demonstrate that administration of phenobarbital to rats previously exposed to 2-acetylaminofluorene increased the carcinoma incidence in comparison with the low incidence in animals given 2-acetylaminofluorene alone. Although the additional application of phenobarbital renders this system more sensitive, it remains a matter of debate whether this approach allows classification of chemical carcinogens into two categories, namely "initiators" and "promoters."[7,20] It should be noted that high doses of phenobarbital have been shown to induce hepatic neoplasms in both rats[116,117] and mice[118] in the absence of additional experimental manipulation. The same applies to most other compounds that can induce hepatocarcinogenesis in two-stage protocols.[7] Since phenobarbital and many other chemicals inducing hepatocarcinogenesis do not appear to interact with DNA, it has been suggested that these compounds promote preneoplastic FAH initiated fortuitously by unidentified exogenous or endogenous factors.[24,100,119] Two studies showed that phenobarbital enhances the development of certain types of FAH in rats only when administered after and not before treatment with N-nitrosomorpholine[120] or 2-acetylaminofluorene.[121] However, since only one marker for FAH was used in each of the two studies (γ-glutamyltransferase and iron deficiency, respectively) a reinvestigation of this problem using a larger number of phenotypic markers for FAH appears to be necessary. In addition, only phenobarbital has been investigated in regard to the order in which the two chemicals are administered, as noted by Williams.[100] Enhancement of hepatocarcinogenesis by many other compounds administered after the initiating carcinogen has been reported uncritically as "promotion" in the absence of appropriate controls. Thus, the possibility that the effects are additive rather than promotive cannot be excluded.

A separation of initiating and promoting effects on the liver parenchyma remains difficult and is frequently impossible. In discussions of the postulated role of pre-existing initiated cell populations in hepatocarcinogenesis induced by nongenotoxic compounds, however, the significance of such altered cell populations for the carcinogenic effect of genotoxic compounds is frequently ignored.[20] At present, there is no way of excluding the possibility that genotoxic compounds might likewise promote pre-existing initiated cell populations. Nevertheless, the assumption of "pure" promoting effects appears to be reasonable in some cases such as the enhancement of hepatocarcinogenesis initiated with nitrosamines by sucrose[122] or fructose.[123]

Of particular interest for human hepatocarcinogenesis are studies of the effects of chronic ethanol ingestion on chemical hepatocarcinogenesis.[37] The majority of these experiments were conducted with nitrosamines as initiators. Nitrosamine-induced hepatocarcinogenesis was only enhanced when ethanol was given subsequent to administration of nitrosamine[124,125] or when a methyl-deficient diet was fed simultaneously.[126] However, when ethanol was given prior to, or together with, the carcinogens, hepatocarcinogenesis was not affected[127] or even inhibited.[127–130] A fourfold increase in vinyl chloride-induced hepatic cancer was observed when ethanol was given at a concentration of 5% in the drinking water prior to, and simultaneously with, exposure to the carcinogen.[131] When AFB_1 was used for initiation of hepatocarcinogenesis in the rat, no effect on the induction of hepatocellular neoplasms by chronic ethanol ingestion was observed,[132,133] but in one experiment a significant increase in the occurrence of sinusoidal peliosis hepatis (which represents an early stage in the development of vascular liver tumors) was found.[132] It is evident from these findings that the influence of chronic alcohol ingestion on experimental chemical hepatocarcinogenesis is variable, depending on the time of ethanol ingestion and other factors. Thus, an extrapolation of these experimental observations to the risk of HCC in humans abusing alcoholic beverages is fraught with many uncertainties.

INTERACTIONS BETWEEN CHEMICAL HEPATOCARCINOGENS AND CHRONIC HEPATITIS

A strong association between chronic hepatitis, particularly due to infection with hepatitis B virus (HBV) and hepatitis C virus, and the development of human HCC is well established, although the precise mechanisms of action of these viruses in human hepatocarcinogenesis remain to be elucidated.[134] In the case of HBV infection, it has been postulated that an interaction with chemical hepatocarcinogens, especially with the mycotoxin AFB_1, might play an important role in the carcinogenic process.[5,135] The assumption that aflatoxins represent additional risk factors for hepatocarcinogenesis is based on their marked hepatocarcinogenicity in various animal species,[32] on classic epidemiologic studies,[32,136] and on molecular epidemiologic evidence for mutational hot spots in codon 249 of the p53 gene,[137–140] as well as the presence of certain urinary metabolites of aflatoxin in exposed populations.[135,141]

In two different lineages of HBV transgenic mice both overexpressing the HBV large surface antigen and developing hepatocellular neoplasms,[142,143] intraperitoneal injection of several chemical carcinogens, including AFB_1, diethylnitrosamine, and 4-dimethylaminoazobenzene, resulted in an earlier appearance and higher incidence and size of liver neoplasms than in nontransgenic mice.[144,145] A combination of various factors, such as altered metabolic activation of the chemicals by induction of hepatocellular enzymes in transgenic mice and HBV-mediated necroinflammation eliciting regenerative cell proliferation, were discussed as possible explanations for the synergistic effects.[5] In ducks chronically infected with the duck hepatitis virus (DHBV), which belongs to the same family of DNA viruses (hepadnaviridae) as HBV, the combination of viral hepatitis and AFB_1 administered intraperitoneally did not result in an increased incidence of HCC.[146–148] In any case, the significance of these experiments for human hepatocarcinogenesis is unclear.[32]

The influence of AFB_1 in woodchucks (*Marmota monax*) chronically infected with the woodchuck hepatitis virus (WHV), another member of the hepadnaviridae, has been the subject of two studies, one inconclusive[149] and one showing a synergistic hepatocarcinogenic effect of hepadnaviral infection and dietary AFB_1.[150] In the latter study, oral administration of low doses of AFB_1 to WHV carriers resulted in a significantly earlier appearance of hepatocellular neoplasms and a higher incidence of HCCs compared with WHV carriers not treated with AFB_1. Striking similarities in altered cellular phenotypes of preneoplastic FAH emerging after both hepadnaviral infection and exposure to AFB_1 suggest closely related underlying molecular mechanisms.[150] A synergistic hepatocarcinogenic effect of chronic hepadnaviral infection and AFB_1 was also demonstrated in tree shrews (*Tupaia belangeri chinensis*).[151,152] The incidence of HCC was significantly higher in the animals both infected with HBV and exposed to AFB_1 (53%) than in those solely infected with HBV (11%) or exposed to AFB_1 alone (13%); in all groups, the development of HCC was preceded by emergence of preneoplastic FAH positive for γ-glutamyltransferase.[152]

Infestation with certain liver flukes has long been considered to play an important role in the development of liver neoplasms, particularly cholangiocellular carcinomas in humans.[5,153] Treatment of hamsters infected with *Opisthorchis viverrini metacercaria* with dimethylnitrosamine has been shown to produce a high yield of cholangiocellular carcinomas and hepatocellular adenomas.[154–156] Although the precise mechanism of the interaction between flukes and chemicals is unclear, the development of cholangiocarcinomas in hamsters treated with nitrite and aminopyrine (precursors of endogenous nitrosamine formation)[157] and the potentiation of this effect in *Opisthorchis viverrini*-infested animals[158] support the hypothesis[153] that endogenous nitrosation and nitrosamine formation occur during parasite infestation.[5]

STAGES OF NEOPLASTIC DEVELOPMENT IN THE LIVER

Conventionally, the process of hepatocarcinogenesis is subdivided into the stages of initiation, promotion, and progression.[6,7,114,159,160] This concept had originally been inferred from experiments in which two- or three-stage protocols were used to induce tumors of the skin, liver, or other tissues.[54] However, an unequivocal explanation of these operationally defined stages in biologic terms has never been proffered. The more recent approach to separate several stages of neoplastic development in terms of genetic and epigenetic alterations, which has particularly been applied to colon carcinogenesis,[161] cannot be applied to hepatocarcinogenesis at present. Although a variety of molecular genetic events have been described in animal models of chemical hepatocarcinogenesis, a consistent sequence of molecular genetic changes has hitherto not been established.[6,16,162] Adaptive cellular responses have been suggested to play a crucial role.[78,163,164]

The discovery of characteristic sequential cellular changes during neoplastic development in the liver (and some other tissues) has opened a new approach for the distinction of stages of carcinogenesis, which can now be defined on the basis of biologic rather than operational criteria.[16,165] Preneoplasia has been defined in this context as the presence of phenotypically altered cell populations that have no obvious neoplastic nature but that represent an increased risk of the development of both benign and malignant neoplasia.[22] As a rule, preneoplasia and neoplasia are successive stages in a biologic continuum leading from the normal to the malignant state (Fig. 15-3). However, neoplasia may also arise directly from preneoplastic lesions without passing through the benign intermediate stage in the continuum.[166,167] Another exception to the rule is that some specific types of epithelial neoplasm, such as cystic cholangiomas, are benign end stages that do not progress to malignancy. Focal preneoplastic lesions frequently persist over long periods without giving rise to overt neoplasia, but this observation does not detract from their well-established significance as early indicators of neoplastic development.[20,21]

CELLULAR ORIGIN OF LIVER NEOPLASMS

The epithelial compartment of the liver is composed of long-living hepatocytes and biliary epithelial cells, the replacement of which, under normal conditions or during physiologic regeneration after liver resection, is attained by the proliferation of residual differentiated cells of each type; this obviates the need for stem cells to renew hepatocellular and cholangiocellular lineages.[168] Recent studies on the location of genetically tagged hepatocytes[169] and on the size of patches in livers of genetically mosaic, chimeric animals[170] provided compelling evidence for a clonal or quasiclonal proliferation of hepatocytes during normal liver growth, which does not follow the liver cell plates in a linear pattern. Despite the fact that stem cells do not appear to be needed under physiologic conditions, it has been a matter of debate for decades whether oval cells, which derive from the epithelia of the cholangioles[171] and often appear early during hepatocarcinogenesis in rodents,[172] may represent facultative liver stem cells that may give rise to both cholangiocelullar and hepatocellular neoplasms.[173–178]

Figure 15-3. Schematic diagram of the stages of neoplastic development as defined in terms of phenotypic cellular changes. (From Bannasch,[19] with permission.)

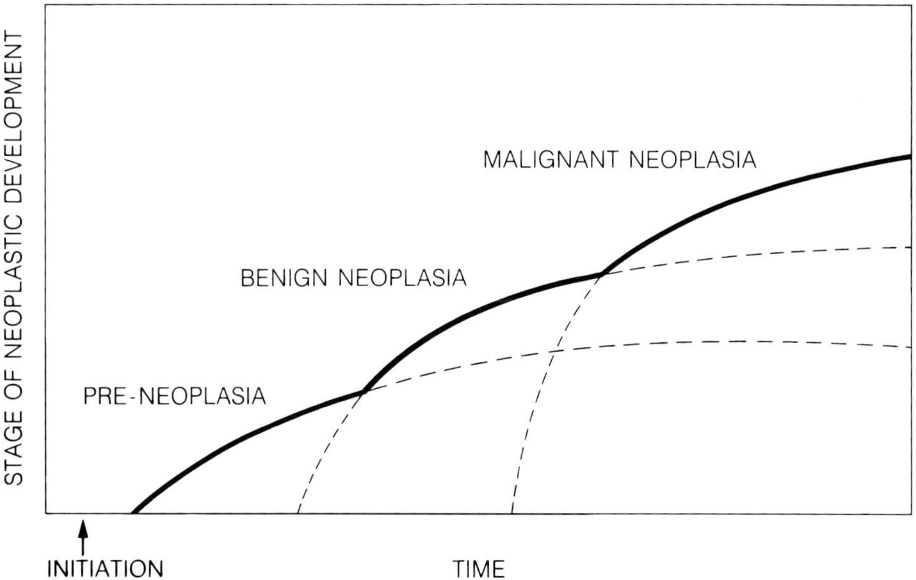

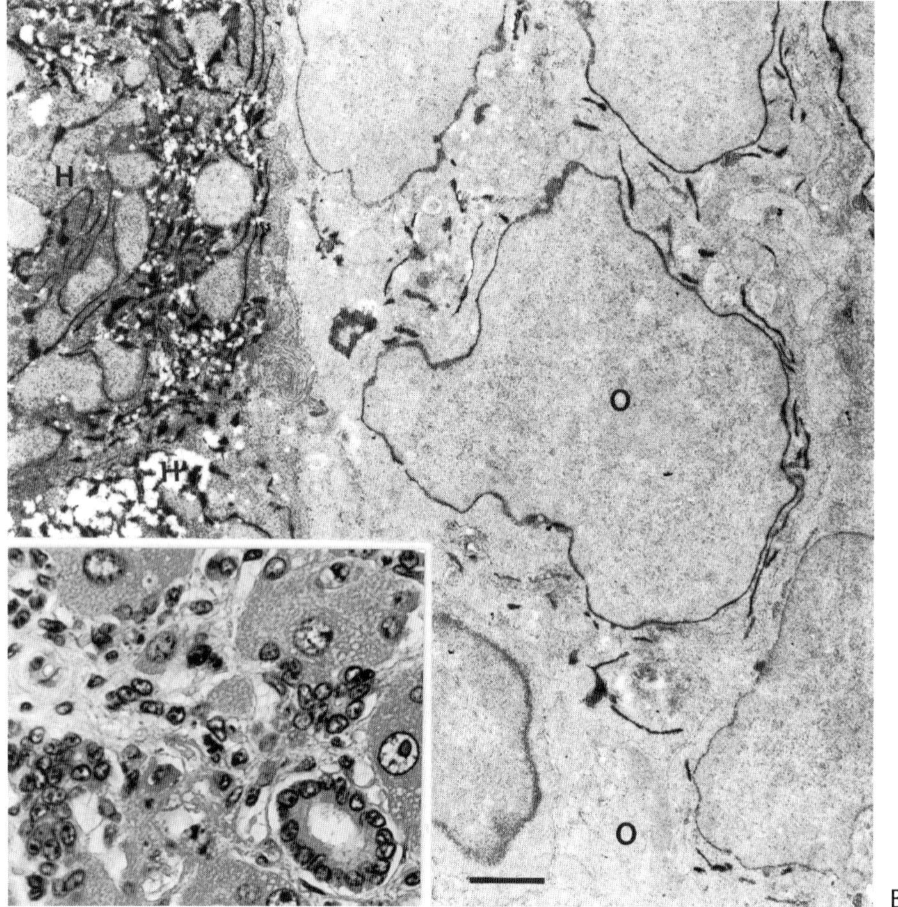

Figure 15-4. Cholangiolar (oval) cell proliferation induced in rat liver with *N*-nitrosomorpholine. (*A*) Light micrograph of oval cell proliferation with formation of ductule. (H&E, ×570.) (*B*) Electron micrograph of oval cells (O) and portions of hepatocytes (H) with enzyme histochemical demonstration of activity of glucose-6-phosphatase in membranes of endoplasmic reticulum and nuclear envelope. (Original magnification ×14,000.)

Oval cell proliferation (Fig. 15-4) develops only after high doses of chemical carcinogens and results in pronounced toxic damage of parenchymal liver cells.[77,80,179–181] Although many of the proliferated oval cells undergo necrotic changes and subsequently disappear,[181–185] persisting oval cell populations may proceed to preneoplastic cholangiofibrosis and neoplastic cholangiocellular lesions in rat liver.[80,179,186–193] Similar sequential changes were observed in other species treated with chemical carcinogens, particularly in hamsters[155,194,195] with and without additional infestation by the liver fluke *Opisthorchis viverrini*. The term *cholangiofibrosis*[196] is in line with the concept that the epithelial component of this preneoplastic lesion derives from duct-type cells that in turn originate from the terminal branches of the biliary system, the cholangioles.[80,176,197] Some authors called the same lesion *adenofibrosis*, implying that its ductular component derives from hepatocytes.[198,199] Recently, Jamison et al[200] proposed retention of this designation, although they regard a stem-like cell, possibly identical with the oval cell, as the site of origin of this pathomorphologic entity, for which they explicitly claim a "non-bile duct origin." However, since nearly all findings favor the notion of an origin of the oval cell compartment from the cholangioles, the classification of this preneoplastic lesion as cholangiofibrosis appears to be most appropriate.

The hypothesis that a subpopulation of the oval cell compartment represents committed precursor cells capable of differentiating into hepatocytes and hepatoma cells remains controversial.[16,175,176] An obligatory role of oval cells in the evolution of hepatocellular neoplasms has been excluded by the experimental finding that with low doses of strong hepatocarcinogens HCC develops without any preceding oval cell proliferation.[77,180] This finding does not completely rule out the possibility, however, that oval cells might be precursors of HCC under other experimental conditions.[201–209] Phenotypic plasticity of oval cells, which may acquire several features similar to those of hepatocytes (e.g., expression of albumin, α-fetoprotein and glucose-6-phosphatase; formation of peroxisomes and smooth endoplasmic reticulum), has been demonstrated.[176–178,210,211] However, using similar methodologic approaches other groups did not observe transitions from oval cells to parenchymal cells or HCC.[179,180,184,185,193,212–214] For example, in rats receiving a choline deficient/ethionine supplemented diet, unequivocal evidence for a differentiation of oval cells to hepatocytes and hepatoma cells was obtained neither in situ[179,193] nor after subcutaneous transplantation of oval cells in vitro.[213] Doubts about the existence of such a differentiation pathway have also been expressed by a number of other authors in the last few years.[180,214–216] There is abundant evidence, however, that the opposite process, namely, a transdifferentiation (metaplasia) from a hepatocellular to a cholangiocellular phenotype, may occur during neoplastic transformation in rodents.[18,217,218]

The assumption of a differentiation process during neoplastic development contrasts with the concept of a progressive dedifferentiation of mature hepatocytes during hepatocarcinogenesis. The most compelling new evidence for this old hypothesis has been provided by the observation that the manifestation of HCC induced in various species by chemicals, viruses, transgenes, or radiation is always preceded by FAH. The earliest emerging types of FAH are composed of differentiated hepatocytes that show characteristic metabolic and molecular aberrations and gradually progress via various intermediate forms to the malignant phenotype.[16,78,166] Similarly, a progressive dedifferentiation appears to take place during the evolution of cholangiocellular neoplasms from preneoplastic cholangiofibrosis[80,179,188] and during the development of angiosarcomas[17,219] or perisinusoidal cell sarcomas[220,221] from the sinusoidal endothelial and the perisinusoidal cells, respectively. Distinction between these cell lineages has been assisted by immunohistochemical demonstration of different types of intermediate filaments of the cytoskeleton (Fig. 15-5) that are characteristics of the cells of origin, including cytokeratins, vimentin, and desmin (Fig. 15-6).[179,213,220,222,223]

Figure 15-5. Electron micrograph showing peripheral regions of HCC cells from rat liver treated with *N*-nitrosomorpholine. Note bundles of intermediate filaments of the cytokeratin type, many of which are attached to desmosomes. Bar = 1 μm. (Original magnification $\times$35,000.) (From Bannasch et al.,[223] with permission.)

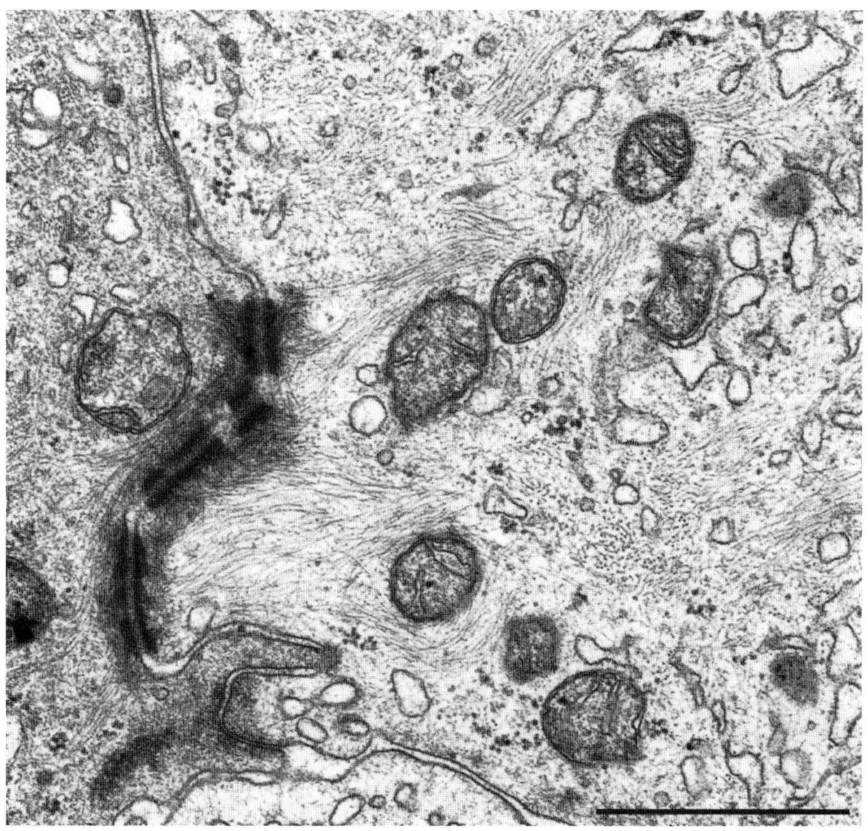

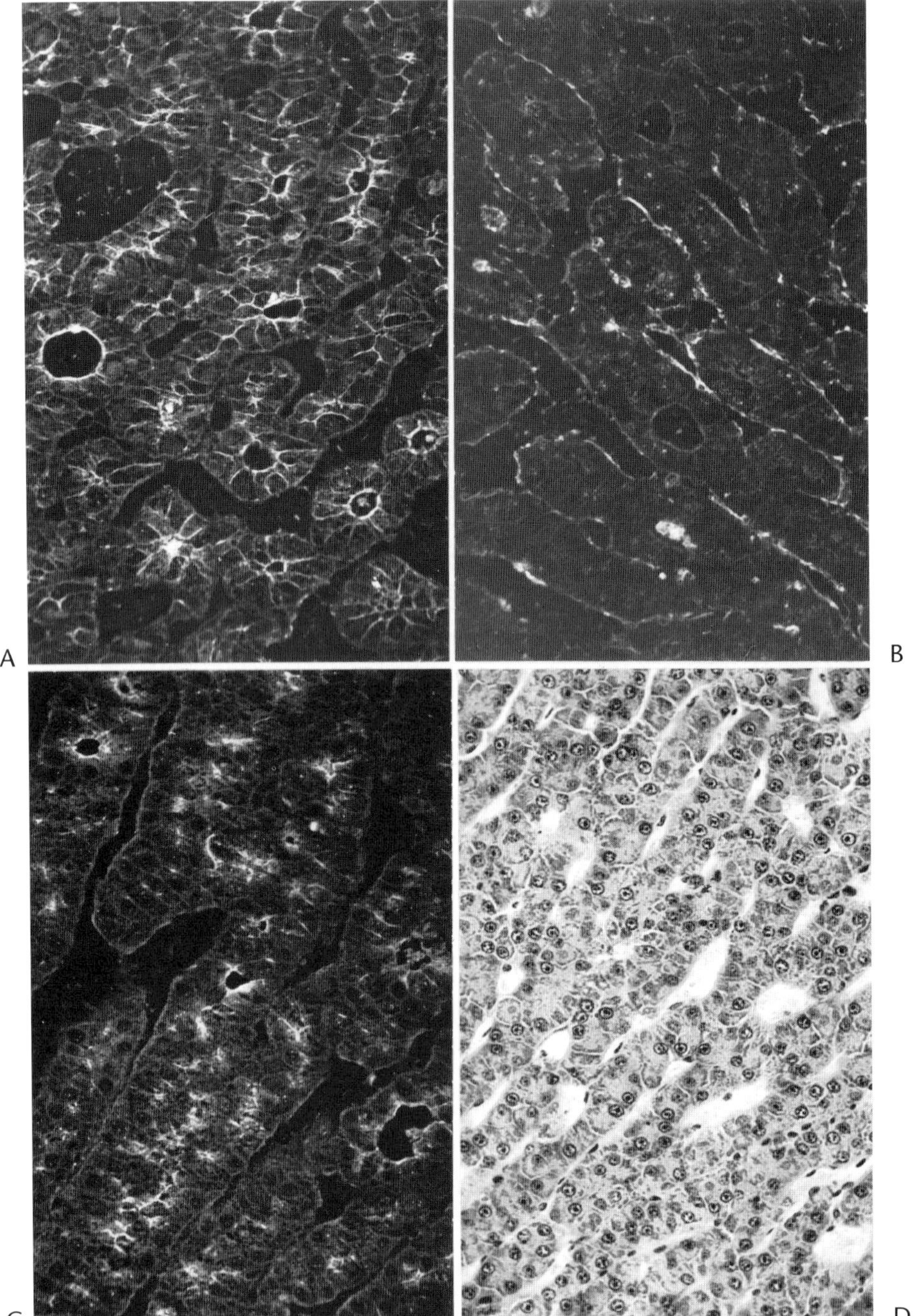

Figure 15-6. Light micrographs of trabecular hepatocellular carcinomas prepared as frozen (*A–C*) or (*D*) paraffin sections from rat liver treated with *N*-nitrosomorpholine. Immunofluorescence microscopic demonstration of (*A*) cytokeratins in carcinoma cells, (*B*) vimentin in sinusoidal lining cells, and (*C*) actin by antibodies to the specific proteins. (*D*) Histologic pattern as shown by staining with H&E. (Original magnification *A–C*, ×270; *D*, ×200.) (From Bannasch et al.,[223] with permission.)

HEPATOCELLULAR CHANGES DURING NEOPLASTIC DEVELOPMENT

Preneoplastic FAH (Fig. 15-7) precede the manifestation of both benign and malignant hepatocellular neoplasms by weeks or months. They were discovered more than three decades ago in rat livers treated with nitrosamines[224,225] and have since been described in a large number of species including primates after administration of virtually all classes of chemical carcinogens.[20–22,159,160,226–228] The main cytomorphologic and cytochemical alterations initially found in early FAH were a clear or acidophilic cytoplasm associated with an excessive storage of glycogen (glycogenosis)[78,224] and a reduction in the activities of glucose-6-phospha-

Figure 15-7. Enzyme histochemical pattern of glycogen storage focus induced in rat liver with *N*-nitrosomorpholine (serial frozen sections). (*A*) Excessive storage of glycogen (PAS). (*B*) Reduced activity of glucose-6-phosphatase. (*C*) Reduced activity of adenylate cyclase. (*D*) Reduced activity of adenosine triphosphatase. (*E*) Increased activity of glutathione S-transferase placental form. (*F*) Increased activity of glucose-6-phosphate dehydrogenase. (Original magnification ×300.) (Courtesy of Dr. H. J. Hacker.)

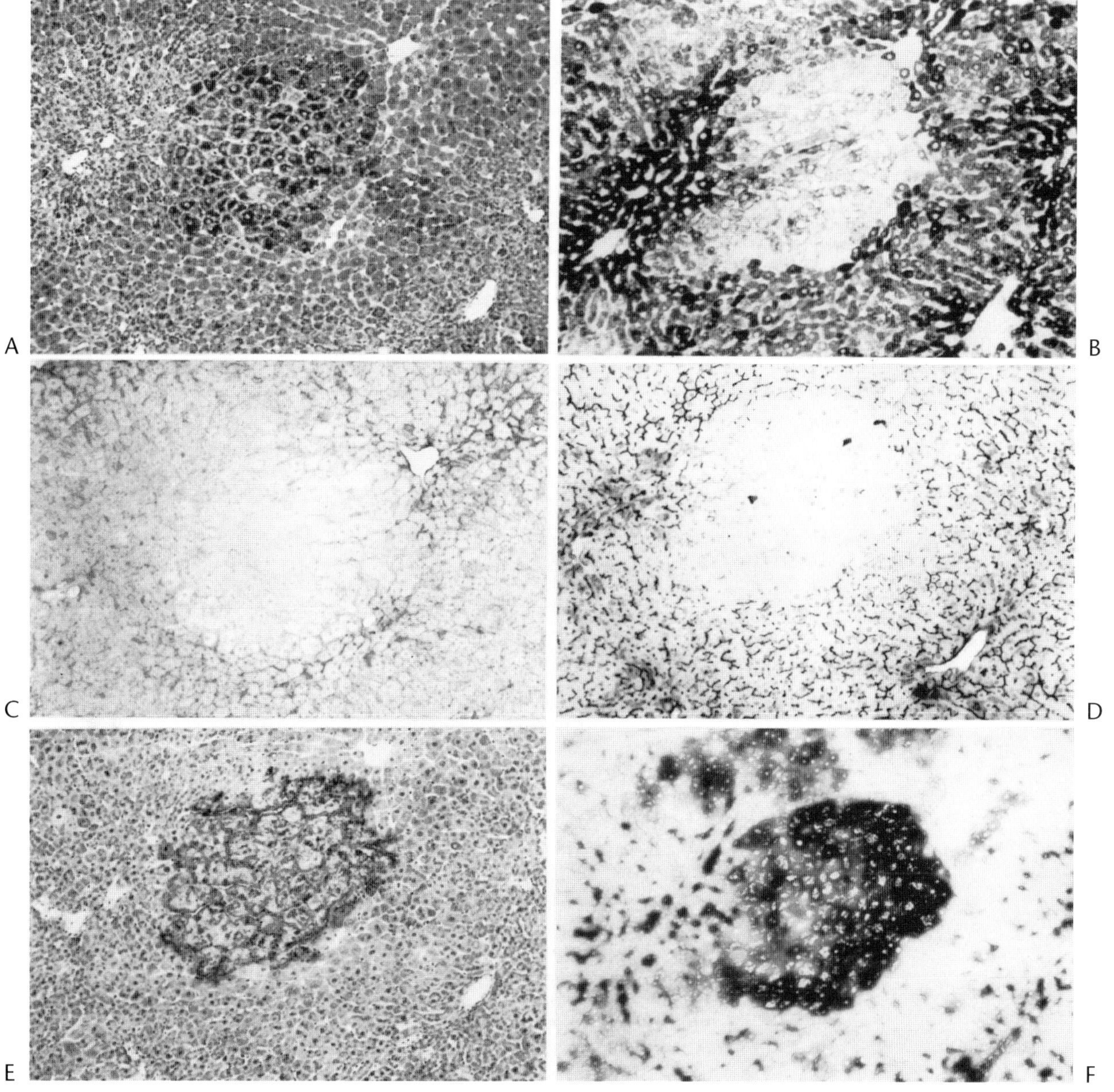

tase[225,229] and the plasma membrane-bound adenosine triphosphatase.[230,231] Additional aberrations of enzymes of carbohydrate metabolism,[16,232], drug metabolism,[21,90] iron metabolism,[233–236] and different components of intracellular signaling pathways[16,237–239] have been observed. The morphologic and the biochemical phenotypes of FAH are neither uniform nor stable. Despite a marked heterogeneity in the cellular phenotype within many FAH, observations in several laboratories suggest a clonal origin of the focal lesions.[240–244] The results of morphometric studies do not exclude this possibility for the earliest foci, but they argue in favor of alterations of many hepatocytes running parallel in larger cell populations rather than repeated clonal selection during the progression of hepatocarcinogenesis.[96,245]

Cellular Metamorphosis

Based on cytomorphologic and simple cytochemical criteria, at least eight types of preneoplastic FAH may be distinguished in rodent liver, that are integrated within three cell lineages (Fig. 15-8) leading to hepatocellular neoplasms.[16,19,227,246] The foci are usually located in peripheral or intermediate parts of the liver lobule corresponding to zones 1 and 2 as defined by Rappaport (see Bannasch[78] and Maguire and Rabes[247]), but after continuous administration of low doses of carcinogens they may start to develop in perivenular regions.[248] Persistent (neoplastic) nodules,[166] which have been classified as hepatocellular adenomas more recently,[18,249] and partially remodeling hepatocyte nodules[250] are frequent interim lesions in the development of HCC from FAH. However, malignant neoplasms may also derive directly from FAH without passing through a benign nodular intermediate stage.[166,167] The predominant sequence of cellular changes (Fig. 15-8) commences with clear and acidophilic cell foci excessively storing glycogen and progresses through mixed cell populations to glycogen-poor, basophilic (ribosome-rich) neoplastic formations.[78,163] The (reticular) cytoplasmic acidophilia of many cells of this lineage is due to a proliferation of the smooth endoplasmic reticulum (Fig. 15-9)[78,163,251] that may be transformed into rough endoplasmic reticulum during neoplastic progression.[78,163] The second cell lineage (Fig. 15-8) is characterized by tigroid basophilic cells (endowed with abundant and highly ordered stacks of the rough endoplasmic reticulum) that may eventually transform into homogeneously basophilic cell populations[252]; these probably represent a variant of the predominant lineage, appearing mainly after low-dose treatment.[97–99,252] The third cell lineage (Fig. 15-8) consists of amphophilic cells with a combination of densely packed granula acidophilic and homogeneously distributed or scattered basophilic cytoplasmic components.[227,253] The amphophilic cell foci are extremely rare after administration of most chemical hepatocarcinogens but are the main phenotype of FAH produced in rats by nongenotoxic agents that induce peroxisomal and mitochondrial proliferations.[59,253–255] Recent investigations on the sequential appearance and ultrastructure of amphophilic cell foci, adenomas, and carcinomas produced by the adrenal hormone dehydroepiandrosterone, which is also a peroxisomal proliferator, revealed that the amphophilic character of these lesions is due to a pronounced proliferation of mitochondria wrapped in rough endoplasmic reticulum, mixed with variable numbers of peroxisomes (Fig. 15-10).[59] An increased number of mitochondria in the hepatocytes is also a consistent feature in early stages of hepatocarcinogenesis induced by administration of methapyrilene to rats.[256]

The phenotype of tigroid and amphophilic cells is often maintained in the neoplasms so that the relationship between the preneoplastic FAH and the respective hepatocellular neoplasms can be inferred without great difficulty. The recognition of the cell lineage leading from glycogenotic clear and acidophilic cell foci to glycogen-poor, basophilic neoplasms is much more difficult, but this sequence in the rat liver has been substantiated in a series of morphometric studies after treatment with *N*-nitrosomorpholine.[95–99] An early increase in the number of small glycogenotic foci is regularly followed by a gradual increase in the number of larger, mixed and basophilic cell lesions, the appearance of which correlates significantly with the later emergence of HCC. Such a sequence is not only evident after continuous administration of the carcinogenic agent[99] but also in stop experiments.[95,96,98] In this experimental approach, the carcinogen is given for a limited time (e.g. 3–7 weeks), which is too short to produce neoplasia during the treatment phase but long enough to result in neoplasia (without any additional experimental manipulation) within the lifespan of the animal.[78] An additional argument for the proposed sequence is the gradual increase in cell proliferation (as determined by the incorporation of ^{3}H-thymidine in the stop model of hepatocarcinogenesis) from glycogenotic through mixed cell foci to hepatocellular adenomas and carcinomas, among which glycogen-poor lesions proliferate much faster than glycogen-rich forms.[257,258] It is evident from these results that there is an inverse correlation between glycogen accumulation and cell proliferation during the progression from the glycogenotic preneoplastic to the malignant neoplastic phenotype. Alterations in the phenotype of hepatocytes persisting for a long time after stopping treatment with hepatocarcinogens may also occur in the extrafocal parenchyma. Thus, a marked increase in cell and nuclear size[163,259] and a reduction in the number of binucleate hepatocytes[259] were found in rats treated for 7 weeks with *N*-nitrosomorpholine. Although FAH are the most striking and probably also the most important phenotypic alterations in early stages of hepatocarcinogenesis, a participation of persisting extrafocal changes

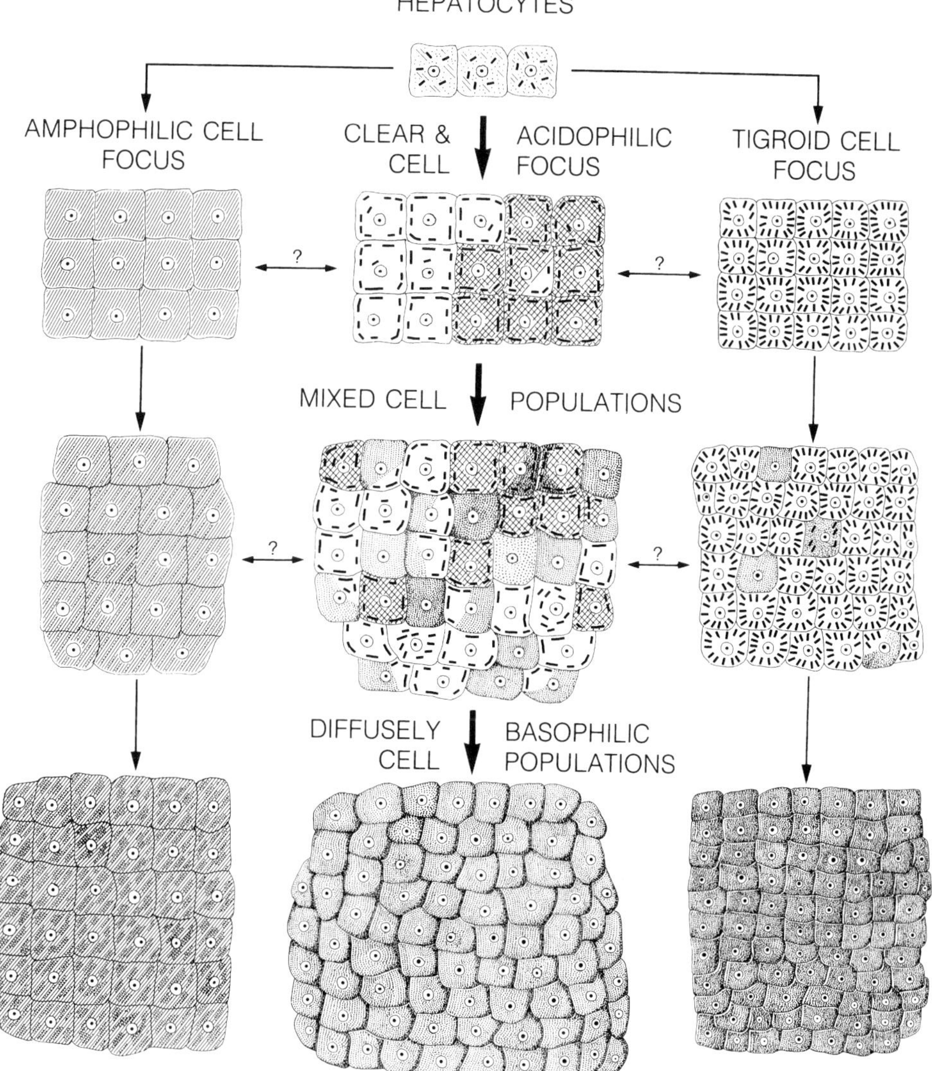

Figure 15-8. Schematic diagram of sequential cellular changes during the development of hepatocellular neoplasms in rodent liver. The predominant sequence of cellular changes (center) commences with glycogenotic clear and acidophilic (reticular cytoplasmic acidophilia due to a proliferation of the smooth endoplasmic reticulum) cell foci and progresses through intermediate phenotypes in mixed cell populations to glycogen-poor, homogeneously basophilic (ribosome-rich) cellular phenotypes prevailing in undifferentiated HCCs. The tigroid basophilic cell lineage (right) is initially characterized by cells with abundant highly ordered stacks of the rough endoplasmic reticulum and seems to represent a variant of the glycogenotic-basophilic cell lineage, occurring especially after low-dose treatment with hepatocarcinogens. The amphophilic cell lineage (left), which has hitherto mainly been described in rats treated with nongenotoxic peroxisome proliferators and in woodchucks chronically infected with the WHV, consists of cells with a glycogen-poor cytoplasm containing both abundant granular-acidophilic (mitochondria and peroxisomes) and basophilic (ribosomes) components. (From Bannasch,[19] with permission.)

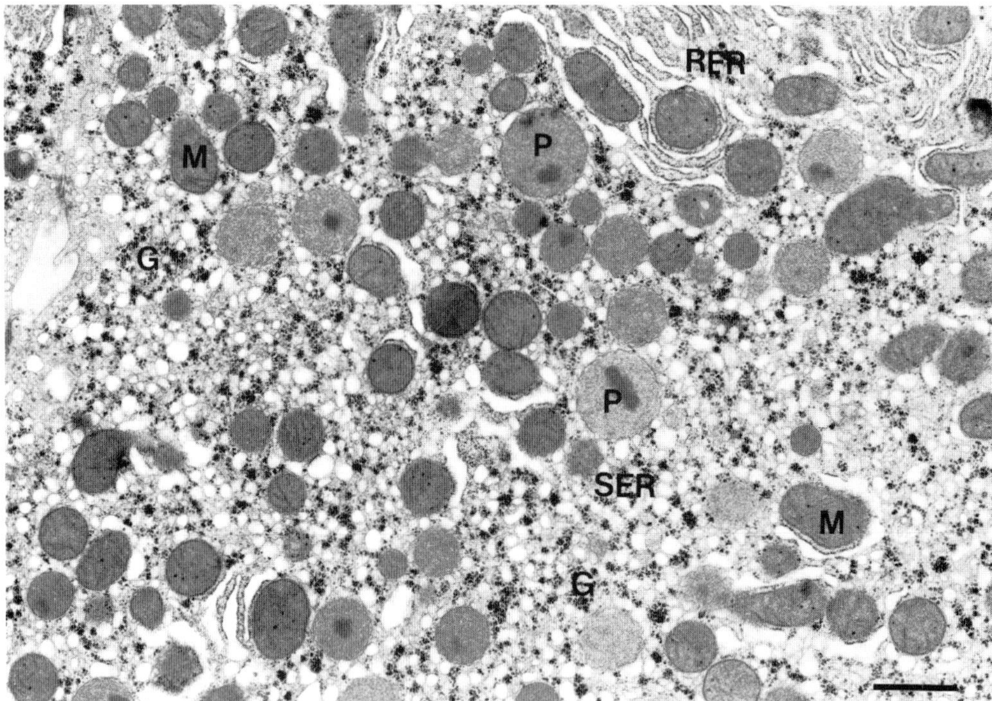

Figure 15-9. Electron micrograph of portion of acidophilic glycogen storage cell induced in rat liver with *N*-nitrosomorpholine. Glycogen (G), abundant smooth endoplasmic reticulum (SER), rough endoplasmic reticulum (RER), mitochondria (M), and peroxisomes (P). Lead citrate and uranyl acetate. Bar = 1 μm. (Original magnification ×14 200.)

cannot be excluded.[254] This holds especially true for the so-called X-cells (enlarged hepatocytes containing abundant glycogens as well as smooth and rough endoplasmic reticulum),[163,260] which are a possible precursor of tigroid cell foci and of hepatocellular neoplasms arising from these foci.[252]

The sequential cellular changes involved in neoplastic development are associated with a progression-linked phenotypic instability that is characterized by irreversible morphologic and biochemical alterations.[20,22,261] However, during the repeated administration of high but sublethal doses of one carcinogenic agent, a reversion-linked phenotypic instability, admitting the reappearance of less altered cellular phenotypes after withdrawal of these agents may occur.[20,22,97–99,159,160,226,261] The cause of reversion-linked phenotypic instability is poorly understood. However, this phenomenon is by no means only associated with agents considered to promote rather than initiate hepatocarcinogenesis. It may appear after withdrawal of high doses of unequivocal complete carcinogens such as *N*-nitrosomorpholine.[261,262] At lower dose levels of *N*-nitrosomorpholine, FAH are elicited without any indication of reversibility.[95,98] Reversion-linked phenotypic instability does not seem to result in a reconstitution of the normal phenotype but in a replacement of a more advanced phenotype (e.g., mixed cell populations) by less altered phenotypes (e.g., clear or acidophilic cell populations).[98] When the administration of the complete carcinogen is continued, instead of a reversion a rapid progression of FAH to HCC takes place.[99] This progression is associated with the frequent emergence of acidophilic and acidophilic/basophilic cell populations well known from many "promoting" regimens. The similarity in the effects exerted by complete carcinogens (so-called initiators) and "promoters" suggests that the differences between their mechanisms of action are quantitative rather than qualitative.[99]

Cell Proliferation and Cell Death (Apoptosis)

Cell proliferation is considered to play an important role in hepatocarcinogenesis,[160,263,264] with a number of authors postulating that it is a prerequisite for initiation of hepatocarcinogenesis by chemicals. In many animal experiments it has been shown that the carcinogenic effect of chemicals can be increased considerably by using a preceding partial hepatectomy to cause a strong regenerative cell proliferation.[263,265] Such an enhancing effect of a previous partial hepatectomy has also been

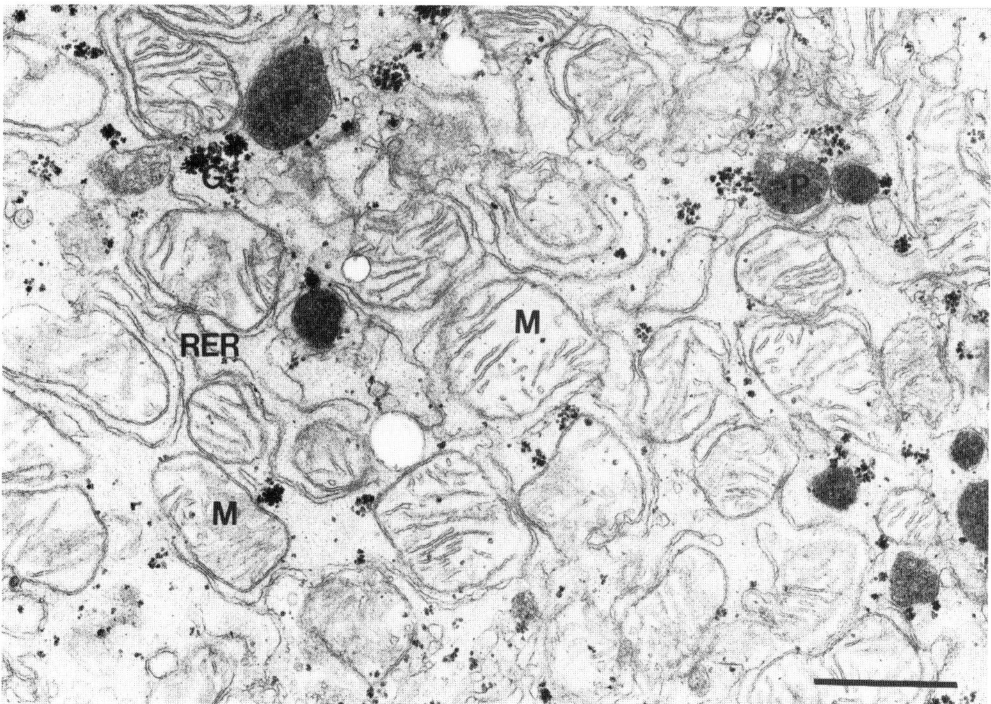

Figure 15-10. Electron micrograph of portion of amphophilic cell induced in rat liver with dehydroepiandrosterone. Abundant mitochondria (M) wrapped with rough endoplasmic reticulum (RER), some peroxisomes (P) stained by the DAB method, and rare glycogen particles (G). Lead citrate. Bar = 1 μm. (Original magnification ×24,000.) (Courtesy of C. Metzger.)

demonstrated for the induction of FAH.[83,265] Partial hepatectomy carried out after administration of the carcinogen has been reported either to have no effect[265] or to enhance the appearance of FAH.[266–269] Consistent with the latter observation, a significantly higher incidence of FAH has been reported in the rapidly proliferating neonatal rodent liver than in the adult rodent liver after treatment with various carcinogens.[270–274] When proliferation of rat hepatocytes was synchronized by hydroxyurea after partial hepatectomy, they had the highest risk of being initiated when they traversed the early S phase of the cell cycle.[275,276] The mechanism of the enhancing effect of partial hepatectomy on hepatocarcinogenesis is not entirely clear, but it is generally assumed that alterations in DNA brought about by the carcinogen are "fixed" and hence become persistent during cell replication. An alternative explanation proposed by Tanaka et al.[265] is that reduced liver mass might lead to a higher dose per unit liver tissue in hepatectomized rats. However, both explanations fail to explain the observation reported by Bartsch et al.[277] that an enhancing effect of partial hepatectomy is still demonstrable when the carcinogen is given 8 to 10 weeks after the operation, when both the liver mass and cell replication should be back to the normal state.

Columbano et al.[278] and Ledda-Columbano et al.[279] found that the cell proliferation induced by "mitogens" such as lead nitrate or cyproterone acetate, unlike compensatory cell replication induced by partial hepatectomy, did not result in increased number of FAH despite the fact that the extent of cell proliferation at the time of carcinogen administration, as determined by the examination of labeled cells, was similar with both types of proliferative stimuli.[278,279] Repeated proliferative stimuli induced in rat liver by lead nitrate or ethylene dibromide also did not exert any enhancing effect on the development of FAH initiated with diethylnitrosamine.[280] It is evident from these observations that DNA synthesis per se is not sufficient to enhance hepatocarcinogenesis.[264] An elevated expression of a mitosis-associated polypeptide with a molecular weight of 14,000 Da, which was shown previously to be a target for 2-acetylaminofluorene and 3′-methyl-4-dimethylaminoazobenzene in rat liver, was detected by immunohistochemical methods in proliferating FAH, partly basophilic hepatocellular adenomas and carcinomas but not in predominantly acidophilic adenomas induced in rats by these chemicals.[281]

FAH are characterized by enhanced cell proliferation, which increases with time[230,263] and is correlated with increasing expression of different marker enzymes.[25,282,283] However, autoradiographic studies of different types of FAH induced in the stop model revealed that incorporation of ^{3}H-thymidine is only slightly enhanced in the clear and acidophilic glycogen storage foci, but increases gradually with increasing appearance of basophilic cells in mixed and basophilic cell foci and in adenomas and carcinomas.[257,258] Inhibition of cell replication in the extrafocal parenchyma as described in the Solt-Farber and related experimental models of hepatocarcinogenesis[284,285] is by no means a prerequisite of hepatocarcinogenesis in general, since it does not occur in the "stop model" of hepatocarcinogenesis.[257,258] These findings are at variance with the resistance hepatocyte concept of hepatocarcinogenesis proposed by Farber and Sarma,[160] which is based on the assumption that carcinogens are mitoinhibitors for normal but not for initiated preneoplastic cells. The mitoinhibitory effect of hepatocarcinogens has usually been observed after high doses, and in this case the relative resistance of preneoplastic cell populations to toxic effects of the carcinogen[160] obviously accelerates the carcinogenic process.

An increase in cell proliferation from preneoplastic hepatic foci to hepatocellular adenomas and carcinomas has been reported to be associated with a progressive decrease in the expression of connexin 32,[286] a major liver gap junction protein, which had previously been shown to be reduced in preneoplastic and/or neoplastic hepatic lesions.[287,288] The gradual increase in cell proliferation during hepatocarcinogenesis is also accompanied by an increase in the number of cells undergoing apoptosis.[258,289–291] Whereas some authors feel that apoptosis might represent an important protective mechanism slowing the growth of FAH and hepatocellular neoplasms,[289,291] others emphasize that cell death occurs more frequently in the course of hepatocarcinogenesis, as neoplastic development advances.[258,290] It has been suggested that the ability of chemicals to enhance hepatocarcinogenesis in a two-stage protocol may be the consequence of inhibition of apoptosis and not necessarily their stimulatory effect on cell replication.[291] Small nonpersisting FAH that apparently disappear due to cellular necrosis have been observed in stop experiments with *N*-nitrosomorpholine.[292]

Nuclear Morphology and Ploidy

A great variety of changes in nuclear morphology and ploidy have been described during chemical hepatocarcinogenesis in rodents, particularly in FAH, but these may be facultative rather than obligatory events in the neoplastic conversion of the hepatocytes.[224,293–295] Controversial results have been published on the ploidy distribution during chemical hepatocarcinogenesis in rodents. Whereas some authors emphasize the emergence of diploid cell populations early in hepatocarcinogenesis,[296–302] others have found a variable ploidy distribution in FAH.[24,303–310] In accordance with previous interpretations,[197,306,309] these findings indicate that changes in ploidy distribution are not of essential significance to hepatocarcinogenesis. The appearance of aneuploidy in FAH has, however, been regarded by several authors as a risk factor that increases their probability of progression.[303,305,309,310] A striking reduction in binucleate cells has been reported[308] but with an increase in mononucleate cells in FAH, suggesting an altered mitotic mechanism. Dose-dependent nuclear enlargement in hepatocytes has recently been reported as a possible early indicator of carcinogenic effects in embryonal turkey liver after in ovo exposure to diethylnitrosamine.[311]

Oncogenes, Tumor Suppressor Genes, and Growth Factors

Changes in the structure and/or function of proto-oncogenes have been observed in hepatocellular neoplasms induced by chemicals.[6,162,227,312–315] Activation of *ras* oncogenes, particularly c-H-*ras*, is a frequent, albeit not ubiquitous event during spontaneous and chemically induced hepatocarcinogenesis in mice[315] and may appear early in this process.[316,317] In rats, however, hepatocellular neoplasms produced by chemicals rarely show *ras* gene activation, except in those elicited by AFB_1[6,314,316,318] Although changes in a number of proto-oncogenes have been described in liver cell tumors of rodents treated with chemicals, we were unable to detect mutations in c-*myc*, c-*fos*, and c-*raf* in hepatocellular carcinomas induced in rats by limited exposure (stop model) to *N*-nitrosomorpholine.[16] There is little information about the behaviour of oncogenes in early stages of chemical hepatocarcinogenesis. Overexpression of c-*myc* was demonstrated by in situ hybridization in FAH[16] and in hepatocellular adenomas induced in rats by nitrosamines.[319] Preneoplastic hepatic foci produced in rats by the Solt-Farber procedure and identified by their immunohistochemically demonstrated expression of the placental form of glutathione S-transferase showed some overexpression of c-*myc*[320] and c-*jun*.[321,322] The product of the c-*myc* proto-oncogene acts as a transcription factor that, according to studies in transgenic mice, regulates hepatic glycolysis.[323] Overexpression of c-*raf* was also found in different types of preneoplastic hepatic foci[16] and in hepatocellular adenomas and carcinomas[287]; c-*raf* occupies a central position in signal transduction pathways regulating glycogen metabolism, in addition to playing a general role in control of cell proliferation and differentiation.[324] Thus, although mutational activation of proto-oncogenes does not seem to be essential for chemical hepatocarcinogenesis, overexpression of such genes may be of importance to neoplastic transformation of hepatocytes.

In experimental chemical hepatocarcinogenesis, the tumor suppressor gene *p53* has been studied in some detail. In preneoplastic FAH[325] and in oval cells[326] an accumulation of the *p53* protein was demonstrated immunohistochemically in rat liver. However, in hepatocellular neoplasms produced by a number of chemicals in mice, mutations were not detected in any tumors.[327–330] In mice with a targeted disruption of one or both alleles of *p53*, there was no increase in the incidence of either hepatocellular neoplasms or preneoplastic FAH after diethylnitrosamine compared with mice with wild-type *p53*.[331]

The role of growth factors in chemical hepatocarcinogenesis[6,313,332] include an overexpression of transforming growth factor α (TGF-α). Immunohistochemical approaches revealed an increased expression of TGF-α in advanced chemical-induced preneoplastic hepatic foci positive for glutathione S-transferase P and progressing to hepatocellular neoplasms[333,334] or in those induced by the Solt-Farber protocol.[335] With other models of chemical hepatocarcinogenesis, TGF-α immunoreactive cells have not been identified in preneoplastic hepatic lesions.[336] This also holds true for the majority of focal lesions (which most probably correspond to the amphophilic cell foci) produced by the peroxisomal proliferator Wy-14,643. On the other hand, enhanced expression of human TGF-α in the livers of transgenic mice has been shown to be associated with neoplastic development leading to well-differentiated HCCs 8 to 12 months after birth.[337]

Metabolic Aberrations

Fundamental metabolic aberrations appear in hepatocellular neoplasms[338–341] and in preneoplastic foci of altered hepatocytes. The early metabolic changes are closely related to neoplastic cell conversion.[16,159,232]

The most striking early metabolic change that characterizes the prevailing glycogenotic-basophilic cell lineage leading to HCC is a focal excessive storage of glycogen.[78,163,179] In rat liver, the focal lesions occupy a maximum of 5% to 10% of the parenchyma, too small a fraction to permit biochemical analysis in liver homogenates. However, assay of individual glycogen storage foci composed of clear and acidophilic cells and dissected with a laser beam from freeze-dried tissue sections from animals treated with chemical carcinogens reveal twice the glycogen concentration in these lesions compared to the parenchyma of untreated controls.[342] Studies on the glycogenotic foci permit outlining of a predominant metabolic pattern of these lesions. Hepatocellular glycogenosis is usually associated with a disturbance in phosphorylytic glycogen breakdown,[343] which is not due to the loss of phosphorylase protein[344] but is apparently the consequence of alterations such as a dysfunction of signal transduction, as demonstrated by a reduction in the activity of adenylate cyclase.[345] In addition, a reduction in the glucose transporter protein GLUT2, which is typically expressed in the liver of adult rats and facilitates glucose transport at the plasma membrane, has recently been demonstrated immunohistochemically in glycogenotic foci.[346] Many glycogenotic foci show reduced activity of the microsomal enzyme glucose-6-phosphatase[229,347] and of the lysosomal α-glucosidase.[348] Thus, phosphorylytic and hydrolytic glycogen breakdown, and a disturbance of glucose transport at the plasma membrane, appear to act together to produce an accumulation of glycogen in preneoplastic hepatocytes. An increase in the concentration of glucose-6-phosphate, the central metabolite of carbohydrate metabolism, was detected in homogenates of livers treated with nitrosomorpholine.[349] This finding correlates with the development of large glycogen-rich areas of the liver parenchyma, but could not be confirmed for pronounced glycogenotic foci analyzed by microbiochemical methods in laser-dissected specimens (Klimek et al., personal communication). Increases in the activities of key enzymes in the pentose phosphate and glycolytic pathways (i.e., glucose-6-phosphate dehydrogenase[342,343,350,351] and pyruvate kinase,[352] respectively) within the glycogen storage foci indicate the beginning of a metabolic shift toward alternative metabolic pathways. The increased activity of glucose-6-phosphate dehydrogenase is associated with changes detectable by immunohistochemistry[351] and in situ hybridization.[353]

When glycogen storage foci give rise to mixed or basophilic cell foci, adenomas, and carcinomas, additional metabolic changes occur. Glycogen, initially stored in excess, decreases.[224,342] At the same time, the storage of glycogen is frequently replaced by an accumulation of neutral lipids.[166] While the expression of the glucose transporter protein GLUT2 remains reduced, the fetal isoform GLUT1 is frequently re-expressed.[346] The activities of glyceraldehyde-3-phosphate dehydrogenase[343] and α-glucosidase[348] usually increase, while the content and activity of pyruvate kinase decrease.[352,354,355] Microbiochemical studies have shown that these changes are accompanied by a decrease in glucokinase and an increase in hexokinase activities, which thus are not early but rather late events[356] in hepatocarcinogenesis. Microbiochemical investigations also revealed that glucose-6-phosphate dehydrogenase activity progressively increases from glycogenotic foci through the mixed and basophilic cell populations that prevail in adenomas and carcinomas.[342] The growth rate of preneoplastic liver lesions gradually increases from glycogenotic to mixed/basophilic cell foci[257,258] and is associated with increasing expression of different marker enzymes.[25,282,283] A positive correlation between the incorporation of ^{3}H-thymidine in the DNA of preneoplastic liver lesions and glucose-6-phosphate dehydrogenase activity has been reported,[283,351,357] indicating that the expression of this enzyme is proliferation linked. It is unlikely, however, that the strong overexpression of glucose-6-phosphate dehydrogenase in the majority of preneoplastic and neoplastic lesions merely reflects increased cell proliferation, since only a slight increase in enzyme activity is related to the rapid cell replication after partial hepatectomy.[353] The production of reducing equivalents (NADPH), which are utilized in reductive processes, the formation of deoxyribose, and onset of cholesterogenesis may be important prerequisites for cell proliferation.[283,351,357] In later stages of hepatocarcinogenesis, metabolites such as glucose-6-phosphate are apparently no longer used for glycogen synthesis but are predominantly channeled to alternative pathways of energy metabolism such as the pentose phosphate pathway and glycolysis, providing the energy and precursors for nucleic acid synthesis associated with an increase in cell proliferation.[16,163]

It has become increasingly evident that the metabolic pattern and proliferative behavior characterizing the preneoplastic focal glycogenosis (and lipidosis) resemble in many ways the effects of insulin.[348,356] This hormone stimulates signal transduction pathways involved in a variety of metabolic processes including glycogen synthesis, lipogenesis, and the regulation of cell proliferation.[358,359] Indeed, Dombrowski et al.[360,361] have recently shown that hepatic foci emerging in the streptozotocin-induced diabetic rat liver after isologous pancreatic islet cell transplantation biochemically resemble the glycogenotic foci induced by oncogenic agents. This observation suggests that high levels of insulin (and possibly other secretory products) derived from the transplanted islets are able to produce phenotypic changes in hepatocytes similar to those caused by hepatocarcinogens.

A glycogenotic prestage has not been demonstrated for amphophilic cell foci, which are poor in glycogen from the beginning and represent the prevailing type of FAH after exposure of rats to peroxisome proliferators,[59,253,254] but are apparently also a frequent preneoplastic phenotype in mice treated with various chemical hepatocarcinogens.[362] In rats treated with the peroxisomal proliferator dehydroepiandrosterone, it has been shown by histochemical[253] and ultrastructural[59] investigations that the amphophilic cell foci are mainly characterized by mitochondrial proliferation associated with variable changes in peroxisome numbers. This observation points to the mitochondrion as a new subject for the analysis of hepatocarcinogenesis produced by peroxisomal proliferators, consistent with reports of the thyromimetic action of peroxisomal proliferators such as clofibrate and acetylsalicylic acid on mitochondrial genes in rat liver.[363] The significance of microsomal and mitochondrial lipid peroxidation found in the dehydroepiandrosterone model of hepatocarcinogenesis remains to be clarified.[364,365] Mitochondrial proliferation induced in the hepatic parenchyma by the nongenotoxic hepatocarcinogen methapyrilene has also been shown to be associated with mitochondrial lipid peroxidation,[366] but the same phenomenon was observed after administration of chemical analogs that are not carcinogenic.[367]

The biochemical phenotype of amphophilic cell foci differs in many respects from that of the glycogenotic foci. Thus the glucose-6-phosphate dehydrogenase activity is usually unchanged or reduced, while the activities of glucose-6-phosphatase, acid phosphatase, and succinate dehydrogenase are often increased in amphophilic cell foci induced in rats by dehydroepiandrosterone (Clinstal Metzger et al., personal communication), in contrast to glycogenotic foci. Dehydroepiandrosterone exerts a number of effects on carbohydrate metabolism in the liver resulting in a pattern that is in direct contrast to that observed in FAH,[368,369] which may at least in part be responsible for the inhibition of hepatocarcinogenesis by dehydroepiandrosterone under certain experimental conditions.[370–372] In spite of these obvious differences in the phenotype of glycogenotic and amphophilic cell foci, there is circumstantial evidence for a close relationship between these two types of focal preneoplastic lesion. Glycogenotic clear cell foci induced by nitrosomorpholine or by dimethylaminoazobenzene in rats were found frequently to undergo phenotypic modulation toward amphophilic cell foci after additional administration of dehydroepiandrosterone.[370,373] A phenotypic modulation in the opposite direction was described by Marsman and Popp,[374] who induced focal lesions resembling amphophilic cell foci (but called *homogeneous basophilic foci*) by the peroxisomal proliferator Wy-14,632, which were replaced by clear cell populations after withdrawal of the chemical insult. Finally, a close spatial relationship between glycogenotic clear cell foci and amphophilic cell foci including a variety of intermediate cellular phenotypes frequently occurs in early stages of hepadnaviral hepatocarcinogenesis in woodchucks with and without oral administration of AFB_1.[150] It is tempting to speculate that interactions between altered signal transduction pathways, such as the insulin-stimulated raf-MAP kinase signaling cascade and the cAMP-dependent protein kinase A signaling pathway, may take place.

Unusual enzymatically hyperactive foci are sometimes observed in the liver parenchyma of rats treated with hepatocarcinogens.[375] This is particularly true for glycogen phosphorylase hyperactive foci with and without increased levels of glycogen, which may be encountered in the livers of carcinogen-treated[193,344] or of untreated aged rats,[376] and have been demonstrated in embryonal turkey liver after administration of diethylnitrosamine in ovo.[377] The significance of these phenomena for hepatocarcinogenesis remains obscure.

There are few detailed studies of other metabolic pathways comparable to those of carbohydrate metabolism and taking into account the various cellular subpopulations of preneoplastic and early neoplastic lesions. Many observations have been made on altered metabolic parameters in FAH or nodular liver lesions produced by the Solt-Farber procedure and, hence, belong mainly to the reversion-linked category of carcinogen-induced lesions.[159,160,234,313,341] An ordered pattern of metabolic changes during hepatocarcinogenesis has also been described for a number of enzymes involved in drug metabolism, such as various cytochrome P_{450} isoenzymes and epoxide hydrolase.[90,378] Histochemical investigations of the activity of several dehydrogenases in focal hepatic lesions induced in rats with a hepatocarcinogenic nitrosamine revealed an increase in NADPH-generating potential in FAH, and particularly in hepatocellular adenomas[379] including increases in glucose-6-phosphate dehydrogenase, malic enzyme, and isocitrate dehydrogenase, and a decrease in β-hydroxybutyrate dehydrogenase. These alterations in enzyme activity again indicate an adaptive metabolic shift in hepatocarcinogenesis[379]; the increased levels of enzymes responsible for generation of NADPH possibly result in increased drug detoxification[160,341] or biosynthetic potential for cholesterogenesis and DNA synthesis.[357] In line with these considerations, Olsson et al.[380] concluded that activation of several enzymes and metabolites of the mevalonate pathway (which mainly produces cholesterol, dolichol, and ubiquinone) in persistent nodules induced in rats with 2-acetylaminofluorene contributes to the increase in detoxification and cell proliferation in the premalignant stages of HCC. Glycogenotic and amphophilic cell foci differ not only in the content or activity of several enzymes of carbohydrate and energy metabolism but also in the content or activity of drug metabolizing enzymes. Whereas glycogenotic foci often exhibit increased content of the placental form of the glutathione S-transferase[341,381] and elevated activity of γ-glutamyltransferase,[226,382] amphophilic cell foci usually do not express these enzymes.[254] This has previously been described for preneoplastic and neoplastic hepatic lesions induced in rats by peroxisomal proliferators.[383,384]

FAH, including glycogenotic foci, are resistant to experimentally induced hemosiderosis,[233,385] and a decrease in a number of iron-containing or iron-dependent enzymes in FAH has been observed.[234] Reduced uptake of iron has also been found in hepatocellular nodules induced by the Solt-Farber procedure, although the number of transferrin receptors was increased.[234] Alterations in intracellular vesicular acidification and in the redox capacity on the cell surface, and possibly also in the endosomes, were proposed as being responsible for the reduced iron uptake. Sequential changes in the expression of transferrin, which is an essential growth factor in many cell systems, have been observed in FAH.[235] Using in situ hybridization, increased levels of transferrin mRNA in glycogenotic foci have been demonstrated,[235] and the loss of glycogen in the more advanced mixed cell foci was usually accompanied by a decrease in transferrin mRNA levels, as demonstrated in the majority of HCCs. These results suggest a close relationship between the decreased expression of the transferrin gene and cellular dedifferentiation emerging during hepatocarcinogenesis. A transcriptional suppression of the transferrin gene in rat liver and in human hepatoma cell lines by hypolipidemic peroxisome proliferators has been reported.[236] Reduced iron availability and modulation of transferrin-dependent differentiation processes have been discussed as possible consequences.[236]

CHOLANGIOCELLULAR CHANGES DURING NEOPLASTIC DEVELOPMENT

With the exception of the extensively studied early proliferation of cholangiolar (oval) cells, our knowledge concerning cholangiocellular changes during neoplastic development is much more limited than that regarding hepatocellular changes. It has been known, however, that cholangiofibrosis (Fig. 15-11) is closely related to

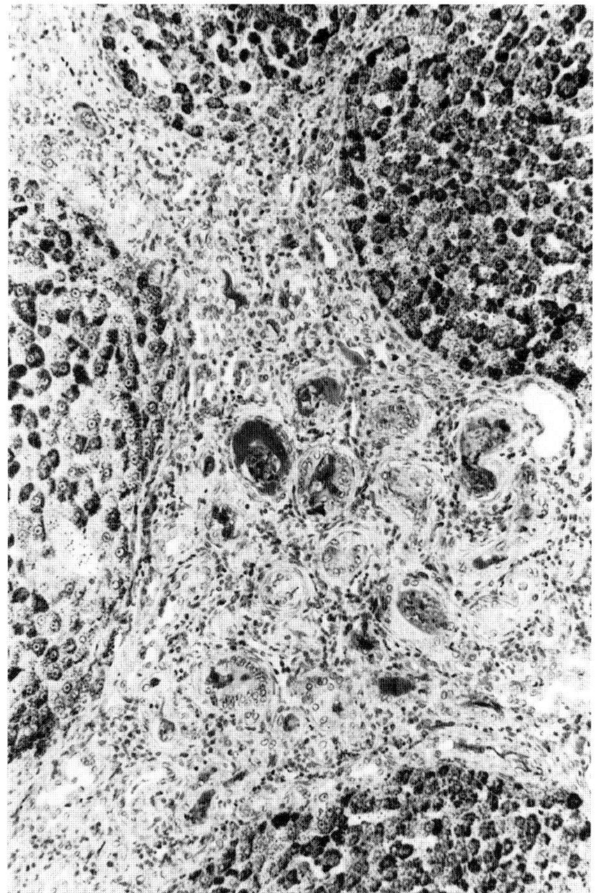

Figure 15-11. Light micrograph of cholangiofibrosis induced in rat liver with *N*-nitrosomorpholine. Note atypical ductules accumulating mucous substances, surrounded by collagen-rich connective tissue. (PAS; original magnification ×140.)

the development of cholangiocellular neoplasms induced by chemicals.[18,196,386] One of the main reasons for the relative infrequency of studies on the whole process of cholangiocarcinogenesis appears to be that it predominantly develops after administration of high doses of hepatocarcinogens and requires a long lag period.[77,80] In livers of rats treated with high doses of *N*-nitrosomorpholine, a sequence with four distinct stages (Fig. 15-1) has been shown, which starts with a cholangiocellular (oval) cell proliferation and proceeds to cholangiofibrosis, cholangiofibroma, and cholangiocarcinoma.[188] Similar sequential cellular changes leading to cholangiocellular neoplasms were observed in rats treated with other chemicals, including methapyrilene,[189] coumarin,[190] the mycotoxin phomopsin,[191] furan,[192,387] or a choline deficient/ethionine supplemented diet,[179,193] and in hamsters administered nitrosamines with and without additional infestation by the liver fluke *Opisthorchis viverrini*.[194,195]

Cellular Metamorphosis

The first stage in the complex sequence of cellular changes resulting in cholangiocellular neoplasms is characterized by a proliferation of cholangiolar (oval) and mesenchymal cells (Fig. 15-4). This seems to be a reactive response to toxicity-dependent parenchymal necrosis rather than an autonomous neoplastic process.[186–188] In the second stage, cholangiofibrosis develops from persisting proliferated cholangiolar and mesenchymal cells. Cholangiofibrosis is well demarcated and is composed of abnormal bile ductules embedded in abundant collagen-rich tissue.[186,187,196,387] The abnormal cholangioles are made up of a single layer of cuboidal or columnar cells that show many similarities to but also some striking differences from normal bile ductular cells.[18,80] The cytoplasm of epithelial cells in cholangiofibrotic lesions is often intensely basophilic due to a well-developed rough endoplasmic reticulum. At the luminal pole, the columnar cells exhibit a brush border, and there are juxtaluminal junctional complexes.[387] Necrotic cells, mitotic figures, and mitotic abnormalities are frequent. An outstanding feature of cholangiofibrosis is the appearance of goblet cells storing and secreting excessive amounts of mucus (Fig. 15-12) containing both acid and neutral mucopolysaccharides.[186,388] This early accumulation of mucus, called *cholangiolar mucopolysaccharidosis*[186] or *intestinal metaplasia*,[185,187,194,387] appears to be specific for cholangiocellular proliferation induced by hepatocar-

Figure 15-12. (*A*) Light micrograph and (*B*) electron micrograph of goblet cells in cholangiofibrotic lesions induced in rat liver with *N*-nitrosomorpholine. (*A*) Portion of atypical duct lined by cuboidal cells and goblet cells accumulating and secreting abundant mucus. (H&E, ×1,800.) (*B*) Selective staining of mucus in goblet cell with silver proteinate. Bar = 1 μm. (Original magnification ×11,000.)

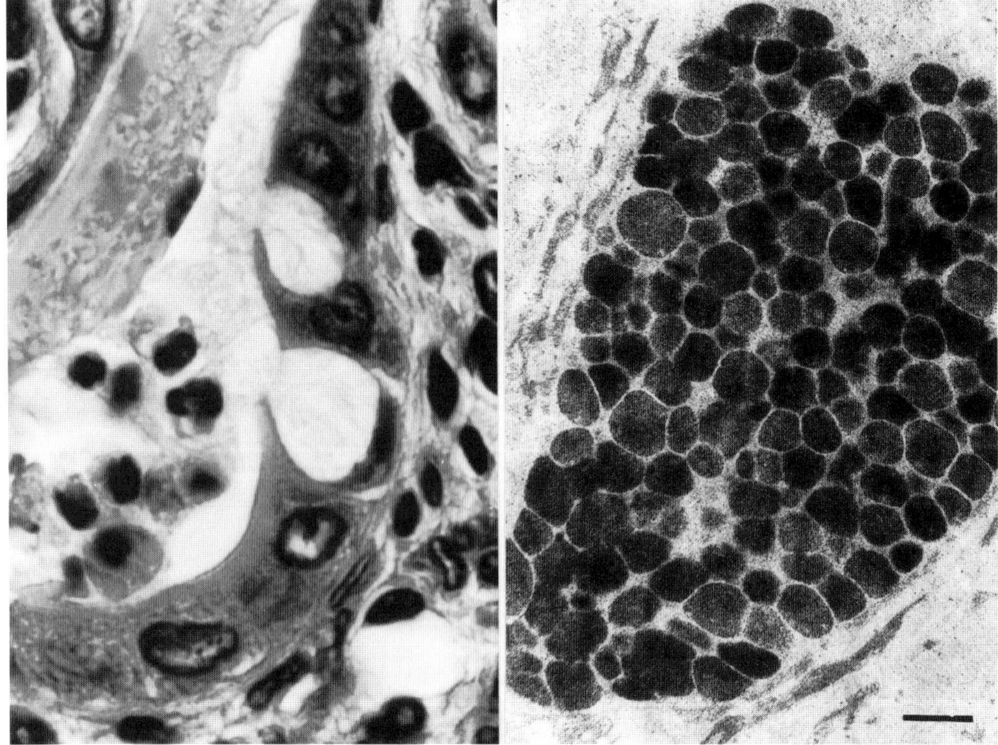

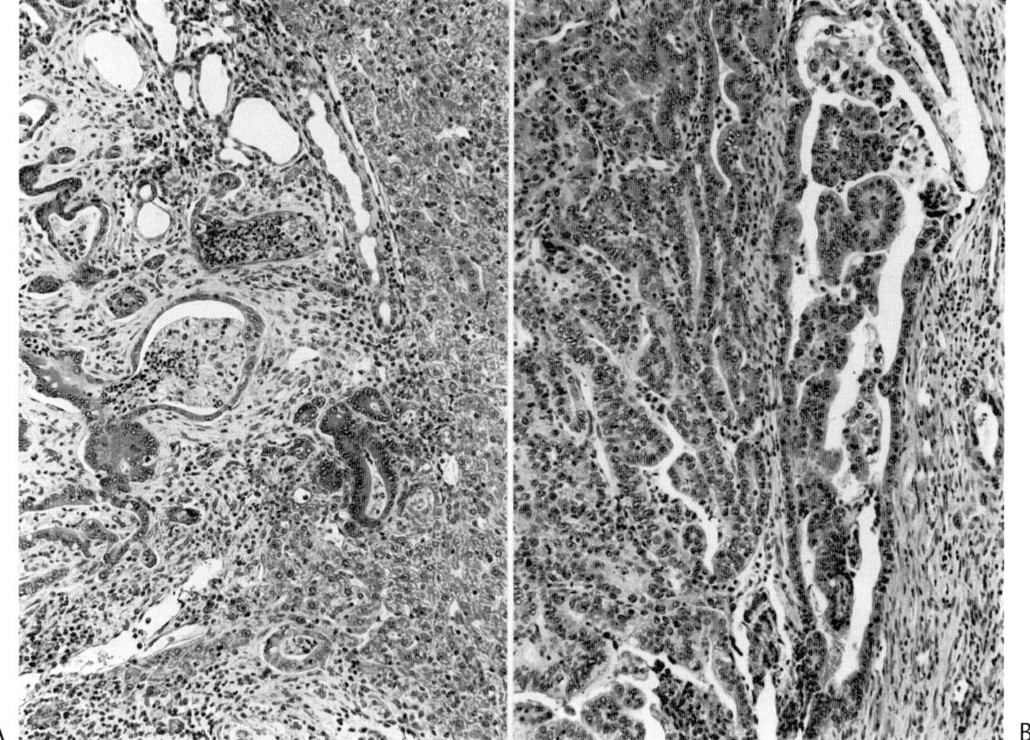

Figure 15-13. Light micrographs of portions of cholangiocellular neoplasms induced in rat liver with *N*-nitrosomorpholine. (*A*) Cholangiofibroma. (H&E, ×150.) (*B*) Cholangiocarcinoma. (H&E; original magnification ×140.)

cinogens. Occasional neuroendocrine-like cells have been described in cholangiofibrotic lesions induced by furan.[387]

Cholangiofibrosis has been considered a non-neoplastic lesion by most authors[186,187,196,386,389]; its epithelial component rarely may undergo degeneration and involution, leaving a scar-like alteration.[190,191] It has been shown in different experimental models, however, that cholangiofibrosis represents a preneoplastic stage with potential for progression to benign cystic cholangioma,[186,390] cholangiofibroma (Fig. 15-13),[179,188–190,193,391] and eventually also cholangiocarcinoma (Fig 15–13b).[188,189,191,194,196,392–394] In line with the interpretation of cholangiofibrosis as a preneoplastic lesion, Ohshima et al.[189] failed to produce tumors by transplantation of mucous cholangiofibrosis induced in rats with methapyrilene into the fat pad of syngeneic animals. However, Maronpot et al.[192] questioned the preneoplastic nature of cholangiofibrosis and considered this lesion to be essentially malignant or premalignant, since they did not observe qualitative differences between furan-induced mild cholangiofibrosis and neoplasms diagnosed as cholangiocarcinomas, some of which were transplantable into syngeneic rats and metastasized after serial passages. These findings support the concept of a precursor relationship between cholangiofibrosis and cholangiocarcinoma,[196] but the view of Maronpot et al.[192] does not take into consideration (1) that even extended cholangiofibrosis may only replace lost liver parenchyma without any indication of expansion beyond the confines of the liver lobe[186,191,197] (2) that the ductular component of individual cholangiofibrotic lesions may sometimes undergo involution[190,193] and (3) that progression of cholangiofibrosis frequently leads to cystic cholangiomas that represent a benign end-stage lesion in the rat[186,197,390], while only a second neoplastic derivative of cholangiofibrosis, the cholangiofibroma, is potentially malignant and may actually give rise to cholangiocarcinomas.[80,188,189,191,394]

During transformation of mucous cholangiofibrosis into cystic cholangiomas, the cylindrical epithelium of the ductules becomes flat and no longer produces mucus.[80,186] However, progression of cholangiofibrosis to cholangiofibromas (Fig.15-13a) during the third stage of cholangiocarcinogenesis is associated with even more pronounced accumulation of mucus.[188] At the ultrastructural level, the epithelial component of cholangiofibroma is characterized by tubules that are surrounded by a basal lamina and have an apical brush border (Fig. 15-14).[80,395] The cytoplasm of the epithelial tumor cells is rich in ribosomes and contains large bundles of intermediate filaments corresponding to the cytokeratin 19

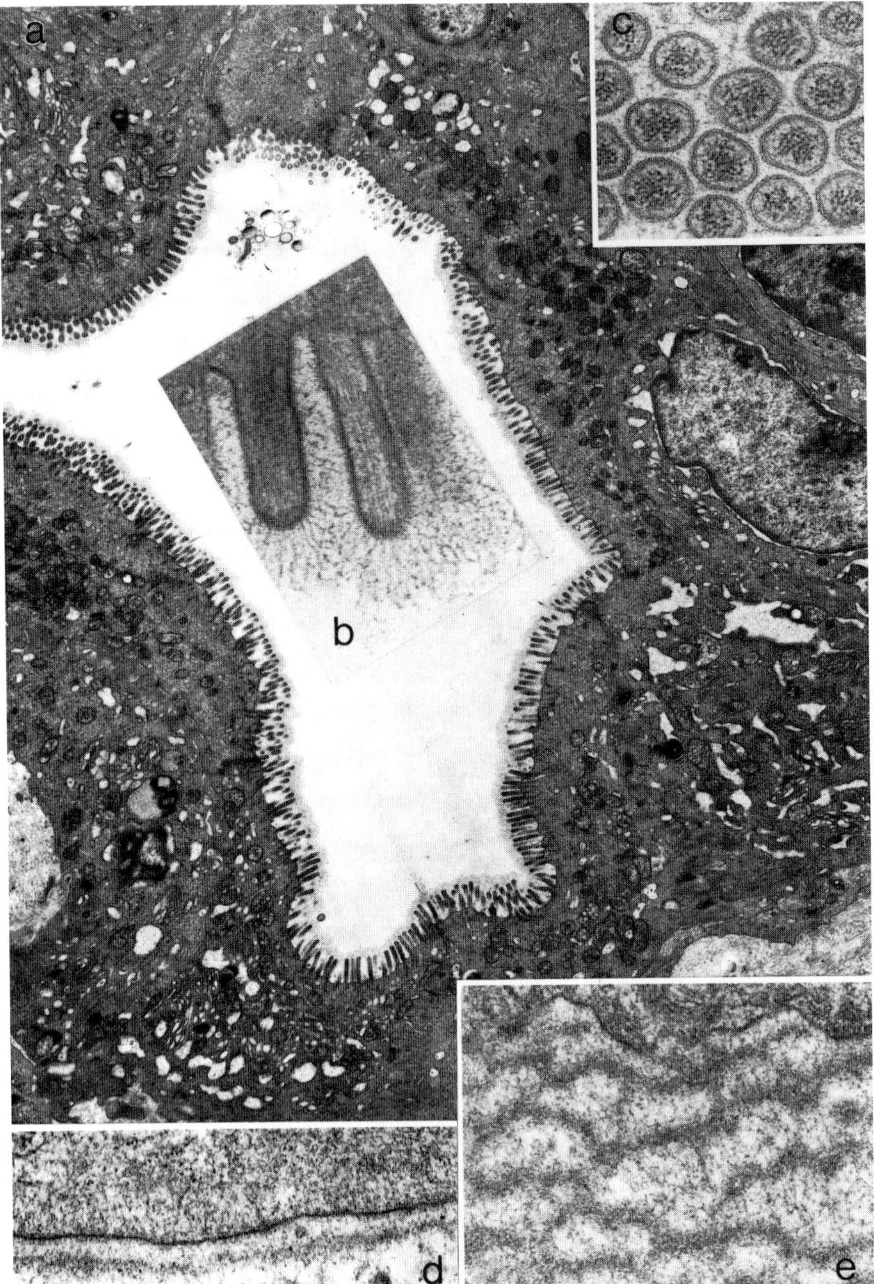

Figure 15-14. Electron micrograph of atypical ductular formation from cholangiofibroma induced in rat liver with *N*-nitrosomorpholine. (*A*) Atypical ductule with luminal brush border and glycocalix. (×5,000.) (*B*) Higher magnification of microvilli covered by glycocalix and containing microfilaments. (×62,500.) (*C*) Cross section of microvilli and microfilaments of the brush border. (×68,000.) (*D*) Lining of neoplastic epithelium by a well-developed basement membrane. (×48,000.) (*E*) Splitting of basement membrane. (Original magnification ×37,500.) (From Bannasch and Massner,[395] with permission.)

as demonstrated immunohistochemically. Although the majority of cholangiofibromas do not metastasize, they are potentially malignant and may give rise to metastasizing cholangiocarcinomas (Fig. 15-14b) after long lag periods.[80,188] During this fourth stage of cholangiocarcinogenesis, a reduction in the number of goblet cells and in the production of mucus takes place (which is sometimes replaced by an accumulation of monoparticulate glycogen); this has also been observed during the progression of cholangiocarcinomas.[394]

It is not yet clear which factors determine whether either benign cystic cholangiomas or cholangiofibromas and cholangiocarcinomas will develop from cholangiofibrosis, but it may be assumed that the degree of cellular injury caused by the carcinogen exposure is different between the two cases. This conclusion is compatible with the observation that cholangiofibromas and cholangiocarcinomas predominate after short-term administration of high doses of hepatocarcinogens, whereas cystic cholangiomas also develop after low doses.[18] However, long-term application of low doses of chemical carcinogens can also lead to cholangiocarcinomas, without producing mucous cholangiofibrosis as an early stage.[77]

Metabolic Aberrations

The pronounced storage and secretion of acid and neutral mucopolysaccharides in mucous cholangiofibrosis and cholangiofibromas indicates a metabolic aberration (mucopolysaccharidosis) that may be analogous to the storage of different polysaccharides or lipids as observed early during the development of a number of other tumor types.[179,186,193,194,396,397] A limited number of enzyme histochemical studies on cholangiocarcinogenesis have been conducted.[179,193,194] Both proliferating and persistent oval cells, as well as cholangiofibroses and cholangiocarcinomas, showed a strong enzyme histochemical reaction for glucose-6-phosphate dehydrogenase, glyceraldehyde-3-phosphate dehydrogenase, glycerol-3-phosphate dehydrogenase, malic enzyme, alkaline phosphatase, and γ-glutamyltransferase; low activities of glycogen synthase and phosphorylase and of glucose-6-phosphatase were also detected. Although more studies on metabolic changes during cholangiocarcinogenesis are needed, the available data suggest that a metabolic shift toward glycolysis and the oxidative pentose phosphate pathway takes place in this process similar to that in the neoplastic conversion of hepatocytes.[179,193,194]

CHANGES OF THE SINUSOIDAL LINING CELLS DURING NEOPLASTIC DEVELOPMENT

In different species, the sinusoidal lining cells of the liver may give rise to three types of vascular lesions occurring after treatment with various chemical carcinogens,

Figure 15-15. Light micrographs of early angiosarcoma induced in rat liver with *N*-nitrosomorpholine and prepared as (*A*) paraffin or (*B*) frozen sections. Note atypical sinusoidal lining cells stained with hematoxylin and eosin (*A*) or with antibody to vimentin (*B*) along the hepatic cords, which are negative for vimentin. (Original magnifications: A, ×420, B, ×670.) (From Bannasch et al.,[223] with permission.)

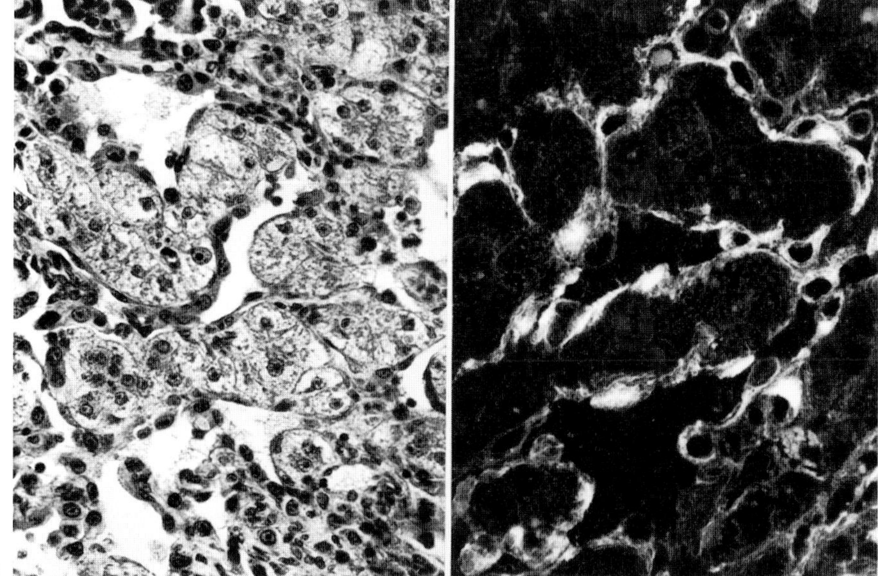

namely, sinusoidal peliosis hepatis, benign hemangioendothelioma, and angiosarcoma.[17,18,219] Sinusoidal peliosis hepatis is characterized by an irregular focal dilatation of the sinuses. The sinusoidal lining cells may at most show some minor alterations such as nuclear enlargement. Most of the peliotic lesions are distributed at random in the liver tissue, but their localization with hepatic adenomas is quite common.[17,398] Peliosis hepatis has been induced in rodents by a number of chemicals including vinyl chloride, vinyl carbamate, nitrosamines, nitrosamides, and nitrosomethylurea.[17,219] Sinusoidal peliosis hepatis as well as benign hemangioendotheliomas and angiosarcomas may be produced by administration of a relatively low single dose of dimethylnitrosamine (10 mg/kg body weight) to rodents.[399] In this experiment, benign hemangioendotheliomas developed later, and angiosarcomas were only seen after long lag periods. These observations are in line with the notion that the carcinogen-induced peliotic lesions coated by a single-layered endothelium are the result of an autonomous growth process.[17,399–401] The most important indication of the neoplastic nature of sinusoidal peliosis hepatis is its occasional joint occurrence with unequivocal benign hemangioendotheliomas or even angiosarcomas.[399] These findings indicate that perisinusoidal peliosis hepatis, benign hemangioendothelioma, and angiosarcoma are only different stages of a uniform pathogenetic process that is sometimes operative.[219]

After administration of relatively high doses of strong carcinogens such as *N*-nitrosomorpholine, angiosarcomas usually develop without a preceding benign stage.[18,219] Immunohistochemical studies with antibodies to the cytoskeletal protein vimentin revealed that the majority of neoplastic cells in early (Fig. 15-15) and particularly in advanced stages of angiosarcomas accumulate excessive amounts of vimentin filaments (Fig. 15-16), sometimes in combination with glycogen.[222,223] The cause of the accumulation of vimentin in the sarcoma cells is not known, but it may be that metabolic aberrations similar to those that lead to storage of polysaccharides or lipids in epithelial preneoplastic or neoplastic cells are responsible.[223]

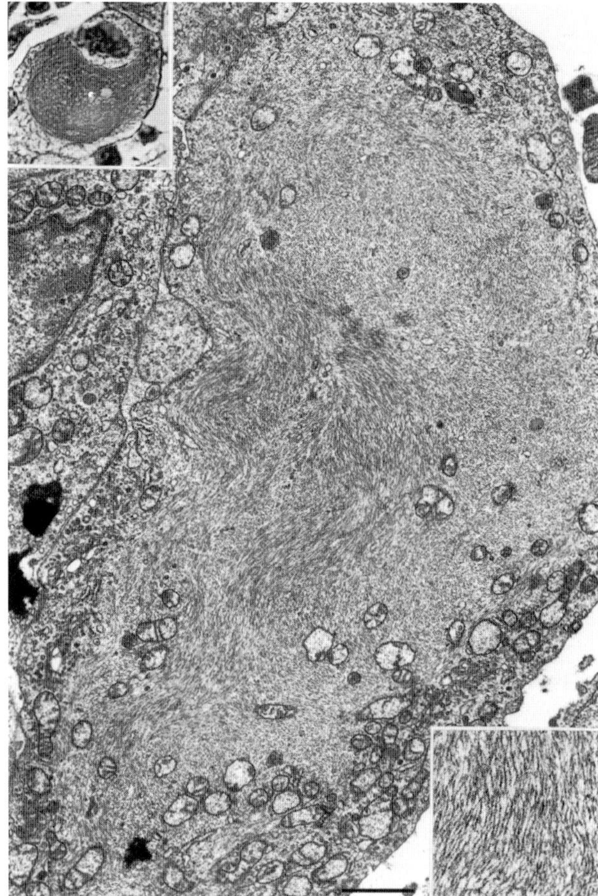

Figure 15-16. Electron micrograph showing a large array of densely packed intermediate filaments in an angiosarcoma cell induced in rat liver with *N*-nitrosomorpholine. (×15,000.) (*Upper inset.*) Light micrograph of a vimentin storage cell of an angiosarcoma exhibiting a large fibrillar cytoplasmic inclusion. (H&E, ×650.) (*Lower inset*) Detail of intermediate filaments. Bar = 1 μm. (Original magnification ×39,000.) (From Bannasch et al.,[223] with permission.)

CHANGES OF THE PERISINUSOIDAL CELLS DURING NEOPLASTIC DEVELOPMENT

The perisinusoidal cells have been identified as frequent targets of chemical hepatocarcinogens in rats[79,220,221,391,402,403] and fish.[404–408] After exposure of rats to various chemicals such as *N*-nitrosomorpholine, dimethylnitrosamine, nitrosopyrrolidine, and 2-acetylaminofluorene, characteristic cyst-like lesions (spongiosis) often develop from the perisinusoidal cells, as demonstrated by electron microscopy (Fig. 15-17). Immunohistochemical methods can show desmin in these lesions, a protein that is specifically expressed in this cell type in the normal liver and accumulates in the cells of spongiosis.[220,402] Initially, these lesions were called *spongiosis hepatis* and were considered to be a preneoplastic lesion that may give rise to pericytomas[79,402]; their neoplastic nature was suggested by Couch.[408] The holes within the spongiosis are lined by neither epithelial nor endothelial cells. In contrast to peliosis hepatis, the multilocular formations of spongiosis are not filled with blood but with a finely flocculent material that is rich in proteoglycans. The walls of the sponge-like formation are composed of fibroblast-like cells that sometimes look like typical fat storage cells but are usually free of fat droplets.

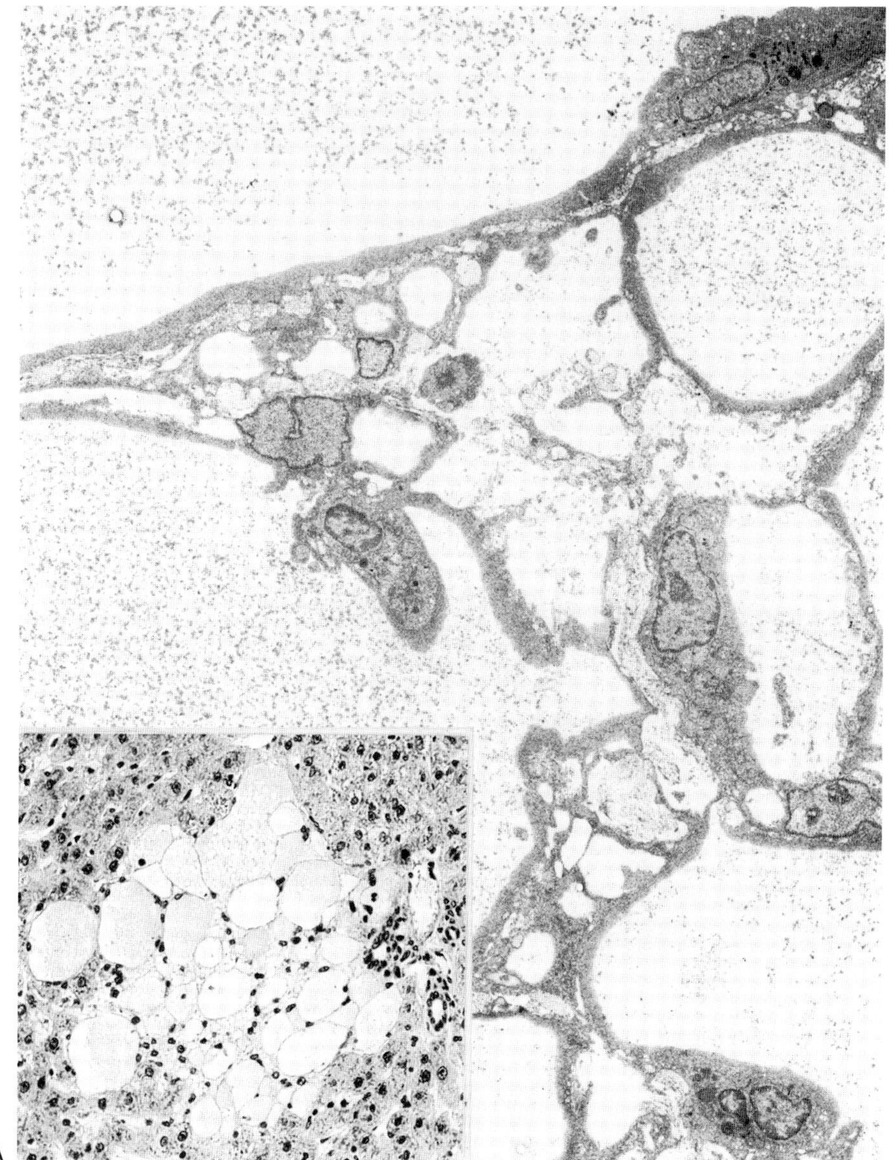

Figure 15-17. (*A*) Light micrograph and (*B*) electron micrograph of spongiotic pericytoma induced in rat liver with *N*-nitrosomorpholine. (*A*) Spongiotic formations surrounded by hepatic parenchyma of normal appearance and closely associated with a portal tract (to the right). (H&E, ×150.) (*B*) Fibroblast-like cells with long cytoplasmic extensions forming a loose sponge. (Original magnification ×2,000.)

In rats treated with *N*-nitrosomorpholine, convincing evidence was found for a regular integration of the spongiotic formations into larger proliferative lesions (Fig. 15-18a), a benign neoplasm classified as spongiotic pericytoma.[220] Because the latter can only be identified by specific immunohistochemical demonstration of desmin in the constituent cells, it appears to be appropriate to retain the designation *spongiosis hepatis* for the spongiotic lesions visible in conventional hematoxylin and eosin-stained sections.[221]

There is circumstantial evidence for a possible progression of the benign spongiotic pericytoma to a malignant neoplasm,[79] for which the term *perisinusoidal (Ito) cell sarcoma* (Fig. 15-18b) has been proposed.[220] During this process the proteoglycans that have accumulated in the cavities of the benign lesions appear to become gradually reduced.[79] It is conceivable that this change in the accumulation of extracellular proteoglycans indicates a metabolic shift similar to the gradual disappearance of intracellular excessive storage of polysaccharides or lipids during progression from the preneoplastic to the neoplastic lesions in epithelial cells of the liver.

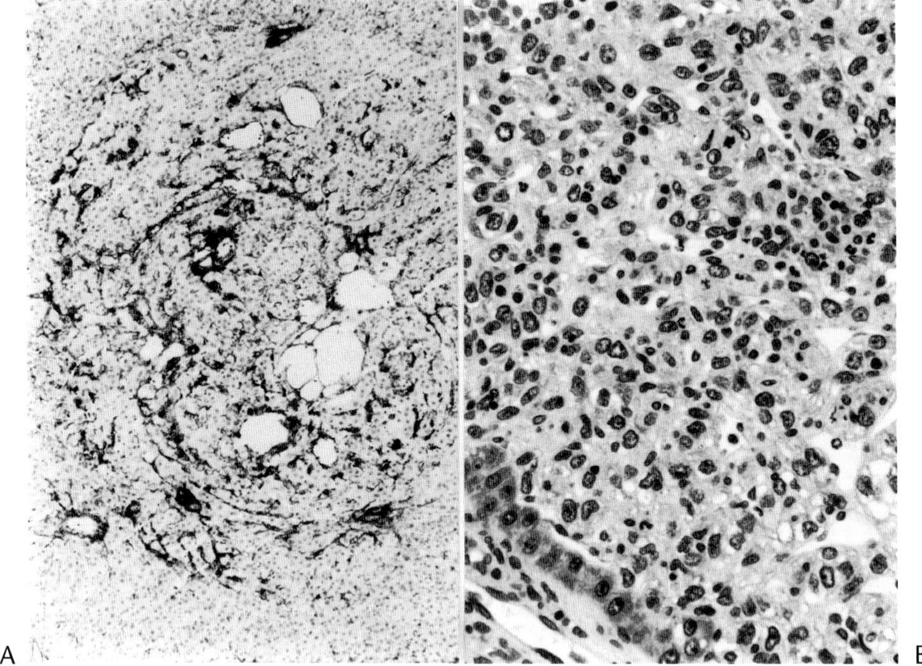

Figure 15-18. Light micrographs of (*A*) spongiotic pericytoma and (*B*) perisinusoidal (Ito) cell sarcoma induced in rat liver with *N*-nitrosomorpholine. (*A*) Demonstration of proliferated perisinusoidal cells with antibody to desmin. (×80.) (*B*) Pleomorphic perisinusoidal (Ito) cell sarcoma containing remnants of hepatic parenchyma. (H&E; original magnification ×340.)

ACKNOWLEDGMENTS

The authors express their appreciation for helpful critical comments to Drs. Heinz Werner Thielmann and Harald Enzmann and gratefully acknowledge the typing of the manuscript by Brigitte Pétillon and the preparation of the illustrations by Joachim Hollatz.

REFERENCES

1. Schmidt MB. Über vitale Fettfärbung in Geweben und Sekreten durch Sudan und geschwulstartige Wucherungen der ausscheidenden Drüsen. Virchows Arch Pathol Anat 1924; 253:432–451
2. Sasaki T, Yoshida T. Experimentelle Erzeugung des Lebercarcinoms durch Fütterung mit *o*-Amidoazotoluol. Virchows Arch Pathol Anat 1935;295:175–200
3. Wogan GN. The induction of liver cell cancer by chemicals. In: Cameron HM, Linsell DA, Warwick GP (eds): Liver Cell Cancer. Elsevier Scientific Amsterdam, 1976, pp. 121–152
4. Preussmann R. Hepatocarcinogens as potential risk for human liver cancer. In Remmer H, Bolt HM, Bannasch P (eds): Primary Liver Tumors. MTP Press Lancaster, 1978; pp. 11–29
5. Montesano R, Kirby GM. Chemical carcinogens in human liver cancer. In Bréchot C (ed): Primary Liver Cancer: Etiological and Progression Factors. CRC, Boca Raton, 1994, pp. 57–77
6. Pitot HC, Dragan YP. Chemical induction of hepatic neoplasia. In Fausto N, Jakoby WB, Schachter DA (eds): The Liver Biology and Pathobiology. 3rd Ed. Raven, New York, 1994, pp. 1467–1495
7. Schwarz M. Tumor promotion in liver. In Arcos JC (ed): Chemical Induction of Cancer. Birkhäuser, Boston, 1995, pp. 161–179
8. IARC Monographs on the Evaluation of Carcinogenic Risks to Humans. Vols 1–65. International Agency for Research on Cancer, Lyon; 1972–1996
9. Stewart HL: Comparative aspects of certain cancers. In Becker FF (ed): Cancer. A Comprehensive Treatise. Vol. 4. Plenum Press, New York, 1975, pp. 303–374
10. Bannasch P. Strain and species differences in the susceptibility to liver tumor induction. In Turusov V, Montesano R (eds): Modulators of Experimental Carcinogenesis. Vol. 51. IARC Scientific Publications, Lyon, 1983, pp. 9–38
11. Thorgeirsson UP, Dalgard DW, Reeves J, Adamson RH. Tumor incidence in a chemical carcinogenesis study of nonhuman primates. Regul Toxicol Pharmacol 1994;19: 130–150
12. Jones TC, Mohr U, Hunt RD (eds): Monographs on Pathol-

ogy of Laboratory Animals: Digestive System. 2nd Ed. Springer, Berlin, 1996

13. Druckrey H. Quantitative aspects of chemical carcinogenesis. In Truhaut R (ed): Potential Carcinogenic Hazards from Drugs. UICC Monograph Vol. 7. Springer, Berlin, 1967, pp. 59–77
14. Peto R, Gray R, Brantom P, Grasso P. Nitrosamine carcinogenesis in 5120 rodents: chronic administration of sixteen different concentrations of NDEA, NDMA, NPYR and NPIP in the water of 4440 inbred rats, with parallel studies on NDEA alone of the effect of age of starting (3,6 or 20 weeks) and of species (rats, mice or hamsters). IARC Sci Publ 1984;57:627–665
15. Aterman K. Hepatic neoplasia: reflections and ruminations. Virchows Arch 1995;427:1–18
16. Bannasch P. Pathogenesis of hepatocellular carcinoma: sequential cellular, molecular, and metabolic changes. In: Boyer JL, Ockner, RK (eds): Progress in Liver Diseases. WB Saunders, Philadelphia, 1996, pp. 161–197
17. Popper H, Maltoni C, Selikoff IJ et al. Comparison of neoplastic hepatic lesions in man and experimental animals. In Hiatt HH, Watson JD, Winsten JA (eds): Origin of Human Cancer, Book C, Human Risk Assessment. Cold Spring Harbor Conferences on Cell Proliferation, Vol 4. Cold Spring Harbor Laboratory Press, Cold Spring Harbor, NY 1977, pp. 1359–1382
18. Bannasch P, Zerban H. Tumours of the liver. In Turusov VS, Mohr U (eds): Pathology of Tumours in Laboratory Animals. Vol. I, Tumours of the Rat. 2nd Ed. International Agency for Research on Cancer, Lyon, 1990, pp. 199–240
19. Bannasch P. Experimental liver tumours. In MacSween RNM, Anthony PP, Scheuer PJ et al. (eds): Pathology of the Liver. Churchill Livingstone, New York, 1994; pp. 681–709
20. Bannasch P, Zerban H. Predictive value of hepatic preneoplastic lesions as indicators of carcinogenic response. IARC Sci Publ 1992;116:389–427
21. Hasegawa R, Ito N. Hepatocarcinogenesis in the rat. In Waalkes MP, Ward JM (eds): Carcinogenesis. Raven, New York, 1994; pp. 39–65
22. Bannasch P. Preneoplastic lesions as end points in carcinogenicity testing. I. Hepatic preneoplasia. Carcinogenesis 1986;7:689–695
23. Williams GM. The significance of chemically induced hepatocellular altered foci in rat liver and application to carcinogen detection. Toxicol Pathol 1989;17:663–672
24. Pitot HC, Campbell HA, Maronpot R et al. Critical parameters in the quantitation of the stages of initiation, promotion, and progression in one model of hepatocarcinogenesis in the rat. Toxicol Pathol 1989;17:594–612
25. Ito N, Tatematsu M, Hasegawa R, Tsuda H. Medium-term bioassay system for detection of carcinogens and modifiers of hepatocarcinogenesis utilizing the GST-P-positive liver cell focus as an endpoint marker. Toxicol Pathol 1989;17: 630–641
26. Ito N, Shirai T, Hasegawa R. Medium-term bioassays for carcinogens. IARC Sci Publ 1992;116:353–388
27. Bannasch P, Jahn U-R, Zerban H. Preneoplastic lesions as early indicators of neoplastic development. In Bannasch P (ed): Cancer Diagnosis. Early Detection. Springer, Berlin, 1992 pp. 178–190
28. Altmann HW. Hepatic neoformations. Pathol Res Pract 1994;190:513–577
29. Graeves P, Goonetilleke R, Nunn G et al. Two year carcinogenicity study of tamoxifen in Alderly Park Wistar-derived rats. Cancer Res 1993;53:3919–3924
30. Hard G, Iatropoulos M, Jordan K et al. Major difference in the hepatocarcinogenicity and DNA adduct forming ability between toremifene and tamoxifen in female Crl: CD (BR) rats. Cancer Res 1993;53:4534–4541
31. Hirsamaki P, Hirsamaki Y, Niemineu L, Payne B. Tamoxifen induces hepatocellular carcinoma in rat liver: a one year study with two antiestrogens. Arch Toxicol 1993;67: 49–54
32. Some naturally occurring substances: food items and constituents, heterocyclic aromatic amines and mycotoxins. In IARC Monographs of the Evaluation of Carcinogenic Risks to Humans, Vol. 56. International Agency for Research on Cancer, Lyon, 1993, pp. 41–524
33. Chemicals, Occupational Exposures and Cultural Habits Associated with Cancer in Humans. Vols. 1–42. In IARC Monographs on the Evaluation of Carcinogenic Risks to Humans. Suppl. 7. International Agency for Research on Cancer, Lyon, 1987, pp. 37–400
34. Huff J, Haseman J, Rall D. Scientific concepts, value and significance of chemical carcinogenesis studies. Annu Rev Pharmacol Toxicol 1991;31:621–652
35. Smith AH, Hopenhayen-Rich C, Bates MN et al. Cancer risks from arsenic in drinking water. Environ Health Perspect 1992;97:259–267
36. Alcohol drinking. In IARC Monographs on the Evaluation of Carcinogenic Risk to Humans, Vol. 44. International Agency for Research on Cancer, Lyon, 1988, pp. 35–378
37. Seitz HK, Simanowski UA, Hoerner M, Kommerell B. Alcohol and liver carcinoma. In Bannasch P, Keppler D, Weber G (eds): Liver Cell Carcinoma. Kluwer, Dordrecht, 1989 pp. 227–241
38. Farber E. Alcohol and other chemicals in the development of hepatocellular carcinoma. Clin Lab Med 1996;16: 377–394
39. Miller EC. Some current perspectives on chemical carcinogenesis in humans and experimental animals. Cancer Res 1978;38:1479–1496
40. Oesch F, Schladt L, Glatt HR, Thomas H. Metabolism of chemical carcinogens. In Bannasch P, Keppler D, Weber G (eds): Liver Cell Carcinoma. Kluwer, Dordrecht, 1989, pp. 243–249
41. Miller JA, Cramer JW, Miller EC. The *N*- and ring-hydroxylation of acetylaminofluorene during carcinogenesis in the rat. Cancer Res 1960;20:950–962
42. Wogan GN. Aflatoxins as risk factors for hepatocellular carcinoma in humans. Cancer Res 1992;52(suppl): 2114s–2118s
43. Bolt HM. Role of etheno-DNA adducts in tumorigenicity of olefines. Crit Rev Toxicol 1988;18:299–309
44. Hemminki K. Nucleic acid adducts of chemical carcinogens and mutagens. Arch Toxicol 1983;52:249–285

45. Enzmann H, Kühlem C, Löser E, Bannasch P. Damage of mitochondrial DNA induced by the hepatocarcinogen diethylnitrosamine in ovo. Mutat Res 1995;329:113–120
46. Beland FA, Poirier MC. DNA adducts and carcinogenesis. In Sirica AE (ed): Pathobiology of Neoplasms. Plenum Press, New York, 1989, pp. 57–80
47. Swenberg JA. The role of DNA damage, repair and replication in hepatocarcinogenesis. In Bannasch P, Keppler D, Weber G(eds): Liver Cell Carcinoma. Kluwer, Dordrecht, 1989, pp. 261–269
48. Bedell MA, Lewis JG, Billings KC, Swenberg JA. Cell specificity in hepatocarcinogenesis: preferential accumulation of O^6-methylguanine in target cell DNA during continuous exposure of rats to 1, 2-dimethylhydrazine. Cancer Res 1982;42:3079–3083
49. Swenberg JA, Dyroff MC, Bedell MA et al. O^4 Ethyldeoxythymidine, but not O^6-ethyldeoxyguanosine, accumulates in hepatocyte DNA of rats exposed continuously to diethylnitrosamine. Proc Natl Acad Sci USA 1984;81:1692–1695
50. Singer B. In vivo formation and persistence of modified nucleosides resulting from alkylating agents. Environ Health Perspect 1985;62:41–48
51. Loechler EL. The role of adduct site-specific mutagenesis in understanding how carcinogen- DNA adducts cause mutations: perspective, prospects and problems. Carcinogenesis 1996;17:895–902
52. Castro GD, Diaz Gomez Ml, Castro JA. Species differences in the interaction between Cl_4 reactive metabolites and liver DNA or nuclear protein fractions. Carcinogenesis 1989;10:289–294
53. Reddy JK, Lalwani ND. Carcinogenesis by hepatic peroxisome proliferators: evaluation of the risk of hypolipidemic drugs and industrial plasticizers to humans. CRC Crit Rev Toxicol 1983;12:1–58
54. Vainio H, Magee P, McGregor D, McMichael AJ. Mechanisms of Carcinogenesis in Risk Identification. International Agency for Research on Cancer Lyon, 1992
55. Ramel C. Genotoxic and nongenotoxic carcinogens: mechanisms of action and testing strategies. IARC Sci Publ 1992; 116:195–209
56. Reddy JK, Rao MS. Oxidative DNA-damage caused by persistent peroxisome proliferation: its role in hepatocarcinogenesis. Mutat Res 1989;214:63–68
57. Nilsson R, Beije B, Préat V et al. On the mechanisms of the hepatocarcinogenicity of peroxisome proliferators. Chem Biol Interact 1991;78:235–250
58. Denda A, Sai K, Tang Q et al. Induction of 8-hydroxydeoxyguanosine but not initiation of carcinogenesis by redoxenzyme modulations with or without menadione in rat liver. Carcinogenesis 1991;12:719–726
59. Metzger C, Mayer D, Hoffmann H et al. Sequential appearance and ultrastructure of amphophilic cell foci, adenomas and carcinomas in the liver of male and female rats treated with dehydroepiandrosterone (DHEA). Toxicol Pathol 1995;23:591–605
60. Counts JL, Goodman Jl. Hypomethylation of DNA: an epigenetic mechanism that can facilitate the aberrant oncogene expression involved in liver carcinogenesis. In Jirtle RL (ed): Liver Regeneration and Carcinogenesis. Academic Press, San Diego, 1995, pp. 227–255
61. Newberne PM, de Camargo JLV, Clark AJ. Choline deficiency, partial hepatectomy, and liver tumors in rats and mice. Toxicol Pathol 1982;10:95–106
62. Mikol YB, Hoover KL, Craesia D, Poirier LA. Hepatocarcinogenesis in rats fed methyl-deficient, amino-acid defined diets. Carcinogenesis 1983;4:1619–1629
63. Goshal AK, Farber E. The induction of liver cancer by dietary deficiency of choline and methionine without added carcinogens. Carcinogenesis 1984;5:1367–1370
64. Locker J, Reddy TV, Lombardi B. DNA methylation and hepatocarcinogenesis in rats fed a choline-devoid diet. Carcinogenesis 1986;7:1309–1312
65. Dizik M, Christman JK, Wainfan E. Alterations in expression and methylation of specific genes in livers of rats fed a cancer promoting methyl-deficient diet. Carcinogenesis 1991;12:1307–1312
66. Zapisek WF, Cronin GM, Lyn-Cook BD, Poirier LA. The onset of oncogene hypomethylation in ther livers of rats fed methyl-deficient, amino-acid defined diets. Carcinogenesis 1992;13:1869–1872
67. Wainfan E, Poirier LA. Methyl groups in carcinogenesis: effects on DNA methylation and gene expression. Cancer Res 1992;52(suppl):2071s–2077s
68. Hernandez L, Allen PT, Poirier LA, Lijinski W. S-adenosylmethionine, S-adenosylhomocysteine and DNA methylation levels in the liver or rats fed methapyrilene and analogs. Carcinogenesis 1989;10:557–562
69. Randerath K, Reddy MV, Disher RM. Age and tissue-related DNA modifications in untreated rats: detection by ^{32}P-postlabeling assay and possible significance for spontaneous tumor induction and aging. Carcinogenesis 1986;7: 1615–1617
70. Randerath K, Lu L-JW, Li D. A comparison between different types of covalent DNA modifications (I-compounds, persistent carcinogen adducts and 5-methylcytosine) in regenerating rat liver. Carcinogenesis 1988;9:1843–1848
71. Li D, Randerath K. Modulation of DNA modification (I-compound) levels in rat liver and kidney by dietary carbohydrate, protein, fat, vitamin, and mineral content. Mutat Res 1992;275:47–56
72. Randerath K, van Golen KL, Dragan YP, Pitot HC. Effects of phenobarbital on I-compounds in liver DNA as a function of age in male rats fed two different diets. Carcinogenesis 1992;13:125–130
73. Li D, Chandar N, Lombardi B, Randerath K. Reduced accumulation of I-compounds in liver DNA of rats fed a choline-devoid diet. Carcinogenesis 1989;10:605–607
74. Liehr J, Avitts T, Randerath E, Randerath K. Estrogen-induced DNA alterations: possible mechanism of hormonal cancer. Proc Natl Acad Sci USA 1986;83:5301–5305
75. Li D, Xu D, Randerath K. Species and tissue specifities of I-compounds as contrasted with carcinogen adducts in liver, kidney and skin DNA of Sprague-Dawley rats, ICR mice and Syrian hamsters. Carcinogenesis 1990;11:2227–2232
76. Drinkwater NR, Lee G-H. Genetic susceptibility of liver cancer. In Jirtle RL (ed): Liver Regeneration and Carcinogenesis. Academic Press, San Diego, 1995; pp. 301–321

77. Bannasch P. Dose-dependence of early cellular changes during liver carcinogenesis. Arch Toxicol 1980;3:(suppl 2)111–128

78. Bannasch P. The cytoplasm of hepatocytes during carcinogenesis. Electron and light microscopical investigations of the nitrosomorpholine-intoxicated rat liver. Rec Res Cancer Res 1968;19:1–100

79. Bannasch P, Zerban H. Pathogenesis of primary liver tumors induced by chemicals. Rec Res Cancer Res 1986;100:1–15

80. Bannasch P, Zerban H. Cholangiofibroma and cholangiocarcinoma, liver, rat. In Jones TC, Mohr U, Hunt RD (eds): Monographs on Pathology of Laboratory Animals, Digestive System. 2nd Ed. Springer, Berlin, 1997, pp. 63–82

81. Druckrey H. Quantitative Grundlagen der Krebserzeugung. Klin Wochenschr 1943;22:532

82. Druckrey H, Schmähl D, Preussmann R, Ivankovic S. Quantitative Analyse der carcinogenen Wirkung von Diäthylnitrosamin. Arzneimittel Forsch 1963;13:841–851

83. Scherer E, Hoffmann M, Emmelot P, Friedrich-Freksa H. Quantitative study on foci of altered liver cells induced in the rat by a single dose of diethylnitrosamine and partial hepatectomy. J Natl Cancer Inst 1972;49:93–106

84. Schieferstein G, Pirschel J, Frank W, Friedrich-Freksa H. Quantitative Untersuchungen über den irreversiblen Verlust zweier Enzymaktivitäten in der Rattenleber nach Verfütterung von Diäthylnitrosamin. Z Krebsforsch 1974;82: 191–208

85. Kunz W, Schaude G, Schwarz M, Tennekes H. Quantitative aspects of drug-mediated tumour promotion in liver and its toxicological implications. In Hecker E, Fusenig NE, Kunz W, et al. (eds): Carcinogenesis—A Comprehensive Survey, Vol. 7. Raven, New York, 1982, pp. 111–125

86. Vesselinovitch SD, Mihailovich N. Kinetics of diethylnitrosamine hepatocarcinogenesis in the infant mouse. Cancer Res 1983;43:4253–4259

87. Scherer E. Neoplastic progression in experimental hepatocarcinogenesis. Biochim Biophys Acta 1984;738:219–236

88. Zerban H, Preussmann R, Bannasch P. Dose-time-relationship of the development of preneoplastic liver lesions induced in rats with low doses of *N*-nitrosodiethanolamine. Carcinogenesis 1988;9:607–610

89. Zerban H, Preussmann R, Bannasch P. Quantitative morphometric comparison between the expression of two different "marker enzymes" in preneoplastic liver lesions induced in rats with low doses of *N*-nitrosodiethanolamine. Cancer Lett 1988;43:99–104

90. Schwarz M, Buchmann A, Schulte M et al. Heterogeneity of enzyme-altered foci in rat liver. Toxicol Lett 1989;49: 297–317

91. Williams GM, Gebhardt R, Sirma H, Stenbäck F. Nonlinearity of neoplastic conversion induced in rat liver by low exposure to diethylnitrosamine. Carcinogenesis 1993;14: 2149–2156

92. Enzmann H, Zerban H, Kopp-Schneider A et al. Effects of low doses of *N*- nitrosomorpholine on the development of early stages of hepatocarcinogenesis. Carcinogenesis 1995; 7:1513–1518

93. Umemura T, Tokumo K, Sirma H et al. Dose-response effects of 2-acetylaminofluorene on DNA damage, cytotoxicity, cell proliferation and neoplastic conversion in rat liver. Cancer Lett 1993;73:1–10

94. Lijinsky W, Kovatch RM, Riggs CW, Walters PT. Dose-response study with *N*-nitrosomorpholine in drinking water of F-344 rats. Cancer Res 1988;48:2089–2095

95. Moore MA, Mayer D, Bannasch P. The dose dependence and sequential appearance of putative preneoplastic populations induced in the rat liver by stop experiments with *N*-nitrosomorpholine. Carcinogenesis 1982;3:1429–1436

96. Enzmann H, Bannasch P. Potential significance of phenotypic heterogeneity of focal lesions at different stages in hepatocarcinogenesis. Carcinogenesis 1987;8:1607–1612

97. Weber E, Bannasch P. Dose and time dependence of the cellular phenotype in rat hepatic preneoplasia and neoplasia induced by single oral exposures to *N*-nitrosomorpholine. Carcinogenesis 1994;15:1219–1226

98. Weber E, Bannasch P. Dose and time dependence of the cellular phenotype in rat hepatic preneoplasia and neoplasia induced in stop experiments by oral exposure to *N*-nitrosomorpholine. Carcinogenesis 1994;15:1227–1234

99. Weber E, Bannasch P. Dose and time dependence of the cellular phenotype in rat hepatic preneoplasia and neoplasia induced by continuous oral exposure to *N*-nitrosomorpholine. Carcinogenesis 1994;15:1235–1242

100. Williams GM. Interactive carcinogenesis in the liver. In Bannasch P, Keppler D, Weber G (eds): Liver Cell Carcinoma. Kluwer, Dordrecht, 1989, pp. 197–216

101. Berger MR. Synergism and antagonism between chemical carcinogens. In Arcos JC (ed): Chemical Induction of Cancer. Birkhäuser, Boston, 1995, pp. 23–49

102. Nakahara W. Mode of origin and characterization of cancer. In Nakahara W (ed): Chemical Tumor Problems. Japanese Society for the Promotion of Science, Tokyo, 1970, pp. 287–330

103. Schmähl D. Syncarcinogenesis: experimental investigations. In Nakahara W (ed): Chemical Tumor Problems. Japanese Society for the Promotion of Science, Tokyo, 1970, pp 1–8

104. Schmähl D. Combination effects in chemical carcinogenesis. Arch Toxicol 1980; (suppl 4): 29–40

105. MacDonald JC, Miller EC, Miller JA. The synergistic action of mixtures of certain hepatic carcinogens. Cancer Res 1952;12:50–54

106. Steiner PE. Carcinogenicity of multiple chemicals simultaneously administered. Cancer Res 1955;15:632–635

107. Berger MR, Schmähl D, Zerban H. Combination experiment of very low doses of three genotoxic *N*-nitrosamines with similar organotropic carcinogenicity in rats. Carcinogenesis 1987;8:1635–1643

108. Berger MR, Schmähl D, Edler L. Implications of the carcinogenic hazard of low doses of three hepatocarcinogenic *N*-nitrosamines. Jpn J Cancer Res 1990;81:598–606

109. Angsubhakorn S, Bhamarapravati N, Romruen K, Sahaphong S. Enhancing effects of dimethylnitrosamine on aflatoxin B_1 hepatocarcinogenesis in rats. Int J Cancer 1981; 28:621–626

110. Nakahara W, Fukuoka F. Summation of carcinogenic ef-

fects of chemically unrelated carcinogens, 4-nitroquinoline *N*-oxide and 20-methylcholanthrene. Gann 1960;51: 125–137

111. Takayama S, Imaizumi T. Sequential effects of chemically different carcinogens, dimethylnitrosamine and 4-dimethylaminoazobenzene, on hepatocarcinogenesis in rats. Int J Cancer 1969;4:373–383
112. Williams GM, Katayama S, Ohmori T. Enhancement of hepatocarcinogenesis by sequential administration of chemicals: summation versus promotion effects. Carcinogenesis 1981;2:1111–1117
113. Peraino C, Fry R, Staffeldt E. Reduction and enhancement by phenobarbital of hepatocarcinogenesis induced in rat by 2-acetylaminofluorene. Cancer Res 1971;31:1506–1512
114. Pitot HC, Sirica AE. The stages of initiation and promotion in hepatocarcinogenesis. Biochim Biophys Acta 1980;605: 191–215
115. Schulte-Hermann R. Tumor promotion in the liver. Arch Toxicol 1985;57:147–158
116. Rossi L, Ravera M, Repetti G, Santi L. Long-term administration of DDT or phenobarbital-Na in Wistar rats. Int J Cancer 1977;19:179–185
117. Feldman D, Swarm RL, Becker J. Ultrastructural study of rat liver and liver neoplasms after long-term treatment with phenobarbital. Cancer Res 1981;41:2151–2162
118. Tomatis L, Partensky C, Montesano R. The predictive value of mouse liver tumour induction in carcinogenicity testing—a literature survey. Int J Cancer 1973;12:1–20
119. Schulte-Hermann R, Timmermann-Trosiener l, Schuppler J. Promotion of spontaneous preneoplastic cells in rat liver as a possible explanation of tumor production by non-mutagenic compounds. Cancer Res 1983;43:839–844
120. Schwarz M, Bannasch P, Kunz W. The effect of pre- and post-treatment with phenobarbital on the extent of gamma-glutamyl transpeptidase positive foci induced in rat liver by *N*-nitrosomorpholine. Cancer Lett 1983;21:17–21
121. Williams GM, Furuya K. Distinction between liver neoplasm promoting and syncarcinogenic effects demonstrated by exposure to phenobarbital or diethylnitrosamine either before or after *N*-2-fluorenylacetamide. Carcinogenesis 1984;5:171–174
122. Hei TK, Sudilovsky O. Effects of a high-sucrose diet on the development of enzyme-altered foci in chemical hepatocarcinogenesis in rats. Cancer Res 1985;45:2700–2705
123. Enzmann H, Ohlhauser D, Dettler T, Bannasch P. Enhancement of hepatocarcinogenesis in rats by dietary fructose. Carcinogenesis 1989;10:1247–1252
124. Takada A, Nei J, Takase S, Matsuda Y. Effects of ethanol on experimental hepatocarcinogenesis. Hepatology 1986; 6:65–72
125. Driver HE, McLean AEM. Dose-response relationship for initiation of rat liver tumors by diethylnitrosamine and promotion by phenobarbitone and alcohol. Food Chem Toxicol 1986;24:241–245
126. Porta AE, Markell N, Dorado RD. Chronic alcoholism enhances hepatocarcinogenesis of diethylnitrosamine in rats fed a marginally methyl-deficient diet. Hepatology 1985;5: 1120–1125
127. Teschke R, Minzlaff M, Oldiges H, Frenzel H. Effect of chronic alcohol consumption on tumor incidence due to dimethylnitrosamine administration. J Cancer Res Clin Oncol 1983;106:58–64
128. Griciute L, Castegnaro M, Bereziat JC. Influence of ethyl alcohol on the carcinogenesis with *N*- nitrosodiethylamine. Cancer Lett 1981;13:345–352
129. Griciute L, Castegnaro M, Bereziat JC, Cabral JRP. Influence of ethyl alcohol on the carcinogenic activity of *N*-nitrosonornicotine. Cancer Lett 1986;31:267–275
130. Habs M, Schmähl D. Inhibition of the hepatocarcinogenic activity of diethylnitrosamine (DENA) by alcohol in rats. Acta Gastroenterol 1981;28:242–244
131. Radike MJ, Stemmer KL, Brown PB et al. Effect of ethanol and vinyl chloride on the induction of liver tumors. Environ Health Perspect 1977;21:153–155
132. Mendenhall CL, Chedid LA. Peliosis hepatis: its relationship to chronic alcoholism, aflatoxin B_1 and carcinogenesis in male Holtzman rats. Dig Dis Sci 1980;25:587–592
133. Misslbeck NG, Campbell TC, Roe DA. Effect of ethanol consumed in combination with high or low fat diets on the postinitiation phase of hepatocarcinogenesis in the rat. J Nutr 1984;114:2311–2323
134. Hepatitis viruses. In IARC Monographs on the Evalutation of Carcinogenic Risks to Humans, Vol 59. International Agency for Research on Cancer, Lyon, 1994, pp. 45–253
135. Qian G-S, Ross RK, Yu MC et al. A follow-up study of urinary markers of aflatoxin exposure and liver cancer risk in Shanghai, People's Republic of China. Cancer Epidemiol Biomarkers Prev 1994;3:3–10
136. Bosch FX, Munoz N. Epidemiology of hepatocellular carcinoma. In Bannasch P, Keppler D, Weber G (eds): Liver Cell Carcinoma. Kluwer, Dordrecht, 1989, pp.3–14
137. Bressac B, Kew M, Wands J, Ozturk M. Selective G to T mutations of *p53* gene in hepatocellular carcinoma from southern Africa. Nature 1991;350:429–431
138. Hsu IC, Metcalf RA, Sun et al. Mutational hotspot in the *p53* gene in human hepatocellular carcinomas. Nature 1991;35:427–428
139. Hollstein M, Sidransky D, Vogelstein B, Harris CC. *p53* Mutations in human cancers. Science 1991;253:49–53
140. Ozturk M et al. *p53* Mutation in hepatocellular carcinoma after aflatoxin exposure. Lancet 1991;338:1356–1359
141. Groopman JD. Molecular epidemiology of aflatoxin exposures. In Eaton DL, Groopman JD (eds): The Toxicology of Aflatoxins: Human Health, Veterinary and Agricultural Significance. Academic Press, New York, 1993; pp. 259–280
142. Chisari FV, Pinkert CA, Milich DR et al. A transgenic mouse model of the chronic hepatitis B surface antigen carrier state. Science 1985;230:1157–1160
143. Babinet C, Farza H, Morello D et al. Specific expression of hepatitis B surface antigen (HBsAg) in transgenic mice. Science 1985;230:1160–1163
144. Dragani TA, Manenti G, Farza H, et al. Transgenic mice containing hepatitis B virus sequences are more susceptible to carcinogen-induced hepatocarcinogenesis. Carcinogenesis 1989;11:953–956

145. Sell S, Hunt JM, Dunsford HA, Chisari FV. Synergy between hepatitis B virus expression and chemical hepatocarcinogens in transgenic mice. Cancer Res 1991;51:1278–1285

146. Uchida T, Suzuki K, Esumi M et al. Influence of aflatoxin B_1 intoxication on duck livers with duck hepatitis B virus infection. Cancer Res 1988;48:1559–1565

147. Cullen JM, Marion PL, Sherman GJ et al. Hepatic neoplasms in aflatoxin B_1- treated, congenital duck hepatitis B virus-infected, and virus-free Pekin ducks. Cancer Res 1990;50:4072–4080

148. Cova L, Wild CP, Mehrotra R et al. Contribution of aflatoxin B_1 and hepatitis B virus infection in the induction of liver tumors in ducks. Cancer Res 1990;50:2156–2163

149. Tennant BC, Hornbuckle WE, Yeager AE, et al. Effects of aflatoxin B_1 on experimental woodchuck hepatitis virus infection and hepatocellular carcinomas. In Hollinger FB, Lemon SM, Margolis H (eds): Viral Hepatitis and Liver Disease. Williams & Wilkins, Baltimore 1990, pp. 599–600

150. Bannasch P, Imani Koshkou N, Hacker HJ et al. Synergistic hepatocarcinogenic effect of hepadnaviral infection and dietary aflatoxin B_1 in woodchucks. Cancer Res 1995;55:3318–3330

151. Yan RQ, Su JJ, Huang DR et al. Human hepatitis B viruses and hepatocellular carcinoma. I. Experimental infection of tree shrews with hepatitis B virus. J Cancer Res Clin Oncol 1996;122:283–288

152. Yan RQ, Su JJ, Huang DR et al. Human hepatitis B virus and hepatocellular carcinoma. II. Experimental induction of hepatocellular carcinoma in tree shrews exposed to hepatitis B virus and aflatoxin B_1. J Cancer Res Clin Oncol 1996;122:289–295

153. Srivatanakul P, Ohshima H, Khlat M, et al. *Opisthorchis viverrini* infestation and endogenous nitrosamines as risk factors for cholangiocarcinoma in Thailand. Int J Cancer 1991;48:821–825

154. Flavell DJ, Lucas SB. Promotion of *N*-nitrosodiethylamine initiated bile duct carcinogenesis in the hamster by the human liver fluke, *Opisthorchis viverrini*. Carcinogenesis 1983;4:927–930

155. Thamavit T, Moore MA, Hiasa Y, Ito N. Enhancement of DHPN induced hepatocellular cholangiocellular and pancreatic carcinogenesis by *Opisthorchis viverrini* infestation in Syrian golden hamsters. Carcinogenesis 1988;9:1095–1098

156. Thamavit T, Moore MA, Hiasa Y, Ito N. Generation of high yields of Syrian hamster cholangiocellular carcinomas and hepatocellular nodules by combined nitrite and aminopyrine administration and *Opisthorchis viverrini* infestation. Jpn J Cancer Res 1988;79:909–916

157. Bergman F, Wahlin T. Tumour induction in Syrian hamsters fed a combination of aminopyrine and nitrite. Acta Pathol Microbiol Scand A 1981;89:241–245

158. Thamavit W, Ngamying M, Boonpucknavig V et al. Enhancement of DEN-induced hepatocellular nodule development by *Opisthorchis viverrini* infestation in Syrian golden hamsters. Carcinogenesis 1987;8:1351–1353

159. Moore MA, Kitagawa T. Hepatocarcinogenesis in the rat; the effect of the promoters and carcinogens in vivo and in vitro. Int Rev Cytol 1986;101:125–173

160. Farber E, Sarma DSR. Hepatocarcinogenesis: a dynamic cellular perspective. Lab Invest 1987;56:4–22

161. Fearon ER, Vogelstein B. A genetic model for colorectal tumorigenesis. Cell 1990;61:759–767

162. Mehta R. The potential for the use of cell proliferation and oncogene expression as intermediate markers during liver carcinogenesis. Cancer Lett 1995;93:85–102

163. Bannasch P, Mayer D, Hacker HJ. Hepatocellular glycogenosis and hepatocarcinogenesis. Biochim Biophys Acta 1980;605:217–245

164. Farber E, Rubin H. Cellular adaptation in the origin and development of cancer. Cancer Res 1991;51:2751–2761

165. Bannasch P. Phenotypic cellular changes as indicators of stages during neoplastic development. In Iversen OH (ed): Theories of Carcinogenesis. Hemisphere Publishing Corporation, Washington, 1988, pp. 231–249

166. Bannasch P. Cytology and cytogenesis of neoplastic (hyperplastic) hepatic nodules. Cancer Res 1976;36:2555–2562

167. Williams GM. Functional markers and growth behaviour of prenoplastic hepatocytes. Cancer Res 1976;36:2540–2543

168. Grisham JW. Hepatic epithelial stem-like cells. Verh Deutsch Ges Pathol 1995;79:47–54

169. Bralet MP, Branchereau S, Bréchot C, Ferry N. Cell lineage study in the liver using retroviral mediated gene transfer. Am J Pathol 1994;114:896–905

170. Ng YK, Iannacone PM. Fractal geometry of mosaic pattern demonstrates liver regeneration is a self-similar process. Dev Biol 1992;151:419–430

171. Grisham JW, Hartroff WS. Morphologic identification by electron microscopy of "oval" cells in experimental hepatic degeneration. Lab Invest 1961;10:317–332

172. Farber E. Similarities in the sequence of early histological changes induced in the liver of the rat by ethionine, 2-acetylaminofluorene and 3′-methyl-4-dimethylaminoazobenzene. Cancer Res 1956;16:142–148

173. Marceau N. Biology of disease. Cell lineages and differentiation programs in epidermal, urothelial and hepatic tissues and their neoplasms. Lab Invest 1990;63:4–20

174. Sell S. Is there a liver stem cell? Cancer Res 1990;50:3811–3815

175. Aterman K. The stem cells of the liver—a selective review. J Cancer Res Clin Oncol 1992;118:87–115

176. Sirica AE (ed): The Role of Cell Types in Hepatocarcinogenesis. CRC, Boca Raton, 1992

177. Fausto N. Liver stem cells. In Arias IM, Boyer JL, Fausto N et al. (eds): The Liver. Biology and Pathobiology, 3rd Ed. Raven Press, New York, 1994, pp. 1501–1518

178. Thorgeirsson SS. Stem cells in hepatocarcinogenesis. In Jirtle RL (ed): Liver Regeneration and Carcinogenesis. Academic Press, San Diego, 1995, pp. 99–112

179. Steinberg P, Hacker HJ, Dienes HP et al. Enzyme- and immunohistochemical characterization of oval and parenchymal cells proliferating in livers of rats fed a choline-deficient/DL-ethionine-supplemented diet. Carcinogenesis 1991;12:225–231

180. Tarsetti F, Lenzi R, Salvi R et al. Liver carcinogenesis associated with feeding of ethionine in a choline-free diet: evidence against a role of oval cells in the emergence of hepatocellular carcinoma. Hepatology 1993;18:596–603

181. Hutterer F, Rubin E, Singer EJ, Popper H. Quantitative relation of cell proliferation and fibrogenesis in the liver. Cancer Res 1961;21:206–215

182. Grisham JW, Porta EA. Origin and fate of proliferated hepatic ductal cells in the rat; electron microscopic and autoradiographic studies. Exp Mol Pathol 1964;3:242–261

183. Rubin E. The origin and fate of proliferated bile ductular cells. Exp Mol Pathol 1964;3:279–286

184. Tatematsu M, Ho RH, Kaku T et al. Studies on the proliferation and fate of oval cells in the liver of rats treated with 2-acetylaminofluorene and partial hepatectomy. Am J Pathol 1984;114:418–430

185. Tatematsu M, Kaku T, Medline A, Farber E. Intestinal metaplasia as a common option of oval cells in relation to cholangiofibrosis in liver of rats exposed to 2-acetylaminofluorene. Lab Invest 1985;52:354–362

186. Bannasch P, Reiss W. Histogenese und Cytogenese cholangiocellulärer Tumoren bei Nitrosomorpholin-vergifteten Ratten. Zugleich ein Beitrag zur Morphogenese der Cystenleber. Z Krebsforsch 1971;76:193–215

187. Terao K, Nakano M. Cholangiofibrosis induced by short-term feeding of 3′-methyl-4-(dimethylamino)azobenzene: an electron microscopic observation. Gann 1974;65: 249–260

188. Bannasch P, Massner B. Histogenese und Cytogenese von Cholangiofibromen und Cholangiocarcinomen bei Nitrosomorpholin-vergifteten Ratten. Z Krebsforsch 1976;87: 239–255

189. Ohshima M, Ward JM, Brennan LM, Creasia DA. Sequential study of methapyrilene hydrochloride-induced liver carcinogenesis in male F344 rats. J Natl Cancer Inst 1984;72: 759–768

190. Evans JG, Appleby EL, Lake BG, Conning DM. Studies on the induction of cholangiofibrosis by coumarin in the rat. Toxicology 1989;55:207–224

191. Peterson JE. Biliary hyperplasia and carcinogenesis in chronic liver damage induced in rats by phomopsin. Pathology 1990;22:213–222

192. Maronpot RR, Giles HD, Dykes DJ, Irwin RD. Furan-induced hepatic cholangiocarcinomas in Fischer 344 rats. Toxicol Pathol 1991;19:561–570

193. Hacker HJ, Steinberg P, Toshkov I, Bannasch P. Persistance of the cholangiocellular and hepatocellular lesions observed in rats fed a choline-deficient/DL-ethionine-supplemented diet. Carcinogenesis 1992;13:271–276

194. Moore MA, Fukushima S, Ichihara A et al. Intestinal metaplasia and altered enzyme expression in propylnitrosamine-induced Syrian hamster cholangiocellular and gallbladder lesions. Virchows Arch B (Cell Pathol) 1986;51:29–38

195. Thamavit W, Kongkanuntn R, Tiwawech D, Moore MA. Level of *Opisthorchis* infestation and carcinogen dose-dependence of cholangiocarcinoma induction in Syrian golden hamsters. Virchows Arch B (Cell Pathol) 1987;54: 52–58

196. Opie EL. The pathogenesis of tumors of the liver produced by butter yellow. J Exp Med 1944;80:231–246

197. Bannasch P. Die Cytologie der Hepatocarcinogenese. In Grundmann E (ed): Handbuch Allg Pathol, VI/VII. Springer, Berlin, 1975, pp. 123–276

198. Edwards JE, White J. Pathologic changes with special reference to pigmentation and classification of hepatic tumor in rats fed *p*-dimethylaminoazobenzene (butter yellow). J Natl Cancer Inst 1941;2:157–183

199. Stewart HL, Williams G, Keysser CH et al. Histologic typing of liver tumors of the rat. J Natl Cancer Inst 1980;65: 179–206

200. Jamison KC, Larson JL, Butterworth BE et al. A non-bile duct origin for intestinal crypt-like ducts with periductular fibrosis induced in livers of 344 rats by chloroform inhalation. Carcinogenesis 1996;17:675–682

201. Inaoka Y. Significance of the so-called oval cell proliferation during azo-dye hepatocarcinogenesis. Gann 1967;58: 355–366

202. Ogawa K, Minase T, Onoé T. Demonstration of glucose-6-phosphatase activity in the oval cells of rat liver and the significance of the oval cells in azodye carcinogenesis. Cancer Res 1974;34:3379–3386

203. Dempo K, Chisaka N, Yoshida Y et al. Immunofluorescent study of 3′-methyl-4-dimethylaminoazobenzene carcinogenesis. Cancer Res 1975;35:1282–1287

204. Shinozuka H, Lombardi B, Sell S, Immarino RM. Early histological and functional alterations of ethionine liver carcinogenesis in rats fed a choline-deficient diet. Cancer Res 1978;38:1092–1098

205. Sell S, Osborn K, Leffert HL. Autoradiography of "oval cells" appearing rapidly in the livers of rats fed *N*-2-fluorenylacetamide in a choline devoid diet. Carcinogenesis 1981;2:7–14

206. Germain L, Goyette R, Marceau N. Differential cytokeratin and α-fetoprotein expression in morphologically distinct epithelial cells emerging at the early stage of rat hepatocarcinogenesis. Cancer Res 1985;45:673–681

207. Evarts RP, Nagy P, Marsden E, Thorgeirsson SS. A precursor-product relationship exists between oval cells and hepatocytes in rat liver. Carcinogenesis 1987;8:1737–1740

208. Evarts RP, Nagy P, Nakatsukasa H et al. In vivo differentiation of rat liver oval cells into hepatocytes. Cancer Res 1989;49:1541–1547

209. Lemire JM, Fausto N. Multiple α-fetoprotein RNAs in adult rat liver: cell type-specific expression and differential regulation. Cancer Res 1991;51:4656–4664

210. Radaeva S, Steinberg P. Phenotype and differentiation patterns in the oval cell lines OC/CDE 6 and OC/CDE 22 derived from the livers of carcinogen-treated rats. Cancer Res 1995;55:1028–1038

211. Radaeva S, Bannasch P. Changes in catalase and glucose-6-phosphatase distribution patterns within oval cell compartments as possible differentiation markers during viral hepatocarcinogenesis in woodchucks. Differentiation 1996; 60:169–178

212. Makino Y, Yamamoto K, Tsuji T. Three-dimensional arrangement of ductular structure formed by oval cells during

hepatocarcinogenesis. Acta Med Okayama 1988;42: 143–150

213. Steinberg P, Steinbrecher R, Radaeva S et al. Oval cell lines OC/CDE6 and OC/CDE 22 give rise to cholangiocellular and undifferentiated carcinomas after transformation. Lab Invest 1994;171:700–709
214. Anilkumar TV, Golding M, Edwards RJ et al. The resistant hepatocyte model of carcinogenesis in the rat: the apparent independent development of oval cell proliferation and early nodules. Carcinogenesis 1995;16:845–853
215. Farber E. On cells of origin of liver cell cancer. In Sirica AE (ed): The Role of Cell Types in Hepatocarcinogenesis. CRC, Boca Raton, 1992, pp. 1–28
216. Gindi T, Ghazarian DMD, Deitch D, Farber E. An origin of presumptive preneoplastic foci and nodules from hepatocytes in chemical carcinogenesis in rat liver. Cancer Lett 1994;83:75–80
217. Butler WH, Jones G. Ultrastructure of hepatic neoplasia. In Newberne PM, Butler WH (eds): Rat Hepatic Neoplasia MIT Press, Cambridge, 1978, pp 142–179
218. Ruan Y, Hacker HJ, Zerban H, Bannasch P. Ultrastructural and immunocytochemical characterization of the cellular phenotype in primary adenoid liver tumours of the rat. Pathol Res Pract 1989;184:223–233
219. Bannasch P, Wayss K, Zerban H: Peliosis hepatis, rodents. In Jones TC, Mohr U, Hunt RD (eds): Monographs on Pathology of Laboratory Animals. Digestive System. Springer, Berlin, 1997, pp. 154–160
220. Ströbel P, Mayer F, Zerban H, Bannasch P. Spongiotic pericytoma: a benign neoplasm deriving from the perisinusoidal (Ito) cells in rat liver. Am J Pathol 1995;146:903–913
221. Bannasch P, Zerban H. Spongiosis hepatis, rat. In Jones TC, Mohr U, Hunt RD (eds): Monographs on Pathology of Laboratory Animals. Digestive System. Springer, Berlin, 1997, pp. 104–113
222. Bannasch P, Zerban H, Schmid E, Franke WW. Liver tumors distinguished by immunofluorescence microscopy with antibodies to proteins of intermediate-sized filaments. Proc Natl Acad Sci USA 1980;77:4948–4952
223. Bannasch P, Zerban H, Schmid E, Franke WW. Characterization of cytoskeletal components in epithelial and mesenchymal liver tumors by electron and immunofluorescence microscopy. Virchows Arch B (Cell Pathol) 1981;36: 139–158
224. Bannasch P, Müller HA. Lichtmikroskopische Untersuchungen über die Wirkung von *N*-Nitrosomorpholin auf die Leber von Ratte and Maus. Arzneimittel Forsch 1964; 14:805–814
225. Gössner W, Friedrich-Freksa H. Histochemische Untersuchungen über die Glucose-6-Phosphatase in der Rattenleber während der Kanzerisierung durch Nitrosamine. Z Naturforsch 1964;19b:862–863
226. Pitot HC. Altered hepatic foci: their role in murine hepatocarcinogenesis. Annu Rev Pharmacol Toxicol 1990;30: 465–500
227. Bannasch P, Zerban H, Hacker HJ. Foci of altered hepatocytes, rat. In Jones TC, Mohr U, Hunt RD (eds): Monographs on Pathology of Laboratory Animals. Digestive System. Springer, Berlin, 1997, pp. 3–37
228. Thorgeirsson UP, Gomez DE, Lindsay CK et al. Liver tumors and possible preneoplastic lesions, induced by a food-derived heterocyclic amine in cynomolgus monkeys; a study of histology and cytokeratin expression. Liver 1996;16: 71–83
229. Friedrich-Freksa H, Papadopulu G, Gössner W. Histochemische Untersuchungen der Cancerogenese in der Rattenleber nach zeitlich begrenzter Verabfolgung von Diäthylnitrosamin. Z Krebsforsch 1969;72:240–253
230. Schauer A, Kunze E. Enzymhistochemische und autoradiographische Untersuchungen während der Kanzerisierung der Rattenleber durch Diäthylnitrosamin. Z Krebsforsch 1968;70:252–266
231. Rabes HM, Scholze P, Jantsch B. Growth kinetics of diethylnitrosamine-induced enzyme-deficient "preneoplastic" liver cell populations in vivo and in vitro. Cancer Res 1972; 32:2577–2586
232. Bannasch P, Hacker HJ, Klimek F, Mayer D. Hepatocellular glycogenosis and related pattern of enzymatic changes during hepatocarcinogenesis. Adv Enzyme Regul 1984;22: 97–121
233. Williams GM. The pathogenesis of rat liver cancer caused by chemical carcinogens. Biochim Biophys Acta 1980;605: 167–189
234. Eriksson LC, Andersson GN. Membrane biochemistry and chemical hepatocarcinogenesis. Crit Rev Biochem Mol Biol 1992;27:1–55
235. Schiebel K, Stumpf H, Zerban H et al. Altered transferrin gene expression in preneoplastic and neoplastic liver lesions induced in rats with *N*-nitrosomorpholine. Virchows Arch B (Cell Pathol) 1992;62:251–257
236. Hertz R, Seckbach M, Zaki MM, Bar-Tana J. Transcriptional suppression of the transferrin gene by hypolipidemic peroxisome proliferators. J Biol Chem 1996;271:218–224
237. Huber BE, Heilmann CA, Thorgeirsson SS. Poly(A)RNA levels of growth-, differentiation-, and transformation-associated genes in the progressive development of hepatocellular carcinoma in the rat. Hepatology 1989;9:756–762
238. La Porta CAM, Perletti GP, Comolli R. Analysis of calcium-dependent protein kinase C isoforms in the early stages of diethylnitrosamine-induced rat hepatocarcinogenesis. Mol Carcinog 1993;8:255–263
239. Suzuki S, Satoh K, Nakano H et al. Lack of correlated expression between the glutathione S-transferase P-form and the oncogene products c-Jun and c-Fos in rat tissues and preneoplastic hepatic foci. Carcinogenesis 1995;16: 567–571
240. Scherer E, Hoffmann M. Probable clonal genesis of cellular islands induced in rat liver by diethylnitrosamine. Eur J Cancer 1971;7:369–371
241. Rabes HM, Bücher T, Hartmann A et al. Clonal growth of carcinogen-induced enzyme-deficient preneoplastic cell populations in mouse liver. Cancer Res 1982;42:3220–3227
242. Howell S, Wareham KA, Williams ED. Clonal origin of mouse liver cell tumors. Am J Pathol 1985;121:426–432
243. Tsuji S, Ogawa K, Takasaka H et al. Clonal origin of γ-glutamyl transpeptidase-positive hepatic lesions induced by initiation-promotion in ornithine carbamoyltransferase mosaic mice. Jpn J Cancer Res 1988;79:148–152

244. Weinberg WC, Iannaccone PM. Clonality of preneoplastic liver lesions: histological analysis in chimeric rats. J Cell Sci 1988;89:423–431

245. Weber E. Dosisabhängigkeit der Sequenz zellulärer Veränderungen bei der *N*- Nitrosomorpholin-induzierten Hepatokarzinogenese in der Ratte. Thesis (TH Darmstadt), 1989

246. Bannasch P, Zerban H. Preneoplastic and neoplastic lesions of the rat liver. In Bannasch P, Gössner W (eds): Pathology of Neoplasia and Preneoplasia in Rodents. EULEP Color Atlas. Schattauer, Stuttgart, 1994; pp. 18–63

247. Maguire S, Rabes HM. Intralobular distribution of preneoplastic foci in rat liver after a single dose of *N*-methyl-*N*-nitrosourea (MNU) following partial hepatectomy. Carcinogenesis 1989;10:871–874

248. Bannasch P, Hesse J, Angerer H. Hepatocelluläre Glykogenose und die Genese sogenannter hyperplastischer Knoten in der Thioacetamid-vergifteten Rattenleber. Virchows Arch B (Cell Pathol) 1974;17:29–50

249. Maronpot RR, Montgomery CA Jr, Boorman GA, McConnell EE. National Toxicology Program nomenclature for hepatoproliferative lesions of rats. Toxicol Pathol 1986;14: 263–273

250. Farber E. The biology of carcinogen-induced hepatocyte nodules and related liver lesions in the rat. Toxicol Pathol 1982;10:197–205

251. Jack EM, Stäubli W, Waechter F et al. Ultrastructural changes in chemically induced preneoplastic focal lesions in the rat liver, a stereological study. Carcinogenesis 1990; 11:1531–1538

252. Bannasch P, Benner U, Enzmann H, Hacker HJ. Tigroid cell foci and neoplastic nodules in the liver of rats treated with a single dose of aflatoxin B_1. Carcinogenesis 1985;6: 1641–1648

253. Weber E, Moore MA, Bannasch P. Enzyme histochemical and morphological phenotype of amphophilic foci and amphophilic/tigroid cell neoplastic nodules in rat liver after combined treatment with dehydroepiandrosterone and *N*-nitrosomorpholine. Carcinogenesis 1988;9:1049–1054

254. Bannasch P, Enzmann H, Klimek F et al. Significance of sequential cellular changes inside and outside foci of altered hepatocytes during hepatocarcinogenesis. Toxicol Pathol 1989;17:617–628

255. Harada T, Maronpot RR, Morris RW, Boorman GA. Observations on altered hepatocellular foci in National Toxicology Program two-year carcinogenicity studies in rats. Toxicol Pathol 1989;17:690–708

256. Reznik-Schüller HM, Gregg M. Sequential morphological changes during methapyrilene-induced hepatocellular carcinogenesis in rats. J Natl Cancer Inst 1983;71:1021–1031

257. Zerban H, Rabes H, Bannasch P. Sequential changes in growth kinetics and cellular phenotype during hepatocarcinogenesis. J Cancer Res Clin Oncol 1989;115:329–334

258. Zerban H, Radig S, Kopp-Schneider A, Bannasch P. Cell proliferation and cell death (apoptosis) in hepatic preneoplasia and neoplasia are closely related to phenotypic cellular diversity and instability. Carcinogenesis 1994;15: 2467–2473

259. Enzmann H, Bannasch P. Morphometric study of alterations of extrafocal hepatocytes of rat liver treated with *N*-nitrosomorpholine. Virchows Arch B (Cell Pathol) 1987; 53:218–226

260. Wanson J-C, Bernaert D, Penasse W et al. Separation in distinct subpopulations by elutriation of liver cells following exposure of rats to *N*-nitrosomorpholine. Cancer Res 1980; 40:459–471

261. Bannasch P, Moore MA, Hacker HJ et al. Potential significance of phenotypic instability in focal and nodular liver lesions induced by hepatocarcinogens. In Brunner H, Thaler H (eds): Hepatology: A Festschrift for Hans Popper. Raven, New York; 1985, pp. 191–209

262. Moore MA, Hacker HJ, Bannasch P. Phenotypic instability in focal and nodular lesions induced in a short term system in the rat liver. Carcinogenesis 1983;4:595–603

263. Rabes HM. Cell proliferation and hepatocarcinogenesis. In Roberfroid MB, Préat V (eds): Experimental Hepatocarcinogenesis. Plenum Press, New York, 1988, pp. 121–132

264. Ledda-Columbano GM, Shinozuka H, Katyal SL, Columbano A. Cell proliferation, cell death and hepatocarcinogenesis. Cell Death Differ 1996;3:17–22

265. Tanaka T, Mori H, Hirota N et al. Effect of DNA synthesis on induction of preneoplastic and neoplastic lesions in rat liver by a single dose of methylazoxymethanol acetate. Chem Biol Interact 1986;58:13–27

266. Cayama E, Tsuda H, Sarma DSR, Farber E. Initiation of chemical carcinogenesis requires cell proliferation. Nature 1978;275:60–62

267. Pound AW, McGuire LJ. Repeated partial hepatectomy as a promoting stimulus for carcinogenic response of liver to nitrosamines in rats. Br J Cancer 1978;37:585–594

268. Ishikawa T, Takayama S, Kitagawa T. Correlation between time of partial hepatectomy after a single treatment with diethylnitrosamine and induction of adenosinetriphosphatase-deficient islands in rat liver. Cancer Res 1980;40: 4261–4264

269. Columbano A, Rajalakshmi S, Sarma DSR. Requirement of cell proliferation for the initiation of liver carcinogenesis as assayed by three different procedures. Cancer Res 1981; 41:2079–2083

270. Peraino C, Staffeldt EF, Ludeman VA. Early appearance of histochemically altered hepatocyte foci and liver tumors in female rats treated with carcinogens one day after birth. Carcinogenesis 1981;2:463–465

271. Vesselinovitch SD, Koka M, Mihailovich N, Rao KVN. Carcinogenicity of diethylnitrosamine in newborn, infant and adult mice. J Cancer Res Clin Oncol 1984;108:60–65

272. Decloitre F, Lafarge-Frayssinet C, Barros M et al. Effect of rat development stage at initiation on the expression of biochemical markers during liver tumor promotion. Tumour Biol 1990;11:295–305

273. Hasegawa R, Takahashi S, Imaida K et al. Age-dependent induction of preneoplastic liver cell foci by 2-acetylaminofluorene, phenobarbital and acetaminophen in F344 rats initially treated with diethylnitrosamine. Jpn J Cancer Res (Gann) 1991;82:293–297

274. Mathur M, Rizvi TA, Nayak NC. Aflatoxin B_1 induced hepatocarcinogenesis in neonatal rats. Ind J Exp Biol 1992; 30:165–168

275. Rabes HM, Müller L, Hartmann A et al. Cell cycle-dependent initiation of adenosine triphosphatase-deficient populations in adult rat liver by a single dose of *N*-methyl-*N*-nitrosourea. Cancer Res 1986;46:645–650

276. Kaufmann WK, Rahija RJ, MacKenzie SA, Kaufman DG. Cell cycle-dependent initiation of hepatocarcinogenesis in rats (±) 7r, 8t-dihydroxy-9t, 10t-epoxy-7,8,9,10-tetrahydrobenzo(a)pyrene. Cancer Res 1987;47:3771–3775

277. Bartsch H, Préat V, Aitio A, et al. Partial hepatectomy of rats ten weeks before carcinogen administration can enhance liver carcinogenesis: preliminary observations. Carcinogenesis 1988;9:2315–2317

278. Columbano A, Ledda-Columbano GM, Coni P et al. Initiation of chemical hepatocarcinogenesis: compensatory cell proliferation versus mitogen induced hyperplasia. In Roberfroid MB, Préat V (eds): Experimental Hepatocarcinogenesis. Plenum Press, New York, 1987, pp. 133–141

279. Ledda-Columbano GM, Columbano A, Curto M et al. Further evidence that mitogen-induced cell proliferation does not support the formation of enzyme-altered islands in rat liver by carcinogens. Carcinogenesis 1989;10:847–850

280. Columbano A, Ledda-Columbano GM, Ennas MG et al. Cell proliferation and promotion of rat liver carcinogenesis: different effect of hepatic regeneration and mitogen induced hyperplasia on the development of enzyme-altered foci. Carcinogenesis 1990;11:771–776

281. Sorof S, Custer RP. Elevated expression and cell cycle deregulation of mitosis-associated target polypeptide of a carcinogen in hyperplastic and malignant rat hepatocytes. Cancer Res 1987;47:210–220

282. Pugh TD, Goldfarb S. Quantitative histochemical and autoradiographic studies of hepatocarcinogenesis in rats fed 2-acetylaminofluorene followed by phenobarbital. Cancer Res 1978;38:4450–4457

283. Baba M, Yamamoto R, Iishi H et al. Role of glucose-6-phosphate dehydrogenase on enhanced proliferation of preneoplastic and neoplastic cells in rat liver induced by *N*-nitrosomorpholine. Int J Cancer 1989;43:892–895

284. Rotstein J, Sarma DSR, Farber E. Sequential alterations in growth control and cell dynamics of rat hepatocytes in early precancerous steps in hepatocarcinogenesis. Cancer Res 1986;46:2377–2385

285. Tatematsu M, Aoki T, Kagawa M et al. Reciprocal relationship between development of glutathione S-transferase positive liver foci and proliferation of surrounding hepatocytes in rats. Carcinogenesis 1988;9:221–225

286. Tsuda H, Asamoto M, Baba H et al. Cell proliferation and advancement of hepatocarcinogenesis in the rat are associated with a decrease in connexin 32 expression. Carcinogenesis 1995;16:101–105

287. Beer DG, Neveu MJ, Paul DL et al. Expression of c-*raf* protooncogene, gamma-glutamyl transpeptidase, and gap junction protein in rat liver neoplasms. Cancer Res 1986; 46:2435–2441

288. Yamasaki H, Mesnil M, Omori Y et al. Intercellular communication and carcinogenesis. Mutat Res 1995;333:181–188

289. Bursch W, Lauer B, Timmermann-Trosiener et al. Controlled cell death (apoptosis) of normal and putative preneoplastic cells in rat liver following withdrawal of tumour promoters. Carcinogenesis 1984;5:453–458

290. Columbano A, Ledda-Columbano GM, Rao PM et al. Occurrence of cell death (apoptosis) in preneoplastic and neoplastic liver cells: a sequential study. Am J Pathol 1984; 116:441–446

291. Schulte-Hermann R, Timmermann-Trosiener I, Barthel G, Bursch W. DNA synthesis, apoptosis, and phenotypic expression as determinants of growth of altered foci in rat liver during phenobarbital promotion. Cancer Res 1990; 50:5127–5135

292. Enzmann H, Bannasch P. Non-persisting early foci of altered hepatocytes induced in rats by *N*-nitrosomorpholine. J Cancer Res Clin Oncol 1988;114:30–34

293. Romen W, Ross W, Bannasch P. Cytomorphologische und morphometrische Studien der Hepatocarcinogenese II. Die Reversibilität von Kerngrößenänderungen in der Nitrosomorpholin-vergifteten Rattenleber. Z Krebsforsch 1972;77: 134–140

294. Romen W, Bannasch P, Aziz A, Reuss W. Karyokinese und Kernstruktur während der Hepatocarcinogenese. II. Die Feinstruktur des Zellkerns in Hepatozyten und Hepatomzellen der Nitrosomorpholin-vergifteten Rattenleber. Virchows Arch B (Cell Pathol) 1973;13:267–296

295. Abmayr W, Deml E, Oesterle D, Gössner W. Nuclear morphology in preneoplastic lesions of rat liver. Anal Quant Cytol 1983;5:275–284

296. Schwarze PE, Petterson EO, Tolleshaug H, Seglen PO. Isolation of carcinogen-induced diploid rat hepatocytes by centrifugal elutriation. Cancer Res 1986;46:4732–4737

297. Deleener A, Castelain P, Préat V et al. Changes in nucleolar transcriptional activity and nuclear DNA content during the first steps of rat hepatocarcinogenesis. Carcinogenesis 1987;8:195–201

298. Styles JA, Kelly M, Elcombe ER. A cytological comparison between regeneration, hyperplasia and early neoplasia in rat liver. Carcinogenesis 1987;8:391–399

299. Haesen S, Derijicke T, Deleener A et al. The influence of phenobarbital and butylated hydroxytoluene on the ploidy rate in rat hepatocarcinogenesis. Carcinogenesis 1988;9: 1755–1761

300. Saeter G, Schwarze PE, Nesland JM et al. The polyploidizing growth pattern of normal rat liver is replaced by divisional, diploid growth in hepatocellular nodules and carcinomas. Carcinogenesis 1988;9:939–945

301. Sargent L, Xu Y-H, Sattler GL et al. Ploidy and karyotype of hepatocytes isolated from enzyme-altered foci in two different protocols of multistage hepatocarcinogenesis in the rat. Carcinogenesis 1989;10:387–391

302. Gerlyng P, Abyholm A, Grotmol T et al. Binucleation and polyploidization patterns in developmental regenerative rat liver growth. Cell Proliferation 1993;26:557–565

303. Mori H, Tanaka T, Sugie S et al. DNA content of liver cell nuclei of *N*-2-fluorenylacetamide-induced altered foci and neoplasms in rats and human hyperplastic foci. J Natl Cancer Inst 1982;69:1277–1282

304. Digernes V. Chemical liver carcinogenesis: monitoring of the process by flow cytometric DNA measurements. Environ Health Perspect 1983;50:195–200

305. Sarafoff M, Rabes HM, Dormer P. Correlations between ploidy and initiation probability determined by DNA cytophotometry in individual altered hepatic foci. Carcinogenesis 1986;7:1191–1196

306. Danielsen HE, Steen HB, Lindmo T, Reith A. Ploidy distribution in experimental liver carcinogenesis in mice. Carcinogenesis 1988;9:59–63

307. Gil R, Callaghan R, Boix J et al. Morphometric and cytophotometric nuclear analysis of altered hepatocyte foci induced by *N*-nitrosomorpholine (NNM) and aflatoxin B_1 (AFB_1) in liver of Wistar rats. Virchows Arch B (Cell Pathol) 1988;54:341–349

308. Jack EM, Bentley P, Bieri F et al. Increase in hepatocyte and nuclear volume and decrease in the population of binucleated cells in preneoplastic foci of rat liver: a stereological study using the nucleator method. Hepatology 1990;11: 286–297

309. Wang JH, Hinrichsen L1, Whitacre CM et al. Nuclear DNA content of altered hepatic foci in rat liver carcinogenesis model. Cancer Res 1990;50:7571–7576

310. Sudilovsky O, Hei TK. Aneuploidy and progression in promoted preneoplastic foci during chemical hepatocarcinogenesis in the rat. Cancer Lett 1991;56:131–135

311. Enzmann H, Kühlem C, Löser E, Bannasch P. Dose dependence of diethylnitrosamine-induced nuclear enlargement in embryonal turkey liver. Carcinogenesis 1995;16: 1351–1355

312. Bannasch P. Pathobiology of chemical hepatocarcinogenesis: recent progress and perspectives. Part II. Metabolic and molecular changes. J Gastroenterol Hepatol 1990;5: 310–320

313. Saeter G, Seglen PO. Cell biology of hepatocarcinogenesis. Crit Rev Oncol 1990;1:437–466

314. Strom SC, Faust JB. Oncogene activation and hepatocarcinogenesis. Pathobiology 1990;58:153–167

315. Maronpot RR, Fox T, Malarkey DE, Goldsworthy TL. Mutations in the *ras* protooncogene: clues to etiology and molecular pathogenesis of mouse liver tumors. Toxicology 1995;101:125–156

316. Buchmann A, Bauer-Hofmann R, Mahr J et al. Mutational activation of the c-Ha-*ras* gene in liver tumors of different rodent strains: correlation with susceptibility to hepatocarcinogenesis. Proc Natl Acad Sci USA 1991;88:911–915

317. Bauer-Hofmann R, Klimek F, Buchmann A et al. Role of mutations at codon 61 of the c-Ha-*ras* gene during diethylnitrosamine-induced hepatocarcinogenesis in C3H/He mice. Carcinogenesis 1992;6:60–67

318. McMahon G, Davis EF, Huber LJ et al. Characterization of c-Ki-*ras* and N-*ras* oncogenes in aflatoxin B_1-induced rat liver tumors. Proc Natl Acad Sci USA 1990;87:1104–1108

319. Sarafoff M, Rabes HM. Demonstration of temporal and topical c-*myc* expression in regenerating rat liver and in neoplastic nodules by in situ hybridization. J Cancer Res Clin Oncol 1991;S37

320. Simile MM, Pascale R, De Miglio MR et al. Correlation between *S*-adenosyl-L-methionine and production of c-*myc*, c-Ha-*ras*, and c-Ki-*ras* mRNA transcripts in the early stages of rat liver carcinogenesis. Cancer Lett 1994;79:9–16

321. Nakano H, Hatayama I, Satoh K et al. c-Jun expression in single cells and preneoplastic foci induced by diethylnitrosamine in B6C3F1 mice: comparison with the expression of pi-class glutathion S-transferase. Carcinogenesis 1994; 15:1853–1857

322. Suzuki S, Satoh K, Nakano H et al. Lack of correlated expression between the glutathione S-transferase P-form and the oncogene products c-Jun and c-Fos in rat tissues and preneoplastic hepatic foci. Carcinogenesis 1995;6:567–571

323. Valera A, Pujol A, Gregori X et al. Evidence from transgenic mice that myc regulates hepatic glycolysis. FASEB J 1995;9:1067–1078

324. Daum G, Eisenmann-Tappe J, Fries HW et al. The ins and outs of Raf kinases. TIBS 1994;19:474–480

325. Smith MC, Yeleswarapu L, Locker J, Lombardi B. Expression of p53 mutant proteins in diethylnitrosamine-induced foci of enzyme-altered hepatocytes in male Fischer-344 rats. Carcinogenesis 1991;12:1137–1141

326. Wirnitzer U, Enzmann H, Rosenbruch M, Bomhard EM. Accumulation of p53 protein in chemically induced oval cells during early stages of rodent hepatocarcinogenesis. Carcinogenesis 1995;16:697–701

327. Kress S, König J, Schweizer J et al. *p53* mutations are absent from carcinogen-induced mouse liver tumors. Mol Carcinog 1992;6:148–158

328. Goodrow TL, Storer RD, Leander KR et al. Murine *p53* intron sequences 5–8 and their use of polymerase chain reaction/direct sequencing analysis of *p53* mutations in CD-1 mouse liver and lung tumors. Mol Carcinog 1992;5:9–15

329. Rumsby PC, Davies MJ, Evans JG. Screening for *p53* mutations in C3H/He mouse liver tumors derived spontaneously or induced with diethylnitrosamine or phenobarbitone. Mol Carcinog 1994;9:71–75

330. Tokusashi Y, Fukuda J, Ogawa K. Absence of *p53* mutations and various frequencies of Ki-*ras* exon 1 mutations in rat hepatic tumors induced by different carcinogens. Mol Carcinog 1994;10:45–51

331. Kemp Cl. Hepatocarcinogenesis in *p53*-deficient mice. Mol Carcinog 1995;12:132–136

332. Jirtle RL (ed): Liver Regeneration and Carcinogenesis. Academic Press, San Diego, 1995

333. Kaufmann WK, Zhang Y, Kaufman DG. Association between expression of transforming growth factor-alpha and progression of hepatocellular foci to neoplasms. Carcinogenesis 1992;13:1481–1483

334. Dragan Y, Teeguarden J, Campbell H et al. The quantitation of altered hepatic foci during multistage hepatocarcinogenesis in the rat: transforming growth factor α expression as a marker for the stage of progression. Cancer Lett 1995;93:73–83

335. Tanno S, Ogawa K. Abundant TGF α precursor and EGF receptor expression as a possible mechanism for the preferential growth of carcinogen-induced preneoplastic and neoplastic hepatocytes in rats. Carcinogenesis 1994;15: 1689–1694

336. Perez-Tomas R, Mayol Y, Cullere X et al. Transforming growth factor-alpha expression in rat experimental hepatocarcinogenesis. Histol Histopathol 1992;7:754–762

337. Jhappan C, Stahle C, Harkins RN et al. TGF α overexpression in transgenic mice induces liver neoplasia and abnormal development of the mammary gland and pancreas. Cell 1990;61:1137–1146

338. Weber G. Enzymology of cancer cells, part 1 and 2. N Engl J Med 1977;296:486–493, 541–551

339. Farber E. Cellular biochemistry of the stepwise development of cancer with chemicals: G.H.A. Clowes Memorial Lecture. Cancer Res 1984;44:5463–5474

340. Bannasch P, Keppler D, Weber G (eds): Liver Cell Carcinoma. Kluwer, Dordrecht, 1989

341. Sato K. Glutathione transferases as markers of preneoplasia and neoplasia. Adv Cancer Res 1989;52:205–255

342. Klimek F, Mayer D, Bannasch P. Biochemical microanalysis of glycogen content and glucose-6-phosphate dehydrogenase activity in focal lesions of rat liver induced by *N*-nitrosomorpholine. Carcinogenesis 1984;5:265–268

343. Hacker HJ, Moore MA, Mayer D, Bannasch P. Correlative histochemistry of some enzymes of carbohydrate metabolism in preneoplastic and neoplastic lesions in the rat liver. Carcinogenesis 1982;3:1265–1272

344. Seelmann-Eggebert G, Mayer D, Mecke D, Bannasch P. Expression and regulation of glycogen phosphorylase in preneoplastic and neoplastic hepatic lesions in rats. Virchows Arch (Cell Pathol) 1987;53:44–51

345. Ehemann V, Mayer D, Hacker HJ, Bannasch P. Loss of adenylate cyclase activity in preneoplastic and neoplastic lesions induced in rat liver by *N*-nitrosomorpholine. Carcinogenesis 1986;7:567–573

346. Grobholz R, Hacker HJ, Thorens B, Bannasch P. Reduction in the expression of glucose transporter protein GLUT2 in preneoplastic and neoplastic hepatic lesions and reexpression of GLUT1 in late stages of hepatocarcinogenesis. Cancer Res 1993;53:4204–4211

347. Fischer G, Ruschenburg J, Eigenbrodt E, Katz N. Decrease in glucokinase and glucose-6-phosphatase and increase in hexokinase in putative preneoplastic lesions of rat liver. J Cancer Res Clin Oncol 1987;113:430–436

348. Klimek F, Bannasch P. Biochemical microanalysis of α-glucosidase activity in preneoplastic and neoplastic hepatic lesions induced in rats by *N*-nitrosomorpholine. Virchows Arch B (Cell Pathol) 1989;57:245–250

349. Enzmann H, Dettler T, Ohlhauser D, Bannasch P. Elevation of glucose-6-phosphate in early stages of hepatocarcinogenesis induced in rats by *N*-nitrosomorpholine. Horm Metab Res 1988;20:128–129

350. Greaves P, Irisarri E, Monroe AM. Hepatic foci of cellular and enzymatic alteration and nodules in rats treated with clofibrate or diethylnitrosamine followed by phenobarbital: their rate of onset and their reversibility. J Natl Cancer Inst 1986;76:475–484

351. Moore MA, Nakamura T, Shirai T, Ito N. Immunohistochemical demonstration of increased glucose-6-phosphate dehydrogenase in preneoplastic and neoplastic lesions induced by propylnitrosamine in F344 rats and Syrian hamsters. Jpn J Cancer Res (Gann) 1986;77:131–138

352. Klimek F, Bannasch P. Biochemical microanalysis of pyruvate kinase activity in preneoplastic and neoplastic liver lesions induced in rat by *N*-nitrosomorpholine. Carcinogenesis 1990;11:1377–1380

353. Stumpf H, Bannasch P. Overexpression of glucose-6-phosphate dehydrogenase in rat hepatic preneoplasia and neoplasia. Int J Oncol 1994;5:1255–1260

354. Fischer G, Domingo M, Lodder D et al. Immunohistochemical demonstration of decreased L-pyruvate kinase in enzyme altered rat liver lesions produced by different carcinogens. Virchows Arch B (Cell Pathol) 1987;53:359–364

355. Klimek F, Moore MA, Schneider E, Bannasch P. Histochemical and microbiochemical demonstration of reduced pyruvate kinase activity in thioacetamide induced neoplastic nodules of rat liver. Histochemistry 1988;90:37–42

356. Klimek F, Bannasch P. Isoenzyme shift from glucokinase to hexokinase is not an early but a late event in hepatocarcinogenesis. Carcinogenesis 1993;14:1857–1861

357. Ledda-Columbano GM, Columbano A, Dessi S et al. Enhancement of cholesterol synthesis and pentose phosphate pathway activity in proliferating hepatocyte nodules. Carcinogenesis 1985;6:1371–1373

358. Lawrence JC Jr. Signal transduction and protein phosphorylation in the regulation of cellular metabolism by insulin. Annu Rev Physiol 1992;54:177–193

359. Pilkis SJ, Granner DK. Molecular physiology of the regulation of hepatic gluconeogenesis and glycolysis. Annu Rev Physiol 1992;54:885–909

360. Dombrowski F, Lehringer-Polzin M, Pfeifer U. Hyperproliferative liver acini after intraportal islet transplantation in streptozotocin-induced diabetic rats. Lab Invest 1994; 71:688–699

361. Dombrowski F, Filsinger E, Bannasch P, Pfeifer U. Altered liver acini induced in diabetic rats by portal-vein islet isografts resemble preneoplastic hepatic foci in their enzymic pattern. Am J Pathol 1996;148:1249–1256

362. Ruebner BH, Bannasch P, Hinton D, Ward J. Foci of altered hepatocytes, mouse. In Jones TC, Mohr U, Hunt RD (eds): Monographs on Pathology of Laboratory Animals. Digestive System. Springer, Berlin, 1997, pp. 38–49

363. Cai Y, Nelson BD, Li R et al. Thyromimetic action of the peroxisome proliferators clofibrate, perfluorooctanoic acid, and acetylsalicylic acid includes changes in mRNA levels for certain genes involved in mitochondrial biogenesis. Arch Biochem Biophys 1996;325:107–112

364. Swierczynski J, Bannasch P, Mayer D. Increase of lipid peroxidation in rat liver microsomes by dehydroepiandrosterone. Biochim Biophys Acta 1996;1315:199–198

365. Swierczynski J, Mayer D. Dehydroepiandrosterone-induced lipid peroxidation in rat liver mitochondria. J Steroid Biochem Molec Biol 1996;58:599–603

366. Perera MIR, Ktyal SL, Shinozuka H. Methapyrilene induces lipid peroxidation of rat liver cells. Carcinogenesis 1985;6: 925–927

367. Hernandez L, Lijinsky W. Glutathione and lipid peroxide levels in rat liver following administration of methapyrilene and analogs. Chem Biol Interact 1989;69:217–224

368. Mayer D, Weber E, Moore MA et al. Dehydroepiandrosterone induced alterations in rat liver carbohydrate metabolism. Carcinogenesis 1988;9:2039–2043

369. Mayer D, Reuter S, Hoffmann H et al. Dehydroepiandrosterone reduces expression of glycolytic and gluconeogenic enzymes in the liver of male and female rats. Int J Oncol 1996;8:1069–1078

370. Weber E, Moore MA, Bannasch P. Phenotypic modulation of hepatocarcinogenesis and reduction in *N*-nitrosomorpholine-induced hemangiosarcoma and adrenal lesion development in Sprague-Dawley rats by dehydroepiandrosterone. Carcinogenesis 1988;9:1191–1195

371. Moore MA, Thamavit N, Tsuda H et al. Modifying influence of dehydroepiandrosterone on the development of dihydroxy-di-*n*-propylnitrosamine-initiated lesions in the thyroid, lung and liver of F344 rats. Carcinogenesis 1986; 7:311–316

372. Garcea R, Daino L, Frasetto S et al. Reversal by ribo- and deoxyribonucleosides of dehydroepiandrosterone-induced inhibition of enzyme-altered foci in the liver of rats subjected to the initiation-selection process of experimental carcinogenesis. Carcinogenesis 1988;9:931–938

373. Moore M, Weber E, Bannasch P. Modulating influence of dehydroepiandrosterone administration on the morphology and enzyme phenotype of dimethylaminoazobenzene-induced hepatocellular foci and nodules. Virchows Arch B (Cell Pathol) 1988;55:337–343

374. Marsman SD, Popp JA. Biological potential of basophilic hepatocellular foci and hepatic adenoma induced by the peroxisome proliferator, Wy-14,643. Carcinogenesis 1994; 15:111–117

375. Enzmann H, Ohlhauser D, Enzmann H et al. Unusual histochemical pattern in preneoplastic hepatic foci characterized by hyperactivity of several enzymes. Virchows Arch B (Cell Pathol) 1989;57:99–108

376. Enzmann H, Zerban H, Löser E, Bannasch P. Glycogen phosphorylase hyperactive foci of altered hepatocytes in aged rats. Virchows Arch B (Cell Pathol) 1992;13:271–276

377. Enzmann H, Kühlem C, Kaliner G et al. Rapid induction of preneoplastic liver foci in embryonal turkey liver by diethylnitrosamine. Toxicol Pathol 1995;23:560–569

378. Buchmann A, Kuhlmann W, Schwarz M et al. Regulation and expression of four cytochrome P-450 isoenzymes, NADPH-cytochrome P-450 reductase, the glutathione transferase B and C and microsomal epoxide hydrolase in preneoplastic and neoplastic lesions in rat liver. Carcinogenesis 1985;6:513–521

379. Moore MA, Tsuda H, Ito N. Dehydrogenase histochemistry of *N*-ethyl-*N*- hydroxyethylnitrosamine-induced focal liver lesions in the rat—increase in NADPH-generating capacity. Carcinogenesis 1986;7:339–342

380. Olsson JM, Schedin S, Teclebrhan H et al. Enzymes of the mevalonate pathway in rat liver nodules induced by 2-acetylaminofluorene treatment. Carcinogenesis 1995;16: 599–605

381. Sato K, Kitahara A, Satoh K et al. The placental form of glutathione S-transferase as a new marker protein for preneoplasia in rat chemical carcinogenesis. Gann 1984; 75:199–202

382. Kalengayi MMR, Desmet VJ. Sequential histological and histochemical study of the rat liver during aflatoxin B_1-induced carcinogenesis. Cancer Res 1975;35:2845–2852

383. Rao MS, Lalwani ND, Scarpelli DG, Reddy JK. The absence of γ-glutamyltranspeptidase activity in putative preneoplastic lesions and in hepatocellular carcinomas induced in rats by the hypolipidemic peroxisome proliferator Wy-14,643. Carcinogenesis 1982;3:1231–1233

384. Rao MS, Tatematsu M, Subbarao V et al. Analysis of peroxisome proliferator-induced preneoplastic and neoplastic lesions of rat liver for placental form of glutathione S-transferase and γ-glutamyltranspeptidase. Cancer Res 1986;46: 5287–5290

385. Williams GM, Klaiber M, Parker SE, Farber E. Nature of early appearing carcinogen-induced liver lesions resistant to iron accumulation. J Natl Cancer Inst 1976;57:157–165

386. Firminger HJ. Histopathology of carcinogenesis and tumors of the liver in rats. J Natl Cancer Inst 1955;15:1427–1442

387. Elmore LW, Sirica AE. Phenotypic characterization of metaplastic intestinal glands and ductular hepatocytes in cholangiofibrotic lesions rapidly induced in the caudate liver lobe of rats treated with furan. Cancer Res 1991;51: 5752–5759

388. Chou ST, Gibson JB. A comparative histochemical study of rat livers in alpha-naphthyl-iso-thiocyanate (ANIT) and DL-ethionine intoxication. J Pathol 1972;108:73–83

389. Kinosita R. Some recent findings concerning hepatomas induced with *p*-dimethylaminoazobenzene. J Natl Cancer Inst 1955;15:1443–1445

390. Dominis M, Damjanov L. Cystic cholangiofibrosis of the liver. Arch Geschwulstforsch 1977;47:661–669

391. Ito N, Moore MA, Bannasch P. Modification of the development of *N*-nitrosomorpholine-induced hepatic lesions by 2-acetylaminofluorene, phenobarbital and 4,4′-diaminodiphenylmethane: a sequential histological and histochemical analysis. Carcinogenesis 1984;5:335–342

392. Nakano M. Cholangiofibrosis induced in short-term feeding of 3-methyl-4-dimethylaminoazobenzene. Kanzo 1974; 15:292–300

393. Reddy KP, Buschmann RJ, Chomet B. Cholangiocarcinomas induced by feeding 3′-methyl-4-dimethylaminoazobenzene to rats. Am J Pathol 1977;87:189–204

394. Elmore LW, Sirica AE. "Intestinal-type" of adenocarcinoma preferentially induced in right/caudate liver lobes of rats treated with furan. Cancer Res 1993;53:254–259

395. Bannasch P, Massner B. Die Feinstruktur des Nitrosomorpholin-induzierten Cholangiofibroms der Ratte. Virchows Arch B (Cell Pathol) 1977;24:295–315

396. Bannasch P. Carcinogen-induced cellular thesaurismoses and neoplastic cell transformation. Rec Res Cancer Res 1974;44:115–126

397. Bannasch P. Sequential cellular changes during chemical carcinogenesis. J Cancer Res Clin Oncol 1984;108:11–22

398. Ward JM. Morphology of foci of altered hepatocytes and naturally-occurring hepatocellular tumours in F344 rats. Virchows Arch Pathol Anat 1981;390:339–345

399. Wayss K, Bannasch P, Mattern J, Volm M. Vascular liver tumors in *Mastomys* induced by single or twofold administration of diethylnitrosamine. J Natl Cancer Inst 1979;62: 1199–1207

400. Trainin N. Neoplastic nature of liver "blood cysts" induced by urethan in mice. J Natl Cancer Inst 1963;31:1489–1499

401. Maltoni C, Lefime G. Carcinogenicity bioassays of vinylchloride. I. Research plan and early results. Environ Res 1974;7:387–405

402. Bannasch P, Bloch M, Zerban H. Spongiosis hepatis. Specific changes of the perisinusoidal liver cells induced in rats by *N*-nitrosomorpholine. Lab Invest 1981;44:252–264

403. Zerban H, Bannasch P. Spongiosis hepatis in rats treated with low doses of hepatotropic nitrosamines. Cancer Lett 1983;19:247–252

404. Hinton DE, Lantz RC, Hampton JA. Effect of age and exposure to a carcinogen on the structure of the Medaka liver: a morphometric study. Natl Cancer Inst Monogr 1984;65: 239–249

405. Couch JA, Courtney LA. *N*-nitrosodiethylamine-induced hepatocarcinogenesis in estuarine sheephead minnow (*Cyprinodon variegatus*): neoplasms and related lesions compared with mammalian lesions. J Natl Cancer Inst 1987; 79:297–321

406. Myers MS, Rhodes LD, McCain BB. Pathologic anatomy and patterns of occurrence of hepatic neoplasms, putative preneoplastic lesions and other idiopathic hepatic conditions in English sole (*Parophrys vetulus*) from Puget sound, Washington. J Natl Cancer Inst 1987;78:333–363

407. Bunton TE. Hepatopathology of diethylnitrosamine in the medaka (*Oryzias latipes*) following short-term exposure. Toxicol Pathol 1990;18:313–323

408. Couch JA. Spongiosis hepatis: chemical induction, pathogenesis and possible neoplastic fate in a Teleost fish model. Toxicol Pathol 1991;19:237–250

16

SECTION IV
CLINICAL AND PATHOLOGIC FEATURES OF OTHER LIVER TUMORS

FIBROLAMELLAR CARCINOMA: CLINICAL AND PATHOLOGIC FEATURES

JOHN R. CRAIG

DEFINITION

Fibrolamellar carcinoma (FLC) is a variant of hepatocellular carcinoma with distinctive histologic and clinical features.[1] This tumor is composed of large eosinophilic cells arranged in thin or thick trabeculae that are separated by fibrous bands with lamellar stranding. These fibrous strands prompted the name *fibrolamellar*. FLC occurs primarily in young adults, typically arises in the noncirrhotic liver, and has serum biochemical markers that differ from the usual HCC. α-Fetoprotein is usually normal in FLC, but the levels of serum vitamin B_{12} binding globulin (des-γ-carboxyprothrombin, a distinctive prothrombin variant) and neurotensin are usually increased. FLC is more often suitable for resection than the usual HCC, and it may have a better prognosis.[1]

FLC also has been known by several other names since its first recognition by Dr. Hugh Edmondson in 1954, including eosinophilic hepatocellular carcinoma with lamellar fibrosis,[2] polygonal cell carcinoma with fibrous stroma,[3] hepatocellular carcinoma with stromal fibrosis,[4] eosinophilic glassy cell hepatoma,[5] and fibrolamellar oncocytic hepatoma.[6]

INCIDENCE

In the United States, the incidence of FLC is approximately 1% of all HCC, but there is wide variation according to population group. A separate ICD-9 code for FLC was utilized beginning in 1987, and thus separate coding began in that year. In a statewide registry with mandatory cancer reporting in California, FLC was recorded in 27 patients in the 5-year period 1987–1992 (G. W. Halvorson, personal communication, 1995). However, the statewide registry does not utilize a central pathology review system, so the actual number of cases may be lower because of misclassification. A review of a county registry in California indicates 20% to 30% of cases are misclassified (unpublished data). A series of HCC referred to the Armed Forces Institute of Pathology included 1,753 cases over a 13-year period up to 1993, and 4% were FLC.[7]

The incidence of FLC in large liver cancer referral centers varies by geographic location and type of treatment (surgery vs. chemotherapy). FLC comprised 19% of one large chemotherapy series (37 patients).[8] In another series, composed of young adults under age 35 years, between 1963 and 1981, 10 of 23 HCC were FLC (40%)[9]; many of those cases were likely to have had surgery. An extensive nationwide (U.S.) hospital tumor registry survey found 12 cases in a group of 125 cases of HCC (9.6%),[10] all of whom had had surgical treatment over a 1 year period.

FLC has been reported from many countries in addition to the United States, including Israel,[11] Japan,[12–14] Korea,[15] Australia,[16] South Africa (M. Kew, personal communication, 1995), France,[17] Hungary,[18] Spain,[19] Argentina,[20] and India.[21] It appears to be more common in whites, but a systematic survey of many racial groups has not been reported. Although it has been reported to be rare in South African blacks,[18] 124 cases in black patients elsewhere have occurred (unpublished data).

DEMOGRAPHIC AND CLINICAL ASPECTS

FLC occurs with equal frequency in males and females,[22] and the age range is 5 to 85 years, with a median age of 25 to 34 years in 26 reported series. The clinical symptoms are usually nonspecific and often are related to the presence of a large palpable hepatic mass. Abdominal pain is common. A few cases have been identified due to jaundice.[23,24] Gynecomastia has been reported and associated with elevated serum estradiol levels that regressed following tumor resection.[25] Budd-Chiari syndrome has been reported.[26] Even with extensive radiographic evaluation there may be confusion with focal nodular hyperplasia, and a biopsy may not reliably reflect the correct diagnosis because of sampling error and confusion of specific histologic criteria.[27] Hepatic abscess may be suspected.[28] Extensive radiographic study may clarify some cases.[29]

LABORATORY

Although many FLC patients have elevated levels of serum alkaline phosphatase and γ-glutamyltranspeptidase, the bilirubin is typically normal. There is no general association with hepatitis B virus infection, although a few FLC patients have been reported with chronic hepatitis B virus infection. An elevated serum carcinoembryonic antigen has been noted in FLC and correlated with chemotherapy effect as well as recurrence of tumor in one case.[30]

α-Fetoprotein

Serum AFP is often normal in FLC, although elevated levels (up to 24,179 ng/ml)[22] have been found in 15% to 20% of FLC patients tested. In general, an elevated AFP suggests typical HCC.

Neurotensin

A connection between elevated serum neurotensin (NTN) and FLC has been reported in 4 of 5 FLC and one typical HCC.[31] Surgical resection resulted in normal levels of serum NTN, and recurrence of tumor was associated with return of elevated NTN. Also, chemotherapy response correlated with serum NTN levels.[32] This correlation is an elevated NTN that occurred in the presence of FL HCC. After chemotherapy, the serum NTN was lower. Neurotensin is a 13-amino acid peptide found in the central nervous system and the ileal mucosa and secreted by pancreatic endocrine tumors and small cell carcinoma of the bronchus. This peptide stimulates gut contraction and has effects on carbohydrate metabolism (decreased insulin and increased glucagon). Abundant gene expression was documented in a case of FLC and in fetal liver but not in focal nodular hyperplasia.[33] An aberrant form of NTN (called neurotensin 6-13) has also been found in one FLC).[16]

Vitamin B_{12} Binding Globulin

Increased serum B_{12} binding globulin levels occur in HCC patients as well as FLC patients.[34,35] In one case, serum unsaturated vitamin B_{12} binding capacity and transcobalamin I levels rose 18 months before recurrent tumor was detected.[36] Elevated levels of the unsaturated vitamin B_{12} binding globulin has helped identify FLC in a patient with suspected hepatic abscess.[28]

Des-γ-Carboxyprothrombin (DCP)

Des-γ-carboxyprothrombin (DCP) is an abnormal and nonfunctional prothrombin that has been associated with hepatocellular carcinoma[37] (S. Iwatsuki, personal communication, 1995) and has a high association (not previously reported) with FLC. DCP, also called PIVKA-II (for *protein induced by vitamin K absence or antagonist-II*), has a deficiency in a calcium-binding amino acid, des-carboxyglutamic acid (GLA). DCP production in HCC is not the result of vitamin K deficiency but is due to a defect in the molecule. This defect is not caused by a mutation in the prothrombin gene.[38] Research techniques include a chromogenic assay and several ELISA techniques dependent on a monoclonal antibody.[39] Preliminary data from the University of Pittsburgh liver transplant unit indicate that 100% of 19 FLC patients had elevated values of DCP and that the assay may be useful for detection of recurrences. (M. Virji, B. Carr, and S. Iwatsuki, personal communication, 1996). Regular monitoring of the serum DCP may reveal elevations 4 to 6 weeks before detection of the tumor by radiographic means.

RADIOLOGY

In 50% of FLC patients an abdominal plain x-ray reveals minute calcifications within the tumor; these are rarely seen in routine HCC.[40] Such calcifications may be minute, stellate, or nodular. A sulfur-colloid liver-spleen scan reveals a cold area over the tumor, whereas angiography reveals hypervascularity and shunting. Sonograms can be used to evaluate the tumor volume. Computerized tomography (CT) scan of the liver also reveals small calcification in 50% of cases, and the tumor mass is well demarcated and hypodense. An unusual case had "cystic" changes on CT.[41] CT is most accurate for staging.[42] The multiple radiographic procedures do not allow a firm diagnosis of FLC. Open biopsy is recommended if the lesion resembles focal nodular hyperplasia.[43] Confusion of FLC and focal nodular hyperplasia may also occur with MRI.[44] A ^{99m}Tc-HIDA scan demonstrated a bone metastasis in a patient with a focal liver defect, which ultimately proved to be FLC.[27] Intrahepatic tumor recurrence has been detected by CT, ultrasound, and MRI, and it is not clear which technique is superior.[45]

PATHOLOGY

Macroscopic

FLC develops in a normal liver without cirrhosis, although a few cases have been noted in chronic liver disease including congenital hepatic fibrosis. A majority of reported cases occur in the left lobe, and larger tumors involve both lobes. The tumor is sharply demarcated and is a large bulging mass. Satellite nodules (1 to 2 cm diameter) are common. The cut surface often reveals a central dense "scar" with radiating fibrous strands. The softer component surrounding the scar is dark brown, gray, and often green and may be hemorrhagic and necrotic. Gross resemblance to focal nodular hyperplasia is noted in at least 25%. Five cases have been reported in which focal nodular hyperplasia was present in the adjacent liver.[46] In a few cases, the tumor extends within the biliary system. The tumor size in resected specimens ranges from 7 to 20 cm (13.4 cm average).[3] The weight of resected tumors is often large, ranging from 1,200 to 3,600 g.[1]

Microscopic

FLC biopsies reveal large polygonal cells with a granular cytoplasm and large nucleoli. The light microscopic appearance of FLC is distinctive because of the intermixture of lamellar strands of thin collagen fibers with trabeculae of hepatocytes of relatively uniform large size (Figs. 16-1 to 16-3). The mitotic activity is low; multinucleated cells are not common. The cytoplasm is abundant, eosinophilic, finely granular, and often has scattered pale bodies[47] and PAS-positive diastase resistant globules. Pale bodies consist of one or more cells without nuclei and may contain small hyaline droplets that consist of α_1-antitrypsin. Bile plugs are variable in number and are common. From about half of the tumors, large sheets of the epithelial component exist so that needle aspiration or biopsy may not reveal the fibrolamellar component. Within these large epithelial sheets, a "pelioid" pattern may be noted in 25% of patients (unpublished data) with large dilated spaces containing blood. The trichrome stain reveals the lamellar strands very well. Cytoplasmic copper binding protein granules may

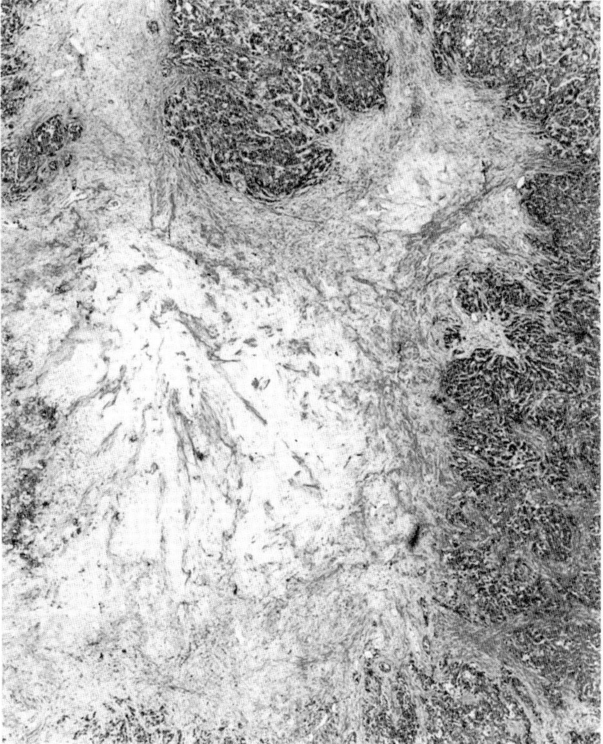

Figure 16-1. Low-power view of central dense fibrous scar with the epithelial component radiating from the central fibrous scar. (H&E.)

be noted.[48] The calcified areas detected radiographically correspond to tumor necrosis with foreign body reaction and dystrophic calcification0 (Fig. 16-4).

Special Immunohistochemistry

Carcinoembryonic antigen immunostaining of canaliculi but not the hepatocellular cytoplasm has been noted. We have observed positive NTN staining in several cases but also noted a positive reaction in non-FLC as well (J. R. Craig and H. Battifora, unpublished results, 1996). The hepatocyte Paraffin 1 antibody is a monoclonal antibody that reacts with hepatocytes and FLC is positive whereas neuroendocrine tumors are negative.[49] These results suggest FLC is not of neuroendocrine lineage. Cytokeratins 8, 18, 7, and occasionally 19 can be detected by immunohistochemistry; thus, FLC does not necessarily retain the cytokeratin expression of normal hepatocytes.[50] The neuron-specific enolase-positive reaction and rare instances of serotonin reaction suggested to one group that the tumor is a "potential carcinoid."[51]

Electron Microscopy

The cytoplasmic organelles of the epithelial component are similar to those of normal hepatocytes. The numerous mitochondria may have reduced cristae, and some con-

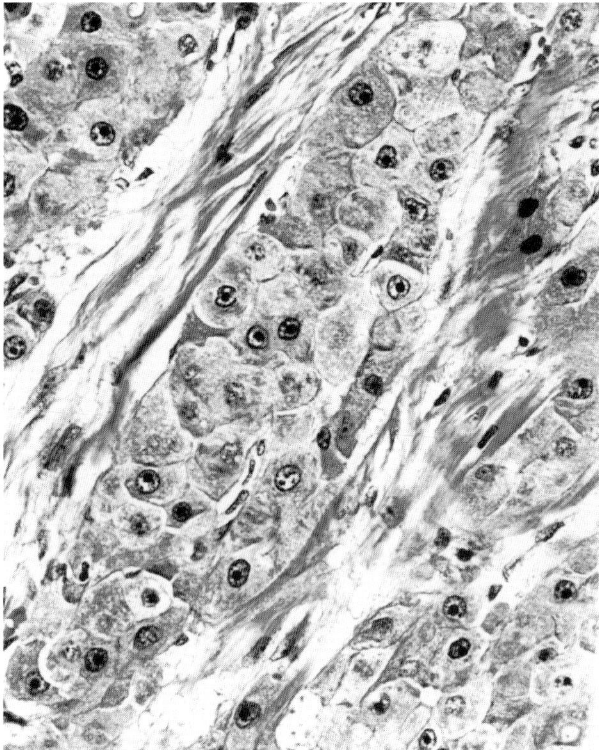

Figure 16-2. Fibromellar carcinoma. Fibrosis is a lamellar pattern (note strands in sinusoids), and the trabeculae are two to four cells in thickness. The epithelial component has large prominent nuclei with large nucleoli. (H&E.)

tain small granular electron-dense deposits in the matrix (Fig. 16-5 and 16-6). Peroxisome-like structures have been reported.[52] Some tumor cells contain highly developed rough endoplasmic reticulum (RER) that fills the cytoplasm and may correspond to the "pale bodies,"[22] which are RER but may also contain distinct droplets, which are α_1-antitrypsin. Abundant round membrane-bound structures about 100 mm in diameter were reported in several cases and appear similar to "neurosecretory granules" or dense-cored granules with uranyl acetate processing.[51] The thin collagen bands noted by light microscopy were confirmed to be homogenous collagen by electron microscopic examination.[6]

Image Analysis

Image cytometry revealed aneuploid or tetraploid DNA distribution in all of 12 FLC cases; this result is similar to HCCs. The mean nuclear area of the tumor cells was larger than the adjacent normal liver.[53] The high frequency of nondiploid tumors in this FLC group contrasts with the relatively favorable prognosis. However, survival data for this group of 12 cases was not available for analysis.

Differential Diagnosis: Other Types of Carcinoma

The differential diagnosis of FLC includes the following:

1. Focal nodular hyperplasia (FNH)
2. Ordinary hepatocellular carcinoma (nonfibrolamellar type)
3. Adenosquamous carcinoma arising in the gallbladder with extension into the liver
4. Metastatic carcinoma with fibrosis such as breast carcinoma and islet cell and other neuroendocrine carcinoma
5. Cholangiocarcinoma with sclerosis

FNH may closely resemble FLC; both are well demarcated with a central scar. Ordinary HCC rarely has significant fibrosis and does not have pale bodies in large numbers and also has more variation in nuclear size and nucleoli size (Fig. 16-7). Adenosquamous carcinoma demonstrates large polygonal cells, but the cytoplasm lacks the fine granularity of FLC; also, pale bodies are absent, and the fibrosis is not lamellar in quality. Several metastatic tumors produce fibrosis but usually not in a lamellar fashion. Neuroendocrine carcinoma may be

Figure 16-3. High-power view of numerous clustered "pale bodies," and the dense round cytoplasmic bodies consist of α_1-antitrypsin as shown by immunohistochemical staining of fibrolamellar carcinoma. (H&E.)

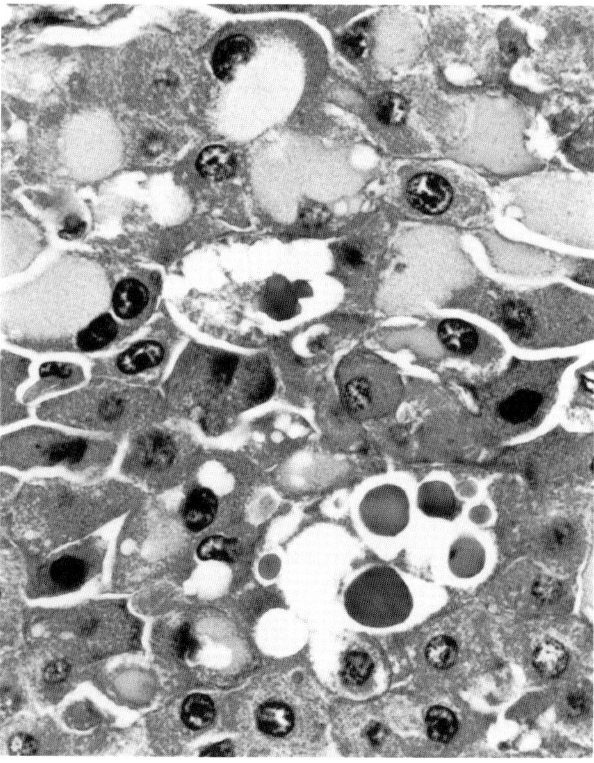

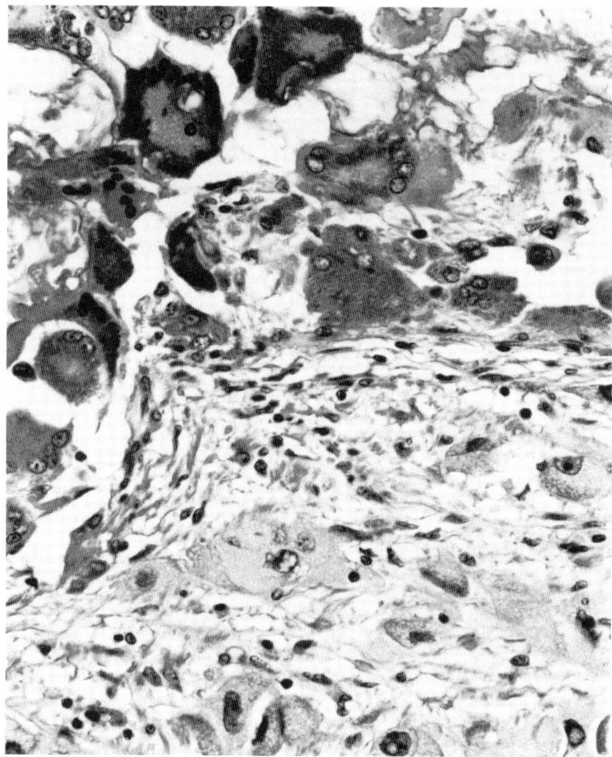

Figure 16-4. Foreign body giant cells and dystrophic calcification in a necrotic area of the FLC surrounded by fibrosis. (H&E.)

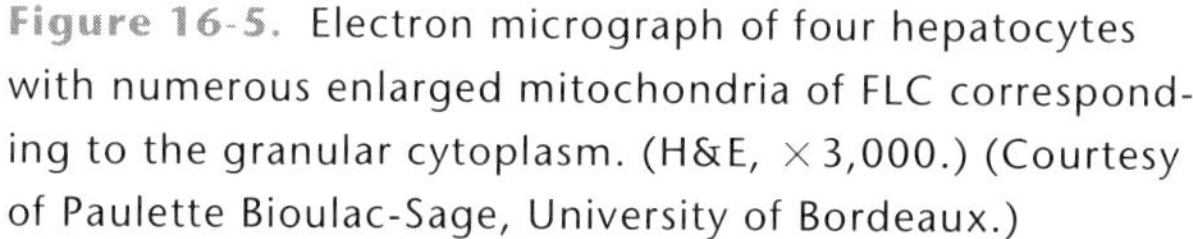

Figure 16-5. Electron micrograph of four hepatocytes with numerous enlarged mitochondria of FLC corresponding to the granular cytoplasm. (H&E, ×3,000.) (Courtesy of Paulette Bioulac-Sage, University of Bordeaux.)

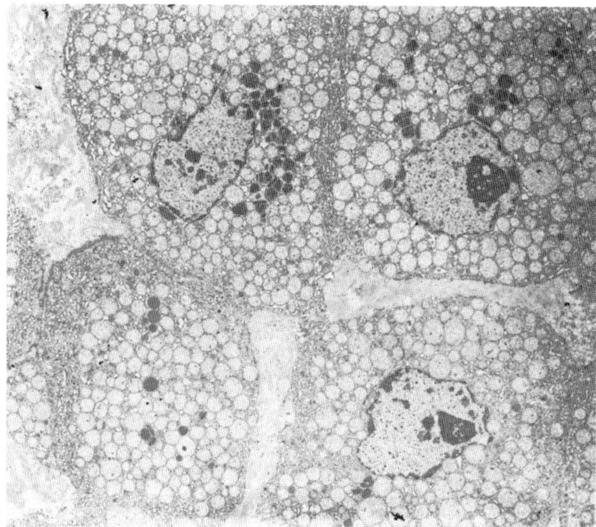

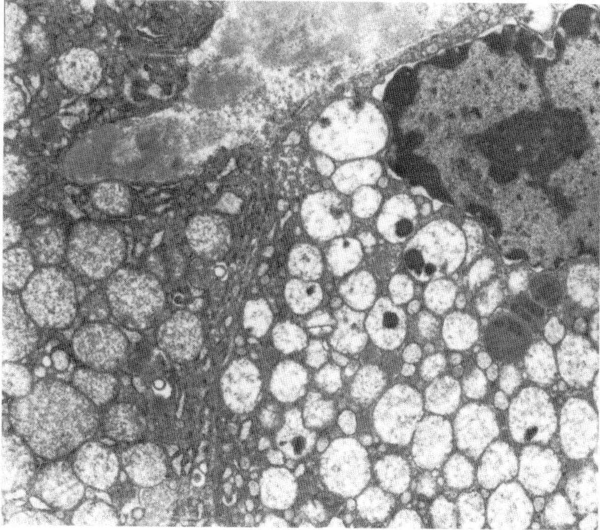

Figure 16-6. Higher power electron micrograph of FLC showing enlarged mitochondria; some contain osmiophilic inclusions. The matrix is foamy and lacks cristae. (×9,000.) (Courtesy of Paulette Bioulac-Sage, University of Bordeaux.)

Figure 16-7. Ordinary HCC with features resembling FLC features: there are thin fibrous strands in the sinusoids. This is not FLC; the epithelial component does not have large nuclei or nucleoli.

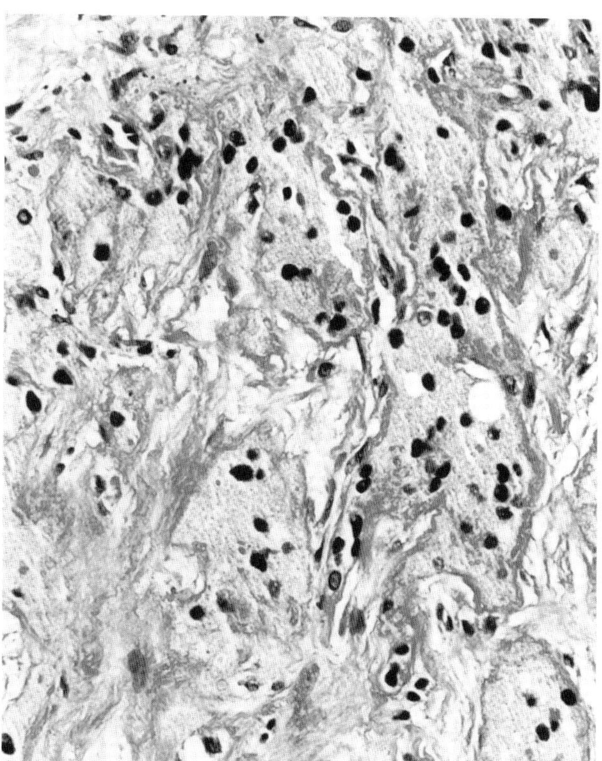

more challenging to exclude, and such tumors may have a trabecular growth pattern. Numerous sections are recommended in order to search for other clues such as "pale bodies," lamellar fibrosis, and bile plugs (which are almost universally present in FLC). Cholangiocarcinoma may be a consideration because of the fibrosis pattern (although not lamellar in quality), but the epithelial component lacks large cells, granular cytoplasm, and large nucleoli.[54] Mitosis is not a prominent feature of FLC, and their presence suggests metastatic carcinoma.

TREATMENT

Complete surgical resection results in a cure in 50% to 75% of cases.[55] Neoadjuvant chemotherapy with 5-fluorouracil via hepatic artery infusion for 1 month can result in tumor shrinkage, allowing resection.[56] Orthotopic liver transplantation can be utilized although the tumor frequently recurs. Survival following resection of FLC (5-year survival of 44.5 months) may be similar to HCC arising in a noncirrhotic liver (5 year survival of 45%).[57] In one series of 87 HCC patients, the survival of 6 FLC patients treated with resection was better than the overall survival of 16 patients with noncirrhotic HCC (5-year survival of 33% vs. 6.3%).[54] Transplantation of liver and associated organs including the duodenum has been reported for 3 patients with lymph node metastasis.[58] Unfortunately, the tumor growth rate appears to be accelerated by liver transplantation.[59] Resection of tumor recurrence in the liver and extrahepatic metastasis may be beneficial.[32] Tumor recurrence in lungs, lymph nodes, peritoneum, and liver are reported after intervals ranging from a few months to 10 years.[60] Surgical resection of the metastatic tumor is commonly performed.[32]

Therapy regimens including doxorubicin with streptozocin[7] or cisplatin,[61] intrahepatic chemoembolization, transcatheter oily chemoembolization (TOCE),[62] and radiation have been performed in some patients, but there has been limited or no benefit.

PATHOGENESIS

There is no recognized association of FLC with hepatitis B virus, alcoholic liver disease, cirrhosis, use of birth control medications, or genetic disorders such as Wilson's disease. The tumor arises typically in a noncirrhotic liver. Chromosome allele loss has been reported.[63]

ACKNOWLEDGMENTS

The author thanks Dr. Paulette Bioulac-Sage for the electron micrographs (Figs. 16-5 and 16-6) and Dr. Jay Packer for the other figures.

REFERENCES

1. Craig JR, Peters RL, Edmondson HA, Omata M. Fibrolamellar carcinoma of the liver: a tumor of adolesecents and young adults with distinctive clinicopathologic features. Cancer 1980;46:372–379
2. Peters RL. Pathology of hepatocellular carcinoma. In Okuda K, Peters R (eds): Hepatocellular Carcinoma. Wiley, New York, 1975, pp. 107–168
3. Berman MM, Libbey NP, Foster JH. Hepatocellular carcinoma polygonal cell type with fibrous stroma—an atypical variant with a favorable prognosis. Cancer 1980;46: 1448–1455
4. Stromeyer WFW, Ishak KG, Gerber MA. Ground-glass cells in hepatocellular carcinoma. Am J Clin Pathol 1980;74: 254–258
5. Christopherson WM. Possible etiologic factors for some malignant hepatic tumors. In Stroehlein JR, Romsdahl MM (eds): Gastrointestinal Cancer. Raven Press, New York, 1981, pp. 257–269
6. Farhi DC, Shikes RH, Silverbery SG. Ultrastructure of fibrolamellar oncocytic hepatoma. Cancer 1982;50:702–709
7. Nzeako U, Goodman ZD, Ishak K. Comparison of tumor pathology with duration of survival of North American patients with hepatocellular carcinoma. Cancer 1995;76: 579–588
8. Ihde DC, Matthews MJ, Makuch RW et al. Prognostic factors in patients with hepatocellular carcinoma receiving systemic chemotherapy. Am J Med 1985;78:399–406
9. Farhi DG, Shikes RH, Murari PJ, Silverberg SG. Hepatocellular carcinoma in young people. Cancer 1983;52: 1516–1525
10. Foster JF, Berman MM. Solid liver tumors: In Ebert PA (ed): Major Problems in Clinical Surgery. Vol. 22. WB Saunders, Philadelphia, 1977, pp. 5–8, 86–97, 111–128
11. Kroll D, Mazor M, Zirkin H et al. Fibrolamellar carcinoma of the liver in pregnancy. A case report. J Reprod Med 1991; 36:823–227
12. Imai T, Yokoi H, Noguchi T et al. Fibrolamellar carcinoma of the liver—a case report. Gastroenterol Jpn 1991;26: 382–389
13. Kohno H, Nagasue N, Taniura H et al. Case report: fibrolamellar carcinoma of the liver—a case report from Japan and a review of the literature. HPB Surg 1988;1:77–80
14. Yoshida K, Amemiya A, Kobayashi S et al. Fibrolamellar carcinoma of the liver in the Orient. J Surg Oncol 1988;39: 187–189
15. Haratake J, Horie A, Lee SD, Huh M. Fibrolamellar carcinoma of the liver in a middle-aged Korean man. JUOEH 1990;12:349–354
16. Read D, Shulkes A, Fernley R, Simpson R. Characterization of neurotensin (6–13) from an hepatic fibrolamellar carcinoma. Peptides 1991;12:887–892
17. Soyer PH, Roche A, Rougier PH, Levesque M. Fibrolamellar hepatocellular carcinoma: report of four cases treated by locoregional intraaterial therapy. JBR-BTR 1992;75:463–468
18. Sarosi I, Kiss A, Schaff Z, Lapis K. Connective tissue con-

tent of fibrolamellar carcinoma and other human liver tumors. Acta Morphol Hung 1991;39:321–331

19. Malondra AB, Picornell MF, Pons JT et al. European cases of fibrolamellar hepatocellular carcinoma. Ann Intern Med 1989;110:324 (letter)
20. Carri J, Peral F, Surreco M et al. Carcinoma hepatocellular fibrolaminar: Presentacion clinica con hipertirosiodismo paraneoplasico. Acta Gastroenterol Latinoam 1989;19: 155–163
21. Karak PK, Mukhopadhyay S, Berry M. Hepatocellular carcinoma—image morphology in 40 patients. Trop Gastroenterol 1992;13:21–26
22. Berman MA, Burnham JA, Sheahan DG. Fibrolamellar carcinoma of the liver: an immunohistochemical study of nineteen cases and a review of the literature. Hum Pathol 1988; 19:784–794
23. Eckstein RP, Bambach CP, Stiel D et al. Fibrolamellar carcinoma as a cause of bile duct obstruction. Pathology 1988; 20:326–331
24. Afroudakis A, Bhuta SM, Ranganath KA et al. Obstructive jaundice caused by hepatocellular carcinoma. Am J Dig Dis 1978;23:609–617
25. McCloskey JJ, Germain-Lee EM, Perman JA et al. Gynecomastia as a presenting sign of fibrolamellar carcinoma of the liver. Pediatrics 1988;82:379–382
26. Lamberts R, Nitsche R, de Vivie RE et al. Budd-Chiari syndrome as the primary manifestation of a fibrolamellar hepatocellular carcinoma. Digestion 1992;53:200–209
27. Reuland P, Aicher KP, Bramabs J et al. Incidental finding of a hepatic lesion: differential diagnostic problems for fibrolamellar hepatic carcinoma. J Nucl Med 1994;35:1342–1346
28. Debray D, Pariente D, Fabre M et al. Fibrolamellar hepatocellular carcinoma: report of a case mimicking a liver abscess. J Pediatr Gastroenterol 1994;19:468–472
29. Belghiti J, Pateron D Panis Y et al. Resection of presumed benign liver tumours. Br J Surg 1993;80:380–383
30. Teitelbaum DH, Tuttle S, Carey LC, Clausen KP. Fibrolamellar carcinoma of the liver. Review of three cases and the presentation of a characteristic set of tumor markers defining this tumor. Ann Surg 1985;202:36–41
31. Collier NA, Bloom SR, Hodgson HJF et al. Neurotensin secretion by fibrolamellar carcinoma of the liver. Lancet 1984;1:538–540
32. Soreide O, Czerniak A, Bradpiece H et al. Characteristics of fibrolamellar hepatocellular carcinoma. A study of nine cases and a review of the literature. Am J Surg 1986;151: 518–523
33. Ehrenfried JA, Zhou Z, Thompson JC, Evers BM. Expression of the neurotensin gene in fetal human liver and fibrolamellar carcinoma. Ann Surg 1994;220:484–491
34. Paradinas FJ, Melia WM, Wilkinson JL et al. High serum vitamin B_{12} binding capacity as a marker of the fibrolamellar variant of hepatocellular carcinoma. BMJ 1982;285:840–842
35. van Tonder S, Kew MC, Hodkinson J, Serum vitamin B_{12} binder in South African blacks with hepatocellular carcinoma. Cancer 1985;56:789–792
36. Wheeler K, Pritchard J, Luck W, Rossiter M. Transcobalamin I as a "marker" for fibrolamellar hepatoma. Med Pediatr Oncol 1986;14:227–229
37. Liebman HA, Furie BC, Tong M et al. Des-γ-carboxy (abnormal) prothrombin as a serum marker of primary hepatocellular carcinoma. N Engl J Med 1984;310:1427–1431
38. Tagawa M, Omata M, Ohto M. Nucleotide sequence of prothrombin gene in abnormal prothrombin-producing hepatocellular carcinoma cell lines. Cancer 1992;69:643–647
39. Fujiyama S, Morishita T, Hashiguchi O et al: Plasma abnormal prothrombin (Des-γ-carboxy prothrombin) as a marker of hepatocellular carcinoma. Cancer 1988;61:1621–1628
40. Friedman AC, Lichtenstein JE, Goodman Z et al. Fibrolamellar hepatocellular carcinoma. Radiology 1985;157: 583–587
41. Pombo F, Rodriguex E, Arnal-Monreal F. Multicystic fibrolamellar hepatocellular carcinoma. CT appearance. Clin Imaging 1993;17:67–69
42. Soyer P, Roche A, Levesque M, Legmann P. CT of fibrolamellar hepatocellular carcinoma. J Comput Assist Tomogr 1991;15:533–538
43. Titelbaum DS, Burke DA, Meranze SG, Saul S. Fibrolamellar hepatocellular carcinoma: pitfalls in nonoperative diagnosis. Radiology 1988;167:25–30
44. Hamrick-Turner JE, Shipkey FH, Cranston PE. Fibrolamellar hepatocellular carcinoma: MR appearance mimicking focal nodular hyperplasia. J Comput Assist Tomogr 1994;18: 301–304
45. Stevens WR, Johnson CD, Stephens DH, Nagorney DM. Fibrolamellar hepatocellular carcinoma: stage at presentation and results of aggressive surgical management. AJR 1995;164:1153–1158
46. Vecchio FM. Fibrolamellar carcinoma of the liver: a distinct entity within the hepatocellular tumors. Appl Pathol 1988; 6:139–148
47. Davenport RD. Cytologic diagnosis of fibrolamellar carcinoma of the liver by fine-needle aspiration. Diagn Cytopathol 1990;6:275–276
48. Vecchio FM, Fedrico F, Dina MA. Copper and hepatocellular carcinoma. Digestion 1986;35:109–114
49. Wennerberg AE, Nalesnik MA, Coleman WB. Technical advances hepatocyte Paraffin 1: A monoclonal antibody that reacts with hepatocytes and can be used for differential diagnosis of hepatic tumors. Am J Pathol 1993;143:1050–1054
50. Van Eyken P, Sciot R, Brock P et al. Abundant expression of cytokeratin 7 in fibrolamellar carcinoma of the liver. Histology 1990;17:101–107
51. Payne CM, Nagle RB, Paplanus SH et al. Fibrolamellar carcinoma of liver: a primary malignant oncocytic carcinoid? Ultra Pathol 1986;10:539–552
52. Caballero T, Aneiros J, Lopex-Caballero J et al. Fibrolamellar hepatocellular carcinoma. An immunohistochemical and ultrastructural study. Histopathology 1985;9:445–456
53. Orsatti G, Greenberg PD, Rolfes DB et al. DNA ploidy of fibrolamellar hepatocellular carcinoma by image analysis. Hum Pathol 1994;25:936–939
54. McPeake JR, O'Grady JG, Zaman S et al. Liver transplantation for primary hepatocellular carcinoma: tumor size and number determine outcome. J Hepatol 1993;18:226–234

55. Starzl TE, Iwatuski S, Shaw B et al. Treatment of fibrolamellar hepatoma with partial or total hepatectomy and transplantation of the liver. Surg Gynecol Obstet 1986;162: 145–148

56. Ringe B, Pichlmayr R, Wittekind C, Tusch G. Surgical treatment of hepatocellular carcinoma: experience with liver resection and transplantation in 198 patients. World J Surg 1991;15:270–285

57. Ringe B, Wittekind C, Weimann A et al. Results of hepatic resection and transplantation for fibrolamellar carcinoma. Surg Gynecol Obstet 1992;175:299–305

58. Alessiani M, Tzakis A, Todo S et al. Gynecol Obstet Assessment of five-year experience with abdominal organ cluster transplantation. J Am Coll Surg 1995;180:1–9

59. Yokoyama I, Carr B, Saitsu H et al. Accelerated growth rates of recurrent hepatocellular carcinoma after liver transplantation. Cancer 1991;68:2095–2100

60. Ang PT, Evans H, Pazdur R. Fibrolamellar hepatocellular carcinoma: therapeutic implications of a ten-year disease free interval. Am J Clin Oncol 1991;14:175–178

61. Carr BI. High-objective response rates of advanced hepatocellular carcinoma (HCC) to intra-arterial (IA) chemotherapy. Proc Annu Meet Am Soc Clin Oncol 1992;11:A470 (abst)

62. Soyer P, Roche A, Rougier P, Levesque M, Nonresectable fibrolamellar hepatocellular carcinoma: outcome of 4 cases treated by intra-arterial chemotherapy. J Belge Radiol 1992; 75:463–468

63. Ding SF, Delhanty JDA, Bowles L et al. Infrequent chromosome allele loss in fibrolamellar carcinoma. Br J Cancer 1993; 67:244–246

17

HEPATOBLASTOMA

J. THOMAS STOCKER
RICHARD M. CONRAN

Hepatoblastoma, the most commonly occurring liver tumor in children, accounts for over 25% of all primary hepatic tumors and nearly 50% of those that are malignant in children (Table 17-1).[1] In children in the first 2 years of life (Table 17-2), hepatoblastomas account for over 40% of the primary liver tumors. As with adults, however, the most frequently occurring malignancies in the liver of children are metastatic tumors, including neuroblastoma, lymphoma, and rhabdomyosarcoma. However, primary liver tumors account for only 0.5% to 2.0% of pediatric tumors, with hepatoblastomas thus accounting for 0.1% to 0.5%,[2] with a prevalance of 1 in 120,000.[3] Hepatoblastomas are observed worldwide. Hepatoblastomas are not unique to humans and have been reported in a number of animal species, including sheep, mice, pigs, cattle, and horses.[4]

EPIDEMIOLOGY

Risk Factors

The etiology of hepatoblastoma is unknown. The risk factors associated with hepatocellular carcinoma, viz., metabolic diseases, hepatitis virus infection, exposure to alcohol and nitrosamines, maternal estrogen use, and smoking, are not risk factors for hepatoblastoma. An increased risk of hepatoblastoma in children whose mothers had occupational exposure to metals, petroleum products, and paints or pigments has been noted.[5] Thus, exposure to environmental agents in utero may be responsible for some hepatoblastomas. Consistent with this observation is the fact that approximately 4% of hepatoblastomas are congenital.[6] Congenital hepatoblastoma has also been found in animals,[4] and hepatoblastoma has been reported in siblings[7] and in identical twins (simultaneously at 7 months of age).[8]

The association of hepatoblastoma with other inherited conditions, such as familial adenomatous polyposis and Beckwith-Wiedemann syndrome, have led researchers to look for chromosomal abnormalities to explain its pathogenesis. A number of studies have focused on insulin-like growth factor 2 (IGF2),[9–12] which is thought to be important in the normal development of the embryonic and fetal liver. Abnormal expression of the IGF2 gene and possible loss of an adjacent tumor suppressor gene may lead to uncontrolled proliferation of cells leading to the development of hepatoblastoma. The IGF2 gene is located at 11p15.5,[9] and it is used as a marker for this region. Abnormalities in chromosome 11 and loss of heterozygosity at the 11p15.5 region have been observed in human hepatoblastomas.[11,13–16] There is also evidence to suggest that the 11p15.5 region codes for a distinct tumor suppressor gene different from the Wilms tumor suppressor gene *WT1*.[13] Abnormal expression of the H19 tumor suppressor gene that is downstream from the IGF2 gene may play a role in tumor growth.[11] Akmal and colleagues[9] have found that expression of IGF2 and

The views of the authors do not purport to reflect the positions of the Uniformed Services University of the Health Sciences or the U.S. Department of Defense.

TABLE 17-1. Hepatic Tumors in Pediatric Patients, Birth to 20 Years (Armed Forces Institute of Pathology, 1970–1995)

Type of Tumor	No. (%)
Hepatoblastoma	167 (26.2)
Hepatocellular carcinoma	123 (19.3)
Infantile hemangioendothelioma	113 (17.7)
Focal nodular hyperplasia	63 (9.9)
Mesenchymal hamartoma	51 (8.0)
Undifferentiated "embryonal" sarcoma	46 (7.2)
Nodular regenerative hyperplasia	31 (4.9)
Hepatocellular adenoma	24 (3.8)
Angiosarcoma	13 (2.0)
Embryonal rhabdomyosarcoma	7 (1.1)
Total	638 (100.0)

(From Stocker et al.,[1] with permission.)

IGF binding protein inversely correlates with tumor differentiation.[9]

Although inactivation of the *p53* tumor suppressor gene is important in a number of tumors, mutation of the *p53* gene was infrequent in hepatoblastoma,[17] and in an animal model no aberrations were present in the *p53* gene in 16 tumors.[18] Oda and colleagues,[19] however, reported that 9 out of 10 hepatoblastomas had mutations in the p53 gene and suggest environmental mutagens may alter the p53 gene and play a role in the pathogenesis of hepatoblastoma.[19] Other reports also suggest abnormal expression of p53 in hepatoblastoma (in three of which immunohistochemistry was used).[20–23] The role of a mutation in the *p53* gene leading to hepatoblastoma is unsettled.

TABLE 17-2. Hepatic Tumors in Pediatric Patients, Birth to 2 Years (Armed Forces Institute of Pathology, 1970–1992)

Type of Tumor	No. (%)
Hepatoblastoma	101 (41.1)
Infantile hemangioendothelioma	97 (39.5)
Mesenchymal hamartoma	33 (13.4)
Nodular regenerative hyperplasia	6 (2.4)
Hepatocellular carcinoma	4 (1.6)
Focal nodular hyperplasia	3 (1.2)
Undifferentiated "embryonal" sarcoma	1 (0.4)
Angiosarcoma	1 (0.4)
Hepatocellular adenoma	0 (0)
Embryonal/rhabdomyosarcoma	0 (0)
Total	246 (100.0)

(From Stocker et al.,[1] with permission.)

Animal Models

Hepatoblastomas have been induced in mice and rats using chemical agents including *N*-nitrosodiethylamine as an initiator followed by different chemical agents as tumor promoters, including phenobarbital,[18,24,25] phenytoin,[26] diazepam, oxazepam,[27] Aroclor-1254, and dichlorodiphenyltrichloroethane (DDT).[24] Hepatoblastoma has been induced in mice exposed to oxazepam for 2 years in their diet.[28] A liver tumor resembling a mixed hepatoblastoma was induced in rats using *N*-methyl-*N'*-nitrosoguanidine.[29] Recently, Suzuki and colleagues[30] established a human hepatoblastoma, designated HBL-2, that secretes α-fetoprotein (AFP) in athymic nude mice. It provides a unique model for investigating the biologic characteristics of this tumor.

Cell Lines

A number of cell lines derived from hepatoblastomas have been developed to study the pathogenesis of this tumor. A hepatoblastoma cell line, designated HB1,[31] expresses AFP, cytokeratins 8 and 18, lactate dehydrogenase, and high levels of the c-*myc* and Ha-*ras* oncogenes. There was no N-*myc* oncogene expression. Cell growth was responsive to hydrocortisone and epidermal growth factor. Two other cell lines derived from hepatoblastomas are HuH-6[32–34] and HB611[33] (which was derived from HuH-6). The Hep G2 cell line[35–42] is widely accepted as derived from human hepatoblastoma.

CLINICAL FEATURES

Hepatoblastomas occur in children under 2 years of age (68% of cases), with 4% of cases present at the time of birth. By 5 years of age, nearly 90% of cases will have presented, and only 3% of cases first present in patients over 15 years of age. There have been reports on 31 adult patients with hepatoblastoma.[43] The oldest reported cases are in a 72-year-old male with macronodular cirrhosis and in an 82-year-old man with a history of chronic hepatitis.[44,45] There is no racial predilection, but there is a male predominance of cases of approximately 1.75:1.

An enlarging abdomen is the most frequently noted symptom, often observed by a parent or discovered by a physician on routine physical examination. Less frequently, weight loss or anorexia may be noted. Other symptoms include nausea, vomiting, and abdominal pain, with jaundice seen in 5% of cases. An irregular, firm mass in the right upper quadrant is present on physical examination and may extend across the midline or down to the pelvic rim.

ASSOCIATED CONDITIONS

The clinical presentation of patients with hepatoblastoma may be influenced by a variety of associated conditions (Table 17-3). One of the most striking is that of precocious puberty in patients whose tumor is producing human chorionic gonadotropin (hCG). Most noticeable in young boys, the hCG, along with serum luteinizing hormone and plasma testosterone, may result in genital enlargement, deepening voice, and the appearance of pubic hair.

Surendran and colleagues[7] have noted the occurrence of hepatoblastoma in a brother and sister, and Riikonen and colleagues[8] report the simultaneous occurrence of hepatoblastoma in identical twins. A familial association between hepatoblastoma and polyposis coli has been described in a number of families,[47–52] and Kurahashi and colleagues[53] suggested that inactivation of the adenomatous polyposis coli gene, as noted in one of their cases of hepatoblastoma, may promote tumorigenesis in familial adenomatous polyposis. Congenital anomalies are present in 5.5% of patients with hepatoblastoma.[54–56] Trisomy 18 has also been associated with hepatoblastoma in four cases.[57] Other recently described associations include the Goldenhar syndrome,[58] Prader-Willi syndrome,[59] and the Beckwith-Weidemann syndrome with opsoclonus-myoclonus.[60] Arico and colleagues[61] have noted a hepatoblastoma in a 4-year-old boy who was infected with human immunodeficiency virus and hepatitis B virus.

LABORATORY FEATURES

Anemia was present in 70% of patients at diagnosis,[6,62] and approximately 50% had an associated thrombocytosis. In a series of 99 patients with hepatoblastoma, 35% of patients had platelet counts greater than 500 × 10^9/L and 29% greater than 800 × 10^9/L.[63] Thrombocytosis in children with a hepatic mass is highly suspicious for hepatoblastoma.

Bilirubin, alkaline phosphatase, and aspartate aminotransferase are elevated in about 20% to 25% of patients. Hypercholesterolemia has been reported as a feature of hepatoblastoma; in one study, four of nine patients had elevated cholesterol levels,[64] but in another, 6 of 50 patients had elevated cholesterol levels.[65] Elevated carcinoembryonic antigen levels have been found in 20% of patients.[6]

Up to 90% of patients with hepatoblastoma have an elevated serum AFP at the time of diagnosis.[66,67] Although the AFP level is not of diagnostic value, the levels do parallel the course of the disease. Mean AFP levels

TABLE 17-3. Clinical Syndromes and Other Conditions Associated with Hepatoblastoma

Absence of right adrenal gland
Alcohol embryopathy
Beckwith-Wiedemann syndrome
Beckwith-Wiedemann syndrome with opsoclonus, myoclonus
Bilateral talipes
Cleft palate, macroglossia, dysplasia of ear lobes
Cystathioninuria
Down syndrome, malrotation of colon, Meckel's diverticulum, pectus excavatum, intrathoracic kidney, single coronary artery
Duplicated ureters
Fetal hydrops
Goldenhar syndrome—oculoauriculovertebral dysplasia, absence of portal vein
Hemihypertrophy
Heterotopic lung tissue
Heterozygous α_1-antitrypsin deficiency
HIV or HBV infection
Horseshoe kidney
Hypoglycemia
Inguinal hernia
Isosexual precocity
Maternal clomiphene citrate and Pergonal
Meckel's diverticulum
Oral contraceptive, mother
Oral contraceptive, patient
Osteoporosis
Persistent ductus arteriosus
Polyposis coli families
Prader-Willi syndrome
Renal dysplasia
Right diaphragmatic hernia
Schinzel-Geidion syndrome[46]
Synchronous Wilms' tumor
Trisomy 18
Umbilical hernia

(Modified from Stocker et al.,[1] with permission.)

as high as 370,260 ng/ml to 10 million ng/ml have been reported.[6,67,68]

CHROMOSOME ABNORMALITIES

Cytogenetic studies performed on hepatoblastoma cells demonstrate a variety of genetic alterations at the chromosomal and molecular level (Table 17-4).[69] High prevalences of trisomy 20 and trisomy of all or part of chromosome 2 have been found.[69–72] A number of oncogenes have been localized to chromosome 2, so abnormal expression may play a role in tumor development. An abnormality in 4q12 was identified recently in hepatoblastomas and was associated with elevated AFP; the AFP gene has been mapped to 4q12–13.[73] Other reported abnormalities include deletions on chromosome 1p[74] and 11p[75] and extra copies of chromosome 8.[76]

DNA content in hepatoblastomas has been analyzed by flow cytometry. No significant correlation between histologic subtype and ploidy was identified in three large series (Table 17-5).[6,77,78]

TABLE 17-5. Distribution of Hepatoblastomas by Ploidy and Histologic Subtype

Author	Fetal	Fetal/Embryonal	Mixed
Conran et al.[6]	2D, 3A	2A	3D, 2A
Hata et al.[77]	6D	3D, 6A[a]	
Schmidt et al.[78]	6D, 1A	11D, 4A	6D, 1A

Abbreviations: D, DNA diploid; A, DNA aneuploid.

[a] Two cases listed as A also contained fetal elements with diploid peak.

IMAGING

Imaging studies are helpful in diagnosing hepatoblastoma and differentiating it from other liver disorders seen in young children. Hepatoblastomas are seen on computed

TABLE 17-4. Cytogenetic Findings in Hepatoblastomas

Case No.	Karyotype	Histologic Type
1	46,XY,−2,der(19) t(4;19),+mar	Epithelial; embryonal
2	47,XY,+20,dmin	Mixed mesenchymal-epithelial; fetal
3	47,XY,+20,dmin	Epithelial; primary embryonal, foci of fetal areas
4	93,XXXX,+i(8q)/93,XXXX,del(1)(p22),+i(8q)	Mixed mesenchymal-epithelial; fetal
5	50,XY,+2,+8,+20,+dic(1)(p12)	Mixed mesenchymal-epithelial; fetal and embryonal
6	47,XX,+20,del(1)(q32.1q32.2)dup(2)(q21q35), dmin/50,XX,+5,+7, +20,+22,del(1),dup(2),i(8q),dmin	Mixed mesenchymal-epithelial; fetal and embryonal
7	47,XX,+20,dup(2)(q23q35)/47,XX,+20,dup(2), dup(6)(p11p24)	Mixed mesenchymal-epithelial; fetal
8	54,Y,der(X)t(X;1)(p22; q21),+2,+6,+8,+8,+12,+15,+17, +20,inv(9)(p11q21)[a]	Mixed mesenchymal-epithelial; fetal and embryonal
9	46,XY,der(4)t(2;4)(q21;q35),t(9;?)(p24;?)/47,XY,+20,der (4),t(9?)	Mixed mesenchymal-epithelial; fetal
10	51,XY,+2,+12,+20,+der(5)t(1;5)(q25;q35),+del(6)(q15)	Epithelial; fetal
11	48,XX,+2,+r/48,XX,+20,+der(2)t(1;2)(q23; p21),inv(5)(q22 q35)/49,XX,+20,+der(2),inv(5),+r	Epithelial; fetal
12	47,XX,+2	Epithelial; primary fetal, foci of embryonal areas
13	47,XX,2q+,t(3;5)(p25;q31),dup(4)(q12q26),+20	Mixed mesenchymal-epithelial
14	46,XY,t(10;22)(q26;q11)	Small cell undifferentiated
15	47,XY,+2	Fetal and embryonal, possible macrotrabecular[70]
16	47,XX,+20	Mixed mesenchymal-epithelial fetal and embryonal[70]
17	46,XX,del(17)(p12)/46,XX	Mixed with teratoid features[70]

[a] inv(9)(p11q21) was constitutional.

(Modified from Stocker et al.,[1] with permission.)

tomography (CT) as a solitary (occasionally multifocal) mass with attenuation values between those of water and normal liver parenchyma[79] and calcification in more than 50% of cases.[80]

Magnetic resonance (MR) imaging with standard spin-echo T_1- and T_2-weighted imaging enhanced by the application of advanced sequences such as gradient-echo, fast spin-echo, and fat suppression techniques can determine tumor extent, help to characterize tissue subtypes of hepatoblastoma, and help to differentiate hepatoblastomas from mesenchymal hamartoma, infantile hemangioendothelioma, and hepatocellular carcinoma (Table 17-2). The "epithelial type" of hepatoblastoma can be differentiated from the "mixed type" by MR, by its homogeneous internal appearance compared to the heterogenous character of the mixed type with its fibrotic bands.[81] Decreased signal intensity compared to normal liver is noted on T_1-weighted images, while on T_2-weighted images the lesion has increased signal intensity (Fig. 17-1). Fibrotic bands are seen as hypointense bands on MR. Gradient-echo MR imaging may detect the presence of vascular invasion.

Ultrasonography displays a mass with increased heterogenous echogenicity, punctate or amorphous calcification, and occasional cystic areas.[80] Using pulsed Doppler ultrasonography, peak systolic Doppler frequency shifts equal to or greater than 4 kHz and antegrade diastolic flow are found.[82]

Angiography shows hepatoblastoma as a hypervascular (rarely hypovascular) lesion with distortion and displacement of vessels, pooling of contrast material, and an ill-defined irregular tumor margin.[56] King and colleagues[83] thought that in patients with advanced hepatoblastomas diagnostic imaging studies provided approximately 80% accuracy in judging whether lesions would be resectable, whereas others conclude that CT scans are not reliable in determining resectability but are of value when used in conjunction with preoperative chemotherapy. CT scans may also be helpful in determining when surgical resection should be attempted.[83]

FIGURE 17-1. (*A*) A large lesion in the right lobe of the liver displays decreased signal intensity relative to the normal liver in this T_1-weighted magnetic resonance (MR) image. (*B*) With T_2-weighted MR, the lesion shows an increased signal intensity as compared to the surrounding normal liver.

A

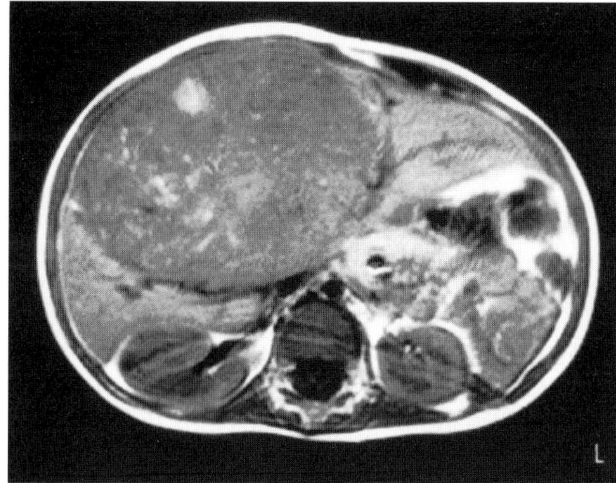

B

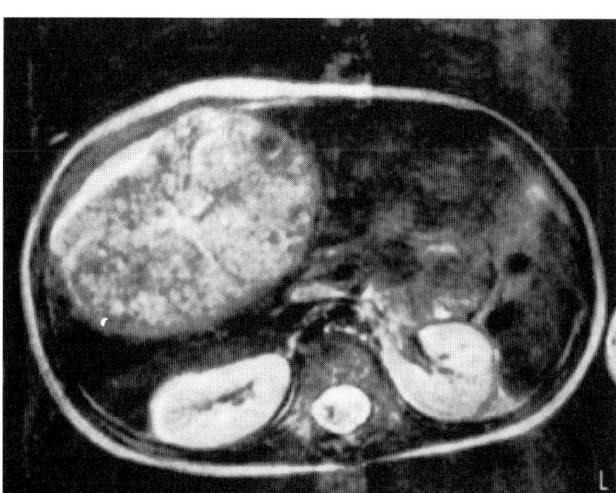

PATHOLOGY

Hepatoblastomas present as single masses in approximately 80% of cases, in the right lobe in 58% of cases, the left in 15%, and the remaining 27% in both lobes (either as a large single lesion extending across the midline or as multiple lesions).[56] These tumors may be up to 15 cm in diameter and can weigh in excess of 1,000 g. Grossly, they are coarsely lobulated and frequently bulge from the surface of the liver. On cut section, the lesions are tan to green and display numerous areas of hemorrhage and necrosis (Fig. 17-2A). The presence of various types of mesenchymal tissues (osteoid, cartilaginous, fibrous) in the mixed type of hepatoblastoma may alter the color and consistency (Fig. 17-2B).

Histologically, the tumor is classified into six patterns (Table 17-6). The four epithelial patterns account for approximately 56% of cases, including pure fetal (31%), embryonal (19%), macrotrabecular (3%), and small cell undifferentiated (3%). The mixed pattern of epithelial and mesenchymal components account for 44% of the cases, including 34% without teratoid features and 10% with components of squamous epithelium or striated muscle.

The fetal pattern includes those cases composed of small, round, uniform cells with abundant cytoplasm and distinct cytoplasmic membranes. The cells are arranged into thin trabeculae, 2 to 3 cells thick, with alternating light and dark areas (Fig. 17-3).

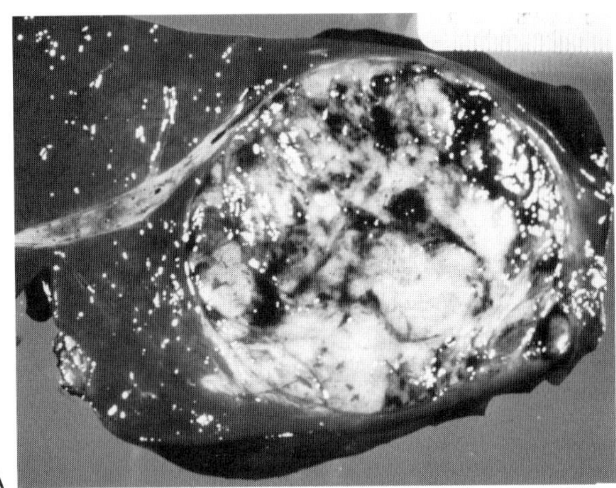

A

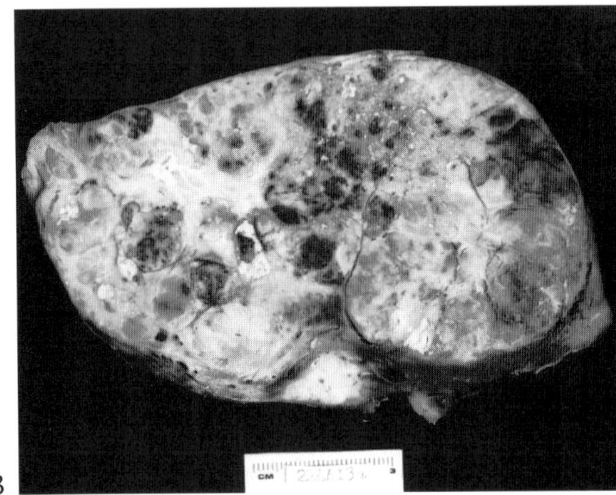

B

FIGURE 17-2. (*A*) A large lesion in the right lobe displays a relatively even light surface interspersed with areas of hemorrhage in this epithelial hepatoblastoma. (*B*) The cut surface of this mixed (epithelial and mesenchymal) hepatoblastoma displays variegated light to dark nodules interspersed with irregular bands of fibrous-like tissue.

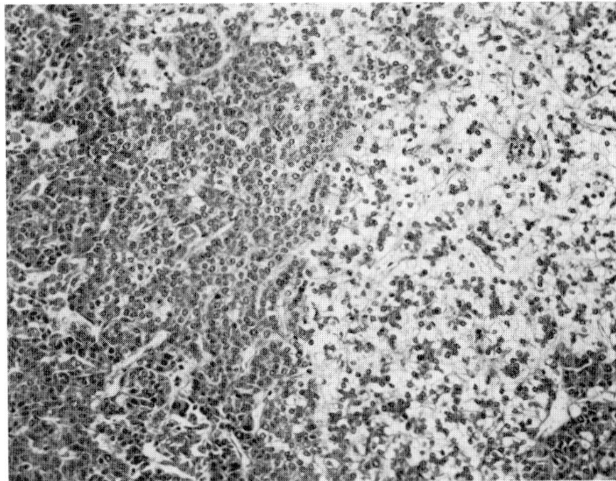

A

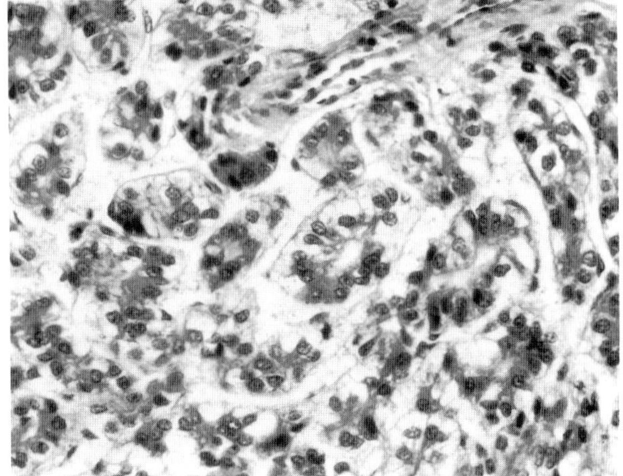

B

FIGURE 17-3. Pure epithelial fetal cell hepatoblastoma. (*A*) Small hepatocyte-like cells with central, regular nuclei form two-cell-thick cords. The presence of cytoplasmic glycogen and lipid imparts a clear or "light" appearance to the cells on the right when compared with the "dark" pattern on the left. (H&E, ×160.) (*B*) The cords of fetal epithelial cells are composed of similar or smaller sized cells than normal hepatocytes and are separated by sinusoids lined by endothelial cells. (H&E, ×400.)

TABLE 17-6. Six Histologic Patterns of Hepatoblastoma

- I. Epithelial type
  - A. Fetal pattern
  - B. Embryonal and fetal pattern
  - C. Macrotrabecular pattern
  - D. Small cell undifferentiated pattern
- II. Mixed epithelial and mesenchymal type
  - A. Without teratoid features
  - B. With teratoid features

The embryonal pattern includes cases in which, in addition to fetal cells, cells are found arranged into sheets of irregular, angulated cells with a high nucleocytoplasmic ratio, increased nuclear chromatin, and indistinct cytoplasmic membranes (Fig. 17-4). Pseudorosette and acinar formation are common features. Foci of extramedullary hematopoiesis are seen in both the fetal and embryonal areas in this pattern.

The macrotrabecular pattern refers to cases where trabeculae more than 10 cells in thickness are present as a repetitive pattern within the tumor (Fig. 17-5). The large trabeculae contain either fetal or embryonal type cells or a third larger cell type with more abundant cytoplasm. Cases with embryonal or mesenchymal cells with an isolated macrotrabecular focus are classified on the embryonal or mesenchymal cell component and not as macrotrabecular.

The small cell undifferentiated or anaplastic pattern is composed of cells resembling neuroblastoma that have scanty cytoplasm and hyperchromatic nuclei (Fig. 17-6). These cells grow in sheets but lack cohesiveness. Mitoses are occasionally present, but the cells do not produce glycogen, fat droplets, or bile pigment. Incompletely formed bile ductules may be present, but electron microscopy and/or immunohistochemical studies may be needed to confirm the diagnosis of hepatoblastoma. Particularly helpful in establishing the diagnosis is the presence of cytoplasmic staining with polyclonal anticytokeratin antibodies.[84] It has been suggested that the small cell form represents the type of pattern with the least differentiation within the highly variable spectrum of hepatoblastomas.[84]

FIGURE 17-4. Epithelial embryonal cell hepatoblastoma. (*A*) While fetal epithelial cells were present in other sections of this patient's tumor, the cells in this area display poor cohesiveness with loss of a cord like pattern. (H&E, ×150.) (*B*) The cells are round to ovoid with tapering ends. Some form gland- or rosette-like structures. The nuclei are hyperchromatic and of varying size. (H&E, ×300.)

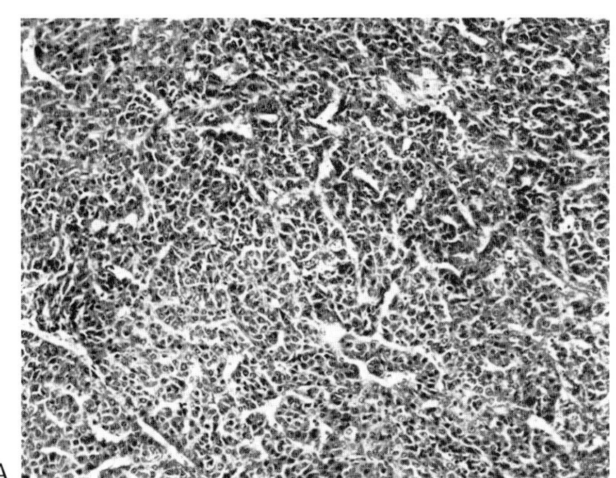

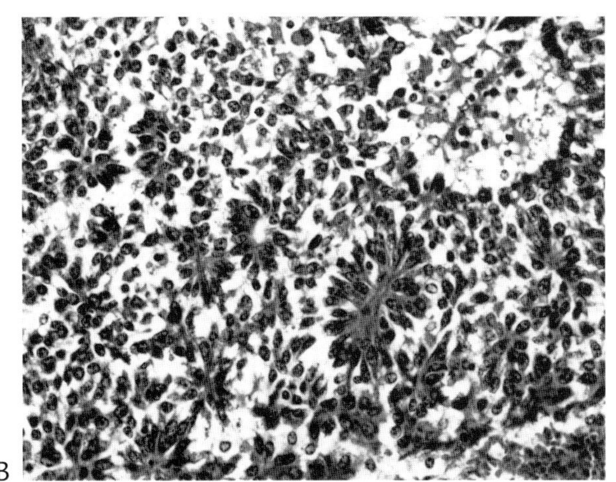

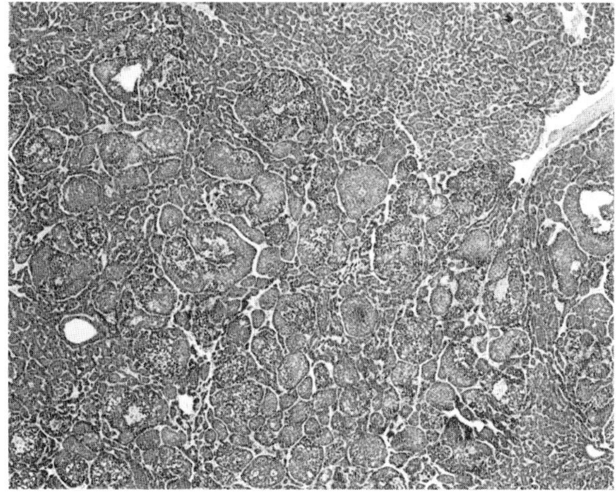

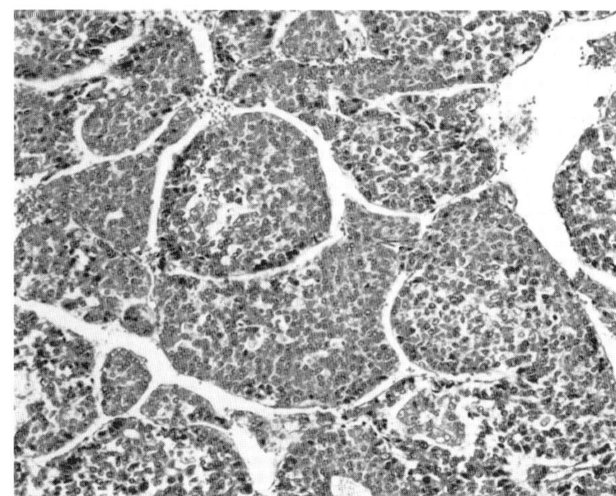

FIGURE 17-5. Macrotrabecular hepatoblastoma. (*A*) Typical cord-like fetal epithelial cells (top and lower right) partially surround an area of this hepatoblastoma composed of trabeculae that are 5 to 20 cells in thickness. (H&E, ×30.) (*B*) Some of the "macro" trabeculae appear as a solid cluster of fetal epithelial cells, while others have a loosely cohesive central core of cells resembling embryonal epithelial cells. (H&E, ×150.)

The mixed epithelial and mesenchymal type contains varying amounts of fetal-type and embryonal-type cells admixed with primitive mesenchyme and various mesenchymally derived tissues (Fig. 17-7A). The highly cellular primitive mesenchyme consists of elongated, spindle-shaped cells with a scanty cytoplasm and elongated plump nuclei with rounded ends. Some areas may display parallel orientation of cells with definite collagen fibers and young fibroblasts, while other areas may have more loosely arranged cells leading to a myxomatous appearance. Mature fibrous septa are also seen along with areas of osteoid and cartilaginous tissue. Cells within the

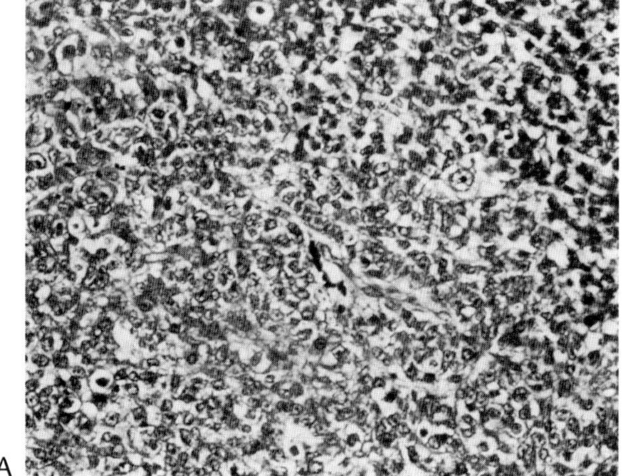

A

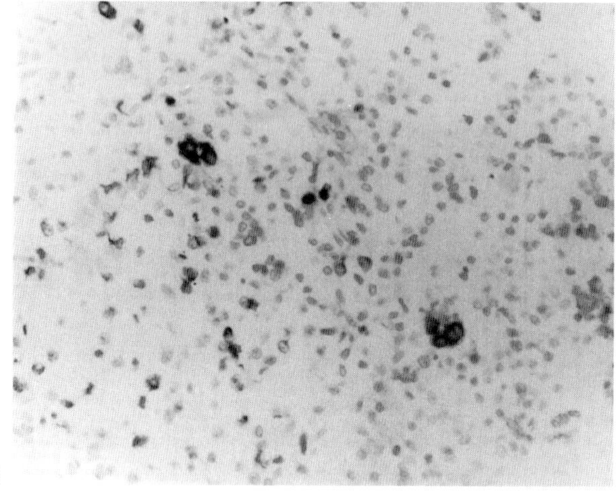

B

FIGURE 17-6. Small cell hepatoblastoma. (*A*) Sheets of small cells with a high nuclear/cytoplasmic ratio are separated by irregular hyalinized septae that do not form distinct trabeculae. (H&E, ×300.) (*B*) Immunoperoxidase staining for a mixture of keratin antigens (Kermix) displays scattered positivity through the sheets of cells. (IP, ×300.)

osteoid foci have an irregular, angular outline and short processes that make them indistinguishable from osteoblasts (Fig. 17-7B). Immunohistochemical studies, however, have identified this osteoid-like material as being produced through a process of epithelial differentiation (Fig. 17-7C).[85] Approximately 20% of the mixed-type hepatoblastomas contain a variety of tissues, including stratified squamous epithelium, melanin pigment, mucinous epithelium, cartilage, bone, and striated muscle, in addition to the epithelial cells, fibrous tissue, and osteoid-like material (Fig. 17-8). These tumors have also been termed *teratoid hepatoblastomas*.[86]

A mixed-type hepatoblastoma that contained elements of yolk sac tumor with rounded papillary structures and with central capillaries surrounded by cuboidal cells, Schiller-Duval bodies and small glandular spaces has been described in a 6-month-old boy.[87] A combined cystic teratoma and hepatoblastoma has been reported.[88] Seventeen hepatoblastomas treated with preoperative chemotherapy have been reviewed in which one could still recognize fetal, embryonal, and mesenchymal cell types.[89]

Immunohistochemical staining is varied for the different cell types but generally reflects the epithelial origin of the tumor.[90–94] The epithelial nature of the osteoid-like material has been established[85,93] by noting the expression of epithelial membrane antigen, cytokeratin, and AFP within the cells of the hyalin matrix. The observation that the small cell undifferentiated pattern showed intense reactivity for vimentin and focal reactivity for α_1-antitrypsin suggested that this pattern is a part of the differentiating spectrum of hepatoblastomas in which only minimal differentiation has occurred.[85] The use of sinusoidal reactivity for CD34 has been noted to show increased staining of hepatoblastoma sinusoids compared to normal liver sinusoids and has been suggested as useful in the differentiation of non-neoplastic liver tissue from highly differentiated fetal hepatoblastoma.[95] Neuroendocrine cells have been identified in the fetal and embryonal areas of hepatoblastoma that were reactive for chromogranin A, serotonin, and somatostatin.[93,96] A number of extracellular matrix proteins were identified in hepatoblastomas.[90] Immunohistochemistry for p53 protein has shown overexpression in hepatoblastomas.[23,90]

Ultrastructural features of hepatoblastomas include well-differentiated cells resembling hepatocytes located in the fetal areas. Other less-differentiated epithelial cells can be seen in the embryonal areas.[93]

Fine-needle aspiration biopsy of four hepatoblastomas provided a diagnosis in only two cases.[97] Fine-needle aspiration was reported to be useful in recognizing fetal and macrotrabecular patterns but could not distinguish the embryonal or small cell patterns from other childhood tumors.[98] Difficulty in distinguishing small cell hepatoblastoma from other small blue-cell childhood tumors, such as neuroblastoma, has been noted.[99]

TREATMENT

Current therapy consists of a combination of surgical resection and chemotherapy. Complete resection of hepatoblastoma at the time of initial laparotomy is the primary goal. Delayed resection increases the chance of postoperative complications and refractoriness of tumor cells to chemotherapeutic regimens. Tumors unresectable at diagnosis can be rendered resectable in the majority of cases with use of preoperative chemotherapy. Orthotopic liver transplantation is a viable option for

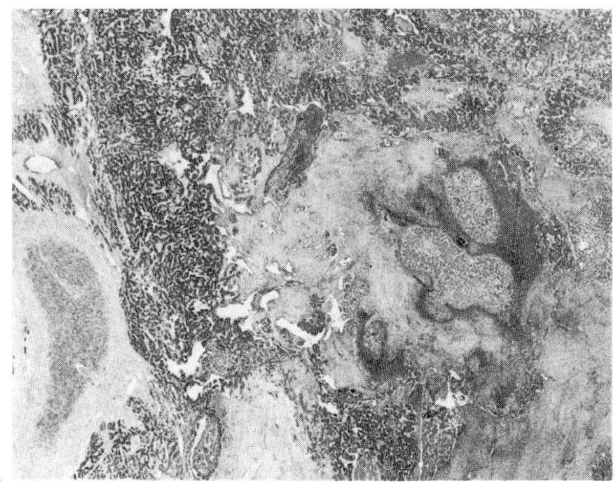
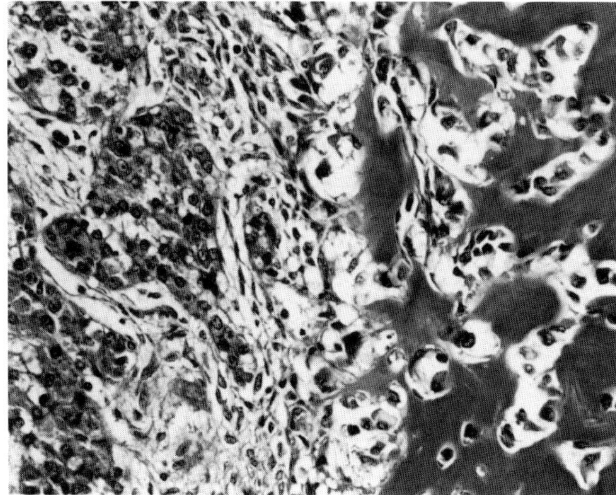
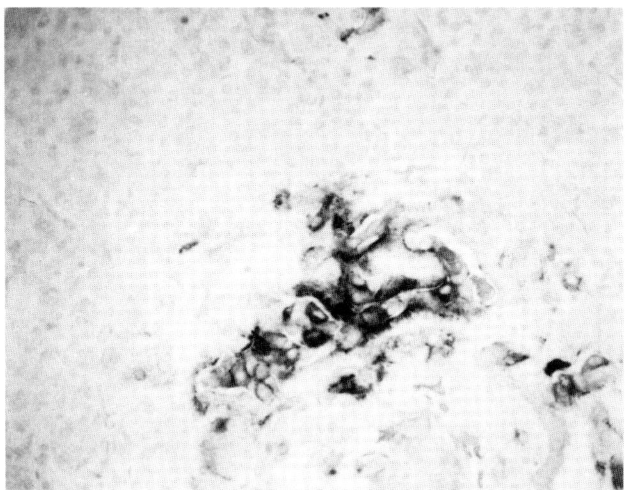

FIGURE 17-7. Mixed (epithelial/mesenchymal) hepatoblastoma. (*A*) Foci of mesenchymal tissue (center) and osteoid-like material (center right) are interspersed with fetal and embryonal epithelial cells. (H&E, ×15.) (*B*) The osteoid-like material (right) contains lacunae filled with ovoid hyperchromatic cells. Note the focus of fetal epithelial cells (left center) surrounded by loose mesenchymal cells. (H&E, ×300.) (*C*) A focus of osteoid-like material stains heavily for epithelial membrane antigen. (IP, ×300.)

unresectable tumors. The combination of preoperative chemotherapy with surgical resection of residual tumor including pulmonary metastases at second and third laparotomies has significantly improved survival.

Resection

For small, solitary tumors localized to one lobe, lobectomy is adequate. For more extensive and multifocal disease, or for tumors that extend across the midline, a trisegmentectomy may be needed. Up to 85% of the liver can be resected safely.[100] Surgical complications have been reported in 14% of primary resections and up to 29% of second resections,[101] with hemorrhage being the most common complication.[102,103] Large size, the involvement of both lobes, and metastatic disease make the tumor unresectable. Multiple studies[6,65,67,102–104] indicate that 40% to 60% of tumors are unresectable at diagnosis; pulmonary metastases are present in about 10% to 20% of patients.[6,105–107]

Significant reductions in tumor volume ranging from 35% to 95% can be obtained by preoperative chemotherapy.[108] Preoperative chemotherapy renders between 80% and 90% of unresectable tumors resectable (Table 17-7). The combination of resection at primary laparotomy or during a second look operation after preoperative chemotherapy renders up to 90% of tumors resectable in some series.[67,101,114] Delayed resection,

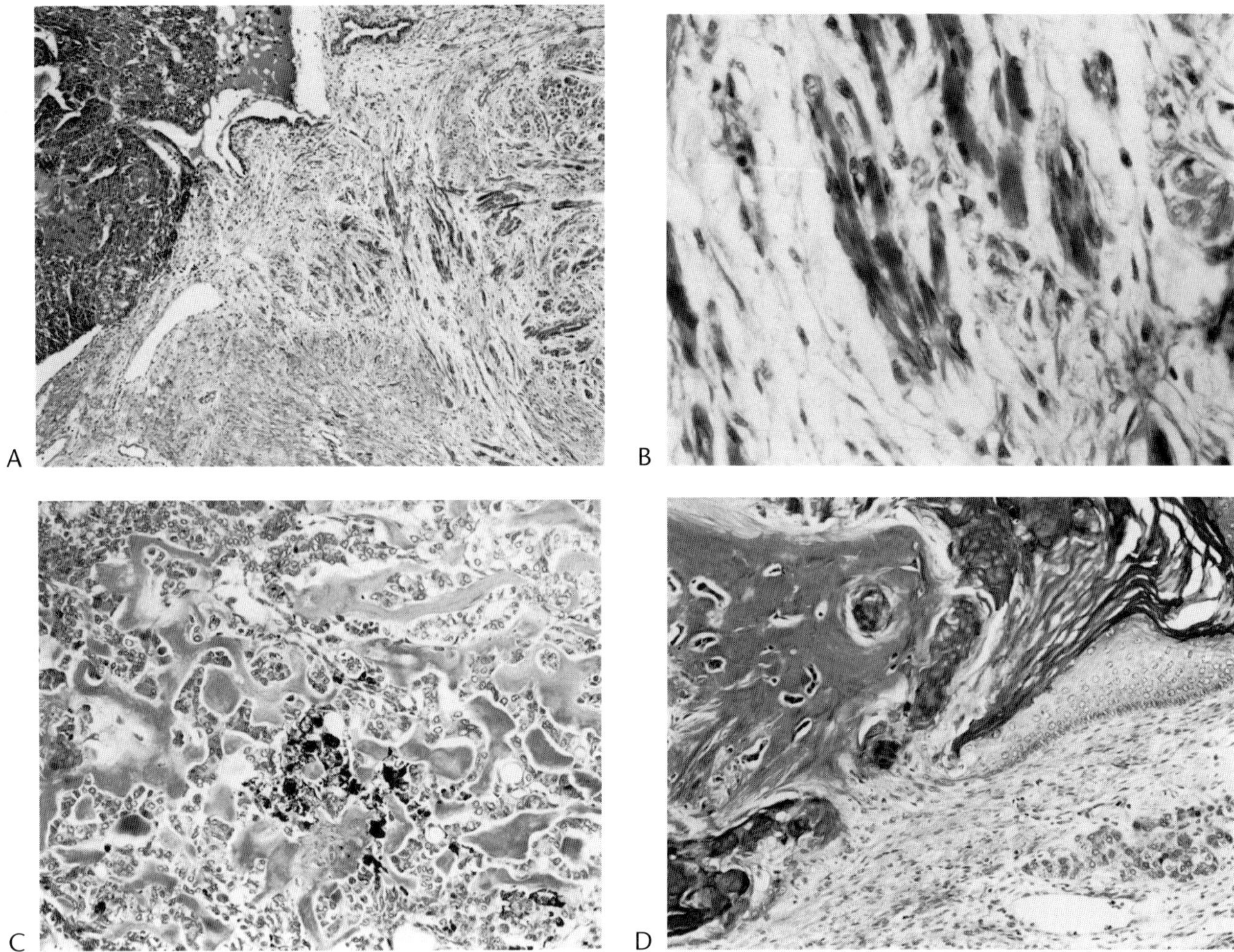

FIGURE 17-8. Mixed hepatoblastoma with teratoid features. Embryonal epithelial cells (upper left in *A*) lie adjacent to mesenchymal tissue composed of fibrous connective tissue and skeletal muscle (*B*). In other areas of the lesion, osteoid-like foci containing melanin pigment (*C*) and squamous epithelium with keratin formation (*D*) were present.

TABLE 17-7. Effect of Preoperative Chemotherapy on Hepatoblastomas Initially Classified as Unresectable

Authors	No. Unresectable (Prior to Chemotherapy)	No. Resectable (After Chemotherapy)	Percent Resected	No. (%) Disease-Free After Resection
Filler et al.[108]	10	10	100	8 (80)
Guglielmi et al.[109]	16	12	75	10 (83)[a]
King et al.[110]	22	17	77	
Pierro et al.[111]	11	8	73	7 (88)[b]
Stringer et al.[112]	26	22	85	16 (73)
Tagge et al.[113]	10	8	80	7 (88)[b]
von Schweinitz et al.[101]	39	34	87	28 (82)
Total	134	111	83	

[a] Two patients lost to follow up.

[b] Intraoperative death.

however, has been reported to increase the risk of postoperative complications and is associated with a poorer survival (41%) compared to subtotal resection at initial laparotomy in some series,[110,115] although others reported no difference in survival between tumors resected at initial laparotomy and those after a course of preoperative chemotherapy.[112]

Metastatic disease is often responsive to chemotherapy. Current protocols, therefore, are directed at excising the primary hepatoblastoma in spite of metastatic disease.[115] Postoperative AFP levels are useful in monitoring patients for metastatic disease and in indicating when a tumor has become resistant to chemotherapy. Surgical excision of pulmonary metastases that are resistant to chemotherapy is advocated.[107,115,116] Black and colleagues[107] list a number of criteria to use in determining when to resect pulmonary metastases resistant to chemotherapy: (1) the primary has been completely resected, (2) the metastases occurred more than 6 months after the primary had been resected, (3) the metastases were initially responsive to chemotherapy, (4), the resection takes place soon after resistance has occurred based on AFP levels, and (5) all gross disease has been excised. Multiple thoracotomies for resection of metastatic disease have been shown to improve long-term survival.[107,117]

Chemotherapy

A number of early studies showed that chemotherapy alone was ineffective in treating hepatoblastoma,[104,118] except for occasional cases.[119] Most current studies report success with a combination of preoperative and adjuvant chemotherapy along with surgical resection. For children with incompletely resected hepatoblastoma, continuous infusion of doxorubicin and cisplatin every 21 days for four courses is effective in reducing tumor burden. Twenty-five of 33 patients with hepatoblastoma (76%) responded to this chemotherapy regimen in a recent study.[67] Complications of chemotherapy in that study included neutropenia, sepsis, and hypomagnesemia. Drug resistance to chemotherapy is another potential problem[68] and may require that a different chemotherapeutic regimen be employed such as high-dose cisplatin[120] or low-dose methotrexate.[121]

Transplantation

Orthotopic liver transplantation is accepted as a treatment modality for hepatic tumors.[113,122–124] In a study of 12 patients with hepatoblastoma, 50% of patients were alive without disease recurrence 24 to 70 months after transplantation, 25% died of tumor recurrence within 24 months, and the remainder died of postoperative complications, such as infection or hepatic artery thrombosis.[124] In another series, 61% (11/18) experienced acute rejection requiring immunosuppression.[113] Bacterial and viral infections were frequent complications.

TABLE 17-8. Children's Cancer Study Group Staging Classification[6]

Stage I, complete resection
Stage II, microscopic residual, negative nodal involvement, no spilled tumor
Stage III, gross residual or nodal involvement or spilled tumor
Stage IV, metastatic disease

Radiotherapy

Radiotherapy has a limited role in treating hepatoblastoma. It is used in combination with chemotherapy in treating residual disease after surgical resection and in the management of inoperable tumors.[115,125]

PROGNOSIS

Staging

In the United States, most patients are staged according to the Children's Cancer Study Group (CCSG) classification (Table 17-8). Staging is performed at the time of initial diagnosis and is best performed by the surgeon at laparotomy (Table 17-9). The TNM staging classification has also been used in staging hepatoblastomas.[105,127] In a study at the Armed Forces Institute of Pathology (AFIP), 105 cases were classified the same way using both systems; there was no statistical difference in survival between the two staging classifications (R. M. Conran, C. L. Hitchcock, M. A. Waclawiw, J. T. Stocker, and K. Ishak, unpublished results).

Survival

Prior to 1975, approximately 35% of hepatoblastomas were cured by surgical excision alone.[65,105] With surgery, preoperative and adjuvant chemotherapy, and transplantation, the overall survival is now between 65% and 70% (Table 17-10). Survival rates are not different between

TABLE 17-9. Distribution of Hepatoblastoma by Stage

Study Group	No.	I	II	III	IV
AFIP[6]	105	48	7	27	18
CCSG[126]	168	33	—[a]	—[a]	20
POG[103]	140	29	11	21	39

Abbreviations: AFIP, Armed Forces Institute of Pathology; CCSG, Children's Cancer Study Group; POG, Pediatric Oncology Group.

[a] Stages II and III were reported together and represent 47% of cases.

TABLE 17-10. Survival Analysis of Hepatoblastoma

Author	No. of Cases	No./Stage I	II	III	IV	Primary Resection[a]	Delayed Resection[b]	Orthotopic Liver Transplantation	No. of Patients Without Evidence of Recurring Disease (%)[c]
Guglielmi et al.[109]	23	6	1	13	3	7[d] (5/7, 71%)[e]	12 (10/12, 83%)	—	15/23 (65)
Stringer et al.[112]	41			8		14 (11/14, 79%)	22[d] (16/22, 73%)	1	27/41 (66)
Tagge et al.[113]	21	5	1	10	5	6 (2/6, 33%)	8 (7/8, 87%)	6 (5/6, 83%)	14/21 (67)
von Schweinitz et al.[114]	64	18	5	36	5	23 (22/23, 96%)	32 (23/32, 72%)	—	45/64 (70)

[a] Complete resection of tumor at initial laparotomy.

[b] Significant tumor shrinkage occurred prior to resection. Preoperative therapy consisted of combination cisplatin and doxorubicin.

[c] Minimum disease-free interval was 19 months.

[d] Intraoperative death.

[e] Numbers in parentheses indicate those disease free after resection or transplantation.

children with primary resection and children treated with preoperative chemotherapy who later undergo delayed resection.[67] For patients with unresectable tumors, transplantation should be considered. CT scans and other imaging modalities are useful in determining resectability.[83,108]

In approximately 33% of patients, the tumor can be completely resected at initial presentation (stage I). Between 5% and 8% have microscopic residual tumor at the surgical margin (stage II). Between 50% and 60% are not resectable at presentation (stage III), and 8% to 15% have metastatic disease (stage IV). Survival for stage I tumors is reported as 100% in recent studies, 75% to 80% for stage II tumors, 65% to 68% for stage III tumors, and none for stage IV tumors.[66,114] In other studies, up to 14%[6] and 27%[108] of stage IV patients became disease free.

Prognostic Features

Since the initial review of 35 hepatoblatomas by Ishak and Glunz,[128] a number of clinical and pathologic prognostic features have been reported. Stage is a key prognostic factor (Table 17-11).[6,68,105] Children with stages I and II tumors have an excellent prognosis compared to children with more extensive disease. However, with the use of preoperative chemotherapy, transplantation, and improved surgical techniques, survival for stage III and IV patients has improved significantly.

Histologic pattern had been suggested as an important prognostic factor. A number of early studies[106,127,129] suggested improved survival with the pure fetal pattern or at least for stage I tumors.[126] For other stages, survival was independent of histologic subtype. A number of studies[6,68,108,130] demonstrate that survival is independent of histologic subtype when adjusted for age, sex, and stage (Table 17-12).

TABLE 17-11. Hepatoblastoma: Relative Risk of Death for Given Stage[a]

Stage	Relative Risk of Death	p Value
I	0.1637	<0.00001
II	0.5672	0.4375
III	2.8742	0.0013
IV	3.5148	0.0002

[a] Stage of interest compared to other stages combined. Adjusted for age and sex.

(From Conran et al.,[6] with permission.)

TABLE 17-12. Relative Risk of Death by Histologic Type[a] for Hepatoblastoma Cases Classified on Both Epithelial and Mesenchymal Components[b]

Histologic Type	Relative Risk of Death	p Value
Fetal	1.0739	0.8850
Embryonal	1.7409	0.1662
Mixed[c]	0.5292	0.0754
Without teratoid features	0.4685	0.0542
With teratoid features	1.1274	0.8128
Macrotrabecular	1.1980	0.7729
Small cell	3.7096	0.1061

[a] Histologic type of interest compared to other histologic types.

[b] Cases adjusted for age, sex, and stage.

[c] Includes all mixed hepatoblastomas with and without teratoid features.

(From Conran et al.,[6] with permission.)

Other pathologic features of prognostic value are increased mitotic activity (regardless of stage) and the presence of osteoid for stage II to IV tumors.[126] This correlates with the good prognosis observed for the mixed hepatoblastoma reported elsewhere.[6] The pTNM classification system[105] may be of prognostic value. Involvement of more than one lobe, multifocality within the liver, and vascular invasion were important features. This supports the premise that stage is a key factor. Nucleolar organizing regions as a marker of epithelial differentiation were also of prognostic significance.[105] DNA aneuploidy has been reported as a poor prognostic feature but was not confirmed in studies by others.[6,78]

REFERENCES

1. Stocker JT, Conran RM, Selby D. Tumors and pseudotumors of the liver. In Stocker JT, Askin FB (eds): Pathology of Solid Tumors in Children. Chapman and Hall, London (in press)
2. Stocker JT. Hepatic tumors. In Stocker JT (ed): Pediatric Hepatology. Hemisphere Pub. Corp., New York, 1990, pp. 399–488
3. Hartley AL, Birch JM, Kesley AM et al. Epidemiologic and familial aspects of hepatoblastoma. Med Pediatr Oncol 1990;18:103–109
4. Neu SM. Hepatoblastoma in an equine fetus. J Vet Diagn Invest 1993;5:634–637
5. Buckley JD, Sather H, Ruccione K et al. A case-control study of risk factors for hepatoblastoma. A report from the Children's Cancer Study Group. Cancer 1989;64: 1169–1176
6. Conran RM, Hitchcock CL, Waclawiw MA et al. Hepatoblastoma: the prognostic significance of histologic type. Pediatr Pathol 1992;12:167–183
7. Surendran N, Radhakrishna K, Chellam VG. Hepatoblastoma in siblings. J Pediatr Surg 1989;24:1169–1171
8. Riikonen P, Tuominen L, Seppa A, Perkkio M. Simultaneous hepatoblastoma in identical male twins. Cancer 1990; 66:2429–2431
9. Akmal SN, Yun K, MacLay J et al. Insulin-like growth factor 2 and insulin-like growth factor binding protein 2 expression in hepatoblastoma. Hum Pathol 1995;26: 846–851
10. Davies SM. Maintenance of genomic imprinting at the IGF2 locus in hepatoblastoma. Cancer Res 1993;53: 4781–4783
11. Li X, Adam G, Cui H et al. Expression, promoter usage and parental imprinting status of insulin-like growth factor II (IGF2) in human hepatoblastoma: uncoupling of IGF2 and H19 imprinting. Oncogene 1995;11:221–229
12. Rainer S, Dobry CJ, Feinberg AP. Loss of imprinting in hepatoblastoma. Cancer Res 1995;55:1836–1838
13. Albrecht S, von Schweinitz D, Waha A et al. Loss of maternal alleles on chromosome arm 11p in hepatoblastoma. Cancer Res 1994;54:5041–5044
14. Byrne JA, Simms LA, Little MH et al. Three non-overlapping regions of chromosome arm 11p allele loss identified in infantile tumors of adrenal and liver. Genes Chromosom Cancer 1993;8:104–111
15. Montagna M, Menin C, Chieco-Bianchi L, D'Andrea E. Occasional loss of constitutive heterozygosity at 11p15.5 and imprinting relaxation of the IGFII maternal allele in hepatoblastoma. J Cancer Res Clin Oncol 1994;120: 732–736
16. Simms LA, Reeve AE, Smith PJ. Genetic mosaicism at the insulin locus in liver associated with childhood hepatoblastoma. Genes Chromosom Cancer 1995;13:72–73
17. Chen TC, Hsieh LL, Kuo TT. Absence of p53 gene mutation and infrequent over expression of p53 protein in hepatoblastoma. J Pathol 1995;176:243–247
18. Calvert RJ, Tashiro Y, Buzard GS, et al. Lack of p53 point mutations in chemically induced mouse hepatoblastomas: an end-stage, highly malignant hepatocellular tumor. Cancer Lett 1995;95:175–180
19. Oda H, Nakatsuru Y, Imai Y et al. A mutational hotspot in the p53 gene is associated with hepatoblastomas. Int J Cancer 1995;60:786–790
20. Farshid M, Hsia CC, Tabor E. Alterations of the RB tumour suppressor gene in hepatocellular carcinoma and hepatoblastoma cell lines in association with abnormal p53 expression. J Viral Hepatitis 1994;1:45–53
21. Ruck P, Xiao JC, Kaiserling E. p53 protein expression in hepatoblastoma: an immunohistochemical investigation. Pediatr Pathol 1994;14:79–85
22. Schaff Z, Sarosi I, Hsia CC et al. p53 in malignant and benign liver lesions. Eur J Cancer 1995;31A:1847–1850
23. Kennedy SM, Macgeogh C, Jaffe R, Spurr NK. Over expression of the oncoprotein p53 in primary hepatic tumors of childhood does not correlate with gene mutations. Hum Pathol 1994;25:438–442
24. Diwan BA, Ward JM, Kurata Y, Rice JM. Dissimilar frequency of hepatoblastomas and hepatic cystadenomas and adenocarcinomas arising in hepatocellular neoplasms of D2B6F1 mice initiated with *N*-nitrosodiethylamine and subsequently given Aroclor-1254, dichlorodiphenyltrichloroethane, or phenobarbital. Toxicol Pathol 1994;22: 430–439
25. Diwan BA, Henneman JR, Rice JM. Further evidence for promoter-dependent development of hepatoblastoma in the mouse. Cancer Lett 1995;89:29–35
26. Diwan BA, Henneman JR, Nims RW, Rice JM. Tumor promotion by an anticonvulsant agent, phenytoin, in mouse liver: correlation with CYP2B induction. Carcinogenesis 1993;14:2227–2231
27. Diwan BA, Rice JM, Ward JM. Tumor-promoting activity of benzodiazepine tranquilizers, diazepam and oxazepam, in mouse liver. Carcinogenesis 1986;7:789–794
28. Devereux TR, White CM, Sills RC et al. Low frequency of H-*ras* mutations in hepatocellular adenoma and carcinomas and in hepatoblastomas from B6C3F1 mice exposed to oxazepam in the diet. Carcinogenesis 1994;15:1083–1087
29. Tsao M, Grisham JW. Hepatocarcinomas, cholangiocarcinomas, and hepatoblastomas produced by chemically trans-

formed cultured rat liver epithelial cells. A light- and electron-microscopic analysis. Am J Pathol 1987;127:168–181

30. Suzuki T, Watanabe K, Hirota M et al. Establishment of a human hepatoblastoma model in athymic nude mice. Producibility of fatty acid-binding protein, α-fetoprotein, and α_1-acid glycoprotein. Acta Pathol Jpn 1992;42:255–261
31. Manchester KM, Warren DJ, Erlandson RA et al. Establishment and characterization of a novel hepatoblastoma-derived cell line. J Pediatr Surg 1995;30:553–558
32. Doi I. Establishment of a cell line and its clonal sublines from a patient with hepatoblastoma. Gann 1976;67:1–10
33. Miyoshi E, Nishikawa A, Ihara Y et al. Selective suppression of *N*-acetylglucosaminyltransferase III activity in a human hepatoblastoma cell line transfected with hepatitis B virus. Cancer Res 1994;54:1854–1858
34. Oka Y, Murata A, Nishijima J et al. The mechanism of hepatic cellular injury in sepsis: an in vitro study of the implications of cytokines and neutrophils in its pathogenesis. J Surg Res 1993;55:1–8
35. Davit-Spraul A, Pourci ML, Soni T, Lemonnier A. Metabolic effects of galactose on human Hep G2 hepatoblastoma cells. Metabolism 1994;43:945–952
36. Farrants A, Nilsson A, Pedersen JI. Human hepatoblastoma cells (Hep G2) and rat hepatoma cells are defective in important enzyme activities in the oxidation of the C_{27} steroid side chain in bile acid formation. J Lipid Res 1993; 34:2041–2050
37. Hara T, Aramaki Y, Takada S et al. Receptor-mediated transfer of pSV2CAT DNA to a human hepatoblastoma cell line Hep G2 using asialofetuin-labeled cationic liposomes. Gene 1995;159:167–174
38. Hou J, Wang F, McKeehan WL. Molecular cloning and expression of the gene for a major leucine-rich protein from human hepatoblastoma cells (Hep G2). In Vitro Cell Dev Biol 1994;30A:111–114
39. Javitt NB. Hep G2 cells as a resource for metabolic studies: lipoprotein, cholesterol, and bile acids. FASEB J 1990;4: 161–168
40. Kasama K, Utsumi J, Matsuo-Ogawa E et al. Pharmacokinetics and biologic activities of human native and asialo-interferon-s. J Interferon Cytokine Res 1995;15:407–415
41. Schrader M, Baumgart E, Volkl A, Fahimi HD. Heterogeneity of peroxisomes in human hepatoblastoma cell line Hep G2. Evidence of distinct subpopulations. Eur J Cell Biol 1994;64:281–294
42. Aden DP, Fogel A, Plotkin S et al. Controlled synthesis of HBsAg in a differentiated human liver carcinoma-derived cell line. Nature 1979;282:615–616
43. Harada T, Matsuo K, Kodama S et al. Adult hepatoblastoma: case report and review of the literature. Aust NZ J Surg 1995;65:686–688
44. Altmann HW. Epithelial and mixed hepatoblastoma in the adult: histological observations and general considerations. Pathol Res Pract 1992;188:16–26
45. Oda H, Honda K, Hara M et al. Hepatoblastoma in an 82-year-old man: an autopsy case report. Acta Pathol Jpn 1990; 40:212–218
46. Robin NH, Grace K, DeSouza TG et al. New finding of Schinzel-Giedion syndrome: a case with a malignant sacrococcygeal teratoma. Am J Med Genet 1993;47:852–856
47. Bernstein IT, Bulow S, Mauritzen K. Hepatoblastoma in two cousins in a family with adenomatous polyposis. Report of two cases. Dis Colon Rectum 1992;35:373–374
48. Iwama T, Mishima Y. Mortality in young first-degree relatives of patients with familial adenomatous polyposis. Cancer 194;73:2065–2068
49. Giardiello FM, Offerhaus JA, Krush AJ N et al. Risk of hepatoblastoma in familial adenomatous polyposis. J Pediatr 1991;119:766–768
50. Hughes LJ, Michels VV. Risk of hepatoblastoma in familial adenomatous polyposis. Am J Med Genet 1992;43: 1023–1025
51. LeSher AR, Castronuovo Jr JJ, Filippone Jr AL. Hepatoblastoma in a patient with familial polyposis coli. Surgery 1989;105:668–670
52. Li FP, Thurber WA, Seddon J, Holmes GE. Hepatoblastoma in families with polyposis coli. JAMA 1987;257: 2475–2477
53. Kurahashi H, Takami K, Oue T et al. Biallelic inactivation of the APC gene in hepatoblastoma. Cancer Res 1995;55: 5007–5011
54. Khosla A. Hepatoblastoma and congenital dysplastic kidney. J Pediatr Surg 1990;25:924
55. Rao PS, Krishna A, Rohatgi M. Multicystic kidney in association with hepatoblastoma, a case report. Jpn J Surg 1989; 19:583–585
56. Stocker JT, Ishak KG. Hepatoblastoma. In Okuda K, Ishak KG (eds): Neoplasms of the Liver. Springer-Verlag, New York, 1987, pp. 127–136
57. Bove KE, Soukup S, Ballard ET, Ryckman F. Hepatoblastoma in a child with trisomy 18: cytogenetics, liver abnormalities, and literature review. Pediatr Pathol Lab Med 1996;16:253–262
58. Barton JW III, Keller MS. Liver transplantation for hepatoblastoma in a child with congenital absence of the portal vein. Pediatr Radiol 1989;20:113–114
59. Hashizume K, Nakajo T, Kawarasaki H et al. Prader-Willi syndrome with del(15(q11,q13) associated with hepatoblastoma. Acta Paediatr Jpn 1991;33:712–722
60. Wilfong AA, Parke JT, McCrary JA III. Opsoclonus-myoclonus with Beckwith-Wiedemann syndrome and hepatoblastoma. Pediatr Neurol 1991;8:77–79
61. Arico M, Caselli D, D'Argenio P et al. Malignancies in children with human immunodeficiency virus type 1 infection. Cancer 1991;68:2473–2477
62. Gururangan S, O'Meara A, Macmahon C et al. Primary hepatic tumors in children: a 26-year review. J Surg Oncol 1992;50:30–36
63. Shafford EA, Pritchard J. Extreme thrombocytosis as a diagnostic clue to hepatoblastoma. Arch Dis Child 1993;69: 171
64. Muraji T, Woolley MM, Sinatra F et al. The prognostic implication of hypercholesterolemia in infants and children with hepatoblastoma. J Pediatr Surg 1985;20:228–230
65. Exelby PR, Filler RM, Grosfeld JL. Liver tumors in children

in the particular reference to hepatoblastoma and hepatocellular carcinoma: American Academy of Pediatrics, Surgical Section Survey—1974. J Pediatr Surg 1975;10: 329–337

66. Vos A. Primary liver tumors in children. Eur J Surg Oncol 1995;21:101–105.106

67. Ortega JA, Krailo MD, Haas JE et al. Effective treatment of unresectable or metastatic hepatoblastoma with cisplatin and continuous infusion doxorubicin chemotherapy; a report from the Children's Cancer Study Group. J Clin Oncol 1991;9:2167–2176

68. von Schweinitz D, Hecker H, Harms D et al. Complete resection before development of drug resistance is essential for survival from advanced hepatoblastoma—a report from the German Cooperative Pediatric Liver Tumor Study HB-89. J Pediatr Surg 1995;30:845–852

69. Ding SF, Michail NE, Habib NA. Genetic changes in hepatoblastoma. J Hepatol 1994;20:672–675

70. Tonk VS, Wilson KS, Timmons CF, Schneider NR. Trisomy 2, trisomy 20, and del(17p) as sole chromosomal abnormalities in three cases of hepatoblastoma. Genes Chromosom Cancer 1994;11:199–202

71. Bardi G, Johansson B, Pandis N et al. Trisomy 2 as the sole chromosomal abnormality in a hepatoblastoma. Genes Chromosom Cancer 1992;4:78–80

72. Fletcher JA, Kozakewich HP, Pavelka K et al. Consistent cytogenetic aberrations in hepatoblastoma: a common pathway of genetic alterations in embryonal liver and skeletal muscle malignancies? Genes Chromosom Cancer 1991; 3:37–43

73. Anneren G, Nordlinder H, Hedborg F. Chromosome aberrations in an alpha-fetoprotein-producing hepatoblastoma. Genes Chromosom Cancer 1992;4:99–100

74. Douglass EC, Green AA, Hayes FA et al. Chromosome 1 abnormalities: a common feature of pediatric solid tumors. J Natl Cancer Inst 1985;75:51–53

75. Haas OA, Zoubek A, Grumayer ER, Gadner H. Constitutional interstitial deletion of 11p11 and pericentric inversion of chromosome 9 in a patient with Wiedemann-Beckwith syndrome and hepatoblastoma. Cancer Genet Cytogenet 1986;23:95–104

76. Bardi G, Johansson B, Pandis N et al. i(8q) as the primary structural chromosome abnormality in a hepatoblastoma. Cancer Genet Cytogenet 1991;51:281–283

77. Hata Y, Ishizu H, Ohmori K et al. Flow cytometric analysis of the nuclear DNA content of hepatoblastoma. Cancer 1991;68:2566–2570

78. Schmidt D, Wischmeyer P, Leuschner I et al. DNA analysis in hepatoblastoma by flow and image cytometry. Cancer 1993;72:2914–2919

79. Amendola MA, Blane CE, Amendola BS, Glazer GM. CT findings in hepatoblastoma. J Comput Assist Tomogr 1984; 8:1105–1109

80. Miller JH, Greenspan BS. Integrated imaging of hepatic tumors in childhood. Part I. Malignant lesions (primary and metastatic). Radiology 1985;145:83–90

81. Powers C, Ros PR, Stoupis C et al. Primary liver neoplasms: MR imaging with pathologic correlation. Radiographics 1994;14:459–482

82. Bates SM, Keller MS, Ramos IM et al. Hepatoblastoma: detection of tumor vascularity with duplex Doppler US. Radiology 1990;176:505–507

83. King SJ, Babyn PS, Greenberg ML et al. Value of CT in determining the resectability of hepatoblastoma before and after chemotherapy. AJR 1993;160:793–798

84. Gonzalez-Crussi F. Case 1. Undifferentiated small cell ("anaplastic") hepatoblastoma. Pediatr Pathol 1991;11: 155–162

85. Abenoza P, Manivel JC, Wick MR et al. Hepatoblastoma: an immunohistochemical and ultrastructural study. Hum Pathol 1987;18:1025–1035

86. Manivel C, Wick MR, Abenoza P, Dehner LP. Teratoid hepatoblastoma. The nosologic dilemma of solid embryonic neoplasms of childhood. Cancer 1986;57:2168–2174

87. Cross SS, Variend S. Combined hepatoblastoma and yolk sac tumor of the liver. Cancer 1992;69:1323–1326

88. Conrad RJ, Gribbin D, Walker NI, Ong TH. Combined cystic teratoma and hepatoblastoma of the liver. Probable divergent differentiation of an uncommitted hepatic precursor cell. Cancer 1993;72:2910–2913

89. Saxena R, Leake JL, Shafford EA et al. Chemotherapy effects on hepatoblastoma: a histological study. Am J Surg Pathol 1993;17:1266–1271

90. Ruck P, Kaiserling E. Extracellular matrix in hepatoblastoma: an immunohistochemical investigation. Histopathology 1992;21:115–126

91. Sciot R, VanEyken P, Desmet VJ. Transferrin receptor expression in benign tumors and in hepatoblastoma of the liver. Histopathology 1990;16:59–62

92. VanEyken P, Sciot R, Callea F, Desmet VJ. A cytokeratin-immunohistochemical study of focal nodular hyperplasia of the liver: further evidence that ductular metaplasia of hepatocytes contributes to ductular "proliferation." Liver 1989;9:372–377

93. Warfel KA, Hull MT. Hepatoblastomas: an ultrastructural and immunohistochemical study. Ultrastruct Pathol 1992; 16:451–461

94. Pontisso P, Barson M, Basso G et al. Cytokeratin patterns in childhood primary liver tumors. Int J Clin Lab Res 1993; 23:225–227

95. Ruck P, Xiao JC, Kaiserling E. Immunoreactivity of sinusoids in hepatoblastoma: an immunohistochemical study using lectin UEA-1 and antibodies against endothelium-associated antigens, including CD34. Histopathology 1995; 26:451–455

96. Ruck P, Harms D, Kaiserling E. Neuroendocrine differentiation in hepatoblastoma: an immunohistochemical investigation. Am J Surg Pathol 1990;14:847–855

97. Wakely PE Jr, Silverman JF, Geisinger KR, Frable WJ. Fine needle aspiration biopsy cytology of hepatoblastoma. Mod Pathol 1990;3:688–693

98. Sola Perez J, Perez-Guillermo M, Bas Bernal AB, Mercader JM. Hepatoblastoma. An attempt to apply histologic classification to aspirates obtained by fine needle aspiration cytology. Acta Cytol 1994;38:175–182

99. Kaw YT, Hansen K. Fine needle aspiration cytology of un-

differentiated small cell ("anaplastic") hepatoblastoma: a case report. Acta Cytol 1993;37:216–220

100. Newman KD. Malignant liver tumors of children. Semin Pediatr Surg 1992;1:145–151
101. von Schweinitz D, Burger D, Mildenberger H. Is laparotomy the first step in treatment of childhood liver tumors?—The experience from the German Cooperative Pediatric Liver Tumor Study HB-89. Eur J Pediatr Surg 1994;4:82–86
102. Andrassy RJ, Brennan LP, Siegel MM et al. Preoperative chemotherapy for hepatoblastoma in children: report of six cases. J Pediatr Surg 1980;15:517–522
103. Finegold MJ. Tumors of the liver. Semin Liver Dis 1994; 14:270–281
104. Pazdur R, Bready B, Cangir A. Pediatric hepatic tumors: clinical trials conducted in the United States. J Surg Oncol 1993;3(suppl):127–130
105. von Schweinitz D, Wischmeyer P, Leuschner I et al. Clinico-pathological criteria with prognostic relevance in hepatoblastoma. Eur J Cancer 1994;30A:1052–1058
106. Lack EE, Neave C, Vawter GF: Hepatoblastoma. A clinical and pathologic study of 54 cases. Am J Surg Pathol 1982; 6:693–705
107. Black CT, Luck SR, Musemeche CA, Andrassy RJ. Aggressive excision of pulmonary metastases is warranted in the management of childhood hepatic tumors. J Pediatr Surg 1991;26:1082–1086
108. Filler RM, Ehrlich PF, Greenberg ML, Babyn PS. Preoperative chemotherapy in hepatoblastoma. Surgery 1991;110: 591–597
109. Guglielmi M, Perilongo G, Cecchetto G et al. Rationale and results of the International Society of Pediatric Oncology (SIOP) Italian pilot study on childhood hepatoma: surgical resection d'emblée or after primary chemotherapy. J Surg Oncol Suppl 1993;3(suppl):122–126
110. King DR, Ortega J, Campbell J et al. The surgical management of children with incompletely resected hepatic cancer is facilitated by intensive chemotherapy. J Pediatr Surg 1991;26:1074–1081
111. Pierro A, Langevin AM, Filler RM et al. Preoperative chemotherapy in "unresectable" hepatoblastoma. J Pediatr Surg 1989;24:24–29
112. Stringer MD, Hennayake S, Howard ER et al. Improved outcome for children with hepatoblastoma. Br J Surg 1995; 82:386–391
113. Tagge EP, Tagge DU, Reyes J et al. Resection, including transplantation, for hepatoblastoma and hepatocellular carcinoma: impact on survival. J Pediatr Surg 1992;27: 292–297
114. von Schweinitz D, Burger D, Bode U et al. Ergebnisse der Studie HB-89 bei der Behandlung maligner epithelialer Lebertumoren des Kindesalters und Konzept eines neuen Protokolls HB-94 (Results of the HB-89 Study in treatment of malignant epithelial liver tumors in childhood and concept of a new HB-94 protocol). Klin Padiatr 1994;206: 282–288
115. Wheatley JM, LaQuaglia MP. Management of hepatic epithelial malignancy in childhood and adolescence. Semin Surg Oncol 1993;9:532–540
116. Feusner JH, Kraillo MD, Hass JE et al. Treatment of pulmonary metastases of initial stage I hepatoblastoma in childhood. Report from the Children's Cancer Group. Cancer 1993;71:859–864
117. Passmore SJ, Noblett HR, Wisheart JD, Mott MG. Prolonged survival following multiple thoracotomies for metastatic hepatoblastoma. Med Pediatr Oncol 1995;24:58–60
118. Giacomantonio M, Ein SH, Mancer K, Stephens CA. Thirty years of experience with pediatric primary malignant tumors. J Pediatr Surg 1984;19:523–526
119. Yokomori K, Hori T, Asoh S et al. Complete disappearance of unresectable hepatoblastoma by continuous infusion therapy through hepatic artery. J Pediatr Surg 1991;26: 844–846
120. Black CT, Cangir A, Choroszy M, Andrassy RJ. Marked response to preoperative high-dose cis-platinum in children with unresectable hepatoblastoma. J Pediatr Surg 1991;26: 1070–1073
121. Weitman SD, Kato GJ, Barbosa JL, Kamen BA. Low-dose methotrexate therapy for hepatoblastoma. Cancer Chemother Pharmacol 1991;28:233–234
122. Iwatsuki S. Liver transplantation for hepatobiliary malignancy. Gann Monogr Cancer Res 1991;38:217–223
123. Koneru B, Cassavilla A, Bowman J et al. Liver transplantation for malignant tumors. Gastroenterol Clin North Am 1988;17:177–193
124. Koneru B, Flye MW, Busuttil RW et al. Liver transplantation for hepatoblastoma. The American experience. Ann Surg 1991;213:118–121
125. Habrand JL, Nehme D, Kalifa C et al. Is there a place for radiation therapy in the management of hepatoblastomas and hepatocellular carcinomas in children? Int J Radiat Oncol Biol Phys 1992;23:525–531
126. Haas JE, Muczynski KA, Krailo M et al. Histopathology and prognosis in childhood hepatoblastoma and hepatocarcinoma. Cancer 1989;64:1082–1095
127. Hata Y. The clinical features and prognosis of hepatoblastoma: follow-up studies done on pediatric tumors enrolled in the Japanese Pediatric Tumor Registry between 1971 and 1980. Part I. Jpn J Surg 1990;20:498–502
128. Ishak KG, Glunz PR. Hepatoblastoma and hepatocarcinoma in infancy and childhood. Report of 47 cases. Cancer 1967;20:396–422
129. Weinberg AG, Finegold MJ. Primary hepatic tumors of childhood. Hum Pathol 1983;14:512–537
130. Dehner LP, Manivel JC. Hepatoblastoma: an analysis of the relationship between morphologic subtypes and prognosis. Am J Pediatr Hematol Oncol 1988;10:301–307

18

CLINICAL AND PATHOLOGIC FEATURES OF CHOLANGIOCARCINOMA

YASUNI NAKANUMA
MASAHISO HOSO
TADASHI TERADA

Cholangiocarcinoma (CC), also known as intrahepatic cholangiocarcinoma or intrahepatic bile duct carcinoma, is a malignant tumor that develops from the epithelium of the intrahepatic biliary tree.[1,2] The reported frequency of CC among primary liver tumors ranges from none to 26.8%,[3] probably dependent on the precise definition of CC used, with an average of about 10%. CC occurs worldwide, but it is less common than hepatocellular carcinoma (HCC) among primary liver tumors. CC is reportedly endemic in some Asian countries.[4,5]

Most CCs develop in an otherwise normal liver, the factors preceding its development being unclear.[2,6,7] However, approximately 10% of all cases of CC are preceded by some endemic diseases such as hepatolithiasis and liver fluke infection or biliary tract diseases such as primary sclerosing cholangitis (PSC).[6,8] Dysplastic changes in the epithelial cells of the biliary lining are occasionally encountered in bile ducts remote from the primary or metastatic site(s) of CC in the liver or from the inflamed biliary tree of PSC or hepatolithiasis.[2,6] These lesions could be precursor lesions or borderline CC. In the majority of cases of CC, however, the etiology, pathogenesis, and early developmental features of CC remain unclear.

In this chapter, we describe the clinical and pathologic features of CC and the processes involved in its development and spread, focusing on the histopathologic and molecular bases for these features. Combined hepatocellular and cholangiocellular carcinoma and biliary cystadenocarcinoma are not described here.

ANATOMIC CLASSIFICATION AND GROSS FEATURES OF CHOLANGIOCARCINOMA

CC is classifiable into several anatomic, histopathologic, and etiologic types. CC arising at different anatomic locations in the intrahepatic biliary tree can differ in development, spread, and clinicolaboratory features. To facilitate the understanding of this classification, we briefly describe the anatomy of the intrahepatic biliary tree.[9]

The intrahepatic biliary tree, defined as the portion that is proximal to the hepatic duct confluence, consists of the right and left hepatic duct, the segmental ducts (the first major branches of each hepatic duct: left medial and lateral, right anterior and posterior), the area ducts (the first major branches of each segmental duct), and their finer branches (according to Healey and Schroy[10]).

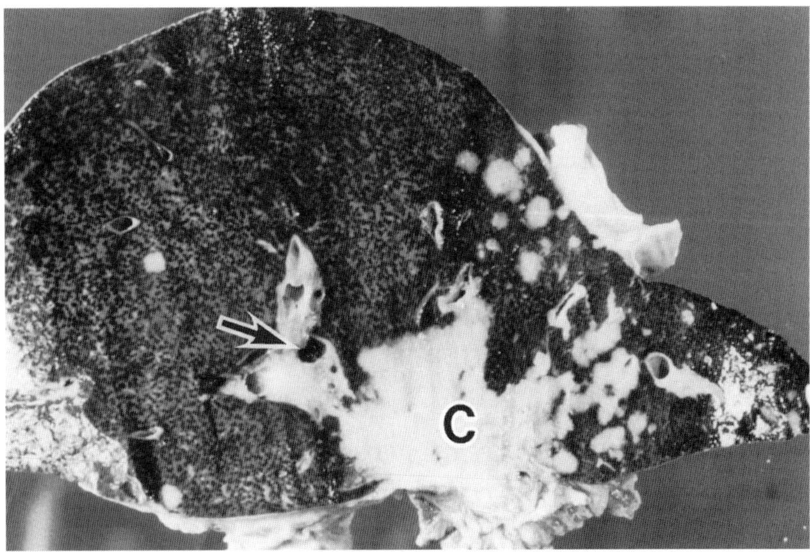

FIGURE 18-1. Cholangiocarcinoma (C) arising at the hepatic hilus (hilar type) forms a whitish mass infiltrating the surrounding liver. The remaining liver is cholestatic, and the bile ducts peripheral to the tumor are dilated (arrow). Autopsy case.

The hepatic, segmental, and area ducts, and their first branches, are collectively called *large intrahepatic bile ducts* here. These ducts are visible macroscopically, and their walls consist of a hypocellular, collagenous band lined by a single layer of columnar duct epithelium. The periductal tissue is a loose, fibrous connective tissue around the bile duct wall. Intramural and extramural peribiliary glands present along the large intrahepatic bile ducts.[11] The extramural glands (in the periductal tissue) can be further divided into serous and mucous glandular acini.

The finer branches of the large intrahepatic bile ducts are divided into septal bile ducts, interlobular bile ducts, and bile ductules, all of which are recognizable by microscopy. Bile ductules, tubular structures found in the peripheral zone of the portal tract, have an external diameter of less than 20 μm; interlobular bile ducts are in the peripheral zone of the portal tract and have an external diameter of 20 to 80 μm. This segment is subdivided into medium-sized (lumen: 40 to 80 μm) and smaller interlobular bile ducts (external diameter 20 to 40 μm). Septal bile ducts are larger than the interlobular bile ducts and are seen in the central or peripheral part of the portal tract.[12] Interlobular and septal bile ducts are not continuous with periportal hepatocytes.

Generally, CCs are defined as carcinomas developing from the epithelium of the intrahepatic biliary tree including the right and left hepatic ducts. CCs are classified as hilar or peripheral types according to their main location along the biliary tree.[2,13,14] Since the surgical approaches to carcinoma at the hepatic hilus outside the liver parenchyma and inside the liver are different, in surgery (particularly in Japan) CC is defined as carcinoma of the biliary tree peripheral to the bifurcation of the right or left hepatic ducts, which are usually located within the liver.[15,16]

In the hilar type, the tumor is located mainly at the hepatic hilus and is usually derived from the right or left hepatic duct or from the segmental duct or its direct finer branches and peribiliary glands around the hilum.[2,14,17] The tumor is not surrounded by a capsule; it can be either a whitish or gray nodule or mass (Fig. 18-1) or an ill-defined fibrous structure along the biliary tree. It is classically seen in a large green liver with collapsed gallbladder and nondilated extrahepatic bile duct. The tumor may be overlooked macroscopically; particularly when the hilar type is small and located at the bifurcation of the hepatic ducts with stenosis of the hilar ducts, the tumor shows unique clinicopathologic features and is termed *Klatskin type* CC.[18]

In the peripheral type, the tumor is located within the liver (by definition, however, excluding the hepatic hilus) and is usually derived from the area ducts and their more peripheral branches, including interlobular bile ducts and bile ductules. This type usually appears as solitary or multiple whitish nodules without a fibrous capsule. These tumors may be unnoticed until the nodules are large.

At an advanced stage, however, in a considerable number of CCs the distinction between peripheral and hilar types, and even the distinction between CC and extrahepatic bile duct carcinoma, is difficult to make or is subjective. In the beginning phases of CC in which the carcinoma is derived from the peribiliary glands, the lumen of the intrahepatic biliary tree is free of carcinomatous changes.[17]

In addition, CCs, particularly those resectable surgically, can be classified macroscopically according to their patterns of growth and invasion patterns.[16] Some cases show intraductal spread and growth in papillary, polypoid, or in situ spreading patterns (papillary or intraluminal type), while other cases show invasion mainly into the hepatic parenchyma, forming a gray or whitish nodule (nodular type). In the papillary or intraluminal type, the involved bile duct shows luminal dilatation. Other cases show preferential spread of carcinoma along the connective tissue of the portal tracts (which can be a periductal spreading, ductal spreading, or stenosing type), resembling sclerosing cholangitis. More advanced CCs may contain several combinations of these growth patterns (Fig. 18-1), and at autopsy some may consist of multiple coalescent nodules or massive tumors.

PRECURSOR LESIONS OF CHOLANGIOCARCINOMA

Although several hepatobiliary diseases are known to precede the development of CC, precursor lesions of the hepatobiliary system are not identifiable in a majority of cases. CC is not a common complication of nonbiliary cirrhosis, thus differing from HCC.

Chronic Cholangitis

Hepatolithiasis,[8,19] PSC, and liver fluke infestation are causes of chronic cholangitis known to be associated with CC. These diseases are found in particular areas of the world.

Hepatolithiasis, which frequently occurs in association with bacterial infection of the biliary tract and bile stasis, is a well-known precursor lesion of CC in the Far East, including Japan.[8] Approximately 10% of hepatolithiasis cases (either of calcium bilirubinate or cholesterol stones) are complicated by CC, and hepatolithiasis is encountered in about 10% of all CC cases in Japan.[8] Chronic proliferative cholangitis, characterized by the proliferation of intramural and extramural peribiliary glands and the proliferation of the epithelial lining, as well as fibrosis of the duct walls, is consistently seen in the stone-containing bile ducts and other nearby ducts.[20] Biliary epithelial dysplasia (or atypical biliary epithelial hyperplasia) is found in these duct lesions (Fig. 18-2). These biliary epithelial lesions variably express oncofetal proteins of the biliary tree, such as carcinoembryonic antigen (CEA), carbohydrate antigen (CA) 19-9, apomucin 1 (MUC 1), and DUPAN-11; the lesions may express gastrointestinal epithelial phenotypes such as histologic features of the pyloric glands or intestinal metaplasia.[21,22]

Biliary epithelial dysplasia near the hepatoliths (Fig. 18-2) shows a higher proliferative activity than in the normal bile ducts when examined by immunohistochemical staining for proliferating cell nuclear antigen (PCNA) or by histochemical staining for argyrophilic nuclear organizer regions (AgNOR).[23] Proliferating and dysplastic biliary epithelial cells and peribiliary glandular cells in hepatolithiasis express immunoreactive c-*met* (a receptor of hepatocyte growth factor [HGF]) and c-*erb*B-2. These cells also express gastric type apomucin (MUC 5/6), which is not present in the normal intrahepatic biliary tree (unpublished observation). Therefore, it seems likely that these proliferative and dysplastic biliary cells are already precancerous and may represent one facet of neoplastic transformation in hepatolithiasis.

PSC is also a well-known precursor lesion of CC, particularly in Western countries,[24,25] and about 10% of PSC is known to be associated with CC. Conversely, about 10% of CC is also known to be associated with PSC. Some cases of ulcerative colitis associated with CC may exhibit microscopic PSC or pericholangitis. Altaee et al.[13] reported that 28.6% of the hilar type and 7% of the peripheral type of CC were associated with ulcerative colitis with or without PSC. This association seems to have been increasing recently in light of the frequent discovery of clinically undetected small CCs in livers resected from PSC patients. Dysplastic and proliferative

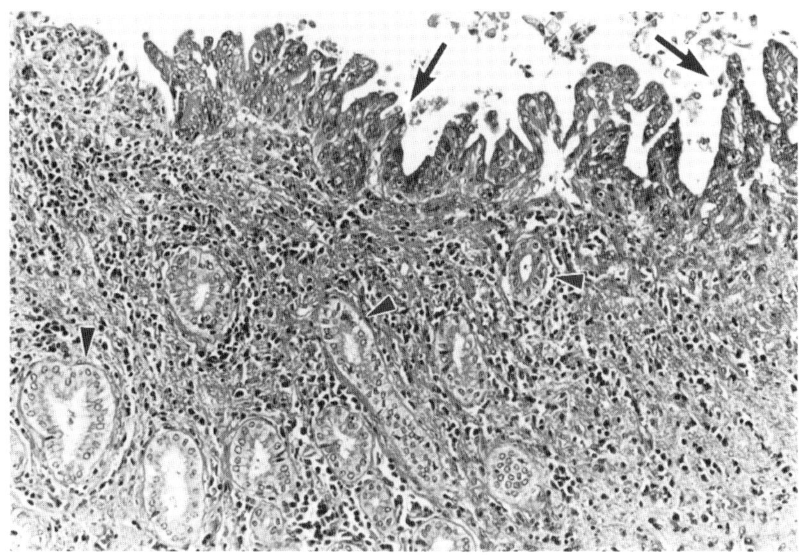

FIGURE 18-2. Biliary epithelial dysplasia (arrows) seen in stone-containing bile duct. Arrowheads show intramural glands that have proliferated in the ductal wall. Hepatolithiasis. (H&E.)

biliary epithelial cells seen in some cases of PSC around the CC or remote from the primary focus in PSC are also sometimes associated with CC. Martins et al.[26] recently reported that biliary epithelial dysplasia preceded the appearance of CC by at least 18 months.

The highest incidence of CC is seen in Southeast Asia, where infestation is common with liver fluke, either *Clonorchis sinensis* in Hong Kong and Canton (China) or *Opisthorchis viverrini* in Thailand.[4–6] The bile ducts harboring such flukes show marked adenomatous proliferation of intramural glands with variable cytologic atypia (prominent invagination of the biliary lining epithelium into the thickened bile duct walls).

Anomalies of the Biliary Tree

Cystic dilatation of the biliary tree, including Caroli's disease and congenital hepatic fibrosis with bacterial infection, or dilatation due to stones (or the resulting cholangitis), increases the risk of CC. Some cases of adenocarcinoma develop from the epithelial lining of polycystic or multicystic livers or from biliary microhamartomas (von Meyenburg's complex). CC may also arise from nonparasitic solitary cysts of the liver. Tumors associated with these congenital anomalies may be partly or wholly squamous.[1,7]

Thorotrast

Worldwide, deposition in the liver of Thorotrast, a radiological contrast medium, can lead to CC. Biliary epithelial dysplasia, which is encountered in non-neoplastic bile ducts, could also be a precursor lesion in this situation.

Some Metabolic Diseases

Genetic hemochromatosis is occasionally associated with CC.[13] In contrast to the association with HCC, heterozygosity of the α_1-antitrypsin type appears not to be associated with an increased risk of CC.[27]

Nonbiliary Cirrhosis

Nonbiliary cirrhosis such as viral or alcoholic cirrhoses is a precancerous condition of HCC. While most CCs arise from noncirrhotic livers, some do develop in nonbiliary cirrhosis.[28] Some cases of CC that arise in nonbiliary cirrhotic livers may correspond to an exuberant proliferation and spread of adenocarcinomatous elements of combined HCC and CC arising in the cirrhotic liver.[29] It is essential to search for HCC elements in such cases by preparing many specimens from several tumor nodules.

Three of 84 autopsy cases of CC studied in our department were associated with nonbiliary cirrhosis; other predisposing factors for CC had been excluded.[28] These three CCs were adenocarcinomas: one case each of adenocarcinoma resembling bile ductules without mucin, adenocarcinoma with broad areas of signet ring cell carcinoma, and adenocarcinoma with extensive sarcomatoid transformation.

Cirrhotic livers have been reported by Taguchi[30] to show a predisposition for the development of cholangiolocellular carcinoma and to have an increased α-fetoprotein level in sera.

Other Etiologies

Smoking, alcohol consumption, and the use of oral contraceptive steroids have been suggested as possible etiologic agents of CC.[13] One case of CC has been reported to be associated with familial polyposis coli and hereditary nonpolyposis colorectal carcinoma.[31] Another case of CC developing after primary biliary cirrhosis has been reported.[32]

HISTOPATHOLOGY AND HISTOLOGIC CLASSIFICATION OF CHOLANGIOCARCINOMA

The majority of CCs are adenocarcinomas with variable differentiation and desmoplasia ("common" CC), while some cases present with uncommon histologic features ("special" or "unusual" CC).

Common Type CC (Adenocarcinoma)

Many cases of CC, either of the hilar or peripheral type, are well-differentiated or moderately to poorly differentiated adenocarcinomas.[7,25] A tubular or glandular structure with a considerable amount of fibrous stroma is usually encountered in these CCs (Fig. 18-3), while occasional tumors are variably composed of small cordlike or compact configurations. In well-differentiated adenocarcinomas these tubules or glands are well formed and similar in size and shape, while the tubules or glands are pleomorphic in moderately to poorly differentiated adenocarcinoma (Fig. 18-4). Some cases consist mainly of a micropapillary configuration. CCs growing within the ductal lumen have a papillary configuration or an in situ pattern of spreading. More than one histologic pattern may be seen even in a single tumor nodule.

The cells of CCs vary in shape; they may be cuboidal, columnar, or polymorphic. The majority of CC cells have a pale or eosinophilic cytoplasm, sometimes vacuolated or finely granular. The production and secretion of acid and/or neutral mucus is demonstrated in one form or another (secreta in the tubular or glandular lumen, along the luminal surface, or in the cytoplasm of the carcinoma). This is a characteristic finding of CC dis-

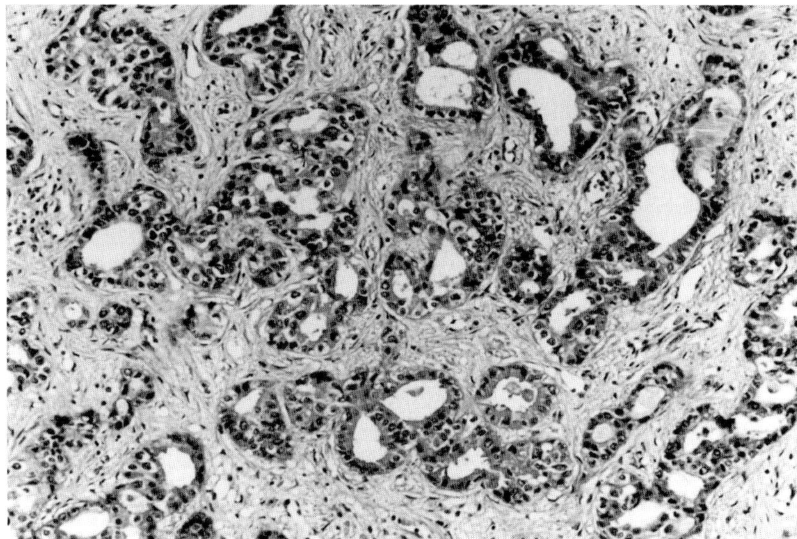

FIGURE 18-3. Well- to moderately differentiated adenocarcinoma forming variable sized tubules with desmoplasia. Peripheral cholangiocarcinoma. (H&E.)

tinct from HCC. A few cases are totally negative for mucin histochemistry.

Abundant fibrous stroma is also an important characteristic of CC. In some cases of CC, particularly the peripheral type, variably shaped tumor cells are widely separated, distorted, and atrophied by the development of a massive, poorly cellular, or hyaline stroma in the center. Some parts may be focally calcified. However, medullary growth with scanty fibrous stroma is seen in some cases, while in a few cases extensive deposition of hyaline fibrosis is seen ("sclerosing carcinoma of the liver").[33]

It is noteworthy that the peribiliary glands and their conduits within or adjacent to CC show variable proliferation and dilatation and their glandular epithelial cells show variable cellular atypia. These features make it difficult to differentiate these glandular elements from well-differentiated CC, especially in frozen sections.

Special (or Unusual) Types of CC

Some cases of the special or unusual types of CC may be derived from the common type, while others appear to arise independently. These include the subtypes adenosquamous and squamous cell carcinomas, mucinous carcinoma, sarcomatous type, signet ring cell carcinoma, cholangiocellular carcinoma, and biliary papillomas.

ADENOSQUAMOUS AND SQUAMOUS CELL CARCINOMA SUBTYPE

Squamous cell carcinoma elements are occasionally found in or admixed with adenocarcinoma in some CCs. This is usually found at an advanced stage of the disease, as indicated by the short survival time, large tumor size, aggressive modes of intrahepatic spread, and frequent metastasis.[10] Histologically, it ranges from focal to exten-

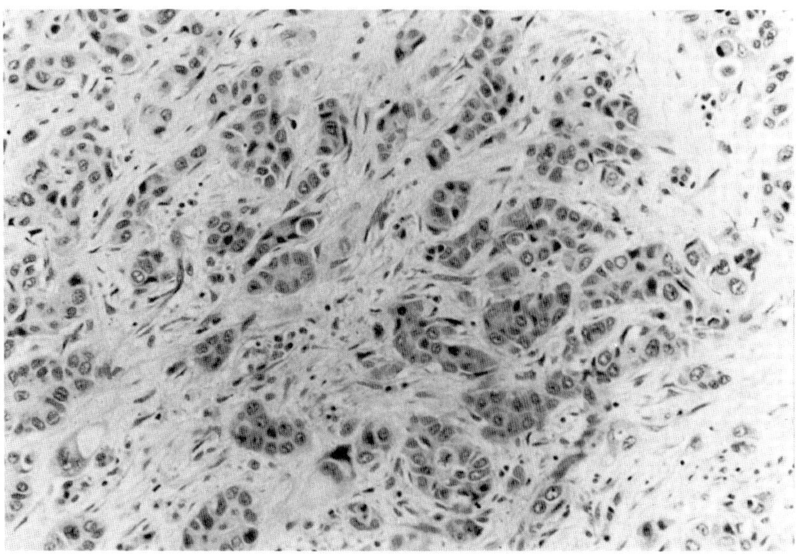

FIGURE 18-4. Poorly differentiated cholangiocarcinoma forming small cords or microacini with desmoplasia. Peripheral cholangiocarcinoma. (H&E.)

sive. Because of the intimate coexistence of adenocarcinomatous and squamous types in the primary and metastatic lesions, squamous elements could be regarded as being the result of metaplastic transformation of adenocarcinoma cells. It has also been suggested that anaplastic carcinoma cells or carcinomatous changes could sometimes be derived from squamous cell carcinomas.[34]

Wholly squamous cell carcinomas, some of which are derived from hepatic cysts and some from bile ducts, are rarely seen in the liver.[7] Squamous cell carcinomas and adenosquamous cell carcinomas complicating hepatolithiasis have been reported,[35] and these probably reflect wholly squamous metaplasia or partially squamous metaplasia of adenocarcinoma, respectively.

No instance of squamous metaplasia of non-neoplastic bile ducts has been demonstrated in cases of squamous cell carcinoma or adenosqamous cell carcinoma in CC; there is thus, at present, no supporting evidence for the possibility of squamous metaplasia of the bile duct epithelium and its subsequent malignant transformation.[36]

MUCINOUS CARCINOMA SUBTYPE

Mucin production is one of the characteristics of CC, but usually only small quantities are demonstrable. In the mucinous subtype, however, large quantities of intracellular and extracellular mucin are present (Fig. 18-5).[34,37] Coalescent mucin lakes are seen within the liver, where carcinoma cells float in the mucin and carcinoma cells with cuboidal or columnar epithelial cells cover the fibrous septa of this carcinoma.[36] Rapid progression and a fatal outcome are common. This subtype is different from mucinous cystadenocarcinoma and also from mucin-hypersecreting bile duct neoplasm (biliary papillomatosis or a mucin-secreting papilloma).[37]

SARCOMATOUS SUBTYPE

Sarcomatous features occur such as those of spindle cell sarcoma or malignant fibrous histiocytoma[34,38] or squamous carcinoma elements.[32] To make a diagnosis of sarcomatous CC, a definite area of adenocarcinomatous elements must be found. In contrast, primary sarcoma of the liver is quite rare.

SIGNET RING CELL CARCINOMA SUBTYPE

In a few CC, some parts are composed mainly of signet ring cells.[38] However, there have been no reports of cases of CC consisting entirely of signet ring cell carcinomas.

CHOLANGIOCELLULAR CARCINOMA SUBTYPE

The cells are arranged as narrow tubular structures resembling bile ductules or canals of Hering with frequent anastomosis to each other. Cirrhosis is common. However, there is as yet no consensus on the criteria for this subtype.

BILIARY PAPILLOMA AND PAPILLOMATOSIS SUBTYPE

These tumors (also called *mucin-hypersecreting biliary neoplasm*) can be solitary or multiple along the intrahepatic and/or extrahepatic biliary tree.[39] They are villous, have a slender fibrovascular core, and tend to secrete much mucin. They frequently obstruct the ductal lumen, causing obstructive jaundice. The tumor is benign, although in a few cases malignant transformation to CC occurs.[6,7]

COMMENTS

It is noteworthy that intrahepatic peribiliary glands can undergo papillary hyperplasia, atypical hyperplasia, and even carcinomatous transformation. Thus, these glands appear to constitute some of the cellular origins of CC.[17]

Neuroendocrine carcinoma, undifferentiated carcinoma, and rare varieties of CC also have been reported.[6,7]

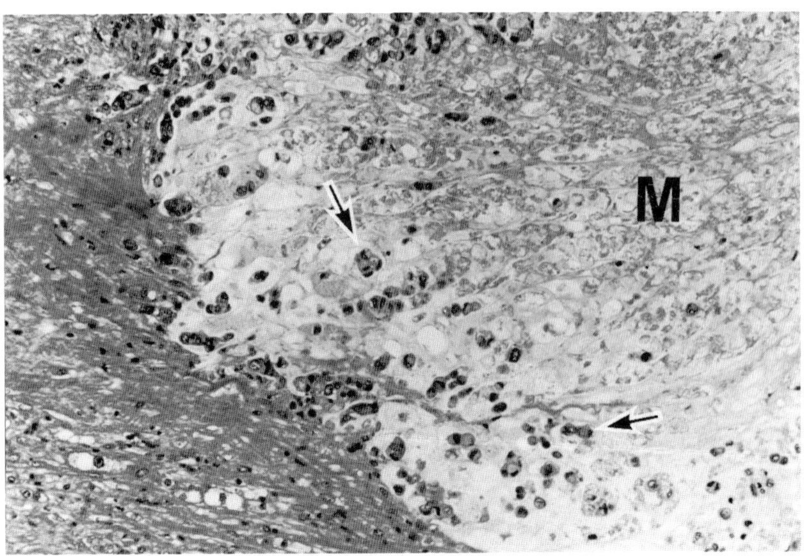

FIGURE 18-5. Mucinous cholangiocarcinoma. Mucin lakes (M) with floating carcinoma cells (arrows) are seen. (H&E.)

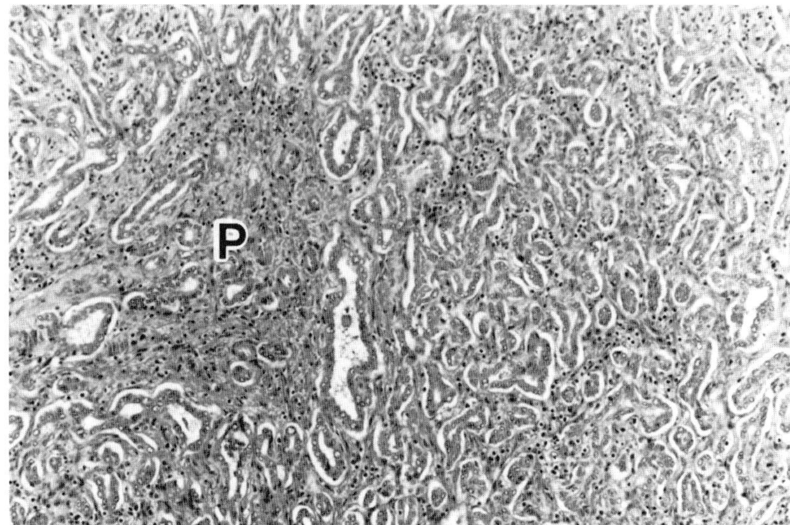

FIGURE 18-6. Very well-differentiated cholangiocarcinoma forming ductular structures. In the tumor, a well-formed portal tract (P) remains. Small peripheral cholangiocarcinoma. (H&E.)

Differential Diagnosis

Bile duct adenoma is a benign neoplasm[40] of the intrahepatic bile ducts and consists of small tubular structures with little or no lumen. Portal tracts are frequently seen within this single, subcapsular lesion.[40] The size is usually less than 1 cm in external diameter. Well-differentiated CC of small size can resemble bile duct adenoma (Fig. 18-6), and a size of more than 1 cm and the presence of nuclear atypia favor a diagnosis of CC.

von Meyenburg's complex is composed of variably dilated small ducts, some of which contain inspissated bile. This lesion is usually multiple and is associated with cystic disease. A few cases reported thus far suggest that this can undergo malignant transformation.[1,5,7]

Biliary epithelial dysplasia (atypical biliary epithelial hyperplasia) (Fig. 18-2) is occasionally encountered in the intrahepatic bile ducts of chronic cholangitis, remote from neoplastic nodules in livers with CC (without other hepatobiliary disease). These dysplastic cells reportedly stain positive for CEA.[8,26] Biliary epithelial dysplasia in large intrahepatic bile ducts in PSC or hepatolithiasis may lead to CC.

BIOLOGIC FEATURES, DEVELOPMENT, AND SPREAD OF CHOLANGIOCARCINOMA

Mutations of oncogenes and tumor-suppressor genes may be responsible for the development and progression of CC as in other tumors.[41] Tada et al.[42,43] reported mutations of the K-*ras* and N-*ras* genes in 45% and 6%, respectively, of CCs.[42,43] These mutations are more prevalent in hilar than in peripheral CC.[42,43] Ohta et al.[39] reported one case of biliary papillomatosis with mutations of the K-*ras* gene.

p53 is a tumor-suppressor gene located on the short arm of chromosome 17. Its coded product is a 53-kd nuclear phosphoprotein, called p53, with cell cycle-regulatory function and putative nuclear transcriptional activity. Mutations of the *p53* gene frequently occur in association with neoplastic transformation in human tissues. These mutations often stabilize the p53 protein, causing it to accumulate within the nucleus to the extent that its overexpression becomes detectable immunohistochemically. Our immunohistochemical study revealed that about 22% of CCs in Japan have *p53* mutations.[44] The reported incidence of *p53* mutation is low in CCs in the United States.[45]

The overexpression of transforming growth factor-α is infrequent in CC, whereas it is frequent in HCC. Other growth factors or oncogene products are also expressed in CC. In our recent study, CCs occasionally contained c-*met* and c-*erb*B-2 oncogene products (unpublished observations). These growth factors and oncogene products may be involved in the proliferation of CC carcinoma cells via autocrine or paracrine mechanisms.[46] C-*met* and c-*erb*B-2 are also expressed in dysplastic and proliferative epithelial cells of the intrahepatic bile ducts in patients with hepatolithiasis. Interestingly, c-*met* and c-*erb*B-2 also are present in primitive biliary cells of the fetal liver. These findings strongly suggest that the HGF/c-*met* system operates in CC and that the c-*erb*B-2 genes may be common to CC cells and to primitive biliary cells of the fetus.

Somatostatin (SS) receptors have been described in various neuroendocrine and epithelial malignancies that arise in the target tissues of SS, such as the anterior pituitary, the endocrine and exocrine pancreas, and the gastrointestinal tract.[47] The normal biliary tract is a target tissue (it has SS-containing cells),[48] and SS receptors have been identified in rodent biliary epithelial cells.[49] Tan et al.[48] recently reported that messenger RNA of

SS receptors is expressed in human CC. SS inhibits the proliferation of CC cells both in vitro and in vivo so that the loss of SS receptors in CC may be related to the aggressive proliferation and spread of CC.

CC cells produce and secrete variable quantities and types of mucin, biliary epithelial cytokeratin (CK9 and CK19), epithelial membrane antigen, CEA, and apomucin type I.[1,21] In addition, CC cells express the genes for pancreatic exocrine enzymes such as pancreatic amylase, lipase, and trypsinogen, as well as blood group antigens such as the ABO group and CA 19-9.[50] In contrast, α-fetoprotein is not detectable in CC cells. Although these phenotypic markers are useful in the differentiation of CC from HCC, at present there are no markers that distinguish CC from metastatic adenocarcinoma, particularly when arising in the extrahepatic bile duct or pancreas.

Gastric and intestine-related mucins and apomucins (MUC 2 and MUC 5/6) are frequently expressed in CC and their precursor lesions (unpublished observations). Markers of gastrointestinal epithelial cells are also expressed in pancreatic duct cancer.[51]

The extracellular matrix around CC consists of tenascin and type IV collagen, which are present in the sinusoids of normal adult livers and are expressed in the stroma of CCs.[49] Their expression may be the result of malignant transformation of intrahepatic biliary epithelial cells. Tenascin in the stroma may stimulate the growth of CC. Tenascin, which is present in the stroma of many cancers, contains epidermal growth factor-like repeats,[52] and may induce tumor growth and progression by an autocrine mechanism.[53] Its expression may have prognostic value. These extracellular matrix components play a central role in the structural support, proliferation, migration, and differentiation of CC. Laminin, another extracellular matrix component, has not yet been identified in the stroma of CC.[54]

α-Smooth muscle actin (α-SMA)-positive stromal cells are frequently noted in CC stroma and in the nontumoral sinusoids around CCs.[55] The α-SMA-positive cells in the sinusoids are activated Ito cells (myofibroblasts). It seems likely that Ito cells proliferate to become α-SMA-positive stromal cells (myofibroblasts) that are incorporated into the stroma of CC. These cells may contribute to fibrosis in CC stroma by secreting extracellular matrix proteins.

Noninvasive Cholangiocarcinoma

CCs that are located mainly within the lumens of the large intrahepatic bile ducts represent the noninvasive phase of CC; they are biliary epithelial cells with malignant features that have spread along the lumen in either a spreading or a papillary pattern. However, it is difficult to differentiate the in situ spread of CC from severe biliary epithelial dysplasia. Carcinoma cells, as well as dysplastic biliary epithelial cells, form fronts that are located against nonmalignant or dysplastic epithelial cells in the lining biliary epithelial layer and also spread in the peribiliary glands and their conduits around the large intrahepatic bile duct. Cases of biliary epithelial dysplasia with microinvasion actually should be diagnosed as CC.

In the noninvasive phase of CC, carcinoma cells show higher proliferative activity than do normal and hyperplastic biliary cells, as determined by PCNA immunostaining and AgNOR histochemistry.[23] Noninvasive CC cells also show immunophenotypic alterations, such as positive staining with CEA and increased staining with CA 19-9 and DUPAN-2. Of particular interest, noninvasive CCs express immunoreactive c-*met* and c-*erb*B-2, and this may represent activation of these oncogenes (unpublished data). In addition, many noninvasive CCs express pancreatic digestive enzymes, such as pancreatic α-amylase, trypsinogen, chymotrypsinogen, and pancreatic lipase. These enzymes may play a role in CC invasion by degrading extracellular matrix proteins.

Invasive Cholangiocarcinoma

Many CCs eventually invade the surrounding tissues of the liver, including the peribiliary glands. CC cells invade the ductal wall and its surrounding connective tissue, finally reaching the hepatic parenchyma and/or the portal tracts. These cells destroy the basement membrane of the bile ducts, invade the extracellular matrix, invade the vessels, and form metastatic foci both within and outside the liver. CC cells also may invade the neural and perineural tissue. Metastases may be found preferentially at lymph nodes at the hepatic hilus. The detection of c-*met*/HGF in CC cells appears to indicate that HGF stimulates c-*met*-positive CC cells via an autocrine or paracrine mechanism during CC invasion. c-*erb*B-2 may be related to the malignant grade and invasive characteristics of the invasive CC.

Proteolytic enzymes, called matrix proteinases, degrade the extracellular matrix proteins and are thus involved in the invasion of cancer cells.[56] Matrix proteinases include metalloproteinases (MMP), serine proteinases, cysteine proteinases, and aspartic proteinases. One of these, cathepsin B, a cysteine proteinase, is a lysosomal enzyme capable of catalyzing extracellular matrix proteins. Recently, tumor-associated trypsinogen, a serine proteinase, has been shown to degrade extracellular matrix proteins. We have found recently that cathepsin B and pancreatic trypsinogen/trypsin are expressed on CC, and they may be involved in the invasion and metastasis of CC.[46] In addition, we found that CCs frequently express immunoreactive MMP (MMP-1, MMP-2, MMP-3, and MMP-9) and tissue inhibitors of MMP (TIMP-1 and TIMP-2) (unpublished data). MMP activators, such as cathepsin B and chymotrypsin, are also expressed in CC cells. Therefore, it seems very likely that MMPs play an important role in CC invasion. This MMP-mediated CC invasion appears to be regulated by TIMP and MMP activator. HCCs do not express MMP and TIMP, and normal biliary cells rarely express MMP and TIMP.

A high recurrence rate of CCs has been reported after orthotopic liver transplantation of both the peripheral and hilar types, even when the CCs were very small or appeared to be at the stage of intraductal spread.[57] These findings strongly suggest that invasion and even micrometastases of CCs are present from the early stages.

CLINICAL FEATURES OF CHOLANGIOCARCINOMA AND DIAGNOSTIC APPROACHES

Compared to HCC, CCs occur infrequently and are usually not associated with cirrhosis. CCs are usually fatal because of the absence of methods for early detection and the lack of effective therapy. It is difficult to select those patients who may be predisposed to develop CCs. To date, subgroup analysis has failed to identify reliable risk factors that distinguish patients in whom CC develops from those in whom it does not.

The symptoms associated with CC are jaundice, weight loss, hepatomegaly, abdominal pain, and pruritus. The clinical features of CC appear to differ according to the location of the tumor along the intrahepatic biliary tree, whether the CC is the hilar or the peripheral type.[7,14] The hilar type tends to present with a slow, relentless, obstructive jaundice or cholangitis, while the peripheral type presents with abdominal pain and weight loss. The development of CCs in patients with PSC or hepatolithiasis is typically associated with rapid clinical deterioration with a distinctively worsened prognosis.

In Japan and the United States, the average age at clinical detection of CC is 60 to 65 years[30,45]; the age of clinical detection of the hilar type is a little younger than that of the peripheral type.[30] In the United Kingdom, the average age at clinical detection of CC is 48 ± 11 years for the peripheral type and 52 ± 12.5 years for the hilar type.[13]

Patients with CC complicated with PSC and/or ulcerative colitis are younger than those without those complications. In Japan and the United Kingdom, both sexes are affected equally, although males are more commonly affected by the hilar type than females. At present, as the number of elderly people in the population is increasing, it is conceivable that the incidence of CC will gradually increase.

Occult CCs are sometimes found in explanted or surgically resected livers. For example, Marsh et al.[57] reported that previously unrecognized CC was found in the explanted livers in 5 of 55 patients with PSC at the University of Pittsburgh who underwent orthotopic liver transplantation.

In addition to elevation of biliary enzymes and serum bilirubin and elevation of CEA, CA 19-9 (the latter being sialosylfucosyl-lactotetraose, corresponding to sialylated blood group antigen Lewis) is increased in 40% to 80% of patients with CC. The measurement of serum CA 19-9 is a particularly promising test for detecting CC in patients with PSC[58] and also for detecting patients predisposed to the development of CC.

Several imaging modalities are available for the detection of CC. CC is usually visible by ultrasound sonography (US), magnetic resonance imaging (MRI), and computed tomography (CT) as a space-occupying lesion in the liver. In addition, secondary hepatic changes due to CC, such as dilatation of the distal biliary tree and portal veins or regional atrophy distal to the CC, are also detectable by these methods. In some cases, only these secondary changes are detectable. In general, the primary tumor mass or nodule is seen with ultrasound in 20% of CC patients and with CT in 40%.[59] MRI may be more sensitive in detecting such masses or nodules. The combination of primary mass and biliary dilatation may be more suggestive of CC. However, in most cases, a precise diagnosis of CC cannot be made with these methods.

Endoscopic retrograde cholangiography, arteriography, and portography are also available to detect and characterize CC, particularly that arising in the large intrahepatic bile ducts including the hepatic hilus. Bile ducts, portal veins, and hepatic arteries show stenosis, occlusion, or replacement by CC using these methods. CC is usually hypovascular, and encasement of arteries around CC is also found. However, these invasive tests cannot be used for routine screening. In addition, the usefulness of these approaches, particularly cholangiography, is limited in patients with chronic cholangitis or bile duct anomalies. CC complicating PSC or hepatolithiasis is often difficult to diagnose because of the preexisting distortion of the biliary tree and the portal and arterial vessels.

CCs can be detected by ordinary nuclear techniques of biliary scintigraphy, using ^{99m}Tc-PMT. In addition, Tan et al.[48] reported that CCs have a receptor for SS, and, using gamma camera imaging with an ^{111}In-SS analog, they localized histologically proven CCs, suggesting that SS analogs may be useful in the diagnosis of biliary tract malignancies.

The combination of cytologic study of the biliary tree with cholangiography may be another useful approach in the diagnosis of CC.[26] The sensitivity of this method varies from as low as 18% when exfoliative cytology is employed to 70% for brush cytology alone or combined brush/exfoliative cytology.[26] The specificity of the diagnosis of CC is reported to be very high for these cytologic approaches.

The differential diagnosis of space-occupying lesions

in the liver should include HCC, metastatic liver cancers, and inflammatory pseudotumors that must be distinguished from CC. The precise differentiation of CC from metastatic carcinoma, particularly that arising from the extrahepatic biliary tree or pancreas, is difficult.

In the past, CC and PSC were considered to be distinct entities and, indeed, the diagnosis of CC specifically excluded PSC. PSC has now been found to be not infrequently complicated by CC. Therefore, the differentiation of CC with infiltration along the portal tract from PSC, as well as the detection of CC inpatients with PSC or hepatolithiasis, is now an important but usually difficult task.

THERAPY

Improvements in surgical techniques have benefited CC patients, although otherwise little progress has been made in recent years. For example, Altaee et al.[13] recently reported that tumor recurrence was frequent in patients who underwent surgical resection or orthotopic liver transplantation; none of the patients who underwent chemotherapy or radiation therapy showed any response. However, CC of the hilar type, especially the Klatskin type, have received considerable attention since the introduction of interventional radiologic techniques aimed at establishing percutaneous or enteric biliary drainage with or without additional local radiation therapy; more aggressive management may be warranted in this type of CC.[13]

Palliative chemotherapy for CC comprises a systemic regimen of 5-fluorouracil, doxorubicin, and mitomycin C, although few good responses have been reported.[13] Several biologically active substances, such as SS and its analogs, have been shown experimentally to inhibit the proliferation of CC both in vivo and in vitro, but they have not yet been tried clinically to the best of our knowledge. Preventative therapy should also be considered; when biliary epithelial dysplasia of the affected bile ducts is found in patients with hepatolithiasis or PSC, surgical resection or orthotopic liver transplantation should be considered, even though the response rate with these therapies also is not satisfactory.

REFERENCES

1. Ishak KG, Anthony PP, Sobin LH. Histological Typing of Tumours of the Liver. 2nd Ed. WHO Series. Springer-Verlag, Berlin, 1994
2. Nakanuma Y, Kida T, Minato H et al. Pathology of cholangiocellular carcinoma. In Tobe T et al. (eds): Primary Liver Cancer in Japan. Springer-Verlag, Tokyo, 1992, pp. 39–50
3. Mizumoto R, Kawarada Y. Diagnosis and treatment of cholangiocarcinoma and cystic adenocarcinoma of the liver. In Okuda K, Ishak K (eds): Neoplasms of the Liver. Springer-Verlag, Tokyo, 1988, pp. 381–396
4. Kurathong S, Lerdverasirikul P, Wongpaitoon V et al. *Opisthorchis viverrini* infection and cholangiocarcinoma. Gastroenterology 1985;89:151–156
5. Belamaric J. Intrahepatic bile duct carcinoma and C. *sinensis* infection in Hong Kong. Cancer 1973;31:468–473
6. Anthony PP. Tumours and tumour-like lesions of the liver and biliary tract. In MacSween RNM et al. (eds): Pathology of the Liver. 3rd Ed. Churchill Livingstone, Edinburgh, 1994, pp. 635–711
7. Craig R, Peters RL, Edmonson AE. Tumors of the Liver and Intrahepatic Bile Duct. Atlas of Tumor Pathology. Second Series, fascicle 26, AFIP, Washington, DC, 1988
8. Nakanuma Y, Terada T, Tanaka Y et al. Are hepatolithiasis and cholangiocarcinoma aetiologically related? A morphologic study of 12 cases of hepatolithiasis associated with cholangiocarcinoma. Virchows Arch Pathol Anat Histol 1985; 406:45–58
9. Nakanuma Y, Hoso M, Terada T et al. Microstructure and development of the normal and pathologic biliary tract in humans, including blood supply. MRT, 1995 (in press)
10. Healey JE, Schroy PC. Anatomy of the biliary ducts within the human liver. Arch Surg 1953;66:599–616
11. Terada T, Nakanuma Y, Ohta G. Glandular elements around the intrahepatic bile ducts in man: their morphology and distribution in normal livers. Liver 1987;7:1–8
12. Nakanuma Y, Ohta G. Histometric and serial section observations of the intrahepatic bile ducts in primary biliary cirrhosis. Gastroenterology 1979;76:1326–1332
13. Altaee MY, Johnson PJ, Farrant JM et al. Etiologic and clinical characteristics of peripheral and hilar cholangiocarcinoma. Cancer 1991;68:2051–2055
14. Okuda K, Kubo Y, Okazaki N et al. Clinical aspects of intrahepatic bile duct carcinoma including hilar carcinoma. A study of 57 autopsy-proven cases. Cancer 1977;39:232–246
15. Hyone PM, Kernohan JW. Primary carcinoma of the liver: a study of 31 cases. Arch Intern Med 1947;79:532–554
16. Liver Cancer Study Group. The General Rules for the Clinical and Pathological Study of Primary Liver Cancer. 3rd Ed. (in Japanese.) Kanehara Publishers, Tokyo, 1992
17. Terada T, Nakanuma Y. Pathological observations of intrahepatic peribiliary glands in 1000 consecutive autopsy livers. II. A possible source of cholangiocarcinoma. Hepatology 1990;12:92–97
18. Klatskin G. Adenocarcinoma of the hepatic duct at its bifurcation within the porta hepatis. Am J Med 1965;38:241–256
19. Nakanuma Y, Yamaguchi K, Ohta G et al. Pathologic features of hepatolithiasis in Japan. Hum Pathol 1988;19: 1181–1186
20. Terada T, Nakanuma Y. Morphologic examination of intrahepatic bile ducts in hepatolithiasis. Virchow Archiv Pathol Anat Histol 1988;413:167–176
21. Sasaki M, Nakanuma Y, Terada T et al. Biliary epithelial expression of MUC1, MUC2, MUC3 and MUC5/6 apomuc-

ins during intrahepatic bile duct development and maturation. An immunohistochemical study. Am J Pathol 1995; 147:574–579

22. Sasaki M, Nakanuma Y. Expression of mucin core protein of mammary type in primary liver cancer. Hepatology 1994; 20:1192–1197
23. Terada T, Nakanuma Y. Cell kinetics analyses and expression of carcinoembryonic antigen, carbohydrate antigen 19-9 and DU-PAN-2 in hyperplastic, pre-neoplastic and neoplastic lesions of intrahepatic bile ducts in livers with hepatoliths. Virchow Arch A Pathol Anat Histol 1992;420: 327–335
24. Wee A, Ludwig J, Coffey RJ et al. Hepatobiliary carcinoma associated with primary sclerosing cholangitis and chronic ulcerative colitis. Hum Pathol 1985;16:719–726
25. Haworth AC, Manely PN, Groll A et al. Bile duct carcinoma and biliary tract dysplasia in chronic ulcerative colitis. Arch Pathol Lab Med 1989;113:434–436
26. Martins EBG, Fleming KA, Garrido MC et al. Superficial thrombophlebitis, dysplasia and cholangiocarcinoma in primary sclerosing cholangitis. Gastroentereology 1994;107: 537–542
27. Berkowitz M, Gavalier JS, Keller RH et al. Lack of increased heterozygous alpha-1-antitrypsin deficiency phenotypes among patients with hepatocellular carcinoma and bile duct carcinoma. Hepatology 1992;15:407–410
28. Terada T, Kida T, Nakanuma Y et al. Intrahepatic cholangiocarcinoma associated with nonbiliary cirrhosis. A clinicopathologic study. J Clin Gastroenterol 1994;18:335–342
29. Harada K, Terada T, Nakanuma Y et al. A case of small combined hepatocellular and cholangiocellular carcinoma arising in a nodule of atypical adenomatous hyperplasia of the liver. Am J Gastroenterol 1993;88:1968–1969
30. Taguchi J. Clinicopathologic study on 26 resected cases of cholangiocarcinoma (in Japanese.) Kanzo 1994;35:737–744
31. Mecklin JP, Jarvinen HJ, Vivolaninen M. The association between cholangiocarcinoma and hereditary nonpolyposis colorectal carcinoma. Cancer 1992;69:1112–1114
32. Ryorin H, Ohta H, Terada T et al. Cholangiocarcinoma associated with primary biliary cirrhosis [in Japanese]. Acta Hepatol Jpn 1995;36:175(abstr)
33. Omata M, Peters RL, Tatter D. Sclerosing hepatic carcinoma: relation to hypercalcemia. Liver 1981;1:33–40
34. Sasaki M, Nakanuma Y, Nagai Y et al. Intrahepatic cholangiocarcinoma with sarcomatous transformation: an autopsy case. J Clin Gastroenterol 1991;13:220–225
35. Song E, Kew MC, Grieve T et al. Primary squamous cell carcinoma of the liver occurring in association with hepatolithiasis. Cancer 1984;53:542–546
36. Nakajima T, Kondo Y. A clinicopathologic study of intrahepatic cholangiocarcinoma containing a component of squamous cell carcinoma. Cancer 1990;65:1401–1404
37. Motoo Y, Sawabu N, Minamoto T et al. Rapidly growing mucinous cholangiocarcinoma. Intern Med 1993;32: 116–121
38. Nakajima T, Tajima Y, Sugano I et al. Intrahepatic cholangiocarcinoma with sarcomatous change. Cancer 1993;72: 1872–1877
39. Ohta H, Yamaguchi Y, Yamakawa O et al. Biliary papillomatosis with the point mutation of *K-ras* gene arising in congenital choledochal cyst. Gastroenterology 1993;105: 1209–1212
40. Govindarajan S, Peters RL. The bile duct adenoma. A lesion distinct from Meyenburg complex. Arch Pathol Lab Med 1984;108:922–924
41. Vogelstein B, Fearon ER, Hamilton SR et al. Genetic alterations during colorectal-tumor development. N Engl J Med 1988;319:525–532
42. Tada M, Omata M, Ohto M. Analysis of *ras* gene mutations in human hepatic malignant tumors by polymerase chain reaction and direct sequencing. Cancer Res 1990;50: 1121–1124
43. Tada M, Omata M, Ohto M. High incidence of *ras* gene mutation in intrahepatic cholangiocarcinoma. Cancer 1992; 69:1115–1118
44. Terada T, Shimizu K, Izumi R et al. p53 expression in formalin-fixed, paraffin-embedded archival specimens of intrahepatic cholangiocarcinoma: retrieval of p53 antigenicity by microwave oven heating of tissue sections. Mod Pathol 1994; 7:249–252
45. Choi SW, Hytiroglou P, Geller SA et al. The expression of p53 antigen in primary malignant epithelial tumors of the liver: an immunohistochemical study. Liver 1993;13: 172–176
46. Terada T, Ohta T, Minato H et al. Expression of pancreatic trypsinogen/trypsin and cathepsin B in human cholangiocarcinomas and hepatocellular carcinomas. Hum Pathol 1995; 26:746–752
47. Kurumaya H, Nakanuma Y, Ohta G. Endocrine cells in intrahepatic biliary tree in normal livers and hepatolithiasis. Arch Patol Lab Med 1989;113:143–147
48. Tan CK, Podila PV, Taylor GA et al. Human cholangiocarcinomas express somatostatin receptors and respond to somatostatin with growth inhibition. Gastroenterology 1995; 108:1908–1916
49. Pham LD, Alpini G, LaRusso NF. Bile duct ligation upregulates the message for the somatostatin receptor in intrahepatic bile duct epithelial cells: implications for somatostatin-induced ductular cholestasis. Gastroenterology 1984;1044: A972(abstr)
50. Terada T, Nakanuma Y. Pancreatic lipase is a useful phenotypic marker of intrahepatic large and septal bile ducts, peribiliary glands and their malignant counterparts. Mod Pathol 1993;6:419–426
51. Sessa F, Bonato M, Frigerio B et al. Ductal cancers of the pancreas frequently express markers of gastrointestinal epithelial cell. Gastroenterology 1990;98:1655–1665
52. Jones FS, Burgoon MP, Hoffman S et al. cDNA clone for cytotactin contains squences similar to epidermal growth factor-like repeats and segments of fibronectin and fibrinogen. Proc Natl Acad Sci USA 1988;85:2186–2190
53. Engel M. EGF-like domains in extracellular matrix proteins: localized signals for growth and differentiation? FEBS Lett 1989;251:1–7
54. Terada T, Nakanuma Y. Expression of tenascin, type IV collagen and laminin during human intrahepatic bile duct de-

velopment and in intrahepatic cholangiocarcinoma. Histopathology 1994;25:143–150

55. Terada T, Makimoto Y, Terayama H et al. Alpha-smooth muscle actin-positive stromal cells in cholangiocarcinomas, hepatocellular carcinomas and metastatic liver carcinomas. J Hepatol, 1996;29:37–43
56. Mignatti P, Rifkin DB. Biology and biochemistry of proteinases in tumor invasion. Physiol Rev 1993;73:161–195
57. Marsh JW, Iwatsuki S, Makowka L et al. Orthotopic liver transplantation for primary sclerosing cholangitis. Ann Surg 1988;207:21–25
58. Nichols JC, Gores GJ, LaRusso NF et al. Predicting cholangiocarcinoma in patients with primary sclerosing cholangitis: an analysis of the serological marker CA1 19-9. Mayo Clin Proc 1993;68:874–879
59. Dachman AH. Primary biliary neoplasm. In Friedman AC, Dachman AH (eds): Radiology of the Liver, Biliary Tract and Pancreas. Mosby, St. Louis, 1994, pp. 611–620

19

MALIGNANT MESENCHYMAL TUMORS AND SOME OTHER NONHEPATOCELLULAR TUMORS OF THE LIVER

KAMAL G. ISHAK

Malignant mesenchymal tumors of the liver are much rarer than epithelial neoplasms of the liver, but figures regarding their incidence are quite limited. Of 405 primary malignant tumors of the liver collected by Edmondson and Peters,[1] 1.2% were sarcomas. A survey of death certificates, a notoriously unreliable method of disease surveillance, disclosed 205 hepatic sarcomas in the United States from 1966 to 1973, including angiosarcoma (36%), leiomyosarcoma (12%), fibrosarcoma (7%), and unspecified sarcomas (44%).[2]

Primary sarcoma of the liver usually develops in a noncirrhotic liver, although fibrosis may be present in cases of angiosarcoma related to prior exposure to Thorotrast or vinyl chloride. Sarcoma and carcinoma occurring simultaneously in a cirrhotic liver are exceptionally rare.[3] The diagnosis should be made with caution since hepatocellular carcinoma can show a spindle cell (pseudosarcomatous) pattern. Carcinosarcomas (admixtures of carcinoma, either hepatocellular or cholangiocellular, and various sarcomatous elements) also are rare.

The clinical course of some sarcomas, such as epithelioid hemangioendothelioma, is unpredictable, but in general they are rapidly growing and uniformly fatal. Therapy remains unsatisfactory, although some progress has been made on the treatment of the childhood sarcomas, such as undifferentiated sarcoma and embryonal rhabdomyosarcoma. Etiologic factors for sarcomas are unknown, except for angiosarcoma, which has been linked to Thorotrast, vinyl chloride, and arsenic exposure.

Malignant mesenchymal tumors include epithelioid hemangioendothelioma, angiosarcoma, Kaposi's sarcoma, fibrosarcoma, malignant fibrous histiocytoma, leiomyosarcoma, embryonal rhabdomyosarcoma, and embryonal (undifferentiated) sarcoma. (Primary lymphomas of the liver and metastases are also briefly covered.)

EPITHELIOID HEMANGIOENDOTHELIOMA

Epithelioid hemangioendothelioma involves the liver[4–20] as well as other organs such as soft tissue and bone.[21–24] Etiologic factors in hepatic hemangioendothelioma are unknown. Some patients had used oral contraceptives,[7,18] and one patient had had prior exposure to vinyl chloride.[25] The average age at presentation is approximately 50 years, but ranges from the second to the eighth decade. Two-thirds of affected patients are women. Symptoms and signs include weakness, anorexia, nausea, episodic vomiting, upper abdominal pain, jaundice, and hepatosplenomegaly.[4] An acute abdomen from rupture of the tumor with hemoperitoneum,[4] a Budd-Chiari-like syndrome,[5] or liver failure[6] are less common presentations.

Serum alkaline phosphatase activity is elevated in about two-thirds of patients.[4] Occasional cases[4,13] have elevated serum factor VIII levels. Hepatic scintigraphy generally reveals "filling defects" throughout the liver. Calcification may be evident in plain films of the abdomen. In computed tomography (CT), tumor nodules have low attenuation, are peripherally based, and are associated with capsular retraction or flattening.[8] Contrast-enhanced CT scans show peripheral enhancement of alternating attenuation values correlating with a hyperemic rim seen on pathologic examination.[14] In one CT study, initially nodular lesions later became diffuse.[15] Ultrasound examination reveals predominantly hypoechoic lesions.[14,15] On magnetic resonance, the tumor signal is low on T_1-weighted and high on T_2-weighted images, with a low signal halo present around the nodules.[14] However, a definitive diagnosis of epithelioid hemangioendothelioma can only be established by liver biopsy.

Gross Features

Epithelioid hemangioendothelioma usually consists of multiple lesions involving the entire liver,[4] but they were described as mostly peripheral in one study.[14] They vary from a few millimeters to several centimeters in diameter (Fig. 19-1). The neoplastic tissue is tan to white in color and firm in consistency, and sometimes a gritty sensation is noted when the specimen is sectioned. The margins of the lesions may be hyperemic. The tumor generally does not arise on a background of chronic liver disease, with the exception of two reported cases that occurred in cirrhotic livers.[4,16] Some cases are associated with nodular regenerative hyperplasia.[4]

FIGURE 19-1. Epithelioid hemangioendothelioma. Section of a solitary tumor (8 cm in diameter) reveals ill-defined margins and a variegated surface.

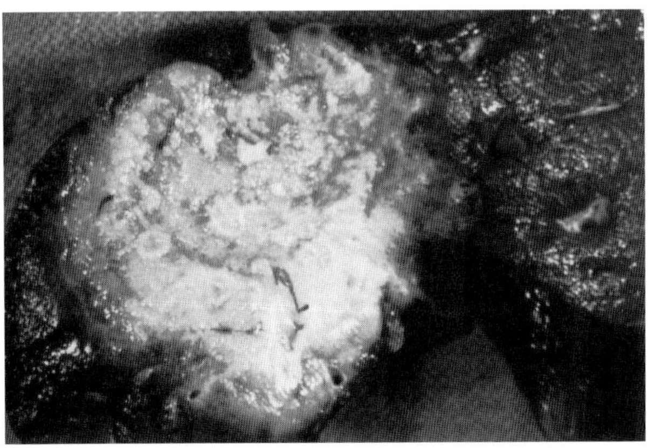

Microscopic Features

The tumor nodules are ill-defined and often involve multiple contiguous acini. In actively proliferating lesions the acinar landmarks, such as terminal hepatic venules (THV) and portal areas, can be recognized despite extensive infiltration by the tumor. The tumor cells grow along pre-existing sinusoids, THV, and portal vein branches and often invade Glisson's capsule (Fig. 19-2). Growth within the acini is associated with gradual atrophy and eventual disappearance of liver cell plates (Fig. 19-2). Intravenous growth may be in the form of a solid plug or a polypoid or tuft-like projection. Neoplastic cells are either "dendritic," with spindle or irregular shapes and multiple interdigitating processes, or "epithelioid," with a more rounded shape and abundant cytoplasm (Fig. 19-3); nuclear atypia and mitoses are mainly observed in the epithelioid cells. Cytoplasmic vacuoles, representing intracellular vascular lumens, are often identified and may contain erythrocytes (Fig. 19-4).

The tumor cells synthesize a factor VIII-related antigen, which can be demonstrated in the cytoplasm or in the neoplastic vascular lumens (Fig. 19-5). Other endothelial cell markers, such as CD31 and CD34 (QB-END/10), have proven useful in diagnosis.[26,27] Tumor cells also express vimentin. The stroma of actively proliferating lesions has a myxoid appearance due to an abundance of sulfated mucopolysaccharide. Basement membrane can be demonstrated around the cells by the periodic acid-Schiff (PAS) stain, as well as immunohistochemically and ultrastructurally.

As the lesions evolve they are associated with progressive fibrosis and calcification. Eventually, tumor cells (and, indeed, the vascular nature of the lesion) may be difficult if not impossible to recognize in the densely sclerosed areas.

The histopathologic differential diagnosis[4,24] includes angiosarcoma, which is much more destructive than epithelioid hemangioendothelioma and obliterates acinar landmarks resulting in cavity formation. The cells are spindle shaped or show considerable pleomorphism, and intracellular lumina are not seen. Cholangiocarcinomas display a tubular or glandular pattern and often produce mucin; their cells are cytokeratin positive and, unlike epithelioid hemangioendothelioma, do not express endothelial cells markers.

Ultrastructural Features

The cells of epithelioid hemangioendothelioma have many of the characteristics of endothelial cells. These include a basal lamina, pinocytotic vesicles, and Weibel-Palade bodies. Intracellular lumina are frequently seen. Unlike normal endothelial cells, these tumor cells con-

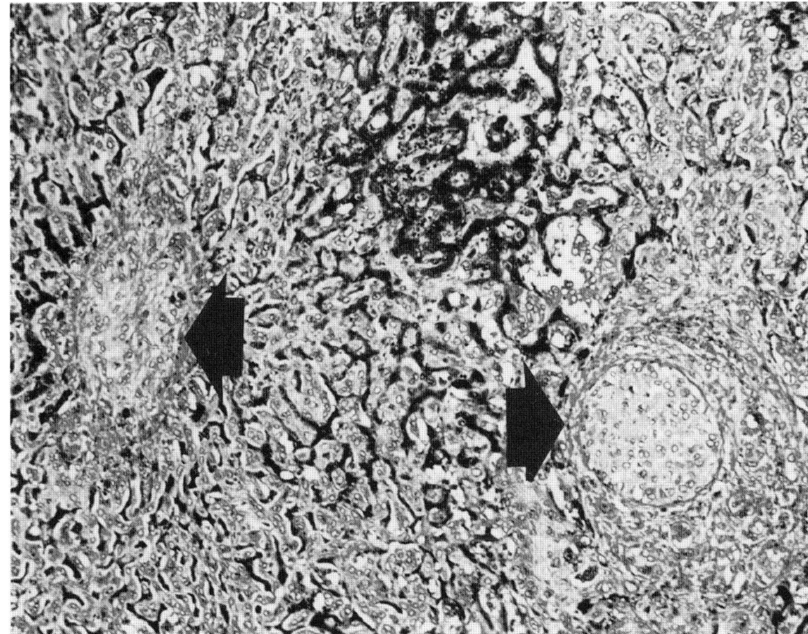

FIGURE 19-2. Epithelioid hemangioendothelioma showing occlusion of terminal hepatic venule (left) and portal vein branch (right) and infiltration of the acini with break up of hepatic cords (darkly stained). (Masson trichrome, ×100.)

tain a large number of intermediate filaments that account for their "epithelioid" appearance by light microscopy; dense bodies may also be present.

Treatment and Course

The prognosis of epithelioid hemangioendothelioma is unpredictable. About 28% of the tumors metastasize,[4] but the development of metastases does not preclude a long survival. Follow-up information on 17 patients[4] revealed that 7 of the 17 patients had died within 2 years of diagnosis and one patient died of metastatic disease 10 years after diagnosis, but only 6 (35%) of the deaths were attributable to the tumor. Twelve of the 17 patients have survived more than 3 years (range 3 to 28 years; average 9.8 years). Only 3 of the 12 surviving patients had been treated—by radiation and chemotherapy, by hepatic lobe resection, and by hepatic transplantation.

Some 30 other cases have since been treated by hepatic transplantation.[8,17,18] In some of the cases, metastatic spread did not correlate with poorer survival.[17,18] In the series of Kelleher et al.,[18] 9 of 10 patients who underwent transplantation were alive 5 to 134 months

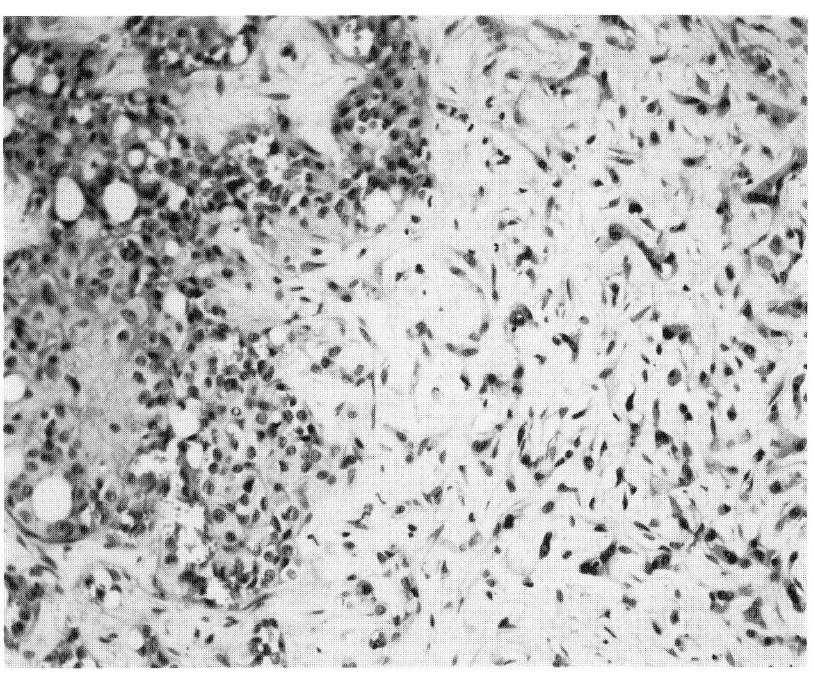

FIGURE 19-3. Epithelioid hemangioendothelioma with loosely arranged spindle and stellate cells (left) and epithelioid cells (right). (H&E, ×160.)

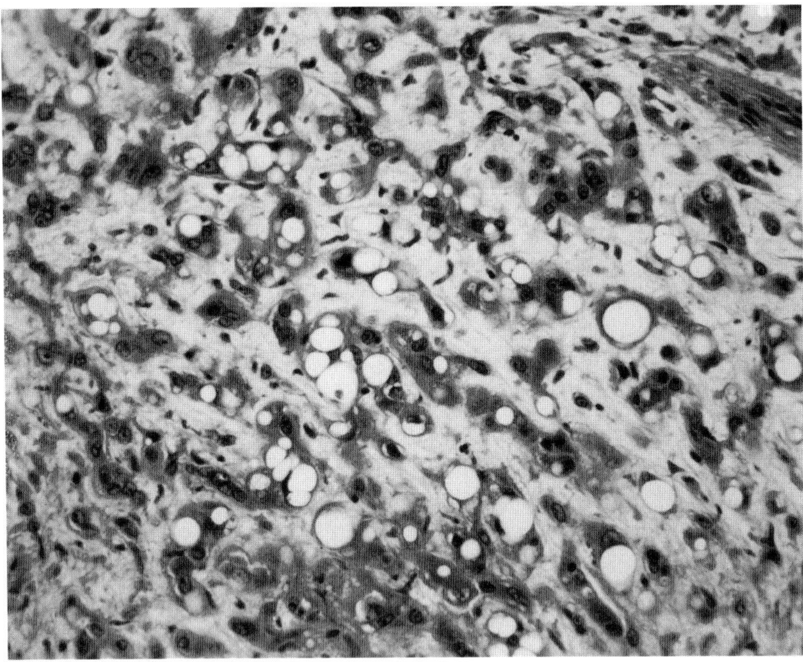

FIGURE 19-4. Epithelioid hemangioendothelioma. Empty spaces are intracellular vascular lumina in epithelioid cells. (H&E, ×250.)

postoperatively (five disease free and four with tumor). In the series of Marino et al.,[17] the projected 5-year actuarial survival was 76%. One patient with unresectable tumor has been reported who survived 4 years after hepatic intra-arterial 5-fluorouracil therapy.[20]

ANGIOSARCOMA

Angiosarcoma is a rare malignant vascular tumor and the most common sarcoma arising in the liver. Worldwide, more than 200 cases are diagnosed annually.[2,28] The peak age of onset is in the sixth and seventh decades, with a male to female ratio of 3 : 1.[29] Angiosarcomas occur rarely in children; most are believed to arise from infantile hemangioendothelioma[30–34] and were referred to in one study as type 2 hemangioendothelioma.[35] Etiologic factors implicated in these childhood angiosarcomas include androgenic/anabolic steroids[36] and possibly environmental exposure to arsenic.[37] A unique case of an angiosarcoma arising in a calcified cavernous hemangioma in an adult has been reported.[38] Angiosarcoma can present with (1) symptoms and signs indicative of liver disease, such as hepatomegaly, ascites, abdominal

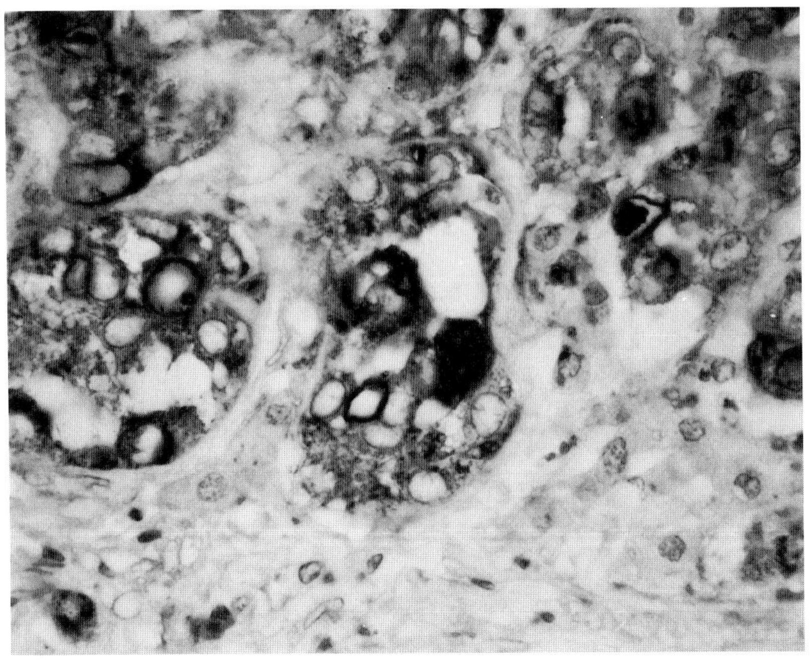

FIGURE 19-5. Epithelioid hemangioendothelioma. Tumor cells show marked expression (black) of von Willebrand factor (factor VIII-related antigen). (Peroxidase antiperoxidase immunostain, ×630.)

pain, anorexia, nausea and occasional vomiting, weight loss, and fever (62% of cases); (2) signs and symptoms of an acute abdomen from hemoperitoneum due to rupture of the tumor (15%); (3) splenomegaly, with or without pancytopenia (5%); (4) symptoms or signs referable to metastases to distant organs such as the skeleton or lungs (9%).[39] Portal hypertension, a recognized complication of vinyl chloride exposure,[40,41] may antedate the development of angiosarcoma.[40] The diagnosis is best established by open liver biopsy following suggestive radiologic studies.

Laboratory findings include anemia and sometimes a microangiopathic hemolytic anemia, leukocytosis or leukopenia, and thrombocytopenia.[39] Disseminated intravascular coagulopathy is a rare complication.[42] Serum liver tests are abnormal in about two-thirds of the patients.[29,39] The most consistent laboratory abnormalities are BSP retention (100%), increased serum alkaline phosphatase activity (83%), and a prolonged prothrombin time (72%). Hyperbilirubinemia develops in about 60% of cases, while mild to moderate aminotransferase elevations are found in less than half the cases.

Radiologic Features

Chest x-rays reveal elevation of the diaphragm (32% of cases) or, much less frequently, right pleural effusions, atelectasis, or pleural masses.[29] Plain films of the abdomen in Thorotrast-related angiosarcomas invariably disclose opacification of the liver, spleen, and abdominal lymph nodes.[43] Hepatic scans are abnormal in the majority of cases, but definite filling defects are recorded in only 70% of cases.[29] Computed tomography (CT) has been utilized in diagnosis,[43–47] as well as in detecting rupture of the tumor,[44] detecting tumors as small as 3 cm in diameter.[45] Nonenhanced scans show hypodense masses. Dynamic scanning during intravenous contrast injection reveal peripheral or central foci of enhancement in the nodules.[47] In delayed postcontrast scans the lesions become wholly or partly isodense.[47] Although the CT findings are nonspecific they are consistent with the findings expected with a vascular tumor. Angiographic studies are valuable[29,48]; the abnormal vascular pattern, with a persistent peripheral tumor stain and a central radiolucent area, is thought to be highly suggestive of angiosarcoma.[48]

Gross Features

The liver involved by angiosarcoma reveals grayish-white tumor tissue alternating with hemorrhagic foci (Fig. 19-6). Large cavities filled with liquid blood may be observed. A reticular pattern of fibrosis is often seen in cases associated with Thorotrast or prior exposure to vinyl chloride. Typically, the entire liver is involved. The spleen is usually large, except in Thorotrast-related angiosarcoma, when it is atrophic. Sections of the spleen and abdominal lymph nodes have a chalky white appearance in cases with a previous history of Thorotrast exposure. A true cirrhosis in patients with angiosarcoma, regardless of the etiology of the cirrhosis, is exceptionally rare in my experience. Angiosarcomas can sometimes occur with one or more other malignant tumors, such as hepatocellular carcinoma and/or cholangiocarcinoma. This has been reported with both Thorotrast[49–53] and vinyl chloride-associated[54,55] angiosarcoma.

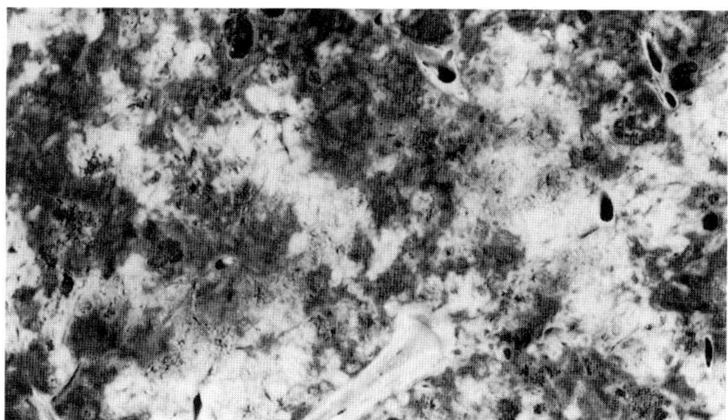

FIGURE 19-6. Angiosarcoma. Section of liver shows diffuse neoplastic infiltration, with a light and dark mottled pattern.

Microscopic Features

Angiosarcoma is composed of malignant endothelial cells that are spindle shaped or irregular in outline and have ill-defined borders (Figs. 19-7 and 19-8). The cytoplasm is lightly eosinophilic, and nuclei are hyperchromatic and elongated or irregular in shape. Nucleoli can be either small or large and eosinophilic. Large, bizarre nuclei and multinucleated cells may be seen, and mitotic figures are frequently identified. Factor VIII-related antigen (von Willebrand factor) can be identified in tumor cells by immunohistologic techniques,[56,57] although reported to be undetected by others.[58] Immunostaining for *Ulex europaeus* lectin is more sensitive though less specific than that for factor VIII.[59] Immunostaining can detect CD31 and CD34.[26,27]

The tumor cells grow along preformed vascular channels, such as sinusoids, THV, and portal vein branches (Fig. 19-8). Sinusoidal growth is associated with progressive atrophy of liver cells and disruption of the plates with the formation of larger and larger vascular channels and, eventually, the development of cavities. These cavities have ragged walls lined by tumor cells, sometimes with polypoid or papillary projections, and are filled with clotted blood and tumor debris. Invasion of THV and portal vein branches leads to progressive obstruction of these vessels and readily explains the fre-

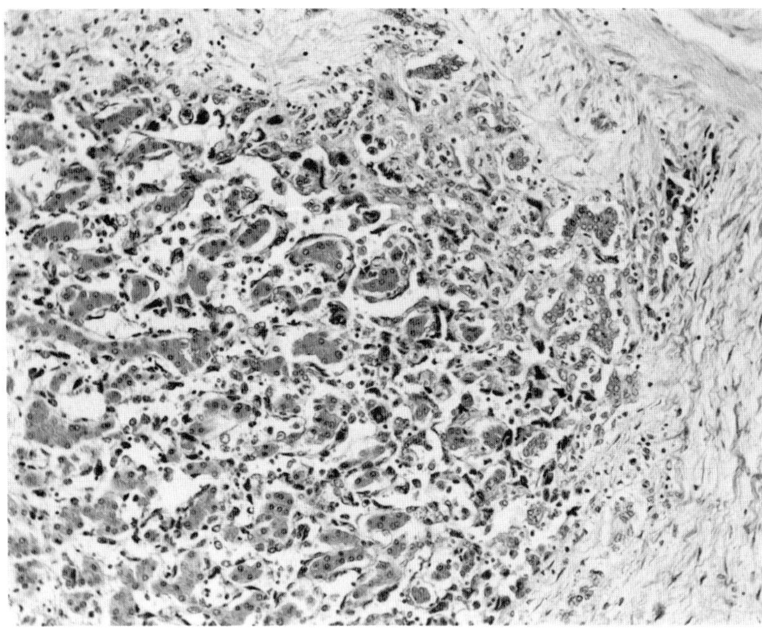

FIGURE 19-7. Angiosarcoma. Tumor cells have grown along existing sinusoids with break up of liver cell plates. (H&E, ×125.)

quently encountered areas of hemorrhage, infarction, and necrosis. The tumor cells are sometimes packed solidly in nodules that resemble fibrosarcoma (Fig. 19-9). Hematopoietic activity is observed in the majority of tumors,[11] although this was considered to be a feature most typical of Thorotrast-related cases in one study.[60]

A precursor stage in the development of angiosarcoma has been observed in cases etiologically related to vinyl chloride, Thorotrast, and arsenic.[61–64] It is characterized by foci of simultaneous hypertrophy of both hepatocytes and sinusoidal lining cells, with associated lesions in the sinusoids and perisinusoidal spaces. Sinusoidal lining cells may be hypertrophied and have large irregular and hyperchromatic nuclei. Vinyl chloride-associated cases in humans resemble those induced experimentally in rodents[65]; and typical changes can be seen in vinyl chloride workers without angiosarcoma.[66,67]

Cases related to Thorotrast and vinyl chloride are often associated with considerable periportal and subcapsular fibrosis, and cirrhosis may result. In Thorotrast-induced angiosarcomas, the Thorotrast deposits are readily recognized in reticuloendothelial cells or lying free in

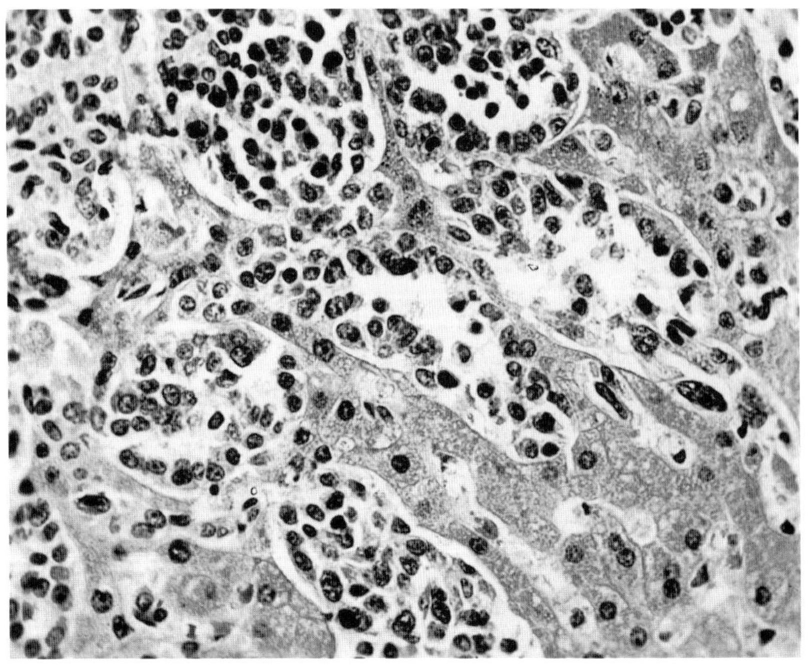

FIGURE 19-8. Angiosarcoma. Tumor cells have extensively infiltrated sinusoids with atrophy and disruption of the hepatic plates. (H&E, ×350.)

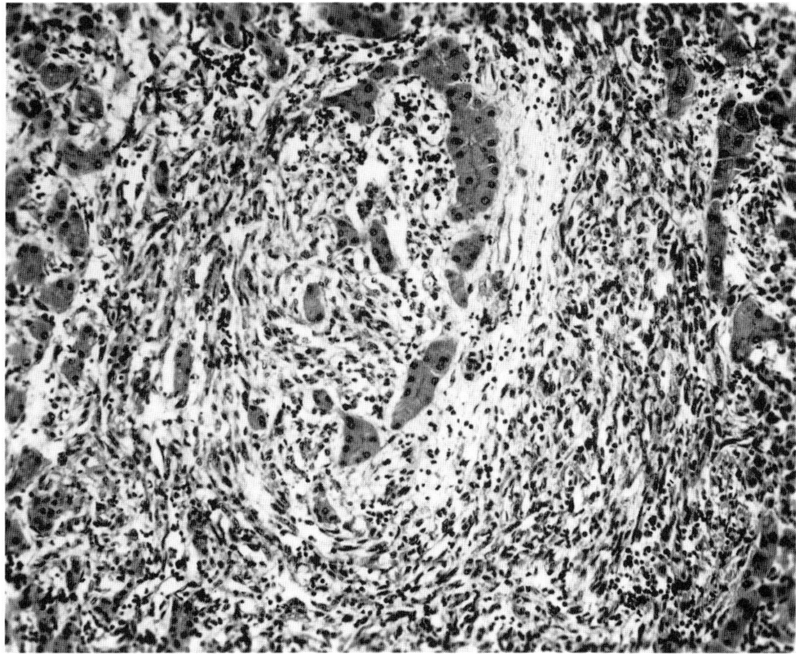

FIGURE 19-9. Angiosarcoma. Solid fibrosarcoma-like pattern. (H&E, ×160.)

portal areas, Glisson's capsule or the wall of THV (Fig. 19-10). The deposits are colorless and refractile, but in an H&E-stained section they usually have a pink-brown hue; they are not birefringent, but can be illuminated by phase contrast microscopy. The alpha emissions of the thorium dioxide in Thorotrast can be visualized by autoradiography, appearing as short, dotted tracks. The particles are readily visualized by scanning electron microscopy of a paraffin section, and the element thorium can be definitively identified by energy dispersive x-ray microanalysis.[68–71]

Treatment and Course

The majority of patients with angiosarcoma die in less than 6 months of diagnosis, usually from liver failure or abdominal bleeding. Surgical excision is generally not feasible, but some prolongation of survival has been achieved by chemotherapy.[29]

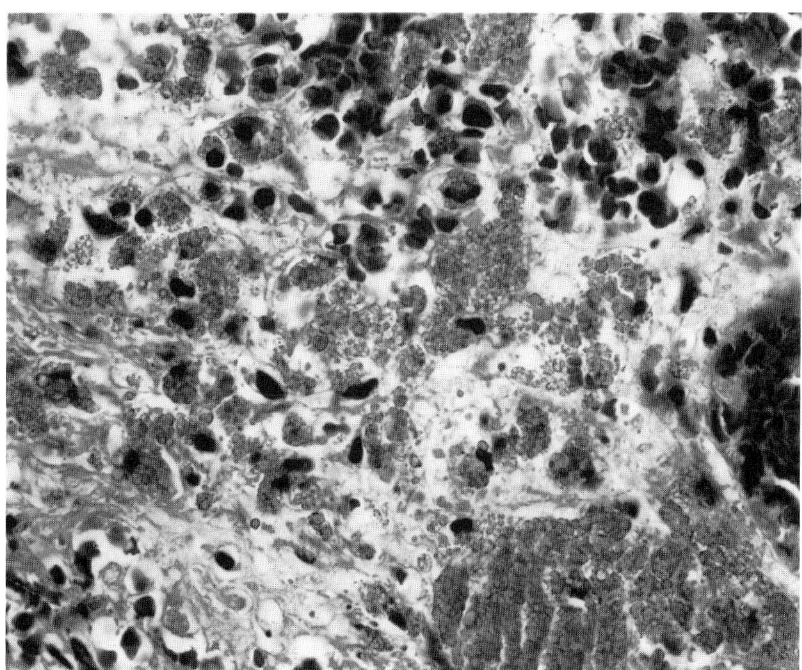

FIGURE 19-10. Angiosarcoma. Numerous granular Thorotrast particles are present in an area of fibrosis. (H&E, ×630.)

TABLE 19-1. Etiology of Angiosarcoma[a]

Physical/Chemical Injury	Circumstances of Exposure	Latent Period (years)	References
Thorotrast	Used as contrast medium for radiographic studies	15–36	39, 45, 58, 60, 209–213
Radium	Radium needle implanted for treatment of breast carcinoma (one case)	3	214
External radiation	Atomic bomb explosion, Hiroshima (one case)	36	215
Vinyl chloride	Industrial exposure during manufacture of polyvinyl chloride; exposure to sprays containing vinyl chloride as propellant	12–28	2, 48, 54, 56, 61–63, 216, 217
Inorganic arsenic	Insecticide for spraying of vineyards; medicinal use of Fowler's solution; high levels of arsenic in drinking water	6–33	37, 218–225
Copper	Use of copper sulfate for spraying of vineyards (one case)	35	226
Pesticides	Farmers exposed to organophosphorous- and organochlorine-containing pesticides	14	227
Iron	Idiopathic hemochromatosis in cirrhotic stage	?	77–79, 228–230
Androgenic/anabolic steroids	Treatment of Fanconi's anemia and other disorders	2–35	36, 231
Contraceptive steroids	Birth control (one case)	10	232
Diethylstilbestrol	Treatment of prostatic cancer (one case)	13	233
Phenelzine	Not known (one case)	6	234

[a] Cases arising in pre-existing benign vascular tumor, such as infantile hemangioendothelioma and cavernous hemangioma, are excluded.

Etiology

The etiology of angiosarcoma is unknown in 75% of cases[2]; 25% are associated with vinyl chloride, Thorotrast, inorganic arsenic, or androgenic anabolic steroids.[2] Etiologic factors implicated in angiosarcoma in humans are listed in Table 19-1.

Analysis of angiosarcomas related to vinyl chloride has shown an increased frequency of *p53* mutations, with a mutational spectrum (A:T to T:A transversion) characteristic of chloroethylene oxide, a carcinogenic metabolite of vinyl chloride.[38,72] Mutations are uncommon in sporadic angiosarcomas and in those associated with Thorotrast, suggesting other mechanisms.[73] Angiosarcoma cells produce and secrete vascular endothelial growth factor that binds to its receptor on the tumor cells, thus promoting their proliferation.[74]

KAPOSI'S SARCOMA

Kaposi's sarcoma involves the liver in 12% to 25% of fatal cases of acquired immunodeficiency syndrome (AIDS),[75–79] but its presence in the liver does not appear to contribute to the morbidity and mortality of AIDS. Functional hepatic impairment has not been recorded in these cases.

Kaposi's sarcoma in the liver is an irregular, variably sized, red-brown spongiform lesion that resembles capillary hemangioma (Fig. 19-11). Histopathologically, the lesions are generally confined to the portal connective tissue, but the tumor may infiltrate the adjacent parenchyma for short distances (Figs. 19-12 and 19-13). Seven histologic patterns, forming a spectrum of cellular differentiation, have been described.[79] The least differentiated

FIGURE 19-11. Kaposi's sarcoma. Autopsy section of liver of patient with acquired immunodeficiency syndrome shows dark infiltrates.

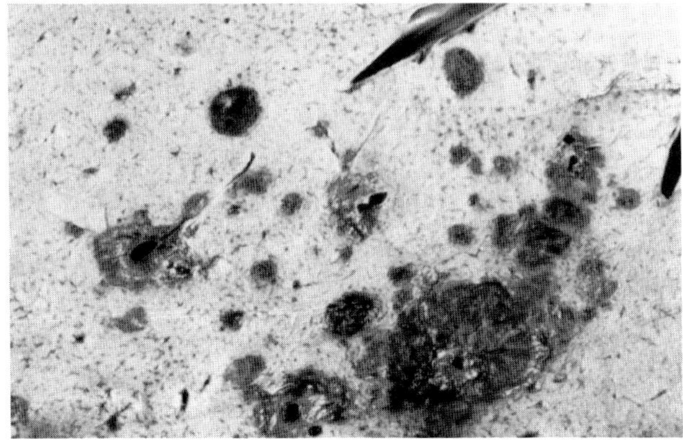

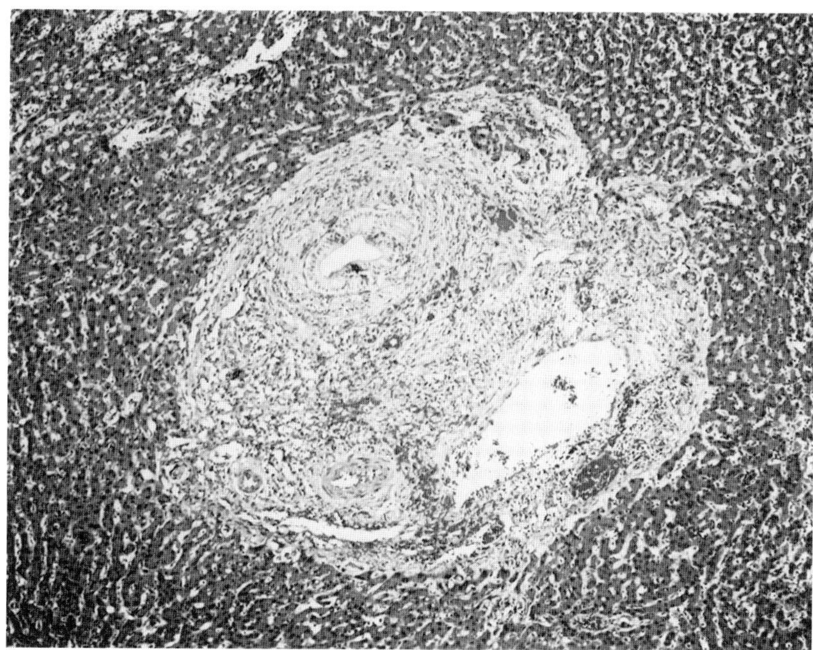

FIGURE 19-12. Kaposi's sarcoma. Sarcomatous infiltrate is mostly confined to a portal area. (H&E, ×400.)

consist of spindle cells that have large, sometimes irregular nuclei. Hyaline globules, thought to be ingested erythrocytes, are found in the majority of cases.[80] The spindle cells express endothelial cell markers (CD31, CD34, von Willebrand factor), thrombomodulin, and endothelial adhesion molecule-1 and are therefore considered to be of vascular origin.[79,81,82] A Kaposi's sarcoma-associated herpesvirus has been reported that may play a causative role in the etiology of the disease.[83–86] It has not been detected in other vascular lesions, such as angiosarcoma.[86]

Treatment of Kaposi's sarcoma includes radiotherapy, chemotherapy, antiviral agents (zidovudine, interferon), and granulocyte-macrophage colony-stimulating factor.[87]

EMBRYONAL RHABDOMYOSARCOMA

Embryonal rhabdomyosarcoma arises in the extrahepatic bile ducts but can involve the large septal ducts in the liver. Most patients are less than 5 years of age, but occasionally these tumors have been diagnosed in older chil-

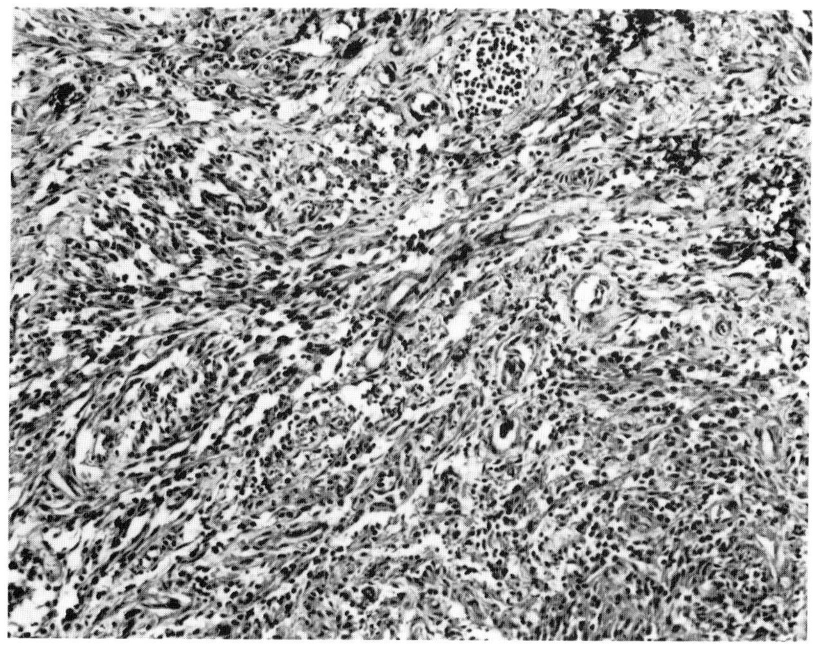

FIGURE 19-13. Kaposi's sarcoma exhibiting spindle cells and slit-like vascular spaces. (H&E, ×150.)

dren and adults.[88–93] In children, embryonal rhabdomyosarcoma affects males and females equally. A primary rhabdomyosarcoma, associated with hepatocellular carcinoma, was reported in a 62-year-old man.[94]

Patients with embryonal rhabdomyosarcoma usually present with intermittent obstructive jaundice, often with fever and hepatomegaly. A mistaken diagnosis of viral hepatitis can lead to delays in therapy.[91] Ultrasonography and CT generally demonstrate a mass in the porta hepatis. Transhepatic cholangiography also has been utilized in preoperative diagnosis.[95]

Treatment and Course

Initial therapy should consist of resection of the mass with only microscopic or minimal gross residual tumor; continuity of bile flow is maintained by variations of Roux-en-Y jejunostomy.[91] Operative cholangiography is useful in demonstrating the site of the obstruction and in verifying a functioning drainage procedure.[91] Postoperative therapy includes multidrug chemotherapy and radiotherapy. Follow-up surgery is useful in evaluating residual or recurrent disease. This regimen has resulted in survival for 2 to 6.5 years in 3 of 10 cases.[91]

Gross Findings

Affected bile ducts have a thick wall with narrowing of the lumen. Sections reveal a white glistening tumor. In some cases, soft or gelatinous grape-like masses (sarcoma botryoides) may project into the lumen. Bile ducts proximal to the occluded segment are dilated, and the liver often has a green color from cholestasis.

Microscopic Findings

The tumor cells are usually set in a loose myxoid stroma containing abundant acid mucopolysaccharide. Areas of inflammation, necrosis, and hemorrhage may be seen. The polypoid tumor masses projecting into the bile duct lumen are covered by bile duct epithelium, but the surface may be ulcerated and inflammatory cells may be present (Fig. 19-14). A dense mass of tumor cells ("cambium layer") lies immediately beneath the epithelium. Tumor cells may be round, spindled, or strap shaped (Fig. 19-15). Nuclei are hyperchromatic, elongated, and have blunt ends. Mitotic figures are usually abundant. Tumor cells may undergo marked cytologic change after chemotherapy.[96] Ultrastructural studies reveal both thick and thin myofilaments, with recognizable Z bands in some cells.[31]

Myoglobin, myosin, muscle-specific actin, and desmin (Fig. 19-16) may be identified in tumor cells by immunohistochemistry. *MYF* (myo D_1) gene expression can be detected and is a specific marker of rhabdomyiosarcoma.[97,98]

EMBRYONAL SARCOMA

Embryonal sarcoma, or undifferentiated sarcoma, has also been called *primary sarcoma* and *malignant mesenchymoma*.[99–101] The latter term is justified only if there is evidence of differentiation into two or more mesenchymal elements other than fibrosarcoma, which is rarely the case.[102–105]

Embryonal sarcoma constitutes 6% to 13%[99] of all

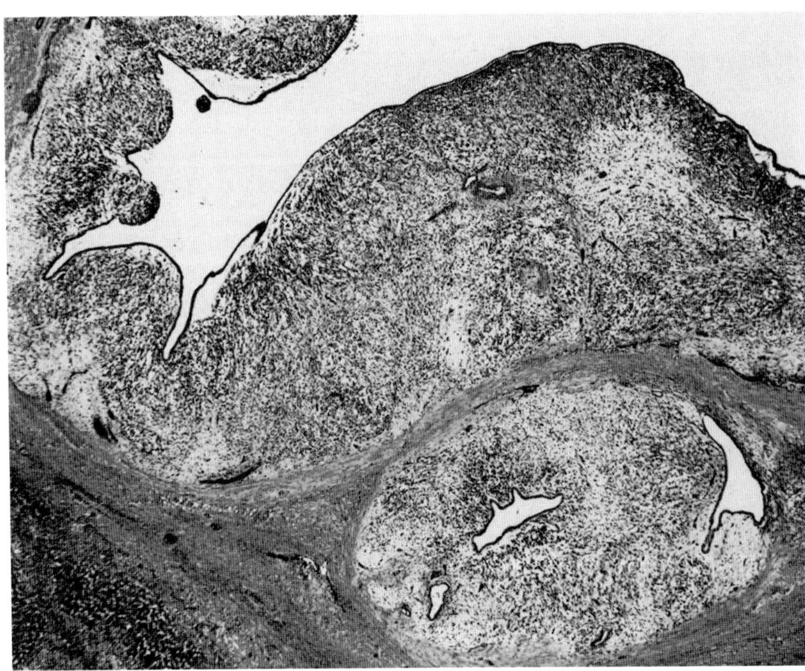

FIGURE 19-14. Embryonal rhabdomyosarcoma. Intrahepatic bile ducts are infiltrated by the tumor, with encroachment on the lumen. (H&E, ×25.)

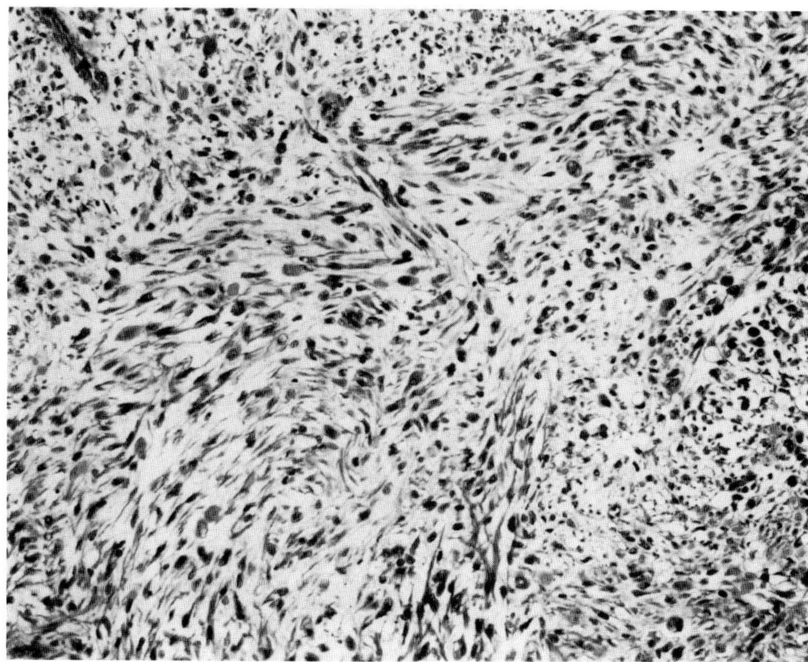

FIGURE 19-15. Embryonal rhabdomyosarcoma. Intersecting bundles of spindle cells. (H&E, ×160.)

primary hepatic neoplasms in the pediatric age group. More than half of patients (52%) with embryonal sarcoma are between 6 and 10 years of age[99]; cases in adults are rare.[106–108]

Abdominal swelling, with or without a palpable mass, and pain are the usual presenting findings. Some patients complain of nonspecific gastrointestinal symptoms, fever, and weight loss. Rarely, the tumors invade the inferior vena cava and grow into the right atrium, presenting clinically as a primary intracardiac tumor.[104] Leukocytosis with a shift to the left is a common finding. Liver tests are abnormal in one-third to one-half of patients, the most frequent abnormality being a slight increase in serum alkaline phosphatase activity.

Radiologic findings reflect the spectrum of solid and cystic features characteristic of the tumor.[109] Sonography typically demonstrates a large mass that may be predominantly solid (with many small anechoic spaces) or cystic. CT reveals a hypodense mass with hyperdense septa of variable thickness and a dense peripheral rim corresponding to the fibrous pseudocapsule. Angiographically, the tumor is usually hypovascular, but hypervascular and avascular patterns occur infrequently. The radiologic differential diagnosis from mesenchymal hamartoma may

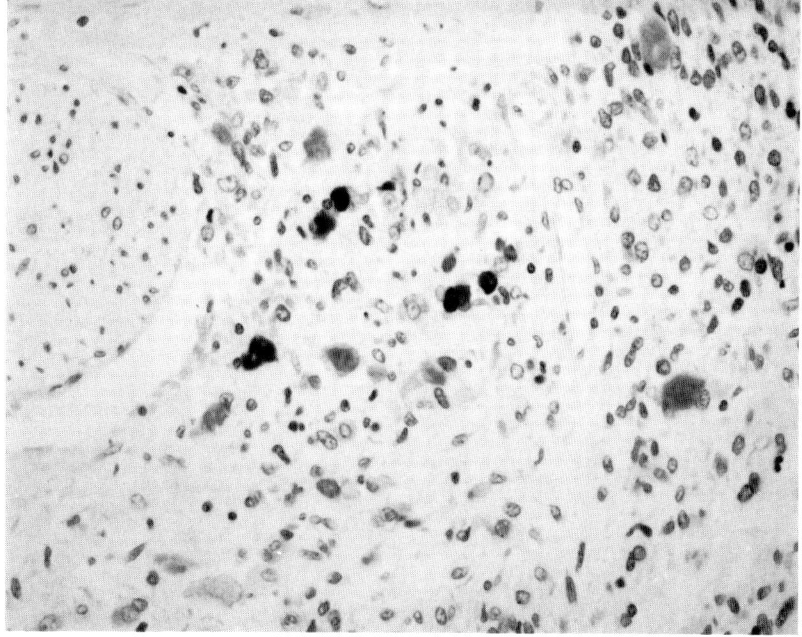

FIGURE 19-16. Embryonal rhabdomyosarcoma. Darkly stained tumor cells are expressing desmin. (Peroxidase antiperoxidase immunostain, ×300.)

be difficult. The older age and more frequent symptomatic presentation of patients with embryonal sarcoma are helpful in the differential diagnosis. A definitive diagnosis requires liver biopsy, which is generally performed at laparotomy. One reported case was diagnosed at peritoneoscopy by guided biopsy.[110]

Treatment and Course

Compared to earlier studies, the prognosis of embryonal sarcoma has greatly improved, with some patients surviving 5 or more years after combined modality treatment.[111–118]

Gross Findings

The majority of embryonal sarcomas are located in the right lobe of the liver. Most measure 10–20 cm in diameter, with an average weight of 1,310 g.[99] They are usually globular and well demarcated, but encapsulation is uncommon. The cut surface is variegated, with solid, glistening, grey-white tumor tissue, alternating with cystic gelatinous areas, and/or red and yellow areas of hemorrhage and necrosis (Fig. 19-17).

Microscopic Findings

A fibrous pseudocapsule may separate the tumor from the adjacent compressed parenchyma. The more peripheral areas typically contain entrapped bile ducts, which can be dilated (Fig. 19-18), and sometimes hepatic parenchymal elements. The tumor cells are stellate or spindle shaped and have ill-defined outlines (Fig. 19-19). They may be compactly or loosely arranged, with an abundant mucopolysaccharide matrix, but areas with a more fibrous stroma are also seen in most tumors. Tumor cells often show marked anisonucleosis with hyperchromasia and sometimes bizarre giant cells; mitoses are usually abundant. A characteristic feature is the presence of multiple, varying-sized eosinophilic globules in the cytoplasm; these are PAS positive and resist diastase digestion (Fig. 19-20). Hematopoietic activity is present in half the tumors. Hemorrhages and necrosis are often present. The neoplastic cells may be reactive to antibodies to α_1-antitrypsin, α_1-antichymotrypsin, and vimentin.[119–122] Occasional cases express cytokeratin.[122,123] There is no evidence of cellular differentiation under the light microscope, but ultrastructural and immunohistochemical studies in isolated cases have shown fibroblastic, rhabdomyoblastic, and/or leiomyoblastic differentiation.[103–105,121–126] In view of these findings, it has been suggested[126] that the term *embryonal sarcoma* is preferable to *undifferentiated sarcoma*, since these tumors may display partial differentiation.

Etiology

Little is known of possible inducing or promoting factors in embryonal sarcoma other than one report of a 19-year-old patient who had been exposed prenatally to phenytoin.[127] The possibility of origin of embryonal sarcoma from mesenchymal hamartoma, first suggested by

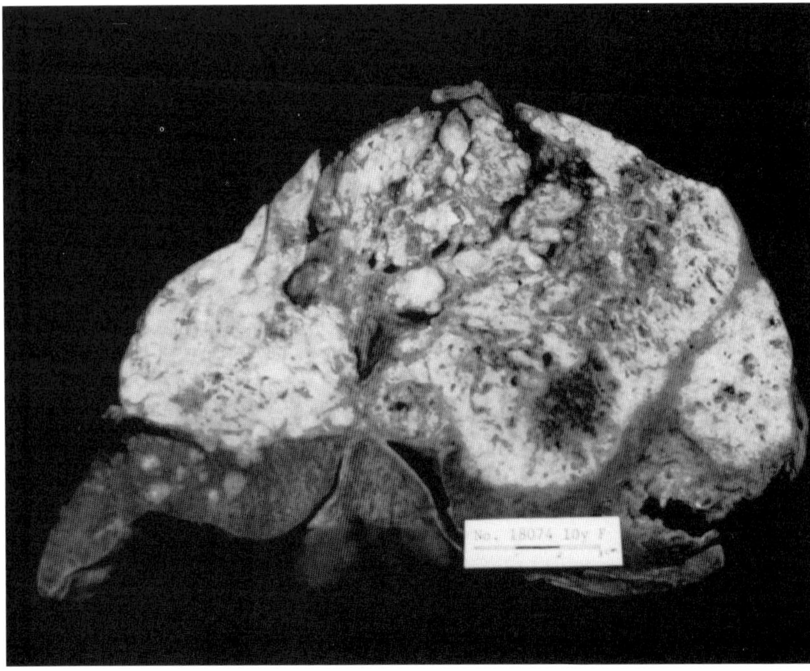

FIGURE 19-17. Embryonal sarcoma. The tumor has replaced most of the liver and displays scattered hemorrhages. Several small satellite tumor nodules are visible below and to the left of the main mass.

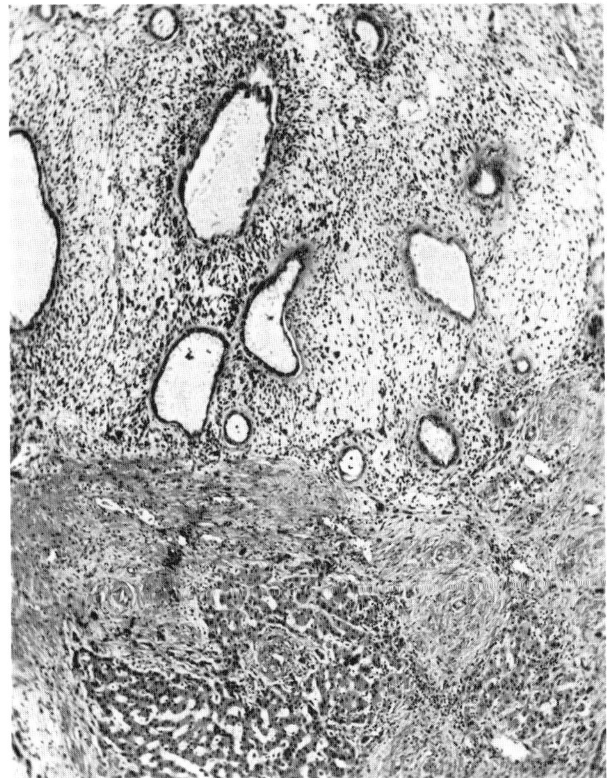

FIGURE 19-18. Embryonal sarcoma. The tumor (upper half of figure) contains several dilated bile ducts. It is sharply demarcated from the hepatic parenchyma (below). (H&E, ×50.)

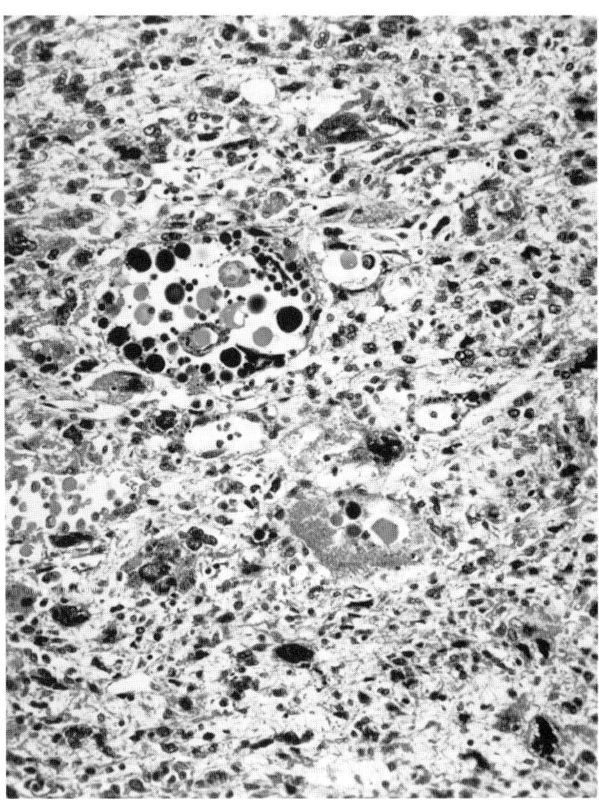

FIGURE 19-20. Embryonal sarcoma. Multiple, darkly stained globules are present in several tumor cells. (PAS after diastase digestion, ×160.)

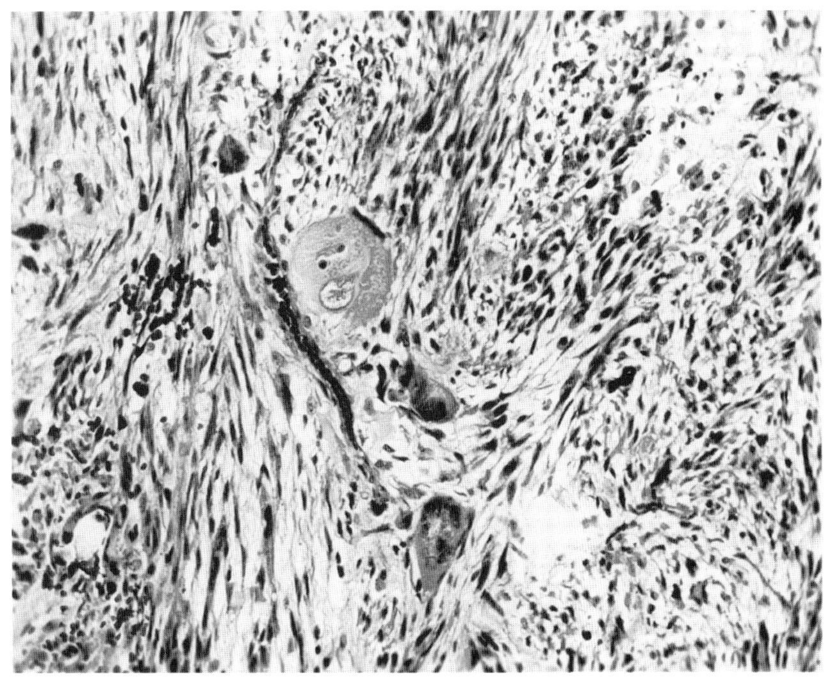

FIGURE 19-19. Embryonal sarcoma. Tumor cells are spindled and arranged in fascicles. Several tumor giant cells are present in the center. (H&E, ×165.)

Stanley et al.,[100] appears to have been confirmed in at least one case.[128]

OTHER MALIGNANT MESENCHYMAL TUMORS

Fibrosarcoma

Fibrosarcoma is a rare tumor of the liver,[39,129–140] occurring at ages 30 to 73 years (median 55 years) and most commonly in males (85%). One tumor developed in the donor liver of a 4-year-old girl who had been transplanted 2 years previously and had been treated with cyclosporine.[140] Symptoms and signs are nonspecific, and the diagnosis is established by biopsy. Severe hypoglycemia may occur.[129,138] The prognosis is very poor, although several patients have survived from 1 to 3 years following resection and/or radiation therapy.

Fibrosarcomas are often large at the time of diagnosis; one of the largest tumors weighed more than 7 kg.[39] The cut surface reveals grayish-white tissue, which can display a whorled appearance. Foci of necrosis and hemorrhage, sometimes with cystic degeneration, are often seen. Microscopically, the tumor is composed of spindle-shaped cells arranged in interlacing bundles, with the typical "herringbone" pattern in some areas. Varying numbers of collagen and reticulin fibers arise from, and intermingle with, the tumor cells. The nuclei are hyperchromatic and elongated and have pointed ends; mitotic activity is variable. The tumor cells express vimentin. Collagen types I and IV have been demonstrated in the tumor matrix.[141]

Leiomyosarcoma

Leiomyosarcoma is also a rare tumor of the liver. In a review of the literature up to 1992, some 60 cases had been reported,[142] not including over 50 leiomyosarcomas of the inferior vena cava,[143,144] the tumors occurring in children or adults with human immunodeficiency virus infection,[145–148] or those developing in liver allografts in pediatric patients.[149] Intrahepatic leiomyosarcomas occur equally in men and women,[142] but those arising in the inferior vena cava are more frequent in women.[143] The mean age of presentation is 52 years. Symptoms and signs include upper abdominal swelling or mass, abdominal pain, and weight loss. Leiomyosarcomas arising in the hepatic veins or inferior vena cava can lead to Budd-Chiari syndrome.[143] The prognosis of leiomyosarcomas arising in the hepatic outflow tract is worse than those that are intrahepatic; the latter, in turn, have a worse prognosis than leiomyosarcomas arising in the ligamentum teres.[39,150] Metastatic disease occurs in about 40% of cases.[142] The mean survival of untreated intrahepatic leiomyosarcoma is less than 1 year. With a combination of surgery and chemotherapy, the mean survival is 3.3 years.[142]

Primary leiomyosarcomas of the liver are usually solitary and can attain a large size. They are firm to rubbery in consistency. The cut surface is pinkish-white with yellow areas of necrosis or dark red hemorrhagic foci. Histopathologically, the tumor is composed of intersecting bundles of elongated, spindle-shaped cells. The lightly eosinophilic cytoplasm may have faint longitudinal striations. Nuclei are hyperchromatic and elongated and have blunt ends. Mitotic activity is variable. Expression of desmin, muscle-specific actin, and smooth muscle actin can be detected by immunohistochemistry. Immunoreactivity for cytokeratin and epithelial membrane antigen have also been demonstrated in some leiomyosarcomas.[151] Recently, a monoclonal antibody, 1H1, anticortactin, was found useful in diagnosis.[152] Ultrastructurally, the cells have thin myofilaments, cytoplasmic dense bodies, marginal dense plaques, a basal lamina, and pinocytotic vesicles. Chromosomal abnormalities have been described in leiomyosarcoma, but are of little diagnostic relevance.[153]

Etiologic factors in leiomyosarcoma are largely unknown. Cases associated with AIDS are believed to be linked to Epstein-Barr virus infection.[147,148] One leiomyosarcoma, arising synchronously with a cholangiocarcinoma, has been reported to be Thorotrast related.[154]

Malignant Fibrous Histiocytoma

Malignant fibrous histiocytoma (MEH) is a rare tumor of the liver; only a few cases have been reported to date.[155–161] The similarity of this tumor to undifferentiated (embryonal) sarcoma has been noted in one case report.[121] In one study, the tumor cells were found to express several types of intermediate filaments, suggesting heterogeneity of the tumor.[162] In another study, 15 of 22 MFHs expressed markers of smooth muscle differentiation and 7 did not, again suggesting heterogeneity.[163] It has been hypothesized[164] that MFH is the final common pathway for some types of sarcomas and is the result of "dedifferentiation." It appears that the histiocyte-like cells of MFH are not a neoplastic component; rather, they are infiltrated macrophages, attracted by tumor-derived monocyte chemoattractants, while the tumor cells themselves are of fibroblastic lineage and are derived from mesenchymal cells.[165]

Other Primary Sarcomas

Primary sarcomas such as osteogenic sarcoma,[166,167] malignant mesenchymoma,[100,101,168,169] and malignant Schwannoma[170,171] are too rare to warrant discussion.

PRIMARY MALIGNANT LYMPHOMA OF THE LIVER

The liver is one of the more frequently involved organs in lymphoma, but primary lymphomas are rare.[172–176] About 100 non-Hodgkin's lymphomas of the liver have been reported.[174] Primary lymphomas of the liver may present with a mass or hepatosplenomegaly (with most being B-cell lymphomas) or with liver disease without lymphadenopathy (with the majority being T-cell lymphomas), as fulminant hepatic failure with hyperlactasemia (with these being lymphomas of various types),[174] or with fever and weight loss.[176]

There is a male to female preponderance of 4:1, with an age range of 7 to 78 years (mean 46.6).[173]

Gross Features

Most primary lymphomas form solitary or multiple masses that can be located in either lobe, but in about 16% there is diffuse infiltration of the liver.[173]

Microscopic Features

The lymphomatous infiltrates are typically in portal areas but can extend into and destroy the adjacent parenchyma. Portal area involvement is typical of B-cell lymphomas, including the recently described T-cell-rich B-cell lymphoma.[177] Bile ducts and veins in the portal areas may be infiltrated by the lymphoma cells. Sinusoidal infiltration is considered typical of peripheral T-cell lymphoma,[178–182] but has also been described in a large cell lymphoma of B-cell phenotype (Fig. 19-21).[183]

The so-called hepatosplenic T-cell lymphomas are characterized by T cells that have the receptor, in contrast to the majority of T-cell lymphomas that express the receptor.[179–182] Experience is required in the histopathologic diagnosis of the lymphomas, and immunohistochemical studies for determination of B- or T-cell lineage are essential.

Etiology

Primary hepatic lymphomas (mostly B-cell lymphomas) have been reported in immunocompromised patients such as those with AIDS[174,184,185] or those who have been immunosuppressed after liver transplantation.[149] There is a strong association with Epstein-Barr virus infection.[186] More recently, the Kaposi's sarcoma-associated herpesvirus was found in AIDS-related lymphomas.[187]

Course and Prognosis

Surgery alone, or combined with chemotherapy and/or radiotherapy, has been used in treatment of primary hepatic lymphoma with variable results.[173,175,188–189] Chinese patients have a highly aggressive course with a poor response to local and systemic therapy and a short survival.[176] The prognosis in patients with AIDS is determined by the underlying disease and its other complications, particularly infections. In a series of patients who had liver transplants in whom the lymphoma was confined to the liver allograft, complete remission was achieved after treatment in 11 of 28 patients.[149]

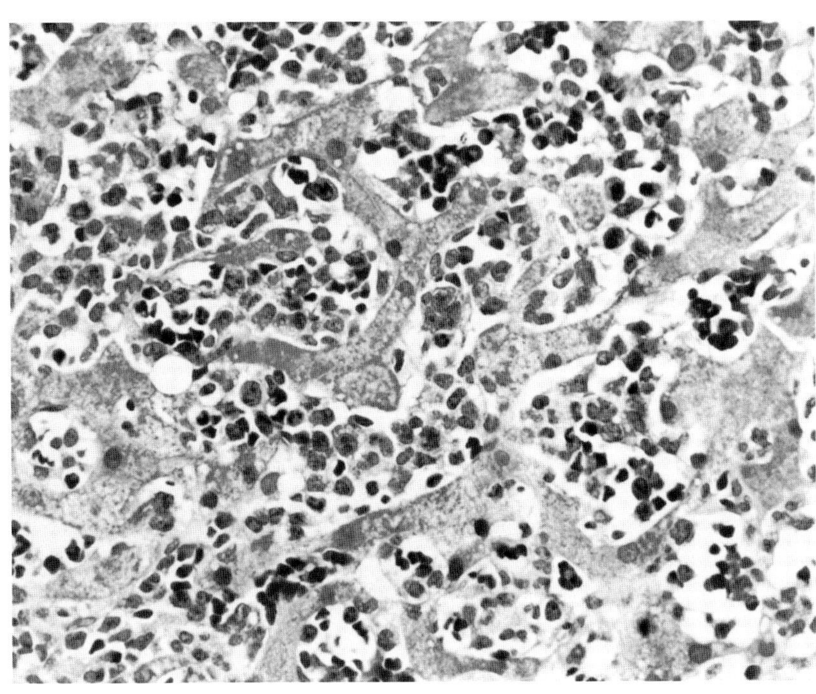

FIGURE 19-21. Large cell lymphoma, B-cell type, with extensive sinusoidal infiltration. (H&E, ×400.)

METASTATIC TUMORS IN THE LIVER

The liver is a frequent site of metastases, particularly from the gastrointestinal tract, pancreas, lung, and breast. Metastases reach the liver by hematogenous spread; the presence of cirrhosis appears to reduce the incidence of metastatic spread. In the United States, and in many other countries, metastatic carcinoma is far more common in the liver than primary malignant tumors; in one large medical center in the United States, metastatic tumors to the liver were 41 times more common than primary hepatic carcinoma.[194]

Metastatic tumors may produce tender hepatomegaly; the liver may be firm and nodular. Serum alkaline phosphatase and lactic dehydrogenase values are often elevated. Uncommon presentations include fulminant hepatic failure,[195–199] obstructive jaundice with hemobilia,[200] and massive intraperitoneal hemorrhage.[201] The diagnosis is established by imaging studies with ultrasound or CT-guided liver biopsy.

Gross Features

The metastases may form solitary nodules or multiple nodules, but can infiltrate the liver diffusely. Umbilication is typical of metastatic adenocarcinoma. Gross examination of tissue specimens can provide clues to the origin of the primary tumor. Metastatic malignant melanoma may be black. Hemorrhagic metastases should suggest metastatic angiosarcoma, choriocarcinoma, or thyroid carcinoma. In Kaposi's sarcoma the tumor infiltrates are red to purple and usually confined to portal areas. Metastatic adenocarcinomas from the gastrointestinal

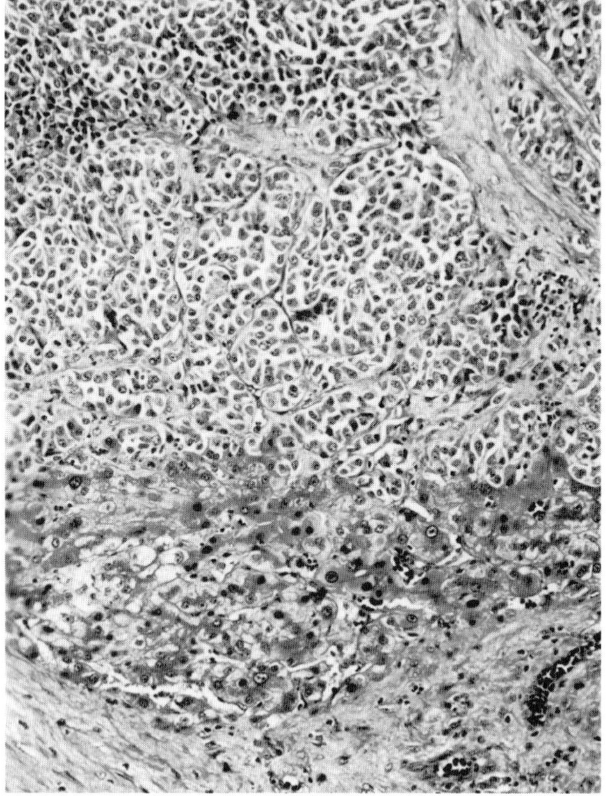

FIGURE 19-23. Metastatic carcinoid tumor. Tumor cells (top two-thirds of field) are arranged in nests. (H&E, ×150.)

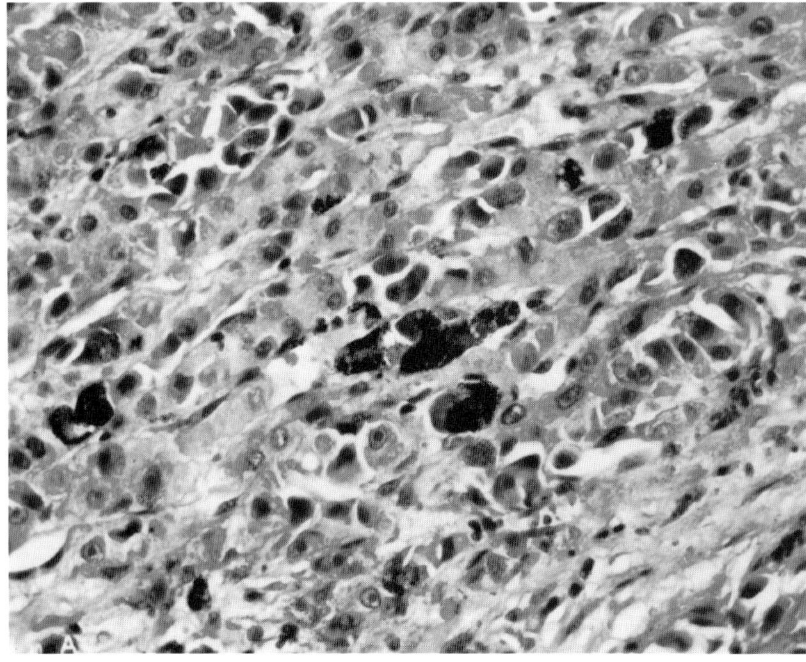

FIGURE 19-22. Metastatic malignant melanoma. Tumor cells in center are black because of their melanin pigment. (H&E, ×400.)

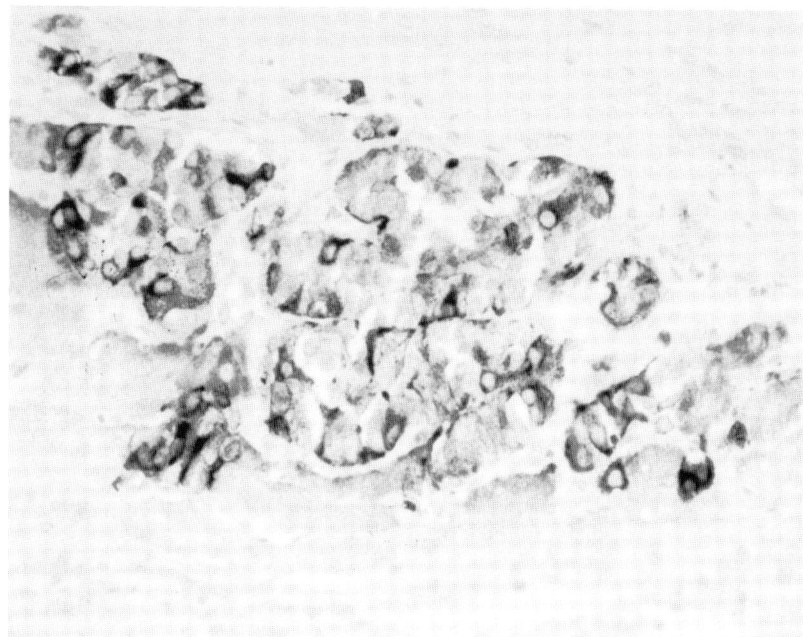

FIGURE 19-24. Metastatic carcinoid tumor (same case as illustrated in Fig. 19-23). Tumor cells show expression of chromogranin (black), a marker of neuroendocrine differentiation. (Peroxidase antiperoxidase immunostain, ×300.)

tract may be glistening and slimy, while metastases from squamous carcinomas are granular and caseous.[202] "Fish-flesh" tumors may be lymphomas, sarcomas, or undifferentiated carcinomas. Metastatic carcinoid tumors can form pseudocysts.[203,204]

Microscopic Features

Metastases from adenocarcinomas of the pancreas, extrahepatic bile ducts or gallbladder, and gastrointestinal tract cannot be distinguished from primary intrahepatic cholangiocarcinoma. Some metastases have distinctive microscopic features, such as Hodgkin's and non-Hodgkin's lymphoma, oat cell carcinoma of the lung, and malignant melanoma (Fig. 19-22). Metastases from clear cell carcinoma of the kidney may be difficult to distinguish from the rare clear cell variant of hepatocellular carcinoma; bile production or demonstration of canaliculi by a polyclonal immunostain for carcinoembryonic antigen is diagnostic of the latter tumor. Metastatic adrenal cortical carcinoma, which may have a trabecular pattern,[205] can also be differentiated from hepatocellular carcinoma by the absence of canaliculi and bile production. Carcinoid tumors are usually metastatic, but rarely can be primary (Fig. 19-23). The diagnosis is confirmed by positive immunostains for chromogranin (Fig. 19-24) and synaptophysin. Immunostains are useful in identifying the origin of other metastatic tumors, for example, prostate-specific antigen for prostatic carcinoma, thyroglobulin for follicular carcinoma of the thyroid, and cytokeratin 20 for tumors of the gastrointestinal tract.[206] Breast carcinoma metastases can be identified by the combined use of zinc-α_2-glycoprotein, gross cystic disease fluid protein 15, and estrogenic receptors.[207] The diagnosis of malignant melanoma can be confirmed by immunostaining for HMB-45 and S-100. Metastatic leiomyosarcoma usually expresses desmin and muscle-specific actin, but metastases from epithelioid leiomyosarcomas (also known as stromal tumors) of the stomach or intestine may not; such tumors express CD34 antigen.[208]

ACKNOWLEDGMENTS

The author is grateful to Ms. Robin-Anne V. Ferris for the excellent photomicrography and to Ms. Fanny Revelo-Chicas for typing the manuscript.

REFERENCES

1. Edmondson HA, Peters RL. Neoplasms of the Liver. In Schiff L, Schiff ER (eds): Diseases of the Liver. 5th Ed. Lippincott, Philadelphia, 1982, pp. 1101–1157
2. Falk H, Herbert J, Crouley S. Epidemiology of hepatic angiosarcoma in the United States: 1964–1974. Environ Health Perspect 1981;41:107–113
3. Shin P, Ohmi S, Sakurai M. Hepatocellular carcinoma combined with hepatic sarcoma. Acta Pathol Jpn 1981;31: 815–824
4. Ishak KG, Sesterhenn IA, Goodman ZD et al. Epithelioid hemangioendothelioma of the liver: a clinicopathologic and follow-up study of 32 cases. Hum Pathol 1984;15: 839–852
5. Fukayama M, Nihei Z, Takizawa T et al. Malignant epithelioid hemangioendothelioma of the liver, spreading through the hepatic veins. Virchows Arch (Pathol Anat) 1984;404:275–287

6. Rojter S, Villamil FG, Petrovic LM et al. Malignant vascular tumors of the liver presenting as liver failure and portal hypertension. Liver Transplant Surg 1995;1:156–161
7. Dean PJ, Haggitt RC, O'Hara CJ. Malignant epithelioid hemangioendothelioma of the liver in young women: relationship to oral contraceptive use. Am J Surg Pathol 1985; 9:695–704
8. Cobden I, Johri S, Terry G et al. Hepatic epithelioid haemangioendothelioma: difficult name, difficult diagnosis? Postgrad Med J 1988;64:128–131
9. Terg R, Bruguera M, Campo E et al. Epithelioid hemangioendothelioma of the liver: a report of two cases. Liver 1988; 8:105–110
10. Scoazec JY, Lamy P, Degott C et al. Epithelioid hemangioendothelioma of the liver: diagnostic features and role of liver transplantation. Gastroenterology 1988;94:1447–1453
11. Dietze O, Davies SE, Williams R, Portmann B. Malignant epithelioid haemangioendothelioma of the liver: a clinicopathological and histochemical study of 12 cases. Histopathology 1989;15:225–237
12. Bancel B, Patricot LM, Caillon P et al. Hémangioendothéliome épithélioide hépatique. Un cas avec transplantation hépatique. Revue de al littérature. Ann Pathol 1993;13: 23–28
13. Kawabe T, Tagawa K, Unuma T et al. Hepatic epithelioid hemangioendothelioma in a young female. Dig Dis Sci 1987;32:1422–1427
14. Miller WJ, Dodd GD III, Federle MP, Baron RL. Epithelioid hemangioendothelioma of the liver: imaging findings with pathologic correlation. AJR 1992;159:53–57
15. Furui S, Itai Y, Ohtomo K et al. Hepatic epithelioid hemangioendothelioma: report of 5 cases. Radiology 1989;171: 63–68
16. Terada T, Nakanuma Y, Hoso M et al. Hepatic epithelioid hemangioendothelioma in primary biliary cirrhosis. Gastroenterology 1989;97:810–812(letter)
17. Marino IR, Todo S, Tzakis AG et al. Treatment of hepatic epithelioid hemangioendothelioma with liver transplantation. Cancer 1988;62:2079–2084
18. Kelleher MB, Iwatsuki S, Sheahan DG. Epithelioid hemangioendothelioma of liver: clinicopathologic correlation of 10 cases treated by orthotopic liver transplantation. Am J Surg Pathol 1989;13:999–1008
19. Yokoyama T, Todo S, Iwatsuki S, Starzl TE. Liver transplantation in the treatment of primary liver cancer. Hepato-Gastroenterology 1990;37:188–193
20. Holley MP, Cuschieri A. Epithelioid hemangioendothelioma of the liver: objective response in hepatic intra-arterial 5-FU. Eur J Surg Oncol 1987;15:73–78
21. Dail DH, Liebow AA, Gmelich JT et al. Intravascular, bronchiolar, and alveolar tumor of the lung: an analysis of twenty cases of a peculiar sclerosing endothelial tumor. Cancer 1983;51:452–464
22. Weiss SW, Enzinger FM. Epithelioid hemangioendothelioma: a vascular tumor often mistaken for a carcinoma. Cancer 1982;50:970–981
23. Ellis GL, Kratichvil FJ. Epithelioid hemangioendothelioma of the head and neck: a clinicopathologic report of twelve cases. Oral Surg Oral Med Oral Pathol 1986;61:61–68
24. Weiss SW, Ishak KG, Dail DH et al. Epithelioid hemangioendothelioma and related lesions. Diagn Histopathol 1986; 3:259–287
25. Gelin M, Van de Stadt J, Rickaert F et al. Epithelioid hemangioendothelioma of the liver following contact with vinyl chloride. J Hepatol 1989;8:99–106
26. Anthony PP, Ramani P. Endothelial markers in malignant vascular tumors of the liver: superiority of QB-END/10 over von Willebrand factor and *Ulex europaeus* agglutinin 1. J Clin Pathol 1991;44:29–32
27. Miettinen M, Lindenmayer E, Chaubal A. Endothelial cell markers CD31, CD34, and BNH9 antibody in H- and Y-antigens: evaluation of their specificity and sensitivity in the diagnosis of vascular tumors and comparison with von Willebrand factor. Mod Pathol 1994;7:82–90
28. Anonymous. Angiosarcoma of the liver: a growing problem? BMJ 1981;282:504–505
29. Locker GY, Doroshow JH, Zwelling LA, Chabner BA. The clinical features of hepatic angiosarcoma: a report of four cases and a review of the English literature. Medicine 1979; 58:48–64
30. Kirchner SG, Heller RM, Kasselberg AG, Greene HL. Infantile hemangioendothelioma with subsequent malignant degeneration. Pediatr Radiol 1981;11:42–45
31. Strate SM, Ruthledge JC, Weinberg AG. Delayed development of angiosarcoma in multinodular infantile hepatic hemangioendothelioma. Arch Pathol Lab Med 1984;108: 943–944
32. Noronha R, Gonzalez-Crussi F. Hepatic angiosarcoma in childhood: a case report and review of the literature. Am J Surg Pathol 1984;8:863–871
33. Alt B, Hafez GR, Trigg M. Angiosarcoma of the liver and spleen in an infant. Pediatr Pathol 1985;4:331–339
34. Selby DM, Stocker JT, Ishak KG. Angiosarcoma of the liver in childhood: a clinicopathologic and follow-up study of 10 cases. Pediatr Pathol 1992;12:485–498
35. Dehner LP, Ishak KG. Vascular tumors of the liver in infants and children. Arch Pathol Lab Med 1971;92:101–111
36. Falk H, Thomas LB, Popper H, Ishak KG. Hepatic angiosarcoma associated with androgenic-anabolic steroids. Lancet 1979;2:1120–1123
37. Falk H, Hervert JT, Edmonds L et al. Review of four cases of childhood hepatic angiosarcoma—elevated environmental arsenic exposure in one case. Cancer 1981;47:382–391
38. Bertrand L, Puyeo JM, Pages A et al. Hemangiosarcoma du foie secondaire à un angiome caverneux calcifié: Mort en coagulopathie de consommation. Ann Gastroenterol Hepatol 1980;18:19–27
39. Ishak KG. Mesenchymal tumors of the liver. In Okuda K Peters RL (eds): Hepatocellular Carcinoma. John Wiley, New York, 1976, pp. 247–307
40. Smith PM, Crossley IR, Williams DMJ. Portal hypertension in vinyl-chloride production workers. Lancet 1976;2: 602–604
41. Blendis LM, Smith PM, Laurie BW et al. Portal hyperten-

sion in vinyl chloride monomer workers: a hemodynamic study. Gastroenterology 1978;75:206–211

42. Truell JE, Peck SD, Reiquam CW. Hemangiosarcoma of the liver complicated by disseminated intravascular coagulation: a case report. Gastroenterology 1973;65:936–942
43. Levy DW, Rindsberg S, Friedman AC et al. Thorotrast-induced hepatosplenic neoplasia: CT identification. AJR 1986;146:997–1004
44. Mahony B, Jeffrey RB, Federle MP. Spontaneous rupture of hepatic and splenic angiosarcoma demonstrated by CT. AJR 1982;138:965–966
45. Van Kaick G, Siegert A, Luhrs H, Lieberman D. Der Beitrag der Computertomographic zur Quantifizierung der Thorotrastose und zur thorotrastinduzierter Lebertumoren. Radiologe 1986;26:123–128
46. White PG, Adams H, Smith PM. The computed tomographic appearances of angiosarcoma of the liver. Clin Radiol 1993;48:321–325
47. Levy DW, Rindsberg S, Friedman AC et al. Thorotrast-induced hepatosplenic neoplasia: CT identification. AJR 1986;146:997–1004
48. Dannaher CL, Tamburro CL, Yam LT. Occupational carcinogenesis: the Louisville experience with vinyl chloride-associated hepatic angiosarcoma. Am J Med 1981;70: 279–287
49. Winberg CD, Ranchod M. Thorotrast induced hepatic cholangiocarcinoma and angiosarcoma. Hum Pathol 1979; 10:108–112
50. Wegener K, Leipoz-Angermuller S. Double tumours of the liver following intravenous Thorotrast injection: patho-anatomic report on two cases. Virchows Arch (Pathol Anat) 1979;382:63–71
51. Kojiro M, Kawano Y, Kawasaki H et al. Thorotrast induced hepatic angiosarcoma, and combined hepatocellular and cholangiocarcinoma in a single patient. Cancer 1982;49: 2161–2164
52. Skai K, Shiina M, Ishihara N, Kato Y. Thorotrast-induced multiple primary malignant tumors of the liver—cholangiocarcinoma and malignant hemangioendothelioma. Jpn J Clin Oncol 1984;14:411–416
53. Jansen TLTA, Meijer JWR, Kesselring FOHW. Synchronous hepatic tumors 60 years after diagnostic thorotrast use. Eur J Gastroenterol Hepatol 1992;4:753–755
54. Pialat JM, Pasquier B, Pahn M, Kopp N. Pathologie hepatique du chlorure de vinyle monomere (CVM): Huit observations anatome-cliniques personnelles. Arch Anat Cytopathol 1979;27:361–375
55. Delore FC. Association d'un angiosarcome du foie et d'un hepatome, chez un ouvrier du chlorure de vinyle. Ann Anat Pathol 1978;23:105–113
56. Fortwengler HP, Jones D, Espinosa E, Tamburro CL. Evidence for endothelial cell origin of vinyl chloride-induced hepatic angiosarcoma. Gastroenterology 1981;80: 1415–1419
57. Manning JT, Ordonez NG, Barton JH. Endothelial cell origin of thorium oxide-induced angiosarcoma of liver. Arch Pathol Lab Med 1983;107:456–458
58. Kojiro M, Nakashima T, Ito Y et al. Thorium dioxide related angiosarcoma of the liver: pathomorphologic study of 29 autopsy cases. Arch Pathol Lab Med 1985;109:853–857
59. Miettinen M, Holhofer H, Lehto V-P. *Ulex euopaeus* 1 lectin as a marker for tumors derived from endothelial cells. Am J Clin Pathol 1983;79:32–36
60. Telles NC, Thomas LB, Popper H et al. Evolution of Thorotrast-induced hepatic angiosarcomas. Environ Res 1979;18:74–78
61. Thomas LB, Popper H, Berk PD et al. Vinyl-chloride induced liver disease. From idiopathic portal hypertension (Banti's syndrome) to angiosarcomas. N Engl J Med 1975; 292:17–22
62. Berk PD, Martin JF, Young RS. Vinyl chloride-associated liver disease. Ann Intern Med 1976;84:717–731
63. Popper H, Thomas LB, Telles NC et al. Development of hepatic angiosarcoma induced by vinyl chloride, Thorotrast and arsenic: comparison with cases of unknown etiology. Am J Pathol 1978;92:349–376
64. Tamburro CH, Makk L, Popper H. Early hepatic histologic alterations among chemical (vinyl monomer) workers. Hepatology 1984;4:413–418
65. Popper H, Maltoni C, Selikoff IJ. Vinyl chloride-induced hepatic lesions in man and rodents. A comparison. Liver 1980;1:7–20
66. Gedigk P, Muller R, Bechtelsheimer H. Morphology of liver damage among polyvinyl chloride production workers: a report of 51 cases. Ann NY Acad Sci 1975;245:278–285
67. Schattenberg PJ, Totovic V, Gedigk P, Marsteller HJ. Die Ultrastruktur der Leberschadigung bei der chronischen Vinylchlorid-Intoxikation. Virchows Arch (Pathol Anat) 1977;373:233–247
68. Terzaki JH, Sommers SC, Snyder RW, Sabbath M. X-ray microanalysis of hepatic thorium depositions. Arch Pathol 1974;98:241–242
69. Bowen JH, Woodward BH, Mossler JA et al. Energy dispersive x-ray detection of thorium dioxide. Arch Pathol Lab Med 1980;104:459–461
70. Irie H, Mori W. Long term effects of thorium dioxide (Thorotrast) administration on human liver: ultrastructural localization of thorium dioxide in human liver by analytical electron microscopy. Acta Pathol Jpn 1984;34:221–228
71. Ishak KG. Applications of scanning electron microscopy to the study of liver disease. Prog Liver Dis 1986;8:1–32
72. Hollstein M, Marion MJ, Lehman T et al. *p53* mutations at A:T base pairs in angiosarcoma of vinyl chloride-exposed factory workers. Carcinogenesis 1994;15:1–3
73. Soini Y, Welsh JA, Ishak KG, Bennett WP. *p53* mutations in primary hepatic angiosarcoma not associated with vinyl chloride exposure. Carcinogenesis 1995;16:2879–2881
74. Hashimoto M, Ohsawa M, Ohnishi A et al. Expression of vascular endothelial growth factor and its receptor in RNA in angiosarcoma. Lab Invest 1995;73:859–863
75. Bergfeld WF, Zemtsov A, Lang RS. Differentiation between AIDS-related and non-AIDS-related Kaposi's sarcoma. Clev Clin J Med 1987;54:315–319
76. Guarda LA, Luna MA, Smith IL. Acquired immune deficiency syndrome: postmortem findings. Am J Clin Pathol 1984;81:549–557

77. Niedt G, Schinella RA. Acquired immunodeficiency syndrome: clinicopathologic study of 56 autopsies. Arch Pathol Lab Med 1985;109:727–734
78. Antinori S, Ridolfo Al, Esposito R et al. Liver involvement in AIDS-associated malignancies. J Hepatol 1994;21: 1145–1146
79. Ioachim HL, Adsay V, Giancotti FR et al. Kaposi's sarcoma of internal organs. Cancer 1995;75:1376–1385
80. Fukunaga M, Silverberg SG. Hyaline globules in Kaposi's sarcoma: a light microscopic and immunohistochemical study. Mod Pathol 1991;4:187–190
81. Regezi JA, MacPhail LA, Daniels TE et al. Human immunodeficiency virus-associated oral Kaposi's sarcoma: a heterogeneous cell population dominated by spindle-shaped endothelial cells. Am J Pathol 1993;143:240–249
82. Zhang J-M, Bachmann S, Hemmer C et al. Vascular origin of Kaposi's sarcoma: expression of leukocyte adhesion molecule-1, thrombomodulin, and tissue factor. Am J Pathol 1994;145:51–59
83. Huang YQ, Li JJ, Kaplan MH et al. Human herpes virus-like nuclei acid in various forms of Kaposi's sarcoma. Lancet 1995;345:759–762
84. Moore PS, Chang Y. Detection of herpes virus-like DNA sequences in Kaposi's sarcoma in patients with and those without HIV infection. N Engl J Med 1995;332:1181–1185
85. Whitby D, Howard MR, Tenant-Flowers M et al. Detection of Kaposi's sarcoma associated herpesvirus in peripheral blood of HIV-infected individuals and progression to Kaposi's sarcoma. Lancet 1995;346:799–802
86. Jin Y-T, Tsai S-T, Yan J-J et al. Detection of Kaposi's sarcoma-associated herpesvirus-like DNA sequence in vascular lesions: a reliable diagnostic marker for Kaposi's sarcoma. Am J Clin Pathol 1996;105:360–363
87. Wang C-Y, Schroeter AL, Su WPD. Acquired immunodeficiency syndrome-related Kaposi's sarcoma. Mayo Clin Proc 1995;70:869–879
88. Davis GL, Kissane JM, Ishak KG. Embryonal rhabdomyosarcoma (sarcoma botryoides) of the biliary tree. Cancer 1969;24:485–491
89. Mori H, Matsubara N, Fuji M. Alpha-fetoprotein producing rhabdomyosarcoma of the adult liver. Acta Pathol Jpn 1979;29:333–342
90. Lack EE, Perez-Atayada AR, Schuster SR. Botryoid rhabdomyosarcoma of the biliary tract: report of five cases with ultrastructural observations and literature review. Am J Surg Pathol 1981;5:643–652
91. Ruymann FB, Raney B, Crist WM. Rhabdomyosarcoma of the biliary tree in childhood: a report from the Intergroup Rhabdomyosarcoma Study. Cancer 1985;56:575–581
92. Aldabagh SM, Shibata CS, Taxy JB. Rhabdomyosarcoma of the common bile duct in an adult. Arch Pathol Lab Med 1986;110:547–550
93. Burrig K-F, Knauers S. Hepatic rhabdomyosarcoma in adulthood. Case report and literature review. Pathology 1994;15:54–57
94. Morimoto H, Takade Y, Akita T. A resected case of the collision tumor of hepatocellular carcinoma and primary liver rhabdomyosarcoma. J Jpn Surg Soc 1986;87:456–463
95. Cannon PM, Legge DA, O'Donnell B. The use of percutaneous transhepatic cholangiography in a case of embryonal rhabdomyosarcoma. Br Radiol 1979;52:326–327
96. d'Amore ESG, Tollot M, Stracca-Pansa V et al. Therapy associated differentiation in rhabdomyosarcomas. Mod Pathol 1994;7:69–75
97. Parham DM. Immunohistochemistry of childhood sarcomas: old and new markers. Mod Pathol 1993;6:133–138
98. Pinkerton R, Pritchard-Jones K, Carter R, Cooper S. Small-round-cell tumours of childhood. Lancet 1994;344: 725–729
99. Stocker JT, Ishak KG. Undifferentiated embryonal sarcoma of the liver. Cancer 1978;42:336–348
100. Stanley RJ, Dehner LP, Hesker AE. Primary malignant mesenchymal tumors (mesenchymoma) of the liver in childhood. Cancer 1973;32:973–984
101. Cuzzutto C, De Bernardi B, Comelli A, Soave F. Malignant mesenchymoma of the liver in children: a clinicopathologic and ultrastructural study. Hum Pathol 1981;12:481–485
102. Lagace R, Delage C, Robert J. Le mesenchymome primitif du foie: etude ultrastructural. Ann Anat Pathol 1974;19: 275–286
103. Gonzalez-Crussi F. Undifferentiated (embryonal) liver sarcoma of childhood: evidence of leiomyoblastic differentiation. Pediatr Pathol 183;1:281–290
104. Gallivan MVE, Lack EE, Chun B, Ishak KG. Undifferentiated ("embryonal") sarcoma of the liver: ultrastructure of a case presenting as a primary intracardiac tumor. Pediatr Pathol 1983;1:291–300
105. Pieterse AS, Smith M, Smith LA, Smith P. Embryonal (undifferentiated) sarcoma of the liver: fine-needle aspiration cytology and ultrastructural findings. Arch Pathol Lab Med 1985;109:677–680
106. Tanner AR, Bolton PM, Powell LW. Primary sarcoma of the liver: report of a case with excellent response to hepatic artery ligation and infusion chemotherapy. Gastroenterology 1978;74:121–123
107. McFadden DW, Kelley DJ, Sigmund DA et al. Embryonal sarcoma of the liver in an adult treated with chemotherapy, radiation therapy, and hepatic lobectomy. Cancer 1992;69: 39–44
108. Reichel C, Fehske W, Fisher HP, Hartlapp JH. Undifferentiated (embryonal) sarcoma of the liver in an adult patient with metastasis of the heart and brain. Clin Invest 1994; 72:209–212
109. Ros PR, Olmstead WW, Dachman AH et al. Undifferentiated (embryonal) sarcoma of the liver: radiologic-pathologic correlation. Radiology 1986;161:141–145
110. Esposito R, Pollavini G, de Lalla F. A case of primary undifferentiated sarcoma of the liver diagnosed by peritoneoscopy and guided biopsy. Endoscopy 1976;8:108–110
111. Smithson WA, Telander RL, Carney JA. Mesenchymoma of the liver in childhood: five-year survival after combined modality treatment. J Pediatr Surg 1982;17:70–72
112. Harris MB, Shen D, Weiner MA. Treatment of primary undifferentiated sarcoma of the liver with surgery and chemotherapy. Cancer 1984;54:2859–2862
113. Horowitz ME, Etcubanas E, Webber BL et al. Hepatic undif-

ferentiated (embryonal) sarcoma and rhabdomyosarcoma in children: results of therapy. Cancer 1987;59:396–402

114. Ware R, Friedman HS, Filston HC et al. Childhood hepatic mesenchymoma: successful treatment with surgery and multiple agent chemotherapy. Med Pediatr Oncol 1988;16: 62–65
115. Leuscher I, Schmidt D, Harms D. Undifferentiated sarcoma of the liver in childhood: morphology, flow cytometry, and literature review. Hum Pathol 1990;21:68–76
116. Walker NI, Horn MJ, Strong RW et al. Undifferentiated (embryonal) sarcoma of the liver: pathologic findings and long-term survival after complete surgical resection. Cancer 1992;69:52–59
117. Kadomatsu K, Nakagewara A, Zaizen Y et al. Undifferentiated (embryonal) sarcoma of the liver: report of three cases. Jpn J Surg 1992;22:451–455
118. Urban CE, Mache CJ, Schwinger W et al. Undifferentiated (embryonal) sarcoma of the liver in childhood: successful combined-modality therapy in four patients. Cancer 1993; 72:2511–2516
119. Abramowsky CR, Cebelin M, Choudhury A, Izant RJ. Undifferentiated (embryonal) sarcoma of the liver with alpha-1-antitrypsin deposits: immunohistochemical and ultrastructural studies. Cancer 1980;45:3108–3113
120. Ellis IO, Cotton RE. Primary malignant mesenchymal tumour of the liver in an elderly female. Histopathology 1983; 7:113–121
121. Keating S, Taylor GP. Undifferentiated (embryonal) sarcoma of the liver: ultrastructural and immunohistochemical similarities with malignant fibrous histiocytoma. Hum Pathol 1985;16:693–699
122. Lack EE, Schloo BL, Azumi N et al. Undifferentiated (embryonal) sarcoma of the liver. Am J Surg Pathol 1991;15: 1–16
123. Chou P, Mangkornkanok M, Gonzalez-Crussi F. Undifferentiated (embryonal) sarcoma of the liver: ultrastructure, immunohistochemistry and DNA ploidy analysis of the two cases. Pediatr Pathol 1990;10:549–562
124. Vetter D, Bellocq JP, Amaral D et al. Sarcomes undifférenciés (ou embryonnaires) hépatiques: problémes diagnostiques et thérapeutiques à propos d'un rhabdomyosarcome botryoide. Gastroenterol Clin Biol 1989;13:98–103
125. Aoyama C, Hachitanda Y, Sato JK et al. Undifferentiated (embryonal) sarcoma of the liver. Am J Surg Pathol 1991; 15:615–634
126. Parham DM, Kelly DR, Donnelly WH, Douglass EC. Immunohistochemical and ultrastructural spectrum of hepatic sarcomas of childhood: evidence for a common histogenesis. Mod Pathol 1991;4:648–653
127. Blattner WA, Henson DE, Young RC, Fraumeni JF. Malignant mesenchymoma and birth defects: prenatal exposure to phenytoin. JAMA 1977;238:334–335
128. de Chadarevian J-P, Pawel BR, Faerber EN, Weintraub WH. Undifferentiated (embryonal) sarcoma arising in conjunction with mesenchymal hamartoma of the liver. Mod Pathol 1994;7:490–493
129. Snapper I, Schraft WC, Ginsberg DM. Severe hypoglycemia due to fibrosarcoma of the liver. Maendschr Kindergenees 1964;32:337–347
130. Ojima A, Sugiyama T, Takeda J. Six cases of rare malignant tumors of the liver. Acta Pathol Jpn 1964;14:95–102
131. Totzke HA, Hutcheson JB. Primary fibrosarcoma of the liver. South Med J 1965;58: 236–238
132. Balouet G, Destombes P. A propos de quelques tumeurs mesenchymateuses hepatiques d'apparence primitive. Ann Anat Pathol 1967;12:273–286
133. Cavallo T, Lichewitz B, Rozov T. Primary fibrosarcoma of the liver: report of a case. Rev Hosp Clin Med Sao Paulo 1968;23:44–69
134. Smith D, Rele SR. A case of primary fibrosarcoma of the liver. Postgrad Med J 1972; 48:62–63
135. Walter VE, Bodner E, Lederer B. Primares fibrosarkom der Leber. Wein Klin Wochenschr 1972;84:808–810
136. Alrenga DP. Primary fibrosarcoma of the liver: case report and review of the literature. Cancer 1974;36:446–449
137. Bodker A, Boiesen PT. A primary fibrosarcoma of the liver. Hepatogastroenterology 1981;28:218–220
138. Gen E, Kusuyama Y, Saito K et al. Primary fibrosarcoma of the liver with hypoglycemia. Acta Pathol Jpn 1983;33: 177–182
139. Nakahama M, Takanashi R, Yamazaki I, Machinami R. Primary fibrosarcoma of the liver. Acta Pathol Jpn 1989; 39:814–820
140. Danhalve O, Ninane J, Sokal E et al. Hepatic localization of a fibrosarcoma in a child with a liver transplant. J Pediatr 1992;120:434–437
141. Hall J, Scheffer C, Tseng G et al. Collagen types in fibrosarcoma: absence of type III collagen in reticulin. Hum Pathol 1995;16:439–446
142. Gates LK, Cameron AJ, Nagorney DM et al. Primary leiomyosarcoma of the liver mimicking liver abscess. Am J Gastroenterol 1995;90:649–652
143. Taylor RW, Sylwestrowicz T, Kossakowska AR et al. Leiomyosarcoma of the inferior vena cava. Liver 1987;7: 201–205
144. Huguet C, Harb J, Gavelli A, Riberi A. Léiomyosarcome de la veine cave inférieure étendu au foie: résection compléte avec reconstruction veineuse. Gastroenterol Clin Biol 1992;16:714–717
145. Ross JS, Del Rosario A, Bui HX et al. Primary hepatic leiomyosarcoma in a child with the acquired immunodeficiency syndrome. Hum Pathol 1992;23:69–72
146. van Hoeven KH, Factor SM, Kress Y, Woodruff JM. Visceral myogenic tumors: a manifestation of HIV infection in children. Am J Surg Pathol 1991;17:1176–1181
147. Prévot S, Néris J, de Saint Maur PP. Detection of Epstein Barr virus in an hepatic leiomyomatous neoplasm in an adult human immunodeficiency virus 1-infected patient. Virchows Arch 1994;425:321–325
148. McLain KL, Leach CT, Jenson HB et al. Association of Epstein-Barr virus with leiomyosarcomas in young people with AIDS. N Engl J Med 1995;332:12–18
149. Penn I. Posttransplantation de novo tumors in liver allograft recipients. Liver Transpl Surg 1996;2:52–59
150. Tomaszewski M-M, Kuenster T, Hartman K. Leiomyosarcoma of ligamentum teres of liver: case report. Pediatr Pathol 1986;5:147–156

151. Miettinen M. Immunoreactivity for cytokeratin and epithelial membrane antigen in leiomyosarcoma. Arch Pathol Lab Med 1988;112:637–640
152. Parham DM, Reynolds AB, Webber BL. Use of monoclonal antibody IHI, anticortactin, to distinguish normal and neoplastic smooth muscle cells: comparison with anti-smooth muscle actin and antimuscle-specific actin. Hum Pathol 1995;26:776–783
153. Sreekantaiah C, Davis JR, Sandberg AA. Chromosomal abnormalities in leiomyosarcomas. Am J Pathol 1993;142: 293–305
154. Shurbaji MS, Olson JL, Kuhajda FP. Thorotrast-associated hepatic leiomyosarcoma and cholangiocarcinoma in a single patient. Hum Pathol 1987;18:524–526
155. Alberti-Flor JJ, O'Hara MF, Weaver F et al. Malignant fibrous histiocytoma of the liver. Gastroenterology 1985;89: 890–893
156. Conran RM, Stocker JT. Malignant fibrous histiocytoma of the liver. A case report. Am J Gastroenterol 1985;80: 813–815
157. Fukayama M, Koike M. Malignant fibrous histiocytoma arising in the liver. Arch Pathol Lab Med 1986;110: 203–206
158. Arends JW, Willebrand D, Blaauw AMM, Bosman FT. Primary malignant fibrous histiocytoma of the liver: a case report with immunocytochemical observations. Histopathology 1987;11:427–431
159. Katsuda S, Kawahara E, Matsui Y et al. Malignant fibrous histiocytoma of the liver: a case report and review of the literature. Am J Gastroenterol 1988;83:1278–1282
160. Hamasaki K, Minura H, Sato D et al. Malignant fibrous histiocytoma of the liver: a case report. Gastroenterol Jpn 1991;26:666–673
161. McGrady BJ, Mirakhur MM. Recurrent malignant fibrous histiocytoma of the liver. Histopathology 1992;21:290–293
162. Miettinen M, Soini Y. Malignant fibrous histiocytoma: heterogeneous patterns of intermediate filament proteins by immunohistochemistry. Arch Pathol Lab Med 1989;113: 1363–1366
163. Roholl PJM, Elbers HR, Prinsen I et al. Distribution of actin isoforms in sarcomas: an immunohistochemical study. Hum Pathol 1990;21:1269–1274
164. Brooks JS. The significance of double phenotypic patterns and differentiation in human sarcomas: a new model of mesenchymal differentation. Am J Pathol 1986;125: 113–123
165. Takeya M, Yamashiro S, Yoshimura T, Takahashi K. Immunophenotypic and immunoelectron microscopic characterization of major constituent cells in malignant fibrous histiocytoma using human cell lines and their transplanted tumors in immunodeficient mice. Lab Invest 1995;72: 679–688
166. Sumiyoshi A, Nicho Y. Primary osteogenic sarcomas of the liver. Acta Pathol Jpn 1971; 21:305–312
167. von Hochstetter AR, Hattenschwiler J, Vogt M. Primary osteosarcoma of the liver. Cancer 1987;60:2312–2317
168. Nakabayashi H, Aiba H, Sakuma S et al. An autopsy case of primary malignant mesenchymoma of the liver with various tissue components. Acta Hepatol Jpn 1985;26:369–375
169. Velilla J, Soler G, Munoz JR et al. Mesenquimoma maligno primitivo hepatico. Gastroenterol Hepatol 1986;9:497–500
170. Young SJ. Primary malignant neurilemoma (Schwannoma) of the liver in a case of neurofibromatosis. J Pathol 1975; 117:151–153
171. Lederman SM, Martin EC, Laffey KT, Lefkowitch JH. Hepatic neurofibromatosis, malignant Schwannoma, and angiosarcoma in von Recklinghausen's disease. Gastroenterology 1987;92:234–239
172. Jaffe ES. Malignant lymphomas: pathology of hepatic involvement. Semin Liver Dis 1987;7:257–68
173. Anthony PP, Sarsfield P, Clarke T. Primary lymphoma of the liver: clinical and pathological features of 10 patients. J Clin Pathol 1990;43:1007–1013
174. Zafrani ES, Gaulard P. Primary lymphoma of the liver. Liver 1993;13:57–61
175. Scoazec JY, Degott C, Brousse N et al. Non-Hodgkin's lymphoma presenting as a primary tumor of the liver: presentation, diagnosis and outcome in eight patients. Hepatology 1991;13:870–875
176. Lei KI-K, Chow JH-S, Johnson PJ. Aggressive primary hepatic lymphoma in Chinese patients. Cancer 1995;76: 1336–1343
177. Khan SM, Cottrell BJ, Milward-Sadler GH, Wright DH T-cell-rich B-cell lymphoma presenting as liver disease. Histopathology 1993;23:217–224
178. Gaulard P, Zafrani ES, Mavier P et al. Peripheral T-cell lymphoma presenting as predominant liver disease: a report of three cases. Hepatology 1986;6:864–868
179. Mastovich S, Ratech H, Ware RE et al. Hepatosplenic T-cell lymphoma: an unusual case of a T-cell lymphoma with a blast-like terminal transformation. Hum Pathol 1994;25: 102–108
180. Krishnan J, Goodman Z, Frizzera G. Primary hepatic sinusoidal presentation of malignant T cell lymphoma. Mod Pathol 1992;5:81(abstr)
181. Wong KF, Chan JKC, Matutes E et al. Hepatosplenic T-cell lymphoma: a distinctive aggressive lymphoma type. Am J Surg Pathol 1995;19:716–718
182. Dommann-Scherrer CC, Kurer SB, Zimmermann DR et al. Occult hepatosplenic T-lymphoma: value of genotypic analysis in the differential diagnosis. Virchows Arch 1995; 426:629–634
183. Trudel M, Aramendi T, Caplan S. Large-cell lymphoma presenting with hepatic sinusoidal infiltration. Arch Pathol Lab Med 1991;115:821–824
184. Caccamo D, Perez NK, Marchevsky A. Primary lymphoma of the liver in the acquired immunodeficiency syndrome. Arch Pathol Lab Med 1986;110:553–558
185. Lisker-Melman M, Pittaluga S et al. Primary lymphoma of the liver in a patient with acquired immune deficiency syndrome and chronic hepatitis B. Am J Gastroenterol 1989;84:1445–1448
186. Rustgi VK. Epstein-Barr viral infection and posttransplantation lymphoproliferative disorders. Liver Transplant Surg 1995;1:100–108

187. Cesarman E, Chang Y, Moore PS et al. Kaposi's sarcoma-associated herpesvirus-like DNA sequences in AIDS-related body-cavity-based lymphomas. N Engl J Med 1995; 332:1186–1191

188. Miller ST, Wollner N, Meters PA et al. Primary hepatic or hepatosplenic non-Hodgkin's lymphoma in children. Cancer 1983;52:2285–2288

189. Osborne BM, Butler JJ, Guarda LA. Primary lymphoma of the liver: ten cases and a review of the literature. Cancer 1985;56:2902–2910

190. Redondo C, Martin L, Cano AL et al. Primary lymphoma of the liver treated with hepatic lobectomy and chemotherapy. Cancer 1987;60:736–740

191. Ryan J, Strauss DJ, Lange C et al. Primary lymphoma of the liver. Cancer 1988;61:370–375

192. Sondenaa K, Stadaas JO. Primary non-Hodgkin's lymphoma treated with liver resection. Acta Chir Scand 1988; 154:681–682

193. Pescovitz MD, Snover DC, Orchard P et al. Primary hepatic lymphoma in an adolescent treated with hepatic lobectomy and chemotherapy. Cancer 1990;65:2222–2226

194. Pickren JW, Tsukada Y, Lane WW. Liver metastasis: analysis of autopsy data. In Weiss L, Gilbert HA (eds): Liver Metastasis. Hall Medical Publishers, Boston, 1982, pp. 2–18

195. Harrison HB, Middleton HM, Crosby JH, Dasher MN. Fulminant hepatic failure: an unusual presentation of metastatic liver disease. Gastroenterology 1981;80:820–825

196. Bouloux PMG, Scott RJ, Goligher JE, Kindell C. Fulminant hepatic failure secondary to diffuse liver infiltration by melanoma. JR Soc Med 1986;79:302–303

197. Green ST, Dutton AH, Bouchier IAD. Occult malignancy presenting as acute fulminant hepatic failure. Scott Med J 1986;31:113–114

198. Trimble MS, Ghent CN, Grant DR, McLean CA. Metastatic breast cancer presenting as fulminant hepatic failure: a case report and literature review. Can J Gastroenterol 1989;3:149–152

199. Ghosh P, Fox IJ, Rader AM, Sorrell MF. Fulminant hepatic failure as the initial manifestation of non-Hodgkin's lymphoma. Am J Gastroenterol 1995;90:2207–2209

200. McArthur MS, Teergarden DK. Metastatic melanoma presenting as obstructive jaundice with hemobilia. Am J Surg 1983;145:830–832

201. Cooperman AM, Weiland LH, Welch JS. Massive bleeding from a ruptured metastatic hepatic melanoma treated by hepatic lobectomy. Mayo Clin Proc 1976;51:167–170

202. Craig JR, Peters RL, Edmondson HA. Tumors of the Liver and Intrahepatic Bile Ducts. Armed Forces Institute of Pathology, Washington, DC, 1989, pp. 123–255

203. Dent GA, Feldman JA. Pseudocystic liver metastases in patients with carcinoid tumors: report of three cases. Am J Clin Pathol 1984;82:275–279

204. Thompson NW, Eckhauser FE, Vinik AI et al. Cystic neuroendocrine neoplasms of the pancreas and liver. Ann Surg 1984;199:158–164

205. Evans HL, Vassilopoulu-Sellin R. Adrenal cortical neoplasms: a study of 56 cases. Am J Clin Pathol 1996;105: 76–86

206. Moll R, Zimbelmann R, Goldschmidt MD et al. The human gene encoding cytokeratin 20 and its expression during fetal development and in gastrointestinal carcinomas. Differentiation 1993;53:75–93

207. Chaubert P, Hurliman J. Mammary origin of metastases: immunohistochemical determination. Arch Pathol Lab Med 1992;116:1181–1188

208. Goldblum JR, Appelman HD, Stromal tumors of the duodenum: a histologic and immunohistochemical study of 20 cases. Am J Surg Pathol 1995;19:71–80

209. Falk H, Telles NC, Ishak KG et al. Epidemiology of Thorotrast-induced hepatic angiosarcoma in the United States. Environ Res 1979;18:152–173

210. Da Motta CL, Da Silva Horta J, Tavares MH. Prospective epidemiological study of Thorotrast-exposed patients in Portugal. Environ Res 1979;18:152–173

211. Baxter PJ, Langlands AO, Anthony PP et al. Angiosarcoma of the liver: a marker tumour for the late effects of Thorotrast in Great Britain. Br J Cancer 1980;41:446–452

212. Van Kaick G, Muth H, Kaul A et al. Results of the German Thorotrast study. Prog Cancer Res 1984;26:253–262

213. Yamada S, Hososda S, Tateno H et al. Survey of Thorotrast-associated liver cancer in Japan J Natl Cancer Inst 1983; 70:31–35

214. Ross JM. A case illustrating the effects of prolonged action of radium. J Pathol Bacteriol 1932;35:899–912

215. Miyake S, Onoue K, Ueda M et al. Clinical studies on two cases of hepatic angiosarcoma. Acta Hepatol Jpn 1982;23: 1326–1333

216. Falk H, Creech JL, Heath CW et al. Hepatic disease among workers at a vinyl chloride polymerization plant. JAMA 1974;230:59–63

217. Forman D, Bennett B, Stafford J, Doll R. Exposure to vinyl chloride and angiosarcoma of the liver: a report of the register of cases. Br J Ind Med 1985;42:750–753

218. Roth F. The sequelae of chronic arsenic poisoning in Moselle vintners. Ger Med Mon 1957;2:211–217

219. Regelson W, Kim U, Ospina J, Holland JF. Hemangioendothelial sarcoma of the liver from chronic arsenic intoxication by Fowler's solution. Cancer 1968;21:514–522

220. Rennke H, Prat GA, Etcheverry RB et al. Hemangioendothelioma maligno del higado y arsenicismo chronica. Rev Med Chil 1971;99:1582–1586

221. Lander JJ, Stanley RJ, Sumner HW et al. Angiosarcoma of the liver associated with Fowler's solution. Gastroenterology 1975;68:1582–1586

222. Brady J, Liberatore F, Harper P et al. Angiosarcoma of the liver: an epidemiologic study. J Natl Cancer Inst 1977;59: 1383–1385

223. Falk H, Caldwell GG, Ishak KG et al. Arsenic-related hepatic angiosarcoma. Am J Ind Med 1981;2:43–50

224. Roat JW, Wald A, Mendelow H, Pataki KG. Hepatic angiosarcoma associated with short-term arsenic ingestion. Am J Med 1982;73:933–936

225. Kasper ML, Schoefield L, Strom RL, Theologides A. Hepatic angiosarcoma and bronchioloalveolar carcinoma induced by Fowler's solution. JAMA 1984; 252:3407–3408

226. Pimentel JC, Menezes AP. Liver disease in vineyard sprayers. Gastroenterology 1977;72:275–283

227. El Zayadi A, Khalil A, El Samny N et al. Hepatic angiosarcoma among Egyptian farmers exposed to pesticides. Hepato-Gastroenterology 1986;33:148–150

228. Baker HC, Paget GE, Davson J. Haemochromatosis of the liver. J Pathol Bacteriol 1956;72:173–182

229. Kwittken J, Tartow LR. Haemochromatosis and Kupffer cell sarcoma with unusual localization of iron. J Pathol Bacteriol 1966;92:571–573

230. Sussman EB, Nydick I, Gray G. Hemangioendothelial sarcoma of the liver and hemochromatosis. Arch Pathol 1974; 97:39–42

231. Nordsten M. Hemangiosarcoma hepatis associeret med brug of androgene steroider. Ugeskr Laeger 1985;147:2615–2616

232. Shi ECP, Fischer A, Crouch R, Ham JM. Possible association of angiosarcoma with oral contraceptive agents. Med J Aust 1981;1:473–474

233. Hoch-Ligeti C. Angiosarcoma of the liver associated with diethylstilbesterol. JAMA 1978;240:1510–1511

234. Daneshmend TK, Scott GL, Bradfied JWB. Angiosarcoma of liver associated with phenelzine. BMJ 1979;6:1679

20

SECTION V
DIAGNOSIS

CLINICAL AND NONIMAGING DIAGNOSIS OF HEPATOCELLULAR CARCINOMA

MICHAEL C. KEW

CLINICAL DIAGNOSIS

Far advanced hepatocellular carcinoma (HCC) usually presents with typical symptoms and physical signs. Before this late stage, however, clinical recognition is often difficult. There are a number of reasons for this. The position of the liver deep beneath the lower ribs makes the liver difficult to feel. Moreover, the tumor must reach a substantial size before it can be discerned or before it invades adjacent organs or structures. The liver's considerable functional reserves ensure that jaundice and other evidence of hepatic dysfunction do not appear until a large part of the organ has been replaced by tumor. None of the symptoms or signs attributable to HCC is pathognomonic. Finally, HCC generally spreads to distant sites late in the course of the disease. In its early stages, therefore, HCC usually runs a silent course, making diagnosis difficult at the very time that the tumor is most amenable to cure.

Ease of clinical recognition of HCC also differs between geographic regions. In countries where HCC occurs frequently, clinicians are alert to the tumor and its diverse presentations. Consequently, they recognize HCC with greater facility than do clinicians in countries where the tumor is rarely seen. Furthermore, HCC often coexists with cirrhosis,[1] and the influence that this associated disease exerts on diagnosis differs between regions of high and low (or intermediate) HCC incidence. In the latter (but also in Japan, a country of high incidence), HCC usually develops as a complication of long-standing, symptomatic cirrhosis resulting from either chronic infection with hepatitis C virus or from alcohol abuse, or both, and the patient has few if any new symptoms.[2,3] If, in addition, the tumor is small (which is often the case in the cirrhotic liver[4]), it may not be obvious in the presence of advanced cirrhosis; it may be discovered only when the liver is imaged, at the time of liver transplantation or other surgical intervention, or at necropsy. One circumstance that should alert the clinician to the possibility that HCC has developed in a cirrhotic liver is a sudden, unexplained change in the patient's condition. These changes can include abdominal pain, weight loss, ascites, liver enlargement or bruit, or hepatic failure.

In contrast, in ethnic Chinese and black African populations, which are at high risk of HCC, the accompanying cirrhosis often does not produce symptoms or is overshadowed by symptoms of the tumor.[5–8] Cirrhosis is then discovered coincidentally during the diagnostic work-up or at necropsy. HCCs are usually appreciably larger at the time of diagnosis in these populations than in those with low or intermediate incidences.[4,9] In these populations, the symptoms and signs of HCC are more florid, facilitating diagnosis.

Unusual Clinical Presentations[2]

One of the most dramatic ways in which HCC presents and one that requires early diagnosis and intervention if there is to be any chance of survival is with an "acute abdomen". This results from sudden intraperitoneal bleeding when the tumor, or the liver tissue overlying the tumor, ruptures. This is a very rare complication in countries with a low incidence of HCC[2]; it is seen more often in high incidence populations.[8–10] In sub-Saharan Africa, it is taught that until proved otherwise, acute hemoperitoneum in a black male is caused by rupture of an HCC. A superficial location of the tumor in the liver is the most important determinant of this complication. Rupture is usually spontaneous,[8–10] but it may follow blunt abdominal trauma (which need not be severe).[11] An abdominal tap yields blood, which, in the presence of an enlarged liver, strongly suggests a diagnosis of HCC, although a number of other, albeit rare, hepatic tumors can have this complication. If necessary, emergency hepatic arteriography will confirm bleeding from the liver into the peritoneal cavity.

Another unusual presentation of HCC is obstructive jaundice. This occurs in less than 10% of patients in high-incidence populations and even less often in other populations.[2,4–9] The symptoms of cholestasis overshadow or accompany other symptoms and signs. Deep jaundice is the outstanding physical finding, and hepatomegaly may be less marked than it commonly is in HCC. Obstruction can result from any of four conditions.[9] Invasion of the biliary tree by the primary tumor with propagation toward the porta hepatis obstructs the major intrahepatic bile ducts. In some instances the tumor plug reaches as far as the common hepatic duct or even the common bile duct (Fig. 20-1).[12] A primary tumor sited near the porta hepatis may compress the major intrahepatic bile ducts (Fig. 20-2), or less often malignant lymph nodes in the porta hepatis may compress the common hepatic duct. The obstruction caused in these ways is unremitting and progressive. Rarely a free-floating tumor plug in the extrahepatic biliary tree may cause intermittent jaundice, and this may be accompanied by colicky pain. Finally, obstruction occasionally results from severe hemobilia.

HCC also has a propensity to invade the hepatic venous system, causing the patient to present with features of the Budd-Chiari syndrome.[9] Tumor in the hepatic veins may propagate along the lumen to the inferior vena cava, where it causes partial or complete obstruction (Fig. 20-3). This results in the sudden appearance of severe pitting edema extending up to the inguinal region. The tumor plug in the inferior vena cava may grow up the lumen and into the right atrium or even into the right ventricle (Fig. 20-4), where it may be re-

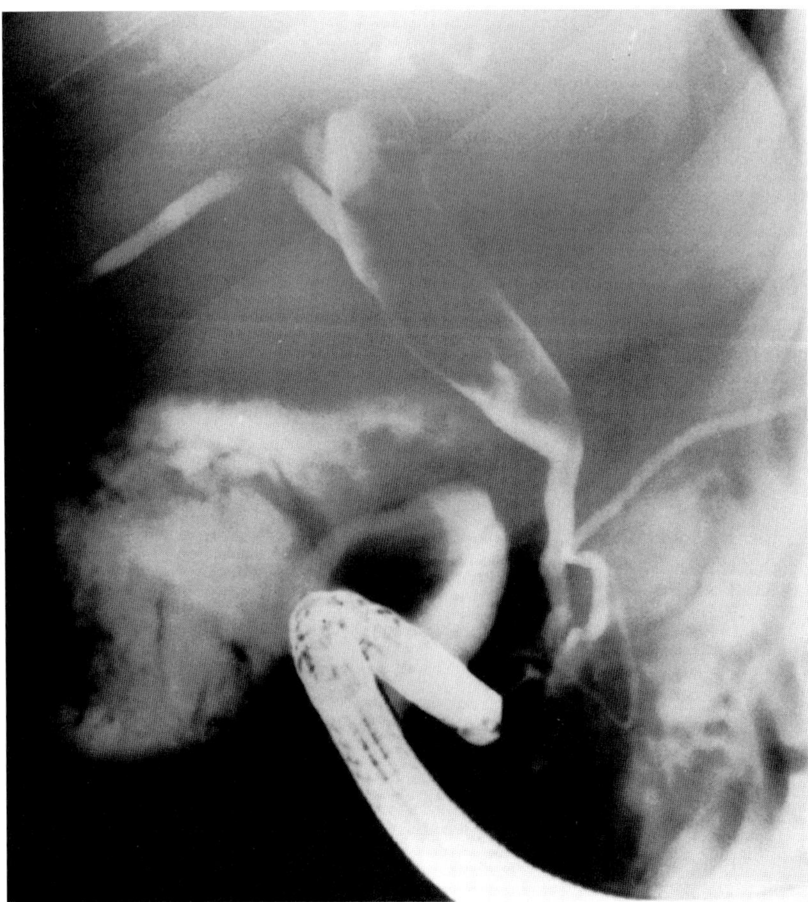

FIGURE 20-1. Endoscopic retrograde cholangiopancreatography showing the presence of HCC in the common bile duct in a patient presenting with obstructive jaundice. (From Moosa et al.,[12] with permission.)

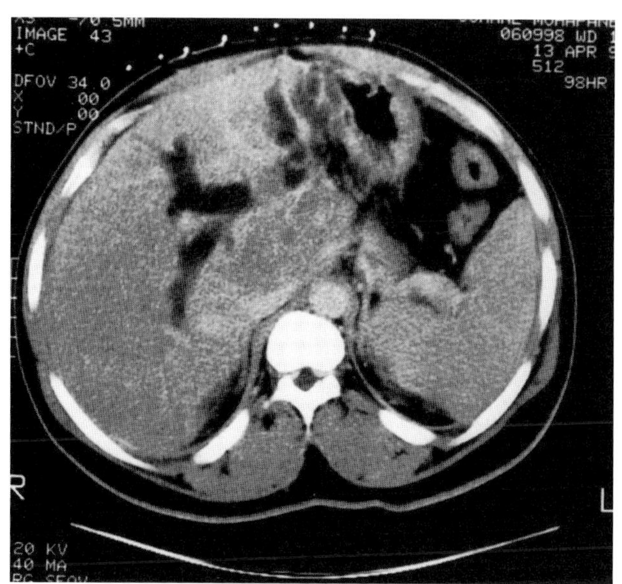

A

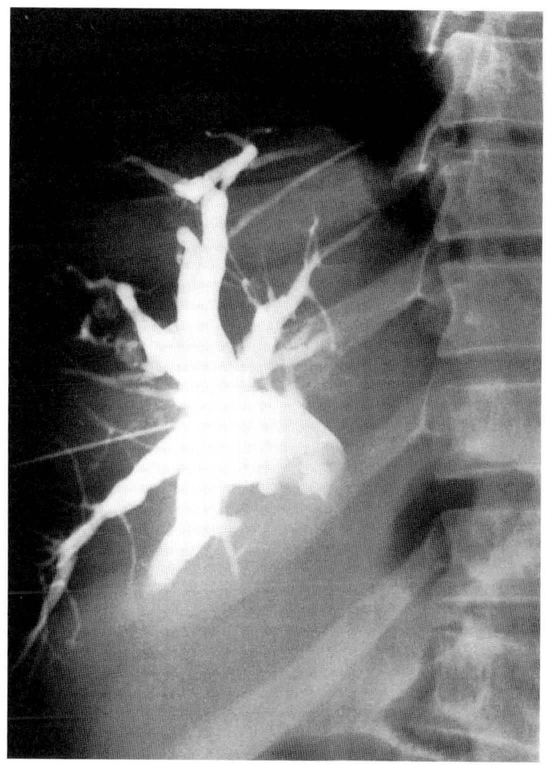
B

FIGURE 20-2. (*A*) Computed tomogram of the liver showing compression of intrahepatic bile ducts by a primary HCC located near the porta hepatis, with gross dilatation of the ducts beyond the obstruction. (*B*) Percutaneous transhepatic cholangiogram demonstrating the grossly dilated ducts and the site of obstruction.

sponsible for acute respiratory distress or sudden death. Changing right-sided cardiac murmurs due to compromise of the function of the tricuspid valve may indicate the presence of this condition. In black patients from rural southern Africa, the incidence at necropsy of invasion of the hepatic veins by HCC is 14% of all HCC patients; of the inferior vena cava, 9%; and of the right atrium, 2%.[9]

The superior vena cava may also be obstructed by HCC. A mass of lymph nodes in the mediastinum enlarged by metastases in rare cases compresses the superior vena cava (Fig. 20-5), causing the patient to present with the symptoms and signs of the superior mediastinal syndrome.[13] A Virchow-Trossier node should be looked for, since it may indicate metastatic HCC in the mediastinum.[14]

Another unusual clinical manifestation of HCC is bone pain resulting from osteolytic metastases with or without pathologic fracture (Fig. 20-6).[9] Skeletal metastases are detected at necropsy in as many as 20% of patients, more often than they are evident during life (in 3% to 12% of patients). An initial presentation with bone pain is rare, however. Bone metastases may be single or multiple; the bones most frequently affected are the neck of the femur, ribs, vertebrae, skull, and sacrum. Destruction of vertebrae (Fig. 20-7) may cause damage to the spinal cord with paraplegia or nerve root compression.

Raised right hemidiaphragm (Fig. 20-8) or multiple pulmonary metastases on x-ray may often be present.[15,16] For example, 19% of black Africans with HCC have radiologically evident pulmonary metastases at the time of first admission, and 30% have a pathologically elevated right hemidiaphragm (more than 2.5 cm above the left hemidiaphragm in a standard posteroanterior chest x-ray).[15] The presence of these two radiologic findings together (in 11% of southern African blacks with HCC) is highly suggestive of a diagnosis of HCC. A pleural effusion may be present, as may linear atalectases in the right lower lobe of the lung. When HCC affects the left lobe of the liver predominantly, the left hemidiaphragm may be elevated. This radiologic sign is present in 2% of black patients with HCC.[15] Very rarely, multiple tumor emboli to the pulmonary microvasculature may be responsible for presentation with pulmonary arterial hypertension.[17] Pulmonary metastases complicating HCC are frequently multiple and of more or less the same size, and they may increase in size surprisingly quickly.[15] The elevated hemi-

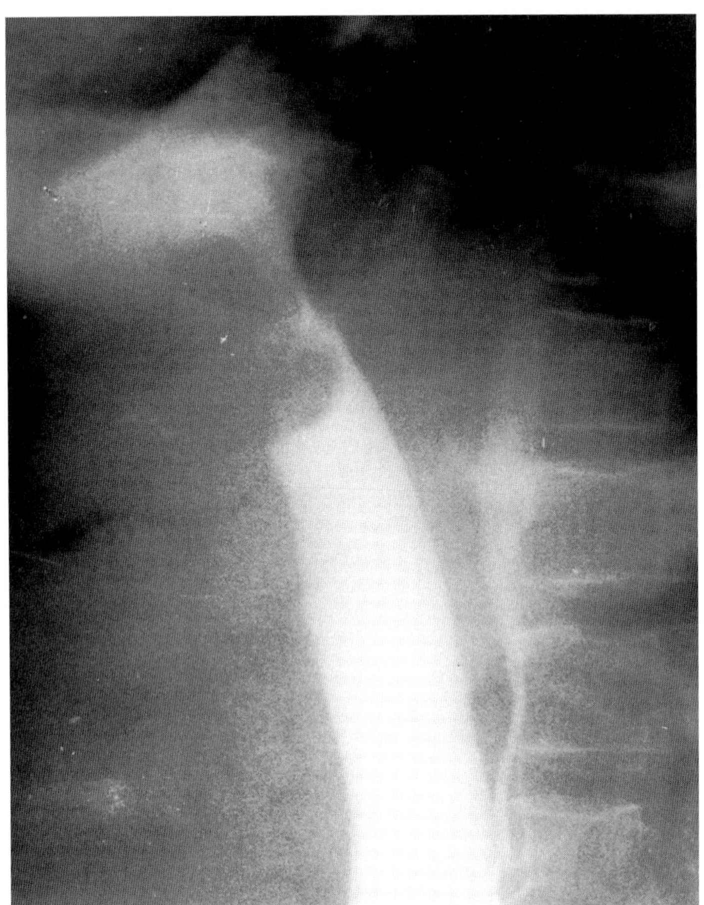

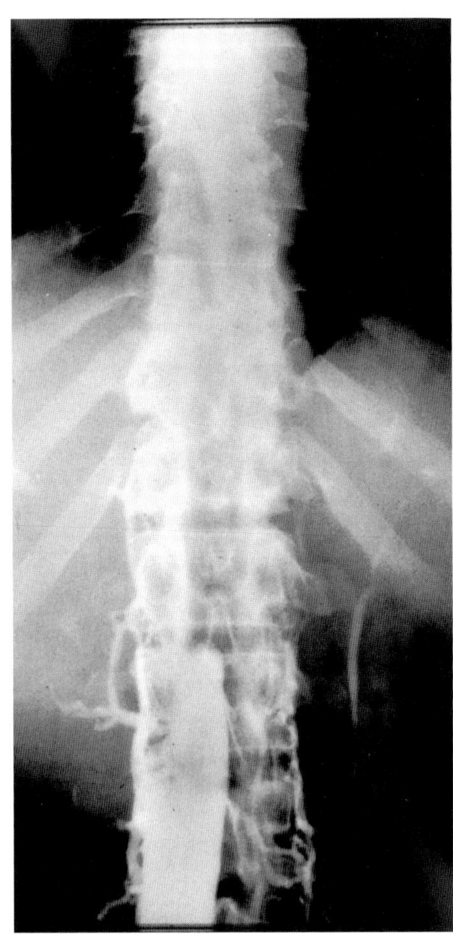

FIGURE 20-3. (*A*) Inferior vena cavogram showing partial obstruction of the lumen of the inferior vena cava by HCC in the region of the entrance of the hepatic veins just below the diaphragm. (*B*) Inferior vena cavogram in another patient with HCC showing complete occlusion of the lumen of the upper portion of the inferior vena cava by tumor, which has propagated down the lumen from the site of entry at the hepatic veins.

diaphragm in HCC may be generalized and follow the upper contour of the liver or have one or more localized bulges in it (Fig. 20-8). Extreme elevation may displace the heart to the left (see Fig. 20-11). However, symptoms that are related to elevation of the diaphragm or the pulmonary metastases such as dyspnea, cough, or hemoptysis are uncommon.

Low or moderate grade, remittent or intermittent fever occurs in 6% to 54% of patients with HCC, particularly in black African and ethnic Chinese patients.[5–8] An occasional patient presents with a "fever of unknown origin."[18] Fever may be accompanied by leukocytosis (which is present in as many as 16% of patients[5]), further misleading the clinician into believing that an infection is present.

Membranous obstruction of the inferior vena cava, a rare congenital or acquired anomaly (Fig. 20-9), is complicated by HCC (with a frequency of approximately 40%) in some populations, notably in black Africans and Japanese.[19,20] Long-standing obstruction of the inferior vena cava is recognized by the dilated and tortuous collateral veins coursing over the trunk (Fig. 20-10 and Plate 20-1), the presence of which, as well as the finding of a dilated vena azygos on a plain chest x-ray (Fig. 20-11), suggests the diagnosis. The presence of the obstruction is confirmed by inferior vena cavography (Fig. 20-9).

The clinical features characteristic of other disorders that have causal associations with HCC, such as hereditary hemochromatosis, Wilson's disease, α_1-antitrypsin deficiency, and ataxia telangiectasia may be evident in addition to those attributable to the tumor.

Among the more peculiar of the unusual ways in which HCC may present are a host of paraneoplastic syndromes (Table 20-1). Because they may antedate the

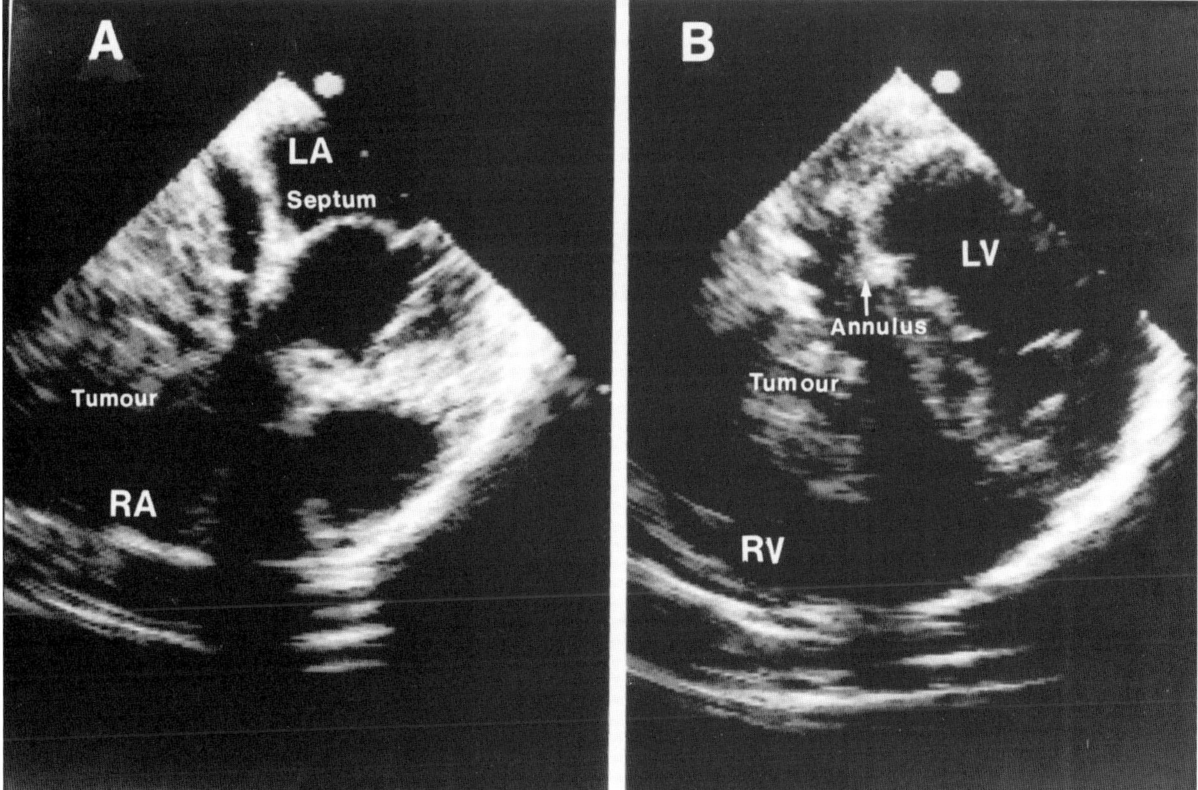

FIGURE 20-4. Echocardiogram demonstrating the presence of HCC in the lumen of the right atrium (*A*) and projecting through the orifice of the tricuspid valve into the right ventricle (*B*).

local effects of the tumor, paraneoplastic syndromes may direct the attention of the initiated to the presence of HCC, or they may mislead the uninitiated into making a wrong diagnosis.

Paraneoplastic Syndromes

Because type B hypoglycemia occurs early in the course of HCC and is severe, it is likely to be the reason why patients with this paraneoplastic complication come to medical attention.[21] (Type A is a mild form of hypoglycemia that occurs as a preterminal phenomenon and is not a paraneoplastic complication.) The patient presents with confusion, drowsiness, epilepsy, acute neuropsychiatric disturbance, stupor, or coma. Under these circumstances, an enlarged liver may easily be overlooked. Drowsiness or confusion in a patient with HCC may also be evidence of severe hypercalcemia.[21] Type B hypoglycemia and hypercalcemia not attributable to osteolytic metastases each occurs in less than 5% of patients with HCC.

In populations with a low incidence of HCC, the tumor is often a late complication of cirrhosis.[2] The expanded plasma volume characteristic of cirrhotic patients falsely lowers the plasma hemoglobin concentration and the hematocrit. The presence of polycythemia (erythrocytosis) in a patient known to have cirrhosis is therefore a very strong diagnostic clue that hepatocellular carcinoma has developed.[21] Polycythemia is present in up to 10% of patients with early HCC, but it is seen less often when the tumor is far advanced.

Male patients with HCC rarely present with features of feminization.[21] In boys this takes the form of isosexual precocity (more commonly seen with hepatoblastoma), while adult males may have gynecomastia alone (which also may be caused by the coexisting cirrhosis) or florid feminization.

Systemic arterial hypertension has recently been reported in a few patients with HCC,[22] as has the syndrome of watery diarrhea, hypokalemia, and achlorhydria.[23] Cutaneous markers of HCC such as dermatomyositis, pemphigus foliaceous, and Leser-Trelat sign (Fig. 20-12 and Plate 20-2) occasionally are seen in an HCC patient. Less rare is pityriasis rotunda (Fig. 20-13 and Plate 20-3), although this rash occurs with any frequency only in black African patients with HCC.[24] It consists of single or multiple, round or oval hyperpigmented, scaly lesions

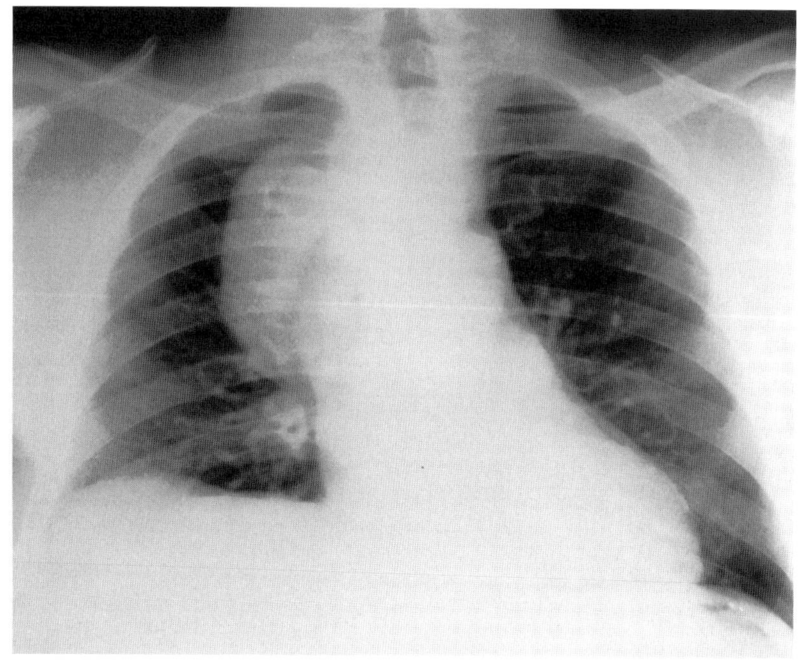

A

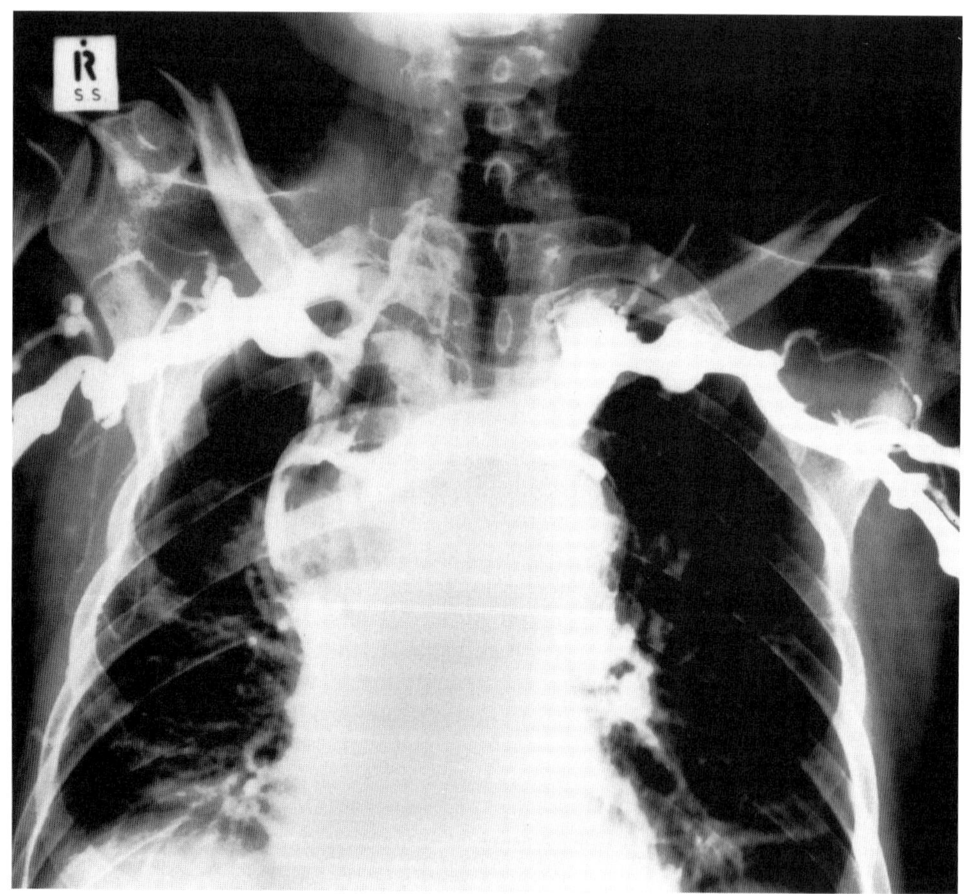

B

FIGURE 20-5. (*A*) Posteroanterior chest x-ray showing a large mass of metastatic mediastinal lymph nodes in a patient with HCC presenting clinically with the superior mediastinal syndrome. (*B*) Venography demonstrating compression of the superior vena cava by metastatic HCC in another patient presenting with the superior mediastinal syndrome. (From Kew,[13] with permission.)

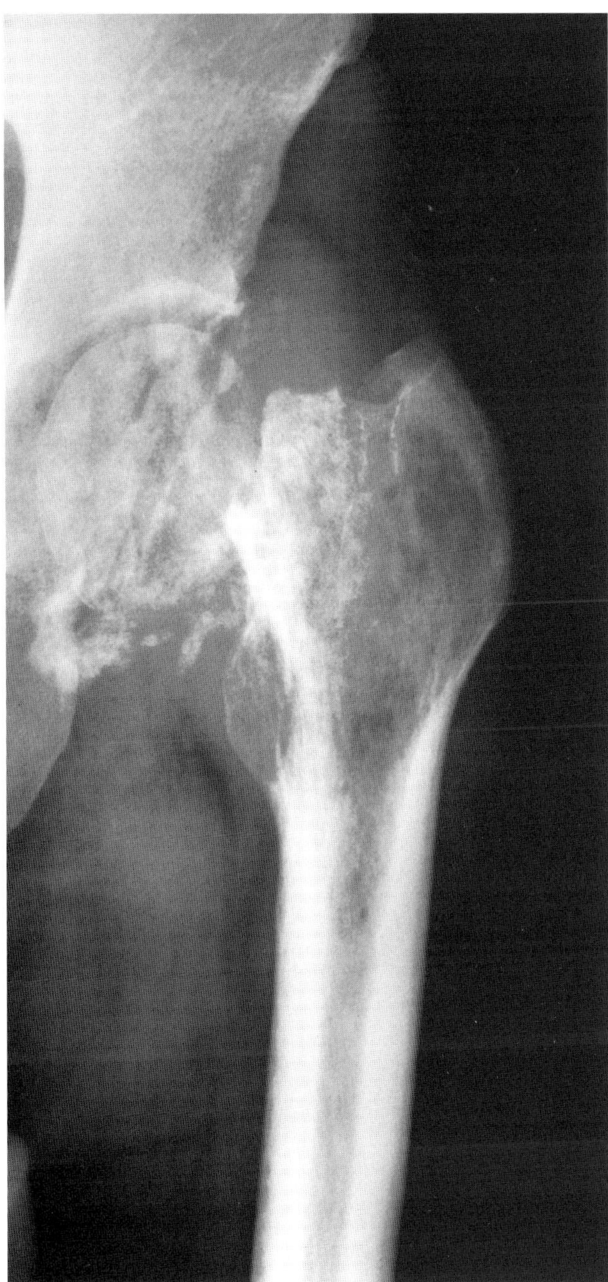

FIGURE 20-6. Osteolytic metastasis of the head and neck of the femur with a pathologic fracture in a patient with HCC.

on the trunk, buttocks, or thighs. The lesions vary in size from 0.5 to 25 cm and may become confluent.

DIFFERENTIAL DIAGNOSIS OF HCC

A number of hepatic diseases may be mistaken for HCC. These belong in two broad categories, mass lesions of the liver and chronic parenchymal or infiltrative diseases of the liver.

Mass Lesions of the Liver

In adults living in geographic regions with low or intermediate incidences of HCC, hepatic metastases outnumber primary malignant tumors of the liver. Hepatic metastases complicate 40% to 50% of all tumors.[25] They generally originate from primary sites within the portal venous drainage system, lung, and breast. Hepatic metastases are often clinically silent, or their symptoms are overshadowed by those of the primary tumor. Symptoms attributed to hepatic metastases are malaise, weight loss, and upper abdominal pain. Depending on the extent of the metastatic disease, the liver may be enlarged, sometimes markedly so. The surface of the enlarged liver may be smooth or irregular, and umbilication may be felt. Umbilication is rare with HCC. A friction rub may be heard when hepatic metastases are subcapsular, but is rarely present with HCC. Wasting is often apparent.

Appreciable elevation of the right hemidiaphragm on chest x-rays is uncommon with hepatic metastases but is often seen with large HCCs.[15,16] Depending on the site of origin, hepatic metastases may be accompanied by a slightly or moderately (and sometimes even a markedly) raised serum α-fetoprotein concentration,[26] whereas very high serum levels favor a diagnosis of HCC. Imaging of the liver may be helpful in distinguishing between HCC and hepatic metastases, but a percutaneous biopsy will often be needed for definitive diagnosis.

An arterial bruit over an enlarged liver is heard in about one-fourth of patients with HCC but virtually never with metastases, abscesses, or cysts in the liver.[2,5,27] Bruits are, however, occasionally heard over other highly vascular malignant or benign hepatic tumors. The sounds most frequently heard over an enlarged liver (from any cause) are transmitted heart sounds. A bruit caused by compression of the aorta in the supine position by an enlarged liver can sometimes be heard, loudest in the midline of the abdomen and progressively softer away from the midline. It disappears if the patient is positioned in such a way that the aorta is no longer compressed. In contrast, the bruit caused by HCC can be heard anywhere over the liver and in all body positions. It is louder, rougher, and longer than the bruit transmitted from the aorta.

Difficulty may be experienced in differentiating between HCC and abscesses in the liver. Pyogenic hepatic abscesses are uncommon in all populations, but amebic abscesses occur frequently in some geographic regions. Upper abdominal pain is almost invariable in patients with hepatic amebic abscess, and pain referred to the right shoulder occurs more frequently than it does in HCC. Between 20% and 33% of patients with amebic hepatic abscess have coexisting dysentery when they present, and between 10% and 33% have had dysentery in the past. The liver is often enlarged with point tenderness or intercostal tenderness. Abscesses located in the

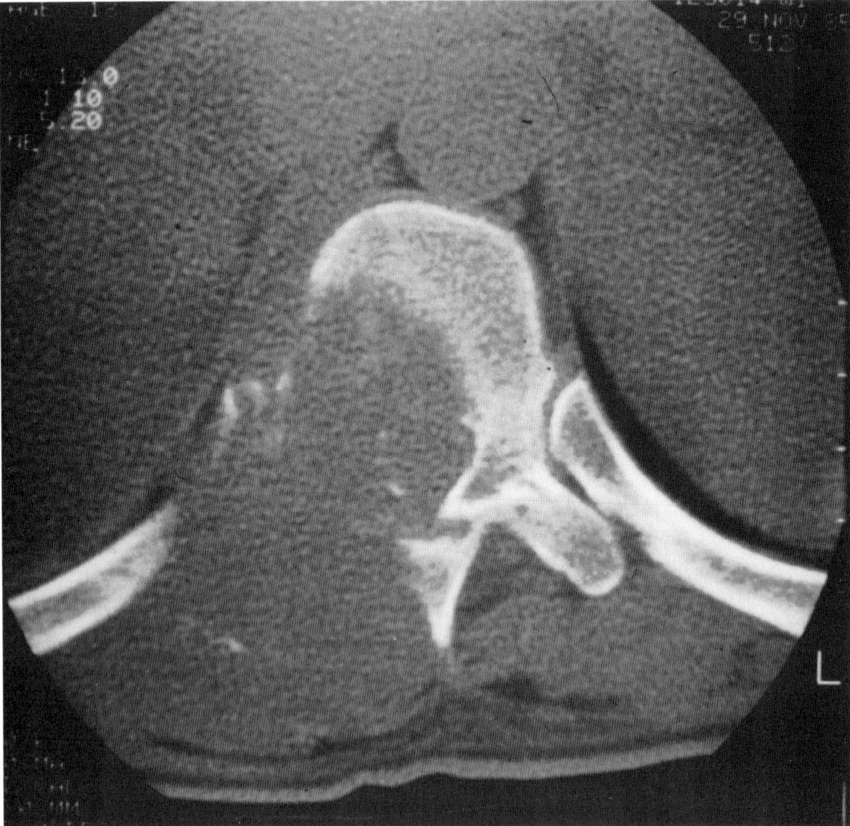

FIGURE 20-7. Computed tomogram showing metastatic destruction of the body and radicle of a vertebra in a patient with HCC complicated by paraplegia.

dome of the liver enlarge upwards; in these patients, the liver edge is not palpable below the costal margin. A friction rub is more likely to be heard over the enlarged liver in hepatic abscess than in HCC.

The right hemidiaphragm may be markedly elevated with both of these "space-occupying lesions." Its outline is frequently hazy, with a small collection of fluid in the costophrenic angle with an abscess; it results from spread of the inflammatory process from the liver to the diaphragm and diaphragmatic pleura. A similar appearance may be seen with HCC, although the outline of the diaphragm is more likely to be distinct,[15] presumably because the tumorous liver pushes up the diaphragm but the tumor seldom infiltrates through it.

Difficulty may occasionally be experienced in differentiating a bulge in the anteromedial portion of the right hemidiaphragm due to HCC from a congenital variation. However, at least in black Africans, the degree of elevation at this site due to HCC, greater than 4 cm, is greater than that due to congenital anatomic variation.[15]

Abscesses of short duration may appear echogenic on ultrasonography and be mistaken for hepatic tumors. If, however, the examination is repeated after about 3 days of treatment with an amebicidal agent, the lesion will have become echolucent and the diagnosis obvious. Serum α-fetoprotein concentrations are occasionally mildly or moderately raised in patients with amebic liver abscesses.[28]

Cholangiocarcinoma occurs frequently in some Far Eastern countries, especially northeastern Thailand. The clinical presentation of the peripheral type of cholangiocarcinoma is similar to that of HCC.[29] Jaundice is, however, earlier, more prominent, and more frequent than in patients with HCC. In addition, the liver is less enlarged, a bruit is not heard over the tumor, ascites is far less likely to be present, and fever and extrahepatic metastases are less frequent. With hilar cholangiocarcinoma (including Klatskin's tumor) jaundice is typically the presenting complaint and may become severe. Serum α-fetoprotein concentrations are sometimes elevated in patients with cholangiocarcinoma.

Hepatoblastoma may be clinically indistinguishable from HCC.[30] However, its occurrence is virtually confined to early childhood, a time when HCC is rare.

Other primary malignant tumors of the liver may mimic the clinical and imaging features of HCC, but they are rare and do not produce raised serum α-fetoprotein levels.

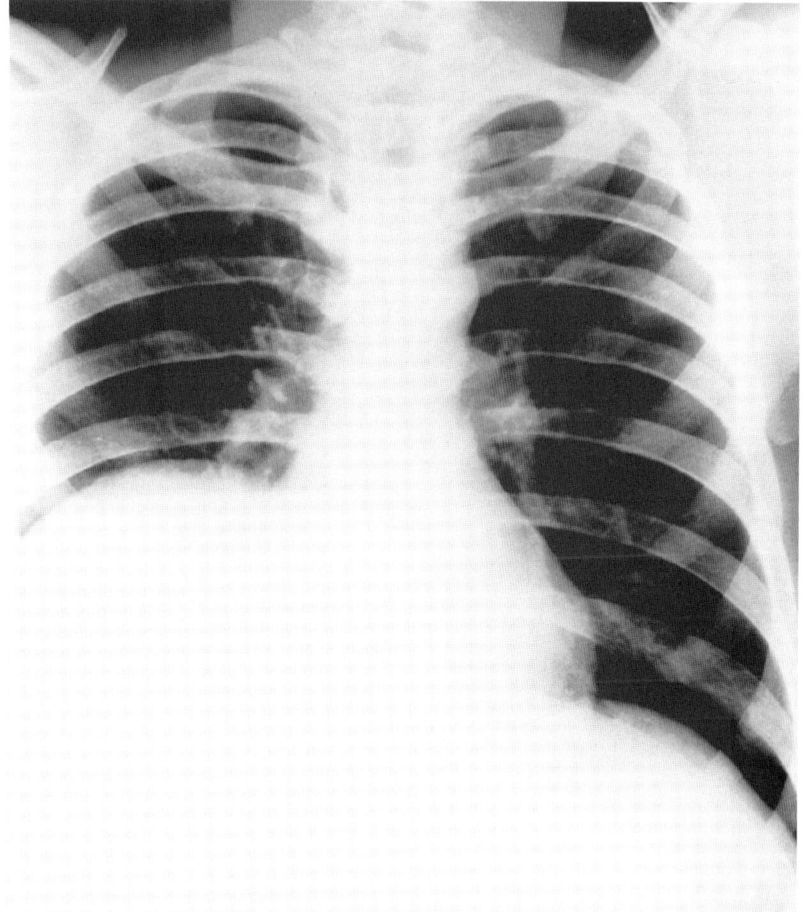

A

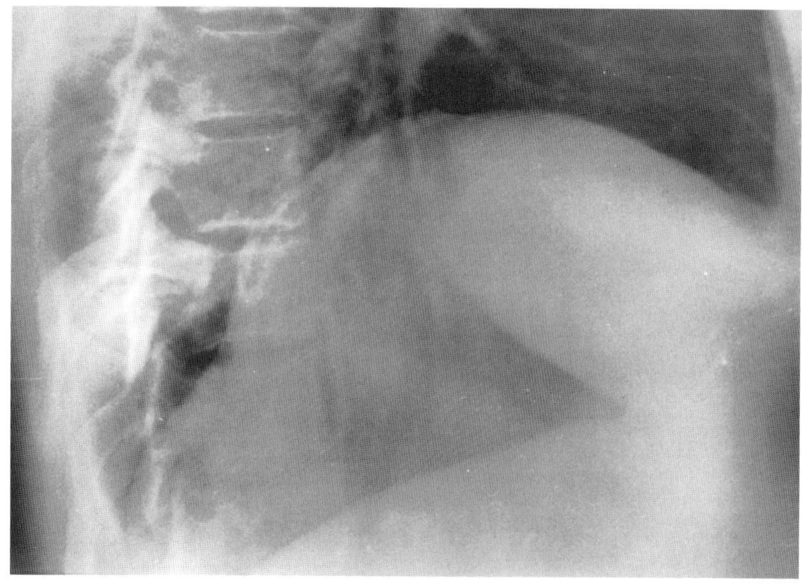

B

FIGURE 20-8. Chest x-rays showing marked elevation of the right hemidiaphragm in a patient with HCC (*A*). Note the well-defined outline of the raised hemidiaphragm. A lateral view (*B*) of another patient shows a localized bulge in the right hemidiaphragm.

Benign hepatic tumors and hepatic cysts, when symptomatic, present with upper abdominal pain and an enlarged liver, but weight loss is unusual. Serum α-fetoprotein concentrations are normal. Some difficulty may be experienced in differentiating between a large hepatocellular adenoma and HCC when the patient is a young woman who has been taking contraceptive steroids. Although contraceptive steroids are best known for their causal association with hepatocellular adenomas,[31] they are also a minor risk factor for HCC.[32] Both hepatocellular adenoma and carcinoma have a propensity to rupture. In adenomas, however, this complication almost always

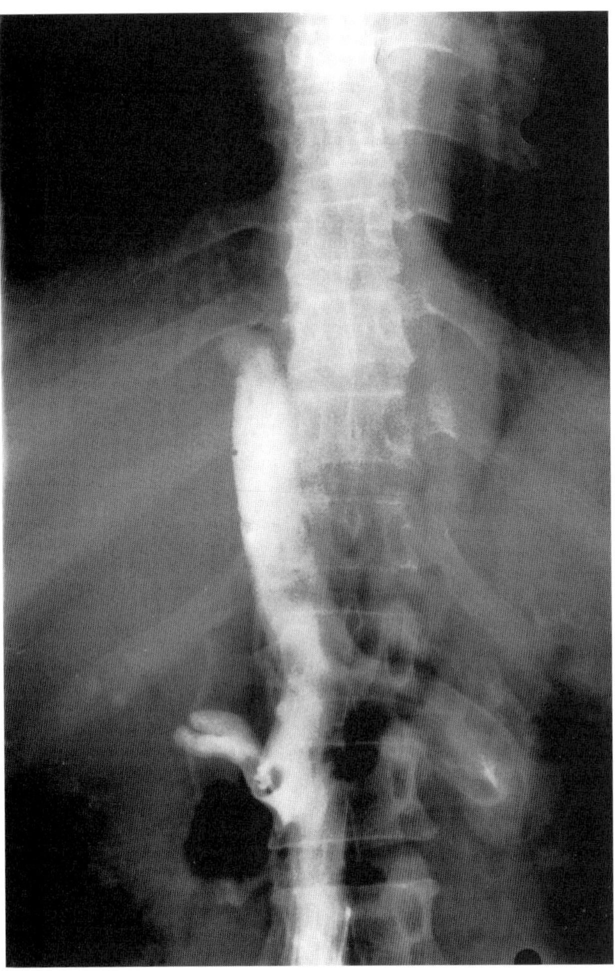

FIGURE 20-9. Inferior vena cavogram in a patient with membranous obstruction of the inferior vena cava. The obstruction occurs at the level of the diaphragm just above the entrance of the hepatic veins into the inferior vena cava. (From Kew et al.,[20] with permission.)

occurs in women taking contraceptive steroids. (Some of the rare malignant hepatic tumors, for example angiosarcomas, may also rupture.)

Diffuse Liver Diseases

In Japan and western populations at low or intermediate risk of HCC, HCC commonly arises as a late complication of cirrhosis.[2] Patients have the symptoms and signs of advanced cirrhosis, and it may be difficult to recognize a small tumor. Imaging of the liver is useful but not infallible in making a diagnosis.

Hepatic tuberculosis in developing countries or in any population in which acquired immunodeficiency syndrome (AIDS) is common may have a clinical presentation similar to that of HCC. Upper abdominal discomfort or pain, malaise, loss of weight, and fever are often present, and the liver is usually enlarged.[33] Ascites may be present. The surface of the liver is smooth, and no bruit is heard. Serum α-fetoprotein levels are not elevated. Imaging will usually distinguish hepatic tuberculosis from HCC. Liver biopsy provides a definitive diagnosis.

NONIMAGING DIAGNOSIS

Liver Function Tests

In a patient with cirrhosis, a sudden and unexplained increase in the serum alkaline phosphatase concentration should suggest the possibility that HCC has developed. In populations in which dietary and familial hypercholesterolemia are rare, such as black Africans, ethnic Chinese, and Japanese, a high serum cholesterol concentration in a patient with noncholestatic liver disease is

FIGURE 20-10. Markedly dilated and tortuous collateral veins in a patient with membranous obstruction of the inferior vena cava. (See also Plate 20-1).

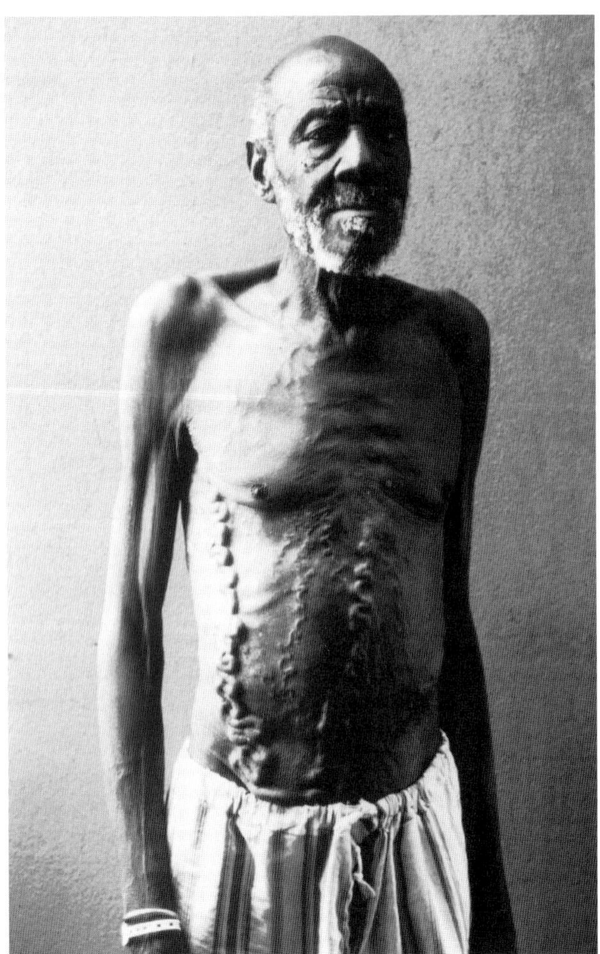

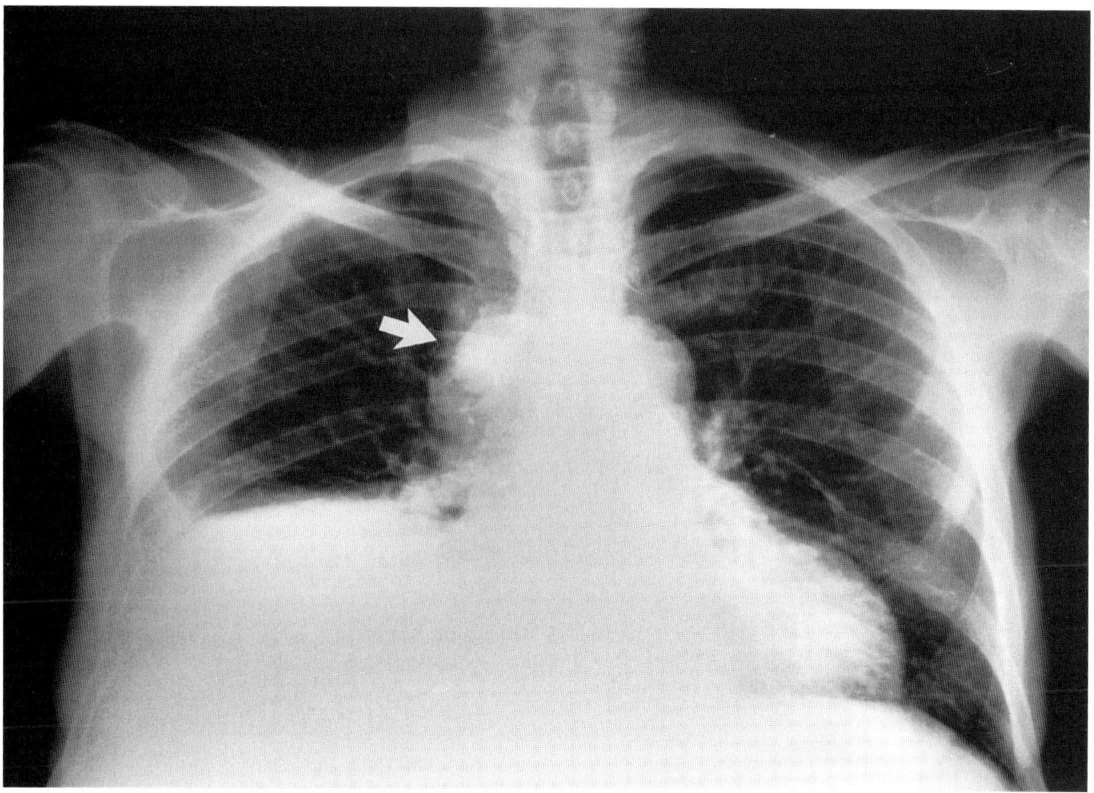

FIGURE 20-11. Dilated vena azygos (arrow) in a patient with HCC complicating membranous obstruction of the inferior vena cava. Note also the raised right hemidiaphragm and the displacement of the heart.

TABLE 20-1. Paraneoplastic Syndromes in HCC

Hypoglycemia
Polycythemia (erythrocytosis)
Hypercalcemia
Sexual changes
Isosexual precocity
Gynecomastia
Feminization
Arterial hypertension
Watery diarrhea syndrome
Porphyria
Carcinoid syndrome
Osteoporosis
Hypertrophic osteoarthropathy
Thyrotoxicosis
Thrombophlebitis migrans
Polymyositis
Neuropathy

a strong indication of HCC. Autonomous de novo biosynthesis of cholesterol by malignant hepatocytes resulting in hypercholesterolemia is one of the more common paraneoplastic phenomena seen with this tumor.[34] For example, 14% to 38% of black Africans with HCC have elevated serum cholesterol levels.[21] Measurement of the serum cholesterol concentration can be useful if a diagnosis of HCC is being considered.

α-Fetoprotein Level

A sensitive and specific serum marker of the tumor would greatly facilitate its diagnosis. Detection of α-fetoprotein, an α_1-globulin, in human fetal serum in 1956 and its subsequent finding in the serum of mice and humans with HCC raised the prospect that such a marker may indeed exist. The diagnostic usefulness of this glycoprotein has since been amply confirmed, although both false-negative and false-positive results do occur. The search for an ideal serum marker of HCC continues, and a list of those substances that have at one time or another been advocated to be useful in this regard is given in Table 20-2.

Serum α-fetoprotein concentrations are elevated in

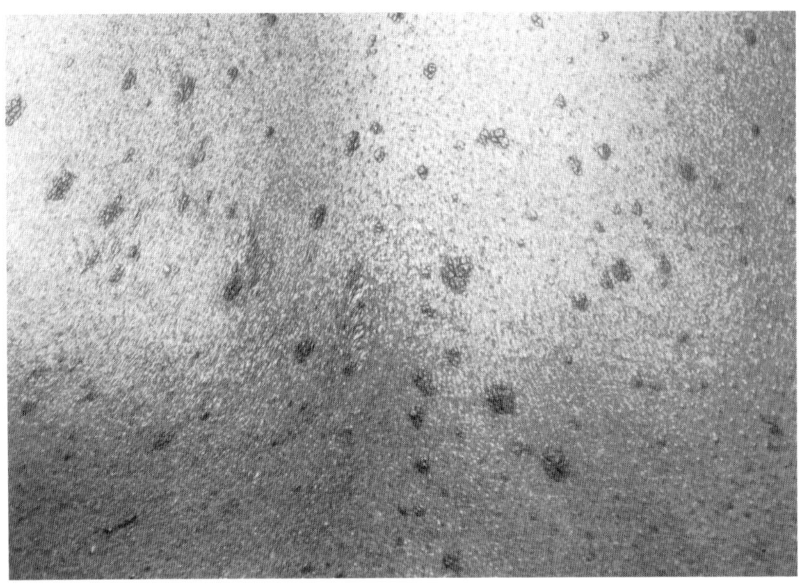

FIGURE 20-12. Leser-Trélat sign. (Sudden onset of seborrheic dermatitis and freckles with rapid increase in the number of the lesions, accompanied by pruritus.) (See also Plate 20-2).

most (but not all) patients with HCC.[26] In high-incidence areas, values are raised in at least 90% of HCC patients, with a mean concentration of around 70,000 ng/ml, compared with 70% to 90% of HCC patients and a mean of around 8,000 ng/ml in patients from areas with low (or intermediate) incidence.[26,35] α-Fetoprotein production by HCC is also age related, younger patients being more likely to have elevated values and to attain higher levels.[36] There is no gender difference.[26] Although synthesis of α-fetoprotein in mice with chemically induced HCC correlates with the degree of differentiation of the tumor, the information available for human HCC is conflicting, with most workers not confirming the association.[26] Nor is there an obvious correlation between serum α-fetoprotein concentrations and any clinical or biochemical indices or with survival time. In countries with a low incidence of HCC, α-fetoprotein levels are higher when the tumor coexists with cirrhosis and in patients with evidence of current hepatitis B virus infection, but this does not apply in countries where the tumor is common.[37]

Serum α-fetoprotein may also be elevated in patients with a variety of benign hepatic diseases, including acute and chronic hepatitis and cirrhosis.[26] The levels attained, however, are almost always substantially lower than those in patients with HCC. Elevated levels are also found in about one-third of patients with undifferentiated teratocarcinoma or embryonal cell carcinoma of the ovary or testis and in approximately 10% of patients with tumors of endodermal origin.[26] If the cut-off value for α-fetoprotein as a marker for HCC is increased to 400 ng/ml (or 500 ng/ml in some studies), most elevations due to other tumors can be eliminated, and 70% to 75% of patients with HCC in high-incidence regions

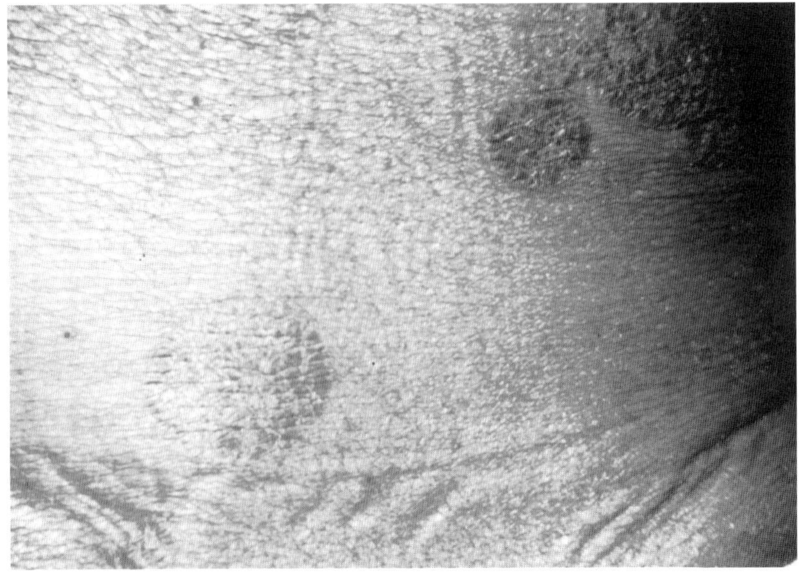

FIGURE 20-13. Pityriasis rotunda (round or oval hyperpigmented scaly lesions) on anterior abdominal wall. (See also Plate 20-3).

TABLE 20-2. Substances Secreted by HCC That Have Been Studied as Potential Serum Markers of the Tumor

α-Fetoprotein
Des-γ-carboxy prothrombin
α-L-Fucosidase
Isoenzymes of γ-glutamyl transferase
Abnormal vitamin B_{12}-binding protein
Abnormal fibrinogen
Antithrombin III
Calcitonin
Neurotensin
Chorionic gonadotropin
Chorionic somatotropin
Thyroxine-binding globulin
α_1-Microglobulin (HC protein)
Isoferritin
Isoenzymes of 5′ nucleotide phosphodiesterase
Variant alkaline phosphatase
Aldolase isoenzyme (type A)
Glutathione S-transferase (type B)
Carcinoembryonic antigen
Tissue polypeptide antigen
CA 19-9; CA 125; CA 50
DU-PAN 2; CSLEX 1; ST-4-39; POA
Liver-specific F antigen
Novel glycosphingolipids
Pseudouridine

remain positive (less than 50% of patients in low incidence regions).

α-Fetoprotein is heterogenous in structure. The microheterogeneity of the molecule results from differences in the asparagine-linked biantennary oligosaccharide side chain and accounts for the differential affinity of this glycoprotein for lectins. Early reports attested to the usefulness of the reactivity of α-fetoprotein with lens culinaris agglutinin A in differentiating between HCC and benign hepatic diseases and, to a lesser extent, reactivity with concanavalin A in distinguishing HCC from other tumors capable of producing this protein.[38,39] Differential reactivity was initially detected by measuring the proportion of α-fetoprotein that reacted with the lectin, but now lectin-affinity electrophoresis coupled with antibody-affinity blotting followed by densitometric analysis is preferred.

Differential lectin reactivity of α-fetoprotein will distinguish HCC from benign hepatic diseases even when the serum levels are only slightly raised.[40,41] Fucosylated α-fetoprotein has also been shown to be useful in the diagnosis of small presymptomatic HCCs in surveillance programs of individuals at high risk for this tumor.[42]

Des-γ-Carboxy Prothrombin Level

Des-γ-carboxy prothrombin (also known as "protein-induced by vitamin K absence, or antagonism-II" [PIVKA-II]), a precursor of prothrombin, has been claimed to be a better marker of HCC than α-fetoprotein.[43] Elevated serum levels have been reported in 60% to 91% of patients from various high- and low-incidence regions of HCC.[26] However, in a direct comparison between the two markers in black African patients, the sensitivity of α-fetoprotein was 83% and the specificity 90.8% compared with 67% and 84.7%, respectively, with des-γ-carboxy prothrombin.[44] In an earlier study, when the diagnostic level for des-γ-carboxy prothrombin was increased in an attempt to eliminate false-positive results, the number of patients with HCC with a diagnostic value decreased from 91% to 67%.[43] Production of des-γ-carboxy prothrombin by HCC is caused by failure of the tumor to express the prothrombin carboxylase gene.[44a] This results in the accumulation in the tumor of des-γ-carboxy prothrombin, which subsequently leaks into the bloodstream.

Tumor-Associated Isoenzymes of γ-Glutamyl Transferase

Serum from normal humans and patients with various forms of benign hepatobiliary disease can be shown on polyacrylamide gradient gel electrophoresis to contain 10 isoenzymes of γ-glutamyl transferase. An additional one to three isoenzymes may be present in the serum of patients with HCC that are not detectable in normal serum.[45,46] The tumor-associated isoenzymes and the normal isoenzymes differ primarily in their carbohydrate composition. One or more of the tumor-associated isoenzymes (I′, I″, or II′) are present in about 60% of patients with HCC. I′ is the most prevalent, being detectable in about 55%; I″ and II′ are each present in about 30%. Although the sensitivity of tumor-associated isoenzymes of γ-glutamyl transferase as a marker for HCC is relatively low, its specificity is excellent. No correlation exists between the presence of the isoenzymes and the age, sex, or tumor burden of the patients.[46] Because the presence of one or more of the isoenzymes is almost invariably accompanied by a raised total serum γ-glutamyl transferase level, it is generally not worth testing for the presence of individual isoenzymes if the latter is normal.

Other Possible Tumor Markers

None of the other substances proposed to be serum markers for HCC (Table 20-2) has a sufficiently high sensitivity and specificity to warrant routine use in the diagnosis of HCC. Serum levels of carcinoembryonic antigen are often slightly or moderately raised in patients with HCC, but similar values are frequently present in patients with benign hepatic disease, particularly alcoholic cirrhosis.[47] CA 125, tissue polypeptide antigen, and tumor-associated isoenzymes of 5′ nucleotide phosphodiesterase have high sensitivities but very poor specificities.[26] CA 19–9 and calcitonin have both a low sensitivity and a low specificity.[26]

α-L-Fucosidase, a lysosomal hydrolase that degrades fucose-containing glycoconjugates, is present in many tissues. Raised serum levels of α-l-fucosidase were reported in European patients with HCC[48]; however, the sensitivity is low, and it is a poorer marker for HCC than α-fetoprotein.[49,50] Serum ferritin concentrations are often raised in patients with HCC.[51] The reason for the elevation is not known, but there is no proof that it reflects secretion of a tumor-associated acidic isoferritin. Variant alkaline phosphatase[26] is detected in the serum of 2% to 18% of patients with HCC.[52–54] Variant alkaline phosphatase is rarely present in other tumors or in benign liver disease, and never in normal serum, but its very low sensitivity limits its usefulness as a tumor marker.

Two tumor markers are particularly associated with the fibrolamellar variant of HCC. They are abnormal vitamin B_{12}-binding protein[55] and neurotensin.[56] When present, they provide useful confirmatory evidence, but both are of low sensitivity.

REFERENCES

1. Kew MC, Popper H. The relationship between hepatocellular carcinoma and cirrhosis. Semin Liver Dis 1984;4: 136–146
2. Kew MC, Dos Santos HA, Sherlock S. Diagnosis of primary cancer of the liver. BMJ 1971;4:408–411
3. Chlebowski RT, Tong M, Weisman J et al. Hepatocellular carcinoma. Diagnosis and prognostic features in North American patients. Cancer 1984;53:2701–2706
4. Steiner PE. Cancer of the liver and cirrhosis in trans-Saharan Africa and the United States of America. Cancer 1960;13: 1085–1145
5. Alpert ME, Hutt MSR, Davidson CS. Primary hepatoma in Uganda. Am J Med 1969;46:794–802
6. Kew MC, Geddes EW. HCC in rural southern African blacks. Medicine (Baltimore) 1982;61:98–108
7. Lai CL, Lam KC, Wong KP, Todd D. Clinical features of HCC: review of 211 patients in Hong Kong. Cancer 1981; 47:2746–2755
8. Sung JL, Wang TH, Yu JY. Clinical study of primary carcinoma of the liver in Taiwan. Am J Dig Dis 1976;12: 1036–1049
9. Kew MC, Paterson AC. Unusual clinical presentations of HCC. Trop Gastroenterol 1985;6:10–22
10. Chearanai O, Plengvanit U, Asavanich C et al. Spontaneous rupture of primary hepatoma. Cancer 1983;51:1532–1536
11. Kew MC, Hodkinson J. Rupture of HCCs as a result of blunt abdominal trauma. Am J Gastroenterol 1991;86:1083–1085
12. Moosa MR, Segal I, Mannell A et al. Biliary obstruction in HCC diagnosed by endoscopic retrograde cholangiopancreatography. S Afr Med J 1984;66:962–964
13. Kew MC. HCC presenting with the superior mediastinal syndrome. Am J Gastroenterol 1989;84:1092–1094
14. Kew MC. Virchow-Troisier's lymph node in hepatocellular carcinoma. J Clin Gastroenterol 1991;13:217–219
15. Levy I, Geddes EW, Kew MC. The chest radiograph in primary liver cancer. S Afr Med J 1976;15:1323–1326
16. Sanders CF. The plain chest radiograph in 75 cases of primary carcinoma of the liver. Clin Radiol 1968;19:341–346
17. Willett IR, Sutherland RC, O'Rourke MF, Dudley FJ. Pulmonary hypertension complicating hepatocellular carcinoma. Gastroenterology 1984;87:1180–1184
18. Okuda K, Kondo Y, Nakano M et al. Hepatocellular carcinoma presenting with pyrexia and leucocytosis: report of 5 cases. Hepatology 1991;13:695–700
19. Simson IM. Membranous obstruction of the inferior vena cava and HCC in South Africa. Gastroenterology 1982;82: 171–178
20. Kew MC, McKnight A, Hodkinson J et al. The role of membranous obstruction of the inferior vena cava in the etiology of HCC in southern African blacks. Hepatology 1989;9: 121–125
21. Kew MC, Dusheiko GM. Paraneoplastic manifestations of HCC. In Chalmers TC, Berk PD (eds): Frontiers of Science in Liver Disease. Thieme-Stratton, New York, 1981: 305–319
22. Kew MC, Leckie BJ, Greeff MC. Arterial hypertension as a paraneoplastic phenomenon in HCC. Arch Intern Med 1989;149:2111–2113
23. Steiner F, Velt P, Gutierrez O et al. HCC presenting with intractable diarrhea. Arch Surg 1986;121:849–851
24. Di Bisceglie AM, Hodkinson HJ, Berkowitz I, Kew MC. Pityriasis rotunda: a cutaneous marker of hepatocellular carcinoma in South African blacks. Arch Dermatol 1986;122: 802–804
25. Pickren JW, Tsukada Y, Lane WW. Liver metastasis: analysis of autopsy data. In Weiss L, Gilbert HA (eds): Liver Metastases. GK Hall, Boston, 1982;2–18
26. Kew MC. Tumor markers in HCC. J Gastroenterol Hepatol 1989;4:373–384
27. Clain D, Wartnaby K, Sherlock S. Abdominal arterial murmurs in liver disease. Lancet 1966;2:516–519
28. Kew MC. Serum alpha-fetoprotein levels in amebic hepatic abscess. Trop Gastroenterol 1988;9:23–25
29. Okuda K, Kubo Y, Okazaki N et al. Clinical aspects of intrahepatic bile duct carcinoma including hilar carcinoma. Cancer 1977;39:232–246
30. Ishak KG, Glunz PR. Hepatoblastoma and hepatocarcinoma in infancy and childhood. Cancer 1967;20:396–422
31. Mays ET, Christopherson W. Hepatic tumors induced by sex steroids. Semin Liver Dis 1984;4:147–157
32. Thomas DB. Exogenous steroid hormones and hepatocellular carcinoma. In Tabor E, DiBisceglie AM, Purcell RH

(eds): Etiology, Pathology, and Treatment of Hepatocellular Carcinoma in North America. Portfolio Publishing Co., The Woodlands, Texas, 1991:77–90

33. Korn RJ, Kellow WF, Hellar P. Hepatic involvement in extrapulmonary tuberculosis. Am J Med 1957;27:60–71
34. Danilewitz MD, Herrera GA, Kew MC et al. Autonomous cholesterol biosynthesis in murine hepatoma. A receptor defect with normal coated pits. Cancer 1984;4:373–384
35. Trichopoulos D, Sizaret P, Tabor E et al. Alpha-fetoprotein levels of liver cancer patients and controls in a European population. Cancer 1980;46:736–740
36. Kew MC, Macerollo P. Effect of age on the etiologic role of the hepatitis B virus in HCC in blacks. Gastroenterology 1988;94:439–442
37. Kew MC. HCC with and without cirrhosis. A comparison in southern African blacks. Gastroenterology 1989;97:136–139
38. Aoyagi Y, Isemura M, Yosizawa Z et al. Fucosylation of serum α-fetoprotein in patients with primary HCC. Biophys Acta 1985;85:217–223
39. Buamah PK, Harris R, James OWF, Skillen AW. Lentil lectin-reactive α-fetoprotein in the differential diagnosis of benign and malignant liver disease. Clin Chem 1986;32: 2083–2084
40. Taketa A, Sekiya C, Namiki M et al. Lectin-reactive profiles of α-fetoprotein characterising HCC and related conditions. Gastroenterology 1990;99:508–518
41. Du M-Q, Hutchinson WL, Johnson PJ, Williams R. Differential α-fetoprotein lectin binding in HCC: Diagnostic utility at low serum levels. Cancer 1991;67:476–480
42. Sato Y, Nakata K, Kato Y et al. Early recognition of HCC based on recognition of altered profiles of alpha-fetoprotein. N Engl J Med 1993;328:1802–1806
43. Liebman HA, Furie BC, Tong MJ et al. Des-gamma (abnormal) prothrombin as a serum marker of HCC. N Engl J Med 1984;310:1427–1431
44. King MA, Kew MC, Kuyl JM, Atkinson P. A comparison between des-gamma-carboxy prothrombin and alpha-fetoprotein as markers of HCC in southern African blacks. J Gastroenterol Hepatol 1989;4:17–24

44a. Shah DV, Engelke JA, Suttie JW. Abnormal prothrombin in the plasma of rats carrying hepatic tumors. Blood 1987; 69:850–854

45. Kojima J, Kanatani N, Nakamura H et al. Electrophoretic fractionation of serum gamma glutamyl transpeptidase in human hepatic cancer. Clin Chim Acta 1980;106:165–172
46. Kew MC, Wolf OP, Rowe P. Tumor associated isoenzymes of gamma glutamyl transferase in the serum of patients with HCC. Br J Cancer 1984;50:451–455
47. Macnab GM, Urbanowicz JM, Kew MC. Carcinoembryonic antigen in HCC. Br J Cancer 1978;38:510–514
48. Deugnier Y, David V, Brissot P et al. Alpha-l-fucosidase as a serum marker for primary liver cancer. Hepatology 1984; 4:889–892
49. Di Coccio RA, Barlow JJ, Motta KL. Evaluation of alpha-L-fucosidase as a marker of primary liver cancer. IRCS Med Sci 1985;13:849–851
50. Bukofzer S, Stass PM, Kew MC et al. Alpha-L-fucosidase as a serum marker of hepatocellular carcinoma. Br J Cancer 1989;59:417–420
51. Kew MC, Torrance JD, Derman D et al. Serum and tumor ferritins in primary liver cancer. Gut 1978;19:294–298
52. Kay PM, Warnes TW, Smith A et al. Tumor markers of HCC—a different diagnostic approach is required in Caucasians and Chinese. Hepatology 1984;4:800
53. Higashino K, Ohtani R, Kudo S. Hepatocellular carcinoma and a variant alkaline phosphatase. Ann Intern Med 1975; 83:74–78
54. Bukofzer S, Kew MC, Rowe P. The presence of variant alkaline phosphatase in HCC in southern African blacks. Cancer 1988;62:978–981
55. Paradinas FJ, Melia WM, Wilkinson ML et al. High serum vitamin B 12 binding capacity as a marker of the fibrolamellar variant of HCC. BMJ 1982;285:840–842
56. Collier NA, Weinbren K, Bloom SR. Neurotensin secretion by fibrolamellar cancer. Lancet 1984;2:538–540

21

ULTRASOUND

MASATOSHI KUDO

The early detection of hepatocellular carcinoma (HCC) has been simplified with recent advances of noninvasive imaging modalities, especially ultrasound. However, the confirmation of HCC is not always possible based on B-mode ultrasonographic findings alone. In this chapter, the efficacy of ultrasound in the screening and diagnosis of small HCC and the capacity of ultrasound angiography to differentiate HCC from other hepatic tumors are described. Furthermore, a description is also presented of the efficacy of color Doppler ultrasound, which provides both B-mode and vascular images, in diagnosing small HCC, with special emphasis on values of spectral analysis, power Doppler, and contrast-enhanced study after intravenous injection of a transpulmonary contrast agent.

ULTRASOUND SCREENING

In patients with small HCC, 2 cm or less in diameter, the surgical prognosis is significantly better than that in patients with larger nodules. In one large study, the patient survival rates at 5 years were 60.5% for nodules 2 cm or less (n = 347), 39.3% for those 2 to 5 cm (n = 1,127), and 26.8% for those more than 5 cm (n = 529).[1] Similarly, the 5-year survival rate for percutaneous ethanol injection therapy, which is widely used as an alternative to resection for HCC less than 3 cm in diameter, is 53.2% (n = 562).[2] Thus, early detection is extremely important for improving the prognosis of HCC.[3]

Modern real-time ultrasound equipment is known to be highly sensitive in the detection of nodular lesions in the liver, as well as highly cost-effective and easy to perform.[4,5] Therefore, ultrasound has been the method of first choice for screening high-risk patient populations, such as cirrhotic patients and patients infected with hepatitis B or C viruses, since hepatitis B and C viruses are known to be closely related to human hepatocarcinogenesis.[6–8]

In Japan, a screening protocol[9,10] was established, including regular follow-up of high-risk patients with ultrasonographic examination every 3 to 4 months and serum α-fetoprotein (AFP) and/or protein induced by vitamin K absence or antagonist II (PIVKA-II) measurements every 1 to 2 months. This resulted in great success in detecting small HCC less than 2 cm in diameter and early-stage well-differentiated HCCs, the prognosis in both of which is very good. Based on this screening protocol, at present in Japan approximately 20% to 30% of the HCC nodules detected are less than 2 cm in diameter, and 50% to 60% are less than 5 cm in diameter. In only 15% to 20% of the small HCC cases (less than 2 cm) is the AFP level increased to more than 20 ng/ml. Thus, regular screening of high-risk patients by ultrasound is undoubtedly important in the early detection of small HCC in the clinical setting, especially in countries where HCC is prevalent. Regular follow-up of HCC high-risk patients with ultrasound is strongly recommended.

ULTRASONOGRAPHIC DIAGNOSIS (B-MODE)

The typical ultrasonographic findings of small HCC are mosaic pattern, septum formation, peripheral sonolucency (halo), lateral shadow produced by fibrotic pseudo-

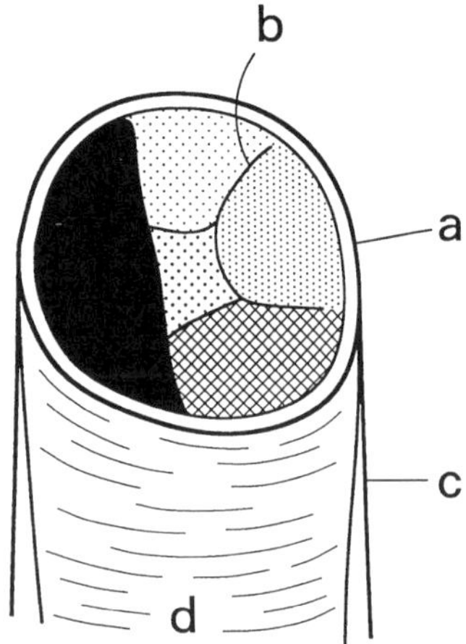

FIGURE 21-1. Scheme of ultrasound findings of typical small HCC. Mosaic pattern is clearly seen. *a*, peripheral sonolucency (halo); *b*, Septum formation; *c*, lateral shadow; *d*, posterior echo enhancement.

capsule, and posterior echo enhancement (Figs. 21-1 to 21-3).[11–13] Posterior echo enhancement is produced by softness of the tumor compared with the surrounding cirrhotic tissues. When the nodule is small, the internal echo pattern tends to be hypoechoic (Fig. 21-4 and Plate 21-1). Sometimes small HCC presents with a hyperechoic pattern (Fig. 21-5 and Plate 21-2), which is indicative of fatty metamorphosis, clear cell change, pseudoglandular arrangement of the cancer cells, periodic changes of the vascular space, or sclerotic change in the tumor. Two-thirds of the nodules present with a hypoechoic pattern, and one-third present with a hyperechoic or bright loop pattern (Fig. 21-6), when the HCC is less than 2 cm in diameter.

In more advanced HCCs, portal tumor thrombi, biliary invasion, and/or hepatic vein invasion are also observed, which strongly indicate the diagnosis of HCC (Fig. 21-7). The detection of multiple nodules is another common finding in HCC.

ULTRASOUND ANGIOGRAPHY

Concept

Although angiography remains the most specific imaging method for confirmation of HCC, small HCCs, which have previously been detected by ultrasound, cannot always be detected as characteristic hypervascular nodules on conventional angiography, digital subtraction angiography (DSA), or computed tomography (CT) after intra-arterial administration of iodized oil (Lipiodol CT).[14–18]

FIGURE 21-2. Mosaic pattern of HCC (arrows) on ultrasound. Halo, septum, and internal mosaic echo are clearly demonstrated.

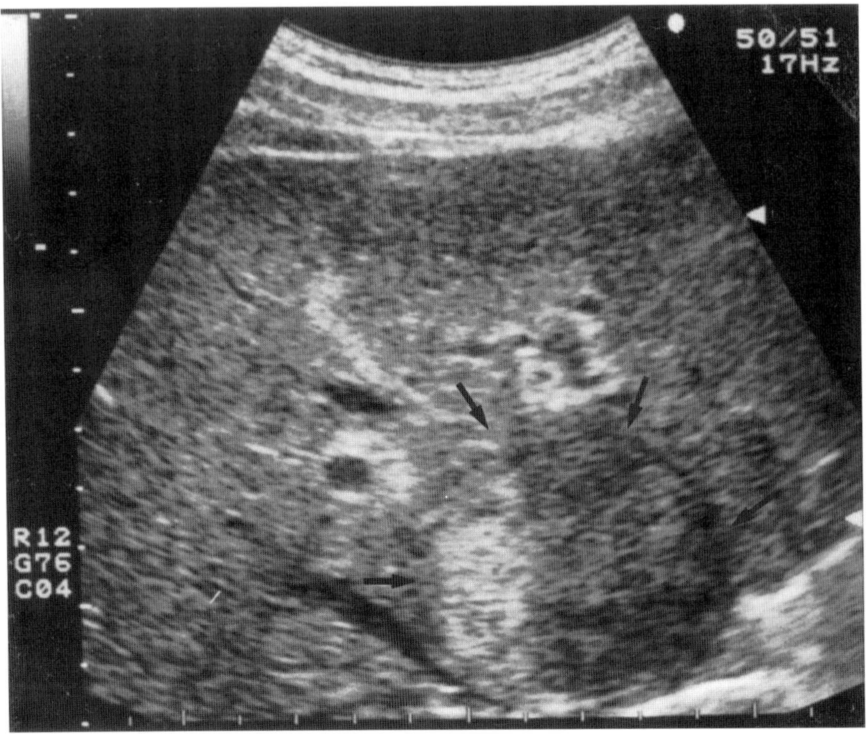

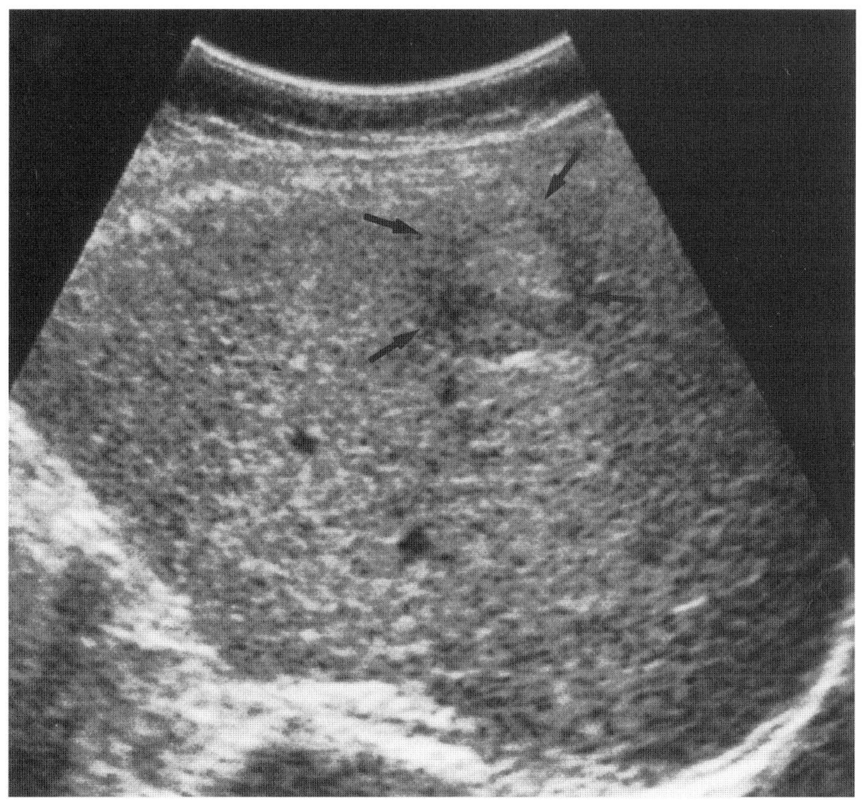

FIGURE 21-3. Small HCC (arrows) on ultrasound. Mosaic pattern, septum, halo, lateral shadow, and posterior echo enhancement are evident.

FIGURE 21-4. (*A*) Hypoechoic HCC (arrows) on ultrasound. (*B*) Resected specimen. (See also Plate 21-1.)

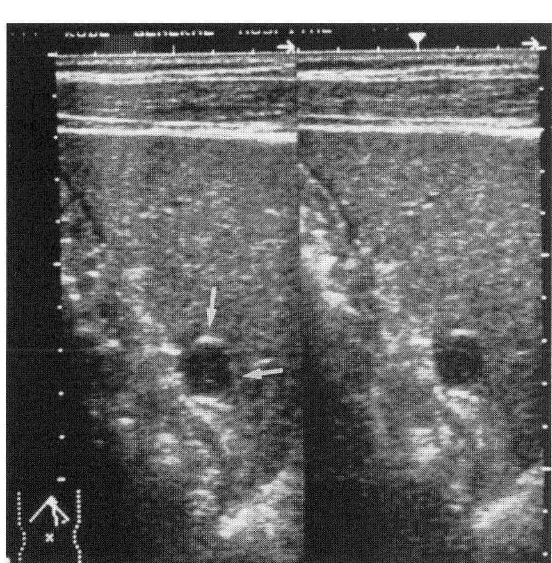

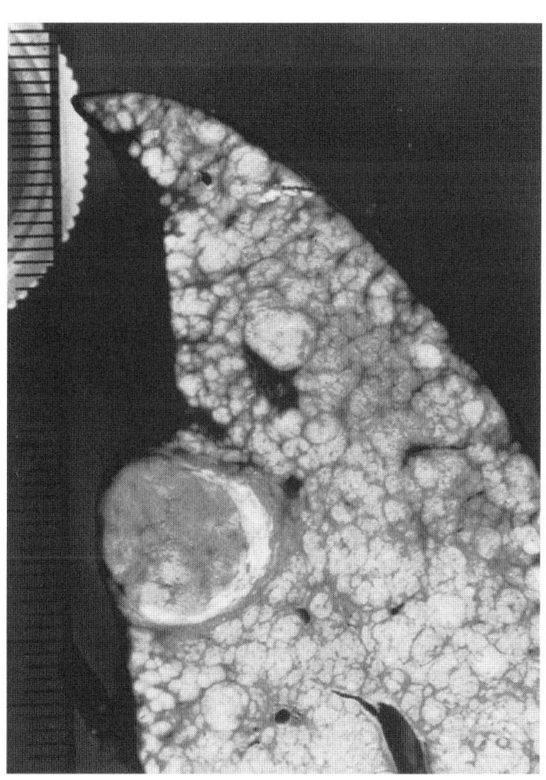

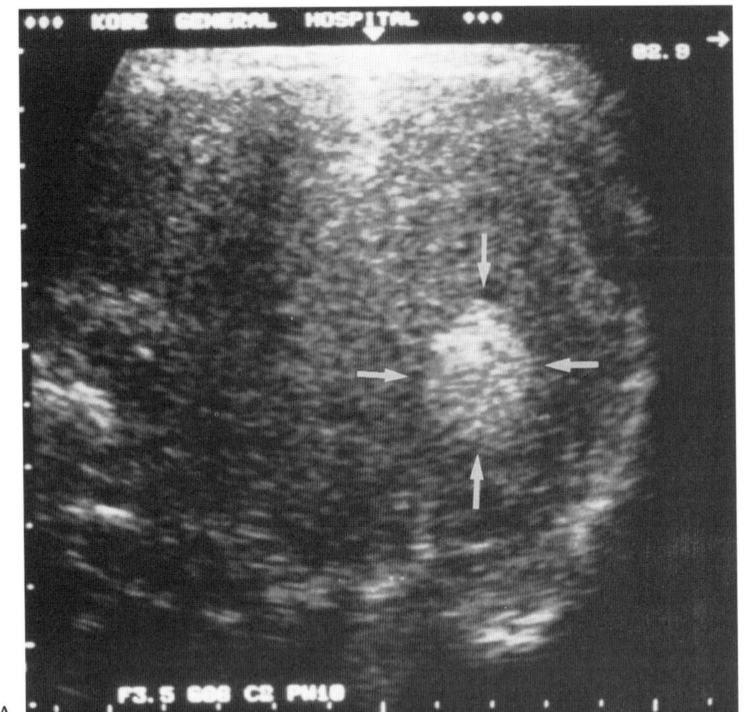

A

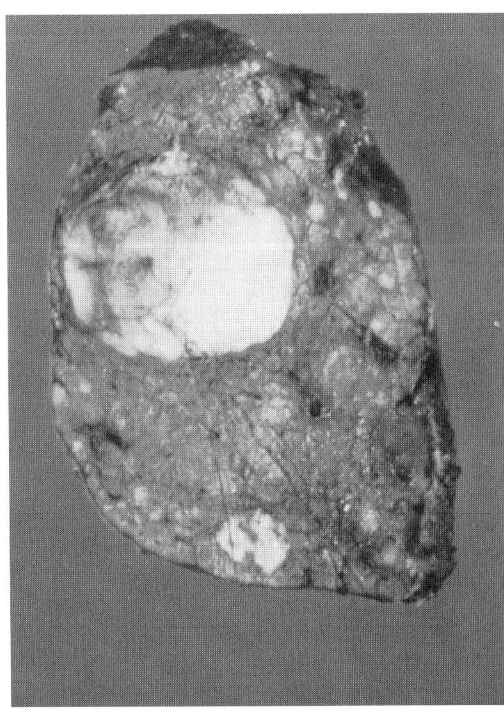

B

FIGURE 21-5. (*A*) Hyperechoic HCC (arrows) on ultrasound. (*B*) Resected specimen. Fatty change can be seen within the nodule. (See also Plate 21-2.)

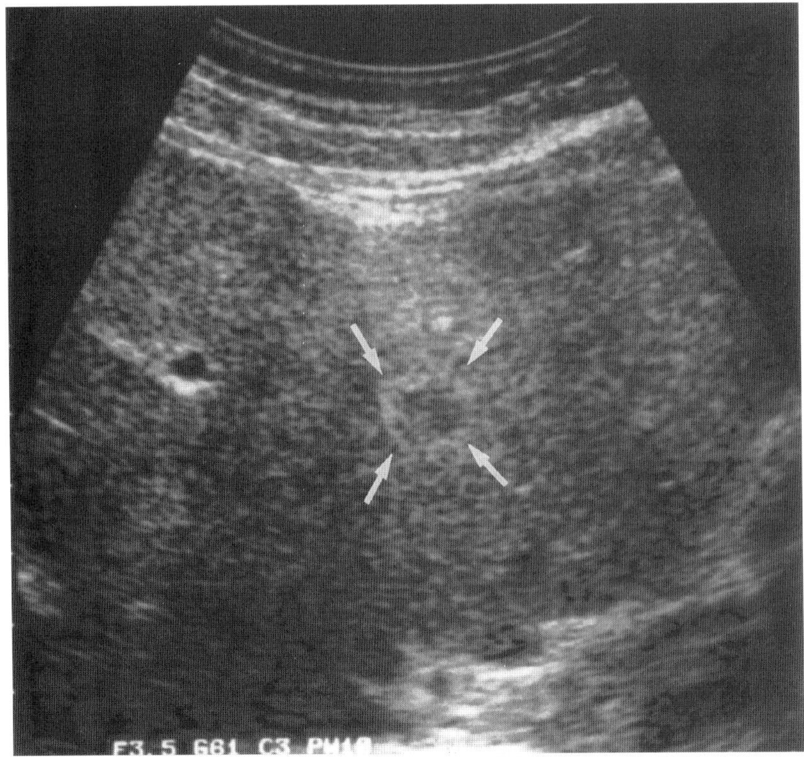

FIGURE 21-6. Bright loop pattern of HCC (arrows) on ultrasound. The hyperchoic loop represents well-differentiated foci with fatty change compared to the internal hypoechoic less differentiated lesion.

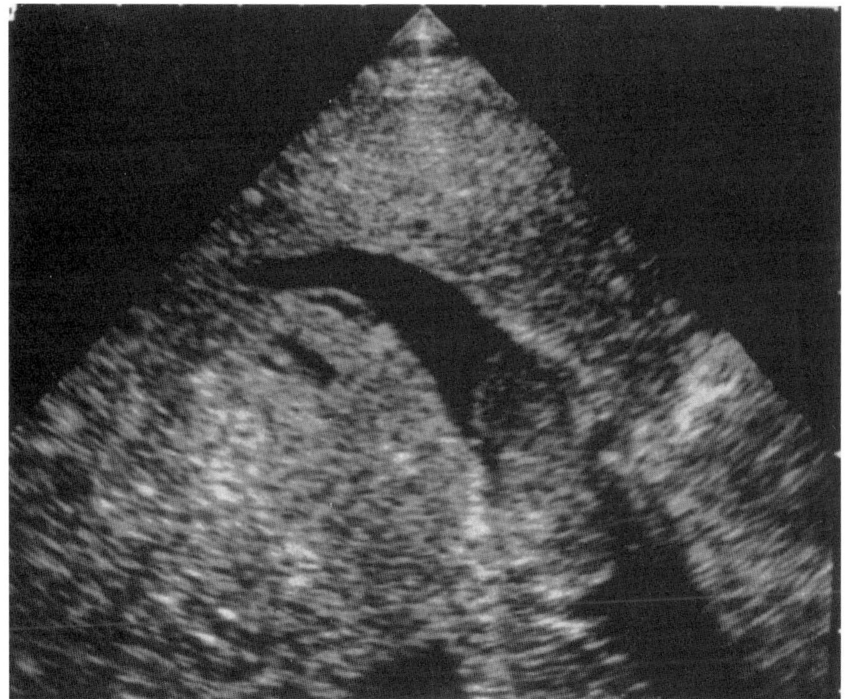
A

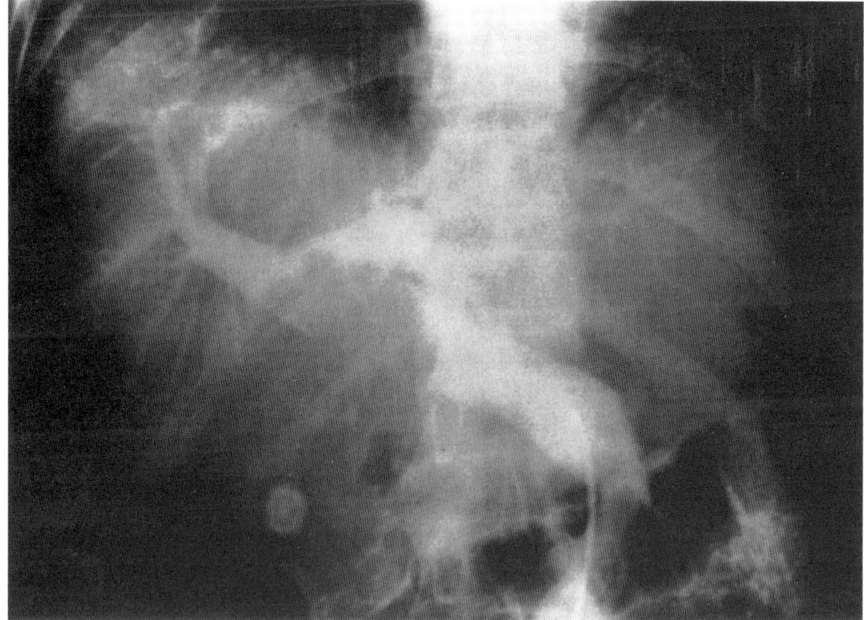
B

FIGURE 21-7. (*A*) Tumor thrombus of HCC is evident by ultrasound in the first branch of the portal vein. (*B*) Portography confirmed the portal tumor thrombus.

The diagnostic approach to recognition of such angiographically undetectable HCCs is currently one of the most important concerns in the fields of radiology and hepatology. Dynamic contrast-enhanced ultrasound (ultrasound angiography) with intra-arterial infusion of CO_2 microbubbles, a contrast material for use in ultrasound examinations, is a newly developed imaging technique that is a combination of ultrasound and angiography.[19,20]

Technique

Ultrasound angiography is performed by injecting microbubbles of CO_2 through a catheter placed into the hepatic artery after conventional hepatic angiography. The

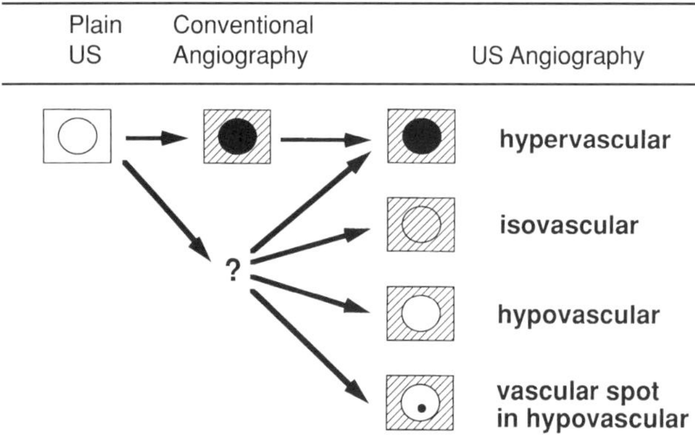

FIGURE 21-8. Vascular patterns depicted on ultrasound angiography as compared with conventional angiography. An angiographically undetected nodule can be demonstrated as any of hypervascular, isovascular, hypovascular, or vascular spot in hypovascular pattern. US, ultrasound.

CO_2 microbubbles are prepared by vigorously mixing by hand 10 ml of CO_2, 10 ml of heparinized normal saline, and 5 ml of the patient's blood.

The total duration of the procedure is classified into the three phases of early, middle, and late in accordance with the degree of enhancement of the liver parenchyma with CO_2 microbubbles. Vascular findings on ultrasound angiography can be classified into four patterns depending on the tumor vascularity compared with the surrounding liver parenchyma: these are hypervascular, isovascular, hypovascular, and vascular spot in hypovascular (Fig. 21-8). The hypervascular pattern is subclassified into four types: a homogeneous or mosaic pattern with peripheral arterial supply; spotty pooling; peripheral hypervascularity; and central arterial supply with dense stain.[20,21]

Tumor Characterization

A typical angiographic finding of HCC is abundant tumor vessels with hypervascular stain, but this finding is not always demonstrated, especially in small HCCs.[14–18]

FIGURE 21-9. Hypervascular HCC (arrow). Sonographically undetected nodule is also demonstrated as a hypervascular lesion (arrowhead) by ultrasound angiography.

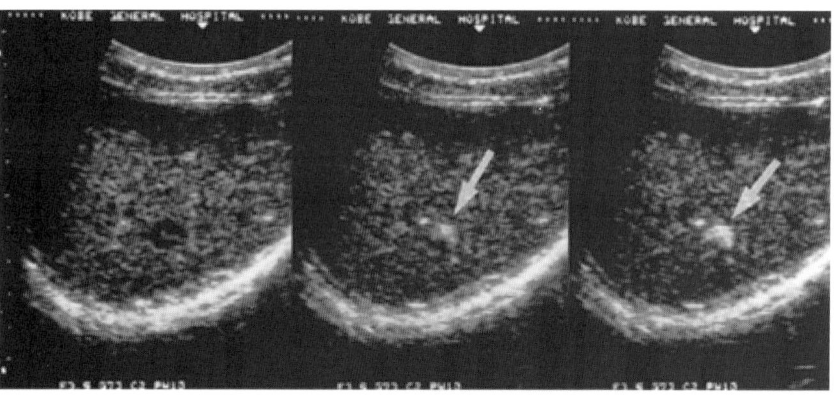

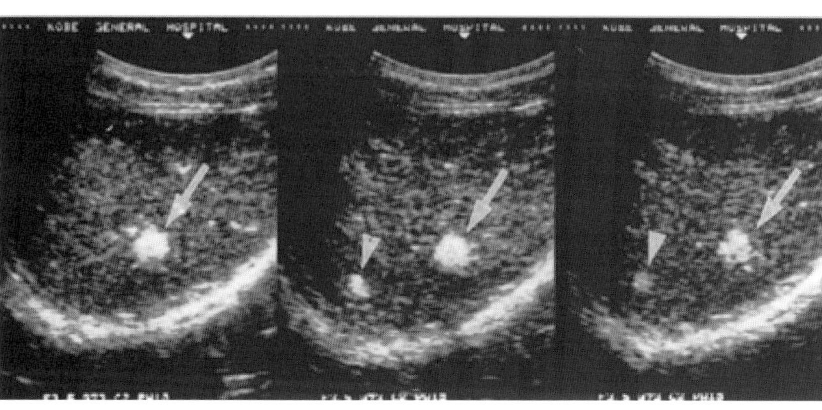

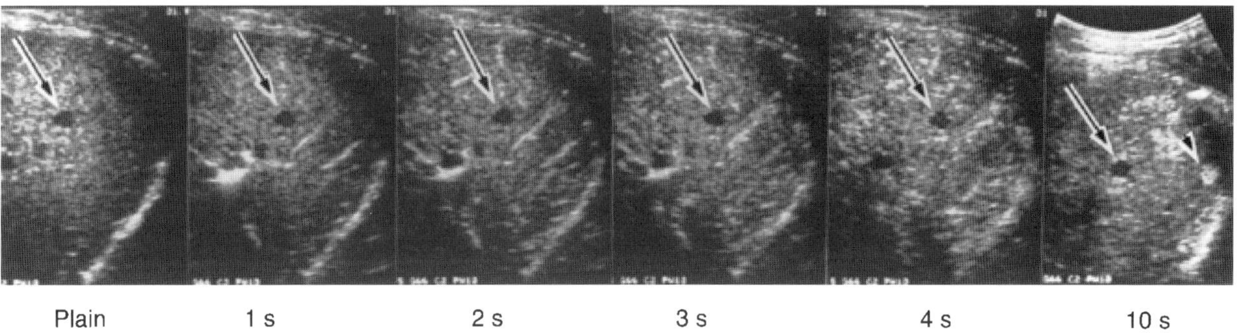

FIGURE 21-10. Concurrent presence of hypovascular HCC (arrow) and hypervascular HCC (arrowhead) on ultrasound angiography. Histopathologically, the hypovascular nodule was identified as well-differentiated HCC and the hypervascular nodule as moderately differentiated HCC.

These angiographically undetected HCCs can be diagnosed by ultrasound angiography as a faint hypervascular (Figs. 21-9, 21-10), isovascular, hypovascular (Fig. 21-10), or a vascular spot in hypovascular (Fig. 21-11) pattern. The typical vascular patterns of HCC demonstrated by ultrasound angiography are a peripheral arterial supply and a homogeneous or mosaic hypervascular pattern. The sensitivity and specificity of this finding in our experience was around 90% (125/139) and 89% (74/83), respectively.

All nodules of adenomatous hyperplasia appear in a hypovascular pattern (Fig. 21-12) on ultrasound angiography and can be accurately differentiated from advanced HCC. Adenomatous hyperplastic nodule (AHN) with malignant foci (HCC within AHN) can be demonstrated as a vascular spot in a hypovascular pattern (Fig.

FIGURE 21-11. HCC with vascular spot in hypovascular pattern on ultrasound angiography. A vascular spot (black arrow) is clearly demonstrated within a hypovascular nodule (bold arrow). A feeding artery supplying a vascular lesion is also depicted as a pulsatile vessel within the hypovascular nodule (arrowhead). Histopathologically, the vascular lesion was identified as well-differentiated HCC and the hypovascular lesion as adenomatous hyperplasia; thus, this nodule is HCC within an adenomatous hyperplastic lesion.

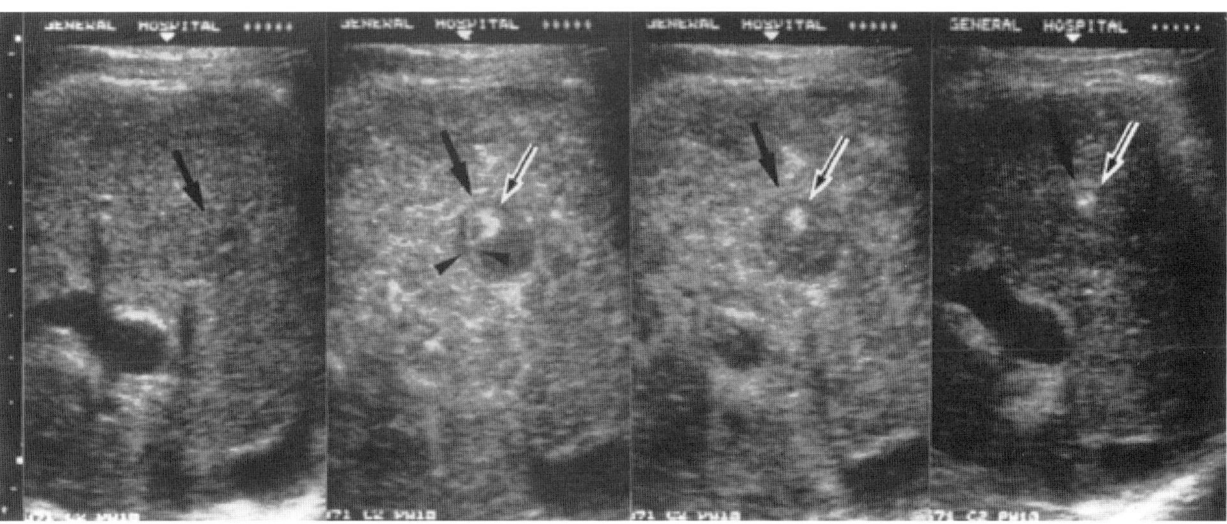

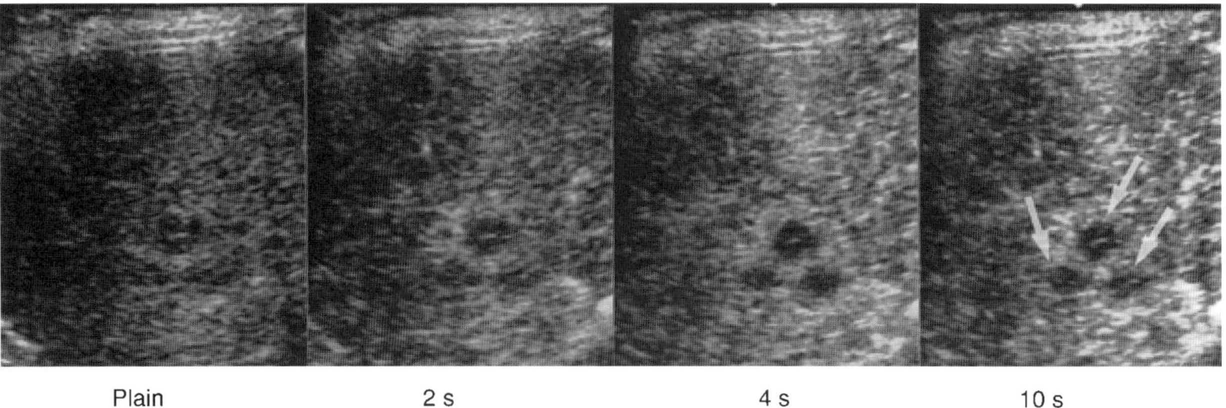

FIGURE 21-12. Ultrasound angiography of adenomatous hyperplasia. Three hypovascular nodules (arrows) are clearly demonstrated by ultrasound angiography.

21-11) (nodule in nodule) on ultrasound angiography. This finding is an extremely specific finding for HCC within AHN.[22]

Hemangioma has an extremely characteristic vascular pattern on ultrasound angiography: central hypovascularity with peripheral echogenic spots in the early arterial phase, gradually infiltrating to the center over time, and spotty pooling in the very late phase, lasting up to 30 to 60 minutes after injection. The sensitivity and specificity of this set of findings are both 100%.

Ultrasound angiography of hepatic metastasis presents a variety of vascular patterns; peripheral hypervascular pattern is seen in 64%, hypovascular pattern in 15%, homogeneous hypervascular pattern in 15%, and mosaic or inhomogeneous hypervascular pattern in 6%.[20] The peripheral hypervascular pattern is characteristic for metastasis; the specificity is 100%.[20]

Focal nodular hyperplasia has an extremely characteristic vascular pattern in all cases: early central hypervascular supply with centrifugal fill-in to the periphery in the arterial phase and a uniform or lobulated dense stain in the parenchymal phase (Fig. 21-13). The sensitivity and specificity of this finding are both 100%.[20,21]

Detection and Diagnosis of Small HCC

The detection rate of small HCCs less than 3 cm in diameter with ultrasound angiography is superior (overall sensitivity of 95%: hypervascular, 82%; isovascular, 8%; vascular spot, 5%) to conventional angiography (62%), digital subtraction angiography (DSA) (65%), or Lipiodol CT (78%) (Table 21-1). Ultrasound angiography detects small hypervascular HCC, especially those less than 1 cm in diameter. Lipiodol CT had been the most sensitive method in the detection of small hypervascular HCC[23] before ultrasound angiography was introduced. However, it has an inherent limitation in the depiction of small hypervascular lesions, since its capacity depends

FIGURE 21-13. Focal nodular hyperplasia diagnosed by ultrasound angiography. Central arterial supply (arrow) with gradual filling toward the periphery (arrowheads) is clearly demonstrated.

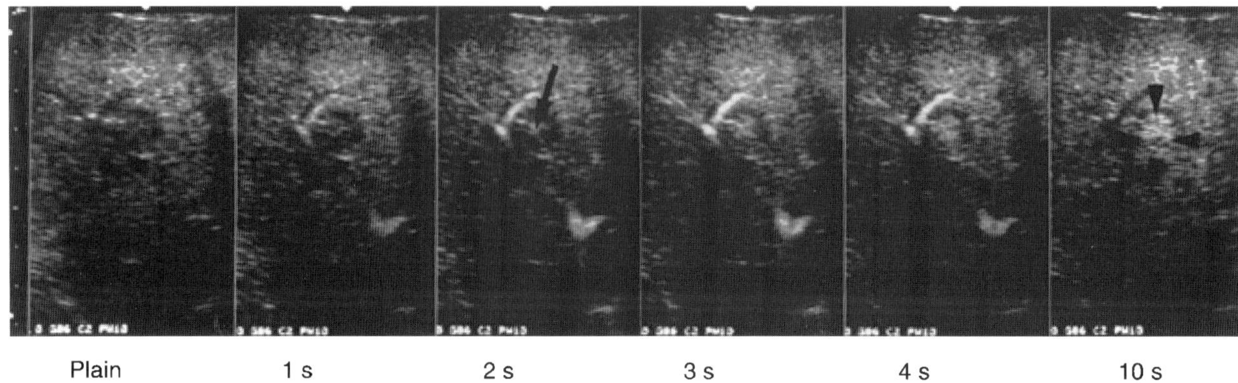

TABLE 21-1. Detection of Tumor Vascularity in 108 HCCs (≦3 cm)

Size (cm)	No. of Nodules	Angiography (n = 108)		Lipiodol CT (n = 96)	Ultrasound Angiography (n = 108)[a]			
		Conventional (n = 71)	DSA (n = 37)		Hypervascular (n = 89)	Isovascular (n = 9)	Hypovascular (n = 5)	Vascular Spot in Hypovascular (n = 5)
≦1	25	25% (3/12)	31% (4/13)	42% (10/24)	56% (14/25)	8% (2/25)	20% (5/25)	16% (4/25)
1–2	45	59% (17/29)	75% (12/16)	85% (33/39)	84% (38/45)	13% (6/45)	—	2% (1/45)
2–3	38	80% (24/30)	100% (8/8)	97% (32/38)	97% (37/38)	3% (1/38)	—	
		62% (44/71)	65% (24/37)		82% (89/108)	8% (9/108)	5% (5/108)	5% (5/108)
	108	63% (68/108)		78% (75/96)		100% (108/108)		

[a] 108 nodules in 100 patients.

(Modified from Kudo et al.,[24] with permission.)

on the dose of iodized oil that is injected, the time that elapses between the injection and CT scanning, the washout speed from the nodule, and the vascularity of the tumor.

Ultrasound angiography seems to be the most sensitive tool in the detection of intranodular vascularity even when the nodule is as small as less than 1 cm in diameter.[24]

Diagnosis of Early-Stage HCC

It is well known that most cases of early-stage HCC do not show tumor stains on an angiogram or retention of Lipiodol within the tumor,[25] which complicates the diagnosis of HCC. Although CT during arterial portography (CTAP)[26] or histologic diagnosis of percutaneous biopsy[27–29] is necessary for the definitive diagnosis, ultrasound angiography is useful in the diagnosis of early-stage HCC since it discloses definitive vascularity in the nodule (Figs. 21-8 to 21-11), theoretically in 100% of the nodules.[24] Concurrent ultrasound angiography and CTAP seems to be the most effective way to obtain imaging diagnosis of early-stage HCC.[30–32] For example, 82% of 17 resected early-stage HCC could be accurately diagnosed as early-stage HCC preoperatively using the combination of ultrasound angiography and CTAP.[30]

Role in Treatment Planning

Real-time observation of tumor vascularity offers information important in treatment selection. When surgical resection is not indicated, transcatheter arterial embolization therapy or intra-arterial infusion of chemotherapeutic agents mixed with iodized oil[33] is effective for treatment of HCCs as long as the HCC is hypervascular, whereas such therapy would not be effective for the treatment of relatively hypovascular HCCs.[25] Percutaneous ethanol injection therapy[34] is indicated for hypovascular nodules. Ultrasound angiography is an extremely valuable method for assessing HCC vascularity.[24,35] In addition, since ultrasound angiography enables depiction of HCC not detected with plain ultrasonography, this technique can also be applicable as a guide to ethanol injection therapy for such sonographically undetected HCCs.[36]

COLOR DOPPLER ULTRASOUND

Tumor Characterization

The typical color Doppler findings in advanced HCC are afferent pulsatile waveform (PW) signals, intratumoral PW signals associated with intratumoral continuous waveform (CW) signals, and efferent CW signals (Fig. 21-14 and Plate 21-3).[37,38] In contrast, the typical findings of early HCC and adenomatous hyperplastic nodule are afferent CW signals, which reflect a feeding portal flow, rarely associated with PW signals (Fig. 21-15 and Plate 21-4).[38] Typical color Doppler findings of focal nodular hyperplasia are centrifugal PW signals originating from the central zone; with these latter findings a differentiation of focal nodular hyperplasia from HCC is possible (Fig. 21-16 and Plate 21-5).[39]

Doppler Spectral Analysis

Prior attempts at differential diagnosis of hepatic tumors using conventional pulsed Doppler ultrasound have been reported to be of value[40–42] but have theoretical limitations. A possible pitfall of pulsed Doppler ultrasound is that flow information is obtained only from the highly

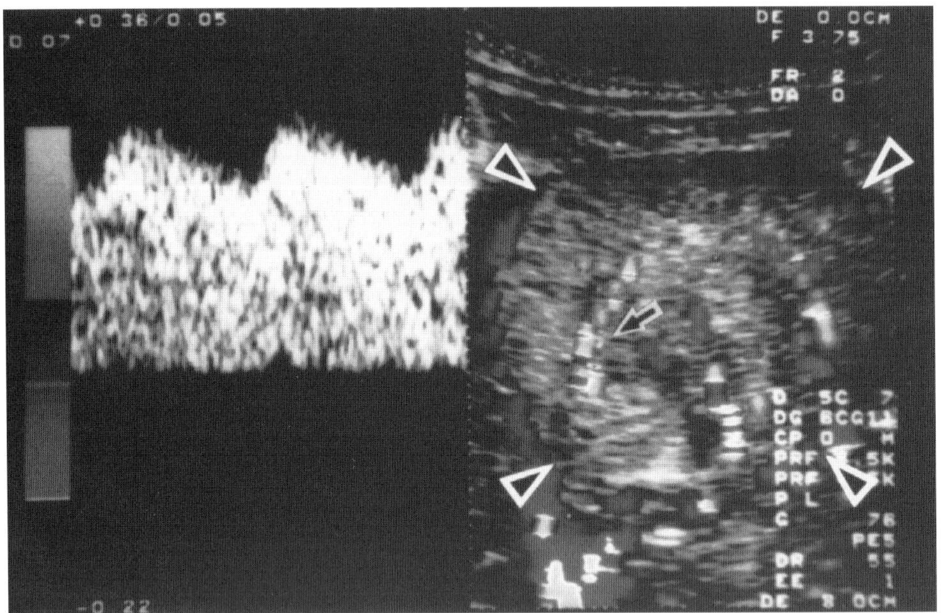

FIGURE 21-14. Color Doppler appearance of typical HCC (arrowheads). Intratumoral pulsatile signal (arrow) is clearly demonstrated. (See also Plate 21-3.)

FIGURE 21-15. Color Doppler appearance of adenomatous hyperplasia. Afferent continuous waveform signal not associated with pulsatile signal can be demonstrated. (See also Plate 21-4.)

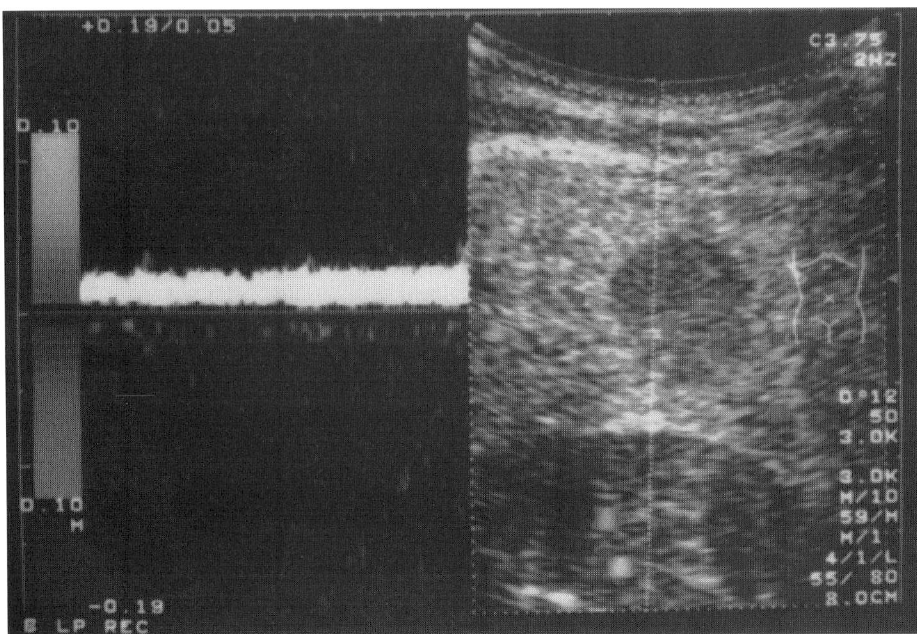

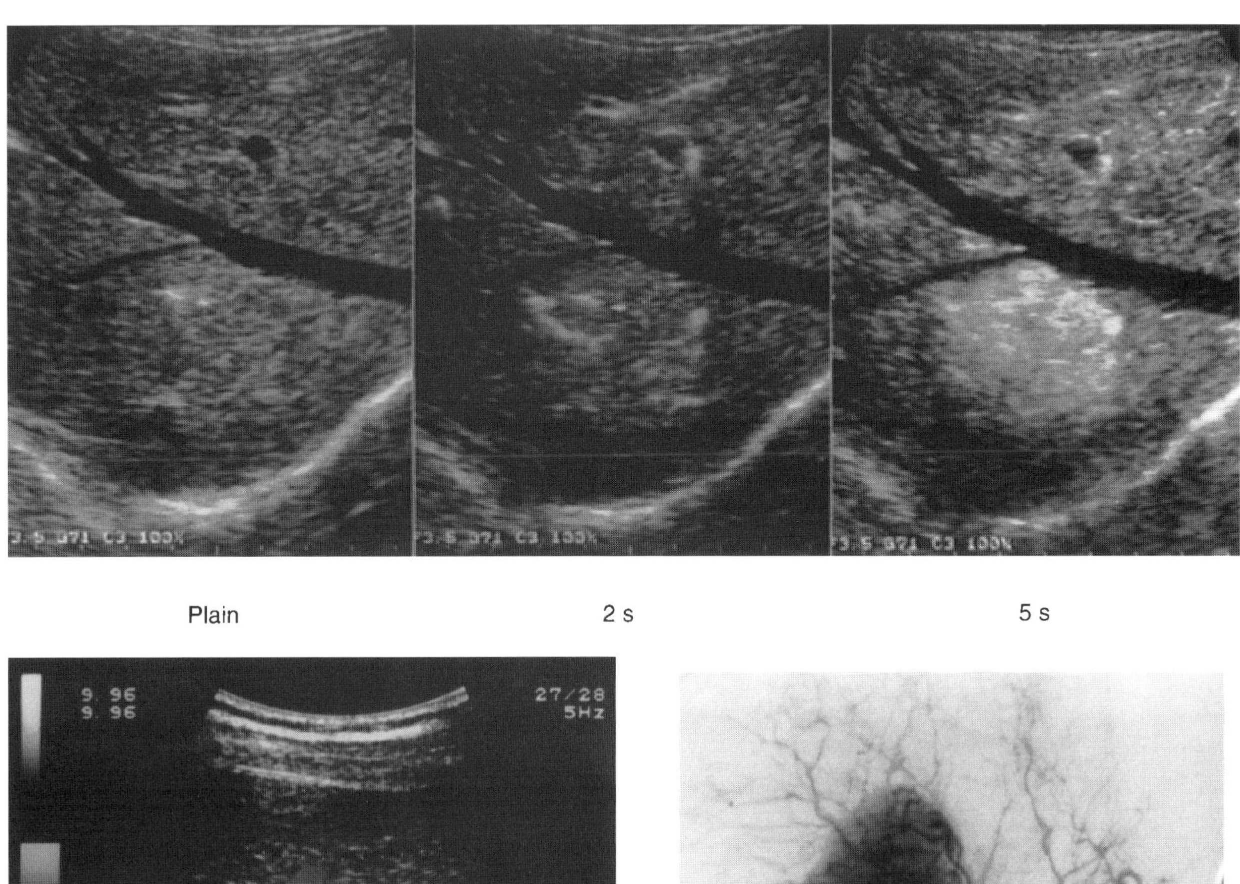

FIGURE 21-16. (*A*) Ultrasound angiography shows typical findings for focal nodular hyperplasia, specifically, central arterial supply with centrifugal flow pattern. (*B*) Color Doppler findings of focal nodular hyperplasia. Centrifugal flow pattern is clearly demonstrated. (See also Plate 21-5.) (*C*) Angiography shows spoke-wheel appearance, which is a typical finding for focal nodular hyperplasia.

restricted region from which the Doppler signals are sampled, and flow is not evaluated in the remainder of the image. However, with the use of color Doppler ultrasound, real-time imaging combined with blood flow imaging, which is depicted in color, is obtained. Consequently, it has become much easier to decide sampling points for performing a subsequent pulsed Doppler study.

Of the several parameters that can be obtained with Doppler spectral analysis, maximum flow velocity (Vmax) and pulsatility index (PI) are very important in the differential diagnosis of hepatic tumors (Figs. 21-17, 21-18).[43] The simultaneous measurement of Vmax and PI increases the diagnostic accuracy of HCC and hemangioma as compared with using the Vmax or PI alone.[43]

Power Doppler Ultrasound

Power Doppler ultrasound is a newly developed technique for depicting a flow signal based on the blood flow, in contrast to the conventional color Doppler, which depicts the flow velocity. Therefore, power Doppler ultrasound is very sensitive in the depiction of intratumoral color signal regardless of the velocity or the direction of the blood flow (Fig. 21-19 and Plate 21-6).

FIGURE 21-17. Maximum velocity (Vmax) obtained by spectral analysis using pulsed Doppler in HCC and hemangioma (Hem). The nodules with Vmax higher than 70 cm can be differentiated from hemangioma with accuracy.

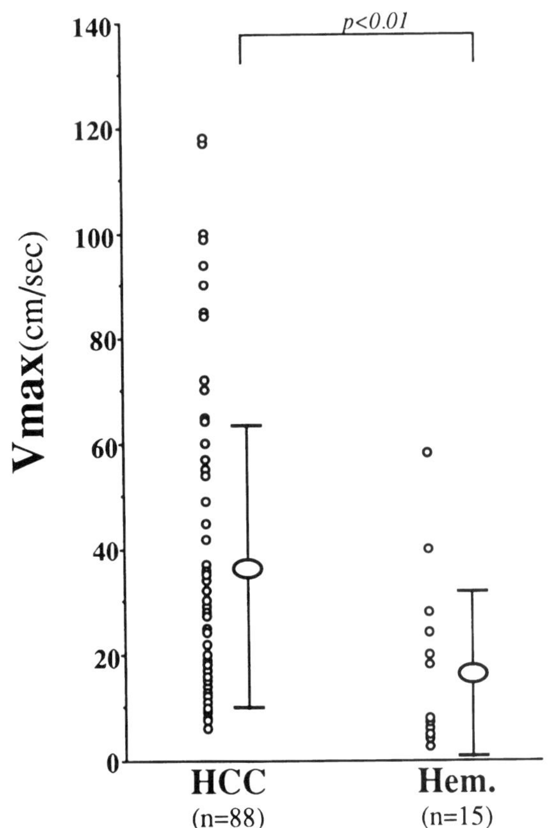

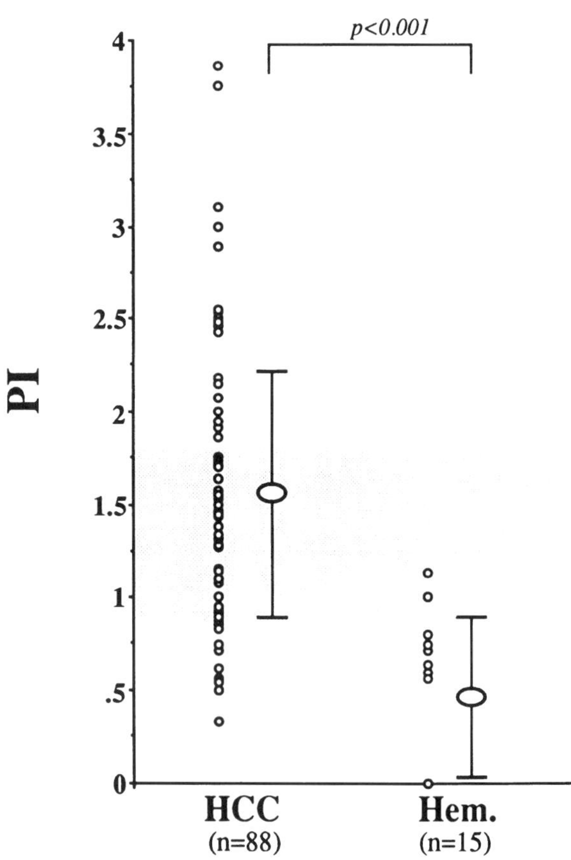

FIGURE 21-18. Pulsatility index (PI) obtained by maximum velocity (Vmax) minus minimum velocity (Vmin) divided mean velocity (Vmean) (Vmax − Vmin/Vmean) in HCC and hemangioma (Hem). The PI in HCC is much higher than that in hemangioma.

INTRAVENOUS CONTRAST-ENHANCED DOPPLER

A galactose-based ultrasound contrast agent for intravenous injection was developed recently[44] and has been applied to various clinical fields including the Doppler study of hepatic tumors. This technique improves the sensitivity of detecting vascularity within the nodule and improves the efficiency of the differential diagnosis by color Doppler imaging (Fig. 21-20 and Plate 21-7).[45] In our experience, the detectability of tumor vascularity by this technique in 18 hepatic tumors was equivalent to that of ultrasound angiography and superior to that of DSA. It is widely believed that the contrast-enhanced color Doppler study is a breakthrough in the color Doppler diagnosis of small hepatic tumors, especially in the early detection and precise evaluation of therapeutic re-

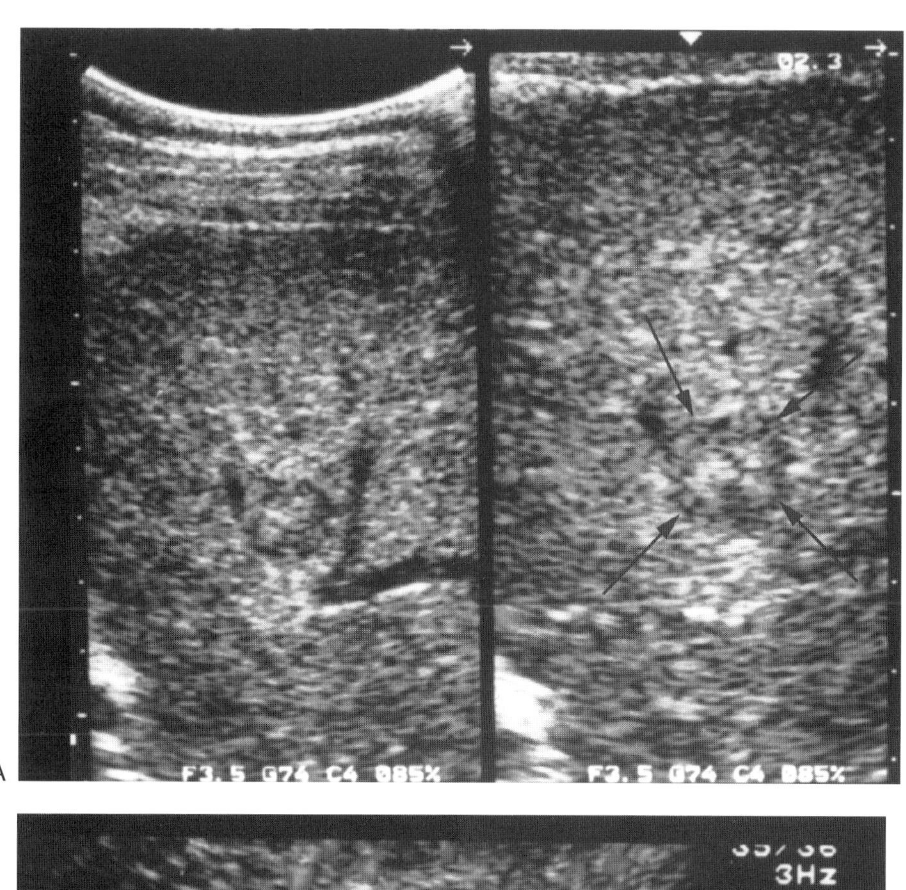

A

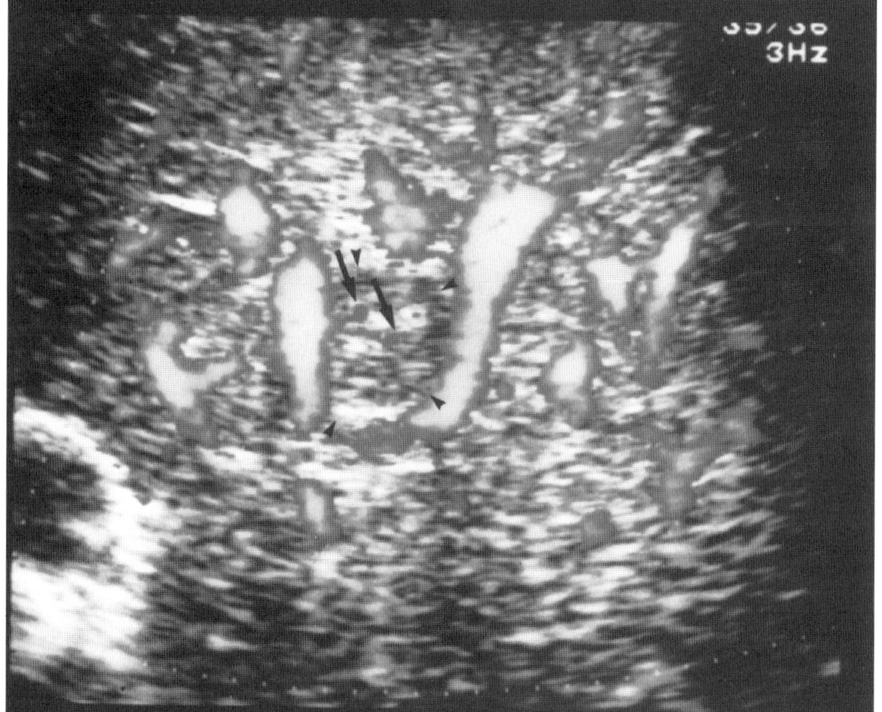

B

FIGURE 21-19. (*A*) Mosaic pattern of 1-cm diameter hepatocellular carcinoma (arrows). (*B*) Apparent color flow signals (arrows) are demonstrated within the nodule (arrowheads) by power Doppler imaging. (See also Plate 21-6.)

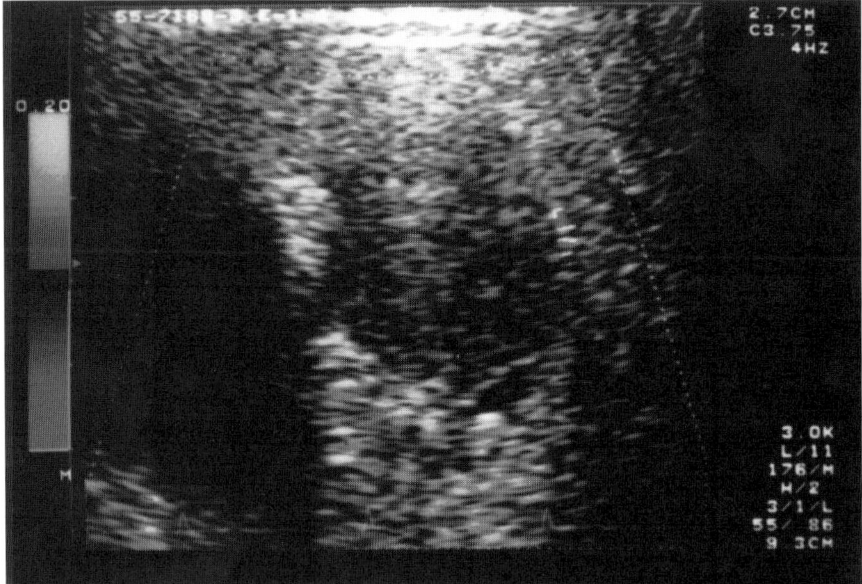

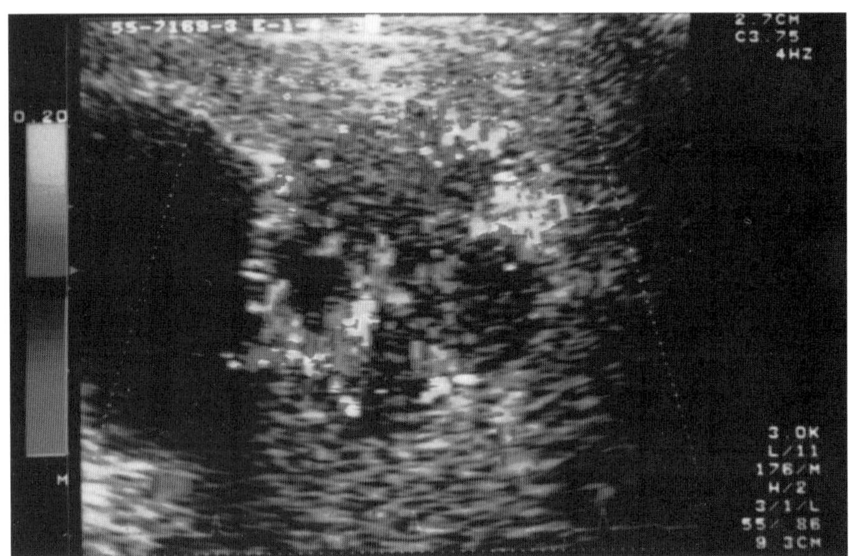

FIGURE 21-20. (*A*) Color signal is not demonstrated within the 5-cm-diameter HCC by plain color Doppler. (See also Plate 21-7A.) (*B*) Abundant color flow signal can be seen upon enhanced color Doppler study with intravenous injection of the contrast medium, Levovist, suggesting HCC. (See also Plate 21-7B.) (*Figure continues.*)

sponse and follow-up of HCC by color Doppler ultrasound.

CONCLUSIONS

Regular monitoring by ultrasound is extremely important in the screening of high-risk patients for HCC. Although ultrasound diagnosis has limitations in characterizing hepatic tumors, the confirmation of HCC is possible by ultrasound if typical findings are demonstrated by B-mode image.

Ultrasound angiography is the most sensitive tool in detecting hypervascularity in small HCCs, and therefore it is useful in the early detection and diagnosis of small HCCs in addition to being useful in the differentiation of HCCs from other hepatic tumors. It is also essential in the diagnosis of early-stage HCC and in formulating treatment plans based on an accurate assessment of vascularity within the nodule.

Color Doppler ultrasound is useful in the noninva-

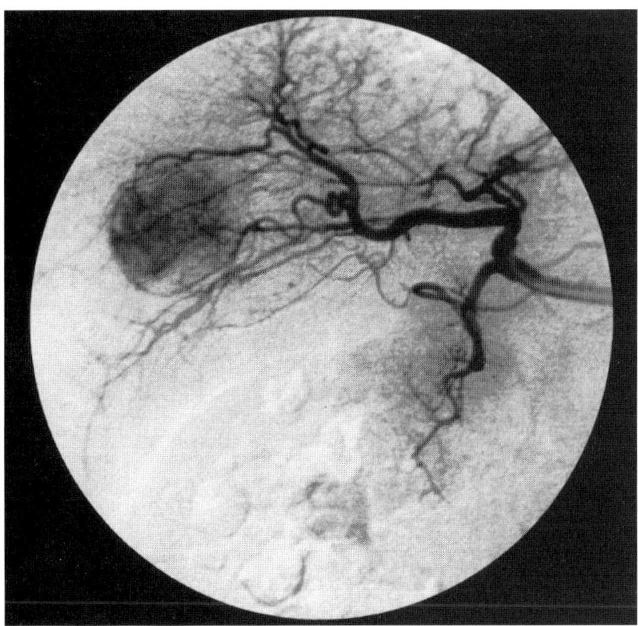

C

FIGURE 21-20 *(Continued)*. (C) Angiography reveals findings similar to those observed using enhanced color Doppler.

sive differentiation of HCC from other hepatic tumors, especially by use of quantitative Doppler spectral analysis, such as Vmax and/or PI and an intravenous transpulmonary contrast agent.

REFERENCES

1. Arii S, Tobe T. Results of surgical treatment. Follow up study by Liver Cancer Study Group of Japan. In Tobe T et al (eds): Primary Liver Cancer in Japan. Spring-Verlag, Tokyo, 1992: 243–255
2. The Liver Cancer Study Group of Japan. Survey and follow-up study of primary liver cancer in Japan. Report 11. Acta Hepatol Jpn 1995;36:208–218
3. The Liver Cancer Study Group of Japan. Predictive factors for long term prognosis after partial hepatectomy for patients with hepatocellular carcinoma in Japan. Cancer 1994;74: 2772
4. Shinagawa T, Ohto M, Kimura K et al. Diagnosis and clinical features of small hepatocellular carcinoma with emphasis on the utility of realtime ultrasonography. A study of 51 patients. Gastroenterology 1984;86:495–502
5. Tanaka S, Kitamura T, Nakanishi K et al. Recent advances in ultrasonographic diagnosis of hepatocellular carcinoma. Cancer 1989;63:1313–1317
6. Beasley RP, Hwang LY, Lin CC, Chien CS. Hepatocellular carcinoma and hepatitis B virus. Lancet 1981;ii:1129–1133
7. Takano S, Yokosuka O, Imazeki F et al. Incidence of hepatocellular carcinoma in chronic hepatitis B and C. A prospective study of 251 patients. Hepatology 1995;21:650–655
8. Bruix J, Calvet X, Costa J et al. Prevalence of antibodies to hepatitis C virus in Spanish patients with hepatocellular carcinoma and hepatic cirrhosis. Lancet 1989;ii:1004–1006
9. Kobayashi K, Sugimoto T, Makino H et al. Screening methods for early detection of hepatocellular carcinoma. Hepatology 1985;5:1100–1105
10. Oka H, Kurioka N, Kim K et al. Prospective study of early detection of hepatocellular carcinoma in patients with cirrhosis. Hepatology 1990;12:680–687
11. Sheu JC, Sung JL, Chen DS et al. Ultrasonography of small hepatic tumors using high-resolution linear-array real-time instruments. Radiology 1984;150:797–802
12. Ebara M, Ohto M, Shinagawa T et al. Natural history of minute hepatocellular carcinoma smaller than three centimeters complicating cirrhosis. Gastroenterology 1986;90: 289–298
13. Tanaka S, Kitamura T, Imaoka S et al. Hepatocellular carcinoma. Sonographic and histologic correlation. AJR 1983; 140:701–707
14. Yoshimatsu S, Inoue Y, Ibukuro K, Suzuki S. Hypovascular hepatocellular carcinoma undetected at angiography and CT with iodized oil. Radiology 1989;171:343–347
15. Sonoda T, Shirabe K, Takenaka K. Angiographically undetected small hepatocellular carcinoma: clinicopathological characteristics, follow-up and treatment. Hepatology 1989; 10:1003–1007
16. Sumida M, Ohto M, Ebara M et al. Accuracy of angiography in the diagnosis of small hepatocellular carcinoma. AJR 1986;147:531–536
17. Takayasu K, Shima Y, Muramatsu Y et al. Angiography of small hepatocellular carcinomas: analysis of 105 resected tumors. AJR 1986;147:525–529

18. Okuda K. Early recognition of hepatocellular carcinoma. Hepatology 1986;6:729–738

19. Matsuda Y, Yabuuchi I. Hepatic tumors. US contrast enhancement with CO_2 microbubbles. Radiology 1986;161: 701–705

20. Kudo M, Tomita S, Tochio H et al. Sonography with intraarterial infusion of carbon dioxide microbubbles (sonographic angiography): value in differential diagnosis of hepatic tumors. AJR 1992;158:65–74

21. Kudo M, Tomita S, Tochio H et al. Hepatic focal nodular hyperplasia. Specific findings at dynamic contrast-enhanced US with carbon dioxide microbubbles. Radiology 1991;179: 377–382

22. Nomura Y, Matsuda Y, Yabuuchi I et al. Hepatocellular carcinoma in adenomatous hyperplasia. Detection with contrast-enhanced US with carbon dioxide microbubbles. Radiology 1993;187:353–356

23. Ohishi H, Uchida H, Yoshimura H et al. Hepatocellular carcinoma detected by iodized oil: use of anticancer agents. Radiology 1985;154:25–29

24. Kudo M, Tomita S, Tochio H et al. Small hepatocellular carcinoma: diagnosis with US angiography with intraarterial CO_2 microbubbles. Radiology 1992;182:155–160

25. Takayasu K, Wakao F, Moriyama N et al. Response of early-stage hepatocellular carcinoma and borderline lesions to therapeutic arterial embolization. AJR 1993;160:301–306

26. Matsui O, Kadoya M, Kameyama T et al. Benign and malignant nodules in cirrhotic livers. Distinction based on blood supply. Radiology 1991;178:493–497

27. Kojiro M, Sugihara S, Nakashima O. Pathomorphologic characteristics of early hepatocellular carcinoma. In Okuda K, Tobe T, Kitagawa T (eds): Early Detection and Treatment of Liver Cancer. Japan Scientific Societies Press, Tokyo, 1991;29–37

28. Sakamoto M, Hirohashi S, Shimosato Y. Early stage of multistep hepatocarcinogenesis. Adenomatous hyperplasia and early hepatocellular carcinoma. Hum Pathol 1991;22: 172–178

29. Okuda K. Hepatocellular carcinoma. Recent progress. Hepatology 1992;15:948–963

30. Kudo M, Tomita S, Tochio H et al. Hemodynamic characteristics of early stage hepatocellular carcinoma. In vivo evaluation with vascular imagings. Acta Hepatol Jpn 1992;33: 283–291

31. Kudo M, Tomita S, Kashida H et al. Tumor hemodynamics in hepatic nodules associated with liver cirrhosis. Relationship between cancer progression and tumor hemodynamic change. Jpn J Gastroenterol 1991;88:1554–1565

32. Muramatsu Y, Nawano S, Takayasu K et al. Early hepatocellular carcinoma. MR imaging. Radiology 1991;181:209–213

33. Takayasu K, Shima Y, Muramatsu Y et al. Hepatocellular carcinoma. Treatment with intraarterial iodized oil with and without chemotherapeutic agents. Radiology 1987;163: 345–351

34. Shiina S, Yasuda H, Muto H et al. Percutaneous ethanol injection in the treatment of liver neoplasms. AJR 1987;49: 949–952

35. Choi BI, Takayasu K, Han MC. Small hepatocellular carcinomas and associated nodular lesions of the liver. Pathology, pathogenesis, and imaging findings. AJR 1993;160: 1177–1187

36. Imari Y, Sakamoto S, Shiomichi S et al. Hepatocellular carcinoma not detected with plain US. Treatment with percutaneous ethanol injection under guidance with enhanced US. Radiology 1992;185:497–500

37. Tanaka S, Kitamura T, Fujita M et al. Color Doppler flow imaging of liver tumors. AJR 1990;143:509–514

38. Tanaka S, Kitamura T, Fujita M et al. Small hepatocellular carcinoma. Differentiation from adenomatous hyperplastic nodule with color Doppler flow imaging. Radiology 1992; 182:161–165

39. Kudo M, Tomita S, Minowa K et al. Color Doppler flow imaging of hepatic focal nodular hyperplasia. J Ultrasound Med 1992;11:553–557

40. Taylor KJW, Ramos I, Morse SS et al. Focal liver masses. Differential diagnosis with pulsed Doppler US. Radiology 1987;164:643–647

41. Yasuhara K, Kimura K, Ohto M et al. Pulsed Doppler in the diagnosis of small liver tumors. Br J Radiol 1988;61:898–902

42. Ohnishi K, Nomura F. Ultrasonic Doppler studies of hepatocellular carcinoma and comparison with other hepatic focal lesions. Gastroenterology 1989;97:1489–1497

43. Tochio H, Minowa K, Tomita S et al. Differential diagnosis of hepatic tumors using color Doppler flow imaging. Value of the Doppler spectral analysis. Jpn J Med Ultrasonics 1992; 19:277–287

44. Nanda NC, Schlief R. Advances in Echo Imaging Using Contrast Enhancement. Kluwer Academic Publishers, Dordrecht, 1993

45. Fujimoto M, Moriyasu F, Nishikawa K et al. Color Doppler sonography of hepatic tumors with a galactose-based contrast agent. Correlation with angiographic findings. AJR 1994; 163:1099–1104

22

HEPATIC ANGIOGRAPHY

KENICHI TAKAYASU

Although the diagnostic value of angiography has become less due to the development of sectional imaging such as ultrasound, computed tomography (CT), and magnetic resonance imaging (MRI), it is still important in preoperative evaluation and in provision of the vascular map. Moreover, angiography can be used for more advanced and detailed examination when combined with CT, namely, CT scanning during arterial portography (CTAP) and CT arteriography (CTA), and when used with Lipiodol CT. Angiography also is an indispensable technique for treatment with transcatheter arterial embolization (TAE).

ANATOMY OF HEPATIC VESSELS

Artery

The origin and course of the hepatic artery can vary from person to person. According to Michels,[1] aberrant hepatic arteries are seen in 45% of individuals, a "normal" anatomy being seen in only 55%. Occasionally there is an accessory artery providing a dual blood supply to an area normally supplied by one artery. When a branch of the posterior artery (Fig. 22-1) has been replaced, or for an accessory left gastric artery, and for some other aberrant arteries, it is important to interpret the branches by comparing the artery with the portal vein system that parallels it.

Portal Vein

The portal vein trunk typically divides into the right and left first-order portal veins in 84% to 92% of individuals. The anterior and posterior branches of the right portal vein and the left portal vein arise independently from the portal trunk without forming a common trunk (trifurcation type) in 4% to 12% of individuals, and the posterior portal vein alone begins early in the portal trunk (posterior independent type) in 3% to 6%. The variation in branching of the intrahepatic portal vein system is thought to be minimal compared to the hepatic artery and hepatic veins. In addition, several rare variations of the portal vein also have been recognized: the anterior portal vein arising from the left portal vein,[2] the portal vein forming a circle at the hepatic hilum,[3] and the right gastric vein directly entering the left lateral and medial portal vein (accessory portal vein) (Fig. 22-2).[4]

Hepatic Vein

The major vessels that drain the liver—the right, middle, and left hepatic veins—open into the inferior vena cava immediately below the diaphragm, and the inferior (right accessory) hepatic vein enters the inferior vena cava 5 to 6 cm caudal to them. Whereas the right hepatic vein joins the inferior vena cava from the right, the middle hepatic vein joins the left hepatic vein near its opening into the vena cava, forming a short common trunk[5] that joins the vena cava anterior and slightly to the left in 85% of cases.

The inferior right hepatic vein is enlarged when the hepatic portion of the inferior vena cava is blocked by a tumor or a membrane (a type of Budd-Chiari syndrome), becoming a collateral route.[6,7] This is an important diagnostic clue to the Budd-Chiari syndrome.

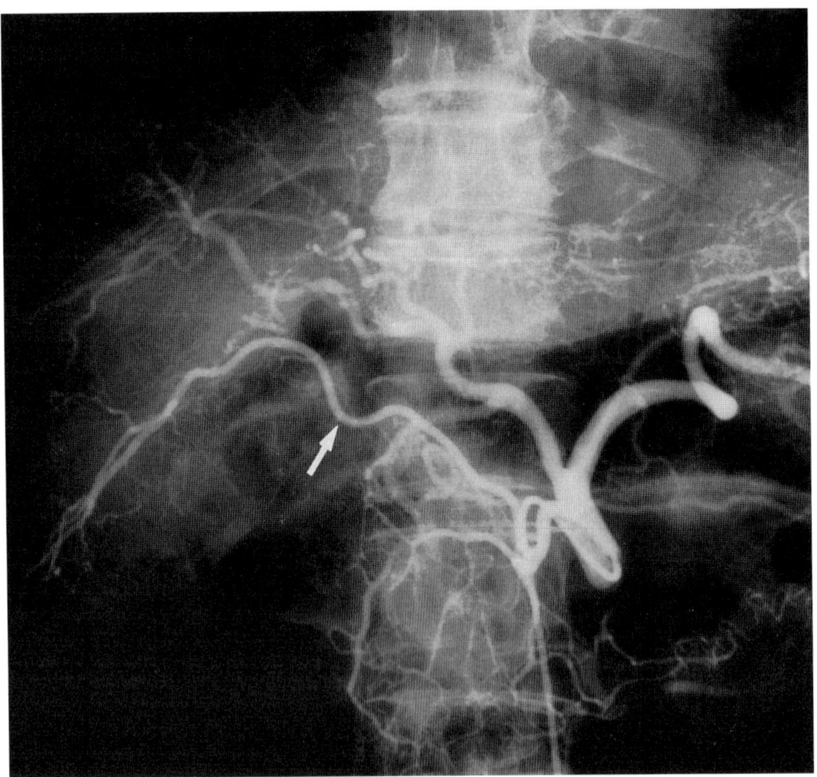

FIGURE 22-1. A replaced hepatic arterial branch (arrow indicates one of the posterior branches) derived from the dorsal pancreatic artery.

HEPATIC SEGMENTATION

The spatial relation between the hepatic artery and the portal vein can be described as "thin arteries creeping on a thick portal vein as ivies do trees" (Fig. 22-3). Therefore, the beginning of the right posterior artery coursing dorsally to the left medial and lateral arteries coursing ventrally seems to be a dense contrast point, which corresponds well to the posterior point (P-point) and umbilical point (U-point) of the portal vein, respectively. To follow these points on the angiogram is important in the identification of the branches, especially in the postoperative liver, and in advancing a microcatheter peripherally.

For hepatic segmentation, the system of Couinaud[8] that divides the liver into eight segments is now widely used. For more specific determination of the location of a small lesion, a more precise segmentation system determined by percutaneous transhepatic portography (PTP) is used.[9]

ANGIOGRAPHY

Hepatic Angiography

The Seldinger technique is commonly used, in which a 5 F sized catheter is advanced through the femoral artery into the hepatic artery. First, celiac angiography is performed to obtain general information regarding the liver and coexisting portal hypertension. It is followed by transmesenteric portography and superselective hepatic angiography. Digital subtraction angiography (DSA) is routinely done to reduce the amount of contrast medium to one-third or one-half of the dose previously used by conventional angiography. Right or left anterior oblique angiography facilitates the diagnosis of a superimposed lesion in the anteroposterior direction and confirmation of the course of vessels.

Recently, a 2.8 to 3 F coaxial catheter system has been developed that facilitates ultrasuperselective catheterization with a high success rate. Some of these catheters are covered by a hydrophilic polymer facilitating advancement in peripheral branches.

Portography

A direct approach to the portal vein system is provided by several procedures such as PTP, transumbilical portography, splenoportography, and transiliac venous portography. Wedged hepatic retrograde portography and postarterial portography are also used as an indirect approach. Currently, postarterial portography is widely carried out because of its ease and low invasiveness.

Venography

To confirm preoperatively the patency of the hepatic vein or inferior vena cava (IVC) or to rule out a tumor thrombus, venography (vena cavography) is performed.

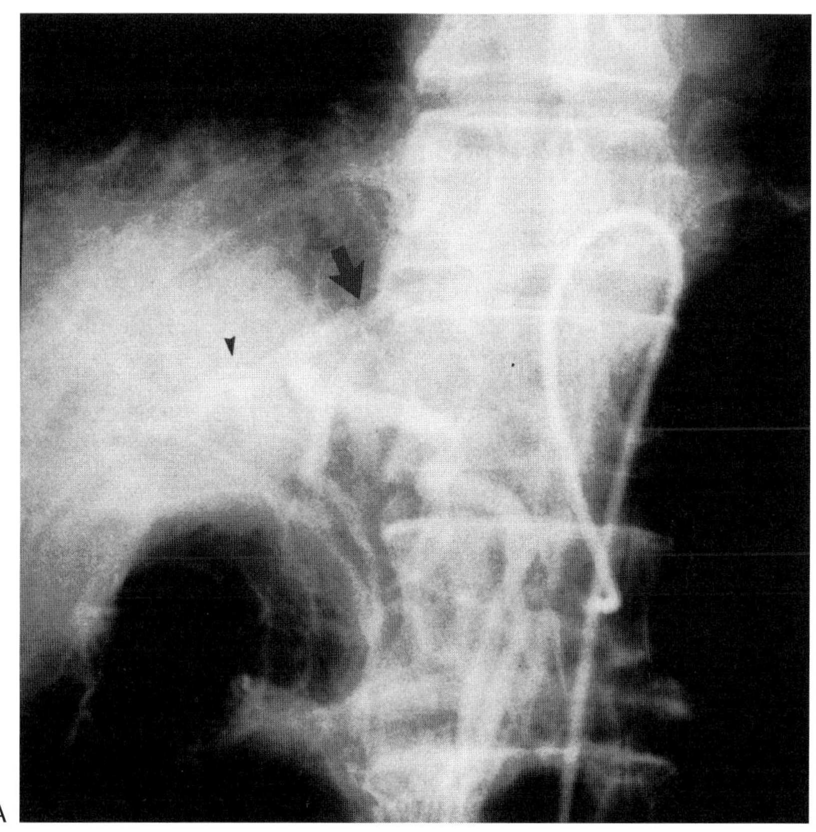

A

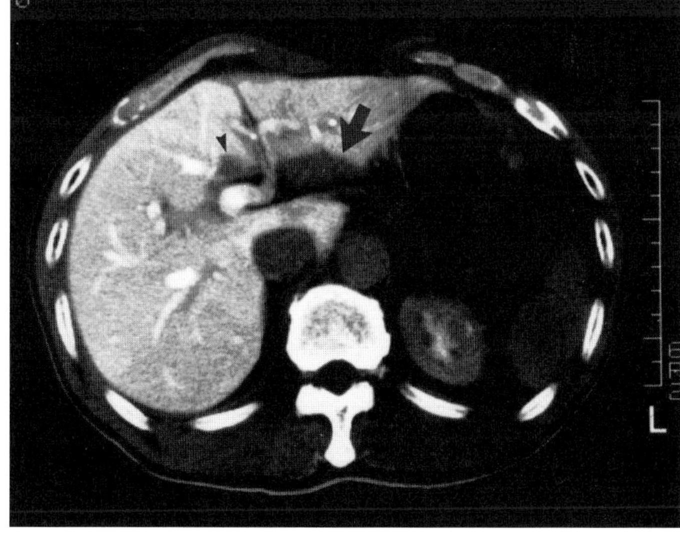

B

FIGURE 22-2. Accessary portal vein. In the late phase of common hepatic angiography (*A*), the right gastric vein is opacified followed by the left lateral superior (arrow) and left medial (arrowhead) portal vein branches. CTAP at the same level (*B*) as in Fig. A discloses a filling defect in the left lateral superior area (arrow) and in the posterior area of the left medial portion (arrowhead).

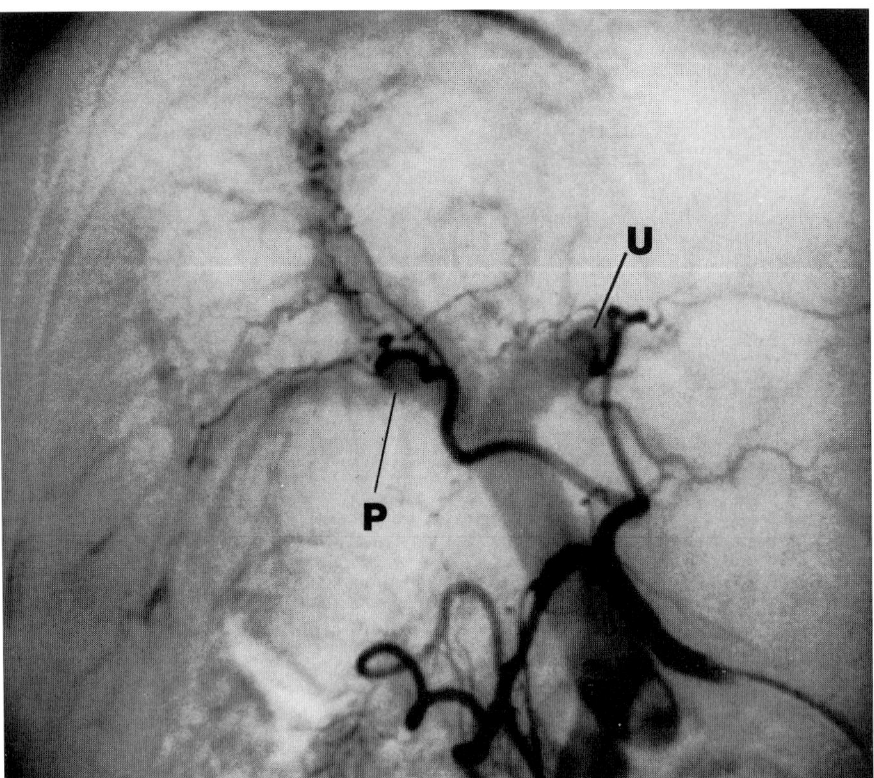

FIGURE 22-3. Relationship of the portal vein and hepatic artery by common hepatic angiography. Interpretation of the ramification and distribution of the artery becomes easier when orientation is made in relation to the dense points along the portal vein, the "posterior" (P) and "umbilical" (U) points.

However, venography is gradually being replaced by ultrasound or CT, and it is now used primarily for portal decompression with transjugular intrahepatic portal shunt (TIPS), combined with TAE, if hepatocellular carcinoma (HCC) is involved. Generally, the compression of the IVC by HCC is not a contraindication for operation (Fig. 22-4). However, operation is contraindicated if compression of the IVC is due to cholangiocarcinoma or metastatic adenocarcinoma.

COMBINATION OF CT AND ANGIOGRAPHY

There are two modalities of CT and angiography, CTAP and CTA. For CTA,[10–12] a catheter is inserted under angiographic visualization into the hepatic artery, for CTAP the superior mesenteric artery,[11,13] and a CT scan is made while contrast medium is injected. This modality is indispensable for preoperative evaluation. Hepatic angiograms are done before the combination study.

CTAP

This modality is very useful for diagnosis and preoperative study, particularly in patients with HCC and metastatic carcinoma. CTAP is the most sensitive technique for detection of HCC[13,14] and metastatic tumor. However, all tumors not supplied by the portal vein are seen as low-density masses, so it has to be preceded by other imaging studies, such as ultrasound, conventional CT, or CTA. It clearly opacifies the intrahepatic vasculature and expedites segment determination, which is necessary for the selection of the operative procedure.

With CTAP, false-positive findings are uncommon, but they do occur. Localized low-density areas, such as segments 1, 2, and 4, may be present if the liver has accessory portal branches that are not derived from the portal trunk and that drain directly into the left portal vein (Fig. 22-2).[9,15–17] A similar false-positive result may be seen if the cystic vein blood flows into the portal vein through the liver.[18] An interpretation based on other imaging findings is necessary. In patients with portal hypertension in whom the bulk of superior mesenteric venous flow goes through collaterals into the systemic circulation, CTAP is not indicated.[19]

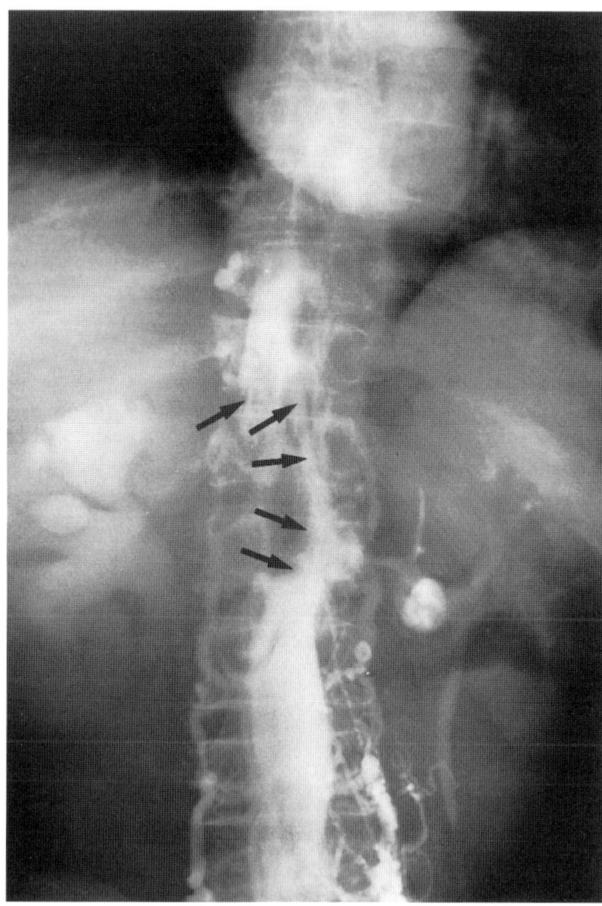

FIGURE 22-4. Inferior venography demonstrating severe compressions (arrows) laterally along the vena cava due to a large HCC and a secondary dilatation of the hemiazygos vein system. In spite of the severe compression, an HCC measuring 5.5 kg was successfully resected.

CTA

CTA was done in the past mainly for the detection of small secondary lesions of HCC. However, CTA is not good for differentiating small HCCs from small areas of arterioportal shunting or from a regenerative nodule. Moreover, CTA cannot be used to evaluate the entire liver because about one-half of patients have anatomic variations in the origin and course of the hepatic artery; repeated catheterization is required for the study of both lobes in such patients. For these reasons, CTA is indicated mainly for patients in whom conventional CT and angiography have failed to make the diagnosis (Fig. 22-5).

Lipiodol CT

This technique was first developed for targeted chemotherapy of HCC[20] and then for the detection of very small HCCs.[21,22] Plain CT at 7 to 10 days after Lipiodol injection into the hepatic artery will disclose very small HCCs, particularly intrahepatic secondary HCCs (Fig. 22-6). A hypervascular cancer, particularly HCC, shows up as a discrete Lipiodol-retaining area on CT. The exact mechanism of Lipiodol disposal by normal tissue is not well understood, but the absence of Kupffer cells and normal lymphatics in cancer tissue may explain Lipiodol retention there.

Lipiodol retention is influenced by vascularity. Lipiodol is retained by HCC and hypervascular metastatic cancer, but it is not well-retained by a hypovascular well-differentiated HCC, cholangiocarcinoma, or metastatic cancer. False-positive findings may occur when Lipiodol is retained in a fan-shaped peripheral area, around the gallbladder, and immediately beneath the liver capsule.

ANGIOGRAPHIC FEATURES OF HEPATIC TUMORS

Hepatic tumors can be classified into hyper-, hypo-, and avascular lesions. Hypervascular primary tumors include HCC, hemangioma, hepatocellular adenoma (HCA), focal nodular hyperplasia (FNH), nodular regenerative hyperplasia (NRH), primary hepatic carcinoid tumor, teratoma, and hepatoblastoma. Hypervascular secondary tumors include (metastatic) islet cell tumor (insulinoma, gastrinoma, somatostatinoma, etc.), renal cell carcinoma, leiomyosarcoma, carcinoid tumor, malignant thymoma, and choriocarcinoma.

Hypo- or avascular primary hepatic tumors include cholangiocarcinoma, necrotic HCC, and early HCC. Most hepatic metastases are hypovascular. The vasculature of combined HCC and cholangiocarcinoma depends on the ratio of the structural components.[23]

HCC

COMMON TYPE

HCC is grossly classified into three groups for the purpose of angiography evaluation: nodular, massive, and diffuse.[24] However, the recent development of screening programs with ultrasound and α-fetoprotein measurement in chronic liver disease now permits detection of small HCCs less than 3 cm in diameter, most of which are of the nodular type.

The typical angiographic findings of HCC are a dilated and markedly tortuous neovasculature seen in the arterial phase and nodular staining in the venous phase (Fig. 22-7). Among a total of 105 small HCCs less than 5 cm in diameter that were resected after angiography at our hospital, 86 (82%) had been diagnosed by angiography.[25] Of the 86 lesions identified, nodular staining was most frequent (76%). Tumor vessels were recognized

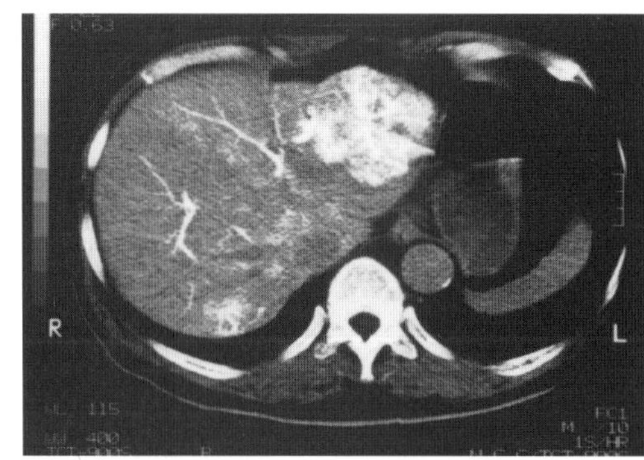

A

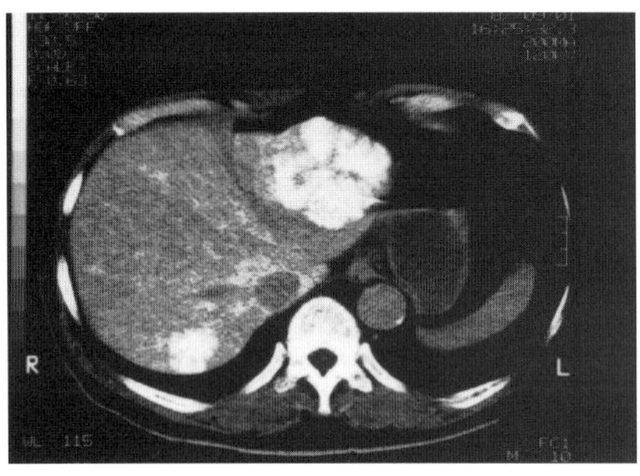

B

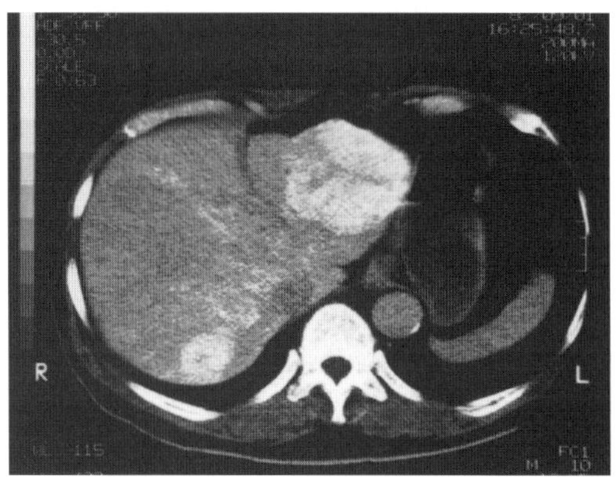

C

FIGURE 22-5. CT arteriography performed at a single slice level. In FNH lesions located in segments 2 to 3 and 7, centrifugal blood flow is seen in the early phase (*A*), and a lobular structure of the mass and a central stellate low-density area corresponding to the central scar are recognized in the intermediate (*B*) and late (*C*) phases.

in only 60 lesions (70%), and an arterioportal shunt was seen in eight lesions (9%). The incidences of tumor vessels and arterioportal shunts were lower in contrast to those of advanced or far-advanced HCCs (95% and 52%, respectively).[26]

SPONTANEOUS RUPTURE AND REGRESSION OF HCC

Spontaneous rupture from an HCC located just beneath the liver surface is initially diagnosed by paracentesis in patients with sudden abdominal pain, abdominal distention, and occasionally a shock state.[27] The bleeding site is diagnosed as extravasation by angiography, and subsequent TAE therapy gives much better results than emergency operation for bleeding control,[28] even though post-TAE abdominal dissemination of the tumor develops in most cases.

Spontaneous regression or disappearance of HCC is extremely uncommon, although there have been several such reports.[29,30] A more common experience is shrinking of the tumor rather than complete disappearance.

FIBROLAMELLAR CARCINOMA

Fibrolamellar carcinoma is usually hypervascular on angiography.[31] Distinction from FNH or HCC by angiography alone is not easy. Although neovasculature appears, arterioportal shunting and intravascular tumor invasion are very rare.

TUMOR THROMBUS IN THE PORTAL AND HEPATIC VEINS AND BILE DUCT

HCC frequently grows into the large vessels such as the portal vein and hepatic vein as well as into the bile duct. Tumor thrombus is directly demonstrated by a parallel, thin neovasculature along the vessels ("thread and streaks" sign[32]) (Fig. 22-8) and indirectly as a filling de-

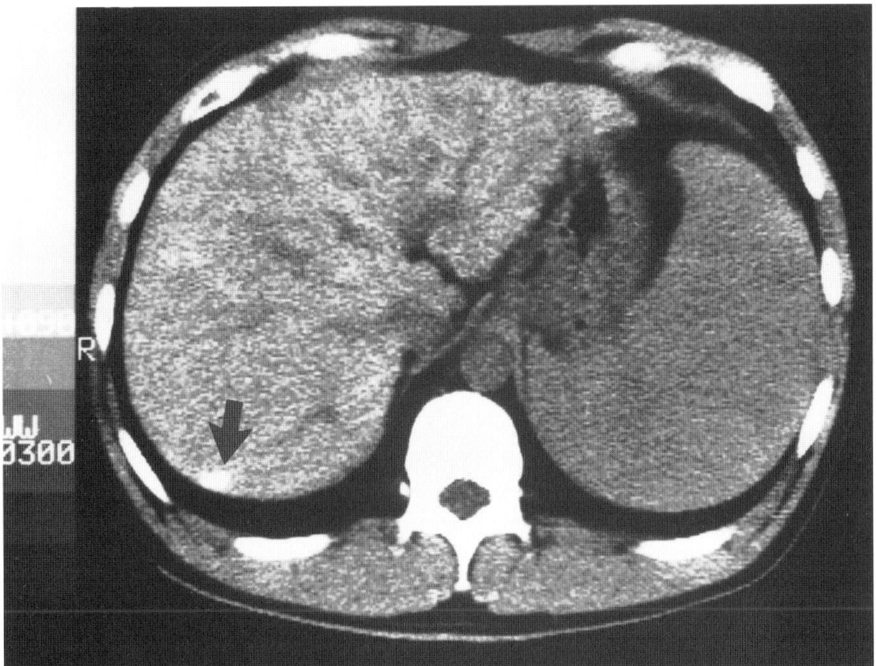

FIGURE 22-6. Lipiodol CT. A small HCC (arrow) is demontrated in segment 7.

FIGURE 22-7. (*A*) A typical HCC demonstrated as a hypervascular lesion with abundant neovasculature in the arterial phase. (*Figure continues.*)

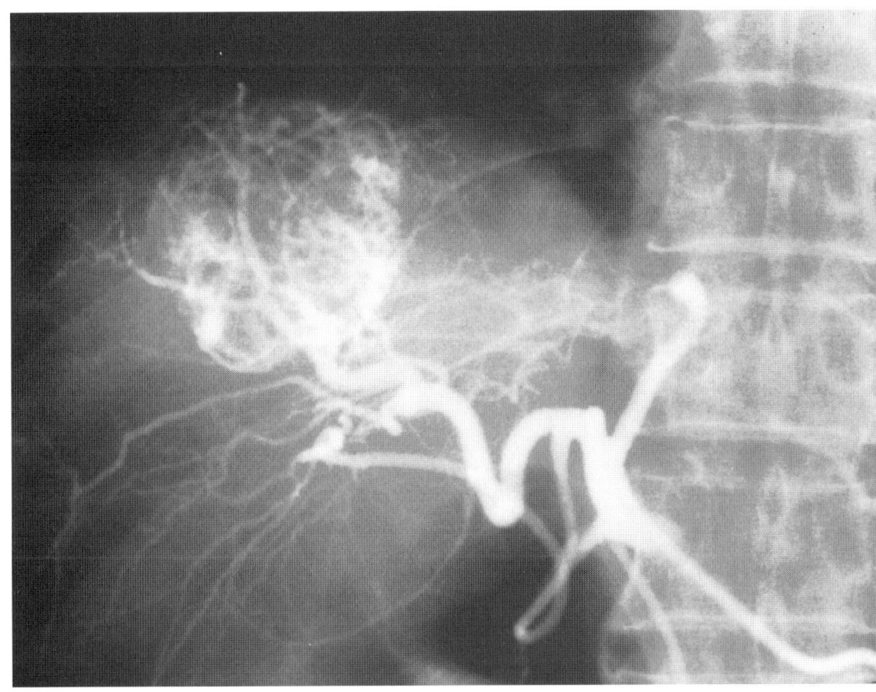

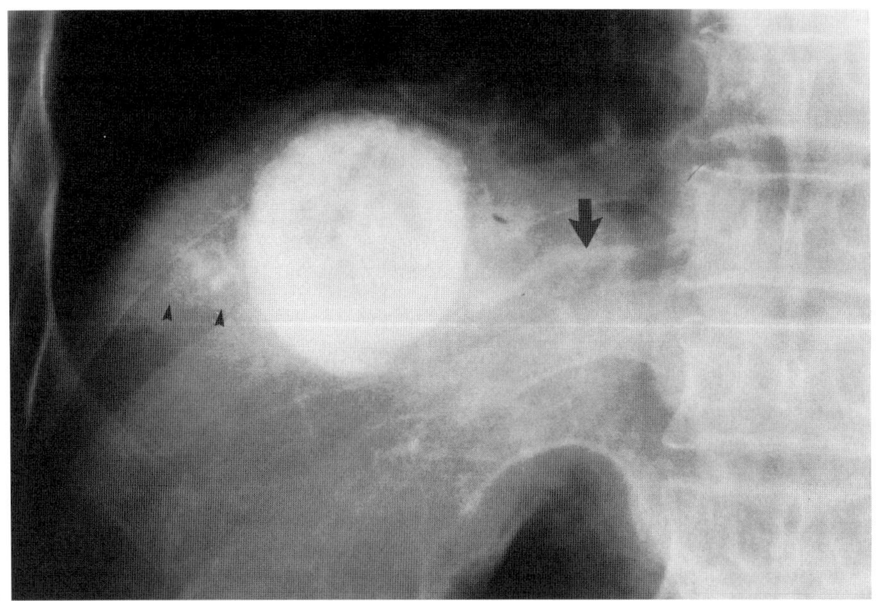

FIGURE 22-7 *(Continued). (B)* A nodular tumor stain and a faint arterioportal shunt (arrowheads) in the venous phase. The arrow indicates the right hepatic vein.

FIGURE 22-8. Tumor thrombi developing in both the right hepatic (thin arrows) and inferior right hepatic veins (thick arrows) are depicted as many parallel thin tumor vessels (''thread and streaks'' sign) on right hepatic angiography. The latter tumor thrombus can be traced into the inferior vena cava.

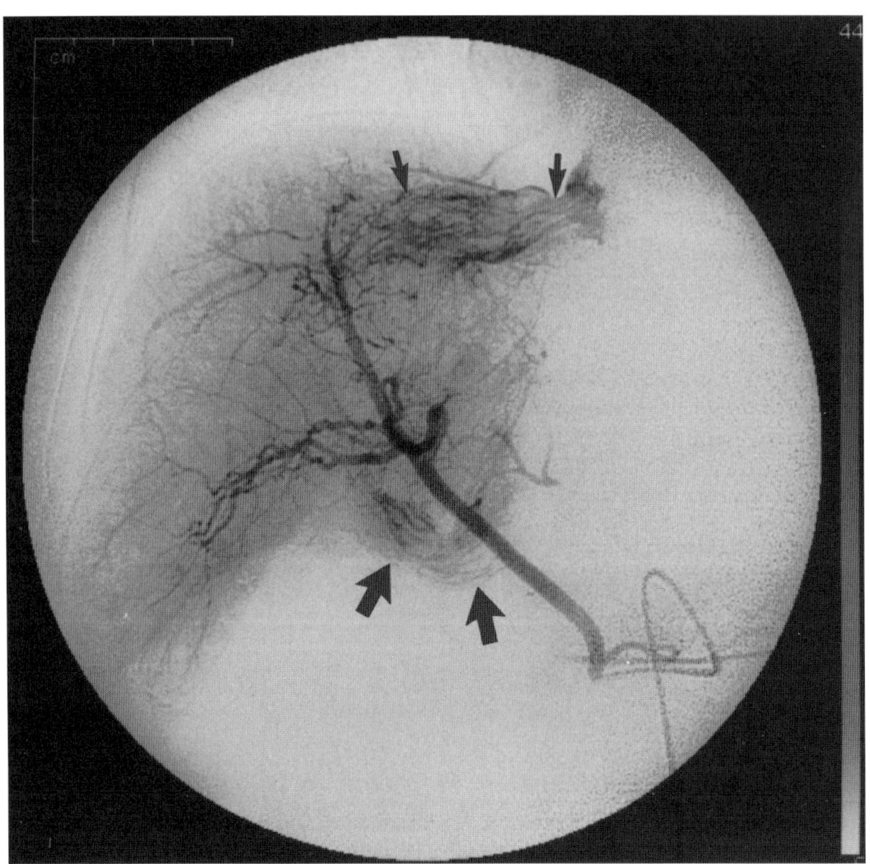

fect in the vessels. Tumor thrombus in the hepatic vein sometimes grows into the right atrium, and its tip moves to and fro like a ball valve. Arterioportal or arteriohepatic shunting is not infrequently associated, and the former frequently elevates the portal pressure, sometimes resulting in the rupture of esophageal varices. Tumor thrombus also can move into the common bile duct, where it is frequently associated with hemobilia, which may cause intermittent jaundice.[33]

EXTRAHEPATIC METASTASIS

Extrahepatic metastases are seen in more than 60% of advanced HCC at autopsy. These are more frequently hematogenous (56%) than lymphatic (27%).[34] In hematogenous spread, metastases to the lung, adrenal, and bone are common, in this decreasing order. A metastatic lesion in the adrenal gland,[35] bone, or lymph node is demonstrated as a hypervascular mass by angiography, unless it is necrotic.

Early HCC and Early Advanced HCC

EARLY HCC

Early HCC is defined here as an adenomatous hyperplastic nodule containing a focus of HCC.[36] Angiography can detect only 9% of early HCCs.[37] Even with the more sensitive CTA, only 15% of such lesions were seen as a hypervascular lesion; in contrast, 93% of small advanced HCCs less than 3 cm were demonstrated as hypervascular masses by the same technique.[38] Early HCC is frequently recognized as a low-density lesion on both CTA and CTAP (Fig. 22-9).

EARLY ADVANCED HCC

Early advanced HCC, a term that sounds contradictory, is a cancerous nodule of advanced HCC (moderately or poorly differentiated cancer cells) that is large enough to be detected at gross examination and surrounded by a rim of early, well-differentiated HCC.[39] On angiography,

FIGURE 22-9. Early HCC, 2.5 cm in size. CTAP (*A*) and CTA (*B*) show early HCC as a hypoattenuating mass (arrow) in segment 8 of the liver. Both the portal vein (seen in Fig. A) and the hepatic artery (seen in Fig. B) cross the mass. The cut surface of the resected specimen showed a yellow color mass with an irregular margin and a portal vein crossing the center (not shown).

A

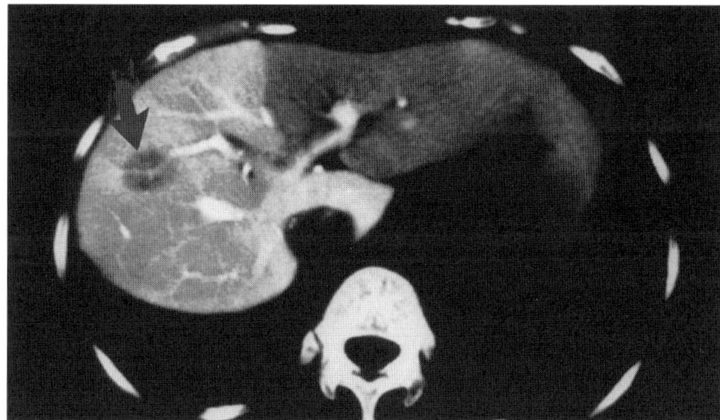

B

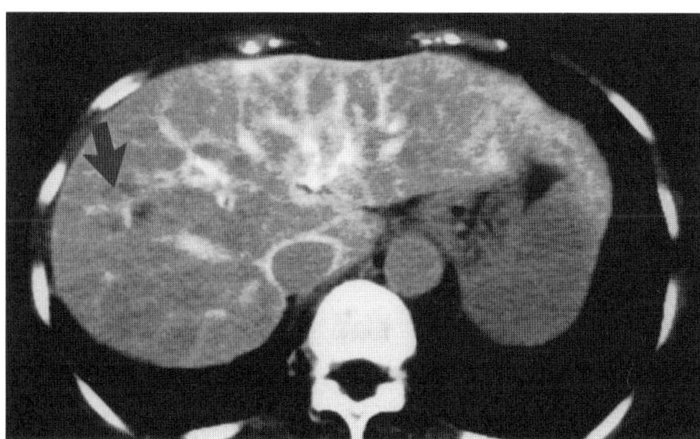

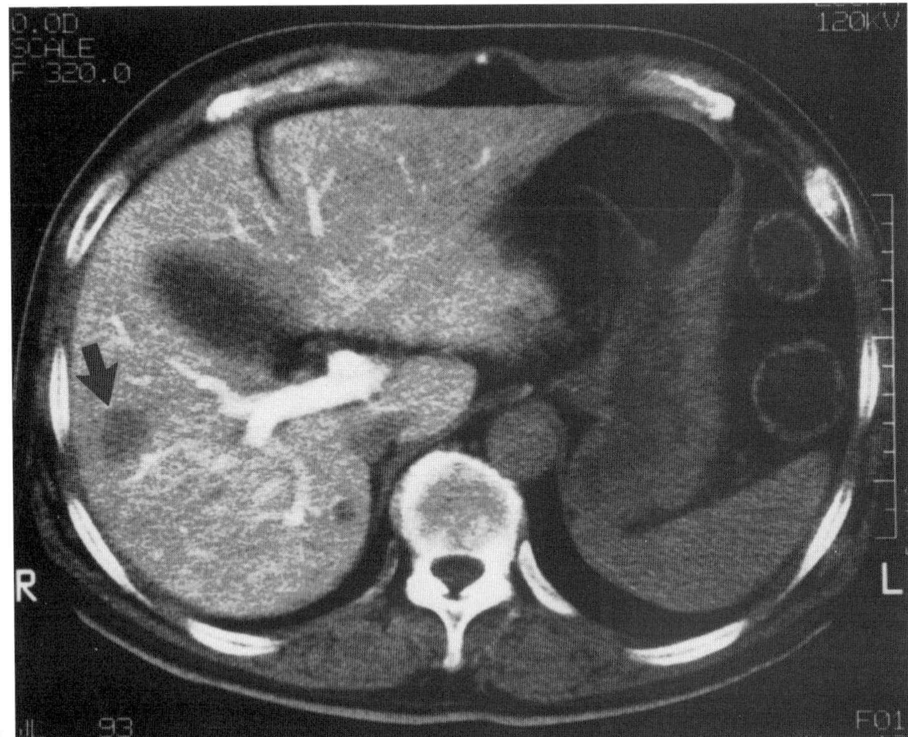

A

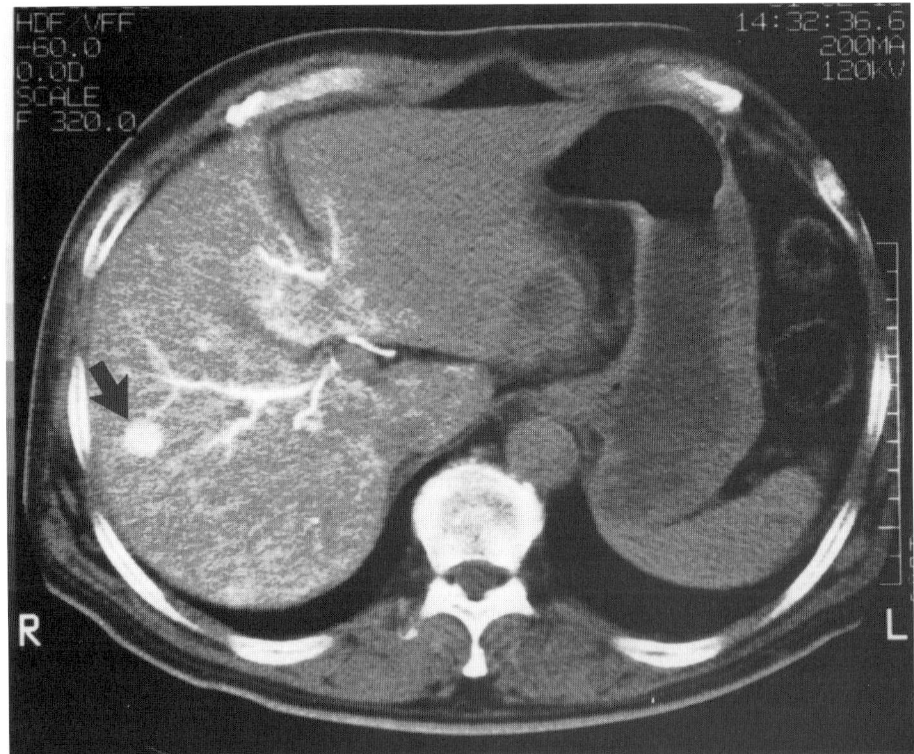

B

FIGURE 22-10. Early advanced HCC, 2.4 cm in size. The 1.8 cm low attenuating mass (arrow) seen by CTAP (*A*) is seen by CTA (*B*) to represent a 1.4-cm homogenous hyperattenuating enhanced mass (arrow). (*Figure continues.*)

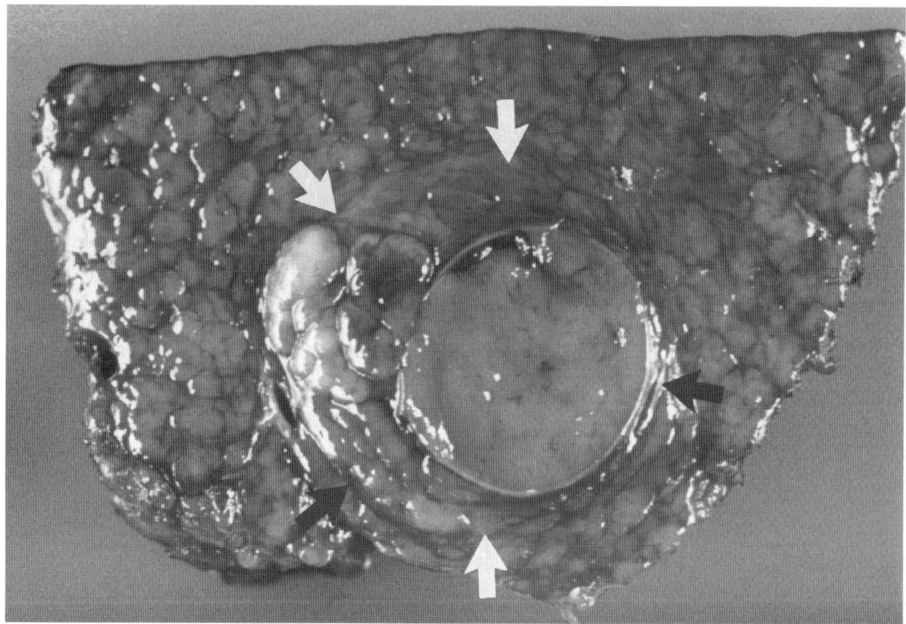

FIGURE 22-10 (*Continued*). (*C*) Cut surface of the resected specimen shows an early advanced HCC that corresponds to the encapsulated central nodule of moderately differentiated HCC, and a peripheral portion (arrows) that consists of differentiated HCC. Presumably, only the central nodule was enhanced by CTA.

only the inner nodule is stained (23%).[37] Therefore, a discrepancy in tumor size between CTA and CTAP is characteristic of this lesion (Fig. 22-10).[40]

Cholangiocarcinoma

Cholangiocarcinoma arises from bile duct cells and is generally hypovascular. However, a small number of lesions are hypervascular, and others show a peripheral vascularity assuming a doughnut-like staining by angiography. Neither an arterioportal shunt nor a translucent rim is recognized. If the portal vein is obstructed due to invasion, a compensatory increase of arterial blood flow is demonstrated as a fan-shaped area in the early phase of the angiogram.

Hemangioma

Cavernous hemangioma is the most frequent benign tumor of the livers, with a frequency of 4% to 8% in adults. Incidental hemangioma is a problem in a cancer-bearing patient. The majority of hemangiomas have a cotton wool appearance, particularly in the late phase of angiography. However, several atypical hemangiomas,[41] (e.g., a nonenhanced hemangioma or a fluid-containing hemangioma) may be encountered.

FNH

FNH is generally considered to be a vascular malformation rather than a neoplasm. The tumor consists of several lobules with a central scar but has no pseudocapsule around the mass. Centrifugal arterial vessels (radiating opacification of tumor vessels from the center to the tumor margin) are one of the characteristics of FNH on angiography, but the frequency of such findings is not high. CTA is helpful in demonstrating the centrifugal arterial vessels (Fig. 22-5). A hypervascular tumor in a patient with normal liver function and lacking hepatitis B or C virus infection suggests the possibility of FNH.

Hepatocellular Adenoma

HCA is a benign tumor that is reported to have close association with the intake of oral contraceptives.[42] On angiography, fine tumor vessels and a homogenous staining are recognized.

SUMMARY

Since angiography has limitations in the detection of HCC because of the existence of hypovascular or avascular HCC, combinations of CT and angiography are indispensable in patients prior to surgery. CTAP and CTA performed at the same time have become easier. CTAP for detection of a lesion followed by CTA for differential diagnosis of the lesion are now routinely performed before conventional superselective angiography. The application of helical CT for CTAP and CTA permits improved diagnosis and shortening of the examination time.

REFERENCES

1. Michels NA. Blood Supply and Anatomy of the Upper Abdominal Organs. Lippincott, Philadelphia, 1955
2. Couinaud C. Le foie: études anatomiques et chirurgicles. Masson, Paris, 1957
3. Sato T, Nimura Y, Kamiya J et al. Interportal communicating branch at the hepatic bifurcation. Report of two cases. Hepato-Gastroenterology 1993;40:180–183
4. Takayasu K, Aoki K, Ichikawa T et al. Aberrant right gastric vein directly communicating with left portal vein system. Acta Radiol 1990;31:575–577
5. Nakamura S, Tuzuki T. Surgical anatomy of the hepatic veins and the inferior vena cava. Surg Gynecol Obstet 1981; 152:43–50
6. Makuuchi M, Hasegawa H, Yamazaki S et al. Primary Budd-Chiari syndrome: Ultrasonic demonstration. Radiology 1984;152:775–779
7. Takayasu K, Muramatsu Y, Moriyama N et al. Radiological study of idiopathic Budd-Chiari syndrome complicated by hepatocellular carcinoma. A report of four cases. Am J Gastroenterol 1994;88:249–253
8. Couinaud C. Lobes et segments hepatiques. Notes sur l'architecture anatomique et chirurgicale du foie. Presse Med 1954; 62:709–712
9. Takayasu K, Moriyama N, Muramatsu Y et al. Intrahepatic portal vein branches studied by percutaneous transhepatic portography. Radiology 1985;154:31–36
10. Prando A, Wallace S, Bernardino MR, Lindell MM Jr. Computed tomographic arteriography of the liver. Radiology 1979;130:697–701.
11. Moriyama N. Angiographic computed tomography [in Japanese]. Jpn J Cancer Clin 1980;26:1037–1040
12. Moss AA, Dean PB, Axel L et al. Dynamic CT of hepatic masses with intravenous and intraarterial contrast material. AJR 1982;138:847–852
13. Matsui O, Kadoya M, Suzuki M et al. Dynamic sequential computed tomography during arterial portography in the detection of hepatic neoplasms. Radiology 1983;146:721–727
14. Takayasu K, Moriyama N, Muramatsu Y et al. The diagnosis of small hepatocellular carcinoma: efficacy of various imaging procedures in 100 patients. AJR 1990;155:49–54
15. Fernandez MP, Bernardino ME. Hepatic pseudolesion: appearance of focal low attenuation in the medial segment of the left lobe at CT arterial portography. Radiology 1991; 181:809–812
16. Nelson RC, Thompson GH, Chezmar JL et al. CT during arterial portography: diagnostic pitfalls. RadioGraphics 1992;12:705–718
17. Matsui O, Takahashi S, Kadoya M et al. Pseudolesion in segment IV of the liver at CT during arterial portography: correlation with aberrant gastric venous drainage. Radiology 1994;193:31–35
18. Matsui O, Takashima T, Kadoya M et al. Staining in the liver surrounding gallbladder fossa on hepatic arteriography caused by increased cystic venous drainage. Gastrointest Radiol 1987;12:307–312
19. Oliver JH III, Baron RL, Dodd GD III et al. Does advanced cirrhosis with portosystemic shunting affect the value of CT arterial portography in the evaluation of the liver? AJR 1995; 164:333–337
20. Konno T, Maeda H, Iwai K et al. Effect of arterial administration of high-molecular weight anticancer agent SMANCS with lipid lymphographic agent on hepatoma. Eur J Cancer Oncol 1983;19:1053–1065
21. Yumoto Y, Jinno K, Tokuyama K et al. Hepatocellular carcinoma detected by iodized oil. Radiology 1985;154:19–24
22. Ohishi H, Uchida H, Yoshimura H et al. Hepatocellular carcinoma detected by iodized oil: use of anticancer agents. Radiology 1985;154:25–29
23. Aoki K, Takayasu K, Kawano T et al. Combined hepatocellular carcinoma and cholangiocarcinoma: clinical features and computed tomographic findings. Hepatology 1993;18: 1090–1095
24. Eggel H. Ueber das primäre Carcinoma der Leber. Beitr Pathol Anat 1901;30:506–604
25. Takayasu K, Shima Y, Muramatsu Y et al. Angiography of small hepatocellular carcinoma: analysis of 105 resected tumors AJR 1986;147:525–529
26. Okuda K, Obata H, Jinnouchi S et al. Angiographic assessment of gross anatomy of hepatocellular carcinoma: comparison of celiac angiograms and liver pathology in 100 cases. Radiology 1977;123:21–29
27. Ong GB, Taw JL. Spontaneous rupture of hepatocellular carcinoma. BMJ 1972;4:146–149
28. Okazaki M, Higashihara H, Koganemaru F et al. Intraperitoneal hemorrhage from hepatocellular carcinoma: emergency chemoembolization or embolization. Radiology 1991;180: 647–651
29. Lam KC, Ho JCI, Yeung RTT. Spontaneous regression of hepatocellular carcinoma. A case study. Cancer 1982;50: 332–336
30. Gottfried EB, Steller R, Paronetto F, Lieber CS. Spontaneous regression of hepatocellular carcinoma. Gastroenterology 1982;82:770–774
31. Friedman AC, Lichtenstein JE, Goodman Z et al. Fibrolamellar hepatocellular carcinoma. Radiology 1985;157: 583–587
32. Okuda K, Musha H, Yoshida T et al. Demonstration of growing casts of hepatocellular carcinoma in the portal vein by celiac angiography: the thread and streaks sign. Radiology 1975;117:303–309
33. Kojiro M, Kawabata K, Kawano Y et al. Hepatocellular carcinoma presenting as intra-bile duct tumor growth. A clinicopathologic study of 24 cases. Cancer 1982;49:2144–2147

34. Nakashima T, Okuda K, Kojiro M et al. Pathology of hepatocellular carcinoma in Japan, 232 consecutive cases autopsied in ten years. Cancer 1983;51:863–877
35. Takayasu K, Muramatsu Y, Moriyama N et al. Surgical treatment of adrenal metastasis following hepatectomy for hepatocellular carcinoma. Jpn J Clin Oncol 1989;19:62–66
36. Arakawa M, Kage M, Sugihara S et al. Emergence of malignant lesions within an adenomatous hyperplastic nodule in a cirrhotic liver. Observations in five cases. Gastroenterology 1986;91:198–208
37. Takayasu K, Wakao F, Moriyama N et al. Response of early-stage hepatocellular carcinoma and borderline lesions to therapeutic arterial embolization. AJR 1993;160:301–306
38. Takayasu K, Muramatsu Y, Furukawa H et al. Early hepatocellular carcinoma: appearance at CT during arterial portography and CT arteriography with pathologic correlation. Radiology 1995;194:101–105
39. Sakamoto M, Ino Y, Fujii T et al. Phenotype changes in tumor vessels associated with the progression of hepatocellular carcinoma. Jpn J Clin Oncol 1993;23:98–104
40. Winter TC III, Takayasu K, Muramatsu Y et al. Early advanced hepatocellular carcinoma: evaluation of CT and MR appearance with pathologic correlation. Radiology 1994; 192:379–387
41. Takayasu K, Moriyama N, Shima Y et al. Atypical radiographic findings in hepatic cavernous hemangioma: correlation with histologic features. AJR 1986;146:1149–1153
42. Edmondson HA, Henderson B, Benton B. Liver-cell adenomas associated with use of oral contraceptives. N Engl J Med 1976;294:470–472

23

MRI DIAGNOSIS OF HEPATOCELLULAR CARCINOMA

MASAAKI EBARA

The clinical application of magnetic resonance imaging (MRI) for studying abdominal organs has some limitations because of artifacts caused by organ movement. However, MRI provides remarkable contrast resolution, multiplanar images, and characterization of lesions based on signal intensities in various pulse sequences.[1–5] Furthermore, contrast-enhanced MRI with gadopentetate dimeglumine (Gd-DTPA) and fast images with gradient-echo sequences provide hemodynamic information that permit the differentiation of hepatic mass lesions.[6,7] More recently, superparamagnetic iron oxide (SPIO) has become available for use as a tissue-specific contrast agent, and it has improved the detectability of hepatic mass lesions.[8,9] MRI is very useful for the differential diagnosis of such mass lesions of the liver as hepatocellular carcinoma (HCC) and hemangioma, because these lesions have characteristic MRI appearances.[10–14] Although it has been reported that fatty change (steatosis) and copper (Cu) within the HCCs are closely related to a high signal intensity on T_1-weighted (T1W) images,[10,15,16] there is still insufficient evidence that they are the definite cause of increased intensity.[17] In this chapter, the usefulness of MRI diagnosis for HCC is discussed in terms of detectability of lesions, characteristic findings, differential diagnosis, tissue characterization, utility of contrast agents, and comparison with computed tomography (CT) based on our experience in Japan. These findings might not apply directly to patients seen in other parts of the world such as South Africa.

TECHNIQUE

From January 1992 we have used a 1.5 T Signa Advantage superconducting system (GE Medical Systems) for MRI. Transverse MRI slices were obtained under the following conditions. Slice thickness was 10 mm with 3-mm gaps. Matrix size was 256 × 192. Spin-echo (SE) pulse sequences were employed with a repetition time (TR) of 500 msec and an echo time (TE) of 11 msec (SE 500/11) for T1W images and SE 2,000/80 for T2W images with two excitations. Gradient echo (GE) pulse sequences were employed with a TR of 35 msec, a TE of 15 msec, a flip angle of 30 degrees (35/15/30), and two excitations. Respiratory compensation, flow compensation, and no-phase wrap techniques were used to reduce artifacts.

CT scanning was performed with a GE 9800 unit as a dynamic study with bolus intravenous injection of contrast agents. Precontrast CT scans of the entire liver were first obtained. Contrast enhanced CT scans were successively obtained as follows. Sequential 10-mm slices, focused on the tumor, were obtained at 10-min intervals during the early phase, from 30 seconds after the start of the intravenous injection of 100 ml of contrast agent at a rate of 2.5 ml/sec, while the table with the patient was being moved. Imaging slices of the entire liver were then obtained during the late phase, from 3 minutes after the bolus injection.

TABLE 23-1. MRI Versus CT in Detectability of HCC

Tumor Size (cm)	MRI (%)	CT (%)
1	40.0 (2/5)	40.0 (2/5)
1.1–2	70.3 (19/27)	63.0 (17/27)
2.1–3	97.1 (34/35)	97.1 (34/35)
3.1–5	100 (9/9)	100 (9/9)
	84.2 (64/76)	81.6 (62/76)

χ^2-test, n.s.

DETECTABILITY OF HCC

In a large series of patients from Western countries, HCC was best detected with T2W images with a higher tumor-liver T2W difference than with a T1W tumor-liver difference.[16] However, in our results from Japan, HCC was more frequently detected with T1W images than proton density weighted (PDW) and T2W images. This difference may depend on tumor size and histologic diagnostic criteria of early stage of HCC.

Here we compared MRI with CT for detectability of HCC according to tumor size (Table 23-1). Of the 76 HCCs, 64 (84.2%) were detected by MRI. In relation to tumor size, 2 of 5 lesions (40.0%) of 10 mm or less in diameter were detected, 19 of 27 (70.3%) of 11 to 20 mm, and 9 of 9 (100%) of 30 to 50 mm were detected. With contrast-enhanced CT scanning performed at the same time, 62 of the 76 lesions (81.6%) were visualized, showing no significant difference in detection rates between MRI and CT. When lesions detected by MRI were compared with those by CT, both MRI and CT were capable of demonstrating the same two lesions of 10 mm or less. Three lesions of 11 to 20 mm were detected by CT but not by MRI, and five were detected by MRI but not by CT; the others were detected by both modalities. Among lesions of 21 to 30 mm, MRI and CT failed to detect one lesion each (not the same lesion).

Although detection rates by MRI according to tumor diameters were generally comparable to those by contrast-enhanced CT, 8 of 32 (25%) lesions of 20 mm or less in diameter could not be detected by either MRI or CT, indicating that improvement in HCC detection requires the complimentary application of both MRI and CT.

MRI SIGNAL INTENSITY PATTERNS AND VISUALIZATION OF THE CAPSULE IN HCC

High signal intensity pattern on T1W images and visualization of the capsule (ring sign) have been noted as the MRI findings characteristic of HCC (Fig. 23-1).[10,11,18] The signal intensity of hepatic masses relative to the surrounding liver parenchyma is classifiable into four patterns as high, iso, low, and mixed. The signal intensity patterns of the 64 HCC lesions were high-intensity, iso-intensity, low-intensity, and mixed-intensity patterns on T1W images in 43 (67.2%), 11 (17.2%), 9 (14.1%) and 1 (1.6%) lesions, respectively (Table 23-2), and in T2W images in 47 (73.4%), 8 (12.5%), 8 (12.5%), and 1 (1.6%) lesions, respectively. Thus, a high-intensity pattern was most frequently observed in both T1W and T2W images. Signal intensity patterns on either T1W or T2W images showed no significant correlation with tumor size. The control lesions, 25 hemangiomas and 9 metastatic liver tumors, all had a low-intensity pattern on T1W images and a high-intensity pattern on T2W images, except for one case of metastasis from gastric cancer that was complicated with hemorrhage. Thus, the high-intensity pattern on T1W images and the low-intensity pattern on T2W images were considered to be characteristic of small HCC. A capsule mostly appears as a low-intensity ring on T1W images[10,11] and occasionally as concentric rings consisting of an internal low-intensity ring and an external high-intensity ring[11] on T2W images. The ring sign, which is usually readily recognized in relatively large encapsulated HCC, was observed in only 15.6% of 64 HCCs smaller than 5 cm and none of the control lesions. However, the ring sign was seen in only 3 of the same 64 HCCs by CT. Other characteristic MRI findings seen with HCC—an intratumoral septum and a nodule-in-nodule pattern (Fig. 23-1)—are rarely observed by MRI and are poorly differentiated from intratumoral necrosis.

DIFFERENTIAL DIAGNOSIS FOR HCC

MRI has been applied to the differential diagnosis of hepatic masses (Table 23-3), and there have been many reports describing its usefulness for the diagnosis of HCC and hepatic hemangioma.[13,14,19] MRI can clearly detect tumor invasion of the portal vein (Fig. 23-2) and other vessels, a finding that is characteristic of HCC.[20]

TABLE 23-2. Intensity Patterns of HCC in MRI

Pulse Sequence	No. of Cases	Intensity Pattern (%)			
		High	Iso	Low	Mixed
T1W	64[a]	67.2	17.2	14.1	1.6
T2W	64[a]	73.4	12.5	12.5	1.6

[a] Same lesions.

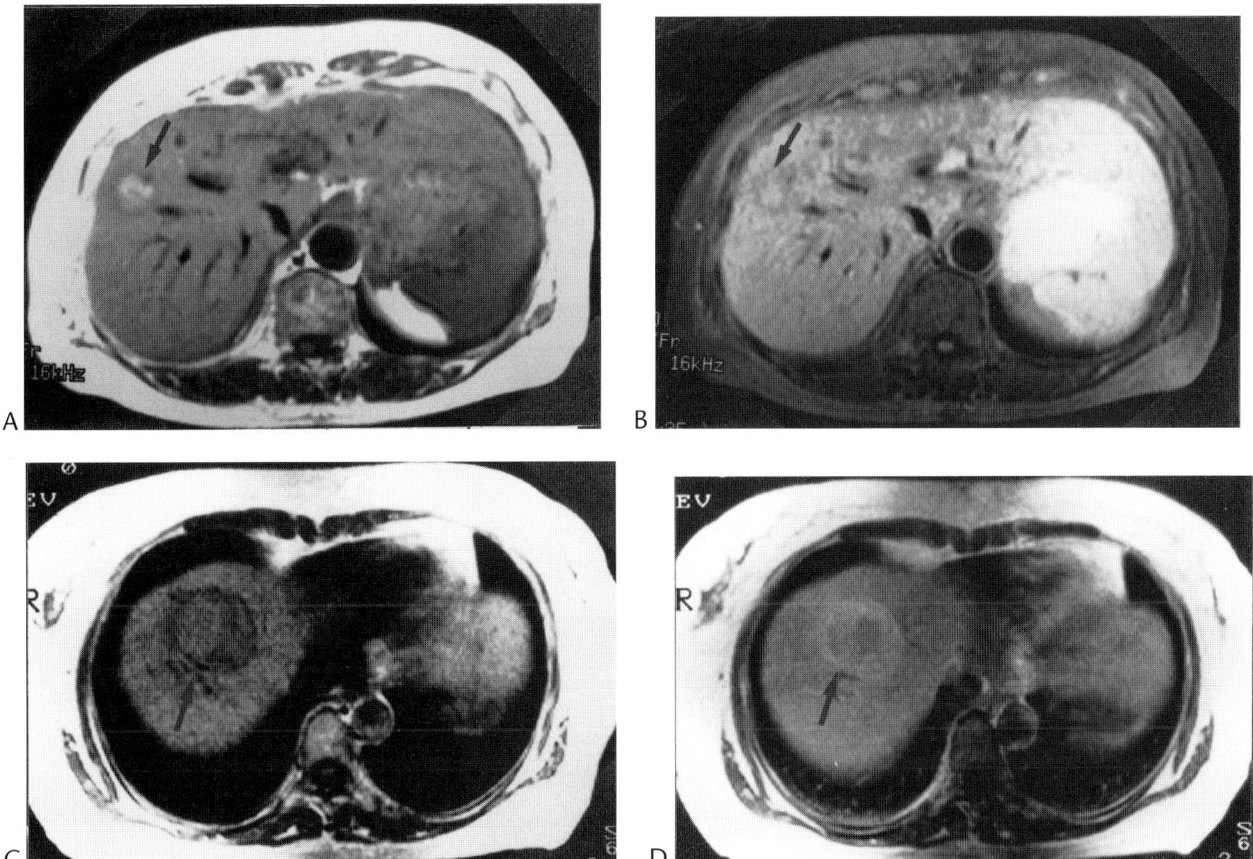

FIGURE 23-1. Characteristic MRI findings of HCC: "ring sign," "nodule in nodule," and "septum." An encapsulated HCC 2 cm in size (arrow) is visualized at S_8 (*A*) as a high-intensity pattern with a peripheral ring of low intensity (ring sign) on a T1W image and (*B*) as an iso-intensity pattern with a low-intensity ring on a T1W fat saturation image. (*C*) Another encapsulated 4-cm HCC (arrow) is demonstrated at S_8 as an iso-intensity pattern with a low-intensity ring and septum on T1W image and (*D*) as a mixed pattern consisting of a round hypointense region and a crescent hyperintense region ("nodule in nodule"). S_8, segment 8 in Couinand's classification.

TABLE 23-3. MRI Versus CT in Diagnostic Capability for HCC

	True-Positive Rate (%)[b]	
Tumor Size (cm)	MRI	CT
1	40.0 (2/5)[a]	0 (0/5)[a]
1.1–2	51.9 (14/27)[a]	33.3 (9/27)[a]
2.1–3	71.4 (25/35)	71.4 (25/35)
3.1–5	77.8 (7/9)	88.9 (8/9)

[a] $p < 0.1$, χ^2-test.

[b] True-positive rates = no. diagnosed as HCC divided by no. with HCC, then multiplied by 100.

MRI Versus CT in Differential Diagnosis of HCC

Although the general ability of MRI to make a definite diagnosis of HCC based on these characteristic features was found not to differ significantly from that of contrast-enhanced CT, MRI seems to be slightly superior in detection of lesions 2 cm or smaller. MRI findings needed for the definite diagnosis of HCC are a high-intensity pattern on T1W images and the presence of the ring sign. True-positive rates were calculated using the following equation: the number of cases with characteristic findings of HCC/the number of cases with HCC × 100. As a result, true-positive cases were observed in 2 of 5 lesions (40.0%) of 10 mm or less in diameter, 14 of 27 (51.9%) of 11 to 20 mm, 25 of 35 (71.4%) of 21 to 30 mm, and 7 of 9 (77.8%) of 31 to 50 mm. A comparison of the

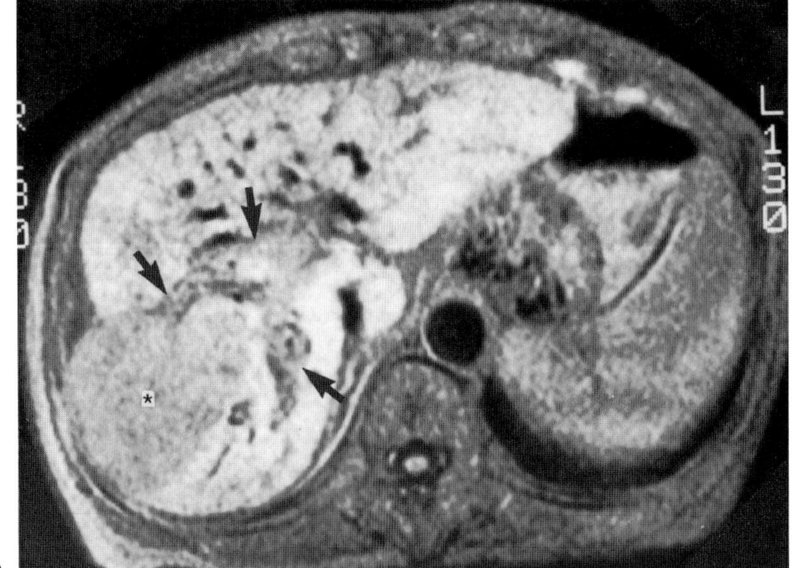

A

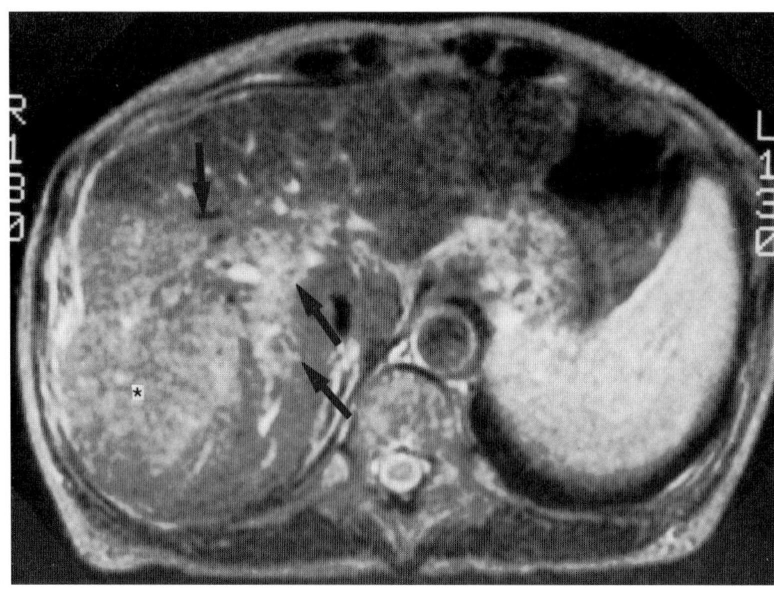

B

FIGURE 23-2. Characteristic MRI findings of an HCC tumor thrombus in the portal vein. A massive HCC measuring 6 × 5 cm in S_8 (*) appears as (*A*) homogeneously hypointense area on a T1W fat saturation image and as (*B*) a hyperintense area on a T2W image. Portal tumor thrombi (arrows) originating from the mass are also visualized.

true-positive rates of MRI and CT revealed no significant differences, but MRI tended to give higher rates for lesions of 20 mm or less in diameter than contrast-enhanced CT ($p < 0.1$).

Cholangiocarcinoma

Cholangiocarcinoma is a malignant neoplasm arising from the epithelium of the intrahepatic bile ducts. These appear grossly as firm masses with large amounts of fibrous tissue; they rarely have small areas of necrosis or hemorrhage. The MRI appearance of cholangiocarcinoma has been described in two reports.[21,22] Cholangiocarcinoma on MRI appears as a large mass with irregular borders, hypointense on a T1W image and hyperintense on a T2W image like many other tumors. However, in some cases of cholangiocarcinoma the mass is seen on a T2W image as a large heterogeneously hypointense area in the center and a homogeneously hyperintense area in the periphery thought to correspond to central fibrosis and viable peripheral tumor. Another characteristic feature of cholangiocarcinoma is encasement of large vessels by the tumor itself without the occurrence of tumor thrombus.

Fibrolamellar Carcinoma

Fibrolamellar carcinoma is a variant of HCC.[23] Its gross appearance is similar to that of focal nodular hyperplasia (FNH) in that it occurs in a noncirrhotic liver and has a central scar and fibrous septa. Few cases of fibrolamellar carcinoma have been reported on MRI,[24,25] though it has been reported that it appears on MRI as a tumor of iso-intensity on T1W images and high intensity on T2W images, with a central scar of low intensity on both. Its MRI differs from that of FNH in that the central scar of FNH appears as a high intensity on a T2W image.

Metastatic Liver Tumor

Metastases are the most common malignancies detected in noncirrhotic livers. On MRI, hepatic metastases are hypointense relative to liver on T1W images and hyperintense on T2W images. Necrosis, seen in 25% to 30% of metastases, appears as central tumor hypo-intensity on T1W images and as hypo-intensity on T2W images.[26] An amorphous appearance, halo, and target sign are also characteristic findings of metastatic tumors.[24] Tumor capsules, tumor scars, vascular invasion, and bile duct dilatation are rarely associated with metastases. The differentiation by MRI between metastases and HCC is possible only when the HCC has characteristic MRI features such as a high-intensity pattern on a T1W image and a ring sign.

Cavernous Hemangioma

Cavernous hemangioma, one of the most common benign liver tumors, has the potential of being characterized by MRI due to both its unusually high intensity on a T2W image and to some morphologic features.[13,14,19] Hemangiomas larger than 6 cm in size are lobulated in 50% of cases, and an internal thrombus or scar tissue can be seen.[27] However, small hemangiomas have few characteristic morphologic features. Dynamic MRI is useful even in small hemangiomas because it shows prolonged enhancement patterns. Hepatic cysts also have extraordinarily high intensity on T2W images and therefore may be difficult to differentiate from hemangioma. Protein density imaging can differentiate hemangioma from hepatic cyst by showing iso- or hypointensity in cysts and hyperintensity in hemangioma.

Regenerative Nodules and Adenomatous Hyperplasia

Differentiating small HCCs from regenerative nodules[24,28,29] or adenomatous hyperplastic nodules (AH)[30] is extremely important. Although AH has been reported to be hyperintense on a T1W image and hypotense on a T2W image,[30] almost all lesions with this pattern were well-differentiated HCCs in our study. This discrepancy might be due to differences in histologic criteria for early stage HCC used in the two studies.

RELATIONSHIP BETWEEN SIGNAL INTENSITY PATTERNS ON T1W AND T2W IMAGES AND HISTOLOGIC DIFFERENTIATION OF HCC

HCCs have microscopic variations with regard to the presence of fat (steatosis), fibrosis, necrosis, and (rarely) bleeding. This variable microscopic composition gives rise to different signal intensity patterns in MRI. Well- and moderately differentiated lesions were significantly more common in the high-intensity than in the low-intensity groups on T1W images ($p < 0.05$), whereas well-differentiated lesions significantly increased in number as signal intensities on T2W images decreased ($p < 0.01$). Although it is generally accepted that almost all HCCs appear with high intensity in T2W image, a considerable proportion of well-differentiated HCCs have low intensity in T2W image.

Steatosis can be a causative factor for the high intensity of HCCs on T1W images.[10] Steatosis was quantified in 47 HCCs; there were no significant differences in intratumoral steatosis rates among the high-intensity, iso-intensity and low-intensity groups. Steatosis was observed to be significantly greater in the cancerous region than in the noncancerous region of the high-intensity group ($p < 0.01$), but not in the iso-intensity or low-intensity group.

Clear cell formation was also greater in the cancerous region than in the noncancerous region in only the high-intensity group, as with steatosis. However, 10 of 32 lesions (31.3%) with the high-intensity pattern on T1W images had both low-grade steatosis and low clear cell formation rates, suggesting the existence of other factors for T1W shortening of MRI signals (Table 23-4).

RELATIONSHIP BETWEEN SIGNAL INTENSITY PATTERNS ON T1W IMAGES AND CONTENT OF HEAVY METALS IN HCCs

Heavy metal content, including Cu, varies among HCCs.[31] The existence of some heavy metals within the tumors has been thought to have a paramagnetic effect. However, the sensitivity and specificity of the measurement of intratumoral heavy metals in earlier reports may have been unreliable, particularly for Cu, because the interpretation depended on qualitative measurements such as rhodamine staining, rubeanic acid staining, and orcein staining.[15,17] In the present study, heavy metals were quantified by particle-induced x-ray emission (PIXE) calculation.[32] Among heavy metals detected from cancerous and noncancerous regions by PIXE analysis, Cu, Fe, and Zn, which were detected in amounts significantly greater than other heavy metals, were quantified and analyzed. The mean Cu content in the cancerous region did not differ between high- and iso-intensity groups, but was significantly greater in the high-intensity groups than in the low-intensity group ($p < 0.01$) (Fig. 23-3). A comparison between cancerous and noncancerous regions showed a greater Cu content in the former only in the high-intensity group ($p < 0.01$).

It has been reported that Cu often binds to metallo-

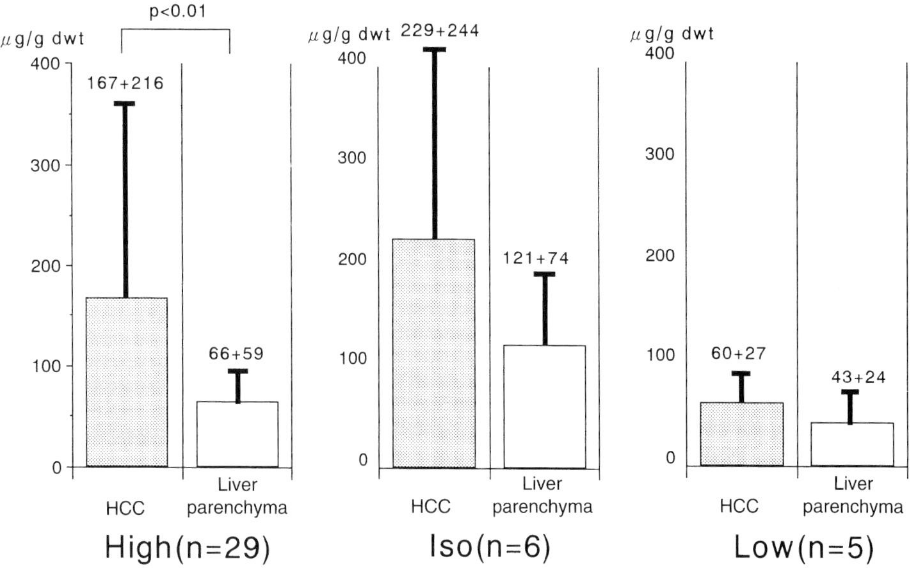

FIGURE 23-3. Copper contents in HCC and liver parenchyma in relation to intensity pattern on T1W images.

thionein to form Cu-thionein in the liver parenchyma, but other forms of Cu or ratios of its different forms, especially in the tumor, have not yet been fully understood.

There were no significant differences in Fe contents between the different signal intensity patterns or between cancerous and noncancerous regions in our study, in contrast to other reports.[33] Similarly, no differences were found for any other heavy metals.

From these results, it was concluded that signal-intensity patterns on T1W images are closely correlated with steatosis, clear cell formation, and Cu content and that T2W images are correlated with differentiation and hemodynamics of HCC. However, further studies will be necessary to determine to what extent individual factors are involved in the signal intensity patterns and what the mechanisms are by which such factors affect the images.

CONTRAST ENHANCEMENT

The use of appropriate contrast agents for enhancing MRI provides an additional advantage. Gd-DTPA is the only intravenous MRI contrast agent approved for human use, and it mainly shortens the T1 relaxation time. Since Gd-DTPA has similar pharmacokinetics to those of the iodinated contrast agents for CT, MRI enhanced with Gd-DTPA can be interpreted in the same way as enhanced CT. Gd-DTPA is used for hemodynamic evaluation of the liver and mass lesions by obtaining multiple rapid images during bolus injection.[6,7] HCC, like other tumors, has similar findings with this method to those seen on enhanced CT: characteristic MRI findings of HCC are uniformly or partially hyperintense in the early phase, with delayed enhancement in capsules and septa (Fig. 23-4).[7] HCC tends to be hyper-

TABLE 23-4. Relationship Between Intensity Pattern and Differentiation

		Differentiation of HCC (%)		
Image	Intensity Pattern	Well-Differentiated	Moderately Differentiated	Poorly Differentiated
T1W	High	45.2^{a} (19/42)	47.6^{a} (20/42)	7.1^{a} (3/42)
	Iso	18.2 (2/11)	72.7 (8/11)	9.0 (1/11)
	Low	12.5^{a} (1/8)	50.0^{a} (4/8)	37.5^{a} (3/8)
T2W	High	$20.0^{b,c}$ (9/45)	$64.4^{b,c}$ (29/45)	$15.6^{b,c}$ (7/45)
	Iso	71.4^{b} (5/7)	28.6^{b} (2/7)	0^{b} (0/7)
	Low	100^{c} (3/8)	0^{c} (0/8)	0^{c} (0/8)

χ^2-test^{a,b}, $p < 0.05$; χ^2-test^{c}, $p < 0.001$.

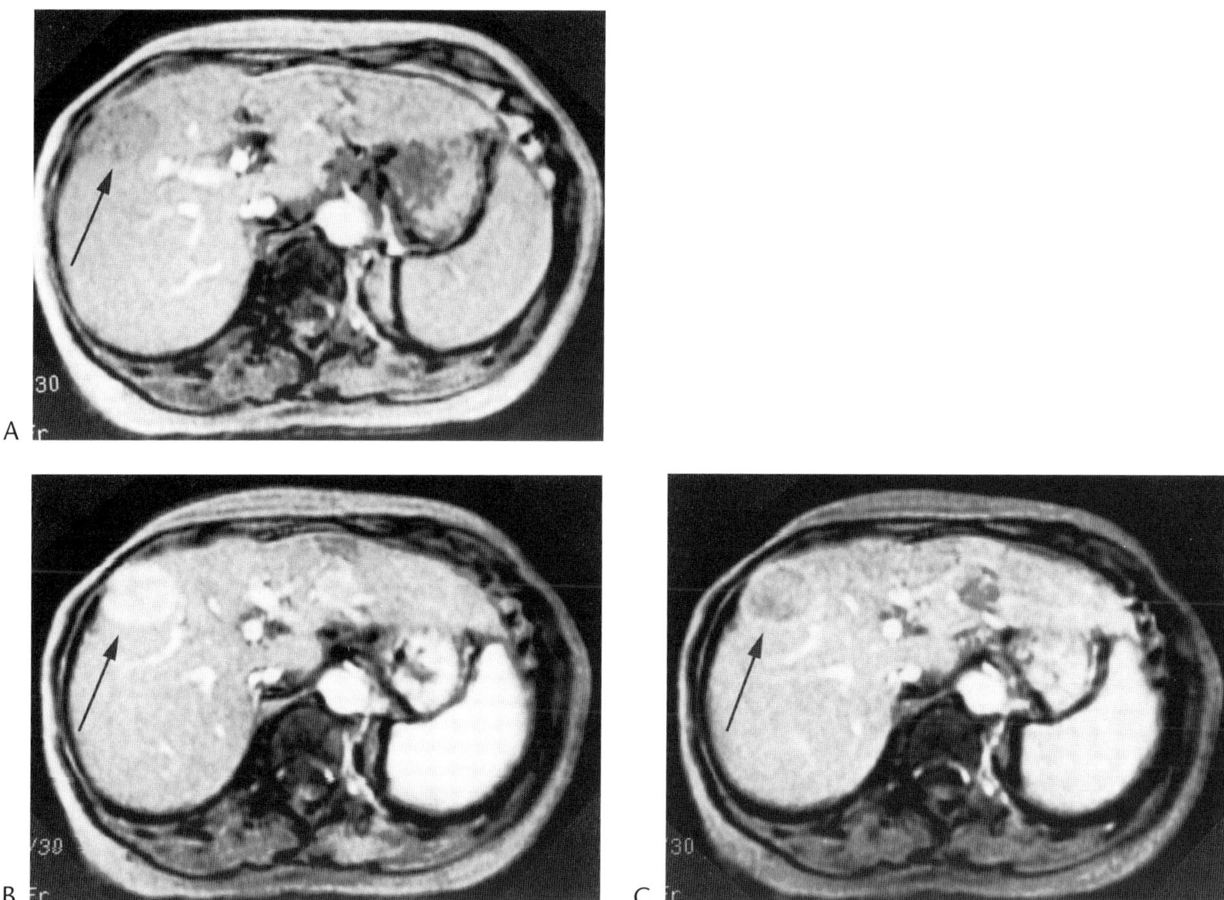

FIGURE 23-4. Dynamic MRI of small HCC (arrow). (*A*) Before bolus injection of 0.05 mmol/kg Gd-DTPA; gradient echo (GRE): TR = 35 msec, TE = 15 msec, flip angle = 30 degrees, two excitations. A low-intensity mass is seen in S_4 on precontrast MRI. (*B*) After 30 seconds. The mass has changed to a homogeneously enhanced one. (*C*) After 3 minutes. The lesion is seen as a hypointense mass with a dense ring enhancement. S_4, segment 4 in Couinand's classification.

intensely visualized by enhanced MRI longer than by enhanced CT. Thus, enhanced MRI with Gd-DTPA is useful for the differential diagnosis of hepatic tumors by revealing their characteristic hemodynamics. Gd-DTPA is also capable of visualizing the presence of a capsule surrounding HCC with higher sensitivity than without intravascular enhancement.

SPIO is another agent used for contrast-enhanced MRI[8] that is useful for HCC.[9,34] SPIO causes marked shortening of the T2 relaxation time, resulting in a loss of signal in the liver and spleen with all commonly used SE images (Fig. 23-5). The introduction of SPIO as a tissue-specific MRI contrast agent for the reticuloendothelial system (RES) offers further improvement in the detection of hepatic mass lesions. Lesions lacking an RES, such as metastatic tumors to liver, are clearly enhanced as hyperintense areas against the remarkably hypointense liver parenchyma because of the liver RES. The smallest hepatic metastasis detected by SPIO has been 0.3 cm in size.[35]

We applied AMI-25 (SPIO) as a contrast agent to 71 patients with hepatic focal mass lesions, including 59 HCC patients.[9] Although there was no significant improvement in detectability of HCC nodules, small HCCs could clearly be detected because of the increase in the signal intensity ratio between lesions and liver parenchyma. Two HCC lesions, seen as hyperintense in precontrast T2W images, were each visualized as a lower intensity mass than the surrounding liver parenchyma after the administration of AMI-25. This unexpected phenomenon may have occurred because of Kupffer cells in the HCC nodules. MRI images with AMI-25 theoretically sometimes may fail to visualize well-differentiated HCC nodules because they often contain Kupffer cells.[36] Nevertheless, most of the HCC nodules were more clearly visualized after the use of AMI-25 in our study.

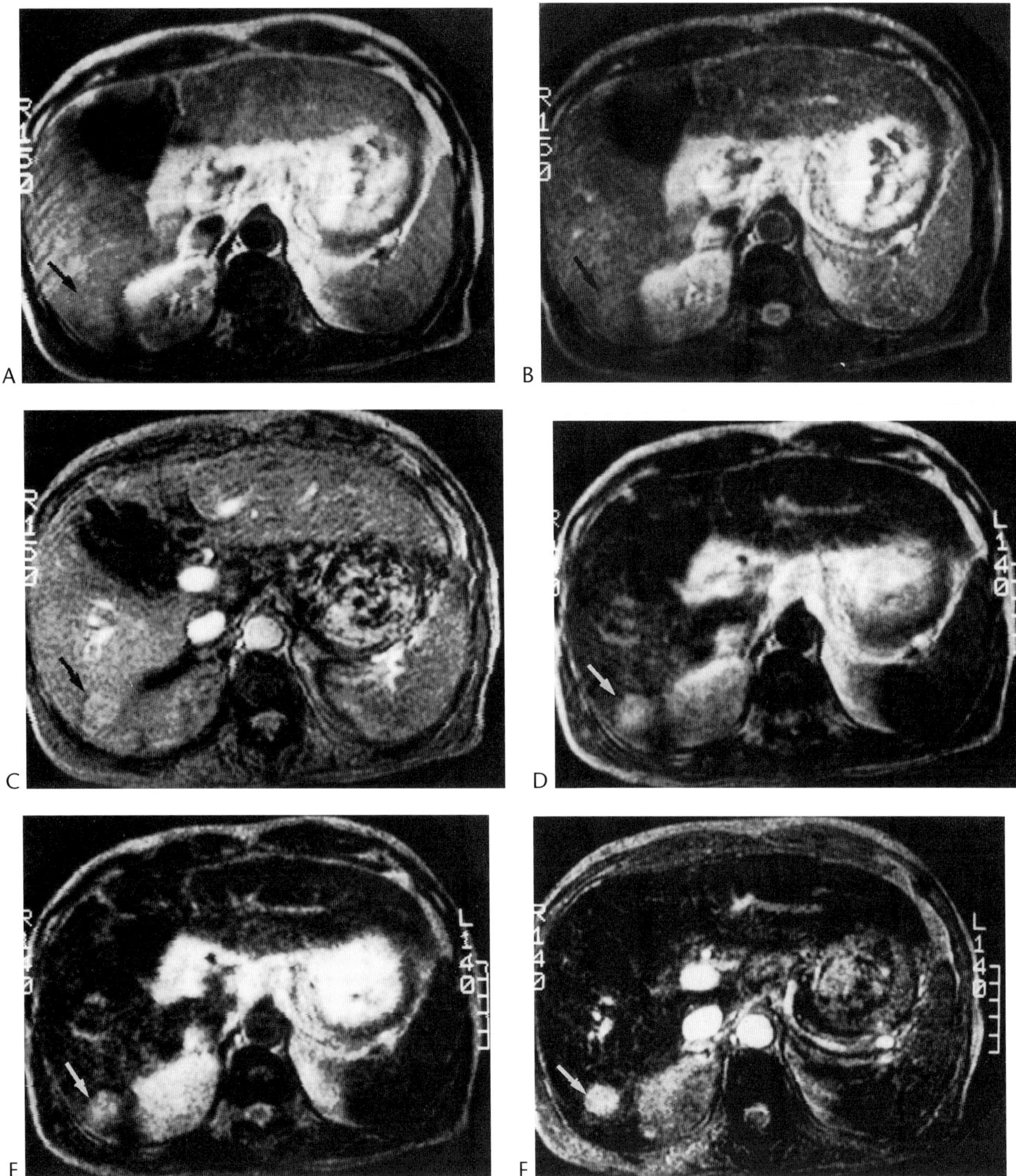

FIGURE 23-5. An HCC (arrow) at S_6 of the liver is more clearly demonstrated as a high-intensity mass lesion in proton density weighted (PDW), T2W, and gradient echo images after administration of AMI-25. Preconstrast images: (*A*) PDW: TR = 2,000 msec, TE = 30 msec; (*B*) T2W: TR = 2,000 msec, TE = 80 msec; (*C*) gradient echo: TR = 35 msec, TE = 15 msec, flip angle = 30 degrees. Postcontrast images: (*D*) PDW, (*E*) T2W, (*F*) GRE. S_6, segment 6 in Couinand's classification.

ACKNOWLEDGMENTS

This work was supported in part by a grant for Scientific Research Expenses for Health and Welfare Programs and the Foundation for the Promotion of Cancer Research and by the Comprehensive 10-year Strategy for Cancer Control.

REFERENCES

1. Smith FW, Mallard JR, Reid A, Hutchinson JMS. Nuclear magnetic resonance tomographic imaging in liver disease. Lancet 1981;1:963–966
2. Dyle FH, Pennock JM, Banks NM et al. Nuclear magnetic resonance tomographic imaging of the liver: initial experience. AJR 1982;138:193–200
3. Glazer GM, Aisen AM, Francis IR et al. Evaluation of focal hepatic masses: a comparative study of MRI and CT. Gastrointest Radiol 1986;11:263–268
4. Heiken JP, Lee JKT, Glazer DL, Ling D: Hepatic metastases studied with MR and CT. Radiology 1985;156:423–427
5. Moss AA, Goldberg HI, Stark DD et al. Hepatic tumors: magnetic resonance and CT appearance. Radiology 1984; 150:141–147
6. Schorner W, Lang P, Bittner R, Felix R: Gd-DTPA enhanced uses for MR imaging of body. Diagn Imaging 1990; 114–119, 153–154
7. Yoshida H, Itai Y, Ohtomo K et al. Small hepatocellular carcinoma and cavernous hemangioma: differentiation with dynamic FLASH MRI with Gd-DTPA. Radiology 1989;171: 339–342
8. Saini S, Stark DD, Hahn PF et al. Ferrite particles: a superparamagnetic MR contrast agent for enhanced detection of liver carcinoma. Radiology 1987;162:217–222
9. Ebara M, Ohto M, Muraoka H et al. Clinical application of AMI-25 for MRI of tumorous lesions in the liver [in Japanese]. Jpn J Med Imaging 1994;13:21–31
10. Ebara M, Ohto M, Watanabe Y et al: Diagnosis of small hepatocellular carcinoma: correlation of MR imaging and histologic studies. Radiology 1986;159:371–377
11. Itoh K, Nishimura K, Togashi K et al. Hepatocellular carcinoma: MR imaging. Radiology 1987;164:21–25
12. Muramatsu Y, Nawano S, Takayasu K et al. Early hepatocellular carcinoma: MR imaging. Radiology 1991;181:209–213
13. Itai Y, Ohtomo K, Furui S et al. Noninvasive diagnosis of small cavernous hemangioma of the liver: advantage of magnetic resonance imaging. AJR 1985;145:1195–1199
14. Ohtomo K, Itai Y, Furui S et al. Hepatic tumors: differentiation by transverse relaxation time (T2) of magnetic resonance imaging. Radiology 1985;155:421–423
15. Ebara M, Watanabe S, Kita K et al. MR imaging of small hepatocellular carcinoma: effect of intratumoral copper content on signal intensity. Radiology 1991;180:617–621
16. Rummeny E, Weissleder R, Stark DD et al. Primary liver tumors: diagnosis by MR imaging. AJR 1989;152:63–72
17. Kitagawa N, Matsui O, Kadoya M et al. Hepatocellular carcinoma with excessive copper accumulation: CT and MR findings. Radiology 1991;180:623–628
18. Ros PR. Encapsulated hepatocellular carcinoma: radiologic findings and pathologic correlation. Gastrointest Radiol 1990;15:233–237
19. Stark DD, Felder RC, Wittenberg J et al. Magnetic resonance imaging of cavernous hemangioma of the liver: tissue-specific characterization. AJR 1985;145:213–222
20. Ohtomo K, Itai Y, Furui S et al. MR imaging of portal vein thrombus in hepatocellular carcinoma. J Comput Assist Tomogr 1985;9:328–329
21. Hamrick-Turner J, Abbitt PL, Ros PR. Intrahepatic cholangiocarcinoma: MR appearance. AJR 1992;158:77–79
22. O'Neil J, Ross PK. Knowing hepatic pathology aids MRI of liver tumors. Diagn Imaging 1989;58–67
23. Craig JR, Peters RL, Edmondson HA. Fibrolamellar carcinoma of the liver. Cancer 1980;46:372–379
24. Mattison GR, Glazer GM, Quint LE et al. MR Imaging of hepatic focal nodular hyperplasia: characterization and distinction from primary malignant hepatic tumors. AJR 1987; 148:711–715
25. Titelbaum DS, Hatabu H, Schiebler ML et al. Fibrolamellar hepatocellular carcinoma: MR appearance. J Comput Assist Tomogr 1988;12:588–591
26. Wittenberg J, Stark DD, Forman B et al. Differentiation of hepatic metastases from hepatic hemangioma and cysts by using MR imaging. AJR 1988;151:79–84
27. Adam YG, Huvos AG, Fortner JG. Giant hemangioma of the liver. Ann Surg 1970;172:239–245
28. Itai Y, Ohnishi S, Ohtomo K et al. Regenerative nodules of liver cirrhosis: MR imaging. Radiology 1987;165:419–423
29. Ohtomo K, Itai Y, Yoshida H et al. Regenerating nodules of liver cirrhosis: MR imaging with pathologic correlation. AJR 1990;154:505–507
30. Matsui O, Kadoya M, Kameyama T et al. Adenomatous hyperplastic nodules in the cirrhotic liver: differentiation from hepatocellular carcinoma with MR imaging. Radiology 1989; 173:123–126
31. Haratake J, Horie A, Nakashima A et al. Minute hepatoma with excessive copper accumulation. Report of two cases with resection. Arch Pathol Lab Med 1986;110:192–194
32. Yukawa M, Kitao K, Terai M. Distribution of element in human kidney by PIXE analysis. Trace Element Anal Chemistry Medicine Biol 1984;3:392–397
33. Stark DD, Mosely ME, Bacon BR et al. Magnetic resonance imaging and spectroscopy of hepatic iron overload. Radiology 1985;154:137–142
34. Ferrucci JT, Stark DD. Iron oxide-enhanced MR imaging of the liver and spleen: review of the first five years. AJR 1990; 155:943–950
35. Stark DD, Weissleder R, Elizondo G et al. Superparamagnetic iron oxide: clinical application as a contrast agent for MR imaging of the liver. Radiology 1988;168:297–301
36. Tobe K, Tsuchiya T, Fujiwara R et al. Kupffer cells in well differentiated tissue of hepatocellular carcinoma [in Japanese]. Acta Hepatol Jpn 1985;26:630–637

24

CT DIAGNOSIS OF LIVER CANCER

BYUNG IHN CHOI

Computed tomography (CT) is useful in the diagnosis of liver cancers in patients in whom ultrasound is unsuccessful. For the early detection of primary liver cancer, the effectiveness of ultrasound has been widely accepted in Asian countries,[1–4] despite the controversies concerning sonographic efficacy.[5,6] However, ultrasound examination of the entire liver is occasionally impossible because of intervening bones, air in the gut or lung, or dense postoperative scar tissue, especially in patients with a small cirrhotic liver. In such patients, CT plays an important role in detecting liver cancer. CT is also useful in differentiating various focal lesions of the liver, evaluating the location and extension of these lesions, and determining the size of liver cancers after treatment. Another advantage of CT is its objectiveness in visualizing the relation between the lesions and the surrounding tissues.[7] CT is now performed in the evaluation of almost all patients with liver cancer and it plays a major role in the treatment of liver cancer.

Several distinct tasks are required of CT of the liver. These are the identification of individual tumors, characterization of individual lesions, and staging to determine resectability. CT may also be used to distinguish hepatic metastatic deposits of tumors such as adenocarcinoma of the colon and visceral sarcomas, which are often possibly amenable to surgical resection or other procedures, from metastases from sites such as the stomach and pancreas, which are more often widespread throughout the liver and therefore are generally only amenable to medical management.[8]

CT TECHNIQUES

General Considerations

CT is one of the most accurate means for noninvasive evaluation of the liver to detect focal lesions. Its accuracy depends on the scanning techniques. Before performing a scan, it is important to consider technical factors such as the size of the x-ray beam controller and the use of intravenous contrast. A CT examination of the liver should be performed initially with either 7-mm or 8-mm collimator. In areas of suspected lesions, thinner collimation may be needed. The slices should be adjacent or nearly contiguous. With increasing gaps between the slices, there is a greater likelihood that small lesions will be missed. Scans can be performed without intravenous iodinated contrast, with contrast, or before and after intravenous contrast.

Intravenous iodinated contrast material, if properly administered, enhances normal tissue to a greater degree than most neoplastic tissues; it determines the course, caliber, and patency of blood vessels, characterizes tissue perfusion patterns, and helps characterize the tumor. If not properly administered, intravenous contrast medium can obscure lesions.[9] Generally, a difference of at least 10 Hounsfield numbers between the abnormal and normal regions of the liver must be present for accurate detection of liver tumors. Although many of these tumors can be detected with unenhanced CT, intravenous contrast media can increase the differences in CT attenuation (absorption degree of x-rays in tissue) between normal liver and hepatic tumors.[10]

Hepatic contrast enhancement can be divided into three phases: bolus, nonequilibrium (redistribution), and equilibrium.[11] When aortic enhancement is plotted against time using either a monophasic or a biphasic injection, a characteristic curve with three phases is obtained. Aortic enhancement increases rapidly during the bolus-injection phase, which may last 1.5 to 2 minutes. During this bolus phase, the initial circulating contrast material is being replenished by a peripheral intravenous injection of contrast material. Vascular enhancement increases progressively until the end of injection. Aortic enhancement decreases steeply during the second "nonequilibrium," or redistribution, phase. During this phase, intravascular contrast material diffuses rapidly into the extravascular space.

The progressive rise of hepatic attenuation that occurs during the bolus and nonequilibrium phases represents both vascular and extravascular contrast material. Peak hepatic enhancement is reached late in the nonequilibrium phase, even when portal venous enhancement is beginning to fall. Most of the hepatic enhancement at this phase is due to extravascular contrast material. When the intravascular and extravascular contrast material equilibrate (the equilibrium phase), enhancement slowly declines at a rate determined by renal filtration.[11–13]

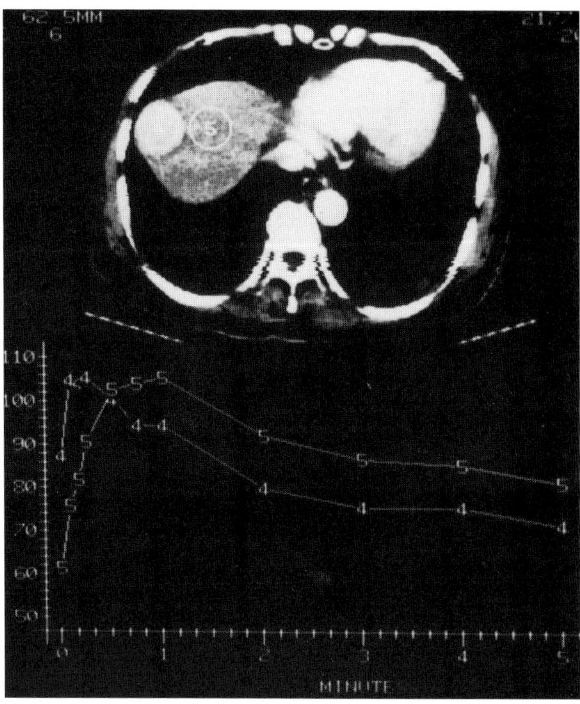

FIGURE 24-1. A nodular encapsulated HCC on single-level bolus dynamic CT scan. Sequential plotting of time-attenuation changes within a mass shows that tumors enhance rapidly but then quickly become less than the nontumorous liver tissue, indicating characteristic hemodynamics of HCC.

Conventional CT

Conventional CT is the mainstay of liver imaging. The incremental bolus dynamic scan method is the preferred CT technique for routine hepatic evaluation, providing rapid acquisition of axial images using automatic table inmovement during the infusion of a large amount of iodinated contrast medium.[9] This has proven valuable in demonstrating in the liver small vascular tumors, arteriovenous shunts and malformations, and vascular invasion from adjacent neoplasms. Although dynamic CT scanning is best performed using fast scanners, satisfactory results can be achieved using scanners with longer scan times. The key principle is to scan only during the bolus and nonequilibrium phases of contrast enhancement, which persist for approximately 2 minutes after the bolus injection.[12]

The drip infusion method, using slow infusion of contrast medium, is the least effective of all CT imaging methods. It only mildly enhances the liver images and provides time for some lesions to accumulate enough contrast medium to become isoattenuating and obscured. This method is actually inferior to unenhanced scans for focal lesion detection.[9]

The single-level bolus dynamic scan method is employed to assess the contrast enhancement characteristics of a single lesion, such as a hemangioma. After injection of iodinated contrast medium, rapid sequential scans are obtained at a single scanning level. Single-level dynamic CT scanning has proven useful to plot time-attenuation changes occurring within a particular lesion (Fig. 24-1).

The delayed high-dose contrast CT (delayed CT) method is useful when the findings of the standard CT study are equivocal or negative. Delayed images obtained 4 to 6 hours after contrast medium injection may be helpful. Delayed scanning provides more discrete definition of the lesion margin and is useful for patients at high risk for metastases who have normal bolus scans. In some studies, delayed scanning has been shown to be superior to dynamic CT; however, time and logistic problems limit its routine use.[14,15]

Unenhanced CT (i.e., scanning without use of contrast material) is generally inferior to contrast-enhanced CT for detecting focal liver neoplasms. There are certain circumstances, however, in which unenhanced images provide more information than dynamic contrast-en-

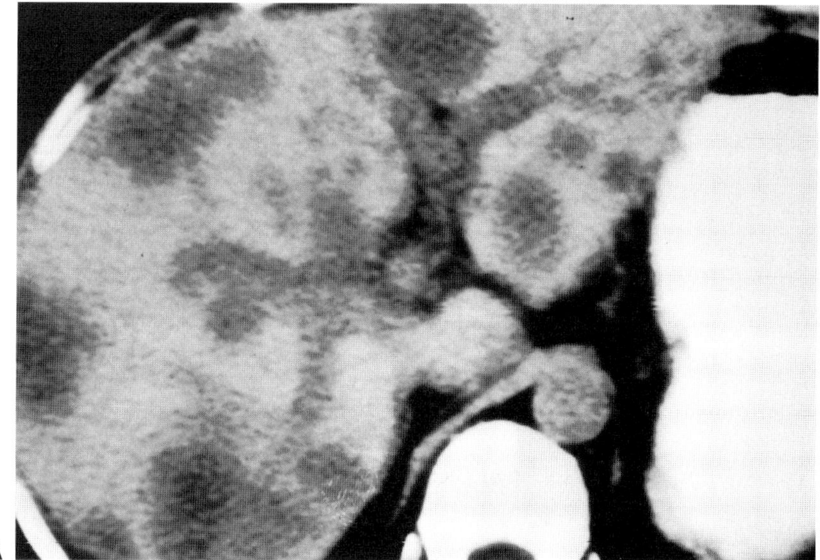

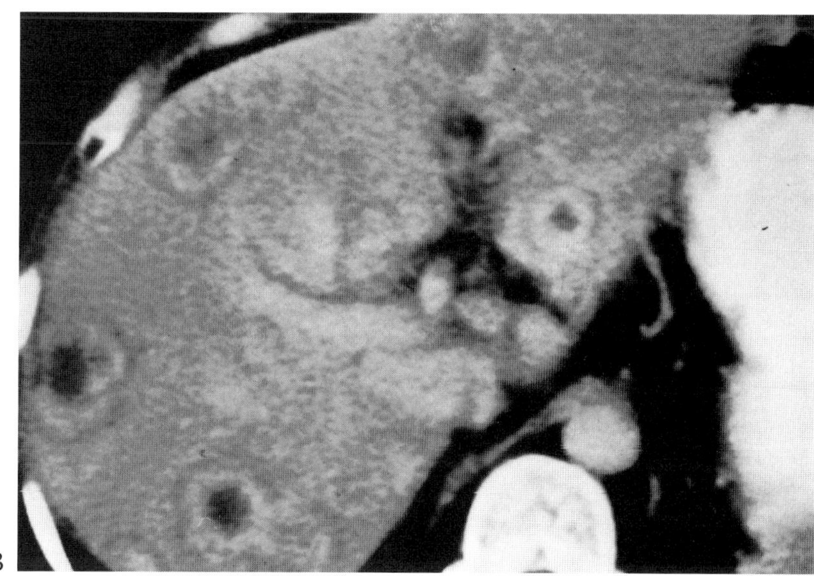

FIGURE 24-2. Metastases of breast cancer to the liver on unenhanced and contrast-enhanced CT scans. (*A*) Unenhanced CT scan shows multiple round masses with low attenuation in both hepatic lobes. (*B*) Contrast-enhanced CT scan shows multiple target-like masses in both hepatic lobes, one of the characteristics of hepatic metastases. The number of hepatic metastatic masses are less than on unenhanced CT scan.

hanced CT scans do. Unenhanced CT is an excellent screening technique for diagnosing metastatic disease (Fig. 24-2), with contrast-enhanced imaging used subsequently for the patients whose scans are negative. In addition, when calcification or hemorrhage within lesions is suspected, unenhanced CT is essential because the contrast material may obscure lesions of higher attenuation.

Angiographically Assisted CT

The combined use of CT and angiography is the most precise imaging method for the diagnosis of hepatic tumors. However, it is an invasive method and its indications should be considered the same as those of hepatic angiography. There are three combinations of CT and angiography: CT arteriography (CTA), CT arterial portography (CTAP) and CT with Lipiodol.

CTA is performed with a catheter placed in the hepatic artery.[16] Its accuracy is derived from the fact that all liver tumors are fed from the hepatic artery. Therefore, tumors have high-attenuation peripheral blushes compared with the surrounding normal liver (Fig. 24-3). Variations in vascular anatomy, flow-related artifacts, altered hemodynamics due to hepatic or systemic disease, and altered anatomy in postoperative patients may significantly change the pattern of enhancement. Familiarity with the hemodynamics and the disease processes, and correlation of the CT findings with those seen on hepatic angiograms, will help avoid these pitfalls.

CTAP consists of rapid CT scans during a bolus injection of contrast material administered through a transfemoral catheter with its tip in the superior mesenteric artery. The superior mesenteric artery injection relies on the fact that no tumors are fed by the portal vein. This procedure produces dense enhancement of portal venous

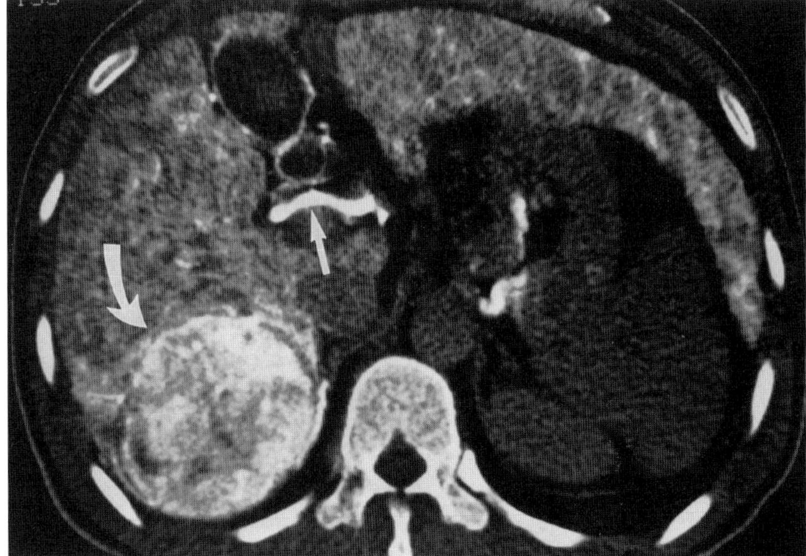

FIGURE 24-3. A nodular HCC on CT arteriogram. CT arteriogram shows high-attenuation tumor blushes (curved arrow) compared with the surrounding liver. Hepatic artery (arrow) is also well visualized.

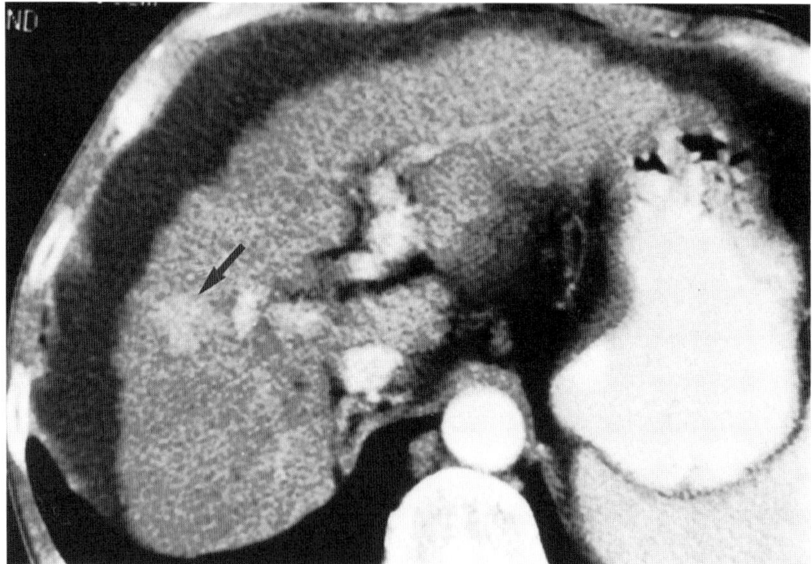

A

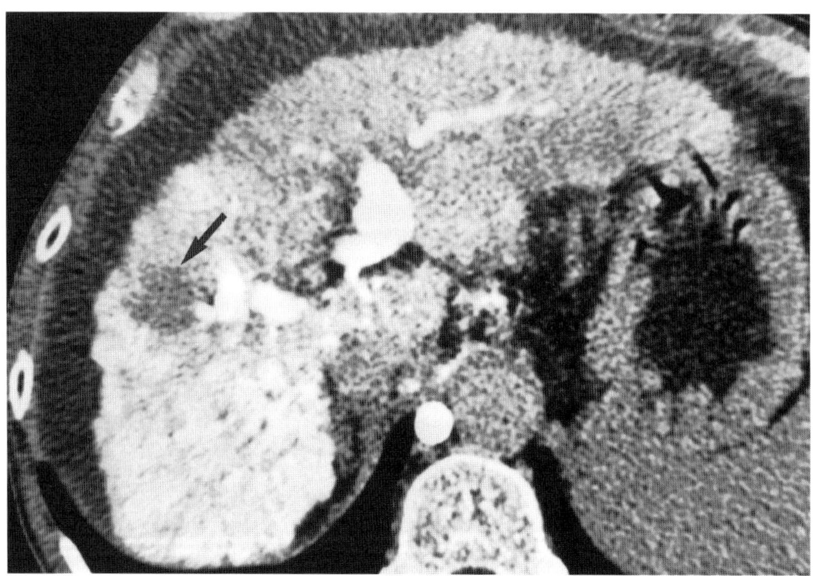

B

FIGURE 24-4. Small advanced HCC on the arterial phase of dynamic CT scan and CT arterial portogram. (*A*) CT scan in the arterial predominant phase of dynamic CT shows high-attenuation tumor (arrow) in right liver, indicating blood supply from the hepatic artery. (*B*) CT arterial portogram shows filling defect (arrow) at the same area as in Fig A, indicating no portal blood supply. Therefore, the tumor is advanced HCC even though the tumor is small.

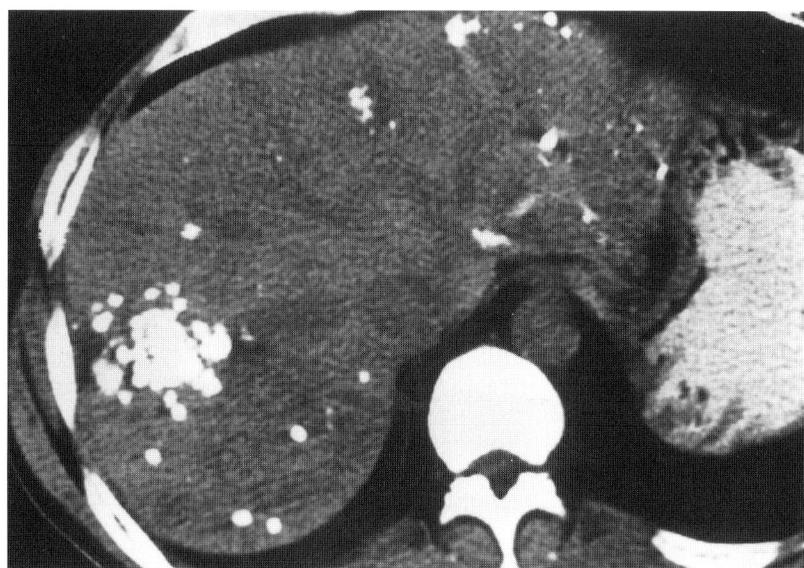

FIGURE 24-5. Multiple intrahepatic metastases of HCC on iodized oil CT scan. Unenhanced CT scan 2 weeks after infusion of Lipiodol shows numerous tiny nodules with retention of iodized oil in entire liver.

blood so that the arterially supplied tumors are highlighted as negative defects. The liver is increased in attenuation, and focal lesions appear as negative defects within the high attenuation hepatic tissue (Fig. 24-4).[17] At present, CTAP appears to be the most accurate approach for detecting focal liver lesions.[18,19]

CT after intra-arterial injection of iodized poppy seed oil (Lipiodol) was introduced for the treatment of hepatocellular carcinoma (HCC), since Lipiodol accumulates in a tumor and can be administered with lipophilic anticancerous agents. It has been reported that iodized oil CT infusion is incidentally useful for the detection of small hepatic nodules, perhaps the most sensitive method in detecting small HCCs. It requires less interpretative skill than hepatic angiography because there is high contrast on CT scans between tumor tissue containing Lipiodol and the adjacent normal liver (Fig. 24-5). Thus, nodules can be identified behind the main tumor or when they are very small.[2] Iodized oil CT has the additional benefit in differentiating small HCCs from regenerating nodules. In the severely cirrhotic liver, small HCCs (particularly those less than 1 cm) and regenerating nodules have similar appearances on sonography and conventional CT scans. With iodized oil CT, small HCCs can usually retain Lipiodol; regenerating nodules do not.[2]

Spiral (Helical) CT

Spiral (helical or volumetric) CT is the latest advance in techniques for rapid scanning. Spiral CT combines continuous tube rotation with continuous table feed, thus permitting volumetric acquisitions to be obtained during a single breath-holding period.[20–22] It allows for faster acquisition of truly volumetric CT data than is possible with conventional scanners. The rapidity with which CT data can be acquired allows completion of scans more rapidly in critically injured patients, and imaging while intravenous contrast material is at its peak level can be easily achieved.

Dynamic incremental scanning of the liver during the nonequilibrium phase is the preferred method for hepatic tumor screening with spiral CT.[23,24] Peak hepatic enhancement does occur during 70 to 120 seconds after the start of the injection, depending on the method of administration.[22] Since conventional state of the art incremental CT scanners require 1.5 to 2.5 minutes to scan the entire liver, it is impossible to scan the entire liver with conventional CT during the optimum liver scanning interval. Spiral CT overcomes this problem because of its relatively short scanning time. With spiral CT, the entire liver can be imaged during the peak of hepatic enhancement without scanning during the equilibrium phase.[22]

The speed of helical CT may make it possible to scan patients both early and late within the nonequilibrium phase (Fig. 24-6). Tumor enhancement on a CT scan may become more analogous to that achieved with an arteriogram (Fig. 24-7). Because of the potential variability in vascularity of primary and metastatic tumors, scanning during the arterial and portal venous phases may provide valuable information. Many investigations are in progress,[25,26] and several reports have described the efficacy of dual-phase spiral CT.[27,28]

The continuous data acquisition with spiral CT makes possible two additional advantages over standard incremental CT: (1) the potential for improved lesion detection due to both elimination of respiratory misregistration and retrospective image reconstruction at arbitrary positions along the z axis[29] and (2) the production of high-quality multiplanar images.[22] Spiral CT with

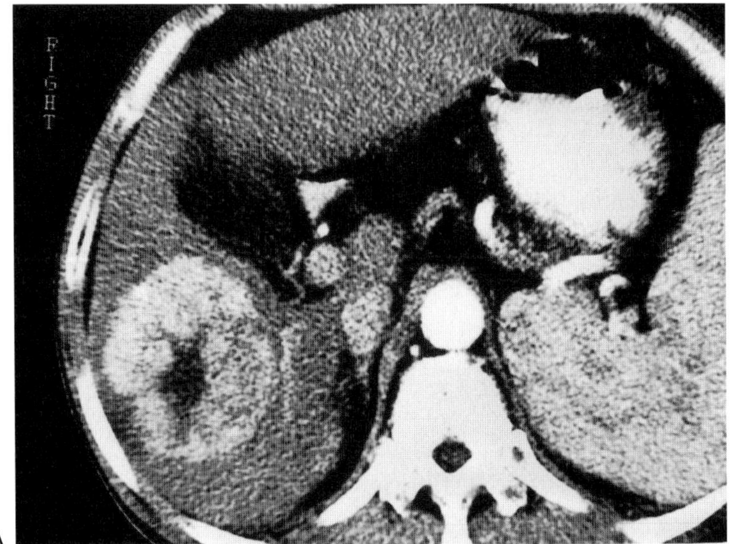

A

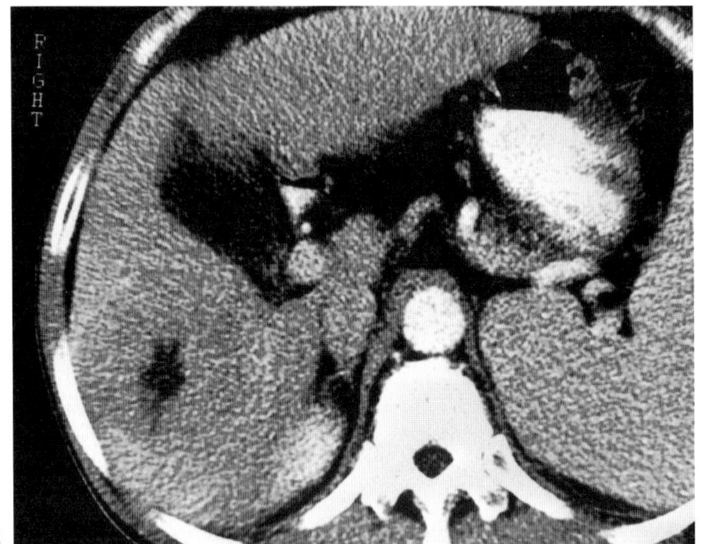

B

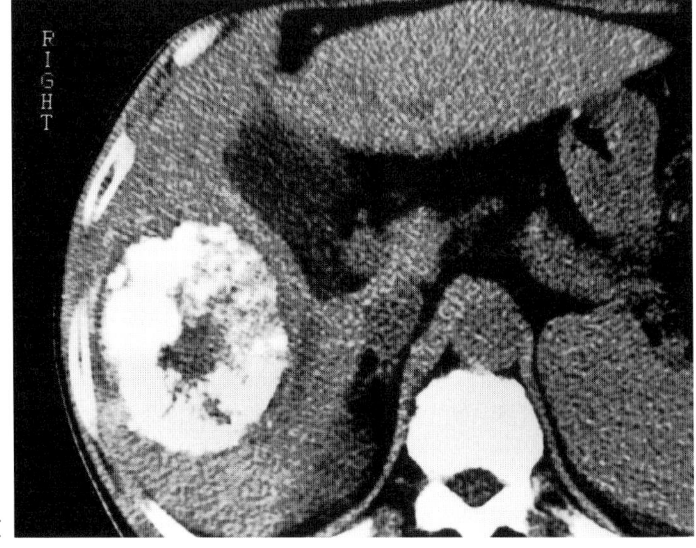

C

FIGURE 24-6. A nodular encapsulated HCC with central necrosis at dual-phase spiral CT and iodized oil CT. (*A*) CT scan in the arterial dominant phase shows nodular high-attenuation tumor with central low-attenuation area, indicating hypervascular mass with necrosis. (*B*) CT scan in the late phase shows low-attenuation tumor, indicating rapid washout of contrast material from the tumor. (*C*) Iodized oil CT scan shows dense retention of Lipiodol in the tumor except in the central necrotic area, indicating successful transcatheter arterial embolization.

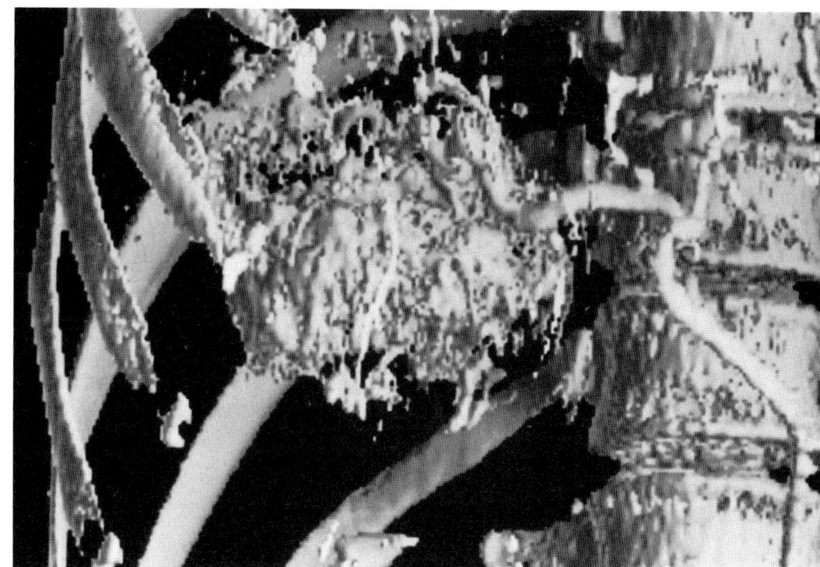

FIGURE 24-7. A hypervascular HCC at CT angiography using a spiral CT. Tumor enhancement with spiral CT becomes more analogous to that seen on a hepatic angiogram.

smaller interscan spacing increases confidence in detection and overall detection rate of focal liver lesions.[30]

CT FOR THE DETECTION OF SMALL TUMORS

Recent advances in liver imaging have made it possible to detect small HCCs by CT scan, and, with the widespread use of these techniques, the number of asymptomatic cases diagnosed has increased considerably.[1–3,31–33] These techniques can detect small tumors not otherwise detected in HCC screening programs, during monitoring of serum α-fetoprotein and ultrasound imaging, and in patients with chronic liver disease.[31–33]

The numerous imaging techniques available for detecting HCCs and regional differences in the techniques have resulted in various diagnostic standards and comparative studies.[34] The relative efficacies of various techniques for detecting HCCs less than 3 cm in diameter have been evaluated. The sensitivity for detecting HCCs less than 3 cm in diameter is 46% to 84% with CT,[2,3,34,35] 82% with CTA,[3] 86% to 91% with CTAP,[3,36] and 71% to 96% with iodized oil CT.[2,3,36,37] In most comparative analyses, the sensitivities of CTAP and iodized oil CT are significantly higher than those of conventional CT.[2,36] The sensitivity for detecting early HCCs is 56% with CT,[38] 70% with CTA,[39] and 66% with CTAP.[39]

CT is important for the detection of peripheral cholangiocarcinoma in the early stages because clinical and laboratory findings are nonspecific and generally minimal. The accuracy of CT for the detection of cholangiocarcinoma is difficult to determine because there are various techniques in performing CT. The detection rate for intrahepatic cholangiocarcinoma is 78% to 100% with conventional CT.[40,41] In our series, the detection rates with magnetic resonance imaging (MRI) and CT were 100% and 91%, respectively.[42] MRI was slightly superior to CT but not statistically significant in detecting these tumors. However, the capability of either CT or MRI to detect small cholangiocarcinomas remains unclear because published reports include few patients and the reported tumors were large in size.[42]

The sensitivities of imaging techniques for the detection of hepatic metastases may vary. The sensitivity for detecting liver metastases using enhanced CT was 51% to 57%; dynamic CT, 67% to 71%; delayed CT, 53% to 72%; CTA, 81%; two-dimensional CTAP, 78% to 91%; and three-dimensional CTAP, 94%.[43–48]

Our approach has been to start with contrast-enhanced CT of the abdomen. Unenhanced scanning may be helpful in certain instances, although Patten et al.[49] concluded that it is unnecessary in patients with hypervascular tumors. Spiral CT performed during the peak level of hepatic parenchymal enhancement is probably the best single noninvasive method, although this has yet to be proved.[50] Furthermore, the usefulness of so-called biphasic spiral CT is unknown.[22,50,51] This technique may be very helpful in detecting hepatic metastasis (Fig. 24-8).[27,28] CT after arterial portography is the most sensitive technique but is reserved for patients who are candidates for surgery, because it is invasive.[18,19]

Over the past several years, many laboratories have attempted to develop an ideal contrast agent for imaging of the liver. Several years ago, EOE-13 (ethiodized oil emulsion) for CT showed considerable promise for disease detection; however, the toxicity of the agent has prevented its widespread use.[52]

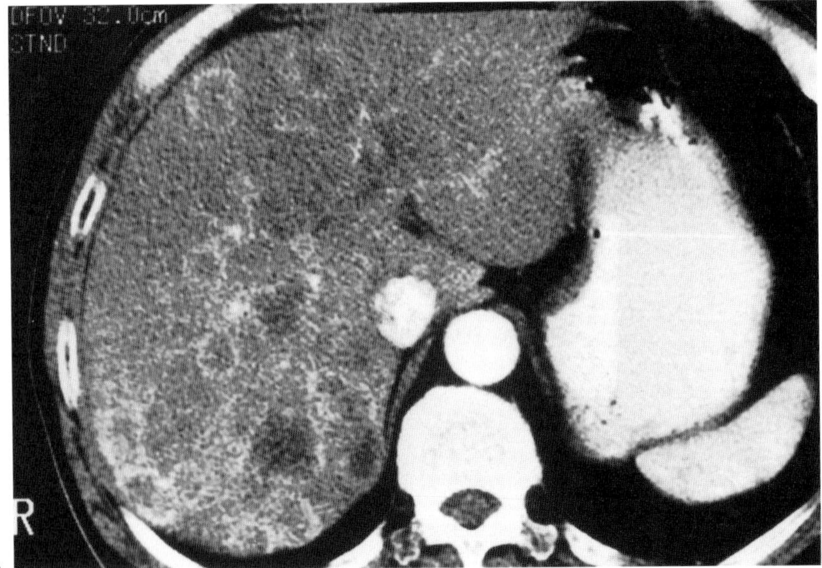

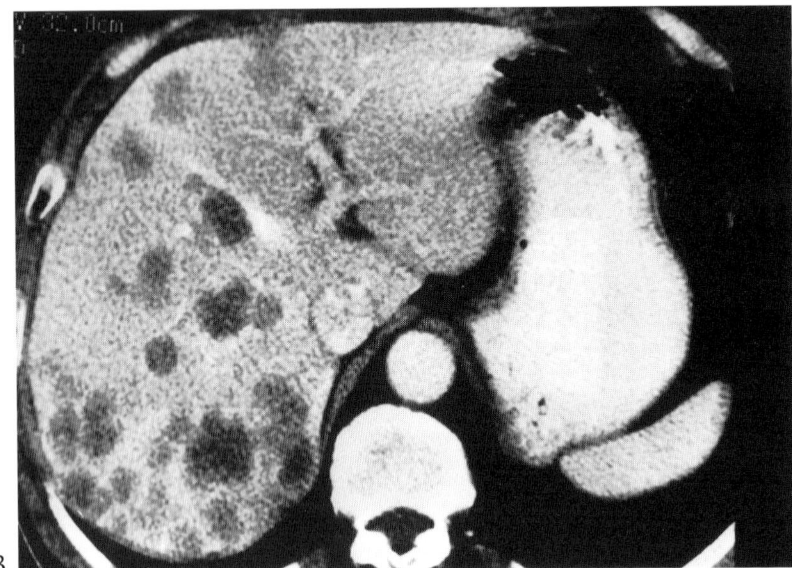

FIGURE 24-8. Metastases to the liver from colon cancer on dual-phase contrast-enhanced CT scans using a spiral CT. (*A*) CT scan in the arterial dominant phase shows multiple tumor nodules with peripheral rim enhancement. The enhancement pattern is indistinct and nonglobular, different from the pattern in hemangiomas. (*B*) CT scan in the portal dominant phase shows multiple tumor nodules with low attenuation in both hepatic lobes. Dual-phase CT scans are complementary to each other in detecting metastatic nodules.

CT FOR THE CHARACTERIZATION OF HEPATIC TUMORS

Tumor Vascularity Versus Contrast Enhancement

Several imaging techniques have been used for differential diagnosis of liver tumors, including CTA, CTAP, iodized oil CT, and sonographic angiography. However, these techniques are too invasive to use for screening procedures. In contrast, incremental dynamic CT, particularly with the spiral technique, is not invasive, is easy to perform, and is rapidly done.

Dynamic incremental hepatic CT scanning protocols are designed to optimize imaging during the portal venous phase of enhancement. Three-fourths of the hepatic parenchymal blood supply is contributed by the portal vein, whereas tumors derive their blood supply entirely from hepatic artery branches. Hepatic arterial enhancement begins approximately 20 seconds after bolus initiation, with portal venous enhancement peaking at 70 to 120 seconds.[22] Most metastatic tumors are hypovascular and appear as low-attenuation lesions during much of the bolus and nonequilibrium phases (Fig. 24-9). However, during the latter part of the nonequilibrium phase and into the equilibrium phase, many of the tumors become isoattenuating compared with the liver. Unlike hypovascular tumors, hypervascular tumors may appear to be high attenuating relative to the hepatic parenchyma during the early bolus phase; they may become isoattenuating compared with the liver in the early nonequilibrium phase. Therefore, such neoplasms are better imaged during the arterial phase of hepatic enhancement (Fig. 24-10).

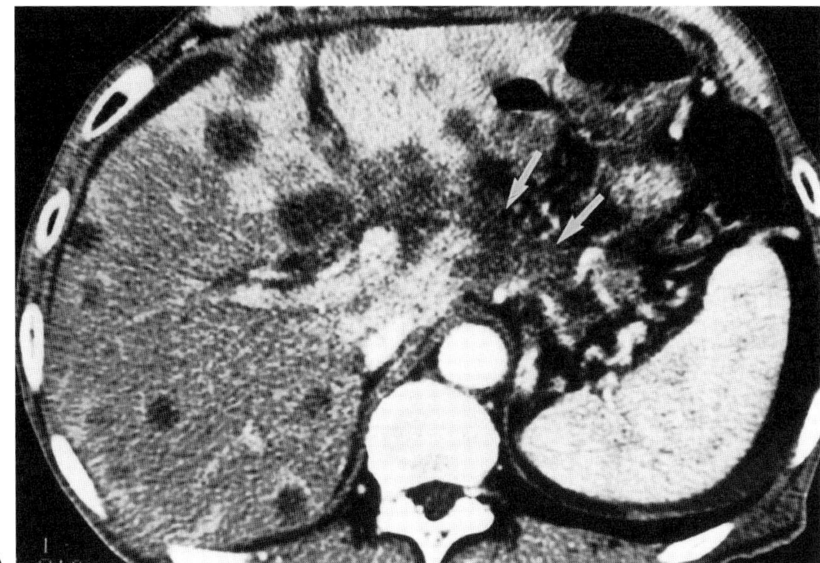

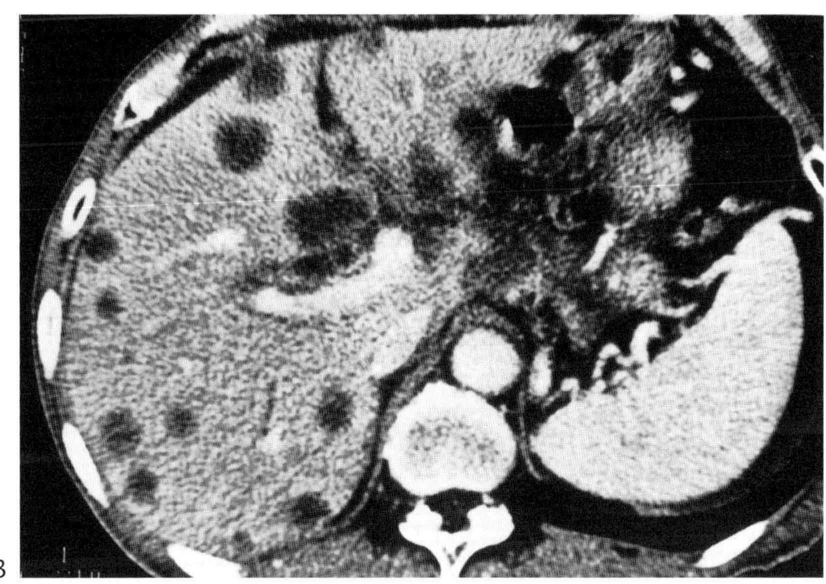

FIGURE 24-9. Metastases from pancreatic cancer on dual-phase contrast enhanced CT scans using spiral CT with phenomenon of transient hepatic attenuation difference (THAD) due to obstruction of the portal vein. (*A*) CT scan in the arterial dominant phase shows multiple metastatic nodules with low-attenuation in both hepatic lobes. The attenuation of the left hepatic lobe is higher than that of the right hepatic lobe, indicating hyperperfusion by the hepatic artery due to the left portal vein obstruction. Pancreatic body and tail cancer (arrows) shows low attenuation. (*B*) CT scan in the portal dominant phase shows multiple metastatic nodules with low attenuation in the liver. The left portal vein is not opacified due to obstruction by tumor nodules. The attenuation difference of both hepatic lobes seen on CT scan in the arterial dominant phase has disappeared.

Advanced HCC

On conventional CT scans, most HCCs appear as relatively well defined, low-attenuation masses. When the HCC is encapsulated, the capsule shows ring-like contrast enhancement. However, the appearance of HCCs on CT scans is often similar to that of other hepatic tumors.[53,54]

Single-level dynamic CT has made possible the analysis of the dynamic distribution of contrast material in the normal liver and in hepatic masses.[55,56] Araki et al.[56] divided hepatic tumors into four types according to the pattern derived from sequential plotting of the attenuation difference between the tumor and the liver parenchyma. In type I, tumor enhancement was high, rapid, and prolonged; in type II, tumors enhanced rapidly but then quickly became less dense than the liver; in type III, no significant change in the attenuation difference between the tumor and the liver occurred; and in type IV, no enhancement or very little enhancement occurred. The majority of HCCs are type II (Fig. 24-1). A type II tumor is hypervascular, but the total extracellular space in the tumor is smaller than in a type I tumor.

Most HCCs of the nodular type associated with cirrhosis have a fibrous capsule and an internal mosaic architecture.[7] In encapsulated nodular HCCs, the fibrous capsule is seen as a thin circular area of low attenuation surrounding the tumor on unenhanced CT and during the arterial dominant phase of dynamic CT and as a high-attenuation ring in the delayed phase (Fig. 24-11).[7,55] The internal mosaic pattern is characterized by multiple components showing different attenuations separated by thin bands with the same CT features as the fibrous capsule (Fig. 24-12). Fatty metamorphosis or steatosis, which is seen on a CT scan as a focal zone of tissue within a tumor that has the same CT appearance

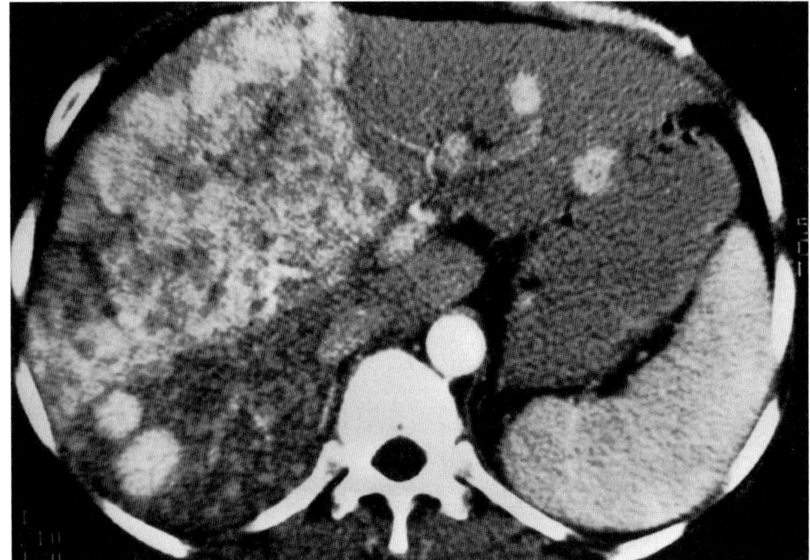

A

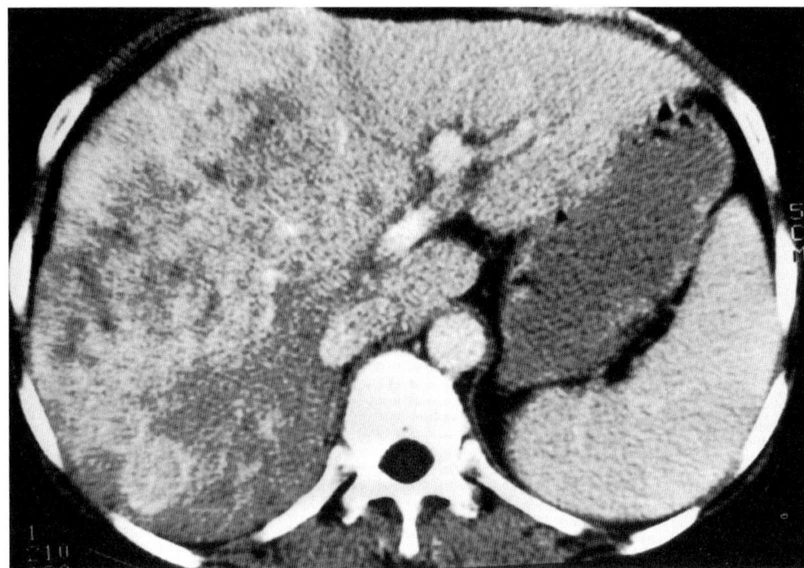

B

FIGURE 24-10. Hepatocellular carcinoma shown better on CT scans in the arterial dominant phase during a dual-phase scan with a spiral CT. (*A*) CT scan in the arterial dominant phase shows massive HCC with high attenuation in right and left medial liver. Several small nodules with high attenuation are also well visualized in both hepatic lobes. (*B*) CT scan in the portal dominant phase shows indistinct margin of a massive HCC and does not show the additional small nodules in left hepatic lobe because tumor and hepatic parenchyma have enhanced to the same degree.

or negative Hounsfield numbers as fat, has been described as a specific feature of HCC.[57,58] Recently, however, Freeny et al.[59] reported a low frequency of typical findings with CT in a non-Asian population. The diffuse type shows numerous small nodules, 0.5 to 1.0 cm in diameter, scattered throughout the liver that do not fuse with each other and are always associated with cirrhosis. Diffuse nodules are visualized as diffusely distributed small low-attenuation areas on both unenhanced and contrast-enhanced CT (Fig. 24-13). This is very similar to the appearance of macroregenerative nodules and diffuse metastases, and it is not easy to differentiate these lesions without dynamic CT.[7]

Another characteristic of HCCs is their tendency to grow into the portal and/or hepatic veins, leading to the formation of tumor thrombi (Figs. 24-13, 24-14).[60] Tumor thrombi appear as solid lesions in the blood vessels with marked hypervascularity, often seen on dynamic CT due to the arteriovenous shunting through them.[61,62]

The value of CTA or CTAP in the detection of HCC lies in the differences in perfusion between normal liver (blood supply from the hepatic artery and portal vein) and HCC (blood supply from the hepatic artery only).[16] Most HCCs are seen as enhancing masses on CT arteriograms and as filling defects on CT scans obtained during arterial portography, because most of these tumors have no portal supply (Fig. 24-4).[63]

Iodized oil CT is useful for detecting small HCCs and for differentiating HCCs from regenerating nodules. Another benefit is that CT with iodized oil can be used to evaluate the therapeutic effect of transcatheter oily chemoembolization therapy of HCCs, particularly in cases of encapsulated nodular HCCs (Fig. 24-6c).[64]

Spiral CT provides the potential to image the entire liver twice, once during the arterial and once during the

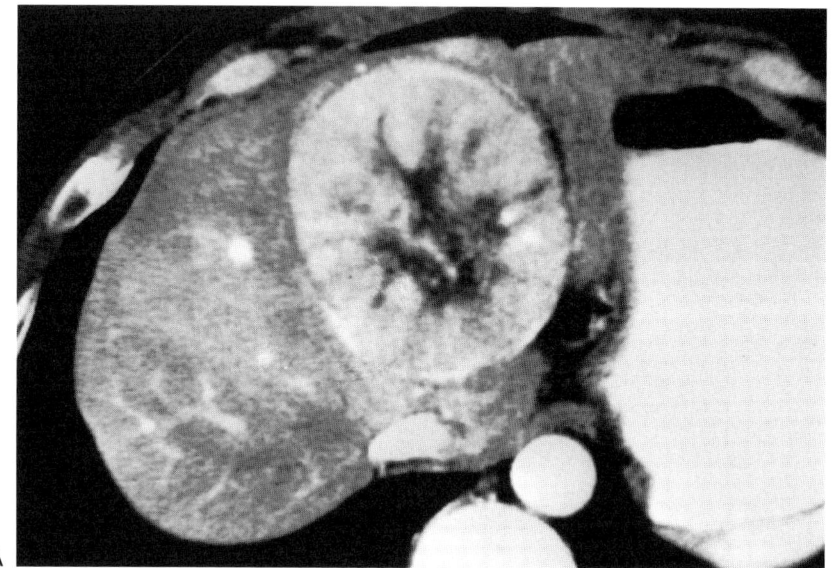

A

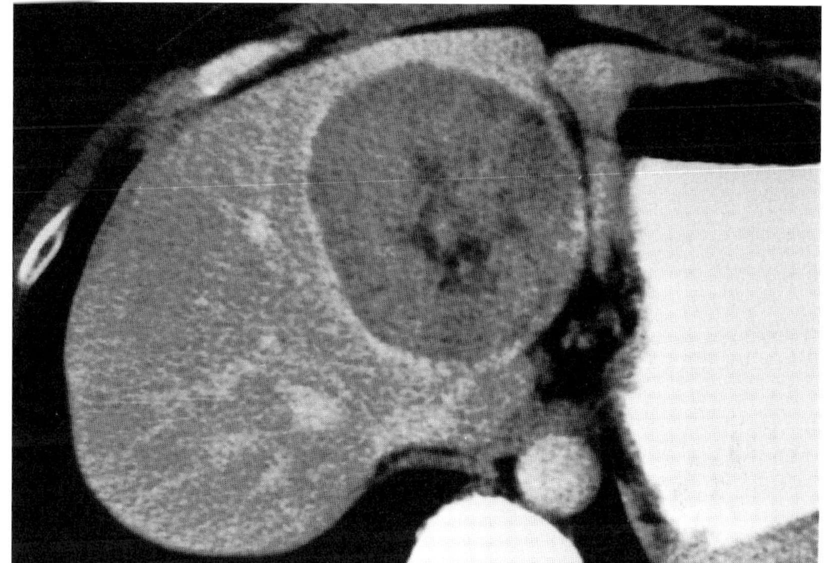

B

FIGURE 24-11. (*A* & *B*) Nodular HCC with fibrous capsule on dynamic CT scans. (*A*) CT scan in the arterial dominant phase shows a large, ovoid, nodular tumor with high attenuation and peripheral hypoattenuating rim in left hepatic lobe. (*B*) CT scan in the late phase shows a mass with low attenuation and peripheral hyperattenuating rim in the same area.

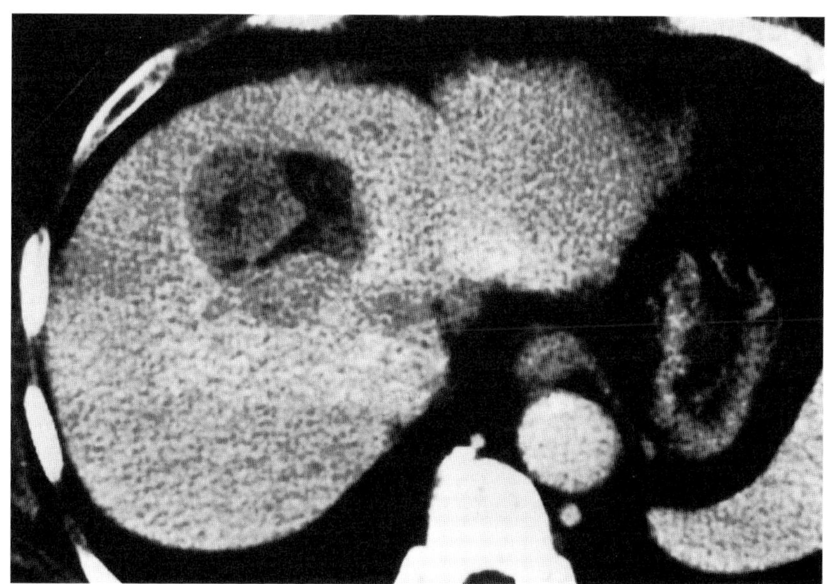

FIGURE 24-12. A mosaic pattern of HCC. Conventional contrast-enhanced CT scan shows a nodular mass with several compartments having different attenuation.

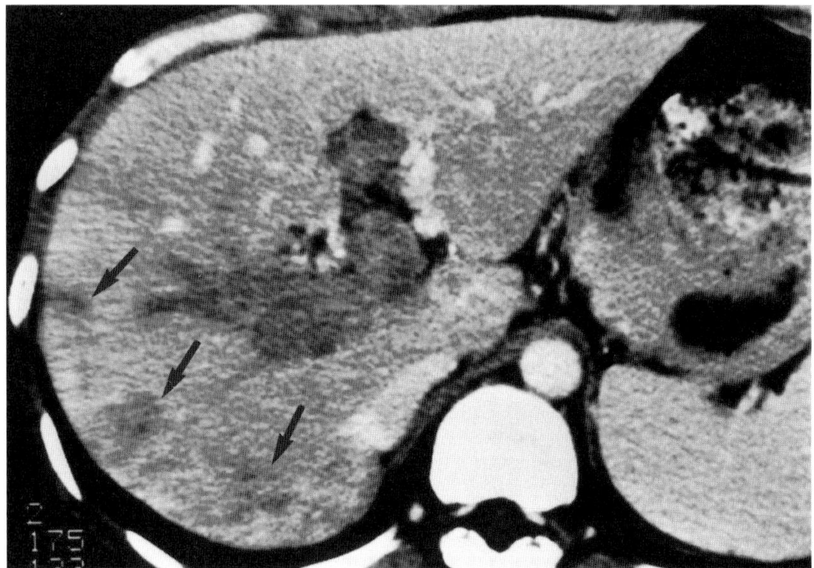

FIGURE 24-13. A diffuse HCC with invasion to the portal vein. Contrast-enhanced CT scan shows multiple indistinct low-attenuation areas (arrows) in the right liver. Intrahepatic portal vein is dilated and not enhanced, indicating diffuse thrombosis.

late phase (Fig. 24-6). Therefore, several distinct patterns of focal hepatic tumors on contrast-enhanced CT scans can be accentuated with this technique.[11,22,26]

Usually hepatic arterial enhancement begins approximately 20 to 30 seconds after bolus initiation,[11,22] when the aorta and hepatic artery first receive contrast material. During this time interval, hypervascular tumors such as HCCs will receive highly concentrated contrast material and will enhance on CT scans without dilution effect by portal venous supply because hypervascular tumors have only hepatic arterial supply and receive little or no flow from the portal vein.[63,65,66] On the other hand, the liver parenchyma will receive little contrast material because the portal vein will not yet have received the contrast material and will not enhance significantly. This maximizes lesion visualization by delivering contrast material to the tumor but not to the liver (Fig. 24-11A).[67] In the arterial phase using fast CT, 60% to 77% of HCCs enhance totally or partially.[26,65,66]

During the late phase, tumors with persistent stain or slow uptake of contrast material theoretically are better imaged. This phase is also useful because a markedly delayed retention of iodinated contrast material is seen within fibrous tumors such as cholangiocarcinoma or metastatic tumor from the gastrointestinal tract,[68,69] and persistent retention of contrast material is seen in the fibrous capsule of nodular HCC (Fig. 24-11B).

Early HCC

Adenomatous hyperplasia can be accompanied by malignant foci, and thus may be an early form of HCC. Early HCCs are small, with mean diameters less than 1.5 cm.[34,70,71] Therefore, detection is difficult, and the efficacy of imaging techniques for evaluation of these lesions has not been well established. A recent study[71] indicates overall sensitivities of 58% for CT, 50% for CTA, and 71% for CTAP.

Early HCC is usually hypovascular. Matsui et al.[63] found that intranodular portal blood flow tends to decrease as the grade of malignancy increases. Unlike adenomatous hyperplasia, almost all HCCs of Edmondson grade II or greater had a definite decrease in the intranodular portal blood supply on CT scans obtained during arterial portography. In early HCCs and well-differentiated HCCs, the intranodular portal blood supply tended to decrease progressively as the grade of malignancy increased, whereas the intranodular hepatic arterial supply increased (Fig. 24-15).

Unlike early HCCs, most ordinary adenomatous hyperplasias without malignant foci are not visualized on CT scans obtained during arterial portography because of portal blood flow in the lesions.[63] The combination of CTA and CTAP is more accurate than either alone in determining the nature of nodular lesions associated with cirrhosis.[63,71]

Cholangiocarcinoma

CT characteristics of cholangiocarcinoma are an irregular large mass with low attenuation, slight contrast enhancement (usually at the periphery), and focal intrahepatic bile ductal dilatation around the tumor (Figs. 24-16, 24-17).[72–76] In addition, an irregular mass with markedly low attenuation, which corresponds to the diffuse, microcystic changes of comedo-type necrosis (Fig. 24-17), may be seen. The CT numbers of these low-attenuation masses vary from +26 to +50 Hounsfield numbers on postcontrast scans. We have rarely encountered this finding in other hepatic tumors. High-attenuation areas within the mass on unenhanced scans can sometimes be seen, corresponding to mucinous substances within the masses. In cholangiocarcinomas, these sub-

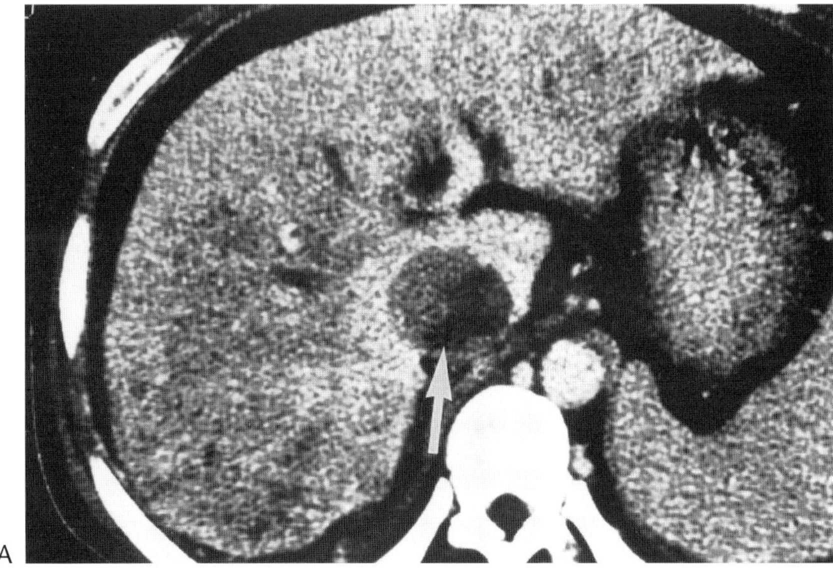

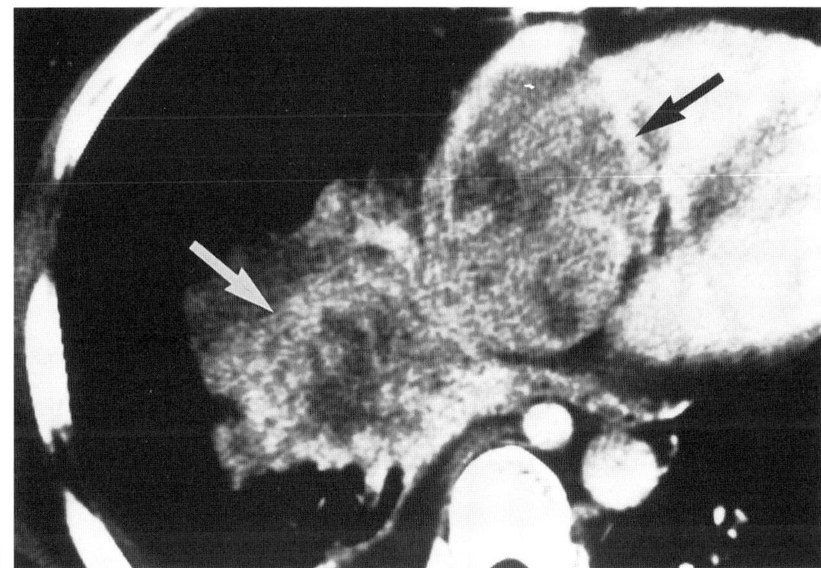

FIGURE 24-14. A diffuse HCC with invasion to the inferior vena cava and right atrium. (*A*) Contrast-enhanced CT scan shows indistinct diffuse HCC with low attenuation in right side of the liver. The inferior vena cava (arrow) is dilated and not enhanced. (*B*) CT scan at the above level shows massive tumor thrombus in the inferior vena cava and right atrium (arrows).

stances are often present within cells in the bile duct lumina.[72]

Peripheral cholangiocarcinoma can be associated with *Clonorchis sinensis* infection (Fig. 24-18). The association of clonorchiasis with cholangiocarcinoma has been debated.[77] Hou[78] found clonorchiasis in many patients with intrahepatic cholangiocarcinoma. In a study of primary liver cancer by Kim,[79] the prevalence of clonorchiasis was significantly higher in cholangiocarcinoma than in HCC. Experimental studies have shown that prolonged severe *Clonorchis sinensis* infection produces adenomatous hyperplasia and bile duct carcinoma.[80,81] The CT appearance of clonorchiasis is a diffuse, mild dilatation of the intrahepatic biliary tree, especially the peripheral portions, without any evidence of obstruction. Cholangiocarcinomas also can be caused by previous exposure to the radiopaque contrast material thorium oxide (Thorotrast).[74]

On dynamic CT, low attenuation is seen in the early phase and increases in the delayed phase (Figs. 24-16b, 24-17).[76] This characteristic enhancement pattern may depend on the presence of a large amount of fibrous tissue and neovascularity in the tumors.[42,82,84] The mechanism of prolonged enhancement of fibrous tumors has not been clarified, but the slow washout of extravascular contrast agents in the fibrous stroma may play a role.[83] Although the CT features are characteristic, they are not specific for cholangiocarcinoma. Metastatic adenocarcinoma of the liver and sclerosing HCC should be included in the differential diagnosis of this tumor.[84]

Metastatic Tumors

CT remains the recommended procedure for metastatic tumors over both ultrasound and MRI since involvement of the bowel and its mesentery can be simultaneously

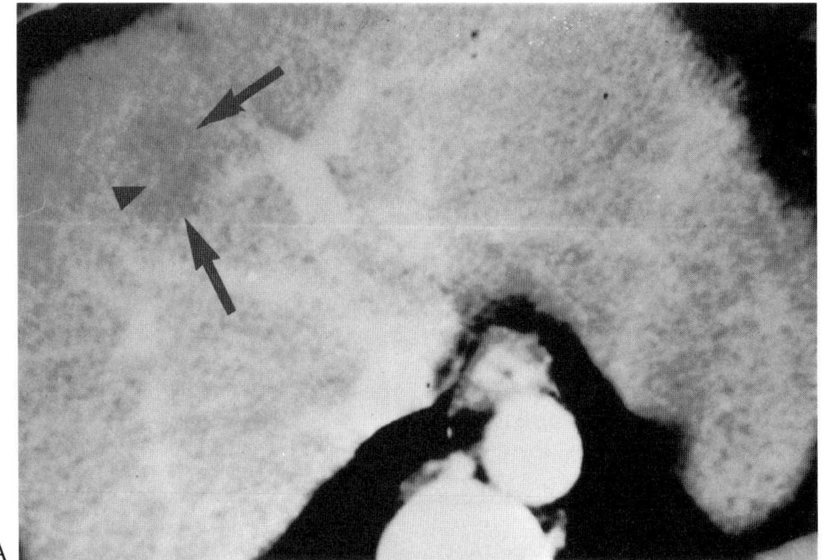

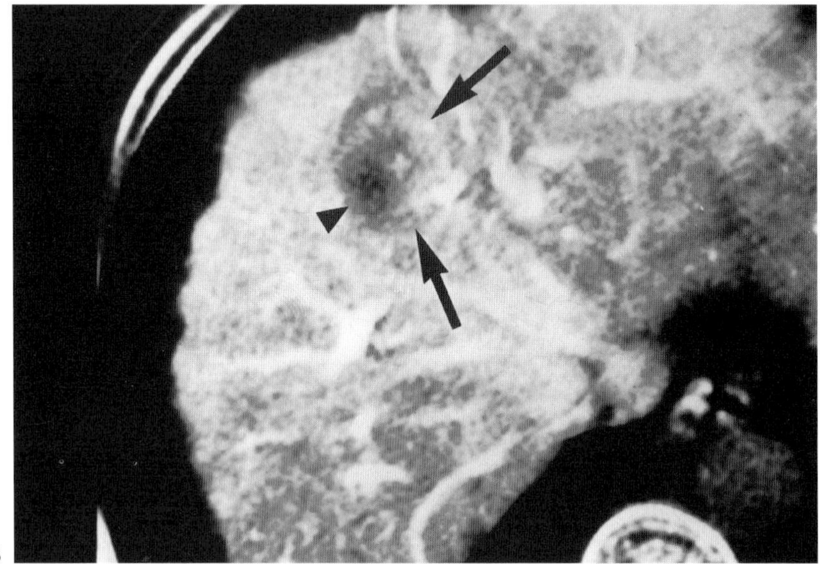

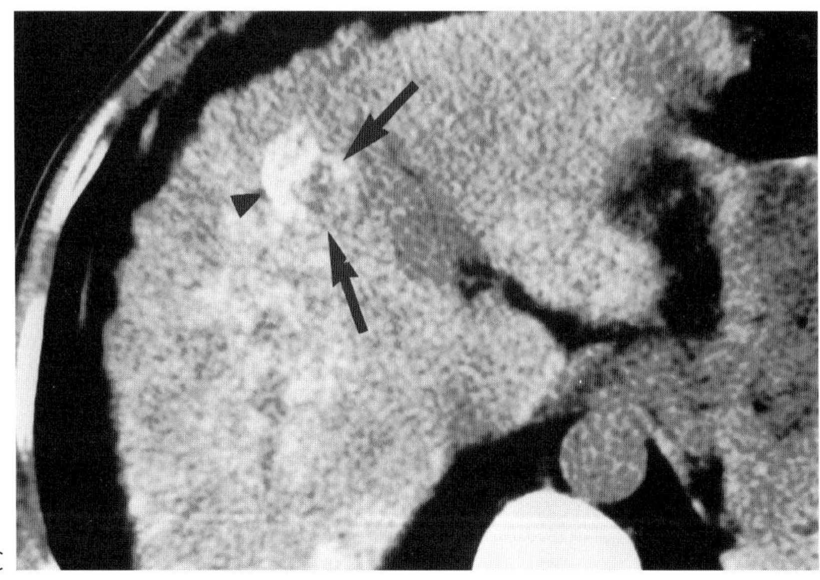

FIGURE 24-15. Early HCC seen on conventional CT, CTAP, and iodized oil CT. (*A*) Contrast-enhanced CT scan shows round hypoattenuating mass (arrows) with inner isoattenuating area (arrowhead). (*B*) CT arterial portogram shows isoattenuating mass (arrows) with inner filling defect area (arrowhead), indicating normal portal perfusion with partial perfusion defect area, corresponding to isoattenuating area seen in Fig. 24-15A. (*C*) Iodized oil CT scan shows retention of Lipiodol in inner area (arrowhead) of the mass, corresponding to filling defect area seen in Fig. 24-15B. Main mass (arrows) shows no retention of Lipiodol, indicating that the tumor is probably adenomatous hyperplasia with malignant focus.

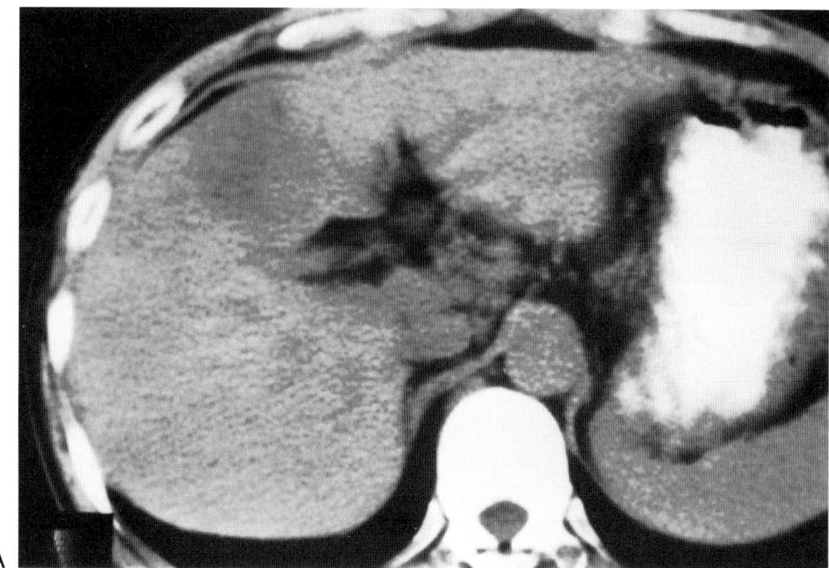

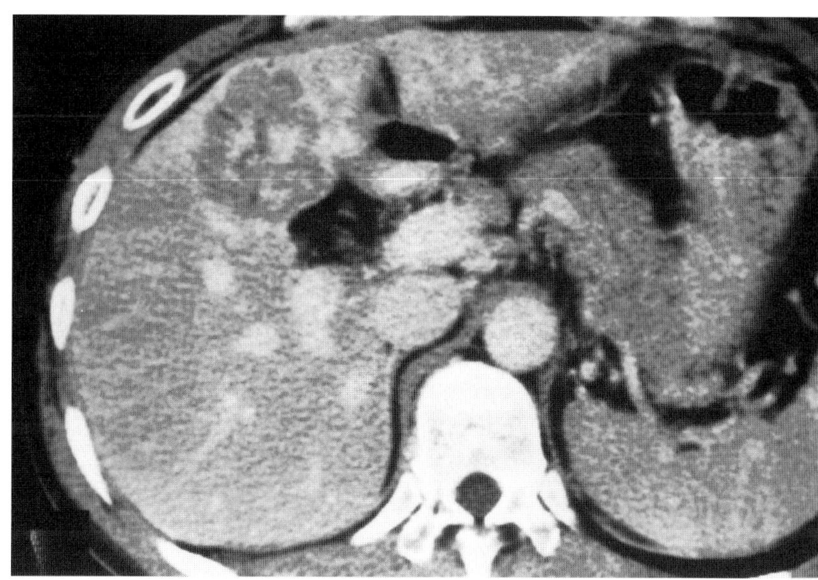

FIGURE 24-16. Cholangiocarcinoma with central fibrotic portion on both the unenhanced and contrast-enhanced CT scans. (*A*) Unenhanced CT scan shows ill-defined, low-attenuation mass in medial segment of the left side of the liver. (*B*) Contrast-enhanced CT scan in the delayed phase shows well-defined, low-attenuation mass with central high attenuation.

evaluated.[85] The CT appearance of metastases to the liver depends on tumor size, vascularity, the degree of hemorrhage and necrosis, and the quality of the intravenous contrast bolus. Thus, individual metastatic lesions within the liver can have different CT findings and metastases from different cell types can appear identical (Fig. 24-19).[10,85] On unenhanced CT scans taken at a narrow window setting, multiple masses appear as round, sometimes confluent, frequently indistinctly demarcated areas of variable low attenuation. Because of possible isoattenuation, a bolus dose of contrast medium is generally necessary for localization of metastases.[10,85,86]

Most metastatic tumors to the liver are hypovascular. Thus, most metastases are detected as low attenuation areas within an enhanced liver parenchyma (Fig. 24-9). Metastases, especially those from adenocarcinomas of the gastrointestinal tract, take up contrast material more slowly.[87,88] Most metastases have better circulation in their periphery, so the low-attenuation center becomes more prominent after contrast medium administration. Therefore, a slight central zone of high-attenuation with a low-attenuation margin appears in the delayed phase (Fig. 24-20).[65] A better understanding of contrast kinetics coupled with newer CT data acquisition systems, such as spiral volumetric CT, may limit contrast-related misinterpretations.[85] In the arterial and late phase images in our study, 25% and 65% of metastasis, respectively, showed low attenuation (Fig. 24-9).[26] Another common CT pattern of metastasis is a peripheral rim enhancement around a less dense central zone (Fig. 24-8a). This reportedly occurs in 29% to 47% of these lesions.[26,69,89]

Even though metastases have many imaging features in common, certain characteristics can help formulate a differential diagnosis. For example, certain metastases, such as mucinous carcinomas arising from the gastroin-

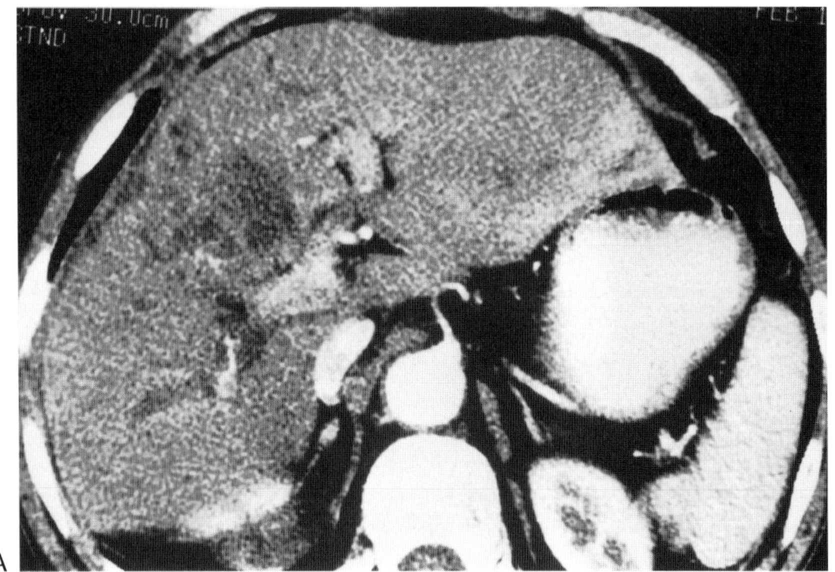

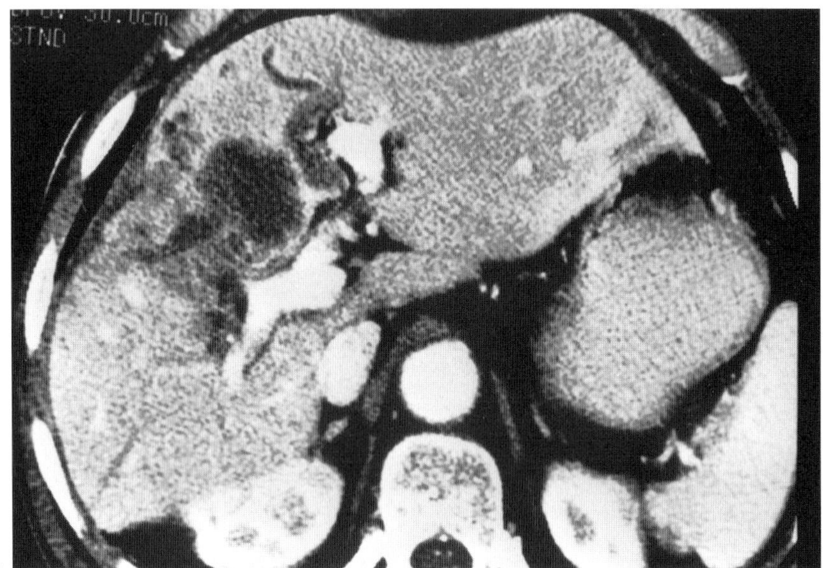

FIGURE 24-17. Cholangiocarcinoma with peritumoral biliary dilatation on dual phase spiral CT. (*A*) CT scan in the arterial dominant phase shows indistinct low-attenuation tumor in right anterior and left medial liver. (*B*) CT scan in the portal dominant phase shows a well-defined, irregular, low-attenuation tumor with intrahepatic bile duct dilatation around the tumor.

testinal tract or medullary thyroid cancer, are more likely to calcify. Other malignant lesions of the liver that occasionally calcify include fibrolamellar HCC, hepatoblastoma, cholangiocarcinoma, cystadenocarcinoma, and numerous metastases. Zones of necrosis do not enhance in metastases with liquefaction, which is one of the characteristics of hepatic metastases from gastrointestinal leiomyosarcoma (Fig. 24-21). Peripheral enhancement is also seen in hemangiomas. However, the enhancing pattern is different. Hemangiomas show nodular, globular enhancement while metastases show indistinct nonglobular enhancement.[90]

Renal cell carcinoma, carcinoid, choriocarcinoma, leiomyosarcoma, pancreatic islet cell tumor, and sarcomatous metastases are characteristically hypervascular and readily detected. The dynamic enhancement patterns of hypervascular metastases differ from those of hypovascular lesions. Hypervascular metastases show high attenuation relative to the liver during the arterial phase, when these tumors are receiving peak delivery of contrast material via hepatic arterial branches. Lesion enhancement begins to diminish during the portal venous phase. At some time during the nonequilibrium phase of maximal hepatic enhancement, the hypervascular metastases may become isoattenuating with enhanced hepatic parenchyma.[49] Therefore, incremental dynamic CT is of limited value in differentiating hypervascular metastases from HCCs and detecting the lesions as well.

CT STAGING OF LIVER CANCER

CT staging of liver cancer defines the extent and location of intrahepatic disease, involvement of surgically critical areas (porta hepatis, portal vein, inferior vena cava,

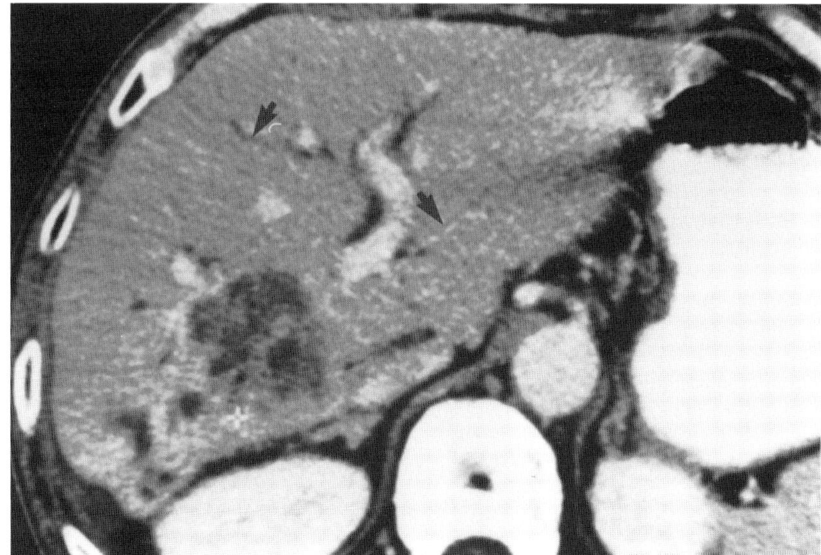

FIGURE 24-18. Cholangiocarcinoma with *Clonorchis sinensis* on conventional contrast-enhanced CT scan. CT scan shows low-attenuation mass with slight peripheral contrast enhancement and peritumoral biliary dilatation. Mild, diffuse, intrahepatic biliary dilatation (arrows) is also seen in other area of the liver, indicating clonorchiasis.

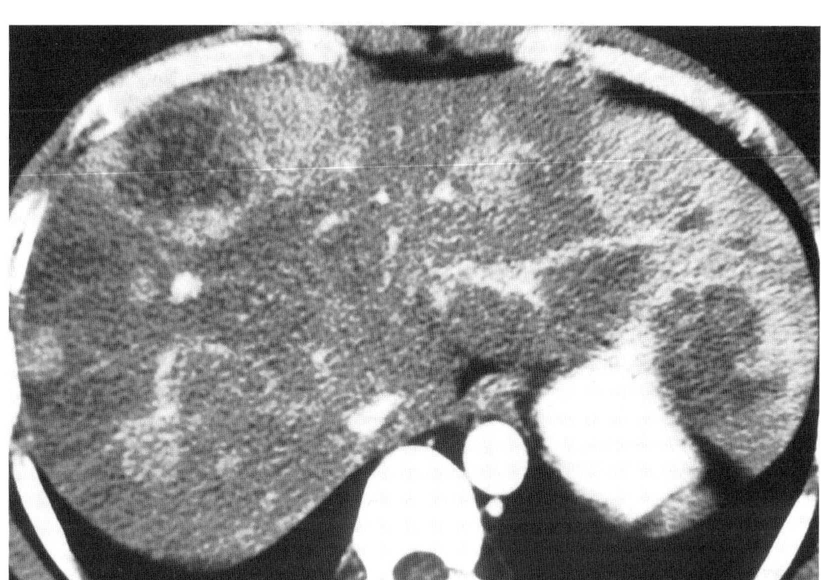

FIGURE 24-19. Metastases to the liver from melanoma with different attenuation. CT scan in the arterial dominant phase shows multiple masses with high and low attenuation in the liver.

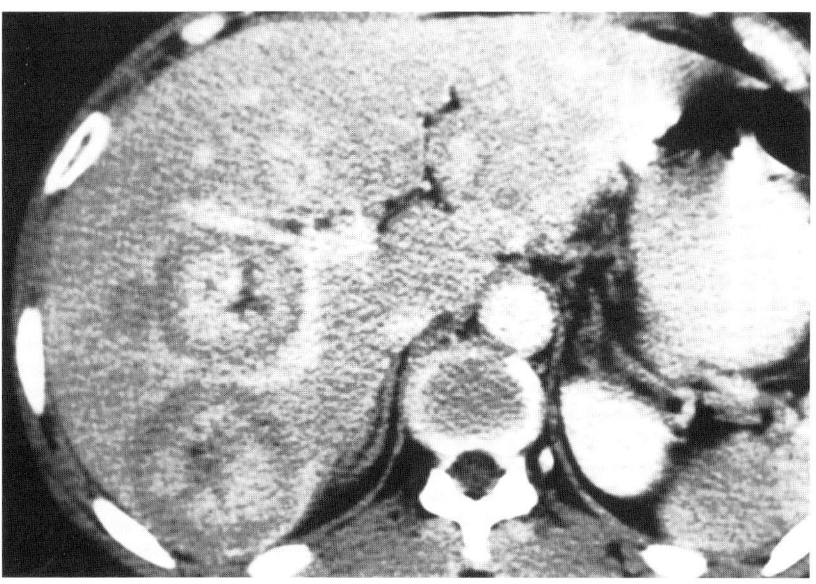

FIGURE 24-20. Metastases from gastric cancer in the delayed phase. Contrast-enhanced CT scan shows multiple round tumors with central high-attenuation and peripheral low-attenuation rim.

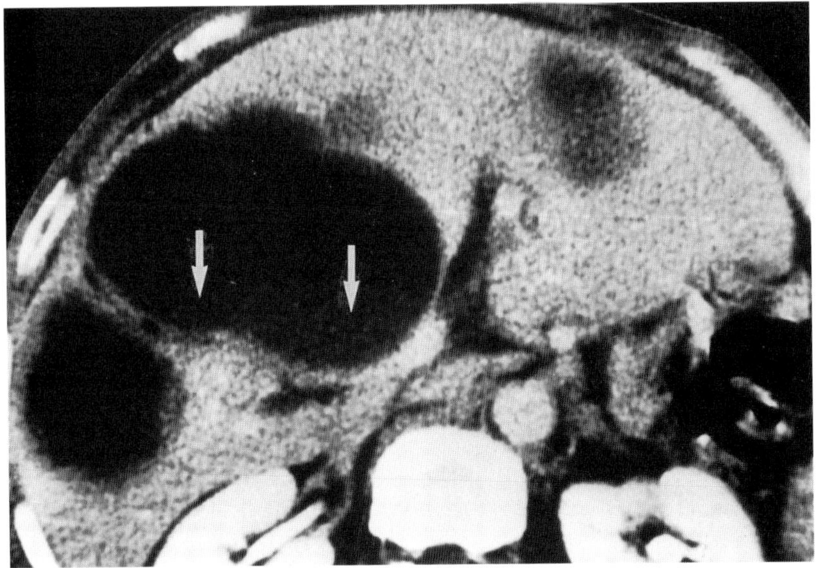

FIGURE 24-21. Metastases to the liver from gastric leiomyosarcoma. Contrast-enhanced CT scan shows multiple low-attenuation tumors with severe necrosis. Fluid-fluid level (arrows) is seen in some tumors.

major bile ducts), and defines the presence of extrahepatic disease.[8] The critical surgical anatomy of the liver is based on the internal vascular skeleton of the liver.[91–93] The French surgical anatomists Couinaud and Bismuth popularized an eight-segment partition based principally on the position of the three major hepatic veins (right, middle, left) and the portal veins. CT descriptions of liver tumor location are now routinely detailed in terms of their Couinaud segment. Whenever possible, subsegmental or wedge excisions are employed; therefore, the principal question is whether other segments of the right and left are truly free of tumor.[8] The portal-dominant phase of dynamic CT, high-dose contrast enhancement CT, and CTAP in which intrahepatic veins are well opacified are valuable for this purpose. Of these three modalities, CTAP is the most accurate in determining the segmental location of the tumor.[17–19,94] Intrahepatic metastases are usually hypervascular in nature and well visualized by dynamic CT, arteriography (especially using digital subtraction angiography), CTA, and iodized oil CT.[2,95,96] When the lesions are extremely hypervascular, nodules less than 0.5 cm in diameter can be detected by these methods, particularly by iodized oil CT (Fig. 24-5). When HCC nodules are hypovascular, they are detected most accurately by CTAP, which can visualize nodules measuring 0.5 cm in diameter or more regardless of their vascularity.[94–96]

REFERENCES

1. Takashima T, Matsui O, Suzuki M, Ida M. Diagnosis and screening of small hepatocellular carcinoma: comparison of radionuclide imaging, ultrasound, computed tomography, hepatic angiography, and alpha-fetoprotein assay. Radiology 1985;145:635–638
2. Choi BI, Park JH, Kim BH et al. Small hepatocellular carcinoma: detection with sonography, computed tomography (CT), angiography and Lipiodol-CT. Br J Radiol 1989;62: 897–901
3. Takayasu K, Moriyama N, Muramastsu Y et al. The diagnosis of small hepatocellular carcinomas: efficacy of various imaging procedures in 100 patients. AJR 1990;155:49–54
4. Tanaka S, Kitamura T, Nakanishi K et al. Recent advances in ultrasonographic diagnosis of hepatocellular carcinoma. Cancer 1989;63:1313–1317
5. Miller WJ, Federle MP, Campbell WL. Diagnosis and staging of hepatocellular carcinoma: comparison of CT and sonography in 36 liver transplantation patients. AJR 1991;157: 303–306
6. Dodd GD III, Miller WJ, Baron RL et al. Detection of malignant tumor in end-stage cirrhotic liver: efficacy of sonography as a screening technique. AJR 1992;159:727–733
7. Matsui O, Itai Y. Diagnosis of primary liver cancer by computed tomography. In Tobe T, Kameda H, Okudaira M et al. (eds): Primary Liver Cancer in Japan. 1st Ed. Springer-Verlag, Tokyo, 1992;129–138
8. Ferrucci JT. Liver tumor imaging: current concepts. Radiol Clin North Am 1994;32:39–54
9. Gore RM. Liver; normal anatomy and examination techniques. In Gore RM, Levine MS, Laufer I (eds): Textbook of Gastointestinal Radiology. 1st Ed. WB Saunders, Philadelphia, 1994;1801–1804
10. Baron RL, Freeny PC, Moss AA. The liver. In Moss AA, Gamsu G, Genant HK (eds): Computed Tomography of the Body with Magnetic Resonance Imaging. 2nd Ed. WB Saunders, Philadelphia, 1992;743–748
11. Dodd GD III, Baron RL. Investigation of contrast enhancement in CT of the liver: the need for improved methods. AJR 1993;160:643–646
12. Foley WD, Berland LL, Lawson TL et al. Contrast enhancement technique for dynamic hepatic computed tomographic scanning. Radiology 1983;147:797–809
13. Cox IH, Foley WD, Hoffman RG. Right window for dynamic hepatic CT. Radiology 1991;181:18–21

14. Bernardino ME, Erwin BC, Steiberg HV et al. Delayed hepatic CT scanning: increased confidence and improved detection of hepatic metastases. Radiology 1986;159:71–74
15. Miller DL, Simmons JT, Chang R et al. Hepatic metastasis detection; comparison of three CT contrast enhancement methods. Radiology 1987;165:787–790
16. Freeny PC, Marks WM. Computed tomographic arteriography of the liver. Radiology 1983;148:193–197
17. Matsui O, Kadoya M, Suzuki M et al. Work in progress; dynamic sequential computed tomography during arterial portography in the detection of hepatic neoplasms. Radiology 1983;146:721–727
18. Heiken JP, Weyman PF, Lee JKT et al. Detection of focal hepatic masses; prospective evaluation with CT, delayed CT, CT during arterial portography, and MR imaging. Radiology 1989;171:47–51
19. Nelson RC, Chezmar JL, Sugarbaker PH, Bernardino ME. Hepatic tumors; comparison of CT during arterial portography, delayed CT, and MR imaging for preoperative evaluation. Radiology 1989;172:27–34
20. Rubin GD, Dake MD, Napel SA et al. Three dimensional spiral CT angiography of the abdomen: initial clinical experience. Radiology 1993;186:147–152
21. Zeman RK, Fox SH, Silverman PM et al. Helical (spiral) CT of the abdomen. AJR 1993;160:719–725
22. Heiken JP, Brink JA, Vannier MW. Spiral (helical) CT. Radiology 1993;189:647–656
23. Bluemke D, Fishman EK. Spiral CT of the liver. AJR 1993;160:787–792
24. Foley WD. Dynamic hepatic CT. Radiology 1989;170:617–622
25. Choi BI, Cho JM, Han JK et al. Spiral CT for the detection of hepatocellular carcinoma: relative value of arterial and late phase scanning. Abdom Imaging 1996;21:440–444
26. Choi BI, Han JK, Cho JM et al. Characterization of focal hepatic tumors: value of two phase scanning with spiral CT. Cancer 1995;76:2434–2442
27. Hollett MD, Jeffrey RB Jr, Nino-Murcia M et al. Dual-phase helical CT of the liver: value of arterial phase scans in the detection of small (< 1.5 cm) malignant hepatic neoplasms. AJR 1995;164:879–884
28. Bonaldi VM, Bret PM, Reinhold C, Atri M. Helical CT of the liver: value of an early hepatic arterial phase. Radiology 1995;197:357–363
29. Choi BI, Shin YM, Han JK et al. Focal hepatic nodules after transcatheter oily chemoembolization: detection with spiral CT versus conventional CT. Abdom Imaging 1996;21:33–36
30. Urban BA, Fishman EK, Kuhlman JE et al. Detection of focal hepatic lesions with spiral CT: comparison of 4- and 8-mm interval spacing. AJR 1993;160:783–785
31. Sheu JC, Sung JL, Chen DS et al. Early detection of hepatocellular carcinoma by real-time ultrasonography: a prospective study. Cancer 1985;56:660–666
32. Tanaka S, Kitamura T, Nakanishi K et al. Effectiveness of periodic checkup by ultrasonography for the early diagnosis of hepatocellular carcinoma. Cancer 1990;66:2210–2214
33. Sheu JC, Sung JL, Chen DS et al. Ultrasonography of small hepatic tumors using high-resolution linear-array real-time instruments. Radiology 1984;150:797–802
34. Choi BI, Takayasu K, Han MC. Small hepatocellular carcinomas and associated nodular lesions of the liver: pathology, pathogenesis, and imaging findings. AJR 1993;160:1177–1187
35. Kudo M, Hirasa M, Takakuwa H et al. Small hepatocellular carcinomas in chronic liver disease: detection with SPECT. Radiology 1986;159:697–703
36. Matsui O, Kameyama T, Yoshikawa J et al. Angiographic diagnosis of hepatocellular carcinoma including CT arteriography and CT arterial portography [in Japanese]. J Med Imaging 1988;8:1289–1300
37. Hayashi N, Yamamoto K, Tamaki N et al. Metastatic nodules of hepatocellular carcinoma: detection with angiography, CT and US. Radiology 1987;165:61–63
38. Takayasu K, Furukawa, Wakao F et al. CT diagnosis of early hepatocellular carcinoma: sensitivity, findings, and CT-pathologic correlation. AJR 1995;164:885–890
39. Takayasu K, Muramatsu Y, Furukawa H et al. Early hepatocellular carcinoma: appearance at CT during arterial portography and CT arteriography with pathologic correlation. Radiology 1995;194:101–105
40. Nesbit GM, Johnson CD, James EM et al. Cholangiocarcinoma: diagnosis and evaluation of resectability by CT and sonography as procedures complementary to cholangiography. AJR 1988;151:933–938
41. Tani K, Kubota Y, Yamaguchi T et al. MR imaging of peripheral cholangiocarcinoma. J Comput Assist Tomogr 1991;15:975–978
42. Choi BI, Han JK, Shin YM et al. Peripheral cholangiocarcinoma: comparison of MRI with CT. Abdom Imaging 1995;20:357–360
43. Soyer P, Roche A, Gad M et al. Preoperative segmental localization of hepatic metastases: utility of three-dimensional CT during arterial portography. Radiology 1991;180:653–658
44. Small WC, Mehard WB, Langmo LS et al. Preoperative determination of the resectability of hepatic tumors: efficacy of CT during arterial portography. AJR 1993;161:319–322
45. Soyer P, Laissy JP, Sibert A et al. Focal hepatic masses: comparison of detection during arterial portography with MR imaging and CT. Radiology 1994;190:737–740
46. Soyer P, Bluemke DA, Zeitoun G et al. Detection of recurrent hepatic metastases after partial hepatectomy: value of CT combined with arterial portography. AJR 1994;162:1327–1330
47. Thoeni RF. Imaging of the liver. Current opinion in radiology 1992;4:44–53
48. Oudkerk M, Ooijen B, Mali SPM et al. Liver metastases from colorectal carcinoma: detection with continuous CT angiography. Radiology 1992;175:157–161
49. Patten RM, Byun JY, Freeny PC. CT of hypervascular hepatic tumors: are unenhanced scans necessary for diagnosis? AJR 1993;161:979–984
50. Baker ME, Pelley R. Hepatic metastases: basic principles and implications for radiologists. Radiology 1995;197:329–337

51. Heiken JP, Brink JA, Sagel SS. Helical CT: abdominal applications. Radiology 1994;14:919–924
52. Miller DL, Vermess M, Doppman JL et al. CT of the liver and spleen with EOE-13: review of 225 examinations. AJR 1984;143:235–243
53. Itai Y, Nishikawa J, Tasaka A. Computed tomography in the evaluation of hepatocellular carcinoma. Radiology 1979;131: 165–170
54. Moss AA, Schrumpf J, Schnyder P et al. Computed tomography of focal hepatic lesions: a blind clinical evaluation of the effect of contrast enhancement. Radiology 1979;131: 427–430
55. Itai Y, Ohtomo K, Kokubo T et al. CT of hepatic masses: significance of prolonged and delayed enhancement. AJR 1986;146:729–733
56. Araki T, Itai Y, Furui S, Tasaka A. Dynamic CT densitometry of hepatic tumors. AJR 1980;135:1037–1043
57. Ebara M, Ohto M, Watanabe Y et al. Diagnosis of small hepatocellular carcinoma: correlation of MR imaging and histologic studies. Radiology 1986;159:371–377
58. Yoshikawa J, Matsui O, Takashima T et al. Fatty metamorphosis in hepatocellular carcinoma: radiologic features in 10 cases. AJR 1988;151:717–720
59. Freeny PC, Baron RL, Teefey SA. Hepatocellular carcinoma: reduced frequency of typical findings with dynamic contrast enhanced CT in a non-Asian population. Radiology 1992; 182:143–148
60. Choi BI. Vascular invasion by hepatocellular carcinoma. Abdom Imaging 1995;20:277–278
61. Suzuki M, Itoh H, Konishi H et al. Hepatocellular carcinoma involving the portal vein. J Comput Assist Tomogr 1982;6: 831–832
62. Itai Y, Furui S, Ohtomo K et al. Dynamic CT features of arterioportal shunt in hepatocellular carcinoma. AJR 1986; 146:723–727
63. Matsui O, Kadoya M, Kameyama T et al. Benign and malignant nodules in cirrhotic livers: distinction based on blood supply. Radiology 1991;178:493–497
64. Choi BI, Kim HC, Han JK et al. Therapeutic effect of transcatheter oily chemoembolization therapy for encapsulated nodular hepatocellular carcinoma: CT and pathologic findings. Radiology 1992;182:709–713
65. Ohashi I, Hanafusa K, Yoshida T. Small hepatocellular carcinomas: two-phase dynamic incremental CT in detection and evaluation. Radiology 1993;189:851–855
66. Honda H, Matsuura Y, Onitsuka H et al. Differential diagnosis of hepatic tumors (hepatoma, hemangioma, and metastasis) with CT: value of two phase incremental imaging. AJR 1992;159:735–740
67. Baron RL. Understanding and optimizing use of contrast material for CT of the liver. AJR 1994;163:323–331
68. Takayasu K, Ikeya S, Mukai K et al. CT of hilar cholangiocarcinoma: late contrast enhancement in six patients. AJR 1990;154:1203–1206
69. Muramatsu Y, Takayasu K, Moriyama N et al. Peripheral low-density area of hepatic tumors; CT-pathologic correlation. Radiology 1986;160:49–52
70. Muramatsu Y, Nawano S, Takayasu K et al. Early hepatocellular carcinoma: MR imaging. Radiology 1991;181:209–213
71. Takayasu K, Makuuchi M, Hirohashi S et al. Imaging of adenomatous hyperplastic lesions containing and not containing hepatocellular carcinoma in the liver [in Japanese]. Nippon Shokakibyo Gakkai Zasshi 1989;86:2404–2412
72. Choi BI, Park JH, Kim YI et al. Peripheral cholangiocarcinoma and clonorchiasis: CT findings. Radiology 1988;169: 149–153
73. Ros PR, Buck JL, Goodman ID et al. Intrahepatic cholangocarcinoma: radiologic-pathologic correlation. Radiology 1988;167:689–693
74. Itai Y, Araki T, Furui S et al. Computed tomography of primary intrahepatic biliary malignancy. Radiology 1983; 147:485–490
75. Yamashita Y, Takahashi M, Kanazawa S et al. Parenchymal changes of the liver in cholangiocarcinoma: CT evaluation. Gastrointest Radiol 1992;17:161–166
76. Honda H, Onitsuka H, Yasumori K et al. Peripheral cholangiocarcinoma: two-phased dynamic incremental CT and pathologic correlation. J Comput Assist Tomogr 1993;17: 397–402
77. Okuda K, Nakashima T. Primary carcinomas of the liver. In Berk JE (ed): Bockus Gastroenterology. WB Saunders, Philadelphia, 1985;3361–3364
78. Hou PT. The relationship between primary carcinoma of the liver and infestation with *Clonorchis sinensis*. J Pathol Bacteriol 1965;72:239–246
79. Kim YI. Liver carcinoma and liver fluke infection. Arzneimittelforschung 1984;34:1121–1126
80. Hou PC. Pathological changes in the intrahepatic bile ducts of cats (*Felis catus*) infested with *Clonorchis sinensis*. J Pathol Bacteriol 1965;89:357–364
81. Hou PC. Hepatic clonorchiasis and carcinoma of the bile duct in a dog. J Pathol Bacteriol 1965;89:365–367
82. Fan ZM, Yamashita Y, Harada M et al. Intrahepatic cholangiocarcinoma: spin-echo and contrast-enhanced dynamic MR imaging. AJR 1993;161:313–317
83. Yoshikawa J, Matsui O, Kadoya Y et al. Delayed enhancement of fibrotic areas in hepatic masses: CT-pathologic correlation. J Comput Assist Tomogr 1992;16:206–211
84. Yamashita Y, Fan ZM, Yamamoto H et al. Sclerosing hepatocellular carcinoma: radiologic finding. Abdom Imaging 1993;18:347–351
85. Kruskal JB, Kane RA. Correlative imaging of malignant liver tumors. Semin Ultrasound CT MRI 1992;13:336–354
86. Ros PR. Malignant liver tumors. In Gore RM, Levine MS, Laufer I (eds): Textbook of Gastrointestinal Radiology. WB Saunders, Philadelphia, 1994;1897–1946
87. Sager EM, Scheel B, Talle K. Increase detectability of liver metastases by the use of contrast enhancement in computed tomography: a comparison between the precontrast, the immediate postcontrast and the one hour postcontrast scan. Acta Radiol 1985;26:369–372
88. Dean PB, Violante MR, Mahoney JA. Hepatic CT contrast enhancement: effect of dose, duration of infusion, and time elapsed following infusion. Invest Radiol 1980;15:158–161

89. Paushter DM, Zeman RK, Scheibler ML et al. CT evaluation of suspected hepatic metastases: comparison of techniques for IV contrast enhancement. AJR 1989;152:267–271

90. Leslie DF, Johnson CK, Johnson CM. Hepatic cavernous hemangioma; re-evaluation of CT criteria. Radiology 1994; 193:358(abstr)

91. Malt RA: Current concepts: surgery for hepatic neoplasms. N Engl J Med 1985;313:1591–1596

92. Sugarbaker PH, Kemeny N: Management of metastatic cancer to the liver. Adv Surg 1989;22:1–56

93. Ward BA, Miller DL, Frank JA et al. Prospective evaluation of hepatic imaging studies in the detection of colorectal metastases: correlation with surgical findings. Surgery 1989;105: 180–187

94. Matsui O, Takashima T, Kadoya M et al. Liver metastases from colorectal cancers: detection with CT during arterial portography. Radiology 1987;165:65–69

95. Merine D, Takayasu K, Wakao F. Detection of hepatocellular carcinoma: comparison of CT during arterial portography with CT after intraarterial injection of iodized oil. Radiology 1990;175:707–710

96. Matsui O, Takashima T, Kadoya M et al. Dynamic computed tomography during arterial portography: the most sensitive examination for small hepatocellular carcinomas. J Comput Assist Tomogr 1985;9:19–24

SECTION VI
SCREENING FOR EARLY DETECTION AND PROSPECTS FOR PREVENTION

25

EARLY DETECTION OF HEPATOCELLULAR CARCINOMA

SHUICHI KANEKO
MASASHI UNOURA
KENICHI KOBAYASHI

Diagnostic strategies for hepatocellular carcinoma (HCC) have made possible the detection of small HCCs prior to the appearance of clinical symptoms. To facilitate the detection of small asymptomatic HCCs, screening strategies for patients with chronic liver diseases have been proposed,[1–8] since HCC is closely associated with chronic liver disease. Close follow-up of patients with cirrhosis by using ultrasonography and serial determinations of α-fetoprotein (AFP) concentrations have led to the identification of HCC at an early stage in patients in Asia. However, in Western countries, screening strategies in patients with cirrhosis have been ineffective in identifying potentially resectable tumors.[5,7,8]

Recent advances in diagnostic modalities also have facilitated the detection of small HCCs. With high-resolution real-time ultrasound, the entire liver of patients with chronic liver disease can be quickly scrutinized, and a hepatic tumor as small as 0.5 cm in diameter can be seen. Computed tomography (CT), magnetic resonance imaging (MRI), and angiography have been used for the diagnosis of hepatic tumors detected by ultrasound, as well as for screening. Ultrasound-guided biopsy to permit histologic examination is sometimes necessary to reach a diagnosis.

THE POPULATION AT HIGH RISK FOR HCC

The survival of patients with clinically apparent HCC is generally limited to a few months. The majority of patients with symptoms of HCC have tumors that are not amenable to curative treatment because of extensive involvement of the liver, invasion of the hepatic or portal vein, the presence of metastases, or, as is frequently the case, advanced underlying disease. Thus, there is growing interest in the use of screening methods for the detection of HCC in patients at a relatively early, asymptomatic stage, when the disease may respond more favorably to treatment. To screen for asymptomatic HCC, high-risk populations must be identified.

HCC and Cirrhosis

An association between cirrhosis and HCC has been recorded in many geographic locations. The majority of patients with HCC have associated cirrhosis caused by hepatitis B virus (HBV) infection, hepatitis C virus (HCV) infection, alcohol abuse, autoimmune hepatitis, primary biliary cirrhosis, genetic diseases, or unknown etiologies.

TABLE 25-1. Prevalence of Hepatocellular Carcinoma (HCC) Among Autopsy Cases With Cirrhosis During Different Time Intervals

Years	No. With Cirrhosis	No. With HCC (%)	Mean Age (Years)
1975–1982	103	61 (59.2)	60.1 ± 12.2
1983–1990	105	69 (65.7)	62.8 ± 9.6
1991–1994	48	38 (79.2)	64.7 ± 9.6

In Japan, between 1982 and 1985, 1,515 of 1,845 (82.1%) autopsy cases and 1,458 of 1,976 (73.8%) operative cases of HCC involved concomitant cirrhosis.[9] One thousand, six hundred seventeen (91.9%) of the autopsy cases and 1,777 (89.9%) of the operative cases involved cirrhosis, fibrosis, or other hepatic changes. Thus, most cases of HCC in Japan are complicated by liver injury, especially cirrhosis. Similarly, a high prevalence of cirrhosis was found in HCC patients elsewhere: Los Angeles, 79% (214 of 292)[10]; other areas of the United States, 74% (50 of 68)[10]; Spain, 93% (231 of 249)[11]; the United Kingdom, 75% (305 of 405)[12]; and Italy, 88% (180 of 205).[13] Cirrhosis was present in 60% of South African patients with HCC.[14] Furthermore, the prevalence of cirrhosis in HCC in Los Angeles County decreased from 79% to 46% if the study population was based on the county cancer surveillance program.[10]

In our recent study of 287 patients with HCC who were admitted to our hospital from 1977 to 1994, 270 (94.1%) had cirrhosis, and the remaining 17 had chronic hepatitis. The increasing incidence of HCC in patients with cirrhosis in recent years also has been demonstrated (Table 25-1). In 256 autopsy cases associated with cirrhosis, 61 of the 103 (59.2%) cirrhotic patients who died from 1975 to 1982 had HCC, as did 69 of 105 (65.7%) during 1983 to 1990 and 38 of 48 (79.2%) during 1991 to 1994. Thus, the majority of cirrhotic patients in Japan have associated HCC at the time of death. The mean age of the patients in successive periods increased, suggesting the lengthening survival time for patients with cirrhosis. If patients with cirrhosis do not die of other causes such as gastrointestinal bleeding or hepatic failure, HCC may occur in most cases.

HCC and the Etiology of Underlying Chronic Liver Diseases

In addition to cirrhosis, chronic HBV and HCV infections, alcohol, aflatoxin, drugs, smoking, and several metabolic disorders have been reported to play a role in the pathogenesis of HCC. The importance of various etiologic factors varies by geographic area and appear to depend on whether the area has a high or low incidence of HCC.

We tested for the presence of the hepatitis surface antigen (HBsAg) and antibodies against HCV (anti-HCV) in 169 patients with HCC who were admitted to our department from 1986 to 1993. Either anti-HCV (second-generation assay) or HBsAg was detected in 95% of these patients. The prevalence of anti-HCV was 74%, and that of HBsAg was 24%. Both HBsAg and anti-HCV were detected in 3% of these patients. Only 5% of the patients had neither HBsAg nor anti-HCV. Moreover, all 169 patients had either cirrhosis or histologic evidence of chronic hepatitis. Thus, chronic liver injury, mainly cirrhosis, caused by HBV and/or HCV infection, is the most important risk factor for the devel-

TABLE 25-2. Characteristics of Patients With Chronic Hepatitis or Cirrhosis Who Were Followed To Detect Hepatocellular Carcinoma

HBsAg	Anti-HCV	No.	Age (Years)	Female:Male Ratio	No. Consuming Alcohol (%)[a]	Histology (%) CPH	CAH2A	CAH2B
Study A[b]								
+	−	100	39.1 ± 12.2	21:79	22 (22)	32 (32)	30 (30)	38 (38)
−	+	124	51.2 ± 10.0	42:82	32 (26)	55 (44)	38 (31)	31 (25)
Total		224	45.8 ± 12.6	63:161	54 (24)	87 (39)	68 (30)	69 (31)
Study B[c]								
+	−	94	50.0 ± 12.0	20:74	21 (22)			
−	+	192	58.0 ± 8.8	89:103	34 (18)			
Total		286	55.4 ± 10.2	109:177	55 (19)			

Abbreviations: CPH, chronic persistent hepatitis; CAH2A, chronic active hepatitis 2A; CAH2B, chronic active hepatitis 2B, according to European classification.[23a]

[a] Alcohol intake >80 g/day for more than 5 years.

[b] Study A consisted of 224 patients with histologically proven chronic viral hepatitis.

[c] Study B consisted of 286 patients with cirrhosis caused by HBV or HCV.

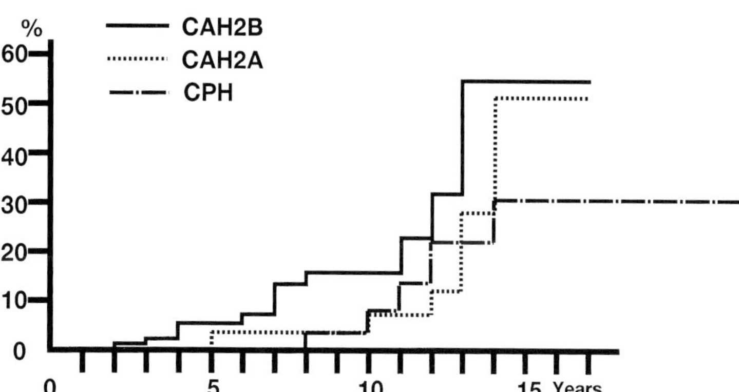

FIGURE 25-1. Cumulative risk of HCC in patients with histologically proven chronic hepatitis (see also Table 25-2, study A) at enrollment, according to the Kaplan-Meier method. There was a significant difference between the chronic active hepatitis 2B (CAH2B) and chronic persistent hepatitis (CPH) groups ($p < 0.01$, generalized Wilcoxon).

opment of HCC in Japan. There were only 8 cirrhotic patients without HBsAg or anti-HCV, and 5 of these had a history of alcohol abuse.

The incidence of HCC without detectable HBsAg or anti-HCV has been calculated to be 1.5 per 100,000 per year in the United States, 1.4 to 2.3 in Italy, 2.5 to 4.8 in France, and 2.6 to 5.0 in Japan.[15–23]

Two hundred twenty-four patients at our hospital with histologically proven chronic viral hepatitis were prospectively studied for the development of HCC (Table 25-2, study A). One hundred of these patients were infected with HBV and 124 with HCV. During a follow-up period of 10.1 ± 3.5 years, 38 patients (17%) developed HCC (after developing cirrhosis) except in 2 cases. Seventeen of 69 (24.6%) patients with chronic active hepatitis 2B[23a] were complicated by HCC within 8.7 ± 3.9 years. This represented a significantly higher rate and within a shorter period than was observed in patients with chronic persistent hepatitis (12.6% within 11.1 ± 1.9 years, respectively). For the first 8 years, there was no HCC found in any patients with chronic persistent hepatitis (Fig. 25-1). Thus, the development of HCC was clearly related to the severity of the chronic hepatitis.

There was no significant difference in the cumulative incidences of HCC between patients with chronic hepatitis B and C using the generalized Wilcoxon test (Fig. 25-2). Takano et al.[24] reported an incidence of new cases of HCC in chronic hepatitis C that was 2.7 times greater than that of chronic hepatitis B with a similar mean follow-up interval (72.6 and 72.9 months, respectively). Although both their study and ours were performed in Japan, the mean patient ages and follow-up periods differed. Indeed, in our study, age was identified as the strongest independent prognostic indicator for the development of HCC by the Cox multivariate proportional hazard model, and after 10 years of follow-up the cumulative incidence clearly increased in our study.

The annual incidence of HCC deaths in chronic hepatitis was 1,679.6 per 100,000 per year in our study, approximately 90 times higher than that in the general Japanese population (Table 25-3). Most patients developed HCC after first developing cirrhosis, although 2 HCCs developed in patients who did not have cirrhosis. The utility of screening for HCC in chronic hepatitis patients without cirrhosis has not been established. However, the careful follow-up of patients with chronic hepatitis to determine whether they develop cirrhosis and subsequent HCC is clearly beneficial.

Two hundred eighty-six patients with cirrhosis

FIGURE 25-2. Cumulative risk of HCC in patients with chronic hepatitis (see also Table 25-2, study A) according to hepatitis virus infection status by the Kaplan-Meier method. There was no difference between the groups (generalized Wilcoxon method).

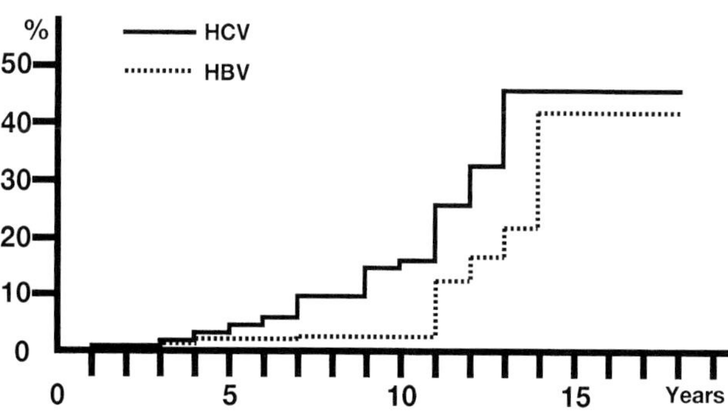

TABLE 25-3. Deaths Due to Hepatocellular Carcinoma

Subjects	HCC Deaths/ 100,000/year	Years of Follow-Up	Relative Risk
Japanese population	19.2[a]		1
Chronic hepatitis	1,679.6	10.1	87.5
Chronic hepatitis B	1,000.0	10.0	52.1
Chronic hepatitis C	2,235.7	10.1	116.4
Cirrhosis	6,019.2	5.2	313.5
Cirrhosis due to hepatitis B	3,596.0	7.1	187.3
Cirrhosis due to hepatitis C	7,708.3	5.0	401.5

[a] Data from Breborowicz et al.[32]

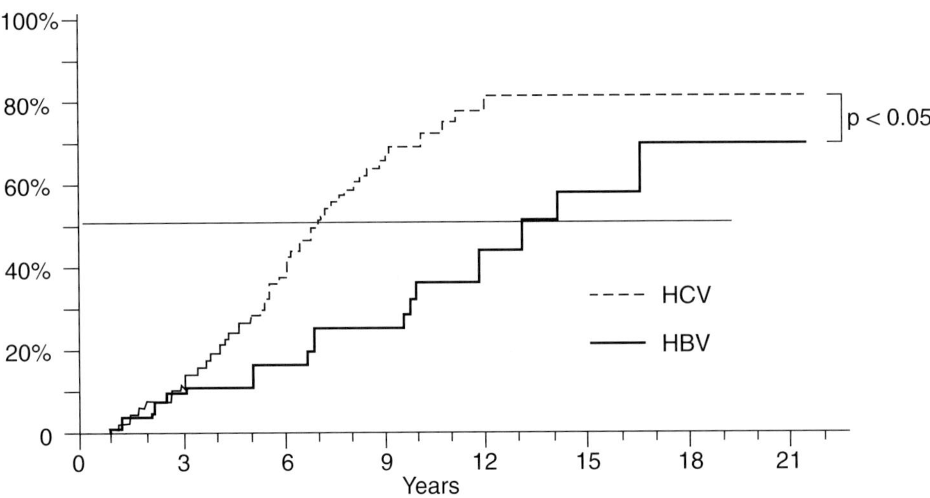

FIGURE 25-3. Cumulative risk of HCC in patients with cirrhosis (see also Table 25-2, study B), according to hepatitis virus infection status by the Kaplan-Meier method. Cirrhotic patients with anti-HCV developed hepatocellular carcinoma at a significantly higher rate than those with HBsAg ($p < 0.05$, generalized Wilcoxon method).

caused by HBV (n = 94) or HCV (n = 192) infections were prospectively followed for 7.1 ± 5.3 and 5.0 ± 2.7 years, respectively (Table 25-2, study B). Twenty-four of the 94 with HBV (25.5%) and 74 of the 192 with HCV (38.5%) developed HCC. The annual incidence of HCC in cirrhotic patients infected with HBV and HCV was 3.6% and 7.7% respectively, approximately 190 and 400 times higher, respectively, than the incidence in the general population in Japan (Table 25-3). The cumulative incidence of HCC in cirrhotic patients with HCV was significantly higher than in those with HBV infection (the generalized Wilcoxon, $p < 0.05$) (Fig. 25-3). Compared with patients with HBV infection, the cumulative incidence of HCC in the patients with HCV infection continued to increase linearly after entry into this study. In the prospective autopsy study (Table 25-1), the course of most of the cirrhotic patients was ultimately complicated by HCC.

Primary biliary cirrhosis (PBC) also is known to be a risk factor for HCC.[25] Seventy-five patients in our department with PBC were retrospectively analyzed (Table 25-4). Anti-HCV was detected in 9 of the 75 patients. During an 11-year period, 4 of the 75 patients with PBC developed HCC, and two of the four patients had anti-HCV. Thus, HCC developed in 2 of 9 (22%) PBC patients with anti-HCV compared with 2 of the 66 (3%) without anti-HCV ($p < 0.05$).[26] Similarly, Floreani et al.[26a] reported that 3 of 4 HCC cases originated in patients with PBC and anti-HCV. Therefore, HCC is a major complication of PBC, especially in those with HCV infection.

TUMOR MARKERS AND EARLY DETECTION

AFP

α-Fretoprotein (AFP) is a glycoprotein produced in the fetal yolk sac and intestine. It is present in the serum in high concentrations during fetal life and the immediate

TABLE 25-4. HCC in Patients With PBC (1981–1991)

HCV[a]	No.	Age (Years)	Female:Male Ratio	Asymptomatic	Symptomatic	Stage[b] I or II	Stage[b] III or IV	HCC
+	9	59.6 ± 11.3	7:2	2	7	5	3	2
–	66	57.1 ± 12.4	55:11	58	8	50	10	2

[a] Seventy-five patients with PBC were retrospectively tested for anti-HCV.

[b] Sheuer's histologic stage. Histologic examination was not performed in 7 patients.

	AFP(ng/ml)		
	>20	>200	AFP 10 20 100 200 1000 10000 ng/ml
Cirrhosis (n=70)	26 (37%)	4 (6%)	
HCC (n=41) (solitary ≤ 2cm)	22 (54%)	8 (20%)	
HCC (n=180) (>2cm or multiple)	128 (71%)	79 (44%)	

FIGURE 25-4. Serum α-fetoprotein (AFP) concentrations in 221 patients with HCC and 70 cirrhotic patients without HCC.

postnatal period. Serum AFP levels are elevated in the majority of patients with HCC, hepatoblastoma, and certain germ cell tumors. Histochemical studies have shown the presence of AFP in HCC cells, and serum AFP levels rapidly normalize after resection of HCC.

Serum AFP levels were assayed in 221 patients in our department with HCC and 70 cirrhotic patients without HCC (Fig. 25-4). One hundred fifty of these 221 patients (68%) had elevated AFP levels of more than 20 ng/ml (the upper level in normal adults), and 87 (39%) had levels greater than 200 ng/ml. Normal AFP levels were encountered in 29% of the patients with large HCCs (more than 2 cm in diameter) and in 46% of patients with small HCCs (2 cm or less). Thus, AFP levels generally correlated with tumor size. It has been reported that many patients with asymptomatic small HCCs have normal serum AFP levels[27]; these may reflect either a smaller number of AFP-producing cells or a tendency for expression later than in larger lesions. Indeed, there is a general correlation between AFP levels and the degree of histologic differentiation and HCC size.[27,28] In some populations, 10% to 20% of HCCs do not produce AFP.[29]

Transient increases in AFP may occur in acute and chronic liver disease, especially during exacerbations of hepatitis.[30] One or more episodes of increased AFP concentrations was reported in approximately 15% of patients with chronic hepatitis B infections in Hong Kong.[31] In our series, 26 (37%) of 70 cirrhotic patients had elevated levels of serum AFP, 4 (6%) at levels greater than 200 ng/ml (Fig. 25-4). Furthermore, patients with nonmalignant liver conditions occasionally have serum levels of AFP in a gray area ranging from 20 to 400 ng/ml, where the results can be difficult to evaluate.

Nonetheless, even minor elevations in the serum AFP level must alert the clinician to the possible presence of a tumor, and an AFP level above 200 ng/ml or that increases from a low level over a few months requires careful evaluation. When exponential growth of an HCC occurs, the increase in the serum AFP level correlates with the increase in size.

The doubling time of HCC was calculated using the serum AFP levels of 61 patients with HCC (Fig. 25-5). All patients demonstrated an increase in AFP during follow-up; the doubling time in 26 cases was less than 60 days, and it was longer than 120 days in 17 cases.

Lectin-Reactive AFP

To solve the problem of AFP elevations in patients without HCC, several groups have attempted to improve the specificity of the test using the different carbohydrate structures found in AFP of different origins.[32–37] The serum AFP of patients with HCC is characterized by greater proportions of AFP that react with *Lens culinaris* agglutin A (LCA) and erythroagglutinating phytohemagglutinin (PHA-E), lectin-reactive AFP, than the serum AFP of patients with benign chronic liver diseases.

Serum AFP samples (above 50 ng/ml) obtained from 86 patients in our department (50 patients with HCC and 36 cirrhotic patients without HCC) were tested for LCA and PHA-E reactivity (Fig. 25-6). Twenty-seven

FIGURE 25-5. Doubling time of serum α-fetoprotein (AFP) concentrations in 61 patients with HCC. AFP concentrations were measured at least at two points during the natural course of the development of HCC in each patient, and the doubling time in days was calculated.

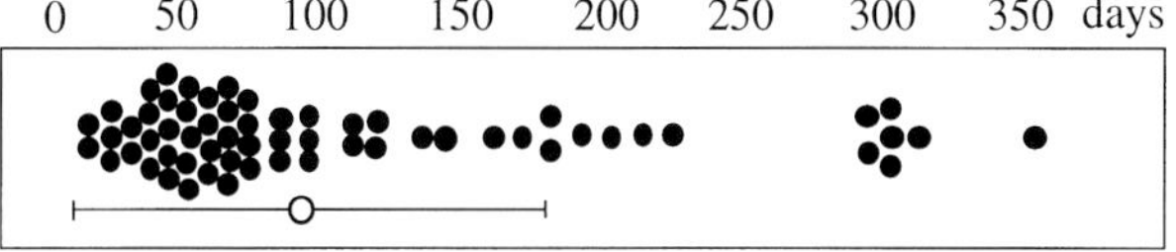

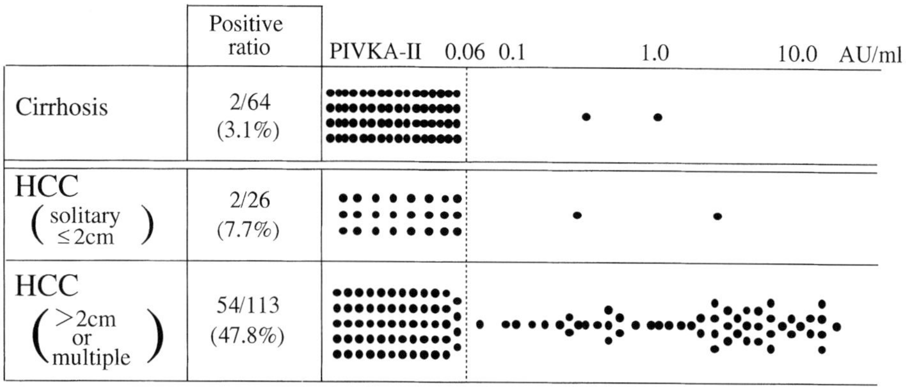

Positive ratio
PIVKA-II 0.06 0.1 1.0 10.0 AU/ml
Cirrhosis
2/64 (3.1%)
HCC (solitary ≤2cm)
2/26 (7.7%)
HCC (>2cm or multiple)
54/113 (47.8%)

FIGURE 25-6. Serum PIVKA-II concentrations in patients with HCC and cirrhotic patients without HCC.

of the 50 patients (54%) with HCC demonstrated reactivity on one or both of the assays, whereas the assays of only 2 (5.6%) of the 36 cirrhotic patients were positive. Thus, these assays allow the differentiation of HCC from cirrhosis in many cases. Seven of 15 (46%) patients with small HCCs (2 cm or less in diameter) were also positive. Furthermore, Sato et al.[38] have reported that an elevation of lectin-reactive AFP was detected in 24 cirrhotic patients with AFP concentrations of 30 ng/ml or more 3 to 18 months prior to detection of the tumor by imaging techniques. Similarly, Taketa et al.[39] also have shown that the assay was positive up to 9 months prior to the detection of HCC by imaging techniques, with a sensitivity of 48% and a specificity of 81%. These data suggest that the lectin-reactive AFP assay may be useful for the early detection of HCC in patients with elevated serum AFP levels.

Des-γ-Carboxy Prothrombin

Prothrombin is the major vitamin K-dependent blood coagulation protein synthesized in the liver. In the absence of vitamin K or in the presence of a vitamin K antagonist such as warfarin, vitamin K-dependent γ-carboxylation in the liver is inhibited and des-γ-carboxy prothrombin is released into the blood. This abnormal prothrombin is referred to by the abbreviation PIVKA-II for "prothrombin induced by vitamin K absence or antagonist-II." Increased PIVKA-II levels have been reported in 67% of patients with HCC.[40]

Serum samples from 139 patients with HCC and 64 cirrhotic patients without HCC were tested for PIVKA-II using enzyme immunoassay (Fig. 25-7). Fifty-six of 139 (40.3%) patients had detectable PIVKA-II. Consistent with reports that the PIVKA-II level correlates with

%
50
40
30
20
10
PHA-E P4 fraction
Cirrhosis
HCC (≤ 2 cm)
HCC (> 2 cm)
0
10
20
30
40
50
60
70 %
LCA L3 fraction

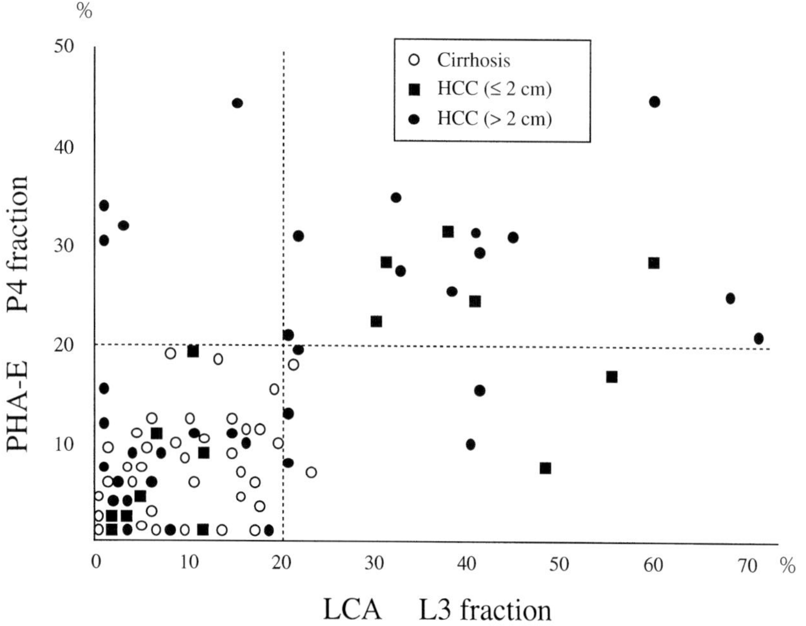

FIGURE 25-7. Serum concentrations of the α-fetoprotein L3 and α-fetoprotein P4 fraction in patients with HCC and cirrhotic patients without HCC.

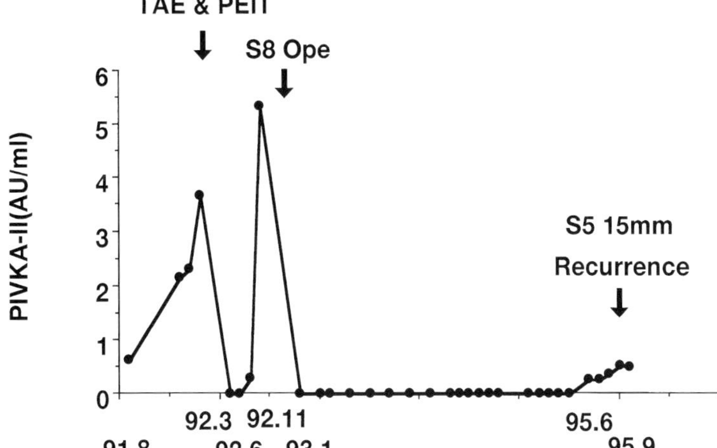

FIGURE 25-8. Utility of serial PIVKA-II measurements in following a patient with treated HCC. After two rounds of treatment for HCC, ultrasound screening and PIVKA-II assay were periodically performed. Because of difficulties in ultrasound screening of the treated liver, a recurrence was not found until an elevation in PIVKA-II occurred.

tumor size, the detection rate in patients with HCCs smaller than 2 cm in diameter was only 7.7% (2/26). Abnormal elevations in PIVKA-II levels have been reported in patients with chronic hepatitis, cirrhosis, obstructive jaundice, and intrahepatic cholestasis.[41] Although the specificity of PIVKA-II for HCC is similar or higher than that of AFP, it is not as sensitive as AFP. Hattori et al.[41] also found that PIVKA-II was a valuable marker for the diagnosis of HCC, especially in patients with a negative or low serum AFP concentration. Therefore, a combination of testing for AFP and PIVKA-II may be useful in the early detection of HCC. A follow-up study comparing ultrasound, AFP, and PIVKA-II assays in one patient showed that PIVKA-II was the first indicator of recurrence of a previously treated HCC (Fig. 25-8). The mechanism of the increase in PIVKA-II seems to differ from that of the increase in AFP, and a possible relation to tumor invasion has been postulated.[42]

Another tumor marker, "novel γ-GTP," caused by sugar chain changes in the HCC, has been demonstrated in approximately 60% of HCC patients.[43] Novel γ-GTP has been found in only 3% of patients with benign liver diseases.

HEPATIC IMAGING AND EARLY DETECTION

Hepatic imaging is used both in the detection of HCC and in its differentiation from other space-occupying lesions. Use of imaging for the screening of asymptomatic patients at high risk for HCC in cirrhotic patients who present to our department for the first time include CT and MRI to evaluate their cirrhosis and to rule out the presence of HCC. These examinations are performed even if ultrasound and tumor marker levels suggest that no HCC is present. Thereafter, they are repeated yearly. In 76 recently diagnosed HCCs, 18 were first detected by CT, 43 by ultrasound, 4 by MRI, and 2 by angiography (Table 25-5).

Detectability by any of the diagnostic modalities was compared in these 76 patients with HCC diagnosed (Table 25-6). Imaging modalities were clearly superior in the detection of large HCCs (larger than 2 cm), and all 31 large HCCs were visualized by ultrasonography, CT, CT during arterial portography (CTAP), MRI, and angiography. In contrast, the small HCCs (2 cm or less) were detectable by all modalities. As the detectability of large HCCs with ultrasound approached 100%, more extensive ultrasound examination may allow the earlier detection of HCC.

Despite the recent advances in imaging technologies, it is still difficult to detect and differentiate HCCs of less than 2 cm. There seems to be a correlation between tumor size and histologic findings, which may explain the low detectability of small HCCs by various imaging modalities and the differences between them. HCC images may differ in different geographic areas[44]; most published studies have been conducted on patients in Asian countries.

Ultrasonography

Real-time ultrasonography permits the easy screening of the entire liver in a noninvasive manner and successfully visualizes hepatic tumors as small as 0.5 cm in diameter. Therefore, ultrasound has been used for screening for asymptomatic HCC along with serum AFP assay in many studies. The results of these screening studies have been encouraging, especially those in Asia where the incidence of HCC is high in patients with cirrhosis and where many HCCs are encapsulated.[1–4,6] The detection rate of potentially curable tumors (less than 3 cm in diameter) was 4 of 8 HCCs in our prospective study,[1] 5 of 7 in the study by Sheu et al.,[2] 28 of 40 in the study by

TABLE 25-5. Modality by Which Hepatocellular Carcinomas Were First Detected

Tumor Size (Diameter)	No.	AFP (%)	PIVKA-II (%)	Ultrasound (%)	CT (%)	MRI (%)	Angiography (%)
≤2cm	45	3 (7)	1 (2)	28 (62)	8 (18)	3 (7)	2 (4)
>2 cm	31	5 (16)	0 (0)	15 (48)	10 (32)	1 (3)	0 (0)

Oka et al.,[3] and 15 of 18 in the study by Okazaki et al.[4] Cottone et al.[8] detected 16 of 30 by ultrasound in Italy, a rate similar to that of Asian studies. However, Colombo et al.[5] detected only 9 unifocal tumors less than 3 cm in diameter among 26 HCCs using ultrasound, and Pateron et al.[7] detected only 3 of 14 HCCs using ultrasound. These differences may be due to different etiologies of liver diseases, pathologic types of HCCs, and/or natural histories of HCC in each area. Furthermore, ultrasound was performed every 3 to 6 months in all Asian studies, but every 6 months to 1 year in the Italian studies. The greater frequency of ultrasound studies at every 3 months might lead to tumor detection at an earlier stage. All screening studies in high-risk populations demonstrated that ultrasound is more sensitive than AFP in the early detection of HCC.

In Japan, many small asymptomatic HCCs (2 cm or less in diameter) have been successfully detected by ultrasound. Many of these lesions are round with homogenous internal echoes (hypo or hyper) and lack the sonographic features of large HCCs such as a hypoechoic halo around the mass, a complex internal structure referred to as a "mosaic pattern," posterior echo enhancement or a posterior shadow, and a lateral shadow. Isoechoic tumors are not easy to detect. Therefore, careful examination by a well-trained person using a machine with a capacity for high resolution is necessary for the early detection of small HCCs.

CT

Although ultrasound has been widely used for the detection of HCC, ultrasound examination of an entire liver is occasionally difficult because of intervening bones, air in the intestine or lung, and the presence of fatty tissue. These do not affect CT of the liver, and an advantage of CT over ultrasound is its objectivity in visualizing the liver.

A yearly CT screening program combined with angiography was reported by Kobayashi et al.[1] in 95 patients with cirrhosis. Okazaki et al.[4] performed yearly CT in patients with atrophied right hepatic lobe and identified 3 cases of HCC with such screening. However, it remains unclear whether CT screening increases the detection rate of HCCs in high-risk patients or improves patient survival.

CT has allowed successful detection of large HCCs (more than 2 cm in diameter) and the differentiation of HCCs from other space-occupying lesions. Advanced HCC has a blood supply mainly from the hepatic artery and a reduced blood supply from the portal vein compared with the surrounding nontumorous liver. Use of spiral CT permits the detectability of small hypervascular tumors (2 cm or smaller) with greater accuracy than conventional CT.[45] However, small HCCs without associated vascularity are still difficult to detect even with contrast medium infused into the artery. Takayasu et al.[46] compared the sensitivity of CT during arterial portography (CTAP) and CT during infusion into the hepatic artery (CTA) in the detection of histologically "early" and "advanced HCCs" of less than 3 cm. "Early" HCCs consisted of well-differentiated cells corresponding to Edmondson grade I, and advanced HCC consisted of moderately or poorly differentiated cells corresponding to Edmondson grade II or III. CTAP detected only 23 of 35 (66%) "early" HCCs as hypoattenuating and CTA only 3 of 20 (15%) "early" HCCs as hypervascular. In contrast, 85 of 88 (97%) "advanced" HCCs were depicted as hypoattenuating by CTAP, and 13 of 14 (93%) "advanced" HCCs appeared hypervascular by CTA.

Thus, even with the usage of CTAP or CTA, small HCCs without dominant hepatic artery vascularity and/or a reduced portal venous supply sometimes are undetected. In addition, differentiation of such small HCCs from nonmalignant nodules such as adenomatous hyperplasia may be difficult.[47]

TABLE 25-6. Diagnostic Accuracy of Various Modalities for Detecting HCC

Size of Tumor (Diameter)	No.	AFP (%)	PIVKA-II (%)	Ultrasound (%)	CT (%)	MRI (%)	CTAP (%)	Angiography (%)
≤2cm	45	34 (76)	7 (16)	36 (80)	31 (69)	27 (60)	40 (89)	25 (56)
>2cm	31	18 (58)	13 (42)	31 (100)	31 (100)	31 (100)	31 (100)	31 (100)

MRI

The signal intensities obtained by MRI reflect multiple factors such as the proton density, longitudinal relaxation time, and transverse relaxation time, whereas CT relies on only one factor. Thus, by changing acquisition techniques, MRI permits the detection and differentiation of most large (greater than 2 cm) HCCs.[48] As with CT, the detectability by MRI is lower when the tumor size is less than 2 cm in diameter. In addition to size, the correlation between MRI and histologic findings of HCC has been studied. Kadoya et al.[49] reported that 0 of 6 Edmondson grade I HCCs were hyperintense on T_1-weighted spin echo images; 4 of the 6 were isointense, and the remaining 2 were hyperintense on T_2-weighted spin echo images. However, 61 of 61 more advanced HCCs (Edmondson grade I + II, II, II + III, III), demonstrated varying signal intensities on T_1-weighted spin echo images and were hyperintense on T_2-weighted spin echo images. Similar MRI findings for "early HCCs" were found by Muramatsu et al.[50] Thus, most advanced HCCs can be detected and differentiated based on findings on T_2-weighted images, but many small HCCs consisting of Edmondson grade I cells do not appear hyperintense on T_2-weighted images. The differentiation of these lesions from nonmalignant nodules is sometimes difficult.[51]

Angiography

Angiography is invasive, expensive, and, when used alone, is not sensitive enough to detect small HCCs. Therefore, it is unsuitable alone for the early detection of

FIGURE 25-9. Utility of ultrasound-guided tumor biopsy. (*A*) Ultrasound showing a small slightly hyperechoic space-occupying lesion (SOL). (*B*) The space-occupying lesion appears isointense on CT during the infusion of contrast medium. (*C*) The space-occupying lesion appears isointense on MRI, including a dynamic study. (*Figure continues.*)

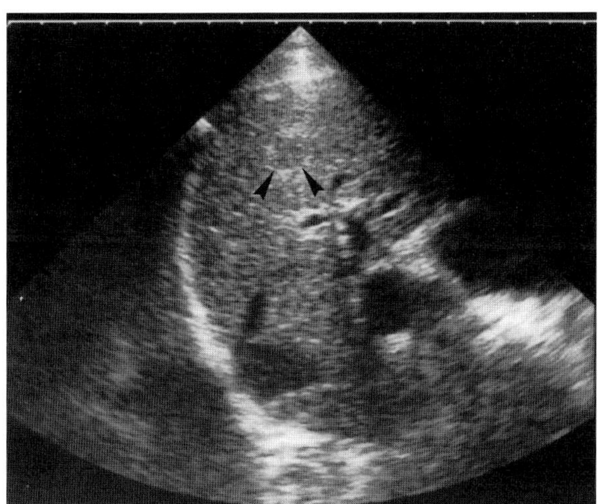
A

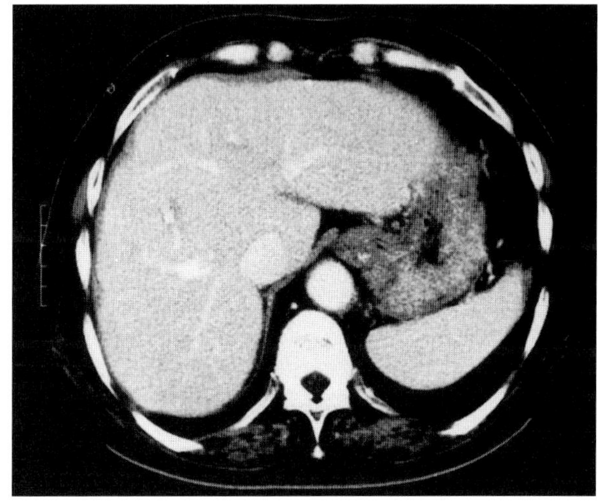
B

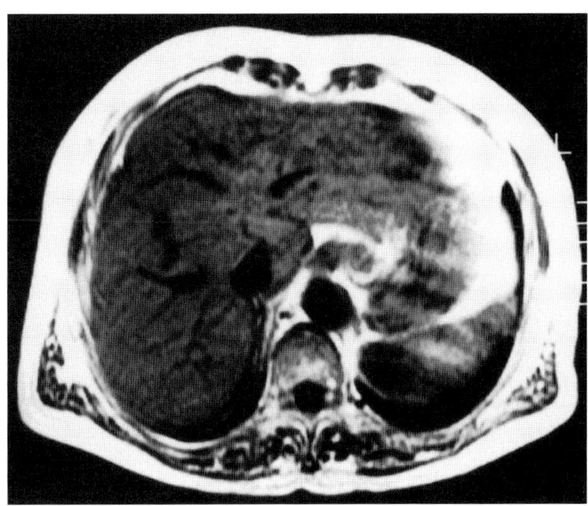
C

D

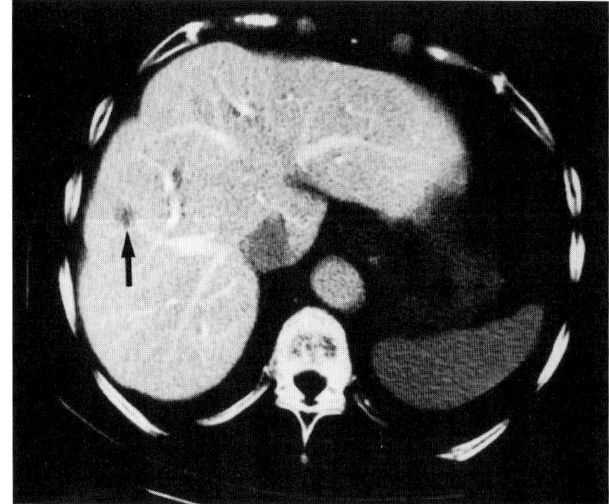

E

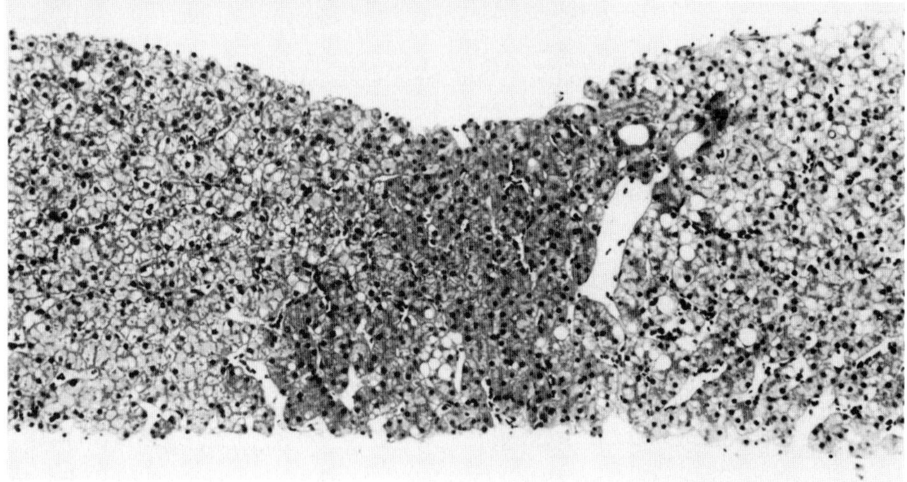

FIGURE 25-9 *(Continued).* (*D*) CT during arterial portography (CTAP) depicts the space-occupying lesion as a partially hypoattenuated tumor. (*E*) A specimen obtained via ultrasound-guided tumor biopsy demonstrating characteristics of a well-differentiated HCC. (H&E, ×124.) This patient was a cirrhotic patient who had undergone periodic screening by ultrasound. Conventional CT, dynamic CT, CTAP, MRI, and angiography were performed after a high-echoic space-occupying lesion was detected by ultrasound. The lesion was isointense on dynamic CT and MRI and partially hypoattenuated on CTAP. These findings indicated similar arterial flow but decreased portal blood flow compared with the surrounding liver. Since this finding is seen in atypical adenomatous hyperplasia, adenomatous hyperplasia with malignant foci, or HCCs consisting of Edmondson grade I cells, tumor biopsy was performed. Histologic examination of the biopsy sample clearly showed HCC, and the tumor was surgically resected. The resected sample showed characteristics of HCC surrounded by adenomatous hyperplasia.

HCC. However, angiography combined with ultrasound, CT, or MRI can be used for the detection and differentiation of HCCs. Recent advances in catheterization have permitted superselective angiography, which permits the use of lower doses of contrast medium with higher resolution. Digital subtraction angiography offers similar advantages.

TUMOR BIOPSY

When a tumor of the liver cannot be diagnosed by imaging modalities and is visible by ultrasound, ultrasound-guided tumor biopsy is performed. A tumor as small as 0.5 cm in diameter can be targeted using this technique.

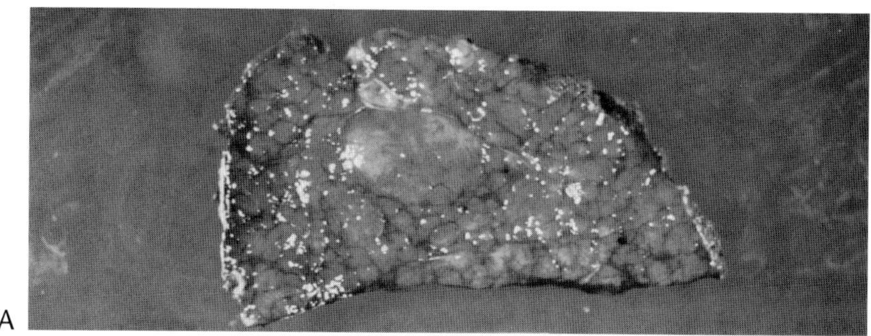

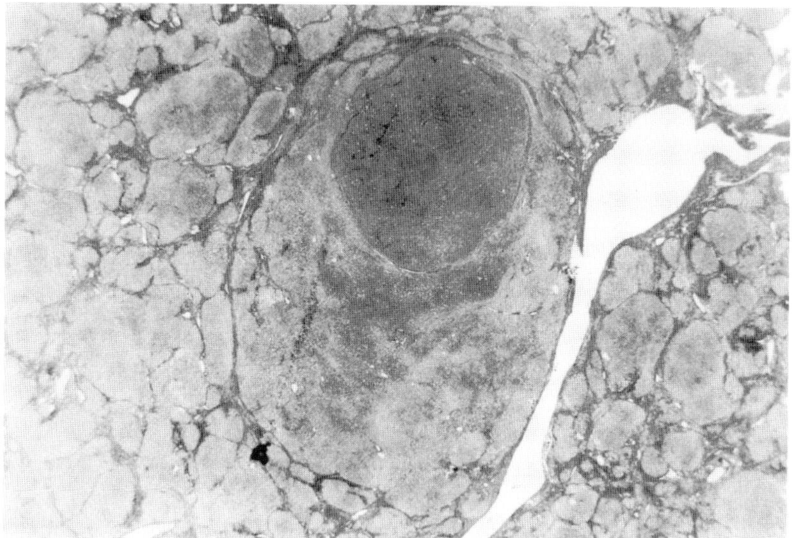

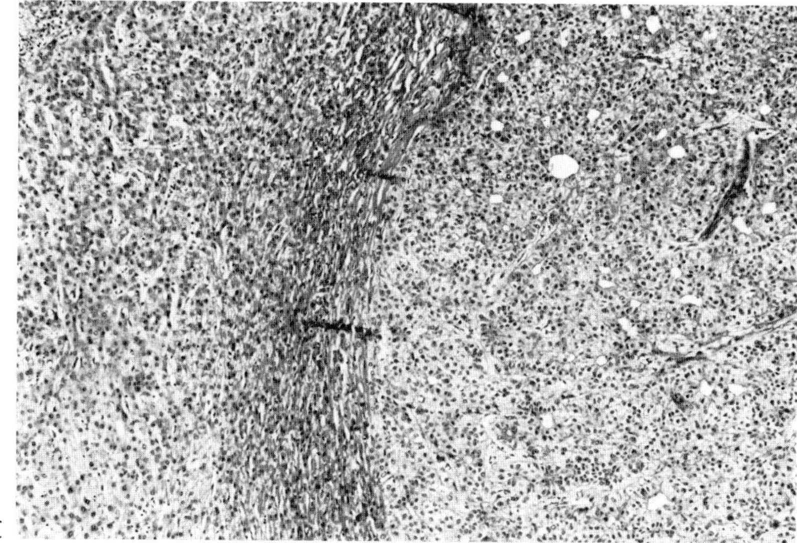

FIGURE 25-10. Example of a nodule originally evaluated by ultrasound-guided biopsy. (*A*) Macroscopic appearance of resected liver. The tumor originated in cirrhotic liver. (*B*) Tumor containing a round nodule. (*C*) The nodule consists of well-differentiated cancer cells. The appearance of the surrounding tissue is consistent with atypical adenomatous hyperplasia. Thus, ultrasound-guided biopsy of the nodule was performed.

A representative case is shown in Figures 25-9 and 25-10.

SCREENING METHODS FOR EARLY DETECTION OF HCC

Recent emphasis has been placed on diagnosing HCC in high-risk patients by screening to detect asymptomatic HCC at a potentially curable stage. Many such asymptomatic HCCs are being detected. In Japan, asymptomatic small HCCs have been successfully detected using several programs.[1,3,4,6,24] However, prospective studies performed in Italy and France failed to demonstrate much benefit of screening programs.[5,7] There are several difficulties in elucidating the utility of screening: (1) The prevalence, incidence, and natural history of HCC differ worldwide, and a different definition of a high-risk popu-

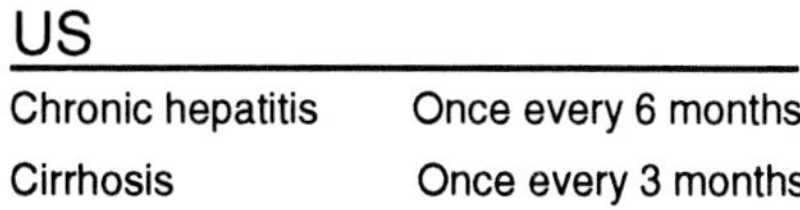

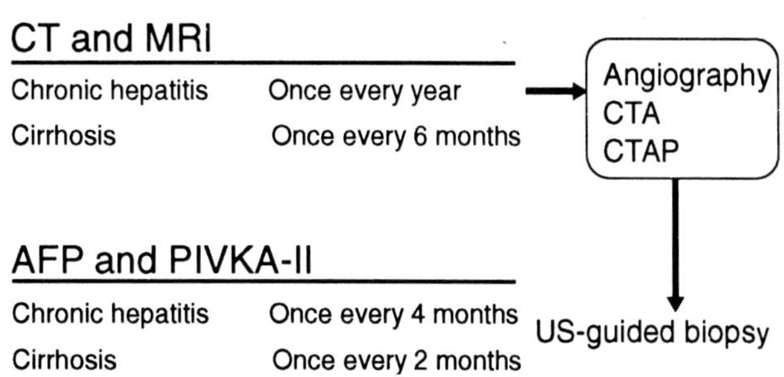

FIGURE 25-11. Screening strategy for patients at high-risk for HCC. US, ultrasonography.

lation may be necessary in each area. (2) The diagnostic tools used for screening have differing sensitivities and are performed at different intervals. (3) It is difficult to assess the benefit of screening in terms of survival. The optimal follow-up interval for effective screening remains unclear. Sheu et al.[52] reported that the doubling time of 31 HCCs (less than 5 cm) ranged from 29 to 398 days, with a median of 117 days. They suggested a suitable screening interval of 4 to 5 months. Similarly, Ebara et al.[53] recommended an interval of approximately 3 months for ultrasound examination for the detection of small HCCs. As described earlier, the doubling time of AFP concentrations in 26 of our cases was less than 60 days (Fig. 25-5). Thus, serum AFP testing once every 2 months would be necessary for the early detection of HCC in our geographic area.

In 1983, we introduced a screening program to detect asymptomatic HCCs (Fig. 25-11). If patients have cirrhosis, they undergo serum AFP testing every 2 months, ultrasound every 3 months, and CT and MRI every 6 months Since a small number of patients with chronic hepatitis without cirrhosis develop HCC, these patients are also enrolled in the program and undergo AFP testing every 4 months, ultrasound every 6 months, and CT and MRI every 12 months. Using this program, we have successively detected many asymptomatic HCCs, and 50% of our patients survived more than 3 years. The cumulative survival rate of 50 patients detected in this program significantly better than that of 70 patients whose HCCs were detected outside the program (Fig. 25-12).

REFERENCES

1. Kobayashi K, Sugimoto T, Makino H et al. Screening methods for early detection of hepatocellular carcinoma. Hepatology 1985;5:1100–1105
2. Sheu JC, Sung JL, Chen DS et al. Early detection of hepatocellular carcinoma by real-time ultrasonography—a prospective study. Cancer 1985;56:660–666
3. Oka H, Kuriola N, Kim K et al. Prospective study of early detection of hepatocellular carcinoma in patients with cirrhosis. Hepatology 1990;12:680–687
4. Okazaki N, Yoshino M, Takayasu K et al. Early diagnosis of hepatocellular carcinoma. Hepato-Gastroenterology 1990; 37:480–483
5. Colombo M, Franchis RD, Ninno ED et al. Hepatocellular carcinoma in Italian patients with cirrhosis. N Engl J Med 1991;325:675–680
6. Unoura M, Kaneko S, Matsushita E et al. High-risk groups and screening strategies for early detection of hepatocellular carcinoma in patients with chronic liver disease. Hepato-Gastroenterology 1993;40:305–310
7. Pateron D, Ganne N, Claude J et al. Prospective study of

FIGURE 25-12. Survival curve of patients with HCC undergoing periodic or nonperiodic follow-up.

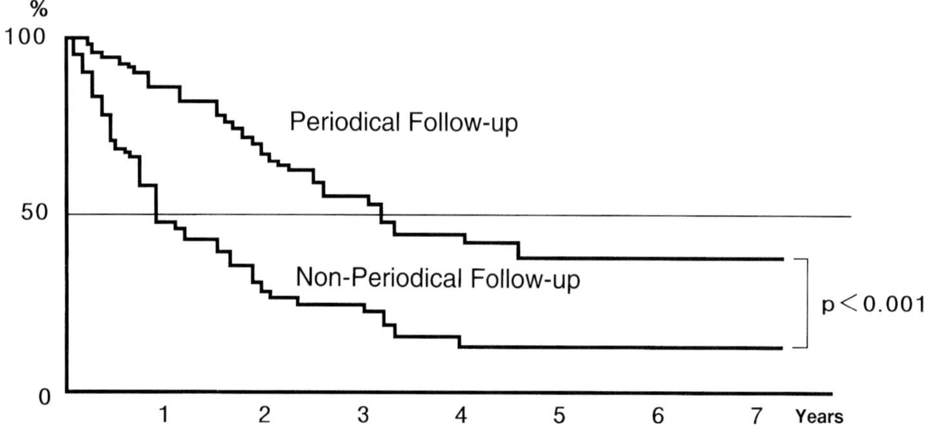

screening for hepatocellular carcinoma in Caucasian patients with cirrhosis. J Hepatol 1994;20:65–71

8. Cottone M, Turri M, Caltagirone M et al. Screening for hepatocellular carcinoma in patients with Child's A cirrhosis: an 8-year prospective study by ultrasound and alphafetoprotein. J Hepatol 1994;21:1029–1034
9. The Liver Cancer Study Group of Japan. Primary liver cancer in Japan—clinicopathologic features and results of surgical treatment. Ann Surg 1990;211:277–287
10. Craig JR, Klatt EC, Yu M. Role of cirrhosis and the development of HCC: evidence from histologic studies and large population studies. In Tabor E, Di Bisceglie AM, Purcell RH (eds): Etiology, Pathology, and Treatment of Hepatocellular Carcinoma in North America. Portfolio, The Woodlands, Texas, 1991:177–190
11. Calvet X, Bruix J, Brú C et al. Natural history of hepatocellular carcinoma in Spain. J Hepatol 1990;10:311–317
12. Zaman SN, Johnson PJ, Williams R. Silent cirrhosis in patients with hepatocellular carcinoma—implications for screening in high-incidence and low-incidence areas. Cancer 1990;65:1607–1610
13. Tiribelli C, Melato M, Crocè LS et al. Prevalence of hepatocellular carcinoma and relation to cirrhosis: comparison of two different cities of the world-Trieste, Italy, and Chiba, Japan. Hepatology 1989;10:998–1002
14. Kew MC, Geddes EW. Hepatocellular carcinoma in rural southern African blacks. Medicine 1982;61:98–108
15. Simonetti RG, Cammà C, Fiorello F et al. Hepatocellular carcinoma—a worldwide problem and the major risk factors. Dig Dis Sci 1991;36:962–972
16. Saito I, Miyamura T, Ohbayashi A et al. Hepatitis C virus infection is associated with the development of hepatocellular carcinoma. Proc Natl Acad Sci USA 1990;87:6547–6549
17. Nishioka K, Tanaka E, Sodeyama T et al. Transition of antibody to hepatitis C virus from chronic hepatitis to hepatocellular carcinoma. Jpn J Cancer Res 1990;81: 1089–1091
18. Colombo M, Kuo G, Choo QL et al. Prevalence of antibodies to hepatitis C virus in Italian patients with hepatocellular carcinoma. Lancet 1989;2:1006–1008
19. Sbolli G, Zanetti AR, Tanzi E et al. Serum antibodies to hepatitis C virus in Italian patients with hepatocellular carcinoma. J Med Virol 1990;30:230–232
20. Chiaramonte M, Farinati F, Fagiuoli S et al. Antibody to hepatitis C virus in hepatocellular carcinoma. Lancet 1990; 335:301–302(letter)
21. Ducreux M, Buffet C, Dussaix E et al. Antibody to hepatitis C virus in hepatocellular carcinoma. Lancet 1990;335: 301(letter)
22. Nalpas B, Driss F, Pol S et al. Association between HCV and HBV infection in hepatocellular carcinoma and alcoholic liver disease. J Hepatol 1991;12:70–74
23. Di Bisceglie A, Order SE, Klein JL et al. The role of chronic viral hepatitis in hepatocellular carcinoma in the United States. Am J Gastroenterol 1991;86:335–338

23a. DeGroote J, Desmet VJ, Gedigk P et al. A classification of chronic hepatitis. Lancet 1968;II:626–628

24. Takano S, Yokosuka O, Imazeki F et al. Incidence of hepatocellular carcinoma in chronic hepatitis B and C: a prospective study of 251 patients. Hepatology 1995;21:650–655
25. Sherlock S, Dooley J. Hepatic tumours. In Sherlock S, Dooley J (eds): Diseases of the Liver and Biliary System. Oxford: Blackwell Scientific Publications, 1993: 503–531
26. Kaneko S, Unoura M, Takeuchi M et al. The role of hepatitis C virus in hepatocellular carcinoma in Japan. Intervirology 1994;37:108–113

26a. Floreani A, Biagini MR, Chiaramonte M et al. Incidence of hepatic and extra-hepatic malignancies in primary biliary cirrhosis. Ital J Gastroenterol 1993;25:473–476

27. Chen DS, Sung JL, Sheu JC et al. Serum α-fetoprotein in the early stage of human hepatocellular carcinoma. Gastroenterology 1984;86:1404–1409
28. Alpert E, Hershberg R, Schur PH et al. Alpha fetoprotein in human hepatoma: improved detection in serum and quantititative studies using a new sensitive technique. Gastroenterology 1971;61:137–143
29. Alpert E. Human alpha-1 fetoprotein. In Okuda K, Peters RL (eds): Hepatocellular Carcinoma. Wiley, New York, 1976: 353–367
30. Bloomer JR, Waldmann TA, McIntire KR, Klatskin G. Serum α-fetoprotein in patients with massive hepatic necrosis. Gastroenterology 1977;72:479–482
31. Lok ASF, Lai CL. α-Fetoprotein monitoring in Chinese patients with chronic hepatitis B virus infection: role in the early detection of hepatocellular carcinoma. Hepatology 1989;9:110–115
32. Breborowicz J, Mackiewicz A, Breborowicz D. Microroheterogeneity of α-fetoprotein in patient serum as demonstrated by lectin affino-electrophoresis. Scand J Immunol 1981;14: 15–20
33. Miyazaki J, Endo Y, Oda T. Lectin affinities of α-fetoprotein in cirrhosis, hepatocellular carcinoma, and metastatic liver tumor. Acta Hepatol Jpn 1981;22:1559–1568
34. Buamah PK, Harris R, James OFW, Skillen AW. Lentil-lectin-reactive alpha-fetoprotein in the differential diagnosis of benign and malignant liver disease. Clin Chem 1986;32: 2083–2084
35. Taketa K, Sekiya C, Namiki M et al. Lectin-reactive profiles of α-fetoprotein characterizing hepatocellular carcinoma and related conditions. Gastroenterology 1990;99:508–518
36. Aoyagi Y, Suzuki Y, Isemura M et al. The fucosylation index of α-fetoprotein and its usefulness in the early diagnosis of hepatocellular carcinoma. Cancer 1988;61:769–774
37. Du MQ, Hutchinson WL, Johnson PJ, Williams R. Differential alpha-fetoprotein lectin binding in hepatocellular carcinoma: diagnostic utility at low serum levels. Cancer 1991; 67:476–480
38. Sato Y, Nakata K, Kato Y et al. Early recognition of hepatocellular carcinoma based on altered profiles of alpha-fetoprotein. N Engl J Med 1993;328:1802–1806
39. Taketa K, Endo Y, Sekiya C et al. A collaborative study for the evaluation of lectin-reactive α-fetoprotein in early detection of hepatocellular carcinoma. Cancer Res 1993;53: 5419–5423
40. Liebman HA, Furie BC, Tong MJ et al. Des-γ-carboxy (ab-

normal) prothrombin as a serum marker of primary hepatocellular carcinoma. N Engl J Med 1984;310:1427–1431

41. Hattori N, Ohmizo R, Unoura M et al. Abnormal prothrombin measurements in hepatocellular carcinoma. J Tumor Marker Oncol 1988;3:207–216
42. Suehiro T, Sugimachi K, Matsushita T et al. Protein induced by vitamin K absence or antagonist II as a prognostic marker in hepatocellular carcinoma—comparison with alpha-fetoprotein. Cancer 1994;73:2464–2471
43. Sawabu N, Ohta H, Motoo Y, Okai T. Immuno-biochemical diagnosis of liver cancer. In Okuda K, Tobe T, Kitagawa T (eds): Early Detection and Treatment of Liver Cancer. Japan Scientific Societies Press, Tokyo, 1991:59–73
44. Freeny PC, Baron RL, Teefey SA. Hepatocellular carcinoma: reduced frequency of typical findings with dynamic contrast-enhanced CT in a non-Asian population. Radiology 1992; 182:143–148
45. Fujita M, Kuroda C, Kumatani T et al. Comparison between conventional and spiral CT in patients with hypervascular hepatocellular carcinoma. Eur J Radiol 1994;18:134–136
46. Takayasu K, Muramatsu Y, Furukawa H et al. Early hepatocellular carcinoma: appearance at CT during arterial portography and CT arteriography with pathologic correlation. Radiology 1995;194:101–105
47. Matsui O, Kadoaya M, Kameyama T et al. Benign and malignant nodules in cirrhotic livers: distribution based on blood supply. Radiology 1991;178:493–497
48. Ebara M, Ohto M, Watanabe Y et al. Diagnosis of small hepatocellular carcinoma: correlation of MR imaging and tumor histologic studies. Radiology 1986;159:371–377
49. Kadoya M, Matsui O, Takashima T, Nonomura A. Hepatocellular carcinoma: correlation of MR imaging and histopathologic findings. Radiology 1992;183:819–825
50. Muramatsu Y, Nawano S, Takayasu K et al. Early hepatocellular carcinoma: MR imaging. Radiology 1991;181:209–213
51. Matsui O, Kadoya M, Kameyama T et al. Adenomatous hyperplastic nodules in the cirrhotic liver: differentiation from hepatocellular carcinoma with MR imaging. Radiology 1989; 173:123–126
52. Sheu JC, Sung JL, Chen DS et al. Growth rate of asymptomatic hepatocellular carcinoma and its clinical implications. Gastroenterology 1985;89:259–266
53. Ebara M, Ohto M, Shinagawa T et al. Natural history of minute hepatocellular carcinoma smaller than three centimeters complicating cirrhosis. Gastroenterology 1986;90: 289–298

26

SCREENING OF PATIENTS WITH CHRONIC LIVER DISEASE

MASSIMO COLOMBO

Screening for hepatocellular carcinoma (HCC) is considered worthwhile in principle for both medical and economic reasons. The medical aim is to improve the health of the general population by early detection and treatment of disease. The economic aims are, in the short term, to save cost by using technicians or automated procedures, and in the long run, to treat the disease in order to lengthen the productive life of the patient.[1] The cost-effectiveness of screening programs for cancer cannot be determined unless the cancer is an important cause of death in the patient population and has an identifiable latent or early symptomatic stage. In addition, persons who are at risk for developing the cancer (high-risk individuals) must be recognizable, the techniques for screening should be effective, and the cost of screening must be acceptable. Since the effectiveness of a screening program is measured in terms of patient survival, the crucial prerequisite is that early detection of patients with cancer must have a favorable impact on survival. While HCC is an important cause of mortality worldwide and the main groups of individuals at risk have been identified, not all aspects of the natural history of this tumor needed for screening are available, and the impact of treatment on patient survival is still debated.

THE PROBLEM OF THE NATURAL HISTORY OF HCC

The natural history of HCC is not fully known, and some aspects of HCC may favor screening programs and others seem to hinder such programs (Table 26-1). In favor of screening is the long-lasting subclinical incubation period of HCC in many cirrhotic patients. During this period, most HCCs grow as a solitary mass to a size at which they can be detected by ultrasound.[2,3] Screening is also helped by the presence of a peritumoral fibrotic capsule. In most Asian and European patients, the peritumoral capsule is associated with an expanding growth pattern. These tumors are less aggressive than the noncapsulated infiltrative forms of HCC.[2]

Other aspects of HCC make screening less helpful. Approximately 20% of all nodules less than 1 cm in diameter when first detected already show microscopic signs of intrahepatic metastases (i.e., tumor cells invading the fibrotic capsule or portal vein branches),[4] which can be detected in some cases by highly sensitive imaging techniques or during surgery.[3] The number of tumors showing microscopic metastases increases with increasing tumor size and approaches 80% for nodules larger than 3 cm. Thus, identification of a small tumor nodule in a cirrhotic patient may not indicate an early lesion in all cases.[3]

This raises the question of whether HCC develops as a single nodule or from multiple, desynchronized neoplastic tumor foci. Data support both interpretations, but the multicentric origin of HCC would be a further factor against screening.

Finally, there are important differences in the growth rates of HCC, even in a single patient with multiple nodules, which might hinder correct prediction of the patient's survival. Expressed as tumor volume doubling time, the doubling time of HCC ranges from 1 to

TABLE 26-1. Controversial Aspects of the Natural History of HCC That May Favor or Attenuate the Cost-Effectiveness of a Screening Program in High-Risk Patients

Favor
- Most nodules have a long-lasting subclinical incubation period.
- Most tumors develop as a single nodule in the liver.
- There are encapsulated expanding tumor nodules.

Attenuate
- There are rapidly growing tumor nodules.
- 20% of nodules < 1 cm have microscopic metastases.
- 20% or more of apparently single encapsulated nodules have ancillary tumors detectable during surgery.

19 months, with a median of 6 months.[2,3] These observations provide the rationale for the 6-month ultrasound screening intervals for patients with cirrhosis. Because of this great diversity of growth rates, the predictive power of the number and size of HCC is not absolute, and survival times are predicted better by the severity of liver impairment.

SCREENING PATIENTS WITH CHRONIC LIVER DISEASE

In numerous case-control studies, the prevalence of HBV was high in the areas of the world in which there is also a high incidence of HCC; the risk for HCC in hepatitis B virus (HBV) carriers was substantially greater than in noncarriers.[2] In prospective studies of cohorts of hepatitis B surface antigen (HBsAg) carriers, for instance in Taiwan, the risk for 3,454 HBsAg carriers of developing HCC was 102 times greater than that of 19,253 noncarriers.[5] The carriers at especially high risk of developing HCC were those with actively replicating infection (HBeAg/HBV-DNA+) and those with cirrhosis (Table 26-2). In a study of 824 native Alaskan males infected with the HBV (HBsAg+), the annual incidence rate of HCC was 387/100,000 men.[6] In the prescreening era, this tumor was the most commonly occurring sequela of cirrhosis in Alaskan natives with chronic HBV infection, accounting for 57% of fatal cancers, compared to the noninfected Alaskan native population, in whom HCC accounted for approximately 2% of cancer-related deaths. In a prospective cohort study of 1,069 persons with chronic HBV infection (HBsAg+) in Toronto, 11 cases of HCC were identified in a 26-month period, an annual HCC incidence of 470/100,000.[7]

In all studies, the incidence of HCC was greater in men than in women, and greater in patients with chronic hepatitis or cirrhosis than in those with chronic HBV infection and persistently normal aminotransferase levels.[5–7] Thus, the differences in the HCC incidence among HBsAg-positive persons ranges from 155 to 3,000/100,000/year.[8,9] In a prospective study of 349 European patients with HBV-related cirrhosis, the probability of developing HCC was 6% in 5 years, highest in elderly patients and those with more advanced liver disease.[10] The higher incidence of HCC in Asians with chronic HBV infection could be due to the fact that most Asians have acquired HBV in infancy or childhood. It is not known whether HBsAg-positive persons with persistently normal aminotransferase levels also are at risk for HCC. The risk of HCC was low in 92 such HBsAg-positive Italians, who were followed prospectively for more than 10 years.[11] However, it should be noted that persons with chronic HBV infection are a heterogeneous group of patients including some with an indolent course and some with cirrhosis. This is the case for many carriers of precore HBV mutants (anti-HBe+/HBV-DNA+), who are common in southern Europe. Liver disease in precore mutant carriers causes a fluctuating pattern of serum aminotransferase levels. However, during the pauses between biochemical flare-ups, these patients are indistinguishable from "healthy" carriers of HBsAg.[12] Thus, all chronic HBsAg-positive patients should be followed at regular intervals, regardless of the pattern of serum aminotransferase levels.

TABLE 26-2. Prospective Study of HCC in 22,707 Chinese Male Government Employees

	HBsAg (+)	HBsAg (−)
No. patients	3,454	19,253
No. HCC	184	10
No. cases/100,000/yr	473.5	4.6
	Relative risk = 102	

(Data from Beasley RP. Hepatitis B virus: the major etiology of hepatocellular carcinoma. Cancer 1987;60:1942–1956.)

CHRONIC HEPATITIS C VIRUS (HCV) INFECTION

The sequential development of cirrhosis and HCC in patients with post-transfusion hepatitis was a clue to the identification of HCV carriers as another important patient population at risk for HCC. Subsequently, the link between HCV and HCC was substantiated by serologic surveys[13] and prospective studies.[14] There are, however, important variations in the HCC risks for antibody to HCV (anti-HCV)-positive patients among continents and also within the same continent[15–22] (Table 26-3).

TABLE 26-3. Anti-HCV as a Risk Factor for HCC

Location		Cases/Controls	Relative Risk	Author
United States	Miami	87/200	134.0	Hasan et al.[15]
	Los Angeles	51/128	10.5	Yu et al.[16]
Africa	South Africa	380/152	61.5	Kew et al.[17]
	Senegal	80/136	19.8	Coursaget et al.[18]
Europe	Italy	212/212	68.1	Simonetti et al.[19]
	Greece	185/467	6.3	Kaklamani et al.[20]
Asia	Japan	91/410	52.3	Tanaka et al.[21]
	Taiwan	128/384	6.9	Chuang et al.[22]

Using the polymerase chain reaction technique, HCV-RNA has been almost invariably detected in serum and tumor tissue of anti-HCV-positive patients with HCC. As a general rule, HCV genotype 1b (HCV1b) is most prevalent in patients with HCC with or without cirrhosis.[23,24] However, evidence against the importance of the association between HCV1b and HCC includes other studies showing similar prevalences of various genotypes in patients with HCC.[25,26] Several methodologic weaknesses in available studies could be responsible for the observed discrepancies, the most important being that they were performed in referral centers where most patients are first seen with advanced liver disease.

It is not clear whether the HCC risk in these patients depends on cirrhosis. There are only a few reports of HCC developing in HCV-infected persons with normal noncirrhotic livers.[24] Thus, one opinion is that HCV may promote cancer through cirrhosis. The fact that HCV is a nonintegrating virus further supports this interpretation.

ALCOHOLIC PATIENTS

Although ethanol has no mutagenic properties per se, chronic alcohol consumption is associated with an increased risk of cancer in several organs, including the oral cavity, pharynx, larynx, and esophagus. The association between ethanol and HCC has been investigated in thousands of patients. The effect of alcohol is dose-dependent, and cirrhosis could be the basis for ethanol-associated HCC cases. In areas such as the United States, in which the prevalence of HBV is low, HCC risk is increased up to 40% by heavy alcohol consumption.[2] The 10-year cumulative occurrence of HCC in Japanese patients with alcoholic cirrhosis is 18.5%.[27] In several European countries and Japan, alcohol has been associated with a higher incidence of HCC among patients with anti-HCV.[2,28] HBV also may contribute to HCC in alcoholics, even when serum markers of infection are not detectable, but integrated HBV-DNA can be found in the hepatocytes.[29]

PATIENTS WITH CIRRHOSIS

Approximately 20% of all patients who die of cirrhosis have associated HCC found at autopsy, and HCC is associated with cirrhosis in more than 90% of cases.[2] Yearly conversion rates from cirrhosis to HCC were 3% in Western patients and up to 6% in Japanese patients[14,30,31] (Table 26-4). Liver cell regeneration in cirrhotic livers could be the crucial oncogenic event, in that it promotes selection and clonal expansion of committed liver cells after damage by genotoxic agents. Whatever the biologic meaning of the association between cirrhosis and HCC, this association provides a formidable tool for screening patients who are at risk for HCC. HCC can appear within adenomatous hyperplastic nodules in posthepatitis cirrhotic livers.[2]

Extremely well-differentiated tumors (grade I of the Edmondson-Steiner classification) are often seen within benign macroregenerative nodules, with cells arranged in layers of nearly normal thickness, showing occasional microacinus formation, nuclear crowding, increased cytoplasmic basophilia, and increased nucleus/cytoplasm ratio (small cell dysplasia). Adenomatous hyperplastic nodules containing small cell dysplasia are defined as

TABLE 26-4. Early Detection of HCC in HBsAg-Positive Alaska Natives,[42] Updated April 1994

Study period:	1982–1992
Study population:	1,400 HBsAg-positive persons
Tumors detected:	20 (19 detected by AFP)
	5 unresectable
	1 refused surgery
	14 resected (6 recurred)
Tumor-free patients:	6 (5 to 11 years postresection).

atypical nodules and are considered precursors of HCC.[2] In a cohort study of 307 consecutive Italian patients with viral cirrhosis who were followed for an average of 46 months, HCC was demonstrated in 45 (15%). Multivariate analysis showed that small cell dysplasia of the liver correlated with tumor development.[32]

OTHER CONDITIONS

HCC has developed in patients with certain rare metabolic conditions. Patients with porphyria cutanea tarda, genetic hemochromatosis, tyrosinemia, hypercitrullinemia, and α_1-antitrypsin deficiency are at high risk for HCC.[2] Patients with glycogenosis types I and III, Wilson's disease, and hereditary fructose intolerance may also develop HCC but have a substantially lower risk. HCC has also been recorded in patients with primary biliary cirrhosis. HCC occurred in 64% of 160 Japanese patients with Budd-Chiari syndrome, the majority of whom had idiopathic obstructing lesions in the inferior vena cava[2] and in 48% of 101 patients in South Africa.[33] (The incidence of Budd-Chiari syndrome among all cases of HCC was less than 1% in the survey made by the Liver Cancer Study Group in Japan.)

SCREENING TESTS

Screening tests must be simple, safe, and reproducible. Serum α-fetoprotein (AFP) and abdominal ultrasound meet these criteria, although their sensitivities and costs differ.

Serum AFP is a potential marker that may help identify patients with cirrhosis who are at increased risk for HCC. In a prospective study of 447 Italian cirrhotics, the cumulative risk of the development of HCC during follow-up study was higher among those with consistently elevated serum levels of AFP than among those with fluctuating levels or those with consistently normal levels.[14] Patients with chronic hepatitis and persistently elevated levels of AFP are also at greater risk for HCC and would benefit from aggressive screening programs.[34]

Serum AFP was the first marker used for screening HCC and is now the most widely used modality for screening patients with cirrhosis. Radioimmunoassays and enzyme-linked immunoassays to detect AFP are commercially available. AFP is a normal serum protein synthesized by fetal liver cells, by yolk-sac cells and in trace amounts by the fetal gastrointestinal tract and in very small amounts by nonfetal liver, with the normal range for serum AFP from 0 to 20 ng/ml for healthy adults. Serum levels equal to or greater than 400 ng/ml are very suggestive of HCC. Unfortunately, two-thirds of patients with small HCCs have AFPs less than 200 ng/ml and up to 30% of HCCs do not produce elevated levels of AFP even in advanced stages. Between the range of 20 and 200 ng/ml, patients with false-positive results are more common than patients with HCC.[6,14] Causes of false-positive results include acute and chronic hepatitis, germ cell tumors, and pregnancy. Screening programs based on a high cut-off level of AFP (400 ng/ml) increase the specificity, but at the expense of sensitivity.

Atypical AFP

In patients with borderline elevations of serum AFP, the microheterogeneity of the sugar component of AFP can be assessed by lectin affinity electrophoresis coupled with antibody-affinity blotting. Serum AFP in patients with HCC is characterized by greater proportions of an AFP that reacts with lens culinaris agglutinin A and erythroagglutinating phytohemagglutinin than the serum AFP of patients with chronic hepatitis or cirrhosis. In a prospective study of 361 patients with viral cirrhosis, atypical AFP 33 had elevated 3 to 18 months before HCC was detected by imaging techniques.[30]

Measuring the microheterogeneity of the sugar component of AFP using lectin-affinity electrophoresis, an elevated percentage of atypical AFP can be detected in patients with HCC or in those who will develop HCC within 12 to 18 months.[30] Thus, patients with altered profiles of serum AFP might be another high-risk group of patients, for whom more aggressive screening is justified.

Serum DCP

Based on the fact that malignant hepatocytes have an acquired defect in the vitamin K-dependent carboxylase system, the serum level of desgamma-carboxy prothrombin (DCP) could be utilized as a serum marker for HCC. Radioimmunoassays and enzyme immunoassays to detect DCP are commercially available. About 55% to 95% of all patients with HCC are DCP-positive, with approximately 27% of positivity among AFP seronegative patients.[35] Unfortunately, only a small proportion of the patients with tumors less than 3 cm were DCP-positive, suggesting that this serum marker is not sensitive enough for the "early" diagnosis of HCCs. False-positive results were observed in 5% of 118 patients with alcoholic cirrhosis.[36]

Ultrasound

As a general rule, a discrete nodule seen in the liver by ultrasound should be presumed to be a preneoplastic lesion or HCC. In expert hands, 80% of small HCCs (less than 2 cm) can be detected by ultrasound only, but some of these may escape detection.[14,37,38] In certain areas of the liver, such as the upper and posterior portion of the right lobe, nodules are difficult to detect by ultrasound; sometimes HCCs are present as isoechoic masses or are too small to be detected. HCC can be suspected when a parenchymal node is larger than 2 cm and is hypoechoic or dysechoic. However, up to 30% of small HCCs have hyperpechoic patterns similar to those of hemangiomas.

SCREENING STRATEGIES

Strategies of HCC screening are adopted according to the local epidemiologic situation and available resources. In population-based studies, either only a few individuals have identifiable risk factors or all the participants have one single risk factor (e.g., HBsAg-positive). Most individuals are asymptomatic. Because of the large number of persons to be screened and the relatively low prevalence of HCC, serum AFP is the screening method of choice.[38] This is not a suitable guideline for clinic-based studies in which participants often have more than one risk factor for HCC (e.g., cirrhosis and HBV) and many are symptomatic. In this setting, both serum AFP and abdominal ultrasound should be used.

Population-based Studies

Population-based screening programs have been successful in Japan, China, Taiwan, and Alaska. In these studies, HBsAg-positive persons with asymptomatic liver disease were screened for elevated AFP levels, and a number of patients with small, subclinical HCCs were detected and treated surgically. In China, beginning in 1971, several surveys were undertaken to screen large populations for HCC. Almost 500 cases of HCC were detected after surveying 1.3 million people.[39,40] In a screening program for Alaskan Natives since 1982,[41] all HBsAg-positive persons identified in previous serosurvey studies or by prevaccination screening were tested semiannually for AFP. Between 1982 and 1992, 18,299 AFP determinations were performed on 2,230 HBsAg carriers.[42] For 371 persons, at least one AFP determination was elevated greater than 25 ng/ml. Elevated AFP levels were found in 318 (30%) of 1,068 HBsAg-positive women (292 of which were due to pregnancy) and 53 (4.6%) of 1,167 HBsAG-positive men. Twenty of these patients developed HCC; 19 had elevated AFP and 5 were found in the first screen to have unresectable tumors. Of the 15 who had resectable tumors, ranging from 1.2 to 6 cm in diameter, 14 were resected (Table 26-4). The sensitivity of AFP screening of HBsAg carriers had 94% sensitivity and 84% specificity.

Clinic-based Studies

Close follow-up study of patients with chronic hepatitis and cirrhosis by AFP and real-time ultrasound has led to the identification of HCC at an early stage.[37,38] In 31% to 60% of the patients, HCC would have gone undetected if the patients had been screened by AFP only (Table 26-5). The yield of single, small HCCs was greater in patients screened at either 3-month or semiannual intervals than in patients who were screened annually. The annual incidence rates of HCC in the studies were 3% to 4%. HCC risk in patients with elevated baseline AFP levels was two to three times greater than that of patients with normal baseline levels[14,31]; thus, prospective AFP determinations were useful. HCC risk in cirrhotic patients with persistently high levels of AFP during a 4-year follow-up period was 13.4 times that of similar patients with persistently normal AFP.[14] HCC risk was also higher in patients with chronic hepatitis and elevated AFP than in patients with chronic hepatitis with persistently normal AFP levels.[34] In a prospective cohort study of 1,069 chronic carriers of HBsAg in Toronto (46% with liver disease), recruited by referral from gastroenterologists and family physicians, with 6-month determinations of AFP and ultrasound examination, 11 patients developed HCC in a 26-month follow-up pe-

TABLE 26-5. Detection of HCC According to Different Screening Intervals in Prospectively Studied Cohorts of Patients With Cirrhosis

Author, year	Screening Interval (months)	Hepatocellular Carcinoma				
		No.	Annual Rate (%)	Single Node (%)	Single Node <3 cm (%)	AFP (−) (%)
Sato et al. 1993[30]	3	33	3.0	88	64	41
Cottone et al. 1994[31]	6	30	4.4	87	53	60
Colombo et al. 1996[a]	12	84	2.8	55	27	33

[a] Unpublished data.

riod, with an incidence of 430/100,000. The sensitivity for ultrasound was 78.8% and the specificity was 93.8%.[7]

ANALYSIS OF PATIENT SURVIVAL

There have been no controlled studies to demonstrate whether screening reduces mortality from HCC. Treatment of single patients after early detection of HCC may prolong the survival in some cases. However, the evaluation of survival of individual HCC cases detected by screening can be biased by several factors: (1) The date of diagnosis is automatically advanced for those cases detected by screening (lead-time bias). (2) Screening detects cancers that stay longer in the asymptomatic state (length bias). (3) Those patients not accepting screening could be at higher or lower risk of dying from cancer than the general population (selection bias).

A recent follow-up study from Shanghai revealed the surprisingly high 10-year rates of survival in HBsAg-positive patients who had resections for subclinical HCC.[39,40] The main reason for the success was related to the biology of HCC in that region, where the tumors tend to be monofocal and encapsulated and the accompanying liver disease tends to be a minimal or a well-compensated cirrhosis.

The best results in terms of both short-term and long-term survival for 347 Japanese patients with single HCCs less than 2 cm in diameter after hepatic resection were a 5-year survival rate of 60.5%, compared to 39.3% for 1,127 patients with 2- to 5-cm tumors and 26.8% for those with 5- to 10-cm tumors.[43] However, the survival of patients who had had resections was greatly influenced by the functional status of the liver. In a study of 72 European patients, the 3-year survival rate was 51% for Child's A patients and 12% for Child's B-C patients.[44] The survival of patients treated with percutaneous ethanol injection (PEI) was influenced by both liver function and tumor size. The 3-year survival rate for patients with two or three HCCs was half that of patients with a single nodule (31% versus 63%) and that of patients with Child's B was half that of those with better liver function (42% versus 76%).[45,46]

The results of three prospective studies carried out in Europe suggest that screening as a modality for reducing mortality from HCC may not be so useful. In a study in Italy,[14] 29% of 59 patients with HCCs that were detected early were judged to be operable. The survival at 1 year for the 12 patients who underwent surgery was 67%, but tumor recurrence rates were 60%. In a study in France,[36] 14 tumors were detected during a prospective follow-up study of 118 patients with alcoholic cirrhosis. Only three patients were judged to be operable, and one ultimately had hepatic resection. In another study in France,[47] HCC was discovered in 7 of 193 patients with cirrhosis (mostly alcoholics), and only one was treated surgically. During the same period, 54 patients with cirrhosis were admitted to the same hospital for symptomatic HCC without having been screened previously. Only two patients underwent surgical treatment. The authors concluded that, since the screened and unscreened patients were comparable for age, sex, cause of cirrhosis, and rates of monofocal tumors smaller than 3 cm, there was no evidence in these studies that screening patients with cirrhosis for HCC prolonged the patient's survival.

COST ANALYSIS OF SCREENING

Several variables determine the cost-effectiveness of screening for HCC: incidence of HCC, sensitivity and specificity of screening tests, screening intervals, growth rates of untreated tumors, results of treatments, and cost of diagnostic and therapeutic procedures.

The proportion of early HCCs detected in HBV-infected patients is directly related to the sensitivity of the screening test and inversely related to the interval between screening tests.[48] Ultrasound is more sensitive but also more costly than AFP. Concurrent use of both tests increases both sensitivity and costs. The cost per early HCC detected also depends on the incidence of the tumor in the population screened. In the United States, HCC incidence was calculated to be 5 cases per 1,000 HBsAg-positive persons per year.[49] Screening with AFP every 4 months and ultrasound every 6 months was calculated to cost US $54,000 per year for screening 1,000 HBsAg.[50] Based on the finding of 5 cases of HCC per year and complete recovery of only half of these cases at most, the cost per person "cured" would be approximately U.S. $216,000. In Hokkaido (Japan), mass screening for HCC based on semiannual ultrasound was carried out in 8,090 individuals, and 91 cases of HCC were identified.[51] The cumulative rates of survival among these patients were similar to those for patients with HCC diagnosed during follow-up study of chronic liver disease and treated surgically (15% at 7 years). The cost for detecting one HCC patient in this program was approximately U.S. $25,000.

CONCLUSIONS

Early diagnosis of HCC in patients with chronic liver diseases is possible with sensitive diagnostic tools. What is still uncertain is whether early diagnosis of HCC also determines an increase in patient survival and whether cost-effectiveness makes the screening worthwhile. Screening may result in some benefits, such as improved prognosis for some cases, less radical treatment needed to cure some cases, and reassurance for those patients

TABLE 26-6. Recommendations for HCC Screening in Italy of the Italian Association for the Study of the Liver AISF

Patients with cirrhosis or with metabolic liver diseases known to be at risk for HCC should be screened by AFP determination and ultrasound *twice a year*.

HBsAg-positive persons older than 35 years or with a family history of HCC should be screened by AFP and aminotransferase determinations *once a year*.

who have negative test results. All these benefits might result in resource savings. However, screening for HCC might also cause disadvantages (for instance, longer morbidity for cases whose prognosis is unaltered, overtreatment of borderline abnormalities, false reassurance for patients with false-negative results, and unnecessary morbidity for those with false-positive results.

In two consensus development conferences held in Anchorage, Alaska,[52] and in Milan, Italy,[53] persons with chronic HBV infection, patients with cirrhosis, and patients with rare metabolic liver diseases were identified as candidates for periodic screening. At the Anchorage conference, it was recommended that healthy HBsAg-positive persons have at least yearly determinations of serum AFP and those with additional risk factors (e.g., cirrhosis) be screened every 6 months by abdominal ultrasound and serum AFP. No specific recommendations were made at either conference for HBsAg-negative patients with chronic liver disease. At the Milan conference, it was recommended that patients with cirrhosis or with certain congenital metabolic conditions be screened by AFP and ultrasound twice a year. It was also recommended that chronically HBsAg-positive persons over age 35 years or with family histories of HCC be screened for HCC by serum AFP and aminotransferase levels once a year (Table 26-6).

REFERENCES

1. Wilson JMG, Jungner G. Principles and practice of screening for disease. World Health Organization, Geneva, 1968 (WHO, public paper 34)
2. Okuda K. Hepatocellular carcinoma: recent progress. Hepatology 1992;5:948–963
3. Colombo M. Hepatocellular carcinoma in cirrhotics. Semin Liver Dis 1993;13:374–383
4. Ebara M, Ohto M, Shinagawa T et al. Natural history of minute hepatocellular carcinoma smaller than three centimeters complicating cirrhosis. Gastroenterology 1986;90: 289–298
5. Beasley RP. Hepatitis B virus. The major etiology of hepatocellular carcinoma. Cancer 1987;61:1842–1856
6. McMahon BJ, Alberts SR, Wainwright RB et al. Hepatitis-B sequelae: prospective study in 1400 hepatitis B surface antigen-positive Alaska native carriers. Arch Intern Med 1990;150:1051–1054
7. Sherman M, Peltekian KM, Lee C. Screening for hepatocellular carcinoma in chronic carriers of hepatitis B virus: incidence and prevalence of hepatocellular carcinoma in a North American urban population. Hepatology 1995;22:432–438
8. London WT, Atleson J, Eto M, Hwang C. Early detection of hepatocellular carcinoma among Asians living in the United States. In Tabor E, Di Bisceglie AM, Purcell RH (eds): Etiology, Pathology, and Treatment of Hepatocellular Carcinoma in North America. Portfolio, The Woodlands, Texas, 1991, pp. 243–253
9. Tong MJ, Schwindt RR, Lo GH, Co RL. Chronic hepatitis and hepatocellular carcinoma in Asian Americans. In Tabor E, DiBisceglie AM, Purcell RH, eds. Etiology, Pathology, and Treatment of Hepatocellular Carcinoma in North America. Portfolio, The Woodlands, Texas, 1991, pp. 15–24
10. Fattovich G, Giustina G, Schalm SW et al. Occurrence of hepatocellular carcinoma and decompensation in Western European patients with cirrhosis type B. Hepatology 1995; 21:77–82
11. de Franchis R, Meucci G, Vecchi M et al. The natural history of asymptomatic hepatitis B surface antigen carriers. Ann Intern Med 1993;118:191–194
12. Bonino F, Brunetto MR. Hepatitis B virus heterogeneity: one of the many factors influencing the severity of hepatitis B. J Hepatol 1991;18:5–8
13. Colombo M, Kuo G, Choo QL et al. Prevalence of antibodies to hepatitis C virus in Italian patients with hepatocellular carcinoma. Lancet 1989;2:1006–1008
14. Colombo M, de Franchis R, Del Ninno E et al. Hepatocellular carcinoma in Italian patients with cirrhosis. N Engl J Med 1991;325:675–680
15. Hasan F, Jeffers LJ, De Medina M et al. Hepatitis C-associated hepatocellular carcinoma. Hepatology 1990;3:589–591
16. Yu MC, Tong MJ, Coursaget P et al. Prevalence of hepatitis B and C viral markers in black and white patients with hepatocellular carcinoma in the United States. J Natl Cancer Inst 1990;82:1038–1041
17. Kew MC, Houghton M, Choo QL, Kuo G. Hepatitis C virus antibodies in southern African blacks with hepatocellular carcinoma. Lancet 1990;335:873–874
18. Coursaget P, Leboulleux D, Le Cann P et al. Hepatitis C virus infection in cirrhosis and primary hepatocellular carcinoma in Senegal. Trans R Soc Trop Med Hyg 1992;86: 552–553
19. Simonetti RG, Cammaà C, Fiorello F et al. Hepatitis C virus infection as a risk factor for hepatocellular carcinoma in patients with cirrhosis. A case-control study. Ann Intern Med 1992;116:97–102
20. Kaklamani E, Trichopoulos D, Tzonou A et al. Hepatitis B and C viruses and their interaction in the origin of hepatocellular carcinoma. JAMA 1992;265:1974–1976
21. Tanaka K, Hirohata T, Koga S et al. Hepatitis C and hepatitis B in the etiology of hepatocellular carcinoma in the Japanese population. Cancer Res 1991;51:2842–2847

22. Chuang WL, Chang WY, Lu SN et al. The role of hepatitis B and C viruses in hepatocellular carcinoma in a hepatitis B endemic area: a case-control study. Cancer 1992;69: 2052–2054
23. Nousbaum JP, Pol S, Nalpas B et al. Hepatitis C virus type 1b (II) infection in France and Italy. Ann Intern Med 1995; 122:161–168
24. De Mitri MS, Poussin K, Baccarini P et al. HCV-associated liver cancer without cirrhosis. Lancet 1995;345:413–415
25. Naito M, Hayashi N, Moribe T et al. Hepatitis C viral quasispecies in hepatitis C virus carriers with normal liver enzymes and patients with type C chronic liver disease. Hepatology 1995;22:407–412
26. Takano S, Yokosuka O, Imazeki F et al. Incidence of hepatocellular carcinoma in chronic hepatitis B and C: a predictive study of 251 patients. Hepatology 1995;21:650–655
27. Yamauchi M, Nakahara M, Maezawa Y et al. Prevalence of hepatocellular carcinoma in patients with alcoholic cirrhosis and prior exposure to hepatitis C. Am J Gastroenterol 1993; 88:39–43
28. Benvegnù L, Fattovich G, Noventa F et al. Concurrent hepatitis B and C virus infection and risk of hepatocellular carcinoma in cirrhosis. A prospective study. Cancer 1994;74: 2442–2448
29. Bréchot C, Nalpas B, Couroucé AM et al. Evidence that hepatitis B virus has a role in liver-cell carcinoma in alcoholic liver disease. N Engl J Med 1982;306:1384–1387
30. Sato Y, Nakata K, Kato Y et al. Early recognition of hepatocellular carcinoma based on altered profiles of alpha-fetoprotein. N Engl J Med 1993;328:1802–1806
31. Cottone M, Turri M, Caltagirone M et al. Screening for hepatocellular carcinoma in patients with Child's A cirrhosis: an 8 year prospective study by ultrasound and alfafetoprotein. J Hepatol 1994;21:1029–1034
32. Borzio M, Bruno S, Roncalli M et al. Liver cell dysplasia is a major risk factor for hepatocellular carcinoma in cirrhosis: a prospective study. Gastroenterology 1995;108:812–817
33. Simon IW. Membranous obstruction of the inferior vena cava and hepatocellular carcinoma in South Africa. Gastroenterology 1982;82:171–178
34. Tsukuma H, Hiyama T, Tanaka S et al. Risk factors for hepatocellular carcinoma among patients with chronic liver disease. N Engl J Med 1993;328: 1797–1801
35. Weitz IC, Liebman HA. Des-gamma-carboxy (abnormal) prothrombin and hepatocellular carcinoma: a critical review. Hepatology 1993;18:990–997
36. Pateron D, Ganne N, Trinchet JC et al. Prospective study of screening for hepatocellular carcinoma in Caucasian patients with cirrhosis. J Hepatol 1994;20:65–71
37. Oka H, Kurioka N, Kim K et al. Prospective study of early detection of hepatocellular carcinoma in patients with cirrhosis. Hepatology 1990;12:680–687
38. Okuda K. Early recognition of hepatocellular carcinoma. Hepatology 1986;6:729–738
39. Sun TT, Wan LC, Chang YL. Radiorocket electrophoresis authography (RREA) through labelled antigen for AFP assay and its application in seroepidemiological investigation on primary hepatocellular carcinoma. Chin Med J 1979;92: 17–22
40. Tang ZY. Subclinical hepatocellular carcinoma-historical aspects and general considerations. In Tang ZY (ed): Subclinical Hepatocellular Carcinoma. China Academic Publishers, Beijing, China, 1985, pp. 1–11
41. Heyward WL, Lanier AP, McMahon BJ et al. Early detection of primary hepatocellular carcinoma. Screening for primary hepatocellular carcinoma among persons infected with hepatitis B virus. JAMA 1985;254:3052–3054
42. McMahon BJ, Wainwright RW, Lanier AP. The Alaska native HCC screening program: a population-based screening program for hepatocellular carcinoma. In Tabor E, Di Bisceglie AM, Purcell RH (eds): Etiology, Pathology and Treatment of Hepatocellular Carcinoma in North America Portfolio, The Woodlands, Texas, 1991, pp. 231–242
43. Tobe T, Arii S. Improving survival after resection of hepatocellular carcinoma: characteristics and current status of surgical treatment of primary liver cancer in Japan. In Tobe T, Kaneda H, Okudaira M et al (eds): Primary Liver Cancer in Japan. Springer, Tokyo, 1992, pp. 219–221
44. Franco D, Capussotti L, Smadja C et al. Resection of hepatocellular carcinomas. Results in 72 European patients with cirrhosis. Gastroenterology 1990;98:733–738
45. Livraghi T, Bolondi L, Lanzarani S et al. Percutaneous injection in the treatment of hepatocellular carcinoma in cirrhosis. A study of 207 patients. Cancer 1992;69:925–929
46. Ebara M, Otho M, Sugiura N et al. Percutaneous ethanol injection for the treatment of small hepatocellular carcinoma. Study of 95 patients. J Gastroenterol Hepatol 1990; 5:616–626
47. Durand F, Buffet C, Pellettier G et al. Hepatocellular carcinoma. N Engl J Med 1993;1:64 (letter)
48. Kang JY, Lee TP, Yaps I, Lun KC. Analysis of cost-effectiveness of different strategies for hepatocellular carcinoma screening in hepatitis B virus carriers. J Gastroenterol Hepatol 1992;7:463–468 (letter)
49. Hoofnagle JH, Shafritz DA, Popper H. Chronic type B hepatitis and the "healthy" HBsAg carrier state. Hepatology 1987;7:758–763
50. Regan LS. Screening for hepatocellular carcinoma in high-risk individuals. Arch Intern Med 1989;149:1741–1744
51. Mima S, Sekiya C, Kanagawa H et al. Mass screening for hepatocellular carcinoma: experience in Hokkaido, Japan. J Gastroenterol Hepatol 1994;9:361–365
52. McMahon BJ, London T. Workshop on screening for hepatocellular carcinoma. J Natl Cancer Inst 1991;83:916–919
53. Colombo M. Early diagnosis of hepatocellular carcinoma in Italy. A summary of a consensus development conference held in Milan, 16 November 1990 by the Italian Association for the Study of the Liver (AISF). J Hepatol 1992;14: 401–403

27

PREVENTION OF HEPATOCELLULAR CARCINOMA WITH VACCINES

B. S. ANAND
F. BLAINE HOLLINGER

OVERVIEW

Hepatocellular carcinoma (HCC) is the seventh most common tumor in humans worldwide, with an estimated annual incidence between 250,000 and over 1 million cases.[1] The association between HCC and hepatitis B virus (HBV) or hepatitis C virus (HCV) infection is well established. However, despite advances in diagnosis and treatment, HCC has one of the lowest survival rates of all malignant tumors. The overall 5-year survival rate for HCC in the United States is only 6% for whites and 5% for blacks.[2] Even when the tumor is diagnosed at a stage when it is localized to the liver, the 5-year survival rates are only 14% for whites and 11% for blacks.[2] Although these percentages show an improvement compared to the results obtained in previous years, they still present a very dismal picture. Clearly, greater efforts are required in other approaches to this problem, including tumor prevention.

Prevention of HCC involves primary and secondary interventions. Secondary prevention includes the use of measures that delay or halt the further progression of liver disease or tumor development. These include using antiviral drugs in patients with HBV and HCV infections,[3,4] removal of excess iron in patients with hemachromatosis, and liver transplantation in end-stage liver disease.

Another approach in the secondary prevention of HCC is the use of imaging studies and tumor markers such as α-fetoprotein (AFP) to screen high risk patients. Screening often permits the diagnosis of HCC at a stage when it is small and limited to the liver. Such tumors are frequently amenable to resection or transplantation, or to other local treatment measures, resulting in a prolonged disease-free survival, as reported from Japan and China.[5] Indeed, early detection through ultrasound and AFP screening, followed by resection of small HCCs less than 5 cm in size, has yielded 5-year survival rates approaching 65%, compared to 25% for untreated patients. However, these results have not been reproduced to the same extent in other countries because of the high cost of screening and a possible difference in the natural history of the tumor.

The development of highly effective and safe hepatitis B vaccines raises the theoretical possibility of complete eradication of HBV infection. There is every reason to believe that protection against HBV will have a profound effect on the incidence of HCC. Many hepatitis B vaccine trials eventually will focus on the efficacy of immunization for the prevention of HCC. Vaccines against HCV and other exciting innovations in vaccine development also may eventually contribute to the prevention of HCC.

VACCINES AGAINST HEPATITIS B VIRUS

Plasma-Derived Vaccines

In the first studies of HBV vaccines in 1973, Krugman and Giles[6] used heat-inactivated (98°C for 1 minute) HBV-containing serum to inoculate 29 individuals who were subsequently challenged with untreated HBV-containing serum. Complete protection was obtained in 17 (59%) subjects, and mild subclinical infection occurred in 3 (10%).

The encouraging results obtained in this pilot study led to the use of more refined techniques for the production of plasma-derived HBV vaccines. The essential aim of these techniques was to harvest hepatitis B surface antigen (HBsAg) free of any infectious virus. The purification process involved a series of steps such as precipitation, ultracentrifugation, gel filtration, and affinity chromatography.

In 1981, a plasma-derived vaccine was approved for marketing in the United States (Heptavax-B, Merck). It used the plasma of asymptomatic persons who were chronically infected with HBV and used a series of purification and inactivation steps, rendering it free of live HBV and all other classes of animal viruses (including retroviruses, such as the human immunodeficiency virus).[7] Postmarketing surveillance for adverse effects between June 1982 and May 1985, evaluating nearly 850,000 vaccine recipients, revealed that 491 persons developed side effects considered to be caused by the vaccine.[8] There were no deaths. Although 41 recipients experienced neurologic complaints including Bell's palsy (10 cases), Guillain-Barré syndrome (11 cases), and convulsions, optic neuritis, or lumbar radiculopathy (5 each), no conclusive association between the vaccine and the neurologic events was found. At present, there are at least five commercially available plasma-derived vaccines produced worldwide, although most of these vaccines are marketed for regional use only.

Recombinant Yeast-Derived Vaccines

The recombinant hepatitis B vaccines currently licensed in the United States are produced by inserting the HBV S gene, which codes for HBsAg, into an expression plasmid. This fragment is then introduced into yeast cells (*Saccharomyces cerevisiae*) and is used to produce large quantities of the antigen. HBsAg is released by disrupting the yeast cells and is then purified.[9]

The recombinant vaccines have several advantages over plasma-derived vaccines: The production process is quicker (12 weeks versus 65 weeks); there is minimal batch-to-batch variability in immunogenicity; the supply is not dependent on the availability of HBV carriers; and the fear of inadvertent contamination by other infectious agents, however unfounded, is eliminated. For these reasons, plasma-derived vaccines are no longer manufactured in the United States, although other regions of the world still use these vaccines for the successful prevention of HBV infection.

In most countries, two recombinant yeast-derived HBV vaccines are currently available: Recombivax HB (Merck) and Engerix-B (SmithKline Beecham). Although these vaccines contain <2% of yeast proteins, the risk of allergic reactions to these has been negligible; anaphylaxis and other symptoms of an immediate hypersensitivity have been exceedingly rare. Both the plasma- and yeast-derived vaccines contain the antigens that are important in inducing protection against HBV infection.[10]

Dose and Immunization Schedules

Dose-response studies show that, in any given individual, higher doses of the vaccine result in more rapid immune responses and greater levels of antibody to HBsAg (anti-HBs) concentrations are achieved.[11–14] The timing of injections also is important in obtaining optimal results. Evaluation of several dose schedules using a single lot of plasma-derived vaccine in weight-matched subjects revealed that the highest anti-HBs responses were obtained with the 0-, 1-, and 6-month or the 0-, 2-, and 4-month schedule.[15] Other regimens, such as 0, 2, and 6 months; 0, 1, and 4 months; and 0, 3, and 6 months were less successful. Two injections are suboptimal and should not be used. At present, the immunization schedule recommended for adults is 0, 1, and 6 months.

The site and route of inoculation also are important in achieving an optimal immune response to the HBV vaccine.[16] Intramuscular injection is the most effective route of administration, and the best results are obtained with inoculation into the deltoid muscle. Experimental inoculation in the gluteal region or intradermally is less immunogenic.[17,18]

Factors Influencing the Response Rate

Several host factors influence the immunologic response to HBV vaccine. The response rate decreases with advancing age. Compared to seroconversion rates of greater than 90% in younger individuals, subjects over 60 years of age have a response rate of less than 70%, and this rate falls below 40% after age 80 years.[19] Obesity, especially in younger individuals, has a negative effect on the response rate, perhaps because obese subjects receive a lower dose of the vaccine per kilogram body weight.[20] Race also may play a role. In one small study, response to the vaccine was better in white children than in Asians and blacks.[13] Certain HLA antigens, such as HLA-A1, B8, and DR3, are associated with a poor immunologic response, perhaps related to alterations in cell-mediated immune activity.[21] Among Chinese, DR14 in association with DR52 appears to correlate with low responsiveness to the hepatitis B vaccine.[22]

Response Rate in Homosexuals

Homosexual populations have a high risk of HBV infection, and HBV vaccine recommendations include them. The current response rate to HBV vaccine in homosexuals is similar to that of the general population, with adequate anti-HBs levels developing in greater than 95%[23,24] of recipients. However, HIV-positive homosexuals show a poor vaccine response rate, with a seroconversion rate of only 31%,[25] as well as a lower concentration of anti-HBs.[26] These findings suggest that HIV-positive individuals should be vaccinated before they develop severe depression of their T-cell-mediated immune functions.

Response Rate in Hemodialysis Patients

Several clinical trials have been carried out on hemodialysis patients and the staff of hemodialysis units.[27] The 95% seroconversion rate in staff members is similar to that of the general population. However, the response rate in patients receiving hemodialysis is markedly reduced (less than 60%). The anti-HBs levels correlate with the severity of uremia and reflect the immunologic abnormalities in these patients. Hemodialysis patients should be vaccinated at an early stage. A higher dose of the vaccine has been recommended in these patients.

Response Rate in Neonates

Perinatal transmission of HBV infection accounts for the existence of 30% to 40% of all chronic HBV infections.[28] The transmission rate to infants is 70% to 90% in hepatitis B e antigen (HBeAg) positive mothers compared with 10% to 12% in HBeAg-negative mothers. Similarly, carrier mothers with higher HBV DNA levels sometimes transmit HBV infection despite use of hepatitis B immune globulin (HBIG) and HBV vaccine in the infants.[29] Perinatal transmission occurs whether the child is delivered vaginally or by cesarean section.[28] The majority of such infants have asymptomatic chronic HBV infection; few develop chronic liver disease and cirrhosis.

Several studies have evaluated the role of immunoprophylaxis in preventing perinatal transmission.[27] Trials of HBV vaccine used alone resulted in protective efficacy rates of 62% to 96%; combination treatment with HBIG and HBV vaccine provided higher overall protective efficacy rates of 80% to 100%.

STRATEGIES FOR GLOBAL CONTROL OF HBV INFECTION

The ideal strategy for the control of HBV infection is universal immunization, starting at birth, regardless of the prevalence of HBV in the region. This is because 70% to 90% of neonates born to HBeAg-positive mothers (versus 10% to 12% of infants born to HBeAg-negative carrier mothers) become persistently infected,[30–33] whereas less than 5% of immunocompetent adults infected with HBV are likely to become chronically infected.[34–36] In high prevalence areas (>7% HBsAg-positive) of the Far East, such as mainland China, Taiwan, and Hong Kong, most infections begin at birth or during infancy. In sub-Saharan Africa, infections usually occur somewhat later in childhood. In high-prevalence areas, the best strategy is vaccination at birth, together with HBIG in infants born to mothers with HBV infection, in particular those who are HBeAg-positive.

In medium prevalence regions of the world (2% to 7% HBsAg-positive), generally in developing countries, it is difficult to pinpoint the most dominant route of infection. In these countries, universal vaccination of infants seems appropriate.

In low prevalence areas (less than 2% HBsAg-positive), such as western Europe and the United States, the major modes of spread of hepatitis B are (1) percutaneous or parenteral transmission, particularly through the use of contaminated needles in injection drug abusers and (2) transmission through unprotected sexual contact, either by homosexual or promiscuous heterosexual lifestyles. Although infection can occur following transfusion of contaminated blood or blood products, this risk has been almost eliminated for most populations through the addition of specific and sensitive testing of donors, the use of all-volunteer blood donors, improvements in assessing the qualifications of donors, and the use of virus-inactivated blood products. Although maternal-infant transmission accounts for less than 4% of reported cases of HBV in the United States, from 20% to 30% of the adult carrier pool is derived from this cohort. In these low prevalence regions of the world, universal immunization of infants has been the goal of public health agencies.

Vaccine Trials in High Prevalence Regions

THE GAMBIA EXPERIENCE

In contrast to the Far East, where HBV transmission is mostly perinatal, in The Gambia and other sub-Saharan countries of West Africa. The infection is usually acquired later in childhood.[37] Horizontal transmission between siblings and playmates by an unidentified route appears to be the predominant mode of spread.[37] The infection rate increases rapidly after birth. Nearly 40% of children are infected by the age of 5 years, and the infection rate is 90% by 15 years; 20% of all children become chronically infected with HBV.[38] The Gambia has one of the highest mortality rates for HCC in Africa, with an age-adjusted incidence in males of 34/100,000 population.[39]

In 1979, the Gambian government initiated a nationwide HBV vaccination program. Fixed and mobile immunization teams visited 104 delivery points at least once every 2 weeks.[40] Follow-up studies have shown that greater than 80% of the children received all HBV vaccination doses.[40] Long-term HBV protection studies in

The Gambia showed that over 95% of children developed a protective level of anti-HBs, and the vaccine was 97% effective in preventing chronic infection in children followed for at least 4 years.[41]

The Gambia Hepatitis Intervention Study (GHIS) was formulated as a collaborative project of the Gambian government, the World Health Organization (WHO), and the Medical Research Council of the United Kingdom to study the impact of HBV vaccination on HBV infection and the development of HCC. Because of the expense of the program, limited quantities of the vaccine, and the desire to document the cancer-protective efficacy of the vaccine, it was decided to have a vaccinated group and a nonvaccinated control group, randomized at the level of health zones. The schedule of vaccination is shown in Table 27-1. Recombinant HBV vaccine was given in 10 μg doses by intramuscular injection, beginning within 24 hours of birth. A four-dose regimen was used because the pilot study found it to be more immunogenic than a three-dose regimen.[42]

By 1990, 124,577 children had been recruited into the study, 50,803 in the vaccinated group and the remaining in the control group. As part of the study, a cohort of 1,000 children was recruited to assess the long-term protection produced by the vaccine.[43] Serologic tests at age 3 years on the 704 children who could be successfully traced showed that 95% had anti-HBs levels greater than 10 mIU/ml, which is considered to be the minimum protective level; over 70% had antibody concentrations greater than 100 mIU/ml. Five children (0.7%) had asymptomatic HBV infection (HBsAg and anti-HBc positive) and 14 others (2%) were found to be anti-HBc-positive but HBsAg-negative. In contrast to these findings, in a survey of 526 nonvaccinated children, 160 (30%) developed HBV infection in a 2-year follow-up period.[40] The impact on prevention of HCC will require a longer follow-up period since the peak age of development of HCC is 30 to 40 years in West Africa.[40]

TABLE 27-1. The Schedule of Hepatitis B Vaccine in the Gambian Expanded Program of Immunization

Age	Routine Vaccines	HBV Vaccine
At birth	BCG, Polio 1	HBV1
2 months	DPT 1, Polio 2	HBV2
3 months	DPT 2, Polio 3	
4 months	DPT 3, Polio 4	HBV3
9 months	Measles, Polio 5, Yellow fever	HBV4

Abbreviations: BCG, bacille Calmette-Guérin; DPT, diphtheria-pertussis-tetanus; HBV, hepatitis B virus.

THE SENEGAL EXPERIENCE

Senegal is a small country that borders Gambia to the south. Most HBV infections in Senegal occur during childhood, and nearly 20% of the children become chronically infected with HBV.[37,44] The annual incidence of HCC in men is 30 to 75/100,000.[45]

In 1978, a trial of plasma-derived HBV vaccine was initiated in one of the districts of Senegal (Niakhar district).[45] All children from birth to 2 years of age were included. Each child received three subcutaneous 10 μg doses of vaccine at 1-month intervals, with a booster dose after 1 year of age in those who showed no evidence of an HBV infection. Among 238 of the vaccinated subjects, anti-HBs developed in 94.5%.[45] The results were slightly better when the initial injection was given to children less than 12 months of age (97%) compared to those immunized initially between the ages of 13 to 24 months (91%). Assessment after a follow-up period of 12 months showed that seven (2.9%) of the participants in the vaccinated group developed HBV infection (HBsAg [1.7%] or anti-HBc without HBsAg [1.2%]) compared to 20 of 195 control subects (10.3%). The protective efficacy rate of the HBsAg vaccine was 85% in this population ($p < 0.0001$). Six years after a booster dose of vaccine at 12 months in 156 subjects, 1.5% per year in the vaccinated group had developed HBV infection compared to 11.5% per year in the unvaccinated children. The protective efficacy rate was determined to be 100% in the first 4 years, but this fell to 67% in the fifth and sixth years based primarily on the detection of anti-HBc in the absence of HBsAg. The authors concluded that a second booster should be given 5 years after the first injection.[46]

THE EXPERIENCE IN ALASKA

The southwestern region of Alaska is a hyperendemic area for HBV infection, with a prevalence of HBsAg in Yupik Eskimos of greater than 6%.[47,48] The annual incidence of HCC in Alaskan males was found to be 11.2 per 100,000, five times greater than that of white males in the rest of the United States.[49]

In 1981, a hepatitis B vaccine project was initiated in the Yukon-Kuskokwim Delta area among 1693 susceptible Alaskan natives.[50,51] Subsequently, over 90% of the susceptible population in southwest Alaska (9840 residents) were immunized, including most infants at birth.[52] The plasma-derived HBsAg vaccine was used at a dose of 10 μg by intramuscular injection for children age 10 years or younger and 20 μg for older participants. The schedule of injections was 0, 1, and 6 months. The study participants were revisited annually by phlebotomy teams for 5 years after the first vaccine. Anti-HBs levels of greater than or equal to 10 mIU/ml were observed in 95% of the study participants, while another 2% had levels between 2.1 and 9.9 mIU/mL. The anti-HBs levels

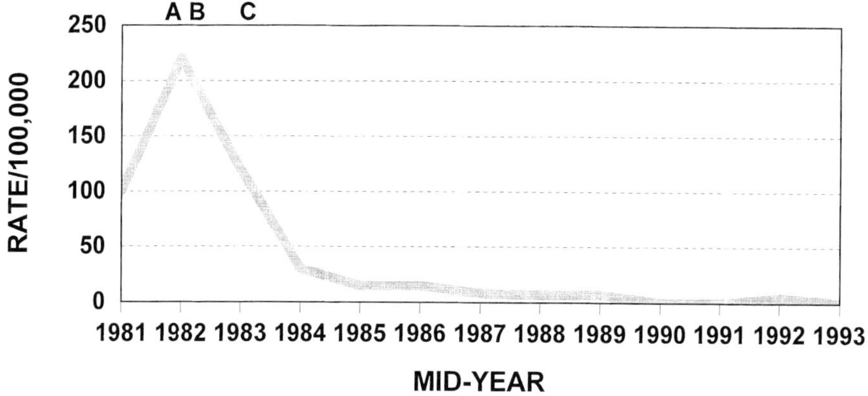

FIGURE 27-1. Incidence of symptomatic HBV infection, Yukon-Kuskokwim Delta area, Alaska. A, CDC IHS immunization program initiated (Nov. '82); B, CDC IHS immunization program completed (Sept. '82); C, Mass immunization program initiated (Mar. '83). (Adapted from McMahon and Wainwright,[52] with permission.)

declined steadily over time, but 81% still maintained anti-HBs concentrations of greater than or equal to 10 mIU/ml for at least 5 years. A higher percentage of younger subjects maintained these anti-HBs levels at 5 years: 84% in the 0 to 19-year age group, 73% in the 20 to 49-year age group, and 63% in those 50 years and older.

The annual incidence of acute symptomatic hepatitis B between 1981 and 1993 among Alaskan natives in southwest Alaska declined from 215 cases per 100,000 to 7 to 14 cases per 100,000[52] (McMahon, personal communication) (Fig. 27-1). Most of the reduction occurred in the first 2 years of the program. Breakthrough infections were observed in only 12 vaccinees, a rate of 0.86 infections per 1,000 person-years of follow-up evaluation. In contrast, the annual incidence of HBV infection was 50 infections per 1,000 person-years observed in this region before the vaccination program was initiated.[53]

THE EXPERIENCE IN ASIA

In countries in the Far East, the prevalence of HBV infection by 40 years of age is nearly 45% in Thailand; over 70% in Taiwan, Hong Kong, and south China; and 70% to 100% in the Philippines.[54] HCC occurs frequently in these countries. Consumption of aflatoxins and other factors appear to contribute to the risk of HCC.

In 1984, a controlled study of universal immunization of newborns was initiated in Qidong, China,[55] on the north shore of the Yangtze River opposite Shanghai. The site was selected because it has a high age-adjusted annual incidence of HCC (86 per 100,000) in a stable population. A standardized cancer registry system is maintained by the local Qidong Liver Cancer Institute, which provides accurate data collection on the epidemiologic and clinical aspects of HCC prevention. All newborns were randomized either to a vaccination group or an age-matched unvaccinated control group. The vaccine in this project was plasma-derived 5 μg intramuscularly at 0, 1, and 6 months after birth. The first dose of vaccine was given half an hour after delivery.

Between 1984 and 1989, a total of 66,840 children had been included in the study, 35,064 in the vaccinated group and 31,776 as controls.[55] The vaccination rate was 98% of all eligible infants, and 90% received all three doses. HBsAg was detected in 2.5% of vaccinees, compared to 12.5% in the unvaccinated group. Anti-HBs was detected in 83% of the vaccinated children. The percentage of children with anti-HBs greater than 10 mIU/ml fell from 80% at 1 year to 63% at 3 years. A booster dose of 5 μg given subsequently raised the anti-HBs prevalence to 83% at 5 years.

In Taiwan, mass vaccination of neonates born to HBsAg-positive mothers was initiated in 1984. In 1986, this program was expanded to include all infants and subsequently was extended to include other high-risk groups. All newborns were given 5 μg of a plasma-derived vaccine intramuscularly in the anterolateral aspect of the thigh within 24 hours of birth and at 5 and 9 weeks of age; a booster dose was administered at 12 months.[56] For neonates of HBeAg-positive mothers, HBIG was administered within 24 hours of birth along with the vaccine.

In a stratified sample of infants recruited for long-term follow-up study,[57] anti-HBs levels exceeded 10 mIU/ml in 93%, 92%, 90%, and 85% of the vaccine responders at 18, 24, 36, and 48 months of age, respectively. HBV infection in vaccinated infants occurred at an annual rate of 2% to 4% compared to a historical control rate of 10% in unvaccinated children more than

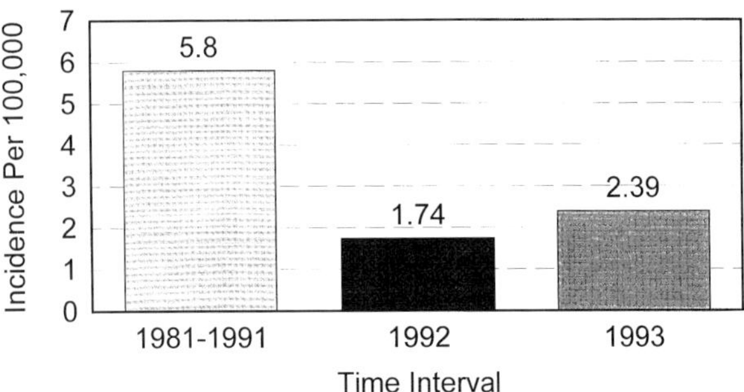

FIGURE 27-2. Hepatitis B vaccine appears to decrease the incidence of HCC in Taiwan among children older than 6 years of age. (Data from Chang et al.[58])

2 years old. Most of the infections occurred in nonresponders or in those with low antibody concentrations, and most were not chronic infections.

In this vaccinated population in Taiwan, the incidence of childhood HCC was evaluated in children 6 years old or younger.[58] Between 1981 and 1991, the annual incidence of HCC ranged from 4.48 to 7.13 cases per 100,000 children (Fig. 27-2), whereas it was 1.74 in 1992 and 2.39 in 1993 ($p < 0.005$). This is the earliest epidemiologic evidence to suggest that HBsAg vaccination can effectively reduce the incidence of HCC in children. Further efforts to document this trend are in progress.

Hong Kong and several other countries in Southeast Asia also have initiated mass vaccination programs. In Hong Kong, vaccination of all children born to HBsAg-positive mothers was started in 1986. In 1988, the program was extended to all neonates.[54] In Thailand, the Ministry of Public Health has decided to include HBV vaccine in its general vaccination program.[54] In Indonesia, HBV vaccinations was included in the general vaccine program in Lombok, an island east of Bali with a population of 2.7 million.[59] Here, more than 90% of the children received all three doses of vaccine, and the prevalence of HBsAg was 1.4% for infants given vaccine within 7 days of birth versus 3.0% for those receiving vaccine more than 7 days after birth.[60]

Strategy in High Prevalence Regions

According to data published in 1991, 22 countries, mainly in the western Pacific and eastern Mediterranean regions, already have a policy of vaccinating all newborns with the hepatitis B vaccine.[61] Another 23 countries have established pilot infant immunization projects in selected regions.

The initial experience of integrating HBV vaccine into the general vaccination program for The Gambia, China, Indonesia, and Taiwan are encouraging. In most of these trials, over 90% of the eligible children were successfully given all three doses of the vaccine and, of those vaccinated, protective titers of anti-HBs usually were present in over 90% of the subjects (Table 27-2). Follow-up studies show that there has been a significant decrease in the incidence of HBV infection.

The introduction of any new health initiative raises the issue of cost, a question of much concern for governmental agencies throughout the world, but particularly in developing countries. A cost-benefit analysis of introducing large-scale immunization programs in countries with a high prevalence rate of HCC[62] showed that the cost of preventing a death from HCC by HBV vaccination ranged from \$150 to \$200, assuming the cost of the vaccine was \$1 per dose. A similar analysis was carried out in Israel, an area of intermediate endemicity for HBV infection.[63,64]

Strategy in Low Prevalence Regions

Compared to HBV infection rates of 0.5% in whites and Hispanics, and 0.7% to 1% in urban blacks, the rate of HBsAg positivity among foreign-born Asian-American women is 8% or greater.[65] Of the approximately 3.9 million women who gave birth in 1988 in the United States, 22,000 were HBsAg-positive and 43% of these were foreign-born Asian women.[65] It has been estimated that nearly 6,000 children of these mothers would become chronic HBV carriers every year if no preventive measures were undertaken. There is also evidence of a high rate of horizontal transmission of HBV infection in children born to immigrant mothers from Southeast Asia.

In 1985, the Advisory Committee on Immunization Practices (ACIP) recommended that prenatal screening for HBV infection be directed toward women who were at high risk of acquiring this infection.[66] High-risk women were those who were injection drug abusers, sexual contacts of HBV carriers, health care workers, and immigrants from high prevalence countries. However, this approach did not result in any appreciable reduction in the incidence of HBV infection,[67,68] and it became clear that a substantial number of HBV carriers (at least 50%) could not be identified by these criteria. In 1988, new guidelines put forward by the ACIP recommended screening all pregnant women for HBsAg, and administration of HBIG and vaccine to all infants born to HBsAg-positive mothers.[69] Universal infant immunization was recommended in 1991. The value of vaccination in low-prevalence areas (and in high-prevalence regions of low-prevalence areas) has been shown in several western countries.[70,71]

Cost-benefit analysis studies show that even in low-prevalence countries such as the United States, universal HBV is cost-effective.[72,73] The estimated cost per year

TABLE 27-2. Comparative Results Between Different Hepatitis B Vaccination Trials

Country	Age at First Vaccine	Dose (μg)	Schedule (months)	Seroconversion Rate (%)
The Gambia	≤1 month	10	1, 2, 3, 9	90
China	at birth	5	0, 1, 6	83
USA (Alaska)	0–>50 yr	10–20	0, 1, 6	95
Senegal	0–24 months	10	0, 1, 2, 12	94
Taiwan	≤1 month	5	0, 1, 2, 12	80

of life saved was $164 after vaccination to prevent perinatal infection, $1,852 for infant vaccination, and $3,739 for adolescent vaccination.[72,73] Finally, the cost-benefit estimates obtained with HBV vaccine compared favorably with other disease-prevention interventions.[65,74]

VACCINE FOR HCV INFECTION

Development of vaccines against HCV infection has been slow.[75] HCV is an RNA virus whose two putative envelope genes (E1 and E2) are thought to induce neutralizing antibodies but are highly divergent between strains.[76] As a result of the variable and inconstant antigenicity of the envelope proteins, responses are restricted to the immunizing strain. The recent observation that HCV may circulate in the bloodstream surrounded by β-lipoprotein could pose an additional obstacle to vaccine development.[77] Experimentally infected animals can be easily reinfected with the same strain of HCV.[78,79] Similarly, in humans, multiple episodes of hepatitis have been observed.[80]

Despite all the difficulties noted, some encouraging observations have been made. First, neutralizing antibodies have been detected in the sera of some HCV-infected patients.[81,82] Second, administration of polyclonal immune globulins, either before or at the time of blood transfusion, appears to reduce the incidence of icteric non-A, non-B post-transfusion hepatitis and the development of chronic hepatitis. Recently, specific hepatitis C immune globulin appeared to modulate HCV infection in a chimpaneze (M. Alter, personal communication).

An experimental envelope protein-based vaccine[83] using an antigen preparation containing an HCV E1/E2 construct was given to seven chimpanzees. They were challenged 2 to 3 weeks after the final booster, using approximately 10 chimpanzee infectious doses (10 CID_{50}) of HCV administered intravenously. Five of the seven chimpanzees were completely protected; none showed biochemical evidence of liver disease or the presence of HCV RNA in the blood. The remaining two animals suffered from very mild disease, and chronicity did not occur in either animal. It is interesting to note that all the chimpanzees with high anti-E1/E2 antibody levels at the time of the challenge were protected, while the two infected animals had lower antibody concentrations. The antibody response was short-lived and most of the animals lost their antibodies within 1 to 3 weeks. In addition, the virus challenge dose was low, and the vaccine used virus sequences that were homologous to those of the challenge virus.

FUTURE DEVELOPMENTS

DNA Vaccines

The difficulties encountered in developing an effective vaccine against viruses such as HIV and HCV has stimulated research into new vaccine strategies that use DNA instead of protein as the antigenic stimulus.[84] Standard vaccines introduce viral proteins into the host that are taken up by phagocytic cells and are processed by major histocompatibility complex (MHC) class II lymphocytes ($CD4^+$ helper T cells), which promote antibody production. By contrast, genes that express viral antigens can be introduced into cells of the host where they produce the corresponding viral protein. These proteins also may activate cytotoxic T lymphocytes through the MHC pathway. Once activated, these cells may not only protect against infection with HCV but the process also may be useful in treating chronic infection.[85] A prototype of such a DNA vaccine against influenza virus has been developed, and studies are underway to produce a DNA vaccine against HIV.[80,87]

Tumor Vaccines

Under normal conditions, tumor cells escape host immune surveillance by down-regulating one or more steps involved in the recognition and elimination of foreign antigens.[88] Nonspecific immune potentiators such as bacille Calmette-Guerin (BCG) and cytokines such as interleukin-2 and interferons, have been used to increase the antitumor effect of host immune cells. Limited success already has been obtained with these measures in renal cell carcinoma and melanoma, but most cancers are not responsive. Guo et al.[89] fused chemical carcinogen-induced hepatoma cells (BEHR-2) with activated rat B lymphocytes (BEHR-2B). Syngeneic rats injected with the hybrid BEHR-2B cells became resistant to challenge with parenterally administered cancer cells (BEHR-2). Furthermore, rats with established hepatomas were cured by subsequent injection of the hybrid cells. Both $CD4^+$ and $CD8^+$ cells were essential for induction of the protective immunity, but only $CD8^+$ cells were necessary for the eradication of BEHR-2 tumors. The effectiveness of this technique in the treatment of spontaneously occurring HCC in humans remains to be determined.

REFERENCES

1. Parkin DM, Stjernward J, Muir CS. Estimates of the worldwide frequency of twelve major cancers. Bull WHO 1984; 62:163–182
2. Parker SL, Tong T, Bolden S, Wingo PA. Cancer statistics, 1996. CA Cancer J Clin 1996;46:5–27
3. Nishiguchi S, Kuroki T, Nakatani S et al. Randomized trial of effects of INF-α on the incidence of hepatocellular carcinoma. Hepatology 1995;22:117A(abstr)
4. Ishibashi K, Kashiwqagi T, Nagasawa M et al. Decreased prevalence of hepatocellular carcinoma in chronic hepatitis type C after interferon therapy: comparison between responders and nonresponders. Hepatology 1995;22: 173A(abstr)
5. Shanghai Coordinating Group for Research on Liver Cancer. Diagnosis and treatment of primary hepatocellular carcinoma in early stage. Chinese Med J 1979;92:810–816
6. Krugman S, Giles JP. Viral hepatitis type B (MS-2 strain): further observations on natural history and prevention. N Engl J Med 1973;288:755–760
7. Centers for Disease Control. Hepatitis B virus vaccine safety: report of an inter-agency group. MMWR Morb Mortal Wkly Rep 1982;31:465–467
8. Shaw FE Jr, Graham DJ, Guess HA et al. Postmarketing surveillance for neurological adverse events reported after hepatitis B vaccination. Experience of the first three years. Am J Epidemiol 1988;127:337–352
9. Ellis RW. Hepatitis B vaccines in clinical practice. Marcel Dekker, New York, 1993
10. Hauser P, Thomas HC, Waters J et al. Induction of neutralizing antibodies in chimpanzees and in humans by recombinant yeast-derived hepatitis B surface antigen particles. In Zuckerman AJ (ed): Viral Hepatitis and Liver Disease. Alan R. Liss, New York, 1988, pp. 1031–1037
11. Hollinger FB, Troisi C, Pepe PE. Anti-HBs response to vaccination with a human hepatitis B vaccine made by recombinant technology in yeast. J Infect Dis 1986;153:156–159
12. Yeoh EK, Lai CL, Chang WK, Lo HY. Comparison of the immunogenicity, efficacy and safety of 10 micrograms and 20 micrograms of a hepatitis B vaccine: a prospective randomized trial. J Hyg 1986;96:491–499
13. Zahradnik JM, Heiberg D, Hollinger FB. Hepatitis B vaccine: immune responses in children from families with an HBsAg carrier. Vaccine 1985;3:407–413
14. Milne A, Moyes C. Response to hepatitis B vaccine in New Zealand children using low doses in a two-month versus six-month schedule. In Zuckerman AJ (ed): Viral Hepatitis and Liver Disease. Alan R. Liss, New York, 1988, pp. 977–979
15. Hollinger FB, Adam E, Heiberg D et al. Response to hepatitis B vaccine in a young adult population. In Szmuness W, Alter HJ, Maynard JE (eds): Viral Hepatitis—1981 International Symposium. Franklin Institute Press; Philadelphia, 1982, pp. 451–466
16. Shaw FE Jr, Guess HA, Roets JM et al. The effect of anatomic injection site, age and smoking on the immune response to hepatitis B vaccination. Vaccine 1989;7:425–430
17. Bryan JA, Sjogren M, Iqbal M et al. Comparative trial of low-dose, intradermal, recombinant- and plasma-derived hepatitis B vaccine. J Infect Dis 1990;162:789–793
18. Clarke JA, Hollinger FB, Lewis E et al. Intradermal inoculation with Heptavax-B: immune response and histological evaluation of injection sites. JAMA 1989;262:2567–2571
19. Denis F, Mounier M, Hessel L et al. Hepatitis-B vaccination in the elderly. J Infect Dis 1984;149:1019
20. Weber DJ, Rutala WA, Samsa GP et al. Obesity is a predictor of poor antibody response to hepatitis B plasma vaccine. JAMA 1985;254:3187–3189
21. Varla-Leftherioti M, Papanicolaou M, Spyropoulou M et al. HLA-associated non-responsiveness to hepatitis B vaccine. Tissue Antigens 1990;35:60–63
22. Hsu HY, Chang MH, Ho HN et al. Association of HLA-DR14-DR52 with low responsiveness to hepatitis B vaccine in Chinese residents in Taiwan. Vaccine 1993;11: 1437–1440
23. Szmuness W, Stevens CE, Harely EJ et al. Hepatitis B vaccine: demonstration of efficacy in a controlled clinical trial in a high-risk population in the United States. N Engl J Med 1980;303:833–841
24. Francis DP, Hadler SC, Thompson SE et al. The prevention of hepatitis B with vaccine: report of the Centers for Disease Control multicenter efficacy trial among homosexual men. Ann Intern Med 1982;97:362–366
25. Collier AC, Corey L, Murphy VL, Handsfield HH. Antibody to human immunodeficiency virus (HIV) and suboptimal response to hepatitis B vaccination. Ann Intern Med 1988; 109:101–105
26. Carne CA, Weller IVD, Waite J et al. Impaired responsiveness of homosexual men with HIV antibodies to plasma derived hepatitis B vaccine. Br Med J 1987;294:866–868
27. Hollinger FB. Hepatitis B virus. In Fields BN, Knipe DM, Howley PM et al (eds): Fields Virology, 3rd Ed. Lippincott-Raven, Philadelphia, pp. 2739–2807
28. Tong MJ, Poovorawan Y, Coursaget P. Immunoprophylaxis of neonates against hepatitis B. In Hollinger FB, Lemon SM, Margolis HS (eds): Viral Hepatitis and Liver Disease. Williams & Wilkins, Baltimore, 1991, pp. 849–855
29. Ip HM, Wong VC, Lelie PN et al. Prevention of hepatitis

B virus carrier state in infants according to maternal serum levels of HBV DNA. Lancet 1989;i:406–410

30. Beasley RP, Hwang LY, Lin CC et al. Hepatitis B immune globulin (HBIG) efficacy in the interruption of perinatal transmission of hepatitis B virus carrier state. Lancet 1981; 2:388–393
31. Beasley RP, Trepo C, Stevens CE, Szmuness W. The e antigen and vertical transmission of hepatitis B surface antigen. Am J Epidemiol 1977;105:94–98
32. Stevens CE, Beasley RP, Tsui J, Lee W-C. Vertical transmission of hepatitis B antigen in Taiwan. N Engl J Med 1975; 292:771–774
33. Stevens CE, Neurath RA, Beasley RP, Szmuness W. HBeAg and anti-HBe detection by radioimmunoassay: correlation with vertical transmission of hepatitis B virus in Taiwan. J Med Virol 1979;3:237–241
34. Beasley RP, Hwang LY, Lin CC et al. Incidence of hepatitis among students at a university in Taiwan. Am J Epidemiol 1983;117:213–222
35. McMahon BJ, Wainwright RB. Protective efficacy of hepatitis B vaccines in infants, children, and adults. In Ellis RW (ed.): Hepatitis B Vaccines in Clinical Practice. Marcel Dekker, New York, 1993, pp. 243–261
36. Seeff LB, Beebe GW, Hoofnagle JH et al. A serologic follow-up of the 1942 epidemic of past-vaccination hepatitis in the United States Army. N Engl J Med 1987;316:965–970
37. Marinier E, Barrois V, Larouse B et al. Lack of perinatal transmission of hepatitis B virus infection in Senegal, West Africa. Trop Paediatr 1985;106:843–848
38. Whittle HC, Bradley AK, McLoughlan K et al. Hepatitis B virus infection in two Gambian villages. Lancet 1983;ii: 1203–1206
39. Bah E, Hall AJ, Inskip HM. The first 2 years of the Gambian National Cancer Registry. Br J Cancer 1990;62:647–650
40. Ryder RW. Hepatitis B virus vaccine in The Gambia, West Africa: synergy between public health research and practice. Mt Sinai J Med 1992;59:487–492
41. Whittle HC, Inskip H, Hall AJ et al. Vaccination against hepatitis B virus and protection against chronic viral carriage in The Gambia. Lancet 1991;337:747–750
42. The Gambia Hepatitis Study Group. Hepatitis B vaccine in the expanded programme of immunization: the Gambian experience. Lancet 1989;i:1057–1060
43. Chotard J, Inskip HM, Hall AJ et al. The Gambia Hepatitis Intervention Study: follow-up of a cohort of children vaccinated against hepatitis B. J Infect Dis 1992;166:764–768
44. Barin F, Perrin J, Chotard J et al. Cross-sectional and longitudinal epidemiology of hepatitis B in Senegal. Prog Med Virol 1981;27:148–162
45. Maupas P, Chiron J-P, Barin F et al. Efficacy of hepatitis B vaccine in prevention of early HBsAg carrier state in children. Controlled trial in an endemic area (Senegal). Lancet 1981;i:289–292
46. Coursaget P, Yvonnet B, Chotard J et al. Seven-year study of hepatitis B vaccine efficacy in infants from an endemic area (Senegal). Lancet 1986;ii:1143–1145
47. Barrett DB, Burks J, McMahon BJ, et al. Epidemiology of hepatitis B in two Alaskan communities. Am J Epidemiol 1977;105:118–122
48. Schreeder MT, Bender TR, McMahon BJ et al. Prevalence of hepatitis B in selected Alaskan Eskimo villages. Am J Epidemiol 1983;118:543–549
49. Heyward WL, Lanier AP, Bender TR et al. Primary hepatocellular carcinoma in Alaskan natives, 1969–1979. Int J Cancer 1981;28:47–50
50. McMahon BJ, Rhoades ER, Heyward WL et al. A comprehensive programme to reduce the incidence of hepatitis B virus infection and its sequelae in Alaskan natives. Lancet 1987;ii:1134–1136
51. Wainwright RB, McMahon BJ, Bulkow LR et al. Duration of immunogenicity and efficacy of hepatitis B vaccine in a Yupik Eskimo population. JAMA 1989;261:2362–2366
52. McMahon BJ, Wainwright RB. Protective efficacy of hepatitis B vaccines in infants, children, and adults. In Ellis RW (ed): Hepatitis B Vaccines in Clinical Practice. Marcel Dekker, New York, 1993, pp. 243–261
53. Heyward WL, Bender TR, McMahon BJ et al. The control of hepatitis B virus infection with vaccine in Yupik Eskimos. Am J Epidemiol 1985;121:914–923
54. Sung JL and the Asian Regional Study Group. Hepatitis B virus eradication strategy for Asia. Vaccine 1990;8(suppl): S95–S99
55. Sun ZT, Zhu Y, Stjernsward J et al. Design and compliance of HBV vaccination trial on newborns to prevent hepatocellular carcinoma and 5-year results of its pilot study. Cancer Detect Prev 1991;15:313–318
56. Chen DH, Hsu NHM, Sung JL et al. A mass vaccination program in Taiwan against hepatitis B virus infection in infants of hepatitis B surface antigen-carrier mothers. JAMA 1987;257:2597–2603
57. Chen D-S. Control of hepatitis B in Asia: mass immunization program in Taiwan. In Hollinger FB, Lemon SM, Margolis HS (eds): Viral Hepatitis and Liver Disease. Williams & Wilkins, Baltimore; 1991, pp. 716–719
58. Chang MH, Chen CJ, Lai MS et al. Hepatitis B mass vaccination program decreases childhood hepatocellular carcinoma in Taiwan. IX Triennial International Symposium on Viral Hepatitis and Liver Disease, 1996, Abstract C243.
59. Gust ID, Ruff TA, Sutanto A et al. Obstacles influencing delivery of hepatitis B vaccine in developing countries: the Lombok experience. In Hollinger FB, Lemon SM, Margolis HS (eds): Viral Hepatitis and Liver Disease. Williams & Wilkins, Baltimore 1991, pp. 708–712
60. Ruff TA, Gertig DM, Otto BF et al. Lombok hepatitis B model immunization project: toward universal infant hepatitis B immunization in Indonesia. J Infect Dis 1995;171: 290–296
61. Kane MA, Ghendon Y, Lambert P-H. Hepatitis B in 1990: Where are we and where are we going? The WHO programme for control of viral hepatitis. In Hollinger FB, Lemon SM, Margolis HS (eds): Viral Hepatitis and Liver Disease. Williams & Wilkins, Baltimore, 1991, pp. 706–708
62. Hall AJ, Robertson RL, Crivelli PE et al. Cost-effectiveness of hepatitis B vaccine in The Gambia. Trans R Soc Trop Med Hyg 1993;87:333–336

63. Ginsgerg GM, Berger S, Shouval D. Cost-benefit analysis of a nationwide inoculation programme against viral hepatitis B in an area of intermediate endemicity. Bull WHO 1992; 70:757–767
64. Ginsberg GM, Shouval D. Cost-benefit analysis of a nationwide neonatal inoculation programme against hepatitis B in an area of intermediate endemicity. J Epidemiol Community Health 1992;46:587–594
65. Shapiro CN, Margolis HS. Impact of hepatitis B virus infection on women and children. Infect Dis Clin North Am 1992;6:75–96
66. Franks AL, Berg CJ, Kane MA et al. Hepatitis B virus infection among children born in the United States to southeast Asian refugees. N Engl J Med 1989;321:1301–1305
67. Alter MJ, Hadler SC, Margolis HS et al. The changing epidemiology of hepatitis B in the United States: need for alternative vaccination strategies. JAMA 1990;263:1218–1222
68. Centers for Disease Control and Prevention. Successful strategies for adult immunization. MMWR Morb Mortal Wkly Rep 1991;40:700–703
69. Advisory Committee on Immunization Practices. Prevention of perinatal transmission of hepatitis B virus: prenatal screening of all pregnant women for hepatitis B surface antigen. MMWR Morb Mortal Wkly Rep 1988;37:341–346
70. Villa GD. Successful mass vaccination against hepatitis B virus in a hyperendemic area in Italy. Res Virol 1993;144: 255–258
71. Dobson S, Scheifele D, Bell A. Assessment of a universal, school-based hepatitis B vaccination program. JAMA 1995; 274:1209–1213
72. Arevalo JA, Washington AE. Cost-effectiveness of prenatal screening and immunization for hepatitis B virus. JAMA 1988;259:365–369
73. Margolis HS, Coleman PJ, Brown RE et al. Prevention of hepatitis B virus transmission by immunization. An economic analysis of current recommendations. JAMA 1995; 274:1201–1208
74. Hollinger FB. Comprehensive control (or elimination) of hepatitis B virus transmission in the United States. Gut 1996; 38 (suppl 2):S24–S30
75. Hollinger FB. Status of HCV vaccine research. In HCV Infection: Epidemiology, Diagnosis, and Treatment. The University of Texas Southwestern Medical Center at Dallas, Dallas, 1995, pp. 10–11
76. Kato N, Ootsuyama Y, Tanaka T et al. Marked sequence diversity in the putative envelope proteins of hepatitis C viruses. Virus Res 1992;22:107–123
77. Thomssen R, Bonk S, Thiele A. Density heterogeneities of hepatitis C virus in human sera due to the binding of beta-lipoproteins and immunoglobulins. Med Microbiol Immunol 1993;182:329–334
78. Farci P, Alter HJ, Govindarajan S et al. Lack of protective immunity against reinfection with hepatitis C virus. Science 1992;258:135–140
79. Prince AM, Brotman B, Huima T et al. Immunity in hepatitis C infection. J Infect Dis 1992;165:438–443
80. Lai ME, Mazzoleni AP, Argiolu F et al. Hepatitis C virus in multiple episodes of acute hepatitis in polytransfused thalassemic children. Lancet 1994;343:388–390
81. Farci P, Alter HJ, Wong DC et al. Prevention of hepatitis C virus infection in chimpanzees after antibody-mediated in vitro neutralization. Proc Natl Acad Sci USA 1994;91: 7792–7796
82. Shimizu YK, Hijikata M, Iwamoto A et al. Neutralizing antibodies against hepatitis C virus and the emergence of neutralization escape mutant viruses. J Virol 1994;68: 1494–1500
83. Choo Q-L, Kuo G, Ralston R et al. Vaccination of chimpanzees against infection by the hepatitis C virus. Proc Natl Acad Sci USA 1994;91:1294–1298
84. McDonnell WM, Askari FK. DNA vaccines. N Engl J Med 1996;334:42–45
85. Vitiello A, Ishioka G, Grey HM et al. Development of a lipopeptide-based therapeutic vaccine to treat chronic HBV infection. I. Induction of a primary cytotoxic T lymphocyte response in humans. J Clin Invest 1995;95:341–349
86. Donnelly JJ, Friedman A, Martinez D et al. Preclinical efficacy of a prototype DNA vaccine: enhanced protection against antigenic drift in influenza virus. Nat Med 1995;1: 583–587
87. Graham BS, Matthews TJ, Belshe RB et al. Augmentation of human immunodeficiency virus type 1 neutralizing antibody by priming with gp160 recombinant vaccinia and boosting with rgp160 in vaccinia-naive adults. J Infect Dis 1993;167:533–537
88. Lanzavecchia A. Identifying strategies for immune intervention. Science 1993;260:937–943
89. Guo Y, Wu M, Chen H et al. Effective tumor vaccine generated by fusion of hepatoma cells with activated B cells. Science 1994;263:518–520

28

HEPATOCELLULAR CARCINOMA: PREVENTION WITH ANTIVIRAL DRUGS

JANICE MAIN
HOWARD C. THOMAS

Chronic viral hepatitis accounts for the majority of hepatocellular carcinoma (HCC) worldwide. It is hoped that vaccination against hepatitis B virus (HBV) will prevent many cases of HCC in future years, but it is likely that the development of an effective vaccine for hepatitis C virus (HCV) will take many years. Therefore, other strategies will be necessary to prevent HCC. With chronic hepatitis B, it is thought that the ongoing liver inflammation and damage leading to cirrhosis also predispose to malignant change. Most cases of hepatocellular carcinoma associated with chronic HBV occur in a cirrhotic liver, but in several cases HCC developed much earlier in the natural history of HBV infection. With HCV, integration of the viral genome is not thought to occur, and the development of chronic inflammation and scarring is thought to be the main factor predisposing to malignant change. HCC also has been reported in patients with noncirrhotic liver disease.

Effective antiviral therapy is now available for many patients with chronic viral hepatitis, and newer agents are being investigated. It is hoped that early recognition and treatment of patients with chronic viral hepatitis can arrest the disease process before malignant change occurs and effectively prevent cancer.

CHRONIC HEPATITIS B

A diagnosis of chronic hepatitis B is established when a patient has at least a 6-month history of biochemical or histologic hepatitis with evidence of ongoing HBV replication. Patients infected with wild-type HBV have detectable hepatitis B e antigen (HBeAg), whereas patients infected with precore variants are HBeAg-negative. A successful response to therapy is demonstrated when there is sustained loss of HBV DNA from the serum with loss of HBeAg and eventually HBsAg in those with wild-type infection. A pretreatment liver biopsy is important to establish the stage of disease (e.g., evidence of cirrhosis) and the level of inflammation, and to exclude other coexistent liver disease. The main aims of antiviral therapy are to clear the virus and to thereby prevent the development of the life-threatening consequences of HBV infection. Eradication of the virus also has public health implications, as the successfully treated patient no longer will infect others. Interferon α is now licensed for the treatment of chronic HBV infection in many countries, and several nucleoside analogs are under investigation as potential antiviral agents for the treatment of HBV infection.

INTERFERON-α

Interferon-α is a glycopeptide of which there are 20 to 30 subtypes found in humans. Interferon-α was first used against HBV in 1976.[1]

The main immunomodulatory effect of interferon-α is the enhancement of the MHC class I display of infected hepatocytes. Hepatocytes have very little class

I display, and it is thought that the enhancement of this by interferon aids immune recognition of the HBV-infected cells. Interferon-α also increases natural killer cell activity and the number of CD4 cells increases. Interferon-α administration leads to an induction of intracellular host enzyme systems that inhibit viral protein synthesis. It is thought that the combination of antiviral and immunomodulatory actions is important in viral clearance.[2] However, interferon-α also has antiproliferative effects and is used to treat malignancies including renal carcinoma, Kaposi's sarcoma, and certain hematologic malignancies.

Interferon α has to be administered by either deep subcutaneous or intramuscular injection. A typical regimen would be 5 to 10 MU administered three times a week for 3 to 4 months. The major side effect is myelotoxicity, and careful monitoring of white cell and platelet counts are required. This is particularly important if the patient has a baseline leucopenia or thrombocytopenia, common in severe chronic liver disease.

Interferons also cause influenza-like side effects with myalgia and fever. This is worse with the initial dosing and can be reduced by administering the interferon doses at bedtime and by giving small doses of acetaminophen. Headaches and lethargy are common side effects. Depression can also occur and may require cessation of the drug. Hair loss, which is usually mild and reversible, may occur. Autoimmune disease can be worsened or precipitated by interferon. Before giving prolonged courses of interferon, it is suggested that autoimmune markers be checked.

Within a few days of commencing treatment, the HBV DNA levels decrease. Six to 8 weeks into the treatment, a surge is noted in the serum aminotransferase values. This is thought to represent immune recognition and lysis of infected hepatocytes. Following this, patients generally become HBeAg negative and positive for antibody to HBeAg (anti-HBe).

Some patients may remain hepatitis B surface antigen (HBsAg) positive, possibly because of integration of HBV DNA within the host genome, but eventually HBsAg may be cleared even in these patients.[3]

The success rate of interferon is 20% to 40% (Table 28-1) in those with HBV infection acquired as adults.[4–7] Unfortunately very few of those with HBV infection acquired from their mothers respond to interferon alone.[8] Predictive factors for a successful response to interferon include low baseline HBV DNA, high baseline aminotranferase values, or active inflammation seen in liver biopsy. Those with coexistent illnesses are less likely to respond, and a poor response rate is seen in those with immunosuppression, particularly for instance those with infection with human immunodeficiency virus type 1 (HIV-1) or immunosuppressive therapy. In one detailed study,[9] 21 pretreatment variables were assessed using data from 114 patients given interferon-α. In those patients who had received a minimum of 90 MU per m^2 total dose over 12 weeks, were negative for antibody to HIV-1, and had active liver disease on biopsy, high alanine aminotranferase value, low HBV DNA level, and a history of acute hepatitis, there was an increased likelihood of response on univariate analysis. This study also showed that the early loss of HBsAg with successful therapy was associated with a short history (less than 2 years) of HBV infection.

It is anticipated that cessation of the chronic HBV-associated inflammation will, if the patient is treated early in the course of disease, lead to long-term clinical benefits with a reduction in the development of cirrhosis and HCC. Long-term follow-up studies of successfully treated patients will be needed to confirm this. In one study,[10] 103 patients with chronic HBV who received interferon were followed up for a mean of 50 months. A total of 53 patients cleared HBeAg or HBV DNA (56%); only 10 patients cleared HBsAg. This compares with a spontaneous clearance rate for HBeAg of 7 of 53 untreated patients (28%) at 5 years. Six of the treated patients (5.8%), all HBeAg-positive, died of liver failure and two more required hepatic transplantation. This compares with 13 patients with severe complications in the untreated group (24.5%). In another study[11] 62 patients with HBV-associated cirrhosis, 34 of whom received interferon-α, were followed for a mean of 49 months. Six of the group developed HCC, but the risk of this did not seem to be modified by interferon-α treatment.

Reactivation of HBV infection can occur following

TABLE 28-1. Treatment of Chronic HBV With Interferon-α Monotherapy

		Treated			Control			
Dose (MU)	Schedule (Frequency; Weeks)	No. of Patients	Loss of HBeAg	%	No. of Patients	Loss of HBeAg	%	Author, Year (Ref.)
5–10/m^2	tiw; 12	37	12	32	24	1	4	Brook et al., 1989[4]
10/m^2	tiw; 24	23	6	26	23	0	0	Alexander et al., 1987[6]
2.5–5/m^2	tiw; 12	37	7	19	23	0	0	Dusheiko et al., 1988[7]
5	tiw; 16	41	15	37	43	3	7	Perrillo et al., 1990[5]

successful therapy but is unusual unless the patient is immunosuppressed.

CORTICOSTEROID PRETREATMENT OF PATIENTS TREATED WITH INTERFERON-α

The observation that cessation of corticosteroid therapy for other conditions led to the clearance of HBV in a number of chronic carriers led to trials of corticosteroid monotherapy or in combination with interferon. The administration of corticosteroid to patients with chronic HBV leads to a decrease in aminotransferase values, associated with an increase in viral replication. Cessation of the corticosteroid leads to an increase in the aminotransferase values thought to be due to improved immune response to HBV.

In a study 8 of 18 patients who received a 6-week tapered course of prednisone followed by interferon-α, 8 (44%) cleared HBeAg.[12] A subsequent study of prednisone priming showed no benefit.

In Taiwan, in one of the largest studies,[13] 120 male Chinese patients were randomized to receive a combination of prednisolone and interferon-α, placebo with interferon, or only placebo. Twelve months after cessation of therapy, clearance of HBeAg was reported in 46% of those who received the combination, 25% who received interferon monotherapy, and 25% of those who received placebo only. Those with lower baseline aminotransferase values (less than 200 U/L) showed a better response to combination therapy than to interferon alone.

In a study in Hong Kong,[14] 17 of 70 treated patients (21.5%) and 3 of 36 controls (8.3%) had partial or complete antiviral responses. In this study, prednisone priming had a marginal benefit compared to interferon alone in those with elevated aminotransferase values.

A fatal outcome has been described following corticosteroid therapy, so corticosteroids are not routinely recommended and are contraindicated in those with severe liver disease.

INTERFERON-β

Results with interferon-β so far appear similar to those achieved with interferon-α.[14a]

INTERFERON-γ

Interferon-γ as monotherapy or in combination with interferon-α has been tried in small studies of patients with chronic HBV and found to confer no benefit.

THYMIC HORMONES

A number of natural and synthetic thymic hormones as potentiators of lymphocyte maturation and function have been investigated as possible therapy for chronic HBV infection. In one of the larger studies,[15] 30 patients were randomized to receive thymopentin or no therapy; no benefit was demonstrated. In a smaller study,[16] nine patients who had failed to respond to interferon monotherapy received thymus humoral factor-γ-2 and interferon-α for 2 months and then interferon-α as monotherapy for a further 2 months. Three of the patients cleared HBeAg.

LEVAMISOLE AND INOSINE PRANOBEX

Levamisole and inosine pranobex, agents with immunostimulatory effects, appear of no clinical benefit for therapy of chronic HBV infection.

VACCINE THERAPY

Reports of 32 patients given three doses of a hepatitis B vaccine containing HBsAg and pre-S2 protein resulted in HBV DNA levels becoming undetectable in 10 (31%) patients and decreased in 4 (13%) at 3 months.[17]

A lipopeptide-based therapeutic vaccine inducing HBV-specific cytotoxic T lymphocyte responses[18] is undergoing investigation.

NUCLEOSIDE ANALOGS: ADENINE ARABINOSIDE AND ADENINE ARABINOSIDE MONOPHOSPHATE

Adenine arabinoside (ara-A) has inhibitory effects on HBV replication and has been studied in patients.[19] It is water insoluble and has to be administered by intravenous injection. This has limited its routine use. In contrast, the monophosphorylated derivative, adenine arabinoside monophosphate (ara-AMP), is water soluble and can be administered intramuscularly, which makes it a more practical option. Neurotoxicity was reported with prolonged use. In one study[20] comparing alternating courses of ara-AMP and interferon with ara-AMP monotherapy and placebo, the clearance rate of HBeAg was highest in the placebo group. Patients who received longer therapy with ara-AMP complained of painful dysesthesia of the peripheries, and discontinuation of ara-AMP did not always lead to a reversal.

In an attempt to circumvent the long-term toxicity, a 1 month course of ara-AMP was administered[20a] and repeated after 6 months. In 60 patients, 17% of those with low levels of viral replication group and none of those in the higher replication group cleared HBeAg. Small studies have reported promising results with the combination of corticosteroid and ara-AMP.[21,22]

ACYCLOVIR

Acyclovir is a nucleoside analog used mainly as therapy for herpes virus infections. It usually requires the herpes simplex or varicella zoster virus thymidine kinase enzyme to convert it to its monophosphate form; subsequent phosphorylations are performed by host enzymes. HBV does not possess thymidine kinase activity, and acyclovir would not be expected to have any inhibitory effect. In high intravenous doses, however, an inhibitory effect on HBV replication has been observed. In a pilot study,[23] few patients cleared HBV. Longer courses of therapy have been limited by the need for intravenous administration because oral acyclovir has only about 30% bioavailability.

FAMCICLOVIR

Famciclovir is the prodrug for penciclovir, which is another nucleoside analog with activity against herpes simplex and varicella zoster viruses. It also requires thymidine kinase activity for the initial phosphorylation. Penciclovir and famciclovir have been shown to inhibit duck hepatitis B viral replication in the Pekin duck model. In a pilot study[24] in patients with chronic HBV, there was a greater than 90% decrease in HBV DNA in 6 of 11 evaluable patients treated with a 10-day course of oral famciclovir. An anecdotal report suggested that famciclovir may be beneficial in controlling HBV viremia after hepatic transplantation.[25]

FIALURIDINE

Preliminary studies with fialuridine (FIAU) appeared promising, with a more sustained reduction in HBV DNA levels than is generally seen with short courses of nucleoside analogs. Trials with more prolonged treatment periods were disbanded when fatalities occurred.[26] One patient developed lactic acidosis and 7 of the 13 patients were found to have severe hepatoxicity. Other symptoms suggestive of peripheral neuropathy or myopathy occurred.

LAMIVUDINE

Lamivudine, 3′-thiacytidine, (3TC) has inhibitory effects on reverse transcriptase activity. This has led to its use against HIV. HBV also has reverse transcriptase activity and within a few days of initiation of therapy, a dramatic fall is seen in the HBV DNA levels. A decrease in aminotransferase values often occurs with treatment for 1 month.[27] A subsequent study with a longer treatment period confirmed that lamivudine is well tolerated in patients with chronic HBV.[28]

Lamivudine appears to be well tolerated. Gastrointestinal symptoms have been reported. Lamivudine has been given prior to and after transplantation. Short-term results appear promising, with reports of some patients clearing HBsAg. However, with long-term term monotherapy in immunosuppressed individuals, there are now reports of development of viral resistance.

Mathematical models suggest that prolonged viral inhibition with antiviral agents such as lamivudine may lead to viral eradication in patients with active liver disease.[2] It was estimated that the plasma half-life of HBV particles in patients receiving lamivudine was about 1 day, implying a 50% daily turnover of the free virus population, with about 10^{11} viral particles being released daily. The half-life of viral producing cells varied from 10 to 100 days depending on the degree of cell lysis in the individual patient. Such studies may help determine the length of future antiviral therapy and whether additional immunotherapy is needed.

RIBAVIRIN

Ribavirin (1-B-D-ribofuranosyl 1,2,4-triazole-3-carboxamide), a guanosine analogue, has broad-spectrum antiviral activity, although its mode of action is not fully understood. In one study of 18 patients with chronic HBV, ribavirin given for 6 months resulted only in a transient reduction in HBV DNA levels.[29]

TREATMENT OF SPECIAL PATIENT GROUPS: DECOMPENSATED LIVER DISEASE

Interferon-α in the standard doses can lead to further hepatic decompensation because of immune lysis of infected hepatocytes. If interferon-α is administered to those patients, lower doses should be used.[30]

HIV INFECTION

The patient with HIV and HBV coinfection is much less likely to respond to interferon-α,[31,4] and the myelotoxicity of interferon-α may complicate therapy with other agents such as zidovudine or ganciclovir. If the patient is prescribed antiretroviral therapy, a combination approach including lamivudine may be necessary.

TRANSPLANTATION

Following transplantation, graft infection by HBV is inevitable for the patient with chronic HBV. High levels of viral replication due to immunosuppression lead to rapid graft failure. Without antiviral intervention, 1-year survival figures are only 50%.

In theory, interferon-α may increase the risk of graft rejection with increased host immune recognition. Although this does not seem to be a major problem in practice, interferon-α as monotherapy is unlikely to lead to the clearance of HBV in this setting, and other approaches are being developed. Famciclovir therapy is under study following the report of a case in Germany[25] and in pilot studies describing the inhibitory effects on HBV replication.[24]

CHILDREN

In one prospective controlled study,[33] 77 children were randomized to receive interferon α at a dose of 3 or 7.5 MU/m^2 three times a week for 6 months or no treatment. Twelve months after the cessation of therapy, HBeAg had been cleared in 30% of those on the higher dose of interferon, 21% on the lower dose, and 13.5% in those who were untreated.

HBeAg-NEGATIVE VARIANTS

It has been recognized for some time that a subgroup of patients with chronic HBV were HBeAg negative and anti-HBe positive with circulating HBV DNA and chronic hepatitis. It was found that these patients were infected with a variant of HBV with a mutation in the precore region.[34] It is unclear how many with this HBV variant were infected de novo by the variant and how many had mutation in an infecting wild-type virus. Interferon-α has been used to treat such patients, but unfortunately there is a very high relapse rate. In one of the largest studies, 50 patients were randomized to receive either low-dose interferon (3 MU three times a week) or no treatment. One year after the initiation of therapy, 11 of the 17 (65%) evaluable patients in the treatment arm had normalization of the aminotransferase values. Subsequent follow-up showed a high relapse rate. Brunetto et al.[35] reported similar results.

CHRONIC HEPATITIS C

Hepatitis C virus (HCV) is the cause of more than 90% of cases of chronic non-A, non-B hepatitis. A successful response to therapy of HCV infection is now generally defined to be the sustained loss (at least 6 months) of HCV RNA from the serum, and this is associated with improvement in the necroinflammatory and fibrosis scores of the liver biopsy.[36] As with chronic HBV, it is hoped that curtailing the hepatic damage with successful antiviral therapy will reduce the lifetime risk of long-term sequelae, including HCC.

INTERFERON-α

Pilot studies for treating chronic HCV infection with interferon-α[37] resulted in a decrease in aminotransferase values within a few days. Larger controlled trials confirmed these findings[38–44] (Table 28-2) and the associated sustained loss of HCV RNA. Histologic improvement also accompanied these findings. Although 50% of those treated responded to interferon, approximately 50% relapsed following discontinuation of therapy, giving an overall sustained response rate of 20% to 25%.

Interferon schedules for treating chronic HCV infection use lower doses and longer duration than those for treating HBV infection. The side effects are generally less than reported with treating HBV infection, but there appears to be a higher risk of the development of autoimmune disease. It is generally recommended that autoantibodies associated with thyroid and liver disease be screened at baseline. Hepatitis C virus is itself associated with autoimmune phenomena that theoretically can be made worse with interferon.

There is increasing evidence that more prolonged courses of interferon (longer than the usual 6 months) are associated with higher sustained response rates in chronic HCV infection. In a study of 40 patients treated with 3 MU three times a week for 60 weeks, alanine aminotransferase (ALT) values were normal in 24 (60%) patients and remained normal in 15 (38%) patients at the end of treatment. HCV RNA was undetectable in 17 of the 24 responders in the follow-up period. In a randomized controlled study[45] of 108 patients, 6 months of interferon was compared with 12 months, and significantly better biochemical results (29% versus 13%) followed the longer treatment period. This study also demonstrated that patients with cirrhosis were less likely to

TABLE 28-2. Treatment of Chronic HCV With Interferon-α Monotherapy

		Treated			Control		
Dose (MU)	Schedule (Frequency; Weeks)	No. of Patients	No. of Patients with Normalization or Near Normalization in ALT (%)	Sustained Remission at Follow-up (%)	No. of Patients	No. of Patients with Normalization or Near Normalization in ALT (%)	Author, Year (Ref.)
3	tiw; 24	58	26 (45)	38	51	4 (8)	Davis et al., 1989[39]
2	tiw; 24	21	13 (62)	10	20	0	DiBisceglie et al., 1989[40]
3	tiw; 24	28	16 (56)	13	29	6 (20)	Causse et al., 1991[41]
3	tiw; 24	26	18 (69)	30	25	1 (4)	Saracco et al., 1990[43]
3	tiw; 24	18	13 (72)	29	18	3 (17)	Marcellin et al., 1991[44]
3	tiw; 24	33	17 (52)	30	33	0	Cimino et al., 1991[42]

respond to interferon (<10%). More recent studies have also confirmed that the relapse rate can be reduced by longer treatment regimens.[46]

In one large randomized trial[47] 174 patients were randomized to receive a 12-month course of interferon at a starting dose of 6 MU three times week and then titrated according to the biochemical response (group A), 3 MU three times a week for 12 months (group B) or 6 MU three times a week for 6 months (group C). Twelve months after cessation of therapy a sustained biochemical response was recorded in 49% of those in group A, 31% in group B, and 28% in group C. In those patients with genotype 1b infection, the response rate was 28% with treatment A, 16% with treatment B, and only 9% with treatment C.

Not all studies support the use of longer treatment courses. In one study,[48] 116 patients with post-transfusion hepatitis C were randomized to receive either 6- or 12-month courses of interferon. The rate of sustained response was lower than reported in other studies with similar results in both groups (18.3% and 18.4%). The predominant genotype in this group was type 1, which has been reported to be associated with a more rapidly progressive outcome and with less chance of responding to interferon.

Re-evaluation of a pilot study of interferon therapy for chronic HCV showed that in a follow-up period of 3 to 6 years, HCV RNA remained undetectable in the six patients with a sustained biochemical response.[49] A sustained virologic response with negative PCR for HCV RNA 6 months after cessation of therapy appears the best predictor of sustained response. Repeat liver biopsies in patients with a successful response to interferon have shown a reduction in the inflammatory and fibrotic activity.[36]

PREDICTIVE FACTORS DETERMINING RESPONSE TO INTERFERON: VIRAL FACTORS

The genotype and pretreatment viremia level may be important in determining the response to treatment. In one Italian study[50] of interferon-α therapy, 74% of 19 patients with genotype 3 HCV had a long-term response compared with 52% of 23 patients with genotype 2 and 29% of 65 with genotype 1 infection. Genotype 1b is particularly associated with a poor chance of sustained response.[51] Patients with type 1b infection tend to be older with more advanced disease and higher levels of viremia, and it has been suggested that host and viral factors also may independently influence outcome. The most recent studies on larger numbers of patients suggest that genotype may be an independent variable.[52]

Lower levels of HCV RNA were found to predict a successful response to interferon.[53] Detailed virologic analysis of the first few weeks of the interferon regimen have shown that a virologic response early in the course of treatment may help predict a sustained virologic response.[54,55] Clearance of HCV RNA by the second or third month of treatment appears to predict a sustained response.

HOST FACTORS

Patients with HIV infection and a CD4 count of greater than 500/mm^3 have a similar chance of responding to interferon as those not infected with HIV.[56] There have been concerns, however, regarding decreases seen in the CD4 count when some patients with HIV/HCV have received interferon-α and the long-term outcome in these patients remains unknown.

Other host factors that may affect a response to interferon-α include cirrhosis; patients with cirrhosis are less likely to respond. Iron stores have also been found to be of importance, and the observation that patients with lower iron stores were more likely to respond to interferon has led to trials with chelating agents and venesection. Obese patients are also less likely to respond to interferon, but presumably this is related to dosing of interferon. Patients with elevated γ-GTP also have a poor sustained response rate.

HEPATOCELLULAR CARCINOMA AFTER INTERFERON TREATMENT

There is now increasing evidence that interferon therapy may reduce or delay the subsequent development of HCC. In one study,[57] 90 patients with HCV-associated cirrhosis were randomized to receive either interferon-α for 12 to 24 weeks (45 patients) or symptomatic therapy (45 patients). The patients were followed for 2 to 7 years. Only 7 (45%) of the treated patients had undetectable HCV RNA at the cessation of therapy. The treatment group had a much lower prevalence of hepatocellular carcinoma (4%) than the control group (38%). The authors suggest that the immunomodulatory effects of interferon and possible enhanced tumor cell recognition by the immune system may be responsible for these results. The direct antiproliferative effects of interferon may also be important.[58]

In another study,[11] the incidence and risk of developing HCC were studied in 385 patients with HCV-associated cirrhosis who were followed for 32 months. Interferon-α resulted in a fourfold reduction in the risk of the development of HCC.

RIBAVIRIN

A pilot study showed that the administration of ribavirin led to a decrease in ALT values in a group of patients with HCV.[59] Subsequent studies have demonstrated only a modest effect on viral replication, with very little change in the HCV RNA levels. In combination with interferon, improvement in the virologic response rates has been reported with ribavirin.[60,61] The main side effect is hemolysis and the hemoglobin therefore has to be carefully monitored.[62]

REFERENCES

1. Greenberg HB, Pollard RB, Lutwick LI et al. Effect of human leucocyte interferon on hepatitis B virus infection in patients with chronic active hepatitis. N Engl J Med 1976;295: 517–522
2. Nowak MA, Bonhoeffer S, Hill AM et al. Viral dynamics in hepatitis B virus infection. Proc Natl Acad Sci USA 1996; 93:4398–4402
3. Korenman J, Baker B, Waggoner J et al. Long term remissions of chronic hepatitis B after alpha interferon. Ann Intern Med 1991;114:629–634
4. Brook MG, Chan G, Yap I et al. Randomised controlled trial of lymphoblastoid interferon alfa in Europid men with chronic hepatitis B virus infection. Br Med J 1989;299: 652–656
5. Perrillo RP, Schiff ER, Davis GL et al. A randomised controlled trial of interferon alfa-2b alone and after prednisone withdrawal for the treatment of chronic hepatitis B. N Engl J Med 1990;323:295–301
6. Alexander GJM, Brahm J, Fagan E et al. Loss of HBsAg with interferon therapy for chronic HBV. Lancet 1987;ii:66–69
7. Dusheiko GM, Kassianides C, Song E et al. Loss of hepatitis B surface antigen in three controlled trials of recombinant interferon alpha-interferon for treatment of chronic hepatitis B. In Zuckerman AJ (ed): Viral Hepatitis and Liver Disease.
8. Lai CL, Lok ASF, Lin HJ et al. Placebo-controlled trial of recombinant alfa-2-interferon (rIFN) in Chinese HBsAg carrier children. Lancet 1987;ii:877–880
9. Brook MG, Karayiannis P, Thomas HC. Which patients with chronic hepatitis B virus infection will respond to alpha-interferon therapy? A statistical analysis of predictive factors. Hepatology 1989;10:761–763
10. Niederau C, Heintges T, Lange S et al. Long-term follow-up of HBeAg positive patients treated with interferon alfa for chronic hepatitis B. N Engl J Med 1996;334:1422–1427
11. Mazzella G, Accogli E, Sottili S et al. Alpha interferon treatment may prevent hepatocellular carcinoma in HCV-related liver cirrhosis. J Hepatol 1996;24:141–147
12. Perrillo R, Regenstein R, Peters M et al. Prednisone withdrawal followed by recombinant alpha interferon in the treatment of chronic type B hepatitis. A randomized controlled trial. Ann Intern Med 1988;109:95–100
13. Liaw Y-F, Lin S-M, Chen T-J et al. Beneficial effect of prednisolone withdrawal followed by human lymphoblastoid interferon on the treatment of chronic type B hepatitis in Asians: a randomised controlled trial. J Hepatol 1994;20: 175–180
14. Lok ASF, Wu PC, Lai CL et al. A controlled trial of interferon with or without prednisone priming for chronic hepatitis B. Gastroenterology 1992;102:2091–2097
14a. Capalbo M, Palmisano L, Bonino F et al. Intramuscular natural beta interferon in the treatment of chronic hepatitis B: a multicentre trial. Ital J Gastroenterol 1994;26:238–241
15. Fattovich G, Giustina G, Alberti A et al. A randomised controlled trial of thymopentin therapy in patients with chronic hepatitis B. J Hepatol 1994;21:361–366
16. Farhat BA, Marinos G, Daniels HM et al. Evaluation of efficacy and safety of thymus humoral factor-gamma 2 in the management of chronic hepatitis B. J Hepatol 1995;23: 21–27
17. Pol S, Driss F, Michel M-L et al. Specific vaccine therapy in chronic hepatitis B infection. Lancet 1994;344:342
18. Vitiello A, Ishioka G, Grey HM et al. Development of a

lipopeptide-based therapeutic vaccine to treat chronic HBV infection. J Clin Invest 1995;95:341–349

19. Bassendine MF, Chadwick RG, Salmeron J. Adenine arabinoside therapy in HBsAg-positive chronic liver disease: a controlled study. Gastroenterology 1981;80:1016–1021
20. Garcia G, Smith CI, Weissberg JI et al. Adenine arabinoside monophosphate (vidarabine phosphate) in combination with human leukocyte interferon in the treatment of chronic hepatitis B. Ann Intern Med 1987;107:278–285

20a. Marcellin P, Pouteau M, Lorrat MA et al. Adenosine arabinoside 5′-monophosphate in patients with chronic hepatitis B: comparison of the efficacy in patients with high and low viral replication. Gut 1995;36:422–426

21. Yokosuka O, Omata M, Imazeki F et al. Combination of short term prednisolone and adenine arabinoside in the treatment of chronic hepatitis B. Gastroenterology 1985;89: 246–251
22. Perrillo R, Regenstein F, Bodicky C et al. Comparative efficacy of adenine arabinoside 5′-monophosphate and prednisone withdrawal followed by adenine arabinoside 5′-monophosphate in the treatment of chronic active hepatitis type B. Gastroenterology 1985;88:780–786
23. Weller IVD, Carreno V, Fowler MJF et al. Acyclovir inhibits hepatitis B viral replication in man. Lancet 1982;i:273
24. Main J, Brown JL, Karayiannis P et al. A double blind placebo-controlled study to assess the effect of famciclovir in virus replication in patients with chronic hepatitis B virus infection. J Viral Hepatitis 1996;3:211–215
25. Boker KH, Ringe B, Kruger M et al. Prostaglandin E plus famciclovir—a new concept for the treatment of severe hepatitis B after liver transplantation. Transplantation 1994;57: 1706–1708
26. McKenzie R Fried MW, Sallie R et al. Hepatic failure and lactic acidosis due to fialuridine (FIAU), an investigational nucleoside analogue for chronic hepatitis B. N Engl J Med 1995;333:1099–1105
27. Tyrrell DLJ, Mitchell MC, De Man RA et al. Phase II trial of lamivudine for chronic hepatitis B. Hepatology 1993; 18(suppl):112A
28. Dienstag JL, Perrillo RP, Schiff ER et al. A preliminary trial of lamivudine for chronic hepatitis B infection. N Engl J Med 1995;333:1657–1661
29. Fried MW, Fong T-L, Swain MG et al. Therapy of chronic hepatitis B with a 6 month course of ribavirin. J Hepatol 1994;21:145–150
30. Kassianides C, Di Bisceglie AM, Hoofangle JH et al. Alpha interferon therapy in patients with decompensated chronic type B hepatitis. In Zuckerman AJ (ed): Viral Hepatitis and Liver Disease. Alan R Liss, London, 1988, pp. 840–843
31. McDonald JA, Caruso L, Karayiannis P et al. Diminished responsiveness of male homosexual chronic hepatitis B virus carriers with HTLV-III antibodies to recombinant alpha-interferon. Hepatology 1987;7:719–723
32. Davies S, Portman B, O'Grady J et al. Hepatic histological findings after transplantation for chronic hepatitis B virus infection including a unique pattern of fibrosing cholestatic hepatitis. Hepatology 1991;13:150–157
33. Barbera C, Bortolotti F, Crivellaro C et al. Recombinant interferon alpha hastens the rate of HBeAg clearance in children with chronic hepatitis B. Hepatol 1994;20:287–290
34. Carman WF, Jacyna MR, Hadziyannis S et al. Mutation preventing formation of hepatitis B e antigen in chronic hepatitis B virus infection. Lancet 1989;ii:588–591
35. Brunetto MR, Oliveri F, Demartini A et al. Treatment with interferon of chronic hepatitis B associated with antibody to hepatitis B e antigen. J Hepatol 1991;13(suppl 1):S8–S11
36. Hiramatsu N, Hayashi N, Kasahara A et al. Improvement of liver fibrosis in chronic hepatitis C patients treated with natural interferon alpha. J Hepatol 1995;22:135–142
37. Hoofnagle JH, Mullen KD, Jones DB et al. Treatment of chronic non-A, non-B hepatitis with recombinant human alpha interferon: a preliminary report. N Engl J Med 1986; 315:1575–1578
38. Jacyna MR, Brooks MG, Loke RHT et al. Randomised controlled trial of interferon alfa (lymphoblastoid interferon) in chronic non-A, non-B hepatitis. Br Med J 1989;298:80–82
39. Davis GL, Balart LA, Schiff ER. Treatment of chronic hepatitis C with recombinant interferon alpha. N Engl J Med 1989;321:1501–1506
40. Di Bisceglie AM, Martin P, Kassianides C et al. Recombinant interferon alfa therapy for chronic hepatitis C: a randomized double blind placebo-controlled trial. N Engl J Med 1989;321:1506–1510
41. Causse X, Godinot H, Chevallier M et al. Comparison of 1 or 3 MU of interferon alfa-2b and placebo in patients with chronic non-A, non-B hepatitis. Gastroenterology 1991; 101:497–502
42. Cimino L, Nardone G, Citarella C et al. Treatment of chronic hepatitis C with recombinant interferon alfa. Ital J Gastroenterol 1991;23:399–402
43. Saracco G, Rosina F, Torrani-Cerenzia MR et al. A randomised controlled trial of interferon alfa 2b as therapy for chronic non-A, non-B hepatitis. J Hepatol 1990;11:S34–49
44. Marcellin P, Boyer N, Giostra E et al. Recombinant human alpha-interferon in patients with chronic non-A, non-B hepatitis. A multi-centre randomised controlled trial from France. Hepatology 1991;13:393–397
45. Jouet P, Roudot-Thorval F, Dhumeaux D et al. Comparative efficacy of interferon alfa in cirrhotic and non-cirrhotic patients with non-A, non-B, C hepatitis. Gastroenterology 1994;106:686–690
46. Poynard T, Bedossa P, Chevallier M et al. A comparison of three interferon alfa-2b regimens for the long-term treatment of chronic non-A, non-B hepatitis. N Engl J Med 1995;332: 1457–1462
47. Chemello L, Bonetti P, Cavalletto L et al. Randomized trial comparing three different regimens of alpha-2a interferon in chronic hepatitis C. Hepatology 1995;22:700–706
48. Craxi A, Di Marco V, Lo Iacono O et al. Transfusion-associated chronic hepatitis C: alpha-n1 interferon for 6 vs 12 months. J Hepatol 1996;24:539–546
49. Shindo M, Di Bisceglie AM, Hoofnagle JH. Long-term follow-up of patients with chronic hepatitis C treated with alpha interferon. Hepatology 1992;15:1013–1016
50. Chemello L, Alberti A, Rose K, Simmonds P. Hepatitis C

serotype and response to interferon therapy (letter). N Engl J Med 1994;330:143

51. Kanai K, Kato M, Okamato H. HCV genotypes in chronic hepatitis C and response to interferon. Lancet 1992;339: 1543
52. Simmonds P, Mellor J, Craxi A et al. Epidemiological, clinical and therapeutic associations of hepatitis C types in western European patients. J Hepatol 1996;24:517–524
53. Yun ZB, Reichard O, Chen M, et al. Serum hepatitis C RNA levels in chronic hepatitis C—importance for outcome of interferon alfa-2b treatment. Scand J Infect Dis 1994;26: 263–270
54. Hino K, Okuda M, Konishi T et al. Serial assay of hepatitis C virus RNA in serum for predicting response to interferon alpha therapy. Dig Dis Sci 1995;40:14–20
55. Booth JCL, Foster GR, Kumar U et al. Chronic hepatitis C virus infection; predictive value of genotype and level of viraemia on disease progression and response to interferon alpha. Gut 1995;36:427–432
56. Soriano V, Garcia-Samaniego J, Bravo R et al. Efficacy and safety of alpha interferon treatment for chronic hepatitis C in HIV infected patients. J Infect 1995;31:9–13
57. Nishiguchi S, Kuroki T, Nakatani S et al. Randomised trial of effects of interferon alpha on incidence of hepatocellular carcinoma in chronic active hepatitis C with cirrhosis. Lancet 1995;346:1051–1055
58. Harada H, Kitagawa M, Tanaka N et al. Anti-oncogenic and oncogenic potentials of interferon regulatory factors-1 and -2. Science 1993;259:971–974
59. Reichard O, Andersson J, Schvarcz R, Weiland O. Ribavirin treatment for chronic hepatitis C. Lancet 1991;337: 1058–1061
60. Chemello L, Cavaletto L, Bernardinello E et al. Response to ribavirin, to interferon and to a combination of both in patients with chronic hepatitis C and its relation to HCV genotypes. J Hepatol 1994;21(suppl 1):S12
61. Brillanti S, Garson J, Foli M et al. A pilot study of combination therapy with ribavirin plus interferon alfa for interferon resistant chronic hepatitis C. Gastroenterology 1994;107: 812–817
62. Di Bisceglie AM, Bacon BR, Kleiner DE, Hoofnagle JH. Increase in hepatic iron stores following prolonged therapy with ribavirin in patients with chronic hepatitis C. J Hepatol 1994;21:1109–1112

29

TREATMENT SELECTION

KUNIO OKUDA
KENICHI TAKAYASU
SHUICHI OKADA

Physicians with patients who have hepatocellular carcinoma (HCC) may need to select treatment. Since subsequent chapters discuss individual treatment modalities, this chapter will focus on what is necessary for selection of treatment. Because each patient differs from others in terms of size, number, and location of tumors, cancer pathology, underlying liver disease, coexisting disease, etc, each patient has to be evaluated without a universal scale. In southern Africa, early diagnosis was almost never achieved in the past among black patients, and treatment was seldom indicated because of the advanced stage of the tumor and the rapidly downhill clinical course. However, the situation is changing for blacks in South Africa. Japanese scientists pioneered in developing screening programs for early detection and treatment of small HCC. Therefore, we will discuss the treatment policy generally used in Japan and, more specifically, at the National Cancer Center Hospital, Tokyo.

GENERAL POLICY FOR TREATMENT SELECTION

Assessment of General Status of the Disease and Patient

The physical examination is used to determine whether the patient is severely ill and cachetic, or physically well enough to tolerate any mode of treatment. The size of tumor may be roughly estimated by palpation of the liver if it is very large, but ultrasound and abdominal computed tomography (CT) are most useful in the assessment of the mass with respect to number, size, and location. If the mass is greater than 4 to 5 cm, one has to make efforts to see whether extrahepatic metastases have already occurred. In the absence of visible signs of metastases, chest radiograph and perhaps abdominal CT scan are desirable. Bone scan and gallium scan of the whole body may be necessary under certain circumstances.

Presence of Extrahepatic Metastasis

When extrahepatic metastasis can be identified, systemic chemotherapy is used. Our study in 105 patients with advanced HCC (Okuda's stage III) demonstrated a significant beneficial effect of systemic chemotherapy; all 62 untreated patients died in 3 months, whereas 43 who were treated with either arterial or systemic chemotherapy had a significantly longer survival.[1] Patients at the brink of death may not benefit from chemotherapy.

In occasional situations, extrahepatic metastasis can be treated surgically. Surgery can be considered if the metastasis is single and the HCC in the liver is under control or will be effectively controlled. We have seen three cases in whom resection was successfully carried out and subsequently an adrenal metastasis was detected. Removal of the adrenal metastasis prolonged survival significantly.[2] In another patient, there was one medium-sized HCC in the liver and a lymph node metastasis behind the head of the pancreas. Both were surgically resected, and the patient lived without recurrence for more than 2 years and 8 months.[3]

Absence of Extrahepatic Metastasis

In the absence of demonstrable extrahepatic metastasis, surgical resection should always be considered as the first line of therapy. It calls for a careful assessment of operative risk based on the functional reserve of the liver and tumor status, as discussed in the chapter on hepatic resection. Not only the size and number of tumors, but location of the tumor has to be considered. If it is located near a large hepatic vein or a junction of large portal veins, even a small HCC may require resection that includes extensive portions of the adjoining liver. In patients with compromised functional reserve, the size of the resection may seriously affect the prognosis. If there is a definite risk, the treatment decision may vary with the physician and surgeon. However, in a situation where the liver function reserve is relatively good and the tumor is small, or where a small HCC is located in an easily resected location such as the lateral portion of the left lobe, then the surgical approach should be chosen.

RESECTION

The liver function tests, the number of tumor nodules and the locations of the tumor(s) are the main factors that determine resectability. Large tumor size is not a contraindication because if the liver is not very cirrhotic, even a huge mass may be removed if it is solitary. A large solitary HCC is often found to be encapsulated in patients in Asia; it may lack intrahepatic spread or portal invasion.[4] Spreading or infiltrating growth[5] portends early recurrence because intrahepatic spread has most likely taken place. Technically, even surgical resection of large tumors is now possible. At our hospital, the resection rate for HCCs greater than 10 cm in diameter was 61.3% (19/31). There was encapsulation in 94.7%, intrahepatic spread in 78.9%, portal tumor thrombosis in 94.7%, and postoperative recurrence in 76.5%. Nevertheless, with multidisciplinary treatment, the 5-year survival was 52.1% compared to a 1-year survival of 10.4% among nonresected cases (n = 12).[6]

Portal vein tumor thrombus is one of the important adverse prognostic factors. However, our study of 104 consecutive cases of HCC with portal vein thrombus in a 9-year period up to 1988 showed a significant difference in survival rate depending on hepatic function and portal invasion. The survival rates for Child A and B patients and Child C patients were 60.8% and 20.0% respectively at 1 year, and 35.4% and 5.5%, respectively at 3 years.[7] If liver function permits, resection excels over nonsurgical treatment in patients with portal vein invasion.

In a study conducted by the Liver Cancer Study Group of Japan, prognostic factors were portal vein invasion, age, cirrhosis, number of tumors, α-fetoprotein (AFP) level, and tumor size.[8] These factors for "resectability" also apply to patients who are treated non-surgically, and should not play a major role in the decision of a surgical vs a nonsurgical approach.

Liver transplantation is possible in a very limited number of patients. It seems best indicated for patients with small HCCs found in livers with very advanced cirrhosis who will die either from cancer or cirrhosis without transplantation.

When surgery is not possible, patients in whom one or two (three at most) small HCCs were detected by the screening program or were detected incidentally are considered separately from patients who have HCC(s) larger than 4 cm.[9]

There are cases in whom the functional reserve is not very good, but surgery may be tolerated if it is a small resection or enucleation of the mass. Such patients can also be treated by transcatheter arterial embolization (TAE).

If the functional reserve of the liver is good and all lesions are in the same lobe, resection is the first choice of treatment. If all lesions are located at sites identifiable by ultrasound, some hepatologists may prefer to treat with percutaneous ethanol injection (PEI). If the patient is in Child C status or the functional reserve is poor, PEI is the best choice. Post-treatment tumor recurrence is almost equally frequent after resection[10] and PEI.[11] Figure 29-1 shows our data at the National Cancer Center Hospital from patients with fewer than 3 HCCs less than 3 cm in diameter who were treated from 1990 to 1994. The disease-free survival was virtually the same between 40 patients treated with PEI (median survival = 21.9 months) and 55 treated with resection (medial survival = 22.8 months). The cause of death was recurrence in the majority of patients. The 3-year survival was slightly better with resection; cancer death was slightly more frequent with PEI. Transcatheter arterial embolization (TAE) or transcatheter arterial embolization in which Lipiodol injection precedes Gelfoam particle embolization is usually less effective compared with PEI. Lipiodol alone has very little anticancer effect.[12] However, with the availability of a very thin catheter and an improved catheter guiding system, subsegmental arteries can now be catheterized.[13] TAE, through the feeding subsegmental artery, is almost as effective as PEI in inducing necrosis of small HCCs. Less commonly, TAE can be used to catheterize the feeding segmental artery and inject a large amount of Lipiodol containing an anticancer agent, so that Lipiodol flows beyond the tumor into the feeding portal vein, augmenting the embolization effect.[14] For a very early HCC that has not yet developed its own neovasculature, TAE has little effect.[15]

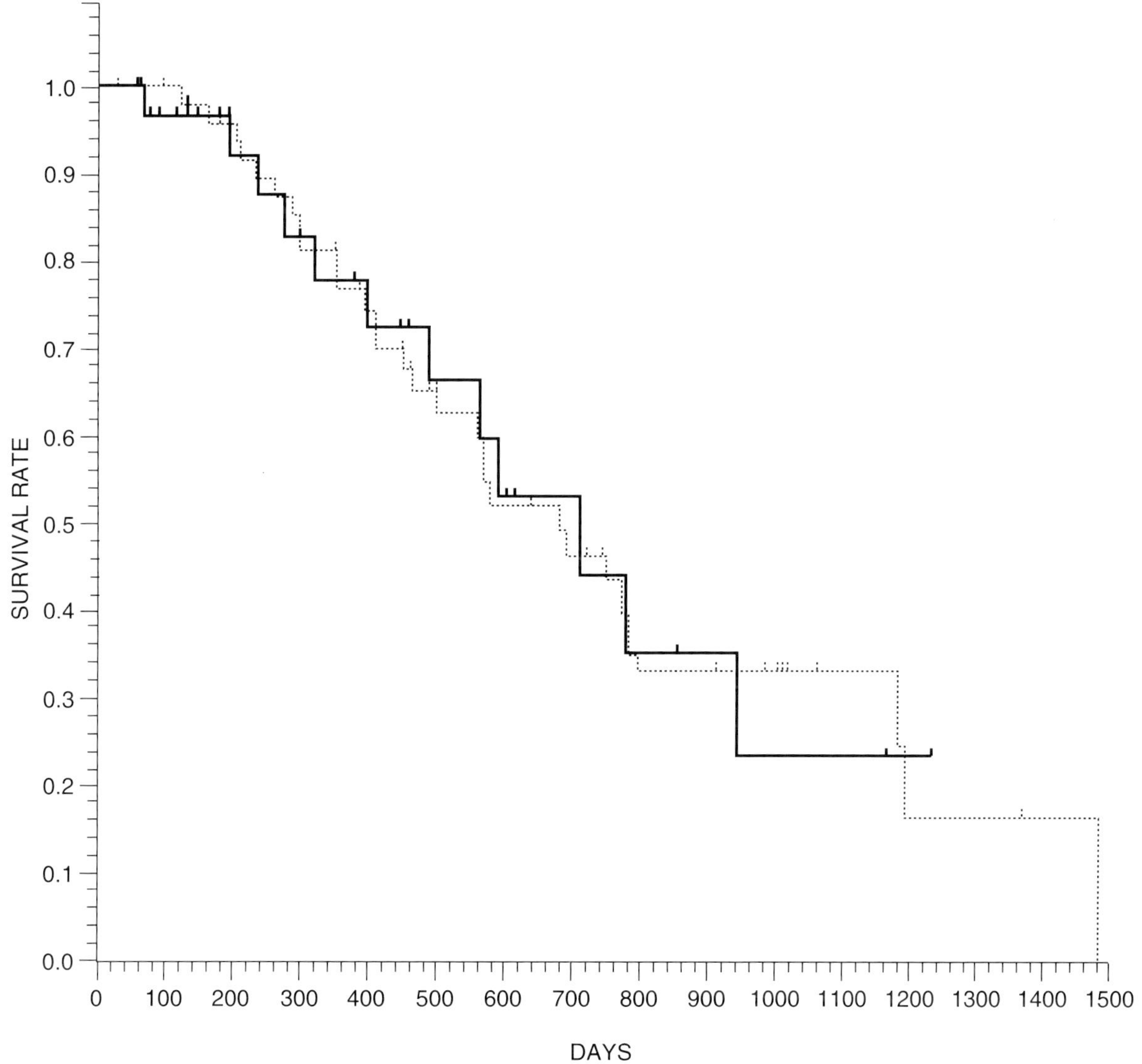

FIGURE 29-1. Disease-free survival for HCC patients treated with percutaneous ethanol injection (PEI) or resection at the National Cancer Center Hospital, Tokyo. (PEI n = 40; resection n = 55). There was no significant difference.

Even when a patient has a tumor greater than 4 cm in diameter or more than four nodules, if the nodules are in one lobe and functional reserve is good, resection is still the first choice of therapy. Otherwise, TAE or transcatheter arterial chemoembolization can be done. There have been attempts to treat large HCCs with PEI alone or in combination with TAE,[16,17] but the results are unclear.

In the case of HCCs greater than 4 cm in diameter or more than four in number, TAE should be attempted unless the tumor is widespread within the liver. Catheterization should be as selective as possible to avoid damage to the liver parenchyma. An important precaution with TAE is a large tumor thrombus in a major (trunk or the first order) portal vein; after embolization in TAE, it will immediately trigger progressive hepatic failure due to lack of blood flow within the liver.

If the disease is so advanced that TAE is deemed ineffective or hazardous, arterial chemotherapy should be chosen whenever possible. A catheter is placed in the common hepatic artery, either surgically (through the gastroduodenal artery) or through the femoral or subclavian artery, with the distal end connected to a subcutaneously implanted reservoir. (The catheter is also in the common hepatic artery, but the gastroduodenal artery has to be occluded by a steel coil to prevent the drug from flowing toward the stomach and duodenum.) Systemic intravenous chemotherapy seldom proves effica-

Smaller than 3 cm, less than 3

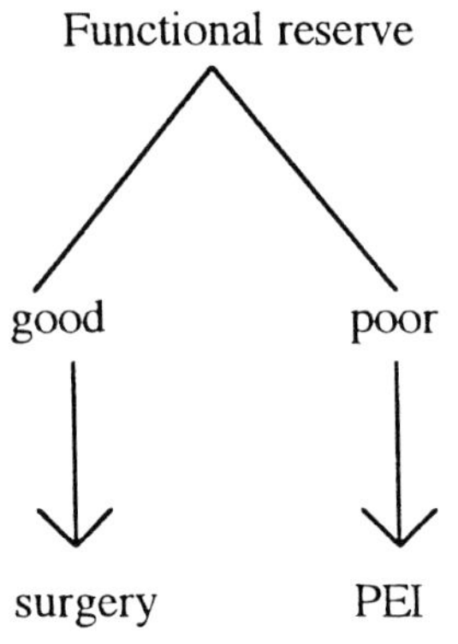

Larger than 4 cm, more than 4

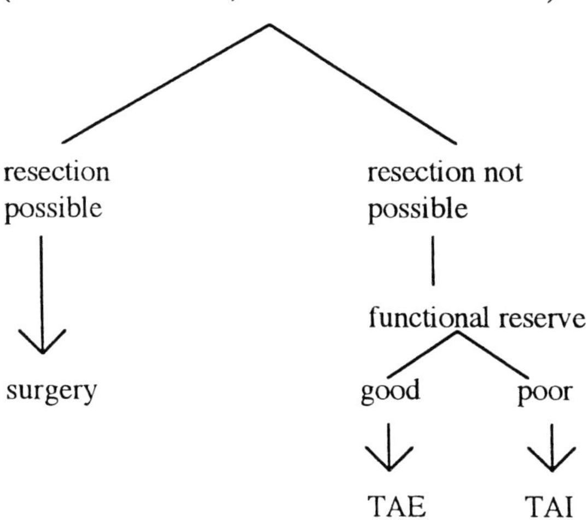

FIGURE 29-2. Flow chart for treatment selection based on HCC size and number (National Cancer Center Hospital, Tokyo). PEI, percutaneous ethanol injection; TAE, transcatheter arterial embolization; TAI, transcatheter arterial chemotherapy.

cious.[18–20] Figure 29-2 and 29-3 are the flow charts currently used at the National Cancer Center Hospital, Tokyo, for a treatment selection based on tumor size and number. The actual distribution of the patients who received the three main treatment modalities, surgery, PEI, and TAE, are depicted in relation to the hepatic functional reserve and stage of tumor progression in Fig. 29-4.

SUMMARY

The three main therapeutic modalities currently used for HCC are hepatic resection, TAE, and PEI. Whenever liver function permits, resection should be considered as first choice. If surgery is not indicated, PEI or TAE should be carried out, depending on tumor size and num-

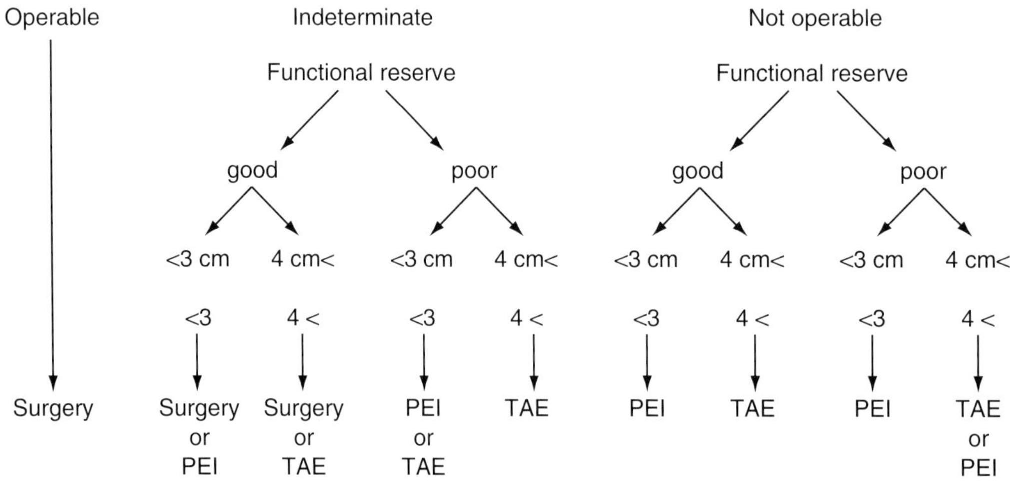

FIGURE 29-3. Flow chart for the treatment selection based on operability and on tumor size. PET, percutaneous ethanol injection; TAE, transcatheter arterial chemotherapy.

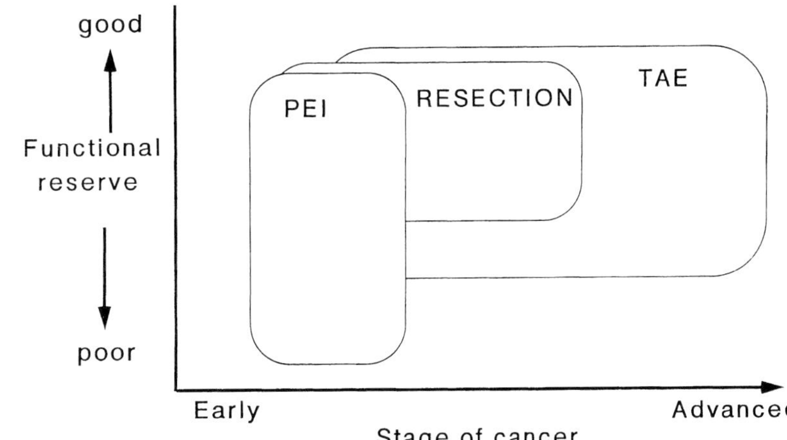

FIGURE 29-4. Schematic representation of the relationship between hepatic functional reserve, stage of cancer, and the choice of the three main treatment modalities for HCC. TAE, transcatheter embolization; TAI, transcatheter arterial chemotherapy. (National Cancer Center Hospital, Tokyo).

ber. If liver function is very poor, PEI is preferred to TAE, because TAE damages not only the cancer but also the liver parenchyma. For patients with very advanced cancer, neither PEI nor TAE is indicated, and only intraarterial chemotherapy can be considered. Systemic chemotherapy seldom proves efficacious.

REFERENCES

1. Okuda K, Ohtsuki T, Obata H et al. Natural history of hepatocellular carcinoma and prognosis in relation to treatment. Study of 850 patients. Cancer 1985;56:918–928
2. Takayasu K, Muramatsu Y, Moriyama N et al. Surgical treatment of adrenal metastasis following hepatectomy for hepatocellular carcinoma. Jpn J Clin Oncol 1989;19:62–66
3. Yokota Y, Takayasu K, Furukawa H et al. Simultaneous resection of hepatocellular carcinoma and solitary parapancreatic lymph node metastasis. Jpn J Gastroenterol Surg 1989;22:2853–2856
4. Okuda K, Musha H, Nakajima Y et al. Clinicopathological features of encapsulated hepatocellular carcinoma. Cancer 1977;40:1240–1245
5. Okuda K, Peters RL, Simson IW. Gross anatomical features of hepatocellular carcinoma from three disparate geographic areas. Proposals of new classification. Cancer 1984;54: 2165–2173
6. Hayashi K, Takayasu K, Moriyama N et al. Clinico-pathological study and selection of treatment of large hepatocellular carcinoma larger than 10 cm. Jpn J Gastroenterol Surg 1989; 22:1782–1790
7. Fujii T, Takayasu K, Muramatsu Y et al. Hepatocellular carcinoma with portal tumor thrombus: analysis of factors determining prognosis. Jpn J Clin Oncol 1993;23:105–109
8. The Liver Cancer Study Group of Japan. Predictive factors for long term prognosis after partial hepatectomy for patients with hepatocellular carcinoma in Japan. Cancer 1994;74: 2772–2780
9. Okuda K. Early recognition of hepatocellular carcinoma. Hepatology 1986;6:729–738
10. Takayasu K, Muramatsu Y, Moriyama N et al. Clinical and radiological assessment of the results of hepatectomy for small hepatocellular carcinoma and therapeutic arterial embolization for postoperative recurrence. Cancer 1989;64: 1848–1852
11. Ebara M, Ohto M, Sugiura N et al. Percutaneous ethanol injection for the treatment of small hepatocellular carcinoma. Study of 95 patients. J Gastroenterol Hepatol 1990; 5:616–626
12. Takayasu K, Shima Y, Muramatsu Y et al. Hepatocellular carcinoma: treatment with intraarterial iodized oil with and without chemotherapeutic agents. Radiology 1987;162: 345–351
13. Matsui O, Kadoya M, Yoshikawa J et al. Small hepatocellular carcinoma: treatment with subsegmental transcatheter arterial embolization. Radiology 1993;188:79–83
14. Nakamura H, Hashimoto T, Sawada S et al. Treatment of hepatocellular carcinoma by segmental hepatic artery injection of adriamycin-in-oil emulsion with overflow to segmental portal vein. Acta Radiol 1990;30:Facs. 4, 347–349
15. Takayasu K, Wako F, Moriyama N et al. Response of early-stage hepatocellular carcinoma and borderline lesions to therapeutic arterial embolization. Am J Roentgenol 1993; 160:301–306
16. Livraghi T, Bolondi L, Buscarini L et al. No treatment, resection and ethanol injection in hepatocellular carcinoma: a retrospective analysis of survival in 391 patients with cirrhosis. J Hepatol 1995;22:522–526
17. Tanaka K, Okazaki H, Nakamura S et al. Hepatocellular carcinoma: treatment with a combination therapy of transcatheter arterial embolization and percutaneous ethanol injection. Radiology 1991;179:713–717
18. Okazaki N. Systemic chemotherapy of hepatocellular. In Okuda K, Peters RL (eds): Hepatocellular Carcinoma. Wiley, New York, 1976, pp. 469–476
19. Falkson G, Coetzer B. Chemotherapy of primary liver cancer. In Okuda K, Ishak KG (eds): Neoplasms of the Liver. Springer, Tokyo, 1987, pp. 321–326
20. Okada S, Okazaki N, Nose H et al. Prognostic factors in patients with hepatocellular carcinoma receiving systemic chemotherapy. Hepatology 1992;16:112–117

30

SECTION VII
THERAPY

CHEMOTHERAPY FOR HEPATOCELLULAR CARCINOMA

SHUICHI OKADA

The recent introduction of screening of high-risk populations for hepatocellular carcinoma (HCC) using ultrasonography and serum α-fetoprotein (AFP) levels has facilitated the early detection of HCC nodules.[1] Standard treatment for HCC nodules includes surgery, percutaneous ethanol injection (PEI), and transcatheter arterial embolization (TAE).[2–4] However, the prognosis for HCC patients is still unsatisfactory, mostly because of post-therapeutic recurrence and multicentric carcinogenesis.[5] Accordingly, to improve the survival rate of HCC patients, it is imperative that new, more effective treatments for this disease be developed.

At present, no established chemotherapeutic regimens have proven effective against HCC. However, according to the 10th National Survey of Primary Liver Cancer in Japan, approximately 90% of the registered HCC patients in Japan received chemotherapy.[6]

Chemotherapy for HCC is administered either intra-arterially or systemically. When the drug is given intra-arterially in Japan, it is usually mixed with Lipiodol, an oily contrast medium, which works as a carrier to deliver the agents and may enhance the antitumor effect.[7,8] Intra-arterial chemotherapy has led to improved tumor responses, but it does not provide a survival advantage over systemic chemotherapy.[9–12]

INDICATIONS

There is no active anticancer agent or chemotherapeutic regimen for HCC that shows a reproducible response rate of more than 20%. Accordingly, only HCC patients in whom the three standard treatments (resection, PEI, and TAE) are contraindicated, who do not have severe hemorrhagic diathesis, jaundice, or risk of hepatic coma, are considered to be candidates for chemotherapy.

Minimum eligibility criteria for any phase II trial of chemotherapy for HCC should include measurable HCC lesions and adequate bodily organic functions, good performance status, and no history of prior anticancer treatment (Table 30-1). In HCC nodules treated with radiotherapy or TAE, the mode of tumor response to chemotherapy has been shown to be modified by the prior treatments.[13] Therefore, any patients previously treated with radiotherapy or TAE should be disqualified from clinical trials to ensure precise evaluation of the chemotherapy.

RESPONSE ANALYSIS

Chemotherapeutic effects are evaluated according to World Health Organization (WHO) guidelines,[14] mainly by using computed tomography and/or ultrasonography. Response is assessed 4 weeks after chemotherapy is started. A complete response (CR) is defined as the complete disappearance of the entire tumor lasting for more than 4 weeks. A partial response (PR) is defined as a 50% or greater reduction in the product of the two greatest perpendicular diameters or at least a 30% reduction in hepatomegaly without the appearance of new le-

TABLE 30-1. Eligibility Criteria for Phase II Trials for HCC at the National Cancer Center, Tokyo

1. Histologically or clinically confirmed HCC
2. Measurable lesions
3. Age: ≥ 15, ≤ 75 years
4. Performance status = 0, 1, or 2
5. No prior anticancer treatment
6. Adequate bone marrow, cardiac, hepatic, and renal function
7. No severe complications of the disease
8. No other active cancer
9. A life expectancy of at least 2 months
10. Informed consent

sions, lasting for more than 4 weeks. Any reduction and/or duration of response insufficient for classification as a PR is classified as a minor response (MR). No change (NC) is defined as no change or up to 25% progression in tumor size 4 weeks after the beginning of chemotherapy. Progressive disease (PD) is defined as a greater than 25% increase in tumor measurements or the appearance of new lesions within 4 weeks after the beginning of treatment.

Serial determinations of the serum AFP level are also a good marker for chemotherapeutic effects in HCC, particularly in the early recognition of tumor response. However, after chemotherapy, a decrease in the serum AFP level does not always indicate tumor reduction, especially in patients who do not have high AFP levels before treatment, and because the correlation with treatment response is otherwise difficult to evaluate.

TABLE 30-2. Anticancer Agents Used in Clinical Trials for HCC

Alkylating agents
- Cyclophosphamide, ifosfamide

Nitrosourea
- Nimustine hydrochloride

Antimetabolites
- Fluorouracil, tegafur, cytarabine, UFT (uracil and tegafur)

Antitumor antibiotics
- Doxorubicin, 4′-epidoxorubicin, mitoxantrone, mitomycin C, SMANCS (zinostatin stimalamer)

Alkaloids
- Vindesine, etoposide

Miscellaneous agents
- Cisplatin, interferon

TREATMENT METHODS

The anticancer agents fluorouracil, doxorubicin, 4′-epidoxorubicin, mitoxantrone, mitomycin C, and cisplatin are the most commonly used agents for HCC in clinical practice, but they have not shown a reliable effect against HCC. Additional agents have been used experimentally in clinical trials (Table 30-2).

If regression of the tumor size and/or a decrease of the serum level of AFP is observed 4 weeks after the start of chemotherapy, the chemotherapy is continued until the development of mild toxicity. If there was any evidence of tumor progression or unacceptable toxicity, the chemotherapy is discontinued.

RESULTS

Tumor Response

In phase II clinical trials at the National Cancer Center Hospital, Tokyo, Japan (Table 30-3),[15–20] all single systemic anticancer agents produced a response rate of less than 10%; the overall response rate for single agents was 7% (95% confidence limits; range: 3% to 11%). All responders listed had a PR (Table 30-3).

The response rate of HCC to cisplatin was 9% (95% confidence limits; range: 3% to 22%), indicating that the clinical value of this drug as a single agent for the treatment of HCC is limited.[20] However, the combination of cisplatin with other anticancer agents may lead to higher response rates and improved survival against

TABLE 30-3. Results of Phase II Trials of Systemic Chemotherapy for HCC at the National Cancer Center Hospital, Tokyo

Regimen	No. of Patients	No. of Responders[a]	Response Rate (%)
Fluorouracil	6	0	0
Tegafur	14	0	0
UFT	15	1	7
Doxorubicin	15	1	7
4′-epidoxorubicin	4	0	0
Etoposide	11	1	9
Mitoxantrone	19	1	5
γ-interferon	14	0	0
Cisplatin	43	4	9
FMP[b]	6	2	33
Total	147	10	7

[a] All responders had a partial response.
[b] Fluorouracil, mitoxantrone, cisplatin.

various cancers, since the activity of cisplatin has been reported to be potentiated by other cytotoxic agents such as fluorouracil.[21–23] Preliminary results of a phase II trial of fluorouracil, mitoxantrone, and cisplatin, which is still in progress at our institute, show a response rate in two of six patients (33%).

Host-related factors did not affect the response rate (Table 30-4). There was no significant difference in response rate depending on the age, sex, hepatitis B surface antigen status, or alcohol abuse history. No patients with jaundice, ascites, or a performance status (PS) of 2 had a response. In regard to tumor-related factors, patients with unilateral HCC had a significantly higher response rate than those with bilateral HCC (Table 30-5). There were no responders among the patients with a tumor size more than 50% of the entire liver or a tumor thrombus in the main portal trunk. Thus, regardless of the chemotherapy regimen used, patients with poor hepatic reserve or with advanced HCC would not be optimal candidates for systemic chemotherapy, although the response is totally unpredictable before chemotherapy.

TABLE 30-4. Tumor Response to Systemic Chemotherapy With Reference to Host-Related Factors

Factors	Response Rate (No. of Responders/No. of Patients)
Age	
<60 yr	6% (4/72)
≥60 yr	8% (6/75)
Sex	
Male	7% (8/123)
Female	8% (2/24)
HBsAg[a]	
Negative	7% (9/122)
Positive	4% (1/25)
Alcohol abuse[b]	
Negative	8% (7/88)
Positive	5% (3/59)
Cirrhosis	
Absent	11% (5/44)
Present	5% (5/103)
Total bilirubin	
<2.0 mg/dl	8% (10/130)
≥2.0 mg/dl	0% (0/17)
Albumin	
<3.5 g/dl	3% (3/86)
≥3.5 g/dl	11% (7/61)
Ascites	
Absent	9% (10/112)
Present	0% (0/35)
Performance status	
0, 1	9% (10/109)
2, 3	0% (0/38)

[a] Hepatitis B surface antigen.

[b] Ethanol intake ≥ 80 g/day for ≥ 5 yr.

TABLE 30-5. Tumor Response to Systemic Chemotherapy With Reference to Tumor-Related Factors

Factors	Response Rate (No. of Responders/No. of Patients)
No. of intrahepatic nodules	
Single	3% (3/93)
Multiple	12% (6/50)
Tumor distribution	
Unilateral	11% (6/56)[a]
Bilateral	3% (3/90)
Tumor size[b]	
<50%	10% (10/99)
≥50%	0% (0/44)
Tumor thrombus in main portal trunk	
Absent	9% (10/113)
Present	0% (0/33)
Extrahepatic metastasis	
Absent	6% (7/109)
Present	8% (3/38)
α-Fetoprotein	
<400 ng/ml	9% (6/69)
≥400 ng/ml	5% (4/78)

[a] $p < 0.05$.

[b] % of liver cross-sectional area.

Responders to systemic chemotherapy[24] (eight patients) were found to survive significantly longer than matched nonresponders (24 patients) (median survival time: 17.5 versus 9.7 months) ($p < 0.05$) (Fig. 30-1).

FIGURE 30-1. HCC: Survival curves of responders and nonresponders to systemic chemotherapy. p = 0.04.

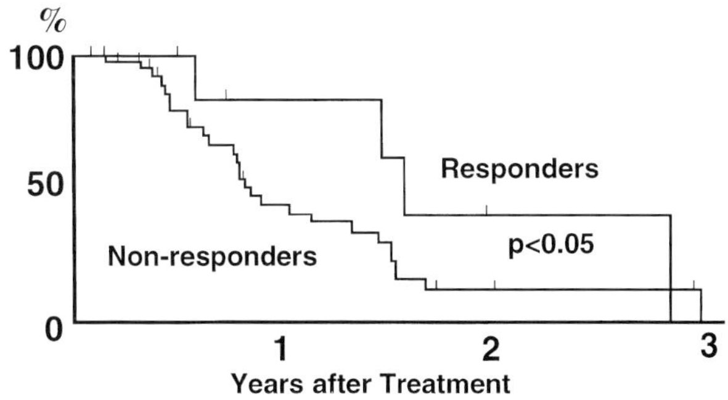

For each responder, three nonresponders matched for age, sex, and various prognostic factors were selected, since there was a difference between these two groups in patient characteristics.

Survival and Prognostic Factors

In the survival curve for 102 patients who received systemic chemotherapy with no other anticancer treatment (Fig. 30-2),[25] the median survival was 5.6 months, and the 1-year and 2-year survival rates were 27% and 8%, respectively. Overall survival rate was not significantly different among patients who received the different chemotherapy regimens.

The relationship of various factors to the survival period was examined using univariate analysis with log-rank tests (Table 30-6, Table 30-7). There was no significant difference in survival depending on the age, sex, hepatitis B surface antigen status, or alcohol abuse history of the patients. The host-related factors identified as significantly favoring longer survival were absence of jaundice, serum albumin of greater than 3.5 g/dl, absence of ascites, and a PS of 0 or 1. The tumor-related factors identified as significantly favoring longer survival were single intrahepatic nodule, unilateral tumor, tumor size less than 50% of the liver cross-sectional area, no tumor thrombus in the main portal trunk, and serum AFP of less than 400 ng/ml.

Multivariate analysis using the Cox proportional hazards model revealed that a PS of 0 to 1, absence of tumor thrombus in the main portal trunk, and age less than 60 years were independent favorable prognostic factors ($p < 0.05$, Table 30-8). For the clinical application of these findings, a prognostic index (PI) was calculated based on the regression coefficients derived from these three variables as follows:

$$
\begin{aligned}
PI = {} & 1.7 \times PS \\
& (0{:}PS\ 0{,}1,\ 1{:}PS\ 2{,}3) \\
& + 1.1 \times \text{Tumor Thrombus} \\
& (0{:}\text{Negative},\ 1{:}\text{Positive}) \\
& + 0.6 \times \text{Age} \\
& (0{:}< 60\ \text{yr.},\ 1{:} \geq 60\ \text{yr.})
\end{aligned}
$$

The PI was defined as natural logarithm ($h_i [t]/h_0 [t]$), where $h_i [t]/h_0 [t]$ was the relative risk of death for the "i-th" patient. The PI in all of the patients ranged from 0 to 3.4. The patients were then assigned to three groups: 48 patients with a PI of 0.6 or less, group A; 33 patients with an PI from 0.6 to 1.7, group B; and 21 patients with PI more

TABLE 30-6. Univariate Analysis of Prognostic Factors Associated With Survival in Patients With HCC

Variable	Median Survival (mo)	1-Year Survival Rate (%)	
Age			
<60 yr	4.8	21.0	
≥60 yr	6.5	33.4	NS[a]
Sex			
Male	5.6	26.1	
Female	5.1	26.9	NS
HBsAg[b]			
Negative	5.6	28.2	
Positive	3.9	19.1	NS
Alcohol abuse[c]			
Negative	5.6	28.5	
Positive	5.6	23.8	NS
Cirrhosis			
Absent	7.3	29.9	
Present	5.3	24.2	NS
Total bilirubin			
<2.0 mg/dl	6.5	31.4	
≥2.0 mg/dl	3.9	0.0	$p < 0.05$
Albumin			
<3.5 g/dl	4.8	21.9	
≥3.5 g/dl	7.3	32.6	$p < 0.05$
Ascites			
Absent	7.5	33.7	
Present	3.1	8.1	$p < 0.001$
Performance status			
0, 1	9.7	41.2	
2, 3	2.6	0.0	$p < 0.001$

[a] Not significant.

[b] Hepatitis B surface antigen.

[c] Ethanol intake ≥ 80 g/day for ≥ 5 yr.

FIGURE 30-2. Actuarial survival curve for 102 patients with HCC.

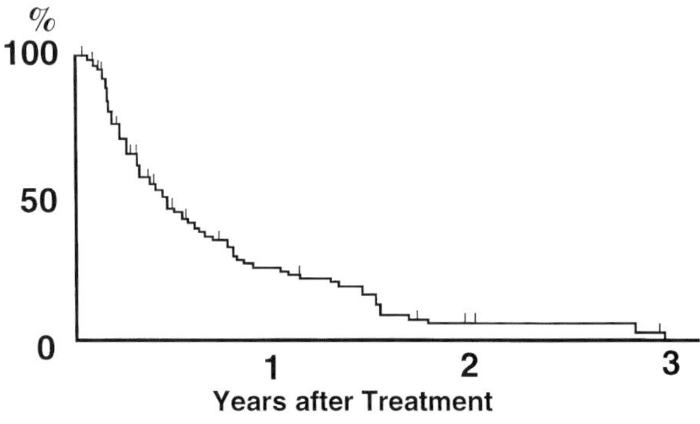

TABLE 30-7. Univariate Analysis of Prognostic Factors Associated With Survival in Patients With HCC

Variable	Median Survival (mo)	1-Year Survival Rate (%)	
No. of intrahepatic nodules			
Single	6.1	35.2	
Multiple	5.6	23.7	$p < 0.05$
Tumor distribution			
Unilateral	8.4	83.3	
Bilateral	3.9	17.7	$p < 0.01$
Tumor size[a]			
< 50%	9.8	42.9	
≥ 50%	3.2	5.1	$p < 0.001$
Tumor thrombus in main portal trunk			
Absent	7.9	34.2	
Present	2.9	10.5	$p < 0.001$
Extrahepatic metastasis			
Absent	5.5	28.8	
Present	6.5	20.7	NS[b]
Alpha-fetoprotein			
< 400 ng/ml	9.8	42.7	
≥ 400 ng/ml	3.9	13.5	$p < 0.01$

[a] % of liver cross-sectional area.

[b] Not significant.

than 1.7, group C (Table 30-9). There was a significant difference among all the three groups in survival ($p < 0.01$) (Fig. 30-3). The median survival period of these groups was 12.6, 3.2, and 2.1 months, respectively. The patients in group C showed the poorest survival; all died within 6 months of starting treatment. Therefore, patients with a PI more than 1.7 can be treated or offered only supportive care. The PI may be helpful in more accurately predicting survival in these patients.

TABLE 30-8. Independent Prognostic Factors for 102 Patients With HCC as Determined by the Cox Proportional Hazard Model

Variable	Coefficient	Risk Ratio	p Value
Performance status	1.7	5.4 (3.2–9.2)[a]	< 0.01
Tumor thrombus[b]	1.1	3.0 (1.8–4.9)	< 0.01
Age	0.6	1.9 (1.2–3.1)	< 0.05

[a] 95% confidence limits.

[b] Tumor thrombus in the main portal trunk.

TABLE 30-9. Survival as a Function of the Prognostic Index Based on Factors Found to Be Significant in the Cox Proportional Hazard Model

	Prognostic Index	No. of Patients	Median Survival (mo)	Rate (%)
Group A	≤0.6	48	12.6	50.2
Group B	0.6<–≤1.7	33	3.2	10.5
Group C	>1.7	21	2.1	0.0

Toxicity

The toxicity of chemotherapy varies with the type of anticancer agent used. The toxicity of fluorouracil derivatives is mostly gastrointestinal and mild.[15,16] The gastrointestinal toxicity of cisplatin, such as nausea and vomiting, is more severe than that of fluorouracil derivatives, but it is still tolerable.[20] The toxicity of anthracyclines and alkaloids is hematologic; white blood cell and platelet counts are lowest 2 weeks after the beginning of treatment, but recover to initial levels within the next 2 weeks.[15,17,18] Leukocytopenia is usually more severe than thrombocytopenia. Severe alopecia is observed with doxorubicin, 4′-epidoxorubicin, and etoposide, but not with mitoxantrone.[17]

DISCUSSION

Systemic chemotherapy for HCC has been of limited value in clinical practice, because only a small portion of patients obtain meaningful palliation, and because the

FIGURE 30-3. Actuarial survival curves for three prognostic groups identified using the prognostic index determined by the Cox proportional hazards model. The categories were defined by prognostic index values of ≤ 0.6 (A, 48 patients), > 0.6 to ≤ 1.7 (B, 33 patients), and > 1.7 (C, 21 patients).

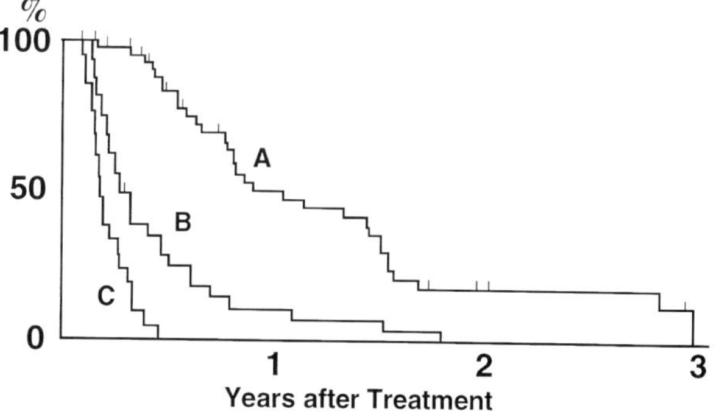

TABLE 30-10. Clinical Trials Reported in the Literature: Systemic Chemotherapy for HCC

Regimen	No. of Patients	No. of Responders	Response Rate (%)
Fluorouracil/leucovorin[29]	29	3	10
Fluorouracil/interferon-α[30]	28	5	18
Doxorubicin Interferon-α[31]	31	1	3
4′-Epidoxorubicin/Interferon-α[32]	30	1	3
Mitoxantrone[33]	17	4	23
Mitoxantrone/Interferon-β[34]	38	9	24
Ifosfamide[35]	15	0	0
Vindesine[36]	14	0	0
Etoposide[37]	15	0	0
Cisplatin[20]	26	4	15
Interferon-α[38]	35	11	31

toxicity of chemotherapy may often outweigh the benefits. The possible explanations for the refractoriness of HCC to chemotherapy include tumor heterogeneity,[26] inadequate dosages of anticancer agents,[10,27] and the inducible overexpression of the multidrug resistance gene.[28] However, in the final analysis, it is clear that an effective agent has not yet been found.

Phase II studies of treatment for HCC[29–38] confirm that there is no effective drug for HCC (Table 30-10),[29–38] although relatively higher response rates were reported in studies of mitoxantrone (23%; 4/17)[33] and interferon-α (31%; 11/35).[38] Inherent biologic differences in HCC among patients from various parts of the world may make the evaluation of chemotherapeutic results difficult.[39,40]

There is no report showing any clinical advantage in using a multidrug combination for HCC, although the synergistic effects of cisplatin and the other anticancer agents have not been fully evaluated in HCC patients. The attempt to increase the therapeutic activity of fluorouracil through biochemical modulation with leucovorin or interferon does not achieve higher response rates, and the toxicity sometimes becomes significant.[29,30] The addition of interferon to anthracyclines such as doxorubicin, 4′-epidoxorubicin, or mitoxantrone does not lead to improved tumor response, although the activity of a variety of cytotoxic agents both in vitro and in animal models has been reported to be synergistically potentiated when interferon is added.[31,32,34]

REFERENCES

1. Tanaka S, Kitamura T, Nakanishi K et al. Effectiveness of periodic checkup by ultrasonography for the early diagnosis of hepatocellular carcinoma. Cancer 1990;66:2210–2214
2. Makuuchi M, Hasegawa H, Yamazaki S. Ultrasonically guided subsegmentectomy. Surg Gynecol Obstet 1985;161: 346–350
3. Ebara M, Ohto M, Sugiura N et al. Percutaneous ethanol injection for the treatment of small hepatocellular carcinoma. Study of 95 patients. Gastroenterol Hepatol 1990;5: 616–626
4. Takayasu K, Suzuki M, Uesaka K et al. Hepatic artery embolization for inoperable hepatocellular carcinoma: prognosis and risk factors. Cancer Chemother Pharmacol 1989;23 (suppl):123–125
5. Okada S, Shimada K, Yamamoto J et al. Predictive factors for postoperative recurrence of hepatocellular carcinoma. Gastroenterology 1994;106:1618–1624
6. Liver Cancer Study Group of Japan. Survey and follow-up study of primary liver cancer in Japan -Report 10-. Acta Hepatol Jpn 1993;34:805–813
7. Nakakuma K, Tashiro S, Hiraoka T et al. Studies on anticancer treatment with an oily anticancer drug injected into the ligated feeding hepatic artery for liver cancer. Cancer 1983; 52:2193–2200
8. Mondazzi L, Bottelli R, Brambilla G et al. Transarterial oily chemoembolization for the treatment for hepatocellular carcinoma: a multivariate analysis of prognostic factors. Hepatology 1994;19:1115–1123
9. Okuda K, Ohtsuki T, Obata H et al. Natural history of hepatocellular carcinoma and prognosis in relation to treatment. Study of 850 patients. Cancer 1985;56:918–928
10. Nerenstone SR, Ihde DC, Friedman MA. Clinical trials in primary hepatocellular carcinoma: current status and future directions. Cancer Treat Rev 1988;15:1–31
11. Kalayci C, Johnson PJ, Raby N et al. Intraarterial adriamycin and lipiodol for inoperable hepatocellular carcinoma: a comparison with intravenous adriamycin. J Hepatol 1990;11: 349–353
12. Kajanti M, Pyrhönen S, Mäntylä M, Rissanen P. Intra-arterial and intravenous use of 4′ epidoxorubicin combined with

5-fluorouracil in primary hepatocellular carcinoma. A randomized comparison. Am J Clin Oncol 1992;15:37–40

13. Okazaki N, Yoshida T, Yoshino M et al. Changes in mode of response to chemotherapy for hepatocellular carcinoma induced by transarterial embolization. A case report. Jpn J Clin Oncol 1991;21:69–74
14. World Health Organization. WHO Handbook for Reporting Results of Cancer Treatment. World Health Organization, Geneva, 1979
15. Okazaki N, Yoshino M, Yoshida T, Hijikata A. A controlled study of intravenous doxorubicin versus oral tegafur in patients with hepatocellular carcinoma. J Jpn Soc Cancer Ther 1985;20:556–561
16. Tokyo Liver Cancer Chemotherapy Study Group. Phase II study of co-administration of uracil and tegafur (UFT) in hepatocellular carcinoma. Jpn J Clin Oncol 1985;15: 559–562
17. Yoshida T, Okazaki N, Yoshino M et al. Phase II trial of mitoxantrone in patients with hepatocellular carcinoma. Eur J Cancer Clin Oncol 1988;24:1897–1898
18. Yoshino M, Okazaki N, Yoshida T et al. A phase II study of etoposide in patients with hepatocellular carcinoma by the Tokyo Liver Cancer Chemotherapy Study Group. Jpn J Clin Oncol 1989;19:120–122
19. Yoshida T, Okazaki N, Yoshino M et al. Phase II trial of high dose recombinant gamma-interferon in advanced hepatocellular carcinoma. Eur J Cancer 1990;26:545–546
20. Okada S, Okazaki N, Nose H et al. A phase 2 study of cisplatin in patients with hepatocellular carcinoma. Oncology 1993;50:22–26
21. Kish JA, Weaver A, Jacobs J et al. Cisplatin and 5-fluorouracil infusion in patients with recurrent and disseminated epidermoid cancer of the head and neck. Cancer 1984;53: 1819–1824
22. Scanlon KJ, Newman EM, Lu Y, Priest DG. Biochemical basis for cisplatin and 5-fluorouracil synergism in human ovarian carcinoma cells. Proc Natl Acad Sci USA 1986;83: 8923–8925
23. Zimm S, Cleary SM, Lucas WE et al. Phase I/pharmacokinetic study of intraperitoneal cisplatin and etoposide. Cancer Res 1987;47:1712–1716
24. Okada S, Okazaki N, Nose H et al. Evaluation of chemotherapeutic effects in hepatocellular carcinoma based on survival analysis. Acta Hepatol Jpn 1992;33:9–14
25. Okada S, Okazaki N, Nose H et al. Prognostic factors in patients with hepatocellular carcinoma receiving systemic chemotherapy. Hepatology 1992;16:112–117
26. Dexter DL, Leith JT. Tumor heterogeneity and drug resistance. J Clin Oncol 1986;4:244–257
27. Lai ECS, Choi TK, Cheng CH et al. Doxorubicin for unresectable hepatocellular carcinoma. A prospective study on the addition of verapamil. Cancer 1990;66:1685–1687
28. Huang C, Wu M, Xu G et al. Overexpression of the MDR1 gene and P-glycoprotein in human hepatocellular carcinoma. J Natl Cancer Inst 1992;84:262–264
29. van Eden H, Falkson G, Burger W, Ansell SM. 5-fluorouracil and leucovorin in hepatocellular carcinoma. Ann Oncol 1992;3:404–405
30. Patt YZ, Yoffe B, Charnsangavej C et al. Low serum alphafetoprotein level in patients with hepatocellular carcinoma as a predictor of response to 5-FU and interferon-alpha-2b. Cancer 1993;72:2574–2582
31. Kardinal CG, Moertel CG, Wieand HS et al. Combined doxorubicin and alpha-interferon therapy of advanced hepatocellular carcinoma. Cancer 1993;71:2187–2190
32. Bokemeyer C, Kynast B, Harstrick A et al. No synergistic activity of epirubicin and interferon-alpha-2b in the treatment of hepatocellular carcinoma. Cancer Chemother Pharmacol 1995;35:334–338
33. Colleoni M, Nole' F, Di Bartolomeo M et al. Mitoxantrone in patients affected by hepatocellular carcinoma with unfavorable prognostic factors. Oncology 1992;49:139–142
34. Colleoni M, Buzzoni R, Bajetta E et al. A phase II study of mitoxantrone combined with beta-interferon in unresectable hepatocellular carcinoma. Cancer 1993;72:3196–3201
35. Lin J, Shiu W, Leung WT et al. Phase II study of high dose ifosfamide in hepatocellular carcinoma. Cancer Chemother Pharmacol 1993;31:338–339
36. Falkson G, Burger W. A phase II trial of vindesine in hepatocellular carcinoma. Oncology 1995;52:86–87
37. Wierzbicki R, Ezzat A, Abdel-Warith A et al. Phase II trial of chronic daily VP-16 administration in unresectable hepatocellular carcinoma (HCC). Ann Oncol 1994;5:466–467
38. Lai CL, Lau JYN, Wu PC et al. Recombinant interferon-alpha in inoperable hepatocellular carcinoma: a randomized controlled trial. Hepatology 1993;17:389–394
39. Okuda K, Peters RL, Simson IW. Gross anatomic features of hepatocellular carcinoma from three disparate geographic areas. Proposal of new classification. Cancer 1984;54: 2165–2173
40. Okuda K. Geographic heterogeneity of hepatocellular carcinoma. Gastroenterol Jpn 1990;25:787–792

31

ARTERIAL EMBOLIZATION

HIRONOBU NAKAMURA
TAKAMICHI MURAKAMI

Recent advances in diagnostic imaging have improved the detection of small hepatocellular carcinoma (HCC); as a result, the number of patients undergoing surgery has increased. However, there are still many patients who cannot undergo surgical resection of HCC because of concurrent cirrhosis or intrahepatic metastases; and among those who can undergo surgical treatment, the rate of postoperative recurrence in the hepatic stump has not decreased. Radiologists often use hepatic arterial embolization to treat HCCs that are difficult to resect, and this has contributed to improved outcome.

Arterial embolization with gelatin sponge for treating HCC was first reported by Doyon et al.[1] from France in 1974, followed by Yamada et al.[2] after a full-scale clinical trial in 1978. Lipiodol (Andre-Gelbe Laboratory, Aulnay-sous-Bois, France), an oily contrast medium, was subsequently used for arterial embolization together with gelatin sponge. It contributed to improvement in both diagnosis and treatment of HCC.[3–8] Regional arterial embolization of the liver has recently been done by placing microcatheters in arteries that supply cancer-bearing regions, and this procedure has greatly improved the outcome of treatment. The results in small HCC are almost equivalent to those of hepatectomy.[9]

Although arterial embolization for metastatic liver cancer has been reported,[10] in our experience, the response in metastatic liver cancer is not good. Hypervascular metastatic lesions respond to some extent,[11] but complete necrosis does not take place because of the absence of tumor capsules, and accordingly the disease recurs earlier. On the other hand, hypovascular metastases respond better to continuous intra-arterial infusion therapy. We therefore use embolization therapy only in exceptional cases of metastatic liver cancer. This chapter is concerned only with its use for treating HCC.

RATIONALE

The liver is supplied by both the hepatic artery and the portal vein. Therefore, it does not become necrotic if only the artery is embolized. However, most HCCs are fed only by the hepatic artery,[12] so the lesion does become necrotic when only the artery is embolized. The liver may be affected differently by various materials used for embolization. The liver of monkeys was shown to be unaffected by Gelfoam, whereas hepatic failure developed due to infarction when silicone was injected.[13] When Lipiodol is given to monkeys by injection at high doses, it flows into the portal vein.[14] Porcine liver became necrotic when Lipiodol or Gelfoam were injected at high doses.[15]

Encapsulated HCCs are totally supplied by the hepatic artery, while extracapsular infiltrative lesions and surrounding satellite lesions are supplied by the portal vein and hepatic artery.[16] Encapsulated HCC therefore becomes completely necrotic after embolization with gelatin sponge, while HCC without a capsule, or extracapsular lesions of HCC, are unlikely to become necrotic.[17,18] Notwithstanding, gelatin sponge plays an important role in making the main tumors necrotic. In addition, this material is absorbed; 2 to 4 weeks later the hepatic artery is recanalized, and noncancerous tissues are less damaged.

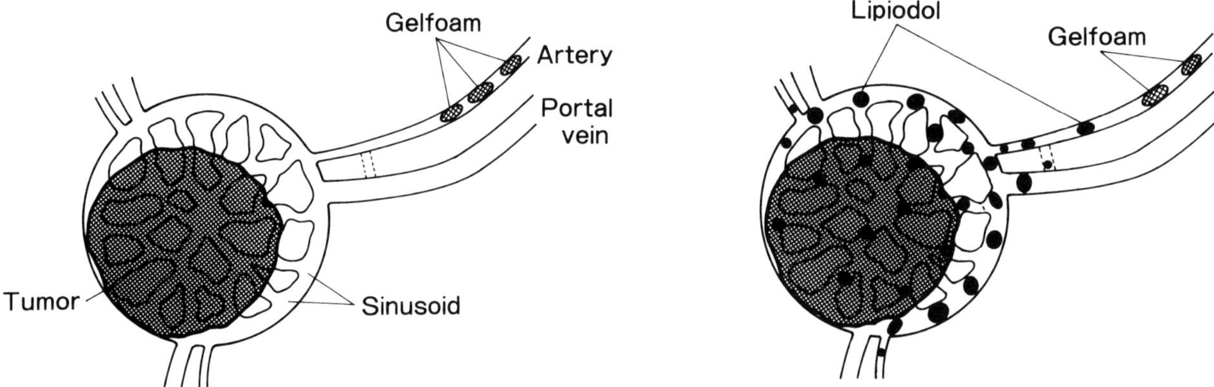

FIGURE 31-1. A mixture of Lipiodol and anticancer drug is retained in the hepatocellular carcinoma and peritumoral sinusoid.

Lipiodol plays an important role as a carrier of anticancer drugs. It is not very effective in blocking arterial blood flow, but it enters the HCC (which has a high blood flow) and is retained there. If a stable mixture of an anticancer drug with Lipiodol is prepared,[7] the drug is retained in the HCC together with the Lipiodol and is slowly released to act locally at high concentrations. The mixture is also retained in the peritumoral sinusoid[19] (Fig. 31-1), and it flows in part into branches of the portal vein via the peribiliary vascular plexus.[14,20] It also works, therefore, in extracapsular lesions that are not responsive to gelatin sponge.[21] However, noncancerous tissues may be more heavily damaged if there is increased backflow of Lipiodol in the portal vein.[14] Therefore, it is strongly recommended that the dose of Lipiodol be adjusted by the size and vascularity of the tumor to minimize the flow of Lipiodol into noncancerous tissues. In contrast, regional injection into a limited area dramatically enhances the antitumor effects of the drug, since the tumor is affected by both arterial and venous supply because of backflow of Lipiodol into the portal vein.

INDICATIONS

Use of arterial embolization in the treatment of HCC depends on both portal blood flow and hepatic function. Since normal hepatocytes are less damaged if sufficient portal blood flow is available, arterial embolization is contraindicated if there is no collateral circulation, as in patients with complete obstruction of the portal trunk. In contrast, it can be used in incomplete obstruction of the portal trunk, in complete obstruction with collateral vasculature, or in complete obstruction of the right main branch of the portal vein, if the dose of embolizing agents is decreased or the extent of embolization is limited. Portal blood flow can be estimated by arterial portography, but more accurate information can be obtained from computed tomography during arterial portography (CTAP).[22] Even if there is no arterial portographic evidence of obstruction due to tumor thrombus, embolization is contraindicated if CTAP suggests that the area of portal perfusion is less than 50% of the whole area (Fig. 31-2).

Another important factor in deciding on embolization is pre-embolization hepatic function. There must be sufficient reserve hepatic function to enable the patient to recover from the damage caused by embolization. It is dangerous to completely embolize the entire liver if the total bilirubin is equal to or greater than 2.0 mg/dl. Embolization can be used without concern if the total bilirubin is equal to or less than 1.0 mg/dl, but it depends on the extent of the portal blood flow when the total bilirubin is between 1.0 to 2.0 mg/dl. Superselective subsegmental arterial embolization can be used even in patients with severe hepatic impairment. Emergency arterial embolization is indicated in ruptured HCC, whether or not portal tumor thrombus is present. However, the prognosis is poor if total bilirubin is equal to or greater than 3.0 mg/dl.[23]

METHODS

Catheterization

Celiac arteriography and superior mesenteric arteriography should first be done to determine the vascular anatomy and the portal blood flow, including the presence or absence of varices. Common hepatic or proper hepatic arteriography then should be done to define the extent of the tumor and to identify the feeding arteries. As nec-

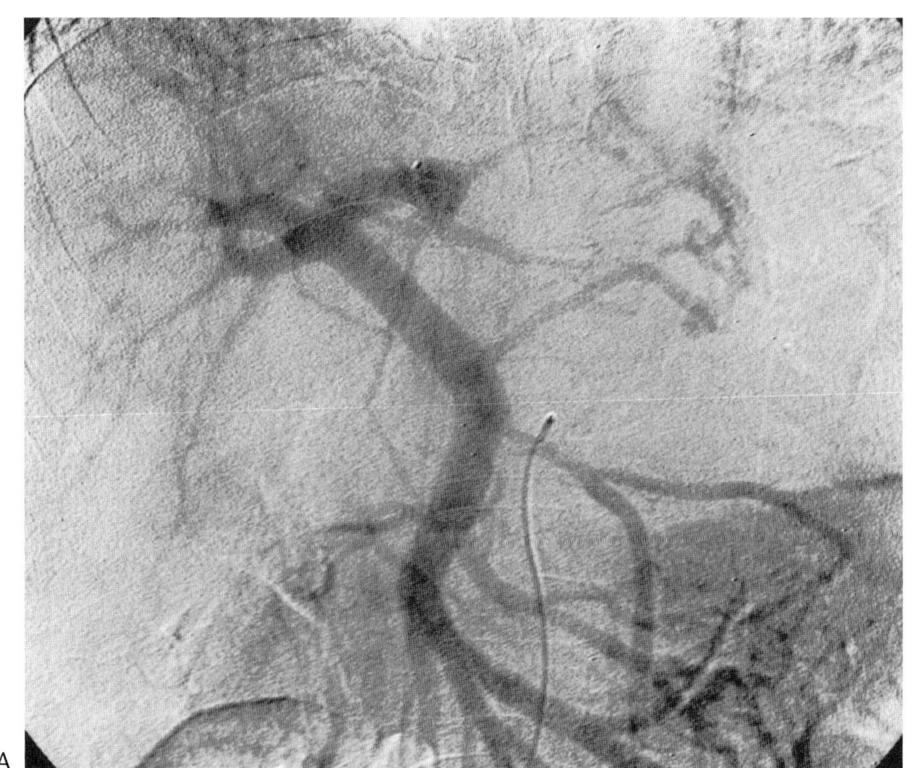

A

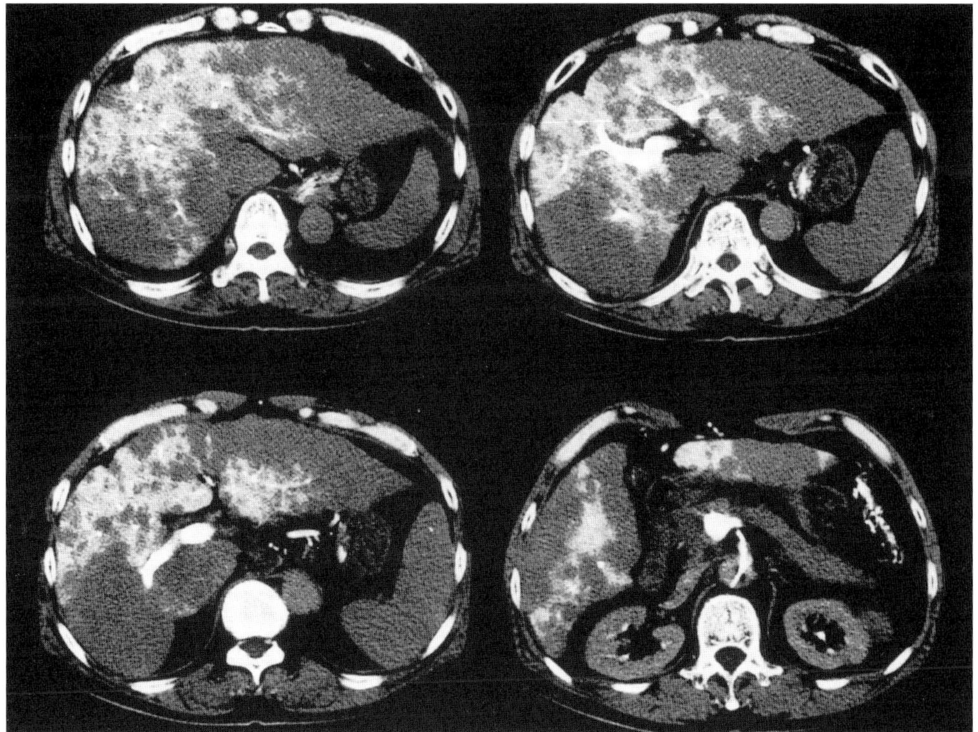

B

FIGURE 31-2. (*A*) Although superior mesenteric arterial portography shows no obstruction of the main portal branches (*B*), computed tomography during arterial portography shows less than 50% of liver parenchyma enhancement.

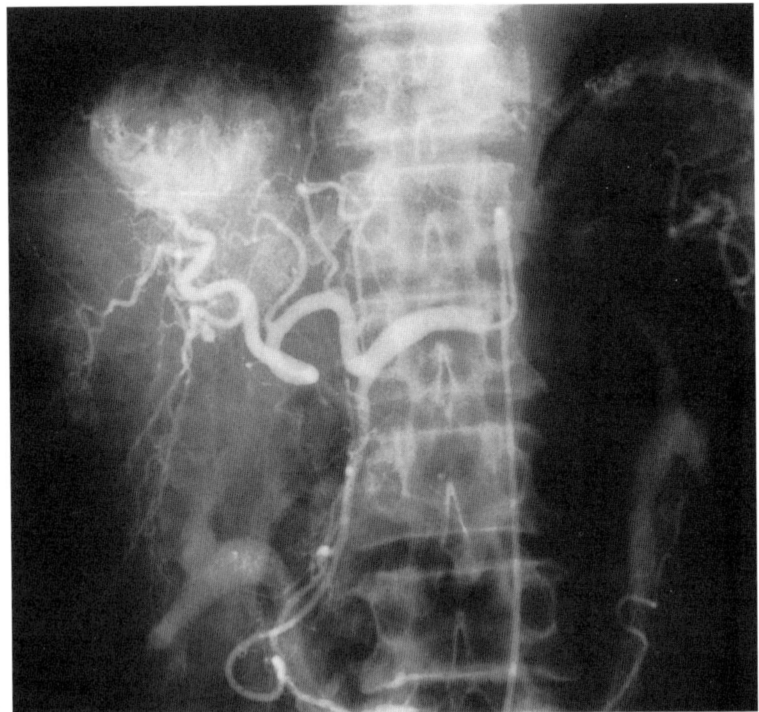

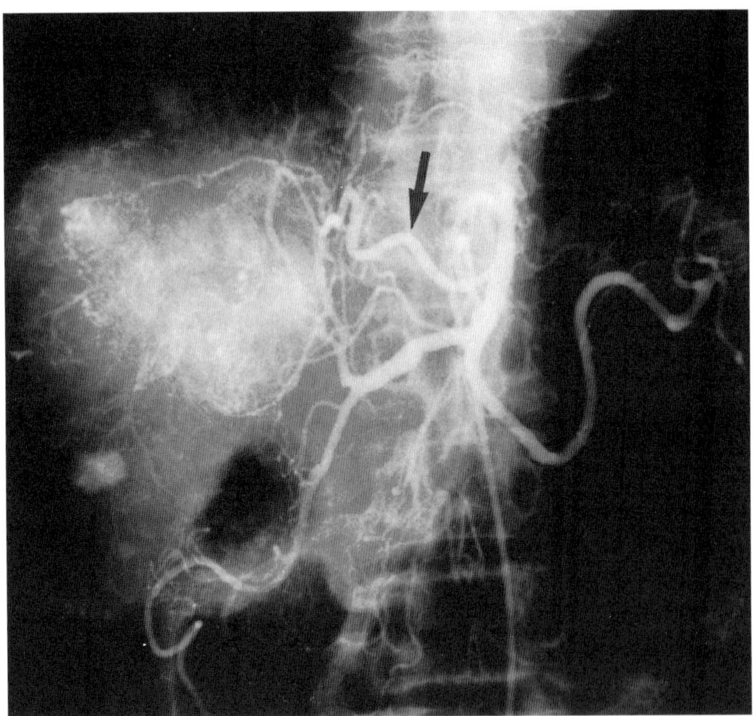

FIGURE 31-3. (*A*) Common hepatic arteriography shows multiple tumors in the right lobe. (*B*) After repeated arterial embolization, celiac arteriography shows occlusion of the right hepatic artery and a massive tumor in the right hepatic lobe mainly fed by the right phrenic artery (arrow). *(Figure continues.)*

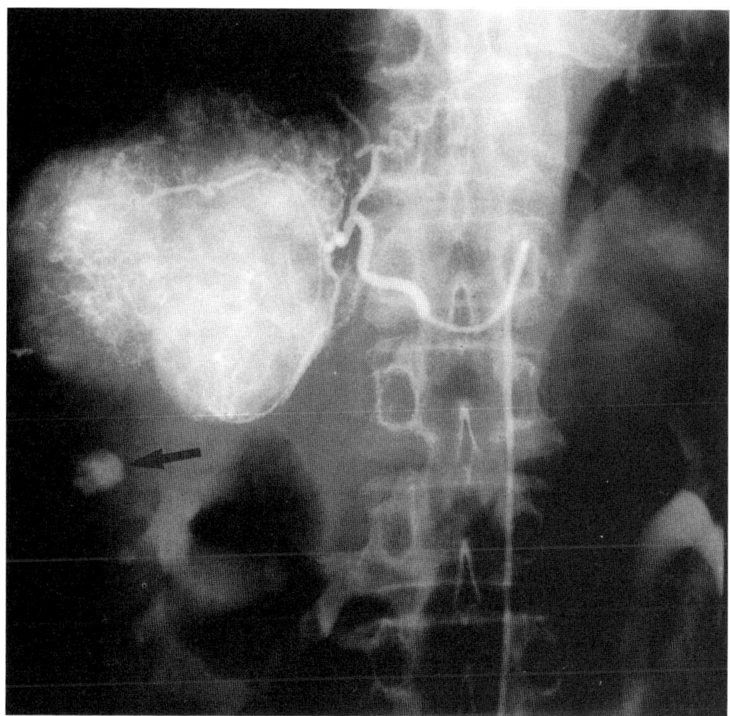

FIGURE 31-3 *(Continued).* (C) Right phrenic arteriography shows a huge tumor in the right hepatic lobe. Lipiodol accumulation from the previous embolization is seen (arrow). (From Nakamura et al.,[52] with permission.)

essary, arteriography should also be done, in the oblique view. The inferior phrenic and intercostal arteries should also be visualized by arteriography to explore collateral supply if the tumor is located on the liver surface, or if there is a history of embolization (Fig. 31-3).

If the tumor is extensive, it is embolized from the common hepatic artery or from the right and left hepatic arteries. If it is difficult to place a catheter in the proper hepatic arteries, a balloon catheter may be used to redirect blood flow so that gastroduodenal arterial blood flow turns to the liver, and the tumor thus may be embolized from the common hepatic artery.[24] This technique can also be applied to the left hepatic artery, which is connected to the left gastric artery. The technique is also effective in cases in which a catheter cannot be placed distally to the accessory left gastric artery[25] originating from the left hepatic artery.[26] If the proper hepatic artery is severely stenotic or obstructed, the tumor can be embolized from periportal collateral vessels by obstructing the common hepatic artery with a balloon catheter.[27]

If the tumor is localized, the catheter can be advanced to the segmental or subsegmental artery to embolize the cancer-bearing region alone. In this technique, it is recommended to use a microcatheter coaxially (Fig. 31-4). Whether the entire tumor area can be embolized from the catheter is generally assessed by angiograms, but it can be more accurately evaluated by computed tomography (CT) hepatic arteriography done during injection of contrast medium from the catheter[28] (Fig. 31-5).

Procedures for Embolization

Gelatin sponge (Gelfoam or Spongel) is often used as an embolic material. Polyvinyl alcohol foam, ethanol, and metal coils may also be used, but with these the hepatic artery is not recanalized, so repeat procedures are impossible. Gelatin sponge powder should not be used because bile duct necrosis is often associated with this material due to obstruction of the peribiliary vascular plexus.[29]

Anticancer drugs should be given as a mixture with Lipiodol if possible. Adriamycin (20 to 40 mg/m^2), epirubicin (30 to 60 mg/m^2), mitomycin C, cisplatin, or Styreae-Maleic Acid-Neocartzinostatin (SMANCS) (4 to 6 mg) can be given individually in this way.[30] Water-soluble anticancer drugs can be placed in stable mixtures by dissolving them in nonionic contrast medium which is almost isotonic with Lipiodol, or in 60% Urografin diluted with distilled water at about one-fifth the volume, isotonic with Lipiodol.[7] The dose of Lipiodol depends on the size and vascularity of the tumor, the site of catheter placement, and the degree of hepatic impairment; doses of 3 to 10 ml are used, 5 ml being the most frequently used. SMANCS, a lipophilic anticancer drug, is suspended in Lipiodol by sonication when used in this way.

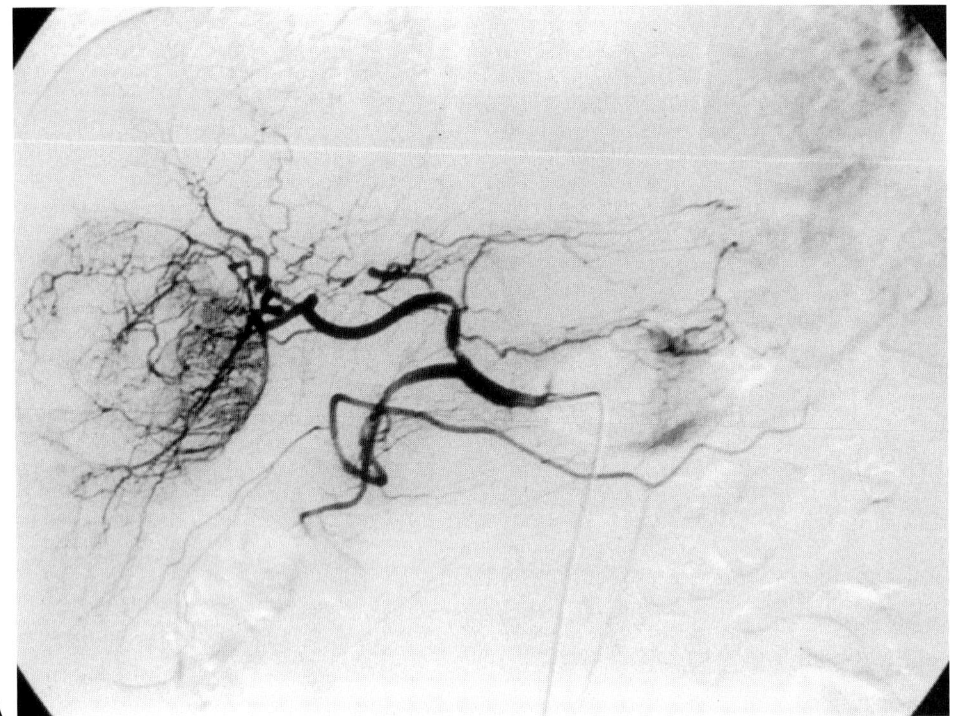

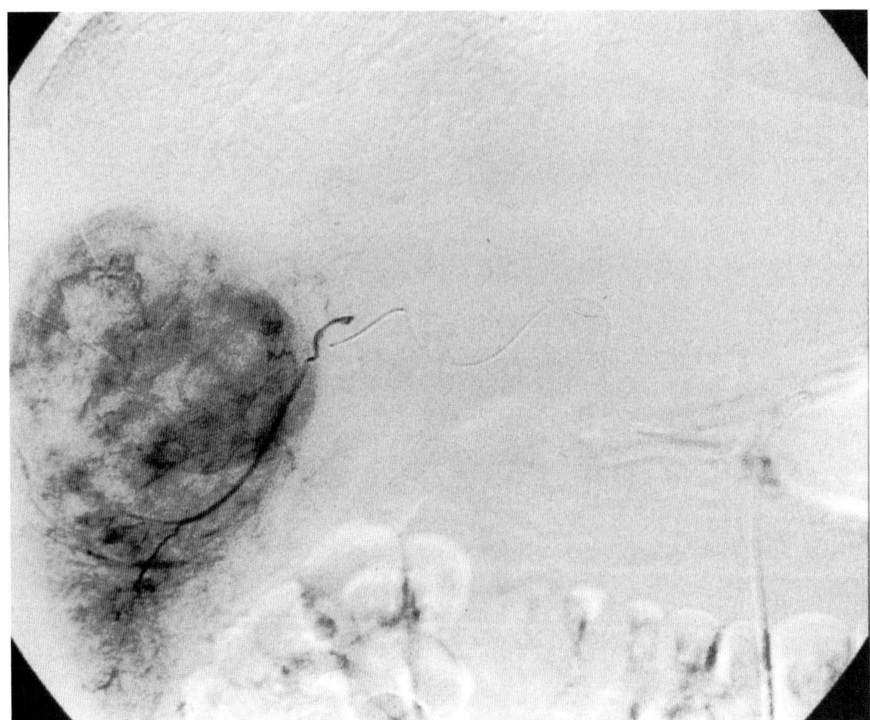

FIGURE 31-4. (*A*) Common hepatic arteriography shows a hypervascular hepatocellular carcinoma in the inferior segment of the right hepatic lobe. (*B*) The tumor is enhanced by contrast injection from the microcatheter advanced to the posterior inferior branch of the right hepatic artery. Arterial embolization with Lipiodol was performed from this microcatheter. *(Figure continues.)*

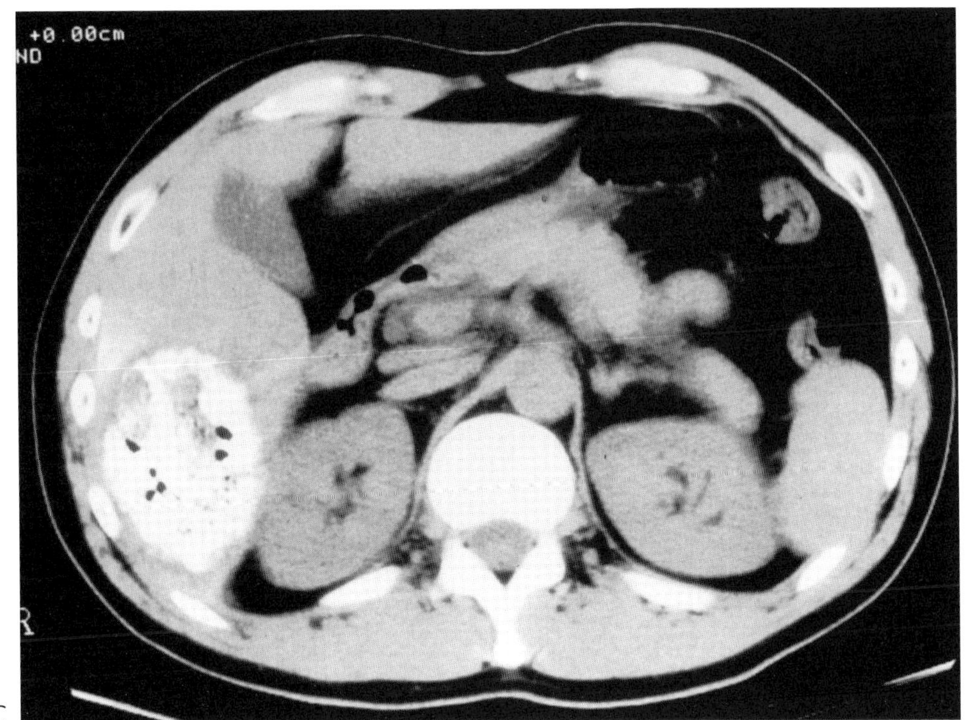

C

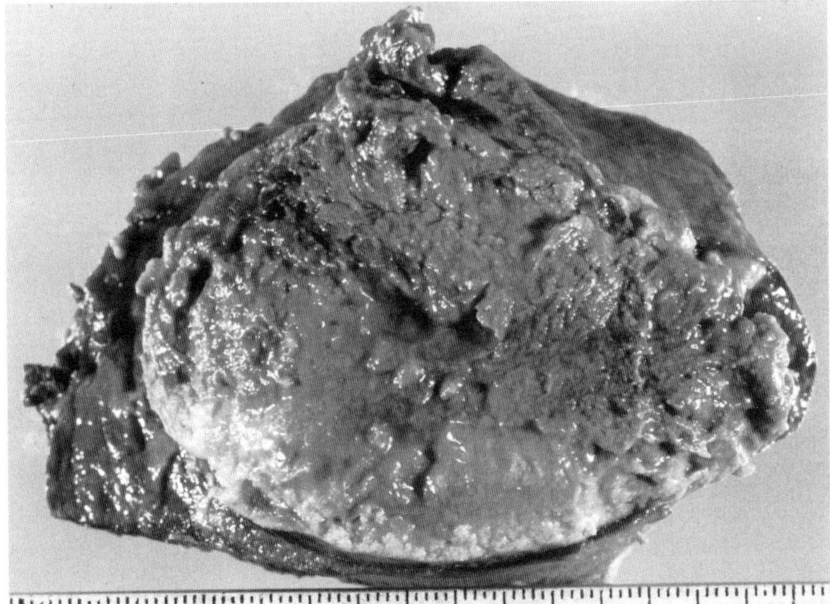

D

FIGURE 31-4 *(Continued).* (C) Lipiodol CT obtained 1 week after embolization shows Lipiodol accumulation and a small amount of gas in the tumor. Partial hepatectomy was performed 3 weeks later. (*D*) Resected hepatic specimen shows complete necrosis of the tumor.

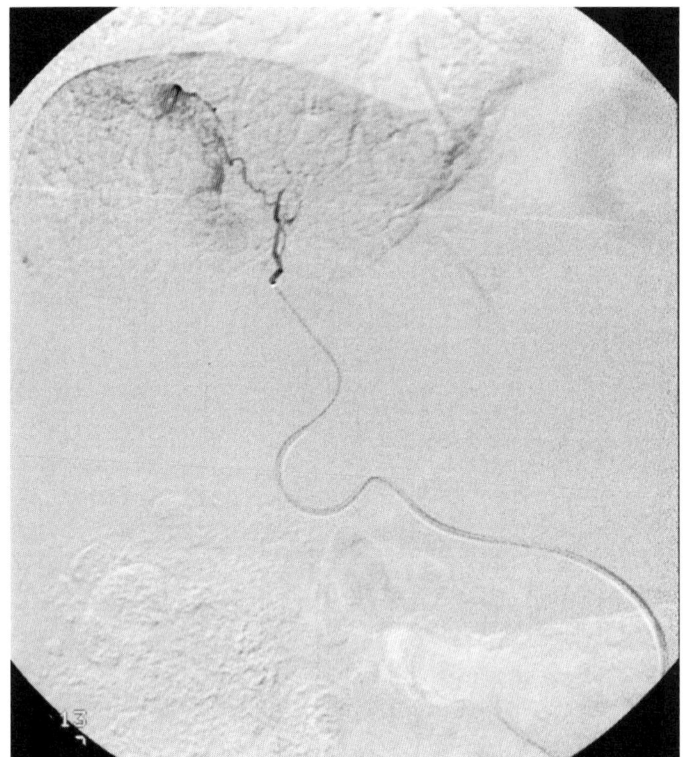

A

FIGURE 31-5. (*A*) Digital subtraction angiography from a microcatheter placed in the subsegmental hepatic artery of the anterior superior liver segment shows only a part of the tumor. (*B*) However, when CT arteriography was obtained during injection of contrast medium from the microcatheter, parts of the main tumor (arrows) and multiple daughter nodules (arrowheads) were seen.

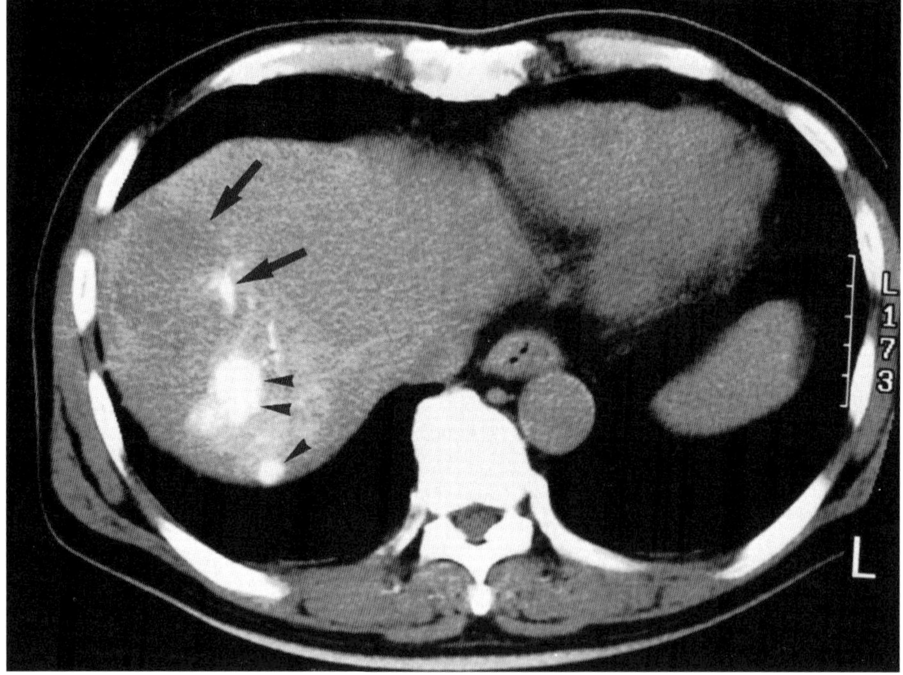

B

Embolization is performed after injecting 2% Xylocaine for intravenous injection into a catheter placed in the target artery. This prevents the severe pain that may develop in the liver during or immediately after the procedure. The mixture of an anticancer drug with Lipiodol is then slowly injected. Lastly, gelatin sponge, which has been cut into small pieces with a scissors, is injected as a mixture with a contrast medium and a small amount of the anticancer drug. When there is an extrahepatic collateral vessel feeding the HCC, a catheter should be placed in the collateral and advanced as close as possible to the tumor.[31] If there is marked arterial-portal shunting, a small amount of gelatin sponge should first be injected to eliminate it, and Lipiodol emulsion should then be administered. Arteriovenous shunts should be similarly treated, but Lipiodol injection should be carefully conducted so as not to flow to the lung directly.

After injection of Lipiodol emulsion, digital subtraction angiography (DSA) should be done to confirm that tumor staining has disappeared (Fig. 31-4). Finally, a plain x-ray film should be taken to confirm retention of the Lipiodol.

Follow-up and Duration of Treatment

After the procedure, the patient should be followed using assays for tumor markers in blood by computed tomography (CT) and/or by magnetic resonance imaging (MRI). The initial response is usually assessed twice by CT, about 1 week and about 1 month after the procedure. The response depends on the retention of Lipiodol in the tumor. If it is retained for 1 month or longer, the tumor often becomes necrotic.[32] If there is any residual tumor or relapse, it is mostly hypervascular, and the site appears dense in the early phase (i.e., arterial phase) of helical dynamic CT (Fig. 31-6). If it is difficult to visualize the state of the tumor interior by CT because of Lipiodol accumulation, MRI should be used. Accumulated Lipiodol does not affect MRI signals, so even relatively small viable tumor masses can be detected at an early phase by dynamic MRI[33] (Fig. 31-7). The procedure is generally performed at intervals of about 6 months. If the initial response is not sufficient or if the tumor is rapidly progressive, repeat embolizations may be done at intervals of 2 to 3 months. If the response is good, a

FIGURE 31-6. (*A*) Precontrast Lipiodol CT of hepatocellular carcinoma obtained 1 month after embolization with Lipiodol. (*B*) Arterial phase image of dynamic helical CT. (*C*) Portal venous phase image. (*D*) Late phase image. Partial washout of Lipiodol accumulation in the tumor is seen in a region that is expected to be a viable region of the tumor. The arterial phase CT image shows hyperenhancement of this region, and the portal venous phase CT image shows isoenhancement to the surrounding liver.

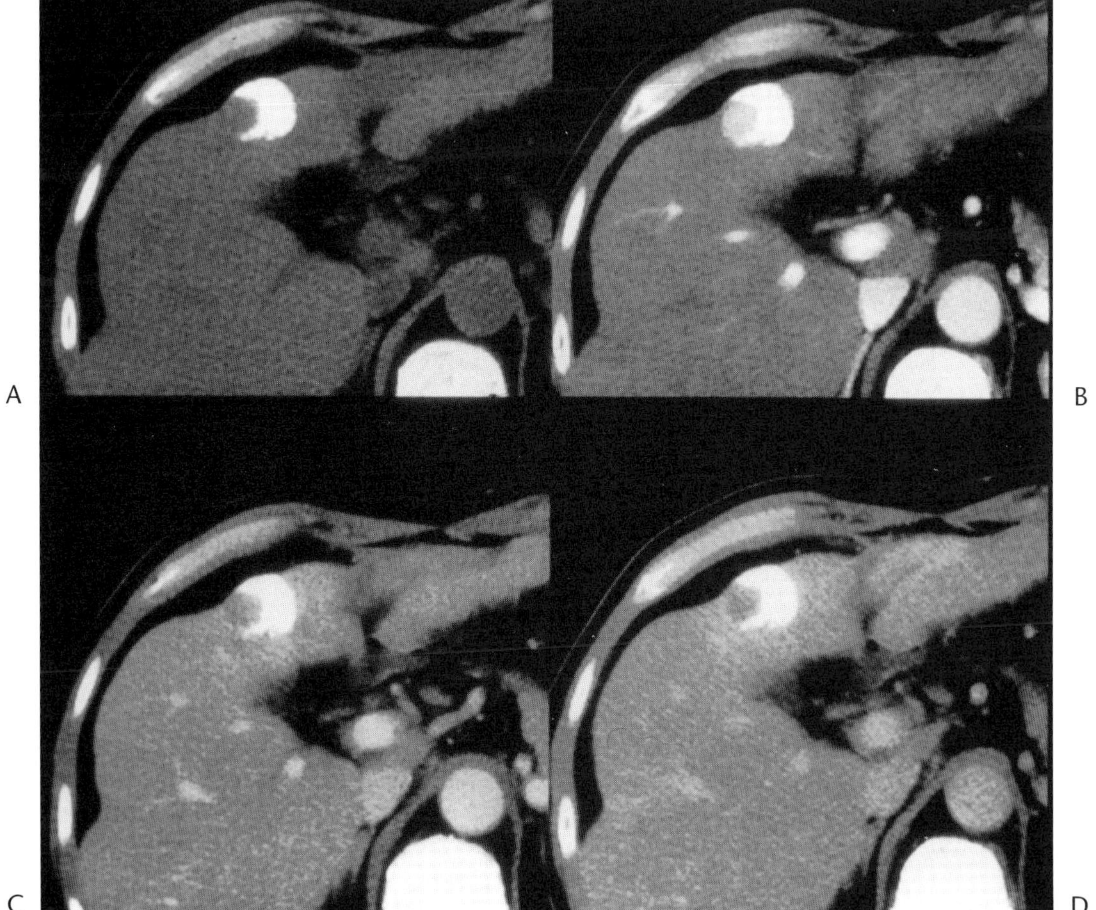

A

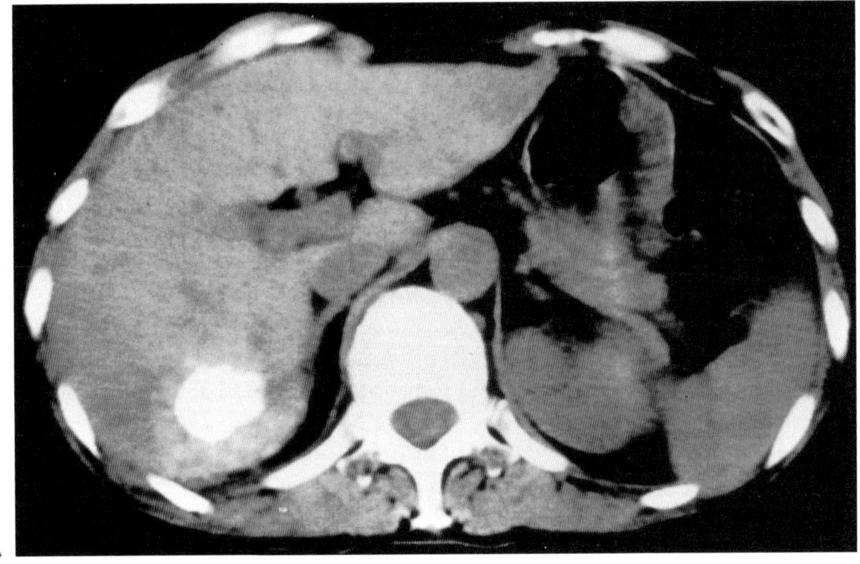

B

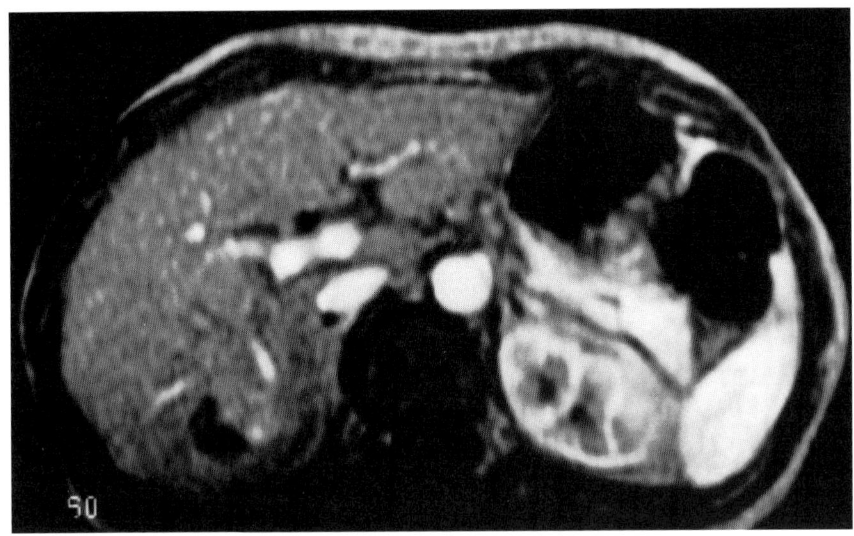

C

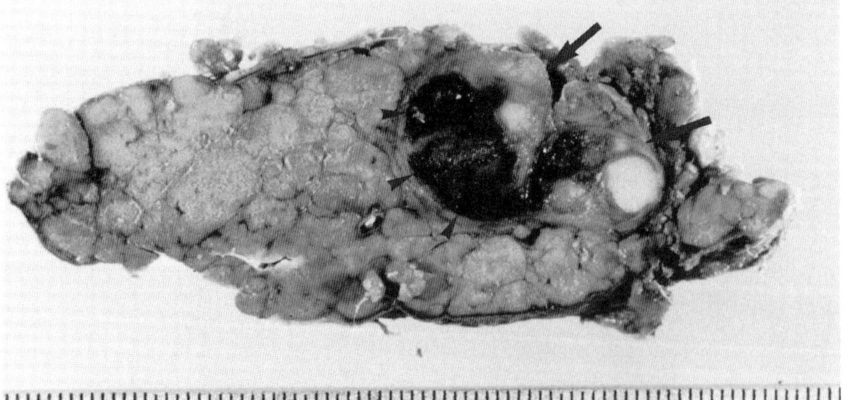

FIGURE 31-7. (*A*) Lipiodol CT, obtained 1 month after arterial embolization with Lipiodol, shows total Lipiodol accumulation in the hepatocellular carcinoma. (*B*) Arterial phase MRI (gradient echo, TR/TE/flip angle = 150 msec/10 msec/60 degrees) with Gd-DTPA shows partial enhancement in the tumor. (*C*) Partial hepatectomy was performed 1 month after embolization. The partial enhancement region seen in the arterial phase MRI corresponds to residual viable tumor (arrows), and the no enhancement region corresponds to hemorrhagic necrosis (arrowheads).

TABLE 31-1. Effect of Arterial Embolization in Microscopic Patterns of Tumor Growth

Growth Pattern	Degree of Necrosis					Total
	100%	99%–95%	94%–80%	79%–50%	<50%	
Expanding	29	13	24	7	6	79
Replacing	0	0	6	5	10	21
Total	29	13	30	12	16	100

(From Hashimato et al.,[36] with permission.)

second embolization may be done more than 1 year later if the tumor remains present.

RESULTS

Tumor Response to Embolization

Direct response to arterial embolization in HCC has been proved by histopathologic examination of patients who underwent hepatectomy after embolization.[34–36] Complete necrosis after embolization was observed in 29 of 100 patients, and necrosis of 80% of tumor tissues occurred in 72 patients.

Tumor response was closely related to tumor growth patterns. More than 80% of tumor tissues became necrotic in 66 of 79 patients (83.5%) with encapsulated tumors of the "expansive growth type." In contrast, more than 80% of tumor tissues became necrotic only in 6 out of 21 with the "replacing growth type" (28.5%) (Tables 31-1 and 31-2).[36] Thus, satellite HCCs and portal tumor thrombi did not respond well.[34–36]

When a group of patients who underwent selective embolization only in subsegments of the liver were analyzed, complete necrosis was found in 60% to 80% of lesions, including extracapsular lesions.[37–39] Response was better if the peritumor portal branches were well visualized with Lipiodol flowing into the portal veins.

In early stage HCCs with angiographic evidence of hypovascularity, Lipiodol was not retained; therefore embolization was virtually ineffective.[40]

Survival Rate

The prognosis of 443 patients with HCC who underwent repeated embolizations without surgical resection after the initial arterial embolization, in our institute and affiliated hospitals up to 1986, included a cumulative survival rate of 56.3% after 1 year, 33.3% after 2 years, 18.3% after 3 years, 11.8% after 4 years, and 8.0% after 5 years.[41] The therapeutic results improved significantly in those patients whose embolization was done with gelatin sponge and Lipiodol. In a subgroup of 228 patients who underwent embolization only with gelatin sponge, the 5-year survival rate was 3.4%, while it was 12.9% in 215 patients who underwent embolization with gelatin sponge and Lipiodol[41,42] (Fig. 31-8).

The prognosis of patients who underwent segmental or subsegmental arterial embolization was better than that of those who underwent less selective embolization. The survival rate of 82 patients who underwent subsegmental embolization, excluding patients with Child C classification and HCC more than 4 cm in diameter, was 100% after 1 year, 93% after 2 years, 73% after 3 years, and 53% after 5 years.[9] In 57 patients with lesions of various sizes (up to 8 cm in diameter) including those

TABLE 31-2. Efficacy of Arterial Embolization in Relation to Macroscopic Characteristics

	Degree of Necrosis					Total
	100%	99%–95%	94%–80%	79%–50%	<50%	
SN	19	7	7	3 (2)	2 (2)	38 (4)
SNE	8	4	16 (1)	5	6 (2)	39 (3)
CMN	1	0	2 (1)	3 (2)	3 (1)	9 (4)
Multiple	1	2	5 (4)	0	1 (1)	9 (5)
Massive	0	0	0	1 (1)	4 (4)	5 (5)
Total	29	13	30 (6)	12 (5)	16 (10)	100 (21)

Abbreviations: SN, single nodular type; SNE, single nodule with extranodular growth type; CMN, contiguous multinodular type; (), number of "replacing growth type."

(From Hashimoto et al.,[36] with permission.)

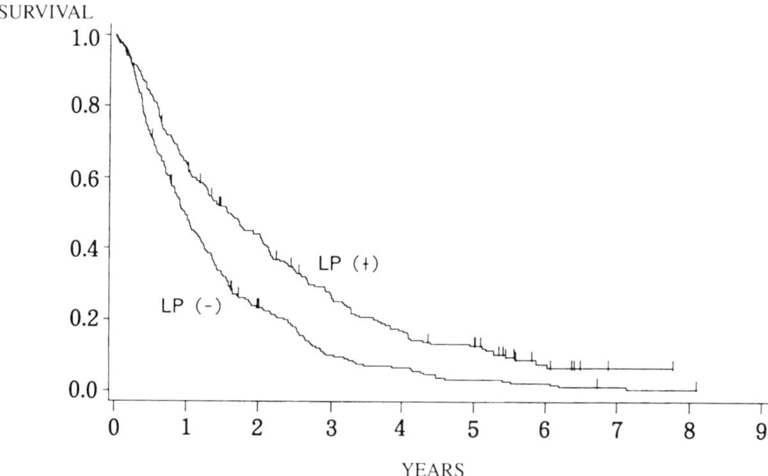

FIGURE 31-8. The cumulative survival rate of hepatocellular carcinoma after arterial embolization with (LP+) and without (LP−) Lipiodol. (From Nakamura et al.,[41] with permission.)

with Child C who underwent embolization in up to 3 subsegments, the survival rate was 87% after 1 year, 66% after 2 years, and 57% after 3 years.[37] Nishimine et al.[43] used similar segmental embolization in 98 cases of various sizes and reported a survival rate of 89% after 1 year, 69% after 2 years, 59% after 3 years, and 30% after 5 years. Patients with nodular lesions 3 cm or less in diameter had a survival rate of 100% after 1 year, 85% after 2 years, and 73% after 3 and 4 years. If catheters can be placed in the artery of the cancerous region, such superselective embolization achieves the best results. These results are comparable with those of hepatectomy.

Adverse Reactions

Transient nausea, vomiting, upper abdominal pain, and fever are associated with embolization. Liver function is also impaired because the noncancerous parenchymal tissue of the liver is also affected. Liver enzymes and total bilirubin often rise immediately after these procedures and return to pretreatment levels in about 10 days. Serum albumin falls gradually after embolization, reaches its lowest level in about 2 weeks, and may return to pretreatment levels after about 4 weeks. Cases with the worse baseline hepatic function and

FIGURE 31-9. Contrast CT obtained 1 month after arterial embolization with Lipiodol shows biloma in the liver.

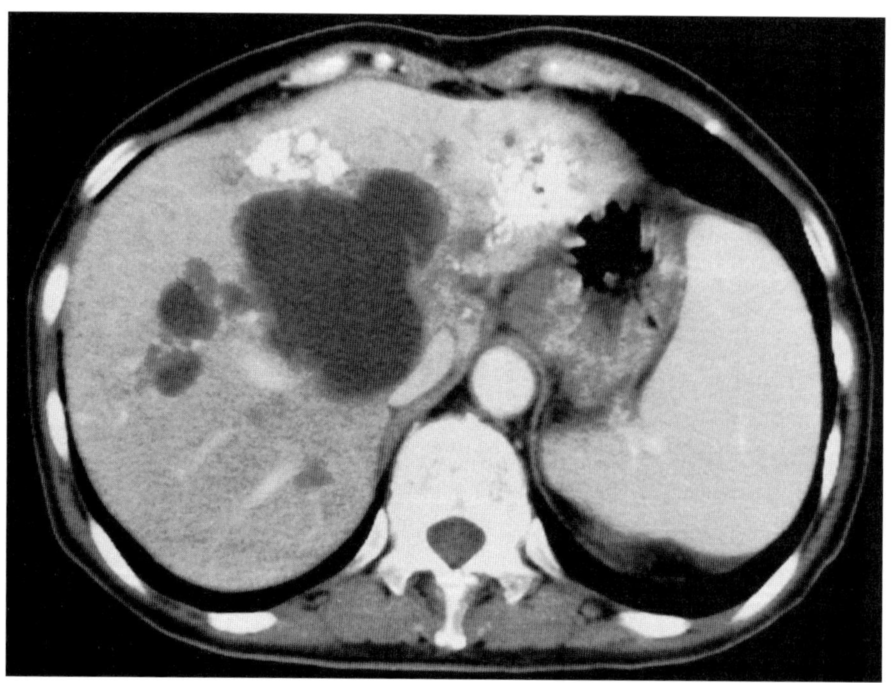

more severe portal invasion may progress to hepatic failure.

Gallbladder infarction related to cystic arterial embolism may often occur with fever and abdominal pain may then develop; however, this is not serious in many cases.[44] Emphysematous cholecystitis may result if gallbladder infarction is complicated by bacterial infection.[45] Biloma may be formed as a result of bile duct necrosis due to embolism in the peribiliary vascular plexus.[46,47] This may progress to abscess if there is concurrent infection (Fig. 31-9). If pneumobilia develops after surgery of the pancreas or the bile duct, necrotic foci in the noncancerous tissues, formed after embolization, may also form abscesses.[48] These possibilities justify the use of prophylactic antibiotics.

Adverse reactions are generally less severe if segmental or subsegmental embolization is used. However, if Lipiodol flows into the portal vein causing infarction or necrosis in the noncancerous hepatic tissues, adverse reactions may be severe. Not only hepatic impairment, but also transient renal failure may develop, because necrotic products may be rapidly released into the circulation. Splenic infarction,[49] pancreatic necrosis,[50] or gastric and duodenal ulcers may be associated with technical errors.

CONCLUSION

Arterial embolization is a useful procedure for the treatment of HCC. It is safe and effective if it is used in the right patients. Subsegmental embolization is at least equivalent to hepatectomy as a treatment of small HCC. The concurrent use of percutaneous ethanol injection or continuous arterial infusion using reservoirs[51] may lead to further improvments in the outcome of arterial embolization.

REFERENCES

1. Doyon D, Mouzon A, Jourde AN et al. L'embolisation artérielle hépatique dans les tumeurs malignes du foie. Ann Radiol 1974;17:593–603
2. Yamada R, Sato M, Kawabata M et al. Hepatic artery embolization in 120 patients with unresectable hepatoma. Radiology 1983;148:397–401
3. Nakamura K, Tashiro S, Hiraoka T et al. Hepatocellular carcinoma and metastatic cancer detected by iodized oil. Radiology 1985;154:15–17
4. Ohishi H, Uchida H, Yoshimura H et al. Hepatocellular carcinoma detected by iodized oil: use of anticancer agents. Radiology 1985;154:25–29
5. Yumoto Y, Jinno K, Tokuyama K et al. Hepatocellular carcinoma detected by iodized oil. Radiology 1985;154:19–24
6. Kasugai H, Kojima J, Tatsuta M et al. Treatment of hepatocellular carcinoma by transcatheter arterial embolization combined with intraarterial infusion of a mixture of cisplatin and ethiodized oil. Gastroenterology 1989;97:965–971
7. Nakamura H, Hashimoto T, Oi H, Sawada S. Transcatheter oily chemoembolization of hepatocellular carcinoma. Radiology 1989;170:783–786
8. Vetter D, Wenger JJ, Bergier JM et al. Transcatheter oily chemoembolization in the management of advanced hepatocellular carcinoma in cirrhosis: results of a western comparative study in 60 patients. Hepatology 1991;13:427–433
9. Masui O, Kadoya M, Yoshikawa J et al. Subsegmental transcatheter arterial embolization for small hepatocellular carcinoma: local therapeutic effect and 5-year survival rate. Cancer Chemother Pharmacol 1994;33(suppl):S84–S88
10. Chuang VP, Wallace S. Hepatic artery embolization in the treatment of hepatic neoplasms. Radiology 1981;140:51–58
11. Kuroda C, Sakurai M, Monden M et al. Transcatheter arterial embolization for metastatic liver tumors: a study in resected cases. Cardiovasc Intervent Radiol 1989;12:72–75
12. Breedis C, Young G. The blood supply of neoplasms in the liver. Am J Pathol 1954;30:969–985
13. Doppman JL, Girton M, Kahn ER. Proximal versus peripheral hepatic artery embolization: experimental study in monkeys. Radiology 1978;128:577–588
14. Nakamura H, Hashimoto T, Oi H, Sawada S. Iodized oil in the portal vein after arterial embolization. Radiology 1988; 167:415–417
15. Kan Z, Sato M, Ivancev K et al. Distribution and effect of iodized poppyseed oil in the liver after hepatic artery embolization: experimental study in several animal species. Radiology 1993;186:861–866
16. Sugihara S, Kojiro M, Nakashima T. Ultrastructural study of hepatocellular carcinoma with replacing growth pattern. Acta Pathol Jpn 1985;35:549–559
17. Nakamura H, Tanaka T, Hori S et al. Transcatheter embolization of hepatocellular carcinoma: assessment of efficacy in case of resection following embolization. Radiology 1983; 147:401–405
18. Kuroda C, Sakurai M, Monden M et al. Limitation of transcatheter arterial chemoembolization using iodized oil for small hepatocellular carcinoma: a study in resected cases. Cancer 1991;67:81–86
19. Miller DL, O'Leary TJ, Girton M. Distribution of iodized oil within the liver after hepatic arterial injection. Radiology 1987;162:849–852
20. Kan Z, Ivancev K, Hagerstrand I et al. In vivo microscopy of the liver after injection of Lipiodol into the hepatic artery and portal vein in the rat. Acta Radiol 1989;30:419–425
21. Nakamura H, Hashimoto T, Oi H et al. Treatment of hepatocellular carcinoma by segmental hepatic artery injection of adriamycin-in-oil emulsion with overflow to segmental portal veins. Acta Radiol 1990;31:347–349
22. Matsui O, Kadoya M, Suzuki M et al. Dynamic sequential computed tomography during arterial portography in the detection of hepatic neoplasms. Radiology 1983;146:721–727
23. Okazaki M, Higashihara H, Koganemaru F et al. Intraperitoneal hemorrhage from hepatocellular carcinoma: emergency

chemoembolization or embolization. Radiology 1991;180: 647–651

24. Nakamura H, Tanaka M, Oi H. Hepatic embolization from the common hepatic artery using balloon occlusion technique. Am J Roentgenol 1985;145:115–116
25. Nakamura H, Uchida H, Kuroda C et al. Accessory left gastric artery arising from left hepatic artery: angiographic study. Am J Roentgenol 1980;134:529–532
26. Nakamura H, Hashimoto T, Oi H et al. Prevention of gastric complication in hepatic arterial chemoembolization: balloon catheter occlusion technique. Acta Radiol 1991;132:81–82
27. Nakamura H, Hashimoto T, Oi H, Sawada S. Hepatic embolization through periportal collaterals using balloon occlusion technique. Am J Roentgenol 1987;148:626–628
28. Murakami T, Kim T, Oi H et al. The detectability of hypervascular hepatocellular carcinoma by arterial phase images of MRI and spiral CT. Acta Radiol 1995;36:372–376
29. Makuuchi M, Sukigara M, Mori T et al. Bile duct necrosis: complication of transcatheter hepatic arterial embolization. Radiology 1985;156:331–334
30. Konno T, Maeda H, Iwai K et al. Effect of arterial administration of high-molecular-weight anticancer agent SMANCS with lipid lymphographic agent on hepatoma. Eur J Cancer Clin Oncol 1983;19:1053–1065
31. Okazaki M, Higashihara H, Ono H et al. Chemoembolization for hepatocellular carcinoma via the inferior pancreaticoduodenal artery in patients with celiac artery stenosis. Acta Radiol 1993;34:20–25
32. Matsui O, Takashima T, Kadoya M et al. Mechanism of lipiodol accumulation and retention in hepatic tumors: Analysis in cases with simple lipiodol injection. Nippon Acta Radiol 1987;47:1395–1404
33. Murakami T, Nakamura H, Tsuda K et al. Treatment of hepatocellular carcinoma by chemoembolization: evaluation with 3DFT MR imaging. Am J Roentgenol 1993;160: 295–299
34. Sasaki Y, Imaoka S, Kasugai H et al. A new approach to chemoembolization therapy for hepatoma, using ethiodized oil, cisplatin and gelatin sponge. Cancer 1987;60:1194–1203
35. Takayasu K, Shima Y, Muramatsu Y et al. Hepatocellular carcinoma treatment with intraarterial iodized oil with and without chemotherapeutic agents. Radiology 1987;163: 345–351
36. Hashimoto T, Nakamura H, Hori S et al. Hepatocellular carcinoma: efficacy of transcatheter oily chemoembolization in relation to macroscopic and microscopic patterns of tumor growth among 100 patients with partial hepatectomy. Cardiovasc Intervent Radiol 1995;18:82–86
37. Nakamura H, Hori S, Kozuka T et al. Transcatheter treatment of localized hepatocellular carcinoma: segmental arterioportal chemoembolization. Reg Cancer Treat 1992;5: 102–105
38. Matsuo N, Uchida H, Nishimine K et al. Segmental transcatheter hepatic artery chemoembolization with iodized oil for hepatocellular carcinoma: antitumor effect and influence on normal tissue. J Vasc Interv Radiol 1993;4:543–549
39. Matsui O, Kadoya M, Yoshikawa J et al. Small hepatocellular carcinoma: treatment with subsegmental transcatheter arterial embolization. Radiology 1993;188:79–83
40. Takayasu K, Wakao F, Moriyama N et al. Response of early-stage hepatocellular carcinoma and borderline lesions to therapeutic arterial embolization. Am J Roentgenol 1993; 160:301–306
41. Nakamura H, Mitani T, Murakami T et al. Five-year survival after transcatheter chemoembolization for hepatocellular carcinoma. Cancer Chemother Pharmacol 1994;33(suppl): S89–S92
42. Nakao N, Uchida H, Kamino K et al. Effectiveness of lipiodol in transcatheter arterial embolization of hepatocellular carcinoma. Cancer Chemother Pharmacol 1992;31(suppl 1): S72–S76
43. Nishimine K, Uchida H, Matsuo N et al. Segmental transarterial chemoembolization with Lipiodol mixed with anticancer drugs for nonresectable hepatocellular carcinoma: follow-up CT and therapeutic results. Cancer Chemother Pharmacol 1994;33(suppl):S60–S68
44. Kuroda C, Iwasaki M, Tanaka T et al. Gallbladder infarction following hepatic transcatheter arterial embolization: angiographic study. Radiology 1983;149:85–89
45. Nakamura H, Kondoh H. Emphysematous cholecystitis: complication of hepatic artery embolization. Cardiovasc Intervent Radiol 1986;9:152–153
46. Doppman JL, Dunnick NR, Girton M et al. Bile duct cysts secondary to liver infarcts: report of a case and experimental production by small vessel hepatic artery occlusion. Radiology 1979;130:1–5
47. Inoue Y, Nakamura H, Takashima S et al. Biloma following transcatheter oily chemoembolization. Radiat Med 1991;9: 57–60
48. Hashimoto T, Mitani T, Nakamura H et al. Fetal septic complication of transcatheter chemoembolization for hepatocellular carcinoma. Cardiovasc Intervent Radiol 1993;16: 325–327
49. Takayasu K, Moriyama N, Muramatsu Y et al. Splenic infarction a complication of transcatheter hepatic arterial embolization for liver malignancies. Radiology 1984;151:371–375
50. Furui S, Otomo K, Itai Y, Iio M. Hepatocellular carcinoma treated by transcatheter arterial embolization: progress evaluated by computed tomography. Radiology 1984;150: 773–778
51. Tateishi H, Kinuta M, Furukawa J. Follow-up study of combination treatment (TAE and PEIT) for unresectable hepatocellular carcinoma. Cancer Chemother Pharmacol 1994; 33(suppl):S119–S123
52. Nakamura H, Hashimoto T, Murakami T et al. Patients with advanced hepatocellular carcinoma (stages III and higher) who survived long periods (more than 5 years) after interventional radiology (IVR). IVR 1995;10:250–252

32

CHEMOEMBOLIZATION OF HEPATOCELLULAR CARCINOMA

JEAN-PIERRE BRONOWICKI
DENIS VETTER
MICHEL DOFFOEL

Chemoembolization, first used by Yamada et al.[1] in the treatment of hepatocellular carcinoma (HCC), is based on the sequential administration of chemotherapy infused into the hepatic artery and hepatic artery embolization. The goal of the combination is to obtain a synergistic effect on the tumors.

PRINCIPLES OF CHEMOEMBOLIZATION

Liver tumors get their blood supply from the hepatic artery while normal liver parenchyma is supplied by both the portal vein and the hepatic artery.[2] Thus, the occlusion of the hepatic artery performs relatively selective tumor ischemia, leading to necrosis. This induced ischemia is able to enhance the cytotoxicity of some antineoplastic agents.[3] Decreasing the arterial flow has also been shown to increase the regional "area under the curve" for the chemotherapeutic agent achieved in the liver tumor bed compared with that achieved in the systemic circulation when chemotherapy is infused into the hepatic artery.[4,5] Moreover, livers resected after chemoembolization showed higher concentration of the drug in the cancer area than that in the intact portions of the same liver.[6,7] This should lead to the reduction of undesirable systemic and hepatic effects of the drug.

TRANSARTERIAL CHEMOEMBOLIZATION

Transarterial chemoembolization (TACE) consists of the intra-arterial infusion of an anticancer agent in the feeding artery of the tumor followed by embolization. To prevent the rapid development of collateral circulation, embolization should be as peripheral as possible in the local circulation. However, because very peripheral hepatic artery occlusion may have deleterious effects on liver function,[8,9] some investigators do not advocate the use of very small embolizing particles (powder; 40 to 50 *m*m in diameter for gelatin powder) as embolizing material.[9] Different embolizing material such as gelatin sponge, starch, polyvinyl alcohol, collagen, and autologous blood clot have been tried.[10] Most investigators have used gelatin sponge in association with the intra-arterial infusion of doxorubicin, mitomycin C, aclarubicin, epirubicin, or cisplatin. This material undergoes degradation and resorption in the circulation, and the vessels recanalize within 48 to 72 hours.[11] Repeated treatments of the same vascular bed can be performed.

CHEMOEMBOLIZATION WITH MICROSPHERES OR MICROCAPSULES

Another approach of chemoembolization consists in the use of microspheres containing an antineoplastic agent. The microspheres measure about 200 μm in diameter and are composed of ethylcellulose, starch, polylactic acid, or albumin. Following intra-arterial injection, the microspheres first embolize small vessels at the level of the third or fourth branch of the hepatic artery and then slowly release the anticancer agent.[5,6,12–15]

TECHNIQUES USING LIPIODOL (TRANSCATHETER OILY CHEMOEMBOLIZATION)

Lipiodol, an oily contrast medium, is an ethyl ester of a fatty acid from poppyseed oil and has been used for lymphography. When Lipiodol is administered through arteries feeding the hepatocellular carcinoma, the oily contrast medium remains selectively in the neoplastic tissue for an extended time, whereas no deposits are evident after 3 weeks in the nontumorous liver tissue. The precise mechanisms of Lipiodol retention are still unclear, but may be due to abnormal vascularity and lack of lymphatics in HCCs.[16] This attribute has led to the investigation of Lipiodol-enhanced computed tomography (CT) aortoportography in the preoperative staging of patients with limited-stage HCC because of its sensitivity in identifying small satellite lesions that may be missed by unenhanced imaging modalities[17,18] (Fig. 32-1).

The therapeutic use of Lipiodol has been explored first with a lipophilic chemotherapeutic agent such as Styrene-Maleic Acid-Neocarzinostatin (SMANCS)[19] and then, more widely, with water-soluble antitumor agents such as doxorubicin, cisplatin, mitomycin C or epirubicin. Often the water-soluble anticancer drug is mixed with a water-soluble contrast medium before the solution is mixed with Lipiodol. This procedure, called by some authors *lipiodolization*, lowers the peak plasma concentration and increases the intratumoral concentration and half-life of the anticancer agent.[4,20–23] Because the intra-arterial injection of Lipiodol alone cannot cause a complete embolization, this iodized oil should not be considered as an embolizing material, but only as a targeting material.[24] Therefore, lipiodolization is usually administered with embolization with gelatin sponge.

RESPONSE TO CHEMOEMBOLIZATION

After chemoembolization with or without Lipiodol, a greater than 50% reduction in size (partial response) was noted by CT scan in 15 to 75% of cases[6,7,11,13–15,23,25–31] and a greater than 50% decrease of α-fetoprotein (AFP) level was observed in 23% to 100% of cases.[6,7,13,14,25–28,31] In one study, transcatheter oily chemoembolization (TOCE) with cisplatin significantly increased the rate of partial necrosis (38%) compared to TOCE with doxorubicin (13%) and TACE with doxorubicin (11%).[31] In another study, TOCE and TACE resulted in partial responses of 21% and 26%, respectively, compared to lipiodolization (9%) and intra-arterial chemotherapy (5%).[29] There is a close relationship between the extent of deposits of Lipiodol in HCC and the antitumor effect.[6] Complete responses are unusual after chemoembolization.[7,24,31–35] Although extensive tumor necrosis can be observed, viable residual tumor cells remain, particularly beneath the tumor capsule, in intracapsular invasion, in daughter tumors, and in portal

FIGURE 32-1. CT scan of an uninodular HCC (arrowhead) *(A)* before and *(B)* after transcatheter oily chemoembolization.

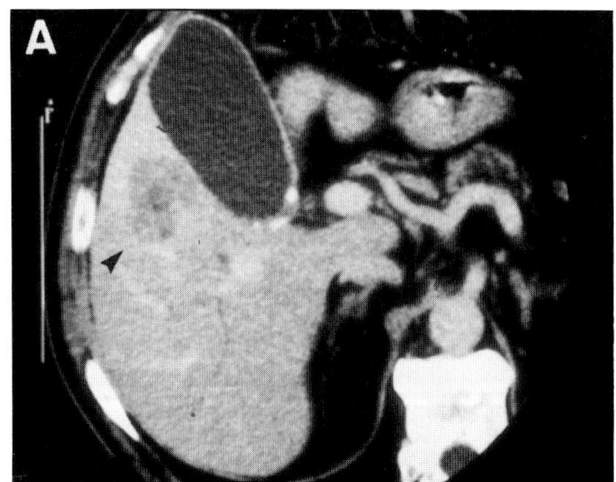

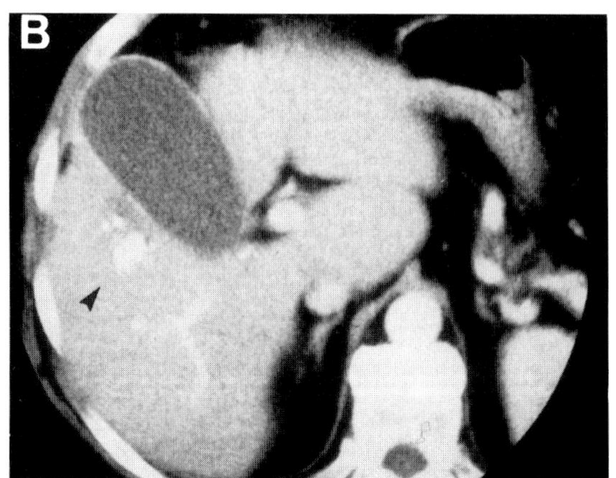

vein tumor thrombi,[24,31,32] due to differences in blood supply from the main tumors[20,36] and probably to the collaterals that develop soon after occlusion.[32,37] Chemoembolization is most effective against encapsulated small HCC without extracapsular invasion.[34,35]

TOCE with cisplatin is significantly better than TACE or than TOCE with doxorubicin in terms of the histologic responses of the main tumor, the daughter tumor, and portal vein thrombi.[31] In the majority of studies this was assessed after a single chemoembolization; therefore, in cases of unresectable HCC, the treatment probably should be repeated. In general, TOCE acts to prevent or delay extension of the cancer, but it has no effect on extrahepatic dissemination.[38,39]

EFFECT ON PATIENT SURVIVAL

Survival after chemoembolization is difficult to assess because of the multiplicity of the techniques used in the different studies, because of the heterogenicity of the disease, and because the majority of the published studies are retrospective (Tables 32-1 and 32-2). The 1- and 2-year survival rates of the 2,094 patients in 15 Asian studies[6,15,20,23,25,26,29,30,31,40–45] were 62% and 41%, respectively. The 1- and 2-year survival rates of 820 patients in 10 Western studies[9,11,14,27,28,39,46–49] were 58% and 35%, respectively.

Few studies compared the survival rate after chemoembolization to the survival rate after symptomatic treatments. In one retrospective study, TOCE significantly increased the survival with Okuda's I and II tumors but was of no effect on survival with Okuda's III tumors.[39] In one prospective randomized study, the probability of survival at 1-year after TACE was not increased (24%) in comparison with the probability of survival after symptomatic treatment (31%).[9] A prospective randomized study found a relative risk of death of 1.3 in the symptomatic management group compared to TOCE group, in patients with Okuda's stage I tumors.[28] In our experience,[39] the probability of survival after TOCE in patients with Okuda's stage I tumor was 85%, 63%, 46% and 46% at 1, 2, 3, and 4 years, respectively, compared to 41%, 19%, 11%, and 0.

Factors predictive of survival after chemoembolization remain unclear. Multivariate analyses showed that

TABLE 32-1. Survival After Chemoembolization According to the Technique, the Okuda's Staging and the Child-Pugh Score, in Asian Studies

			Okuda Staging (%)			Child Score (%)			Survival (%)			
Author (Ref.)	Technique	n	I	II	III	A	B	C	1 yr	2 yr	3 yr	4 yr
Kanematsu et al.[20]	Lip	149	41	55	4	ns	ns	ns	56	29	17	7
Kobayashi et al.[25]	Lip	41	ns	ns	ns	ns	ns	ns	55			
Shibata et al.[23]	Lip	71	ns	ns	ns	ns	ns	ns	55	30		
Yamashita et al.[29]	Lip	135	61	22	17	55	29	16	38	18		
Beppu et al.[15]	MS ' Lip	66	ns	ns	ns	ns	ns	ns	81	64	51	
Ichihara et al.[6]	MS	62	40	29	31	ns	ns	ns	54	25	19	
Ikeda et al.[40]	TACE	158	ns	ns	ns	ns	ns	ns	76	54	41	
Kasugai et al.[31]	TACE	20	ns	ns	ns	ns	ns	ns	40	5		
Nakamura et al.[42]	TACE	228	ns	ns	ns	ns	ns	ns	44	25	12	6
Soga et al.[26]	TACE	40	ns	ns	ns	ns	ns	ns	48	20		
Yamashita et al.[29]	TACE	58	74	26	0	60	33	7	71	55	15	
Gunji et al.[44]	TOCE	22	ns	ns	ns	0	64	36	100	100		
Kasugai et al.[31]	TOCE	77	ns	ns	ns	ns	ns	ns	66	43		
Kawai et al.[45]	TOCE	403	68	32	0	74	24	2	72	50		
Nakamura et al.[42]	TOCE	215	ns	ns	ns	ns	ns	ns	65	44	25	17
Ngan et al.[30]	TOCE or Lip	80	ns	ns	ns	ns	ns	ns	53	38		
Ohishi et al.[43]	TOCE	97	ns	ns	ns	ns	ns	ns	69			
Shijo et al.[41]	TOCE	110	34	66	0	ns	ns	ns	80	50	39	20
Yamashita et al.[29]	TOCE	62	79	21	0	71	24	5	62	44	29	

Abbreviations: Lip, lipiodolization; MS, microsphere; TACE, transarterial chemoembolization; TOCE, transcatheter oily chemoembolization; ns, not specified.

TABLE 32-2. Survival After Chemoembolization According to the Technique, the Okuda's Staging, and the Child-Pugh Score in Western Studies

Author (Ref.)	Technique	n	Okuda Staging (%)			Child Score (%)			Survival (%)			
			I	II	III	A	B	C	1 yr	2 yr	3 yr	4 yr
Kirk et al.[46]	Lip	14	ns	ns	ns	ns	ns	ns	36			
Stefanni et al.[47]	Lip	31	27	60	13	33	50	17	42	0	0	
Audisio et al.[14]	MS	30	47	53	0	60	40	0	36	36		
Pelletier et al.[9]	TACE	21	29	52	19	ns	ns	ns	24			
Venook et al.[11]	TACE	51	ns	ns	ns	ns	ns	ns	40	20	15	
Bismuth et al.[48]	TOCE	291	52	41	7	60	33	7	61	37		
Bronowicki et al.[39]	TOCE	127	39	48	13	57	29	14	64	38	27	27
Mondazzi et al.[49]	TOCE	84	86	14	0	54	46	0	62	31		
Stefanini et al.[47]	TOCE	69	45	49	6	46	45	9	73	44	36	20
Stuart et al.[27]	TOCE	52	ns	ns	ns	ns	ns	ns	60	40	10	
Trinchet et al.[28]	TOCE	50	94	6	0	100	0	0	62	38		

Abbreviations: Lip, lipiodolization; MS, microsphere; TACE, transarterial chemoembolization; TOCE, transcatheter oily chemoembolization; ns, not specified.

age,[49] Child-Pugh score,[49] total serum bilirubin,[29,40,41,49] albumin,[41] tumor size,[29,40,41,49] portal vein invasion,[29,40] degree of Lipiodol labeling,[49] and tumor size change after treatment[49] are independent predictive factors of survival after chemoembolization. The ideal number of procedures and the frequency of procedures remain to be determined. Ikeda et al.[40] showed that a good response during repeated therapy was significantly associated with increased survival.

The angiographic technique that provides the best survival for the majority of patients with HCC remains to be determined. Several teams consider TOCE as the most efficient treatment. However, the benefit of the use of Lipiodol on survival remains unclear. In a retrospective study, Nakamura et al.[42] showed that the survival rate after TOCE was significantly higher than after TACE. This result was confirmed by a prospective randomized trial in which survival after TOCE with cisplatin was significantly higher than after TACE with adriamycin. In this study, patients treated by TOCE with cisplatin tended to survive longer than patients treated by TOCE with adriamycin, but the difference was not statistically significant.[31] In a prospective randomized study, Yamashita et al.[29] showed that there was no statistical difference in survival between TOCE and TACE, but survival differences were significant between TACE or TOCE and lipiodolization.

Recently, several groups compared the results of resection with the results of different techniques of chemoembolization. In one, the survival rate after resection was significantly higher than the survival rate after TACE (5-year survival rate: 55% after resection versus 18% after TACE).[50] Others have shown that for some HCC, especially HCC smaller than 5 cm,[51] the probability of survival was similar after surgery and chemoembolization.[51–53]

SIDE EFFECTS

Fever (usually due to tumor necrosis), abdominal pain, nausea, and/or vomiting are very common after chemoembolization. The frequency of nausea and vomiting depends on the antimitotic agent used. With cisplatin, these side effects are more frequent,[31] and analgesic, antiemetic, and antipyretic drugs should be used to control them. Prophylactic systemic antibiotics are also used.

The major risk of chemoembolization is renal insufficiency, which can be due to the acidosis induced by the necrosis, or to nephrotoxicity of the anticancer agent or the contrast medium. Hyperhydration and forced diuresis should be used to try to prevent this complication.

Cytolysis and the increase of bilirubin are common and transient. Cholecystitis is a rare complication brought about by the use of powder as the embolizing agent. The possibility of pulmonary oil embolism after TOCE can occur in patients who receive more than 20 ml of iodized oil.[54]

INDICATIONS FOR CHEMOEMBOLIZATION

Chemoembolization is indicated in patients who cannot undergo surgery because of insufficient hepatic reserve and/or poor health conditions. Fewer than 10% of HCC patients are eligible for surgery in Western countries; thus a majority of patients with HCC are concerned by this treatment. Complete portal thrombosis and portal flow inversion are absolute contraindications of TACE and TOCE but not of lipiodolization. Lipiodolization can occasionally lead to repermeabilization of the portal trunk.[55] Unilateral intrahepatic vein thrombosis is a relative contraindication. Major hepatic insufficiency (Child C and Okuda's III), hyperbilirubinemia, or severe renal insufficiency are contraindications. The use of autologous blood clot as an embolizing agent has been reported for chemoembolization in Child C cirrhosis.[44]

Chemoembolization is sometimes performed before surgery to obtain a tumor size reduction that will allow a more conservative liver resection[7,32–35,41,48,56–58] or in preparation for liver transplantation.[48,59,60] The benefit of this treatment before surgery has to be evaluated. Some authors feel that chemoembolization before resection should be avoided because it does not improve long-term survival rates,[56–58] possibly because, in patients with partial necrosis, the remaining tumor cells are less firmly attached and more likely to be dislodged into the bloodstream during hepatic resection.[58]

SUMMARY

Chemoembolization can be considered as an effective treatment of unresectable HCC but, in the majority of cases, it remains only palliative. Future improvements may be possible by the combination of chemoembolization with percutaneous ethanol[61] injection, the use of emulsifying agents,[62] or of a membrane-emulsification technique.[63]

REFERENCES

1. Yamada R, Sato M, Kawabata M et al. Hepatic artery embolization in 120 patients with unresectable hepatoma. Radiology 1983;148:397–401
2. Breedis C, Young G. The blood supply of neoplasms in the liver. Am J Pathol 1954;30:969–985
3. Teicher BA, Lazo JS, Sartorelli AC. Classification of antineoplastic agents by their selective toxicities toward oxygenated and hypoxic tumor cells. Cancer Res 1981;41:73–81
4. Raoul JL, Heresbach D, Bretagne JF et al. Chemoembolization of hepatocellular carcinomas. A study of the biodistribution and pharmacokinetics of doxorubicin. Cancer 1992;70: 585–590
5. Andersson M, Aronsen KF, Balch C et al. Pharmacokinetics of intraarterial mitomycin C with or without degradable starch microspheres (DSM) in the treatment of non-resectable liver cancer. Acta Oncol 1989;28:219–222
6. Ichihara T, Sakamoto K, Mori K, Akagi M. Transcatheter arterial chemoembolization therapy for hepatocellular carcinoma using polylactic acid microspheres containing aclarubicin hydrochloride. Cancer Res 1989;49:4357–4362
7. Sasaki Y, Imaoka S, Kasugai H et al. A new approach to chemoembolization therapy for hepatoma using ethiodized oil, cisplatin, and gelatin sponge. Cancer 1987;60: 1194–1203
8. Doppman JL, Girton M, Kahn ER. Proximal versus peripheral hepatic artery embolization: experimental study in monkeys. Radiology 1978;128:577–588
9. Pelletier G, Roche A, Ink O et al. A randomized trial of hepatic chemoembolization in patients with unresectable hepatocellular carcinoma. J Hepatol 1990;11:181–184
10. Venook AP. Treatment of hepatocellular carcinoma: too many options? J Clin Oncol 1994;12:1323–1334
11. Venook AP, Stagg RJ, Lewis BJ et al. Chemoembolization for hepatocellular carcinoma. J Clin Oncol 1990;8:1108–1114
12. Fujimoto S, Miyazaki M, Endoh F et al. Effects of intraarterially infused biodegradable microspheres containing mitomycin C. Cancer 1985;55:522–526
13. Ohnishi K, Tsuchiya S, Nakayama T et al. Arterial chemoembolization of hepatocellular carcinoma with mitomycin C microcapsules. Radiology 1984;152:51–55
14. Audisio RA, Doci R, Mazzaferro V et al. Hepatic arterial embolization with microencapsulated mitomycin C for unresectable hepatocellular carcinoma in cirrhosis. Cancer 1990; 66:228–236
15. Beppu T, Ohara C, Yamaguchi Y et al. A new approach to chemoembolization for unresectable hepatocellular carcinoma using aclarubicin microspheres in combination with cisplatin suspended in iodized oil. Cancer 1991;68: 2555–2560
16. Konno T, Yamashita R, Oda T et al. Targeting cancer chemotherapy used lipiodol as a carrier of anticancer agents for hepatocellular carcinoma. Reg Cancer Treat 1992;5: 110–116
17. Ngan H. Lipiodol computerized tomography: how sensitive and specific is the technique in the diagnosis of hepatocellular carcinoma? Br J Radiol 1990;63:771–775
18. Yumoto Y, Jinno K, Tokuyama K et al. Hepatocellular carcinoma detected by iodized oil. Radiology 1985;154:19–24
19. Konno T, Maeda H, Iwai K et al. Effect of arterial administration of high-molecular-weight anticancer agent SMANCS with lipid lymphographic agent on hepatoma: a preliminary report. Eur J Cancer Clin Oncol 1983;19:1053–1065
20. Kanematsu T, Furuta T, Takenaka K et al. A 5-year experience of lipiodolization: selective regional chemotherapy for 200 patients with hepatocellular carcinoma. Hepatology 1989;10:98–102
21. Konno T. Targeting cancer chemotherapeutic agents by use of lipiodol contrast medium. Cancer 1990;66:1897–1903
22. Nakamura H, Hashimoto T, Oi H, Sawada S. Transcatheter oily chemoembolization of hepatocellular carcinoma. Radiology 1989;170:783–786
23. Shibata J, Fujiyama S, Sato T et al. Hepatic arterial injection chemotherapy with cisplatin suspended in an oily lymphographic agent for hepatocellular carcinoma. Cancer 1989; 64:1586–1594

24. Takayasu K, Shima Y, Muramatsu Y et al. Hepatocellular carcinoma: treatment with intraarterial iodized oil with and without chemotherapeutic agents. Radiology 1987;162: 345–351
25. Kobayashi H, Hidaka H, Kajiya Y et al. Treatment of hepatocellular carcinoma by transarterial injection of anticancer agents in iodized oil suspension or of radioactive iodized oil solution. Acta Radiol Diagn 1986;27:139–147
26. Soga K, Nomoto M, Ichida T et al. Clinical evaluation of transcatheter arterial embolization and one-shot chemotherapy in hepatocellular carcinoma. Hepatogastroenterology 1988;35:116–120
27. Stuart K, Stokes K, Jenkins R et al. Treatment of hepatocellular carcinoma using doxorubicin/ethiodized oil/gelatin powder chemoembolization. Cancer 1993;72:3202–3209
28. Trinchet JC, Groupe d'étude et de Traitement du Carcinome Hépatocellulaire. A comparison of lipiodol chemoembolization and conservative treatment for unresectable hepatocellular carcinoma. N Engl J Med 1995;332:1256–1261
29. Yamashita Y, Takahashi M, Koga Y et al. Prognostic factors in the treatment of hepatocellular carcinoma with transcatheter arterial embolization and arterial infusion. Cancer 1991; 67:385–391
30. Ngan H, Lai CL, Fan ST et al. Treatment of inoperable hepatocellular carcinoma by transcatheter arterial chemoembolization using an emulsion of cisplatin in iodized oil and Gelfoam. Clin Radiol 1993;47:315–320
31. Kasugai H, Kojima J, Tatsuta M et al. Treatment of hepatocellular carcinoma by transcatheter arterial embolization combined with intraarterial infusion of a mixture of cisplatin and ethiodized oil. Gastroenterology 1989;97:965–971
32. Hsu HC, Wei TC, Tsang YM et al. Histologic assessment of resected hepatocellular carcinoma after transcatheter hepatic arterial embolization. Cancer 1986;57:1184–1191
33. Sakurai M, Okamura J, Kuroda C. Transcatheter chemoembolization effective for treating hepatocellular carcinoma. A histopathologic study. Cancer 1984;54:387–392
34. Kuroda C, Sakurai M, Monden M et al. Limitation of transcatheter arterial chemoembolization using iodized oil for small hepatocellular carcinoma. A study in resected cases. Cancer 1991;67:81–86
35. Nakamura H, Liu T, Hori S et al. Response to transcatheter oily chemoembolization in hepatocellular carcinoma 3 cm or less: a study in 50 patients who underwent surgery. Hepatogastroenterology 1993;40:6–9
36. Wakasa K, Sakurai M, Kuroda C et al. Effect of transcatheter arterial embolization on the boundary architecture of hepatocellular carcinoma. Cancer 1990;65:913–919
37. Okazaki M, Yamasaki S, Ono H et al. Chemoembolotherapy for recurrent hepatocellular carcinoma in the residual liver after hepatotectomy. Hepatogastroenterology 1993;40: 320–323
38. Vetter D, Wenger JJ, Bergier JM et al. Transcatheter oily chemoembolization in the management of advanced hepatocellular carcinoma in cirrhosis: results of a western comparative study in 60 patients. Hepatology 1991;13:427–433
39. Bronowicki JP, Vetter D, Dumas F et al. Transcatheter oily chemoembolization for hepatocellular carcinoma. A 4-year study of 127 French patients. Cancer 1994;74:16–24
40. Ikeda K, Kumada H, Saitoh S et al. Effect of repeated transcatheter arterial embolization on the survival time in patients with hepatocellular carcinoma. An analysis by the Cox proportional hazard model. Cancer 1991;68:2150–2154
41. Shijo H, Okazaki M, Higashihara H et al. Hepatocellular carcinoma: a multivariate analysis of prognostic features in patients treated with hepatic arterial embolization. Am J Gastroenterol 1992;87:1154–1159
42. Nakamura H, Mitani T, Murakami T et al. Five-year survival after transcatheter chemoembolization for hepatocellular carcinoma. Cancer Chemother Pharmacol 1994;33: S89–S92
43. Ohishi H, Uchida H, Yoshimura H et al. Hepatocellular carcinoma detected by iodized oil. Use of anticancer agents. Radiology 1985;154:25–29
44. Gunji T, Kawauchi N, Ohnishi S et al. Treatment of hepatocellular carcinoma associated with advanced cirrhosis by transcatheter arterial chemoembolization using autologous blood clot: a preliminary report. Hepatology 1992;15: 252–257
45. Kawai S, Tani M, Okamura J et al. Prospective and randomized clinical trial for the treatment of hepatocellular carcinoma: a comparison between L-TAE with farmorubicin and L-TAE with adriamycin. Preliminary results (second cooperative study). Cancer Chemother Pharmacol 1994;33: S97–S102
46. Kirk S, Blumgart R, Craig B et al. Irresectable hepatoma treated by intrahepatic iodized oil doxorubicin hydrochloride: initial results. Surgery 1991;109:694–697
47. Stefanini GF, Amorati P, Biselli M et al. Efficacy of transarterial targeted treatments on survival of patients with hepatocellular carcinoma. An Italian experience. Cancer 1995;75: 2427–2434
48. Bismuth H, Morino M, Sherlock D et al. Primary treatment of hepatocellular carcinoma by arterial chemoembolization. Am J Surg 1992;163:387–394
49. Mondazzi L, Bottelli R, Brambilla G et al. Transarterial oily chemoembolization for the treatment of hepatocellular carcinoma: a multivariate analysis of prognostic factors. Hepatology 1994;19:1115–1123
50. Kanematsu T, Matsumata T, Shirabe K et al. A comparative study of hepatic resection and transcatheter arterial embolization for the treatment of primary hepatocellular carcinoma. Cancer 1993;71:2181–2186
51. Ohnishi K, Tanabe Y, Ryu M et al. Prognosis of hepatocellular carcinoma smaller than 5 cm in relation to treatment: study of 100 patients. Hepatology 1987;7:1285–1290
52. Yoshimi F, Nagao T, Inoue S et al. Comparison of hepatectomy and transcatheter arterial chemoembolization for the treatment of hepatocellular carcinoma: necessity for prospective randomized trial. Hepatology 1992;16:702–706
53. Bronowicki JP, Boudjema K, Chone L et al. Comparison of resection, liver transplantation and transcatheter oily chemoembolization in the treatment of hepatocellular carcinoma. J Hepatol 1996;24:293–300
54. Chung JW, Park JH, Im JG et al. Pulmonary oil embolism after transcatheter oily chemoembolization of hepatocellular carcinoma. Radiology 1993;187:689–693

55. Derhy S, Bessis L, Atallah R et al. Reperméabilisation portale après chimiothérapie lipiodolée intra-arterielle au cours d'un carcinome hépatocellulaire. A propos de 3 cas. Gastroenterol Clin Biol 1990;14:893–895

56. Nagasue N, Galizia G, Kohno H et al. Adverse effects of preoperative hepatic artery chemoembolization for resectable hepatocellular carcinoma: a retrospective comparison of 138 liver resections. Surgery 1989;106:81–86

57. Wu CC, Ho YZ, Lin Ho W et al. Preoperative transcatheter arterial chemoembolization for resectable large hepatocellular carcinoma: a reappraisal. Br J Surg 1995;82:122–126

58. Adachi E, Matsumata T, Nishizaki T et al. Effects of preoperative transcatheter hepatic arterial chemoembolization for hepatocellular carcinoma. The relationship between postoperative course and tumor necrosis. Cancer 1993;72: 3593–3598

59. Duvoux C, Cherqui D, Tran Van Nhieu J et al. Chemoembolization for hepatocellular carcinoma cirrhotic patients: assessment of efficacy on total hepatectomy specimens. Transplant Proc 1994;26:3572–3573

60. Spreafico C, Marchiano A, Regalia E et al. Chemoembolization of hepatocellular carcinoma in patient who undergo liver transplantation. Radiology 1994;192:687–690

61. Tanaka K, Nakamura S, Numata K et al. Hepatocellular carcinoma: treatment with percutaneous ethanol injection transcatheter arterial embolization. Radiology 1992;185: 457–460

62. Heresbach D, Raoul JL, Bentue-Ferrer D et al. Chimiothérapie couplée au lipiodol. Etude in vitro de la cinétique de libération l'adriamycine. Gastroenterol Clin Biol 1989;13: 775–778

63. Higashi S, Shimizu M, Nakashima T et al. Arterial-injection chemotherapy for hepatocellular carcinoma monodispersed poppy-seed oil microdroplets containing aqueous vesicles of epirubicin. Initial medical application of a membrane-emulsification technique. Cancer 1995;75:1245–1254

33

IMMUNOTHERAPY FOR HEPATOCELLULAR CARCINOMA

DANIEL SHOUVAL

Hepatocellular carcinoma (HCC) is one of the most common neoplasms worldwide. HCC has unique and often heterogeneous biologic properties that are sometimes characteristic for specific geographic regions. For example, unifocal tumors are more frequently reported in east Asia, and especially in Japan and China, compared to Africa or even western Europe and the Americas, where most HCCs are multifocal at clinical presentation. The form of clinical presentation often dictates the treatment strategies for individual patients. Small unifocal tumors should be resected surgically, if possible. Some features are common to most HCCs, regardless of whether they present as unifocal or multifocal tumors, for example, the emergence of transformed cells on a background of chronic inflammatory and regenerating processes in the liver, in association with persistent viral infection with hepatitis B (HBV) or C (HCV) viruses. Regardless of the stimuli or risk factors that lead to the chronic inflammatory process in the liver—viral replication, the host immune response to it, alcohol intake or other toxins—the end result is often emergence of a transformed focus or foci, often resistant to conventional chemotherapy. The failure of systemic chemotherapy to offer even partial acceptable palliation to patients with HCC is an incentive for clinicians and basic scientists to develop more efficacious treatment modalities. However, the heterogeneous etiologies and properties of HCC make it unlikely that a single method of treatment may ever be developed for universal clinical application. Nevertheless, already today a clinician who wishes to offer some palliation to an HCC patient has quite a few options to consider,[1–4] including immunotherapy.

Currently available experimental strategies for immunotherapy of HCC may be divided into two major groups. The first group involves selective and, usually, relatively specific targeting of HCCs by means of monoclonal or polyclonal antibodies. Such antibodies must recognize a signal, usually a protein, on the cell surface of the tumor cell and be able to bind to it. Targeting of such cell surface antigens, ideally present only on the transformed cell, may involve the use of free ("naked") antibodies, or antibodies coupled to chemotherapeutic or biological agents. The second group includes some relatively nonspecific treatment modalities such as interferon-α, interferon-γ, lymphokine-activated killer (LAK) cells, tumor necrosis factor (TNF), or antibodies bound to radioactive isotopes. This review focuses mainly on targeting modalities of immunotherapy for HCC and briefly summarizes the other options for immunotherapy.

POTENTIAL TARGETS FOR IMMUNOTHERAPY: HCC-ASSOCIATED ANTIGENS

Certain tumor cell surface or cytoplasmic antigens and molecules are potential candidates for immunotargeting in HCC. In general, tumor antigens have previously been divided into tumor-specific and tumor-associated antigens, raising the hope that some tumor antigens are so specific that their targeting will enable differential destruction of the tumor cell by delivering a "killer agent" to the transformed liver cell, without harming the surrounding normal tissue.[5,6] It soon became clear that "tumor antigens" are frequently expressed by both transformed and nontransformed cells of similar origin, which differ in the degree and intensity of expression (the expression being much higher in the malignant cells). Thus the term *tumor-associated antigen* was suggested. There are a number of tumor-associated antigens in the gastrointestinal (GI) tract in general and the liver in particular. For example, the oncofetal antigen, carcinoembryonic antigen (CEA), with its subgroups, is frequently expressed in colorectal cancer, but can also be identified in other GI sites and elsewhere.[7] α-Fetoprotein (AFP) is expressed in 40% to 60% of HCCs in humans, but it is also expressed in embryonic tissues, neural and testicular tumors, as well as in regenerating hepatocytes.[8] A relatively newly discovered gastrointestinal tumor-associated antigen, 19/9, is present in many GI tumors.[9] Both AFP and, to a lesser degree, CEA have been shown to be expressed by HCCs. Additional HCC-associated antigens have also been reported.[10–28] Most of these need better definition as to their glycoprotein or glycolipid content, the kinetics of their expression during the cell cycle, and most important, cloning of the genes responsible for synthesizing the antigens. Table 33-1 summarizes the known HCC-associated antigens.

ANTIBODIES TO HCC-ASSOCIATED ANTIGENS

The identification of new HCC-associated antigens became possible following the introduction of the technology for generation of monoclonal antibodies.[29] However, even before the introduction of these, polyclonal antibodies were generated against AFP, CEA, and ferritin.[30–32] Although two of these antigens are also produced by normal hepatocytes, they are highly expressed in transformed liver cells. The hepatitis B surface antigen (HBsAg) can also be categorized as an HCC-associated antigen when present in patients with HCC. In such patients, hepatitis B virus (HBV) DNA sequences integrated into the host hepatocyte genome often code for continuous expression of HBsAg on the membrane of

TABLE 33-1. HCC-Associated Antigens and Their Antibodies[a]

Antigen[a]	MW (kD)	Antibodies		Code
		Polyclonal	Monoclonal	
AFP	70	+	+	anti-AFP
CEA	200	+	+	anti-CEA
Ferritin	450	+	+	antiferritin
HBsAg	27		+	anti-HBs
HCA Ag_1	70		+	anti-PLC_1 (PM4E)
HCA Ag_2	50		+	anti-PLC_2 ($P_2$154)
HCA Ag_3	125		+	anti-PLC_3 (SF-25)
HCA Ag_4	—		+	anti-PLC_4 (XF-8)
HCA Ag_5	120		+	anti-PLC_5 (AF-20)
—	—		+	K-PLC_1
H (II)	>200		+	S_1, S_3
ATM-1	120		+	N 1977
HB4	—		+	—
SB1a	—		+	2 H6G5
—	—		+	4A9E10
—	30		+	YPC2/38.8
Miscellaneous	—		+	—

Abbreviation: MW, molecular weight.

[a] Many of the codes for antigens and antibodies were assigned by the various investigators, and a commonly accepted terminology has not yet been established. Several of these HCC-associated antigens are only partially characterized, although all were detected in transformed hepatocytes.

(From Shouval and Adler,[47] with permission.)

some HCC cells, thus making them a potential target for immune attack.[33,34] Since 1982, quite a number of tumor-associated antigens on the surface of HCC cells have been identified.[10–28,30–32,34] The most common hepatoma cell lines used for immunization to elicit antibodies to tumor-associated antigens were PLC/PRF/5, Focus, SK-Hep 1, Mahlavu, Hep G2, and Hep 3B.[35] These cell lines were also used to generate subcutaneous or intrahepatic HCCs in athymic mice, which were used as a model system for testing the targeting potential of the various MoAbs.[35–38]

Expression of target antigens may vary according to the cell cycle, degree of cell differentiation, and the enhancing influence of some cytokines.[34–43] The fundamental hypothesis behind the targeting concept suggests that tumor-associated surface molecules should be expressed long enough on the cell surface in order to give a killer cell an opportunity to "recognize" it and lyse it. Finally, some hepatic tumor-associated antigens on the HCC surface, such as AFP, HBsAg, and ferritin, may also be shed into the circulation. Would such "floating" circulating antigens serve as a decoy against immune attack, neutralizing its potency before it can reach the transformed hepatocyte target? The available experimental evidence suggests that this is not so.[34,44]

TARGETED IMMUNOTHERAPY OF TRANSFORMED HEPATOCYTES USING MONOCLONAL ANTIBODIES TO HCC-ASSOCIATED ANTIGENS

Free (Uncoupled) Monoclonal Antibodies

Immunization of BALB/c mice with various intact hepatoma cell lines or with purified HBsAg or AFP led to the generation of a panel of ten different monoclonal antibodies to HCC-associated antigens.[10–12] These MoAbs, includings anti-HBs (several IgG and IgM isotypes), anti-AFP, and others were tested for their binding to and cytotoxicity against HCC cells in vitro and in vivo in the presence or absence of complement or lymphocytes.[34,44–46] All ten MoAbs bound specifically to the target cell used for immunization, or to the specific HCC-associated antigens (see Table 33-1 for partial characterization). Three MoAbs to HBsAg have been shown to induce lysis of HCC cell lines that express membrane HBsAg, in the presence of complement. In addition, the MoAb series anti-PLC_1, anti-PLC_3, and anti-PLC_4, generated by immunization of mice against several hepatoma cell lines, as well as some anti-HBs MoAbs, suppressed human HCC xenografts in athymic mice.[38,44,47] Several anti-PLC antibodies were shown to react with biopsies from HCC patients in immunohistochemical assays.[48]

Conjugates of Monoclonal Antibodies to HCC-Associated Antigens With Chemotherapeutic Agents

Successful suppression of HCC tumor growth with antibodies may depend on related immune mechanisms including complement or antibody-dependent, cell-mediated lysis, as well as on possible direct cytotoxic cell activity against as yet undefined transformed cell surface epitopes.[10,38,44,46–53] Other non-immune-mediated mechanism(s) for target cell suppression by MoAbs may also be present.[47] However, regardless of the mechanism(s) involved in target cell suppression or lysis by antibodies, there is a body of evidence suggesting that escape mechanisms do emerge following prolonged exposure of HCC cells, in culture or in vivo (xenografts in athymic mice), to MoAbs of distinct specificity.[44,54]

Another approach for increasing the efficacy of immunotargeting is to couple conventionally used chemotherapeutic agents to antibodies with a distinct specificity.[55–59] Such conjugates may have the advantage of inducing a synergistic effect between the tumor suppression effect of a particular antibody and the cytotoxic effect of the coupled chemotherapeutic agent. If an antibody is used that has a direct antitumor activity, and if this antibody is also active in a complement- or an ADCC-associated mechanism, the use of a conjugate consisting of an antitumor agent may induce a "triple" antitumor effect. The delivery of a cytotoxic agent to a desired site of action should spare normal tissues, as recently reported for four different conjugates of MoAbs against HCC-associated antigens with adriamycin.[38] An example of conjugate treatment reducing AFP levels in athymic mice with intrahepatic human HCC is shown in Figure 33-1.

Direct conjugation of an antibody to a chemotherapeutic agent has been replaced by new methods in which polyclonal or monoclonal antibodies are conjugated to antineoplastic agents using an inert bridge such as dextran, polyglutamic acid, or albumin.[56–62] These bridging agents permit significant amplification of the number of cytotoxic drug molecules that can be coupled to a single antibody molecule. To date, it is possible to conjugate 10 to 30 adriamycin molecules to a single MoAb molecule.[34,47,58] The technique involves oxidation of the bridging agent—for example, dextran (T_{10} or T_{40})—with $NaIO_4$, followed by conjugation with the pharmacologic agent and antibody molecules on the bridge, using the periodate-generated functional aldehyde groups.[34] This technique and others were used for generation of conjugates between adriamycin, cisplatin, methotrexate, 5-fluorouacil, cytosine arabinoside, chlorambucil, bleomycin, vincristine, or ricin and antibodies to HCC-associated antigens or to other tumors.[30,34,56–58,60–69]

Of 17 different conjugates between MoAbs to HCC-associated antigens and adriamycin, 5-fluorouracil, and cytosine arabinoside generated by our groups,[34,60–65] (de-

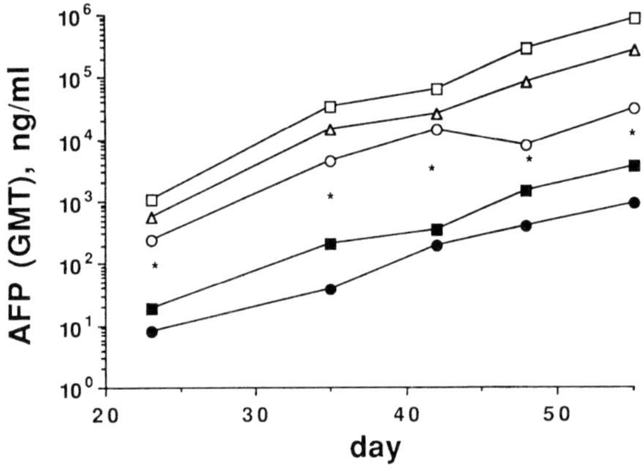

FIGURE 33-1. Effect of MoAb conjugate treatment on serum AFP levels in mice with intrahepatic human HCCs. Hep3B cells (5×10^6), in medium supplemented with fetal calf serum and containing rabbit anti-asialo-GM_1 antibodies, were injected directly into the spleen. The spleen was excised after 1 minute, allowing the tumor to be flushed into the splenic and portal veins. Treatment was started 1 week after tumor cell injection (given twice weekly intravenously). Total dose of adriamycin given was 400 μg, and of MoAb anti-PLC_4, 1780 μg. There were 10 mice per group. Mice were sacrificed 8 weeks after tumor cell injection. Blood samples were taken once a week by retrobulbar puncture. Anti-PLC_4-dex-adr (●), adriamycin (△), mixture of MoAb and adriamycin (■), MoAb (○), PBS (□). Values are given as GMT (geometric mean titer) and expressed in ng/ml. $p < .001$ for values above asterisks, as compared with conjugate-treated animals (below asterisks). The difference between animals treated with a mixture of conjugate components was not statistically significant. (From Adler et al.,[38] with permission.)

spite occasional batch-to-batch variations), most conjugates retained over 70% of their specific binding activity to their HCC target cells in culture when compared to nonconjugated free ("naked") antibodies. In vitro these conjugates were shown to suppress hepatoma cell line growth and to induce cell membrane lysis, as demonstrated through ^{3}H thymidine incorporation and ^{51}Cr release, respectively. In vivo, such conjugates, given intravenously or intraperitoneally, twice or three times a week for 4 to 6 weeks, have been shown to suppress the growth of subcutaneous or intrahepatic human hepatoma cell lines Hep G2, Hep3B, and PLC/PRF/5 tumors transplanted in athymic mice.[34,47] Circulating levels of AFP and HBsAg, as well as tumor weight, were shown to be significantly lower in conjugate-treated mice compared to mice treated with the individual components of the conjugates. Withdrawal of treatment with conjugates was sometimes associated with regrowth of the original tumor. It is interesting to note that circulating HBsAg secreted by some xenografts in athymic mice did not interfere significantly with tumor suppression by the conjugate containing antibodies to HBsAg, although unrecognized interference could not be excluded.

Conjugates Between MoAbs to HCC-Associated Antigens and Radioactive Agents

Radioimmunotherapy utilizes polyclonal or MoAbs against HCC-associated antigens that are labeled with cytotoxic radioisotopes such as ^{131}I, ^{125}I, or ^{90}Y. Radiolabeled antitumor antibodies theoretically could improve the capability to identify tumors smaller than 1 cm in diameter, a technique called radioimmunodetection. Indeed, colorectal tumor xenografts expressing CEA and with a diameter less than or equal to 0.5 to 1 cm can be detected in mice, as well as in humans using these techniques.[70–73] However, modern imaging techniques seem to achieve a similar sensitivity in identifying such lesions. Nevertheless, radiolabeled antibodies could theoretically be useful in distinguishing between regenerative and neoplastic hepatic nodules, which is a common problem in patients with chronic liver disease and cirrhosis. Such techniques may also be useful in identifying residual tumors after surgical resection, or for pretesting whether a particular conjugate is suitable for radioimmunotherapy, as shown by pilot studies in mice and humans, using anti-CEA, anti-AFP, and antiferritin antibodies.[34,47]

The success of radioimmunodetection and radioimmunotherapy depend on qualities of the radioconjugate and its components, including binding affinity and avidity of the antibodies to their target molecules, the radionucleide used, the location of the target tumor, the tumor's vascularity, the presence of necrosis, the stability of the conjugate, and its half-life. In patients who have undergone surgical resection or other treatment for HCC, the basic inflammatory or regenerative process is often still active, and the risk of the emergence of new HCC foci still remains. Radioimmunodetection may be an important tool for post-treatment surveillance in these patients. The development of small Fab fragments, bi-valent antibodies, and recombinant immunoglobulins for radioimmunodetection has in turn led to new developments in radioimmunotherapy.[34,47,68,70–75] Evaluation of radioimmunotherapy in humans with HCC has already been reported.[32,73–81] Order et al.[32] were the first to introduce radioimmunotherapy for patients with HCC using radiolabeled polyclonal or MoAbs to ferritin. Ferritin is a tumor-associated antigen that is produced by a variety of transformed cells, including HCC, Hodgkin's lymphoma, and neuroblastoma. This particular protein, which is also expressed by nontransformed tissues, is synthesized and secreted in much higher quantities by HCCs. Early studies with polyclonal antiferritin antibodies[32] obtained only a 7% complete response, but 48% of patients were believed to have entered remission. Nevertheless, a disappointing median survival of 10.5 months was recorded in AFP-negative patients with HCC, compared to an even worse outcome of 5 months in AFP-positive patients.[32,76,77] Even after refining the technique and introducing tumor volumetric evaluation, the results were essentially similar.[78] The high irradiation dose used in radioimmunotherapy was associated with myelosuppression, which may require autologous bone marrow transplantation.

The relatively low penetration of ^{131}I, its high toxicity, and the difficulties involved in standardizing radioimmunotherapy using polyclonal antiferritin antibodies from heterogeneous sources led to a search for better agents. Klein et al.[17] evaluated the use of high-energy β-emitting radionucleide ^{90}Yttrium (^{90}Y) conjugated to polyclonal antiferritin. ^{90}Y-labeled antiferritin antibody may reach more HCC cells than ^{131}I-labeled antiferritin, and the establishment of murine MoAbs to ferritin offered possible improvement.[17]

Another step forward was reported with selective injection of radiolabeled antibody to the feeding hepatic artery of the tumor in patients who had very large tumors (median diameter 10 × 10 cm). These were treated with high doses of a radioisotope conjugated to antiferritin.[79] This method was developed to minimize the systemic adverse effects of radiotherapy. Tumor shrinkage was reported in 68% of patients treated with intra-arterial radiolabeled antiferritin, compared to 34% with systemic chemotherapy. Furthermore, 61% and 25% 1- and 3-year survival rates, respectively, were recorded in the group receiving radiolabeled antiferritin compared to 37% and 7% for the control subjects. However, the methodology involved requires invasive procedures, including laparotomy and cannulation and ligature of the hepatic artery, and it is associated therefore with potentially significant adverse effects. Thus, although radioimmunotherapy with radiolabeled antibodies to HCC is an experimental therapeutic option, it is still in the early stages of assessment. At this stage, it is doubtful whether the current 25% remission rate after 3 years justifies the introduction of this technology into clinical practice.

ADOPTIVE TRANSFER OF IMMUNITY FOR SUPPRESSION OF EXPERIMENTAL HCC GROWTH

In preliminary experiments[83] immune-competent BALB/c mice were immunized against HBsAg with a recombinant hepatitis B vaccine.[80] Bone marrow from anti-HBs-positive mice was then transplanted to irradiated athymic BALB/c mice carrying HBsAg-positive human HCC xenografts. At approximately 2 months after bone marrow transplantation, tumor volume and serum AFP levels in mice receiving bone marrow transplants were 137- and 52-fold lower than control animals.[81] T-cell depletion of the donor bone marrow reduced, but did not eliminate, this suppression of tumor growth in the bone marrow transplant recipient. In control experiments, this antitumor effect could be distinguished from a nonspecific bone marrow-derived graft-versus-tumor effect. Thus, adoptive transfer of immunity against HBsAg, previously shown to produce immunity to HBV in bone marrow transplant recipients,[80] may also be of value in treatment of HCC. In another study,[82] HBV-transfected murine tumors that express HBsAg or hepatitis B core antigen (HBcAg) on their cell surface transplanted in athymic mice were treated with spleen cells obtained from immunocompetent mice that had been immunized against HBsAg or HBcAg. This form of adoptive transfer of immunity to HBV led to regression of tumor growth.[82]

OTHER FORMS OF IMMUNOTHERAPY FOR HCC

Other forms of adoptive immunotherapy for experimental HCC in mice have been explored in the last decade. These include intratumoral injection with tumor infiltrating lymphocytes (TIL), intrasplenic administration of recombinant interleukin-2 and interferon-α, which caused regression of liver tumors in mice.[83] Pretreatment of Buffalo rats with interferon-γ has attenuated Morris hepatoma tumor growth, associated with significant enhancement of Kupfer cell-mediated tumoricidal activity.[84] Other investigators have suggested intralesional interleukin-2 therapy in experimental murine tumors to induce local cytotoxic activity in the tumor.[85] Tumor-specific cytotoxic T lymphocytes or LAK cells have also been suggested for a similar purpose.[89] Finally, human NK cells injected intravenously or subcutaneously into the spleen of experimental animals with liver metastases can migrate to the tumor site and lead to suppression of tumor cell growth.[84]

Complex protocols using transarterial targeting of interferon-γ and interleukin-2 emulsified in lipiodol-Urografin with a cocktail of chemotherapeutic agents led to some form of remission in patients with unresectable HCC.[87] Another approach was to use a combination of OK-432, recombinant granulocyte colony-stimulating factor, and recombinant interleukin-2, for enhancement of intratumor cytotoxic activity.[88] Other combination protocols between interferon-α and 5-fluorouracil,[89] or with doxorubicin,[90] failed to induce lasting remission in HCC patients; nor had interferon α alone been successful[94] despite promising in vitro studies.

The ability of major histocompatibility complex class I antigens to induce primary proliferative responses in purified allogeneic CD8+ cytotoxic T lymphocytes in the presence of human HCC cells[96] has been studied[92,93] with the intention of "educating" cytotoxic T cells against cells for adoptive transfer therapy. The results suggest that transformed hepatocytes expressing HLA class I and possibly class II molecules participated in induction of cytotoxic T-cell responses partially through ICAM-1-mediated mechanisms. Immune manipulations of these effector cells are now being evaluated for restriction of HCC growth.

The list of experimental protocols under evaluation is constantly enlarging. These protocols include treatment of HCC with adoptive chemoimmunotherapy,[94] transarterial immune embolization,[95,96] injection of allogeneic tumor and lymphokine-activated killer cells (LAK),[97] or MoAbs in liposomes directed against the HCC-associated antigen AF-20.[98]

CRITICAL ASSESSMENT OF EXPERIMENTAL MODES OF IMMUNOTHERAPY FOR HCC

The frequent emergence of HCC on the background of continuous inflammatory activity and persistent viral infection in the liver has made it an even more difficult target for treatment compared with other carcinomas.[99,100] Furthermore, successful suppression or even cure of an HCC focus in a liver with cirrhosis is not a guarantee against emergence of a new focus of transformed hepatocytes. The introduction into clinical practice of targeting techniques, using free MoAbs or MoAbs coupled to chemotherapeutic or radioactive agents, has been slow in view of the many questions still pending regarding safety, efficacy, and cost/benefit analysis.

The success of immunotargeting of HCC depends on a variety of factors. These include vascularity and size of the target tumor, and presence of necrosis (which often reduces vascular access to viable neoplastic cells). Surgical excision of large tumors, followed by targeted immunotherapy, thus may be much more acceptable and successful than immunotherapy alone. On the other hand, HCC shrinkage has been induced with polyclonal ^{131}I-labeled antiferritin antibodies, which made the tumor more amenable to surgical resection.[32,78] Vascular access and permeability of tumor cells to immunotargeting agents may also be improved through use of vasodilating agents and local irradiation.[34,47] The use of some calcium channel blockers may also delay the emergence of multiple drug-resistant tumor cell clones when conjugates between MoAbs and adriamycin are used.[47]

Regardless of the immunotargeting modality used, less than 0.01% of the total amount of injected antitumor antibody binds to its target following intravenous administration.[66] Methods are now being explored to improve the efficacy of targeting by enhancing the expression of tumor-associated antigen(s) on the cell surface of the tumor cell.[39–43] For example, AFP expression on the HCC cell surface may be enhanced through interferon-α treatment, thus making the target more amenable to anti-AFP conjugate treatment.[101] Furthermore, experimental evidence suggests that some cytokines may be useful in synchronizing the cell-cycle-dependent expression of HCC-associated antigens in vitro,[94] and possibly in vivo, which may be important in enhancing the targeting effects of antibody-mediated immunotherapy for HCC.

The "escape" of HCC tumors from MoAb treatment and the generation of breakthrough giant tumors following prolonged in vitro or in vivo use of MoAbs to HCC-associated antigen has been reported.[34,47] To prevent escape phenomena, a combination of two or more antibodies, "naked" or conjugated to chemotherapeutic or radioactive agents, seems to be necessary, as demonstrated for targeting HBsAg-positive HCC xenografts in athymic mice with both IgG and IgM murine-derived monoclonal anti-HBs.[44]

The idea of immunotargeting with antibodies, originally suggested by Paul Ehrlich at the beginning of this century,[101] has indeed been translated into reality in experimental models showing an increased concentration of antibodies at their desired site of action, while minimizing systemic adverse effects, especially adverse effects of the chemotherapeutic agents used. However, much still remains to be learned about the mechanism(s) by which the antibodies and their conjugates suppress or kill the target cells. Ideally, each target cell should come in contact with an antibody and its conjugate, thus enabling either a direct effect of the conjugate and its agent on the cell, or an indirect effect through the action of complement or other mechanisms. However, in reality antibodies and their conjugates do not reach all their potential targets. Therefore, advocates of radioimmunotherapy have suggested the use of ^{90}Y for radioimmunotargeting to improve the effects of local irradiation, since ^{90}Y kills cells beyond the point of binding of the radionucleide.[17]

In the limited experience with treatment of humans with murine-derived MoAbs, it is evident that murine antibodies generate a human antimouse response, which progressively reduces the efficacy of repeated cycles of targeting with the same antibody, especially in patients who have become more immune competent. Several experimental avenues are now being explored to reduce the emergence of a human antimouse response, including immunosuppressive agents such as cyclosporin, Fab fragments without the immunogen Fc component, use of recombinant mouse-human chimera antibodies, or the use of human monoclonal antibodies.[102–104]

CONCLUSION

Successful treatment of HCC remains a difficult challenge. A clinician who wishes to offer palliation to an HCC patient should have the option of offering a battery of complementary treatment modalities, since a single method seems to be effective for only a very small fraction of patients.

An additional potential application of immunotargeting should be evaluated for clearing of residual tumor cells in patients who have undergone liver transplantation for a small HCC, after the removal of the original liver, and even before introduction of the new graft. Thus, although immunotherapy and immunotargeting are still in the early experimental stages, their potential usefulness in improving the survival of patients with HCC stimulates the imagination. Eventually, immunotargeting should find its place among the treatment modalities for HCC

ACKNOWLEDGMENT

The studies cited in this view that were conducted in the Liver Unit, Hadassah University Hospital in Jerusalem were partially supported by the L. Naftali Science Foundation and the Richard Molin Memorial Foundation for Cancer, Inc.

REFERENCES

1. Nerenstone SR, Ihde C, Friedman MA. Clinical trials in primary hepatocellular carcinoma: current status and future directions. Cancer Treat Rev 1988;15:1–31
2. Ellis LM, Demess ML, Roh MS. Current strategies for the treatment of hepatocellular carcinoma. Curr Opin Oncol 1992;4:241–351
3. Falkson G. Treatment for patients with hepatocellular carcinoma: state of the art. Ann Oncol 1992;3:336–337
4. Dusheiko GM, Hobbs KEF, Burroughs AK. Treatment of small hepatocellular carcinomas. Lancet 1992;304: 285–288
5. Reisfeld RA, Cheresh DA. Human tumor antigens. Adv Immunol 1987;40:323–337
6. Carney W. Human tumor antigens and specific tumor therapy. Immunology Today 1988;9:363–364
7. Gold P, Freedman SO. Specific carcinoembryonic antigens of the human digestive system. J Exp Med 1965;122: 467–481
8. Abelev GI. Alpha-fetoprotein in ontogenesis and its association with malignant tumors. Adv Cancer Res 1971;14: 295–358
9. Herlyn M, Sers MF, Steplewski Z et al. Monoclonal antibody detection of a circulating tumor associated antigen. Presence of antigen in sera of patients with colorectal, gastric and pancreatic carcinoma. J Clin Immunol 1982;2: 135–140
10. Shouval D, Eilat D, Carlson RI et al. Human hepatoma-associated cell surface antigen: identification and characterization by means of monoclonal antibodies. Hepatology 1985;5:347–356
11. Carlson RI, Ben Porath E, Shouval D et al. Antigenic characterization of human HCC: development of in vitro and in vivo immunoassays that use monoclonal antibodies. J Clin Invest 1985;76:40–51
12. Wilson B, Ozturk M, Takahashi H et al. Cell-surface changes associated with transformation of human hepatocytes to the malignant phenotype. Proc Natl Acad Sci USA 1988;85:3140–3144
13. Imai K, Sasanami T, Nakanishi T et al. Circulating blood group-related antigen(s) in cancer patients detected by the monoclonal antibodies produced against HCC cell line. Tumour Biol 1985;6:257–272
14. Kaieda T, Imawari M, Yamasaki Z et al. Identification of a tumor-associated target antigen, ATM-1, for a human T-cell clone with activated killer activity and its existence in sera of cancer patients. Cancer Res 1988;48:4848–4854
15. Chang KJ, Finstad CL, Chen PD et al. Serological analysis and biochemical characterization of monoclonal antibodies defining antigens of human HCC. Chung Hua Min Kuo Wei Sheng Wu Chi Mien I Hsueh Tsa Chih 1989;22:1–20
16. Hiraiwa N, Iida N, Ishizuka I et al. Monoclonal antibodies directed to a disulfated glycosphingolipid, SB1a (GgOse4Cer-II3IV3-bis-sulfate), associated with human HCC. Cancer Res 1988;48:6769–6774
17. Klein JL, Nguyen TH, Laroque P et al. Yttrium-90 and Iodine-131 radioimmunoglobulin therapy of an experimental human hepatoma. Cancer Res 1989;49:6383–6389
18. Wiedmann KH, Trejdosiewicz LK, Southgate J, Thomas HC. Human HCC: cross reactive and idiotypic antigens associated with malignant transformation of epithelial cells. Hepatology. 1987;7:543–550
19. Takahashi H, Ozturk M, Wilson B et al. In vivo expression of two novel tumor-associated antigens and their use in immunolocalization of human HCC. Hepatology 1989;9: 625–634
20. Baumann H, Eldredge D. Influence of the liver on the profile of circulating antigens recognized by antiserum against hepatoma membrane glycoproteins. Cancer Res 1982;42: 2398–2406
21. Holmes CH, Hawkey CJ, Gunn B et al. A monoclonal antibody reactive with human hepatocytes. Liver 1983;3: 295–302
22. Sato K, Ikeda T, Katani K, Ogawa H. Preparation of monoclonal antibody to hepatocellular membranes and its application to induction of liver cell membrane damage. Acta Pathol Jpn 1985;5:1375–1383
23. Embelton MJ, Butler PC. Reactivity of monoclonal antibodies to oncoproteins with normal rat liver, carcinogen induced tumours and premalignant liver lesions. Br J Cancer 1988;57:48–53
24. Uotila M, Engvall E, Ruoslahti E. Monoclonal antibodies to human alpha fetoprotein. Molecular Immunol 1980;17: 791–794
25. Moriarity DM, Fox N, Aden DP et al. Identification of human hepatoma defined cell surface molecules. Hybridoma 1983;2:39–47

26. Kataoka T, Chiba J, Ohnuki T et al. New monoclonal antibodies specific for the guinea pig line 10 hepatocarcinoma. Jpn J Cancer Res (Gann) 1987;78:960–967

27. Dunk AA, Brown D, Weidmann K, Thomas HC. In vitro and in vivo tumour localisation with a monoclonal antibody directed against a membrane antigen on the human HCC cell line PLC/PRF/5. J Hepatol 1987;4:52–61

28. Fukuda Y, Imai K, Miura K et al. A monoclonal antibody to the carbohydrate chain on human HCC-associated antigen which suppressed tumor growth in nude mice. Cancer Immunol Immunother 1988;27:26–32.

29. Kohler G, Milstein C. Derivation of specific antibody producing tissue culture and tumor lines by cell fusikon. Eur J Immunol 1976;6:511–519

30. Tsukada Y, Bischof WKD, Hibi N et al. Effect of a conjugate of daunomycin and antibodies to rate α-feto protein on the growth of α-fetoprotein producing tumor cells. Proc Natl Acad Sci USA 1982;79:621–625

31. Blumenthal RD, Sharkey RM, Stephen R et al. Enhanced radioimmunotherapy of human colonic xenografts with antibody mixtures to CEA and colon nspecific antigen-p (CSAp). Cancer Immunol Immunother 1991;32:303–310

32. Order SE, Stillwagon GB, Klein JL et al. ^{131}I anti-ferritin, a new treatment modality in hepatoma: a Radiation Therapy Oncology Group study. J Clin Oncol 1985;3:1573–1582

33. Wands JR, Zurawski VR Jr. High affinity monoclonal antibodies to hepatitis B surface antigen (HBsAg) produced by somatic cell hybrids. Gastroenterology 1981;80:225–232

34. Shouval D, Adler R. Hum,an hepatoma associated antigens: opportunities for immunotherapy. In Thomas HC, Water JA (eds): Immunology of Liver Disease UK, Lancaster, 1993, p-p 69–83

35. Shouval D, Schuger L, Levij IS et al. Comparative morphology and tumorigenicity of human hepatocellular cell carcinoma lines in athymic rats and mice. Virchows Arch A Pathol Anat Histopathol 1988;412:595–606

36. Shouval D, Reid LM, Chakraborty PR et al. Tumorigenicity in nude mice of a human hepatoma cell line containing hepatitis B virus DNA. Cancer Res 1981;41:1342–1350

37. Takahashi H, Carlson R, Ozturk M et al. Radioimmunolocalization of hepatic and pulmonary metastasis of human colon adenocarcinoma. Gastroenterology 1989;96: 1317–1329

38. Adler R, Hurwitz E, Wands JR et al. Specific targeting of Adriamycin conjugates with monoclonal antibodies to hepatoma associated antigens to intrahepatic tumors in athymic mice. Hepatology 1995;22:1482–1487

39. Nakamura K, Kubo A, Hashimoto S. Enhanced tumor targeting and pharmacokinetics change of monoclonal antibody by interferon. Antibody Immunoconj Radiopharmceuticals 1991;4:847–857

40. Carrel S, Schmidt-Kessen A, Giuffre L. Recombinant interferon-gamma can induce the expression of HLA-DR and-DC on DR-negative melanoma cells and enhance the expression of HLA-ABC and tumor-associated antigens. Eur J Immunol 1985;15:118–123

41. Giacomini P, Imberti L, Aguzzi A et al. Immunochemical analysis of the modulation of human melanoma-associated antigens by DNA recombinant immune interferon. J Immunol 1985;4:2887–2894

42. Nakamura K, Kubo A, Hashimoto S. Interferon-induced changes in pharmacokinetics of In-111-labeled anti-CEA antibody. J Nucl Med 1990;31:852–853

43. Nakamura K, Kubo A, Husokawa S et al. Effect of alpha interferon on anti-alpha fetoprotein monoclonal antibody targeting of hepatoma. Oncology 1993;50:35–40

44. Shouval D, Shafritz DA, Zurawski VR Jr et al. Immunotherapy in nude mice of hepatoma using monoclonal antibodies against hepatitis B virus. Nature 1982;298:567–569

45. Takahashi H, Nakada T, Puisieux I. Inhibition of human colon cancer growth by antibody directed human LAK cells in SCID mic. Science 1993;259:1460–1462

46. Shouval D, Wands JR, Zurawski VR Jr et al. Selective binding and complement mediated lysis of human hepatoma cells (PLC/PRF/5) in culture by monoclonal antibodies to hepatitis B surface antigen. Proc Natl Acad Sci USA 1982; 79:650–654

47. Shouval D, Adler R. Tumor site directed therapy for hepatocellular carcinoma using monoclonal antibodies against hepatoma associated antigens. In Boyer JL, Ockner RK (eds): Progress in Liver Diseases. Vol XI. WB Saunders, Philadelphia, 1994, pp. 251–267

48. Shouval D, Livni N, Wands JR. Expression of hepatoma associated antigen in liver biopsies of patients with HCC. Hepatology 1986;6:1111(abstr)

49. Herlyn D, Herlyn M, Ross AH et al. Efficient selection of human tumour growth inhibiting monoclonal antibodies. J Immunol Methods 1984;73:157–167

50. Steplewski Z, Herlyn D, Maul G, Koprowski H. Hypothesis: macrophages as effector cells for human tumor destruction mediated by MoAb. Hybridoma 1983;2:1–5

51. Herlyn D, Herlyn M, Steplewski Z, Koprowski H. Monoclonal anti-human tumor antibodies of 6 isotypes in cytotoxic reactions with human and murine effector cells. Cellular Immunol 1985;92:105–114

52. Shouval D, Wands JR, Zurawski R Jr et al. Protection against experimental hepatoma formation in nude mice by monoclonal antibodies to hepatitis B virus surface antigen. Hepatology 1982;2:128S–133S

53. Shouval D, Wands JR, Shafritz DA. Immunotherapy of human hepatocellular carcinoma: molecular and cellular studies with monoclonal antibodies to hepatitis B virus determinants. In Chadwick CM (ed): Receptors in Tumor Biology. Cambridge University Press, Cambridge, 1986, pp. 221–238

54. Shouval D, Wands JR. Modulation of HBsAg expression and tumorigenicity of human hepatoma cells by monoclonal antibodies to hepatitis B surface antigen. Hepatology 1984;4:1089 (abstr)

55. Byers VS, Baldwin RW. Therapeutic strategies with monoclonal antibodies and immunoconjugates. Immunology 1988;65:329–335

56. Hurwitz E. Attempts at site directed experimental chemotherapy with antibody drug conjugates. In Bundgaard H, Bagger Hansen A, Kofod H, (ed): Optimization of Drug Delivery; Alfred Benzon Symposium no 17. Munksgaard, Copenhagen, 1982, pp. 153–269

57. Schlom J, Hand PH, Greiner JW et al. Innovations that influence the pharmacology of monoclonal antibody guided tumor targeting. Cancer Res 1990;50:820s–827s
58. Pietersz GA. The linkage of cytotoxic drugs to monoclonal antibodies for the treatment of cancer. Bioconjug Chem 1990;1:89–95
59. Tsukada Y, Kato Y, Umemoto N et al An anti-alpha fetoprotein antibody doxorubicin conjugate with a novel poly L-glutamic acid derivate intermediate drug carrier. J Natl Cancer Inst 1984;73:721–729
60. Shouval D, Adler R, Wands JR et al. Doxorubicin conjugates of monoclonal antibodies to hepatoma associated antigen. Proc Natl Acad Sci USA 1988;85:8276–8280
61. Shouval D, Adler R, Wands JR et al. Chemo-immunotherapy of human hepatoma by a conjugate between adriamycin and monoclonal anti-HBs. In Zuckerman A (ed): Viral Hepatitis and Liver Disease. Alan R. Liss, New-York, 1988, pp. 791–794
62. Galun E, Shouval D, Adler R et al. The effect of anti-α-fetoprotein-adriamycin conjugate on a human hepatoma. Hepatology 1990;11:578–584
63. Hurwitz E, Stancovski I, Wilchek M et al. A conjugate of 5-Fluorouridine-poly (L-lysine) and an antibody reactive with human colon carcinoma. Bioconjug Chem 1990;1: 285–290
64. Shouval D, Adler R, Wands JR, Hurwitz E. Conjugates between monoclonal antibodies to HBsAg and cytosine arabinoside. J Hepatol 1986;3(suppl 2):S87–S95
65. Hurwitz E, Adler R, Shouval D et al. Immunotargeting of daunomycin to localized and metastatic human colon adenocarcinoma in athymic mice. Cancer Immunol Immunother 1992;35:186–192
66. Goldenberg DM. Monoclonal antibodies in cancer detection and therapy. Am J Med 1993;94:297–312
67. Tsukada Y, Ohkawa K, Hibi N. Suppression of a human AFP producing hepatocellular growth in nude mice by an anti-AFP antibody-daunorubicin conjugate with a poly-L-glutamic acid derivative as intermediate drug carrier. Br J Cancer 1985;52:111–116
68. Alberici GF, Pallardy M, Marsil L et al. Conjugates of elliptinium acetate with mouse monoclonal α-fetoprotein antibodies or Fab fragments: in vitro cytotoxic effect upon human hepatoma cell lines. Int J Cancer 1988;41:309–314
69. Thomas HC, Montano L, Goodall A et al. Immunological mechanisms in chronic hepatitis B virus infection. Hepatology 1982;2:116S–121S
70. Goldenberg DM. Targeting of cancer with radio-labeled antibodies; prospects for imaging and therapy. Arch Pathol Lab Med 1988;112:580–587
71. Lind P, Lechner P, Eber O et al. A prospective study of CEA immunoscintigraphy with Tc 99m-labelled antibody fragment (IMMU-Fab') in colorectal cancer patients. J Nucl Med 1991;32:1051 (abstr)
72. Munz DL, Alavi A, Koprowski H, Herlyn D. Improved radioimmunoimaging of human tumor xenografts by a mixture of monoclonal antibody $F(ab')_2$ fragments. J Nucl Med 1986;27:1739–1745
73. Markham N, Ritson A, James O et al. Primary hepatocellular carcinoma localized by a radio-labeled monoclonal antibody. J Hepatol 1986;2:25–31
74. Baum RP, Hertel A, Baew–Christow T et al. Initial clinical results with a Tc 99m-labeled anti-AFP monoclonal antibody fragment in germ cell and liver tumors. J Nucl Med 1991;32:1053 (abstr)
75. Ji YY, Liu YF, Chen ZN. Radio immunodetection and autoradiographic localization of monoclonal antibody against human hepatocellular carcinoma in xenografts. Cancer 1992;68:2055–2059
76. Leichner PK, Yang N–C, Frenkel TL et al. Dosimetry and treatment planning for ^{90}Y-labeled anti-ferritin in hepatoma. Int J Radiat Oncol Biol Phys 1988;14:1033–1042
77. Order SE, Sleeper AM, Stillwagon GB et al. Radio-labeled antibodies: results and potential in cancer therapy. Cancer Res 1990;50:1011s–1013s
78. Order S, Pajak T, Leibel S et al. A randomized prospective trial comparing full dose chemotherapy to ^{131}I-ferritin: an RTOG study. Int J Radiat Oncol Biol Phys 1991;20: 953–963
79. Fan Z, Tang Z, Liu K et al. Radioiodinated anti-hepatocellular carcinoma ferritin: Targeting therapy, tumor imaging and anti-antibody response in HCC patients with hepatic aerterial infusion. J Cancer Res Clin Oncol 1992;118: 371–376
80. Shouval D, Ilan Y. Transplantation of hepatitis B immune lymphocytes as means for adoptive transfer of immunity to HBV. J Hepatol 1995;23:98–101
81. Ilan Y, Amit G, Feder R et al. Suppression of experimental hepatocellular carcinoma in mice through adoptive transfer of immunity to HBV. J Hepatol 1993;18:1130A (abstr)
82. Chen SH, Hu C, Lee CK, Chang C. Immune reactions against hepatitis B viral antigens lead to rejection of hepatocellular carcinoma in BALB/c mice. Cancer Res 1993; 53:4648–4651
83. Liu DL, Hakansson CH, Seifert J. Immunotherapy in liver tumors: Intramural injection with activated tumor infiltrating lymphocytes, intrasplenic administration of recombinant IL-2 and interferon alpha cause tumor repression and lysis. Cancer Lett 1994;85:39–46
84. Karpoff HM, Tung C, Ng B, Fong Y. Interferon gamma protects against tumor growth in rats by increasing Kupfer cell tumoricidal activity. Hepatology 1996;24:774–779
85. Den Otter W, De Groot JW, Bernsen MR et al. Optimal regimens for local IL-2 tumour therapy. Int J Cancer 1996; 66:400–403
86. Okada K, Nannmark Y, Vujanovic NL et al. Elimination of established liver metastases by human interleukin-2-activated NK cells after locoregional or systemic adoptive transfer. Cancer Res 1996;56:1599–1608
87. Lygidakis NJ, Kosmidis P, Zinas N et al. Combined transarterial targeting locoregional immunotherapy-chemotherapy for patients with unresectable HCC. J Interferon Cytokine Res 1995;15:467–472
88. Himoto T, Watanabe S, Nishioka M et al. Combination immunotherapy with OK-432, recombinant granulocyte-colony-stimulating factor, and recombinant interleukin-2, for human hepatocellular carcinoma. Cancer Immunol Immunother 1996;42:127–131

89. Stuart K, Tesstare J, Huberman M. 5-fluouracil and alpha interferon in hepatocellular carcinoma. Am J Clin Oncol 1996;19:136–139

90. Lotz JP, Grange JD, Hannoun L et al. Treatment of unresectable HCC with a combination of human recombinant alpha-2b interferon and doxorubicin: results of a pilot study. Eur J Cancer 1994;30A:1319–1325

91. Ilan Y, Eliakim M, Bino T et al. Variable efficacy of interferon alpha treatment on growth of human hepatoma cell lines in vitro. Isr J Med Sci 1988;24:505–511

92. Paroli M, Carloni G, Franco A et al. Human hepatoma cells expressing HLA class I molecules stimulate primary responses of purified CD8+ T lymphocytes. Res Virol 1993;144:327–332

93. Wadee AA, Paterson A, Coplan KA, Reddy SG. HLA expression in hepatocellular carcinoma cell lines. Clin Exp Immunol 1994;97:328–333

94. Cao X, Wang J, Zhang VV et al. Treatment of human hepatocellular carcinoma by fibroblast-mediated human interferon alpha gene therapy in combination with adoptive chemoimmunotherapy. J Cancer Res Clin Oncol 1995;121: 457–462

95. Kanai T, Monden M, Sakon M et al. New development of transarterial immunoembolization (TIE) for therapy of hepatocellular carcinoma with intrahepatic metastases. Cancer Chemother Pharmacol 1994;33:S48–S54

96. Oka M, Hazama S, Yoshino S et al. Intraarterial combined immunotherapy for unresectable hepatocellular carcinoma: preliminary results. Cancer Immunol Immunother 1994;38: 194–200

97. Yasumura S, Higuchi K, Hioki O et al. Induction of allogeneic tumor- and lymphokine-activated lymphocytes against hepatocellular carcinoma. J Gastroenterol Hepatol 1992;7: 136–141

98. Moradpour D, Compagnon B, Wilson BE et al. Specific targeting of human hepatocellular carcinoma cells by immunoliposomes in vitro. Hepatology 1995;22:1527–1537

99. Feitelson M. Hepatitis B virus infection and primary hepatocellular carcinoma. Clin Microbiol Rev 1992;5:275–301

100. Okuda K. Hepatocellular carcinoma: recent progress. Hepatology 1992;15:948–963

101. Ehrlich P. The relationship existing between chemical constitution, distribution and pharmacological action. In Himmelweite F, Marguardt M, Date H (eds): The Collected Papers of Paul Ehrlich, Vol I. Pergamon Press, Elmsford, NY, 1956, pp. 596–618

102. Zebedee SL, Barbas CF, Hom YL et al. Human combinatorial antibody libraries to hepatitis B surface antigen. Proc Natl Acad Sci USA 1992;89:3175–3179

103. Kjeldsen TB, Rasmussen BB, Rose C, Zenthen J. Human-human hybridomas and human monoclonal antibodies obtained by fusion of lymph node lymphocytes from breast cancer patients. Cancer Res 1988;48:3208–3214

104. Nishimura Y, Yokoyama M, Araki K et al. Recombinant human-mouse chimeric monoclonal antibody specific for common acute lymphocytic leukemia antigen. Cancer Res 1987;47:999–1005

34

RADIOTHERAPY

TOSHIAKI OSUGA
YASUSHI MATSUZAKI
TOSHIYA CHIBA
HIROHIKO TSUJII

Hepatocellular carcinoma (HCC) is well recognized as one of the most common malignancies throughout the world, especially in Asia and sub-Saharan Africa. Its prognosis is very poor and median survival is 1.6 months in untreated patients.[1]

Recently, remarkable progress has been made in the detection of small HCCs due to the use of ultrasonography, angiography, or computed tomography (CT). Intensive follow-up of the high risk group, consisting of patients with cirrhosis and chronic hepatitis associated with hepatitis B and C virus infections, has also contributed to the early detection of HCC. Thus, today the natural course of patients with HCCs smaller than 3 cm is such that 90% are alive at 1 year and 12% at 3 years, with an average survival period of 20.7 months.[2]

Surgery offers the best hope for cure of HCC. However, the recurrence rate is about 50% at 5 years. Furthermore, many patients have inoperable tumors at the time of presentation. To palliate inoperable HCCs, many options are available, including transcatheter arterial embolization (TAE), percutaneous ethanol injection (PEI), radiotherapy, cryotherapy, hyperthermia, and liver transplantation.[3] However, none of these can achieve a durable or curative response except in a few cases.

The role of radiotherapy in the treatment of HCC has been of limited use among recently developed therapeutic modalities. For the therapy of 11,397 patients with HCC during 2 years in Japan, treatment was conducted with surgery in 33% (3,803 out of 11,379 cases), chemoembolization in 63.9% (6,518/10,193 cases), and ethanol injection in 16.1% (1,586/9,896 cases), whereas radiation was used only in 0.8% (75/9,644 cases).[4]

Studies of the therapeutic efficacy of radiotherapy are difficult to compare, since study design, patient selection, and criteria of objective response are not uniform. The precise diagnosis, whether primary HCC or metastatic liver cancer, and whether the HCC is nodular, massive, or diffuse, is also important for comparisons between different studies.

Changes of tumor size on images after treatment are not necessarily a useful index of response to radiotherapy, since these do not necessarily reflect the histologic changes of the tumor. Decreased detection by CT scan suggesting devascularization of the tumor, the performance status, or the survival rate are used as objective responses. Survival largely depends on the degree of underlying cirrhosis.

EXTERNAL RADIATION WITH X-RAYS

Radiation Tolerance of the Liver

The use of radiotherapy for HCC has been limited because it has not been capable of curing HCC and because the radiation tolerance of the normal liver is far lower than the tumoricidal dose. In addition, excessive radiation provokes so-called radiation hepatitis. There is a sigmoid relationship between the radiation dose and the tumoricidal effect, and irradiation below the threshold of tolerance cannot stop the tumor growth.

It has long been known that the tolerance dose of the normal liver for x-irradiation is approximately 25 to 30 Gy. Ingold et al.[5] reported that 10 of 21 patients (47.6%) developed radiation hepatitis after 38 to 51 Gy irradiation of whole liver. Tolerance is highly dependent on the dose per fraction. If a dose fraction of 2.5 to 3 Gy is used, whole liver tolerance is limited to 20 Gy in 10 fractions or 21 Gy in 7 fractions. After reviewing the dose volume histogram in 11 patients receiving whole liver irradiation and boost treatment of 53 to 70 Gy equivalent, Austin-Seymour et al.[6] recommended that no more than 30% of the liver be irradiated with doses in excess of 30 to 35 Gy at 2 Gy fractions.

The tolerance of the liver to partial irradiation has been reviewed, and it was suggested that the whole liver can tolerate about 20 Gy, while one-third or one-half of the liver can tolerate 40 Gy without serious complications.[7] Janjan et al.[8] recently reported that transplanted liver exhibits responses to radiation similar to the normal liver. Furthermore, greater than 80% of HCCs are accompanied by cirrhosis. Although the tolerance to radiation of cirrhotic tissue is not precisely known, it is reasonable to speculate that cirrhotic liver can tolerate lesser amounts of irradiation than the normal liver.

Radiation hepatitis is a syndrome characterized by ascites, with elevation of alkaline phosphatase and other serum enzymes, and clinically resembles obstruction of the suprahepatic vein or Budd-Chiari syndrome. It develops about 2 weeks to 4 months after hepatic irradiation. Pathologically, it is a veno-occlusive disease and lacks the characteristics of inflammation, such as exudation of lymphocytes or leukocytes, and recent data suggest that the elevated transforming growth factor-β levels may play a role in its etiology.[9] Schacter et al.[10] reviewed 32 cases of radiation hepatitis in the literature and reported mortality of nearly 50%.

Whole and Partial Liver Irradiation

WHOLE OR LIMITED FIELD IRRADIATION

Whole liver irradiation was used as early as 1940, at a time when the demonstration of the tumor in the liver was technically difficult. It was mostly employed for the palliative care of metastatic liver cancer. However, the experience in the treatment of the metastatic cancer cannot be extrapolated to HCC. HCC is usually more vascular and frequently superimposed on a cirrhotic liver, often associated with portal hypertension and extrahepatic arteriovenous shunting. As techniques such as angiography and CT scan have improved in their abilities to localize the tumor in the liver, therapy with whole or partial liver irradiation has received renewed interest.

Ohto et al.[11] treated 39 patients with HCC using a linear accelerator. The irradiated dose totaled 30 to 50 Gy. A size reduction of more than 25% was observed in 90% of patients with tumors less than 5 cm in diameter. In tumors larger than 5 cm, 7 of 12 (58%) patients had a reduction in size of greater than 50%. Three of four patients with portal tumor thrombosis had a reduction in tumor size, and in the one remaining patient, regrowth was also stopped. Gastroduodenal ulcer was a complication in 10 of the 39 patients. Due to leukopenia, irradiation had to be discontinued in two patients. In terms of prognosis, 73% of patients with tumors larger than 5 cm in diameter died of cancer. In contrast, 80% of those with tumors smaller than 5 cm died of hepatic failure. Recently, Matsuura et al.[12] reported 16 patients with residual or recurrent HCC who were treated with radiation of 58 to 64 Gy (TDF 99 to 113) following TAE. The local tumor control, which is defined as suppression of regrowth of tumor, was achieved in 75% at 6 months, 45% at 1 year, 45% at 2 years, and 36% at 3 years. Survival following initial therapy was 34.3% at 3 years. A dose of 60 Gy was tolerated if the patient was in a mild stage. LePechoux et al.[13] also reported one patient with HCC successfully treated by TAE followed by limited-field irradiation. A total dose of 60 Gy in 30 fractions caused no clinical signs of radiation hepatitis. A 75 mm nodule of tumor was reduced to 42 mm at 6 months after the radiation treatment.

In contrast to these moderately good results, Aoki et al.[14] reported that 50 to 70 Gy of local irradiation caused a partial response (PR) in 33% of 7 patients with HCC, but all seven showed marked shrinkage of the liver at autopsy. Histologic examination revealed apparently viable cancer cells in all cases. One patient developed a serious complication, gastroduodenal ulcer within the irradiated field manifested by melena. They concluded that local radiotherapy of 50 to 70 Gy was not capable of curing HCC.

PORTAL TUMOR INVASION

Portal vein invasion by HCC is a poor prognostic factor. However, as shown in the study of Ohto et al,[11] limited-field irradiation for portal vein invasion may be effective to some extent. Chen et al.[15] performed a study to investigate the effect of external radiation in the control of portal vein invasion. The main HCC nodule was treated with TAE and partial irradiation was performed on nodules involving unilateral portal vein invasion in 10 patients with HCC with cirrhosis of Pugh's classification A. After TAE, portal vein thrombi were irradiated with 30 to 50 Gy; complete disappearance of portal vein thrombus occurred in five patients, and partial shrinkage was seen in the other five patients. However, HCC extended to the contralateral portal vein in two patients. No evidence of postirradiation hepatitis was noted.

^{131}I-Lipiodol embolization was also effective for portal tumor thrombosis as described below.[16]

To enhance further the effect of external irradiation, a variety of approaches has been devised. They are (1) high dose irradiation of limited fields, using the shrinking field technique or boost technique; (2) conformal irradiation; (3) hyperfractionation; (4) use of a radiosensitizer; (5) use of a hypoxic cell sensitizer; and (6) combined irradiation with chemotherapy or hyperthermia.

Conformal Radiotherapy

It has been known that toxicity increases as the volume of normal tissue exposed to irradiation increases, even at the same dose of irradiation. Recently, the development of three-dimensional treatment planning has made it possible to quantify the relationship between dose, volume, and normal tissue complications. Normal tissue tolerance, especially of the liver, depends on the volume of normal tissue irradiated. Therefore, the dose that could be delivered safely to the liver with HCC would depend on the fraction of normal liver that lay outside the high dose volume. For that purpose, a dose volume histogram (DVH) analysis, which depicts a distribution of dose over specifically defined volumes, has been applied for evaluation of tolerance in partial liver irradiation. The goal of this approach is to deliver the maximum possible dose to the tumor within a prescribed normal tissue complication probability.

DVH analysis has been previously used to calculate liver radiation tolerance by Austin-Seymour et al.[6] Lawrence et al.[17] designed a clinical protocol of three-dimensional treatment planning in which the radiation dose was prescribed based on DVH analysis on normal liver. With three-dimensional treatment planning, substantial portions of the normal liver could be spared, somewhat resembling the situation with partial hepatectomy. In this study of 36 patients, 25 (84%) were irradiated to more than 50% of the liver with 45 Gy, and they were irradiated with 60 Gy if more than 75% could be excluded. Applied radiation doses were well above those normally used for whole liver treatment. Thus, HCCs could be treated safely with the high-dose radiation when the dose was guided by DVH concepts.

According to a retrospective review on the use of three-dimensional dose-volume analysis by Lawrence et al.,[18] 9 of 79 patients irradiated developed clinical signs of radiation hepatitis. All patients who developed radiation hepatitis had received whole liver irradiation with a mean dose of more than 37 Gy, suggesting that DVH analysis can be used to quantify the tolerance of the liver to the radiation and to predict radiation hepatitis. The studies by Lawrence et al.[19] and Robertson et al.[20] showed that conformal radiotherapy with or without combined use of intrahepatic arterial chemotherapy attained varying degrees of objective response, whereas subacute or long-term toxicity was observed in some cases. The radiation dose ranged from 48 to 72.6 Gy. Robertson et al.[21] reported that 22 patients with hepatic metastasis from colorectal cancer were treated with conformal radiation therapy in conjunction with intra-arterial hepatic injection of fluorodeoxyuridine (FUDR) with a response in 50% of the patients. However, the response was not durable.

Thus, the availability of three-dimensional treatment planning based on the DVH concept is increasing, and the data of the three-dimensional dose-volume effect for the liver permits one to quantify the tolerance of the liver to radiation. Partial liver irradiation with or without other modalities will be increasingly used in the future.[20]

Hyperfractionation and a Radiosensitizer

Hyperfractionation of the radiation dose to decrease toxicity has failed to demonstrate a significant benefit over standard fractionation. Acute toxicity appeared to be higher and reactions such as thrombocytopenia and esophagitis were increased.[22] Radiotherapy has been combined with the use of anticancer drugs such as 5-fluorouracil (5FU), fluorodeoxyuridine (FUDR), which increases the sensitivity of the liver to radiation, or adriamycin. Whether used in bolus or continuous intravenous infusion, combined therapy showed no significant effectiveness, while bone marrow suppression, nausea, and vomiting increased.[23] Misonidazol, a hypoxic cell radiosensitizer, failed to cause prolongation of survival rate for metastatic cancer.[24]

Summary of External Radiotherapy

External radiotherapy, whole or partial liver irradiation with a high dose including conformal radiation, has been studied, aiming at the delivery of higher radiation doses to the tumor. It has been used either alone or in conjunction with other modalities such as chemotherapy or surgery. Data suggest that tumor regression with a durable response is possible with an adequate dose of radiation, but the therapy is not curative. Rough estimates of these studies showed that the objective response was in the range of 40% to 80%. Mild to serious toxicity was unavoidable in some cases.

INTERNAL RADIOTHERAPY WITH RADIOISOTOPES

The purpose of internal radiotherapy is to irradiate the tumor directly and selectively with a tumoricidal dose of radioisotope. A sealed or an unsealed source is used. Radioisotopes sealed in a needle, seed, or tiny tube are implanted into the tumor (brachytherapy). Unsealed radioisotopes and their carriers are administered by arterial infusion with a catheter, or systemically.

Radioisotopes Used in Internal Irradiation

Radioisotopes such as iodine-131 (^{131}I) and yttrium-90 (^{90}Y) are commonly used in internal radiotherapy. Carriers of these isotopes are antitumor antibody, Lipiodol, or resin microsphere.

Internal irradiation offers several advantages over external beam irradiation. Radioactive seed can be implanted accurately under direct vision or with ultrasound guidance. Localization of unsealed radioisotopes given systemically or infused by catheter can be assessed with use of γ-scintigraphy or a β-detector during laparotomy, which provides some information on dosimetry.

Almost all β-particles are absorbed near the radioactive source, and the radiation penetrates only 2.5 mm (max. 10.3 mm), thus producing a strong, localized tumoricidal effect. In contrast, γ-rays are absorbed by tissues to a lower degree, allowing greater tissue penetration and accurate measurement of dosimetry by scintigraphy with γ-camera.

^{131}I emits both β- and γ-radiation, but mainly γ-rays, whereas ^{90}Y emits purely β-particles. ^{131}I has a physical half-life of 8 days. It accumulates in the thyroid. It has β-energy of 0.6 MeV and γ-energy of 0.3 MeV. Administration of greater than 30 mCi requires hospitalization because of the risk of radiation exposure to other persons. On the other hand, ^{90}Y is a pure β-emitter and no significant external exposure to other individuals. Its physical half-life of 64 hours is shorter, and it has more therapeutic power because of β-emission, with a mean particle energy of 0.9 MeV (max 2.27 MeV) without whole body irradiation. An additional advantage of ^{90}Y is that there is no need for patient isolation because of no γ-emission. However, the potential disadvantage is that ^{90}Y cannot produce a clear tumor scan, and biodistribution for dosimetry cannot be measured by external imaging due to the lack of γ-emission. Another disadvantage is that it is retained within the body indefinitely, concentrated in the bone marrow, sometimes resulting in myelosuppression. Therefore, both ^{131}I and ^{90}Y have advantages and disadvantages for internal radiation.[25–27]

Sealed Sources

^{125}I seeds implanted in the tumor during operation or ^{92}Iridium for remote-controlled after-loading system (RALS) inserted into the tumor guided by ultrasonography are used in selected cases. Side effects are slight, and local control of 75 to 91% was attained for metastatic liver cancer.[22]

Radioimmunotherapy

Ferritin exists in many tissues and is a tumor-associated protein synthesized and secreted by various malignancies. Although it is not specific to HCC, its high concentration in this tumor offers an ideal target for ^{131}I-labeled antiferritin antibody. Hypervascularity within the tumor and ferritin production are essential for selective targetting with radiolabeled antiferritin antibody.

In 1985 Order et al.[28] proposed this treatment of HCC. A total of 105 patients with HCC were treated with ^{131}I antiferritin antibody, all of whom also received external radiation and chemotherapy together. (A dose-escalation study in HCC showed that 30 mCi was sufficient to saturate the tumor and that the tumor-effective half-life was 3.5 to 4 days. This allowed a second infusion within 5, days as well as further repeated administrations.) The delivered dose to the tumor was 10 to 12 Gy, and the estimated total body irradiation was 1 to 1.5 Gy per mCi of ^{131}I. Toxicity was predominantly thrombocytopenia, which was amplified during dose escalation. Complete response (100% size reduction) was achieved in 7% of cases, and partial response in 41%. Notably, in patients who obtained a remission, 1-year survival rate was 45%, and the 2-year survival rate was 15%. The longest partial response continued for 5 years and 8 months.

Subsequently, investigators in Shanghai applied this treatment to unresectable HCC.[29–33] They used ^{131}I-labeled antibody to isoferritin from human HCC, heart, or placenta,[31] iodinated anti-(hepatocellular carcinoma ferritin) antibody (^{131}I- or ^{125}I-labeled)[33] or ^{131}I-labeled anti-HCC monoclonal antibody(Hepma 1),[33] as well as ^{131}I-antiferritin antibody from different species of animals.[28] Usually 10 to 40 mCi of ^{131}I-antiferritin antibody was given by intra-arterial infusion, intravenous injection, or as a part of a multimodality treatment regimen, which might include ligation of the hepatic artery. A total of 60% to 80% of patients had tumor shrinkage. α-Fetoprotein (AFP) levels declined in about 80% of patients. Sequential resection was done in some cases. At sequential resection, surgical specimens revealed massive necrosis of the liver, but residual cancer cells were found at the edge of the specimens. Intrahepatic arterial infusion was superior to intravenous injection.[32] No remarkable toxicity was observed.

Order et al.[34] subsequently studied another newly developed more powerful ^{90}Y-antiferritin antibody. It has a higher energy and higher specific activity. Two of six patients had partial remissions in the preliminary report. One of these patients had complete response of a pulmonary metastasis. Patients had moderate hematologic toxicity. When radioimmunotherapy was compared with systemic chemotherapy in a randomized controlled trial, comparable response and survival rates were observed.[35] Thus, radioimmunotherapy can deliver 10 to 12 Gy to the tumor and convert an unresectable tumor into a resectable one.

Transcatheter Internal Radiotherapy

HCCs derive their blood supply mainly from the hepatic arteries. The development of catheterization techniques permitted intra-arterial infusion of anticancer drugs (chemoembolization) or radioisotopes (radioembolization). Intrahepatic arterial administration of ^{131}I-Lipiodol or ^{90}Y-microspheres has been used with varying degrees of success. Theoretically, transcatheter radiation can be given only where the feeding arteries of an HCC are, whereas radioimmunotherapy can be given even to distant foci of metastasis as well as to the primary cancer. In general, more radioisotope can be delivered to the tumor with transcatheter radiotherapy than with radioimmunotherapy.

^{131}I-LIPIODOL EMBOLIZATION

Biodistribution and Kinetics

Lipiodol is a stable iodine-containing lipid derived from poppy seed oil, with iodine in a concentration of 475 mg/ml (38% by weight). It has been used as a radiologic contrast medium for many years. When Lipiodol is injected into the hepatic end of the hepatic artery, it is retained selectively in foci of HCC.[36] Lipiodol-enhanced arteriography is particularly effective in demonstrating small daughter nodules of HCC that cannot be detected by angiography or CT with TAE.[37]

The iodine moiety of Lipiodol can be changed to radioactive ^{131}I through an atom-for-atom exchange reaction. Since ^{131}I-Lipiodol is both a γ- and β-emitter, its flow can be easily detected by a γ-camera and, therefore, accurate dosimetry is possible. In several studies of dosimetry,[38–40] ^{131}I-Etiodol or -Lipiodol injected at the level of hepatic artery was distributed predominantly in the liver (70% to 80%) and lung (20%). Accumulation of ^{131}I-Lipiodol in extrahepatic or extrapulmonary organs was negligible. Urinary excretion of ^{131}I was 30% to 50% over 8 days, and biliary excretion was 3% over 5 days. In this treatment, uptake of ^{131}I by the thyroid can be blocked easily by administration of potassium iodide (Lugol's solution) before or during the infusion of ^{131}I-Lipiodol.

In 1986 Park et al.[41] and Kobayashi et al.[42] reported that internal radiation with ^{131}I-Lipiodol could deliver a tumoricidal dose to tumors, and biodistribution and dosimetry of ^{131}I-Lipiodol were shown to be satisfactory. The biologic half-life of ^{131}I-Lipiodol depends on blood flow in the liver and the tumor and/or arteriovenous shunting. It is about 4.5 to 6.9 days in HCCs, which is longer than the 3.1 to 4.3 days in adjacent hepatic tissue or in the lung. The tumor : adjacent tissue ratio ranged from 7.5 to 21 in this study.[43] The biodistribution did not change after a second injection.[39]

When 1 mCi (37 MBq) of ^{131}I-Etiodol or -Lipiodol is injected, the estimated delivered dose is 239 cGy to a 4-cm tumor, 31 cGy to normal tissue, and 1.9 cGy to the total body. A 4-cm HCC receives, on average, eight times the radiation dose delivered to the normal liver. Accordingly, it is possible for a 4-cm tumor to receive a dose of almost 100 Gy by giving about 40 mCi (1480 MBq) of ^{131}I-Lipiodol, while the dose to normal liver is still kept at a tolerable level. For tumors larger than 5 cm, a large amount of ^{131}I-Lipiodol (greater than 1,850 MBq) is required, which is technically difficult to give in a single fraction.

Yoo et al.[44] suggested that the mechanism of the therapeutic effect of ^{131}I-Lipiodol embolization of HCC may be attributable to possible destruction of tumor cells by microembolization and to possible radiation fibrosis of tumor vessels.

Clinical Results

In 1985 Ohishi et al.[37] reported that hepatic arterial embolization with Lipiodol in conjunction with mitomycin C or adriamycin followed by embolization with gelform particles caused a tumor size reduction as well as a decrease of serum AFP. This effect is specific to chemoembolization and not Lipiodol alone, because Lipiodol itself does not change hepatic arterial flow and has no therapeutic effect.[45]

Kobayashi et al.[42] treated 7 patients with HCC measuring less than 6.5 cm with a tumor dose of 40 to 190 Gy (281 to 593 MBq) of ^{131}I-Lipiodol. Tumor regression and decrease of serum AFP were seen in all patients. No remarkable side effects were observed. There was necrosis of the tumor at autopsy of a patient who died of hepatic failure after the treatment. Park et al.[41,46] confirmed the feasibility of using ^{131}I-Lipiodol and also reported encouraging results in 47 patients.

In one case of recurrent HCC after surgery studied by Novell et al.[47] ^{131}I-Lipiodol treatment (475 MBq, 12.9 mCi) was administered twice via the hepatic artery. The dose of radioactivity administered to the tumor was calculated to be about 100 Gy. No adverse effects were observed. After treatment, two nodules of recurrent tumor were resected and were found to be completely necrotic and surrounded by a zone of fibrotic but nonmalignant parenchyma. The patient remained well 9 months later, and no evidence of residual tumor was found.

Bretagne et al.[48] reported that an average tumor size reduction of 50% was achieved in 9 of 15 patients with HCC who received 26 to 65 mCi through the hepatic artery, without side effects. A French multicenter group[49] conducted a prospective study of 50 patients with unresectable HCCs of stage I or II by the classification of Okuda et al.[1] The estimated cumulated radiation dose corresponded to 10 to 260 Gy for tumor, 20 to 38 Gy for nontumorous liver, and 0.2 to 10.7 Gy for lungs, reducing the possibility of adverse effects. Tumor size decreased in 73% of 30 patients, but there were no complete responses. Partial response had occurred in 40% of patients 4 months later. Data in this trial confirmed the reproducibility of treatment and the prognostic value of the classification of Okuda et al.[1] for HCC staging and of Maki et al.[50] for grading pf Lipiodol uptake on CT scan.

PORTAL VEIN THROMBOSIS

Portal vein tumor thrombosis is a poor prognostic factor and a contraindication for chemoembolization or gelfoam embolization, since it often induces hepatic insufficiency. A French multicenter group conducted a prospective randomized controlled trial in patients with HCC and portal thrombosis, comparing a ^{131}I-Lipiodol embolization group with a group receiving only medical support.[16] Twenty-seven cases with HCC were administered 60 mCi of ^{131}I-Lipiodol by the intrahepatic artery. The estimated cumulative radiation dose ranged from 10 to 100Gy (43 ± 29 Gy). Survival rates were 71% at 3 months for treated group and 10% for the control group, although survival was only 7% versus 0, respectively, at 9 months.

SUPERSELECTIVE CATHETERIZATION AND IMPLANTED ARTERIAL PORT

For delivering a selectively higher dose to the tumor, Yoo et al.[44] treated 24 patients with nodular HCC of 2.5 to 8 cm size by subsegmental injection under superselective catheterization. ^{131}I-Lipiodol with 15 to 60 mCi (555 to 2,220 MBq depending on tumor size) was given in an attempt to deliver 100 Gy to the tumor. Size reduction occurred in 90% in patients with 4-cm tumors, 66% in 4- to 6-cm tumors, and 25% in tumors greater than 6 cm. Size reduction paralleled the occurrence of devascularization on angiography. However, 8 patients had additional tumor growth or portal vein thrombus within 6 months. Superselective single-injection therapy can deliver high doses in order to cause tumor necrosis. Deep-seated tumors that are unsuitable for PEI can be treated by this method. The limitation is that the best results are obtained only if the tumor is hypervascular, without arteriovenous shunting; homogeneous distribution of ^{131}I-Lipiodol within the tumor is necessary for successful treatment.[40]

Recently, another approach to deliver higher doses was developed by Leung et al.[51] using administration of ^{131}I-Lipiodol from an implantable arterial port, which was placed and inserted into the gastroduodenal artery either during laparotomy or during selective hepatic artery canulation. The dose of ^{131}I-Lipiodol was aimed at 100 Gy to the tumor. Twenty-three patients received a single treatment of 30 to 60 mCi (1,110 to 2,220 MBq) of ^{131}I-Lipiodol and three patients with a large tumor received a dose of 60 to 120 mCi in a three-fractionated fashion. The availability of the arterial port for repeated administration made this possible. An overall 52% response was attained. Two patients (8%) had a complete response, 11 (44%) had a partial response, 5 (20%) had no change, and 7 (28%) had progressive disease. These investigators concluded that a fractionated dose of ^{131}I-Lipiodol is feasible when a large dose is needed for a large tumor. One patient developed liver dysfunction compatible with radiation hepatitis; no bone marrow suppression was observed in any patient.

APPLICATION TO SMALL HCCs

Small HCCs are supplied by feeding arteries originating from subsegmental branches. Yoo et al.[40] treated 18 patients with 25 lesions of nodular, multinodular, or hypervascular tumor measuring less than 4.5 cm in diameter with subsegmental injection of ^{131}I-Lipiodol (10 to 30 mCi; 370 to 1,110 MBq) under superselective intra-arterial catheterization instead of hepatic artery injection. In all, 15 lesions received over 180 Gy (median 168). Tumor to normal liver tissue (T:N) ratio of radioactivity reached up to 22:1 with an average of 15:1. This T:N ratio was higher in comparison with the method used by other investigators.[39,43] In five patients who subsequently underwent surgery, necrosis was found in 65% to 100%. No abnormality of liver function occurred in patients who survived 3 years after treatment. Thus, superselective internal radiation was effective for delivery of a higher dose and long-term control of small HCC.

The safe level of radiation dose to the liver and lungs with internal radiation remains unclear. Liver necrosis was found to occur at more than 120 Gy in dogs.[53]

Comparison with Chemoembolization

An important question is whether radioembolization with ^{131}I-Lipiodol or chemoembolization with anticancer drugs is more effective for treating HCC. The latter is more widely used in Japan today.

Kasugai et al.[53] and Nakamura et al.[54] treated resectable and unresectable HCC by TAE with an anticancer drug. TAE with chemotherapy was safe and effective. In studies of radioembolizations, response was obtained in 40% percent of tumors in the study of Raoul et al.,[49] and 52% in the study of Leung et al[55]; with transarterial oily chemoembolization, responses of 13% to 38%[53,56,57] were reported. However, comparison of the results between these studies is difficult because of different study designs and patient selection criteria.

Recently, Kajiya et al.[58] treated 8 patients with multifocal HCC using transarterial internal radiation with ^{131}I-Lipiodol (TAIR) and 13 patients with TAIR plus diamine dichloroplatinum (CDDP) and/or Adriamycin or Mitomycin C oil suspension. Fifty percent of patients had a 50% or greater decrease in tumor size. Patients treated with TAIR alone had no difference in their survival rate compared with those treated with TAIR plus chemotherapy. Preliminary results of controlled trials suggest that radioembolization and chemoembolization are similar in efficacy, although radioembolization had fewer side effects.[59]

Summary of ^{131}I-Lipiodol Embolization

Using ^{131}I-Lipiodol, it is possible to deliver safely an adequate tumoricidal dose of radiation to HCC. Treatment is well tolerated. Systemic toxicity is minimal. Adverse reactions include fever, mild abdominal pain, nausea, and elevation of serum aminotransferase levels. Long-term local control of the tumor was possible without complications related to the thyroid, lung, gastrointestinal tract, or bone marrow. However, the relatively low energy of ^{131}I limits its use to tumors less than about 5 cm in diameter. If the tumor is larger than 6 cm, multiple administrations are necessary with an adequate interval between them. Also, if arteriovenous shunt is prominent, rapid clearance of ^{131}I-Lipiodol occurs.[43]

^{90}Y-MICROSPHERE EMBOLIZATION

Biodistribution and Dosimetry

^{90}Y incorporated in a glass or resin microsphere is delivered to an HCC through the hepatic artery with superselective catheterization. This technique was first reported by Prinzmetal et al.[60] in 1948. In the early studies, difficulty occurred due to unexpected leaching of ^{90}Y from the surface of the microspheres and right gastric artery radiation gastritis occurred. Also, fatal bone marrow suppression and pulmonary fibrosis occurred due to arteriovenous shunting within the tumor. Production of more stable and safer ^{90}Y, including newer glass microspheres and resin microspheres, has eliminated many of these problems.[26]

The two major side effects of ^{90}Y-microsphere administration are the accumulation of ^{90}Y in the bone marrow with myelosuppression and extrahepatic vascular shunting from liver to lungs and other organs leading to pulmonary fibrosis and gastrointestinal bleeding. The shunting to lungs was recently reported to be due to neoplastic vessels.[55]

To prevent side effects, Gray et al.[61] have developed a technique called selective internal radiation (SIR therapy), which consists of cholecystectomy, ligation of the right gastric artery, and injection of ^{90}Y-microspheres following angiotensin II (which constricts the hepatic artery to avoid leakage of the ^{90}Y-microspheres). However, lack of a specific effect of angiotensin II has been reported. For evaluating the shunting and tumor volume, a technetium-99m-labeled macroaggregated albumin (^{99m}Tc-MAA) scan is performed before administration of ^{90}Y-microspheres for diagnostic scintigraphy. High levels of lung shunting and a poor T:N ratio make a patient unsuitable for this treatment because of excessive irradiation to lungs and nontumorous hepatic tissue. A pretreatment ^{99m}Tc-MAA scan can exclude patients with a T:N ratio of less than 2. For dosimetry, T:N ratio, and percentage shunting of ^{99m}Tc-MAA, scanning of the liver before the treatment correlated well with results using a direct β-probe and liquid scintillation counting of multiple liver biopsies during surgery. ^{99m}Tc-MAA scanning also was useful for selecting a treatment dose.[62]

Clinical Results

In 1989 Houle et al.[63] used a new ^{90}Y glass microsphere in a pilot study of seven HCC patients. No toxicity was found using an absorbed dose of 50 to 100 Gy to the liver and up to 320 Gy to the tumor itself. A tumor response was seen at the higher doses used. Shepherd et al.[64] conducted a dose-escalation study in 10 patients with HCC. Targeted hepatic doses were 50, 75, and 100 Gy with 40 to 180 mCi of ^{90}Y. T:N ratio of the dose ranged from 1 to 10. Significant bone marrow suppression or hepatic toxicity was not seen, although one patient developed a radiation-induced duodenal ulcer. Lau et al.[62] reported 18 patients with inoperable HCC treated using resin-based ^{90}Y-microspheres administered via an intrahepatic arterial port placed during laparotomy. All patients had lung shunting at less than 15% and T:N greater than 2. Treatment was well tolerated; no toxicity of the bone marrow occurred. Serum AFP and ferritin levels fell. Although complete response, defined as disappearance of the lesion, did not occur, partial response, defined as greater than 50% decrease of tumor size, was achieved in 7 of 8 patients among those whose tumors received more than 120 Gy, and in one of eight patients whose tumors received less than 120 Gy. Thus, tumor regression was found to be dose-related. Progressive or static disease occurred in the patients whose tumors received less than 120 Gy. Survival was better in those whose tumors received more than 120 Gy. These authors,[63] as well as Yoo et al.,[65] recommended a tumor dose of greater than 120 Gy.

Rösler et al.[66] reported 20 patients with unresectable HCCs treated with transarterial radioembolization with ^{90}Y-resin particles of 21 to 34 mCi who were followed up to 5 years. Although the authors aimed at a dose of 200 to 300 Gy, the majority of patients received a smaller dose. The mean dose to the tumor ranged from 152 to 213 Gy. Doses absorbed by the liver remained as small as 6 to 35 Gy, making the T:N ratio high. The survival rate was correlated with the absorbed dose, but recurrence occurred even after greater than 300 Gy tumor doses. The overall survival rates were 56%, 38%, and 14% after 1, 2, and 3 years, respectively. However, survival rates of 83%, 67%, and 40% at 1, 2, and 3 years, respectively, were achieved in the patients with a unifocal tumor and a single feeding artery (n = 7). Quality of life improved in all patients, and post-treatment symptoms were minimal. Morbidity was severe only in one patient, who had gastric necrosis.

Summary of Internal Radiotherapy

Among modalities of internal radiotherapy, radioimmunotherapy showed a potential of converting an unresectable tumor to resectable one. From 10 to 140 mCi of ^{131}I-antiferritin antibody delivers about 10 to 12 Gy to the tumor. Tumors less than about 5 cm in diameter, even with portal invasion, were effectively treated with ^{131}I-Lipiodol embolization; 40 mCi of ^{131}I-Lipiodol delivers about 100 Gy to the tumor and 180 Gy by superselective catheterization. ^{90}Y-microsphere embolization may be a preferable modality for a tumor larger than about 5 cm; 30 mCi of ^{90}Y-microsphere delivers 200 Gy to the tumor. All of these modalities were well tolerated. The tumor response rate was similar to that seen with external radiation. However, side effects of internal radiotherapy were minimal.

PROTON BEAM RADIOTHERAPY

Proton beam radiotherapy for the treatment of HCC provides superior dose distribution compared to conventional radiotherapy. It is an external radiotherapy, with resulting local tumor control almost equivalent to surgery.

Protons, being charged particles, travel in practically straight lines in tissue and lose most of their energy by ionization near the end of their range. Hence, their range is finite. This physical characteristic allows a low entrance dose (plateau) followed by a sharp peak (the Bragg peak) and provides a favorable distribution in cancer tissue (Fig. 34-1). The very sharp distal fall-off of the Bragg peak and the sharp lateral penumbra of the energy range permit selective irradiation of the target while avoiding nearby critical structures. This differs from γ-rays, which lose their energy exponentially inside the body tissue. In general, relative biologic effectiveness (RBE, relative to x-rays) is different for different beam energies or biologic systems, and the RBE of protons used for therapy is in the range of 1.0 to 1.3. The Bragg peak can be designed so as to conform to a targeted focus in width and depth according to the shape of tumor.[61] Figure 34-2 shows a dose distribution for a patient with HCC irradiated with proton beams (see also Plate 34-1).

In 1990, Loma Linda University set up a hospital-based proton beam treatment center for the first time,

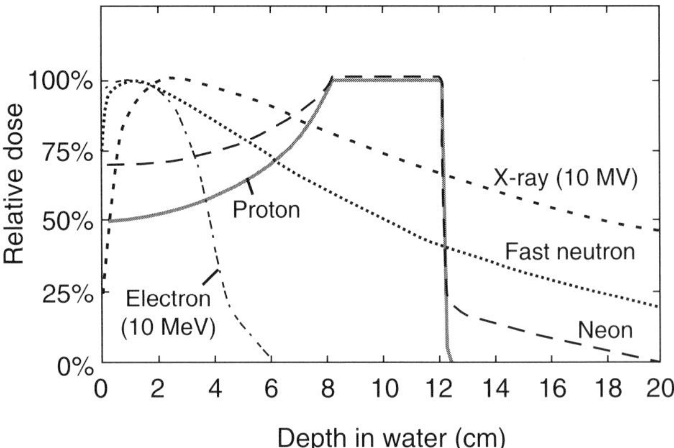

FIGURE 34-1. Comparison of depth dose curve of proton beam with other radiation beams. High-dose peak area of proton beam (Bragg peak) is formed in the deep site inside the body tissue before proton stops and loses its energy.

which was dedicated to medical service and research.[68] Currently, proton therapy is being carried out in 16 facilities in the world, and over 15,000 patients have been treated to date. Proton beam therapy has been applied mainly for small lesions of the eye and the brain, with good results.[69] In 1983, the Proton Medical Research Center, University of Tsukuba, started proton radiotherapy for multi-site malignancies in collaboration with the National Laboratory for High Energy Physics[70,71] including treatment of HCCs.

Protons are provided by a booster synchrotron of the National Laboratory for High Energy Physics. For use in cancer therapy, energy is reduced to 250 MeV from the original 500 MeV. For calculation of dose distribution, CT scans are taken at intervals of 5 to 10 mm across the lesion. Automatic extraction of the body contours on the CT scan and the outlines of the target volume are entered manually to permit the determination of irradiation parameters such as portal numbers, beam directions, and dose calculations. Field outlines, the width of the extended Bragg peak and the design of the beam-shaping compensator (bolus) are determined. It is relatively easy to determine the location of the tumor for the patient who had previously received Lipiodol angiography. For other patients, irridium seeds are implanted around the tumor edge under ultrsonographic guidance as a marker that can be verified by CT. By using these methods, localization errors, if any, are minimized to ± 1 mm. Setup time is usually 5 to 10 minutes, and actual exposure time is 2 to 5 minutes. To minimize irradiation to the surrounding normal tissues, a respiratory synchronized system was developed.[72]

For defining a target volume, the smallest possible margin was added around the tumor volume, and 5 to 10 mm of grossly normal tissue around the radiographically

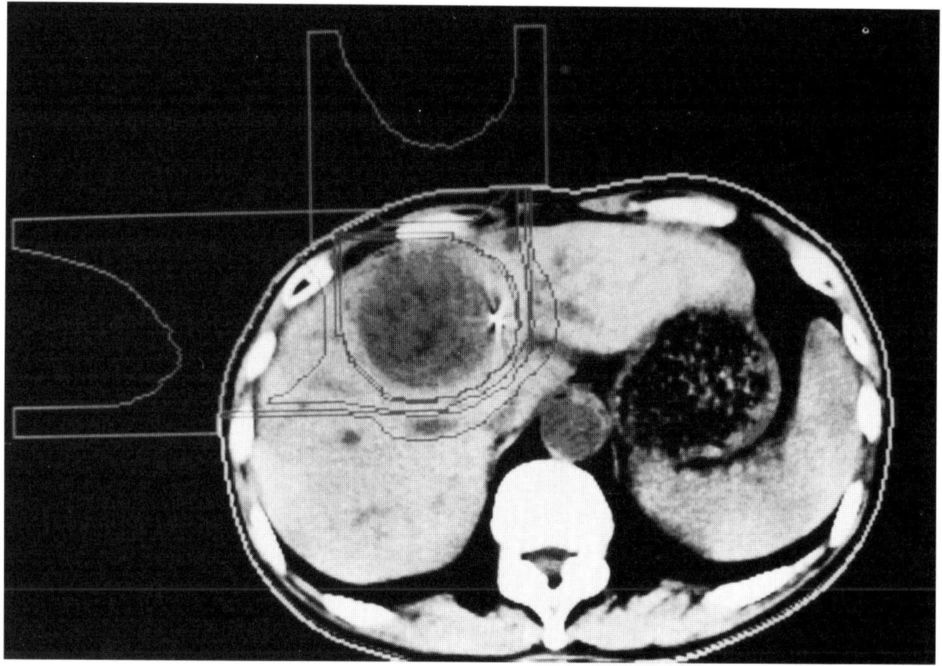

FIGURE 34-2. Dose contour of proton beam in a patient with HCC who was irradiated with proton beam. Iso-dose curves of proton beams show that radiation dose deposited in the normal tissue of the liver surrounding the tumor is minimal. If x-ray were used in this case, over one third of liver would receive more than 35 Gy, which may be beyond the tolerance of the normal liver tissue. (See also Plate 34-1.)

demonstrable tumor was included in the treatment volume. In a patient whose HCC has daughter lesions, all of the visible tumors were included in one radiation field. The dose contour around the target volume was set at the prescribed 100% dose level. A relative biologic effectiveness (RBE) of 1.0 relative to ^{60}Co was used. One course of treatment consisted of daily fraction sizes ranging from 3.0 to 4.5 Gy (median 3.5 Gy) and the treatment period was 13 to 56 days (median 33 days). Total doses ranged from 50 to 87 Gy (median 72 Gy).

Clinical Results of Proton Beam Radiotherapy

PATIENT SELECTION

In the early phase of our study,[73–75] a total of 32 lesions in 25 patients with single or multinodular tumors were treated, selected from those who refused surgery or had unresectable HCC. The reasons for unresectability were multiple tumors, vessel invasions, complications with advanced cirrhosis or chronic renal failure, and myelodysplastic syndrome. Also, patients with insufficient accumulation of Lipiodol in the lesion were included. All patients had accompanying cirrhosis graded as Child A (11 patients), Child B (7 patients) and Child C (6 patients). Three patients had portal invasion of the tumor. For 15 lesions in 11 patients, Lipiodol-targeted chemotherapy was not available because of pre-existing cirrhosis, chronic renal failure, or myelodysplastic syndrome. Tumor size ranged from 1.0 to 12.0 cm in all, and the average size was about 4 cm.

RESULTS

Complete response (100% size reduction), partial response (50% to 99% size reduction), no change (less than 50% size reduction), and progressive disease were found in 16% (5 of 32 cases), 31%, 53%, and 0 respectively at 3 weeks after completion of the treatment course. At 1 year after the treatment, they were 43% (10 of 23 cases), 35%, 22% and 0, respectively. Further, after 2 years, they were 36% (4 of 11 cases), 36%, 18%, and 1%, respectively. Tumors that were larger than 3 cm before therapy responded more poorly than smaller tumors of less than 3 cm. However, this was interpreted as indicating that a fixed volume of tumor had been destroyed by the same irradiation amount, irrespective of tumor size.

With regard to tumor control, almost 100% of local tumor control was accomplished at 3 weeks, 1 year, and 2 years after completing the treatment. Fourteen patients died of causes not attributable to proton therapy, but rather to complications of cirrhosis within the observation period of 2 years. Thus, despite its use in patients with unfavorable conditions, proton therapy appeared to be effective enough in achieving tumor control. AFP significantly decreased after completion of the treatment.

Follow-up biopsies obtained 3 weeks after proton therapy did not show any viable cancer cells in 9 of 12 lesions biopsied. In one patient with viable cancer cells, the tumor disappeared 5 weeks after biopsy. Hence, there was a discrepancy and time lag between the changes in tumor size and the histologic findings. Therefore, effectiveness of treatment should be judged both from tumor size and histology, devascularization of the tumor on angiography should also be taken into consideration. As is often seen in the case of TAE, it is not infrequent that the content of the tumor is completely necrotic even though tumor size on CT remained unchanged. This situation also may be observed in the tumor with proton therapy.

SIDE EFFECTS

It is noteworthy that the side effects are very low in proton therapy. No patients experienced any serious adverse reactions. Elevation of aspartate aminotransferase or alanine aminotransferase more than twice the baseline level up to 500 IU/L was observed in 7 of 24 patients (29%), rapidly returning to pretreatment levels within 1 to 2 weeks in most patients. Transient elevation of serum aminotransferases might have been due to local radiation hepatitis in the area by proton beam before

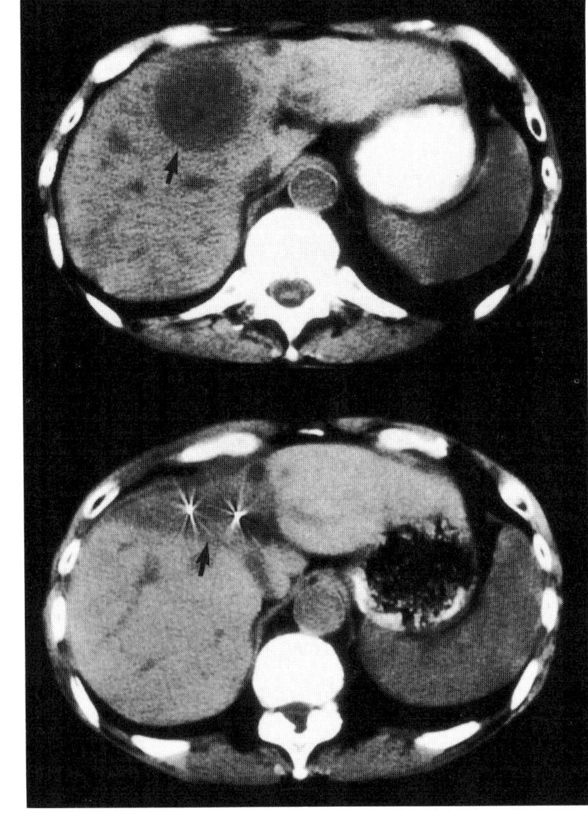

FIGURE 34-3. *Case 1.* A 67-year-old man who had a 5 × 5-cm HCC with cirrhosis (Child's grade B) received 83 Gy of proton irradiation in 23 fractions in 45 days. Lipiodol chemoembolization was not applied because of accompanying severe chronic renal failure. The irradiated tumor was completely necrotic by biopsy 3 weeks after finishing the treatment. It disappeared after 1 year. Radiographic CT images (*A*) before and (*B*) 3 weeks after proton therapy. Arrow shows the irradiated tumor. Cited from ref. 74.

TABLE 34-1. Side Effects in Proton Beam Radiotherapy

Side Effects	No. of Patients (n = 24) (%)
Fever (>38°C)	0
Abdominal pain	0
Pleural effusion	0
Elevation of aminotransferase levels[a]	7 (29)
Elevation of bilirubin (>3.0 mg/dl)	0
Anemia (hemoglobin >2 g/dl more than baseline level)	1 (4)
Leukocytopenia (<3,000/mm^3)	7 (29)
Thrombocytopenia (<5 × 10^4/mm^3)	5 (21)

Note: There was a transient elevation of aspartate or alanine aminotransferase, decreased blood cell counts, and decreased hemoglobin levels, all of which returned to baseline levels 1 or 2 weeks postirradiation.

[a] More than twice baseline levels.

(From Matsuzaki et al.,[74] with permission.)

reaching the target tumor. Leukocytopenia (less than 3,000/mm^3) was seen in 7 of 27 cases (29%), thrombocytopenia (less than 5 × 10^4/mm^3) in 21%, and decreased hemoglobin (greater than 2 g/dl more than baseline value) in 4%, all of which returned to normal by 2 weeks after irradiation. (Table 34-1). All patients maintained their usual lifestyle, and there were no restrictions in physical activity.

To date, 139 lesions in 117 patents with HCC have been treated with proton irradiation in our study and 114 lesions were assessable. They were followed for 3 months to 6 years. According to preliminary analysis, local tumor control was obtained in 97.2% at 1 year and 87.5% at 3 years; thereafter, this rate was maintained up to 6 years without regrowth of tumor. Overall survival rates were approximately 78% at 1 year, 48% at 3 years, and 37% at 5 years. These survival rates were largely dependent on the Child's grade of the underlying cirrho-

A 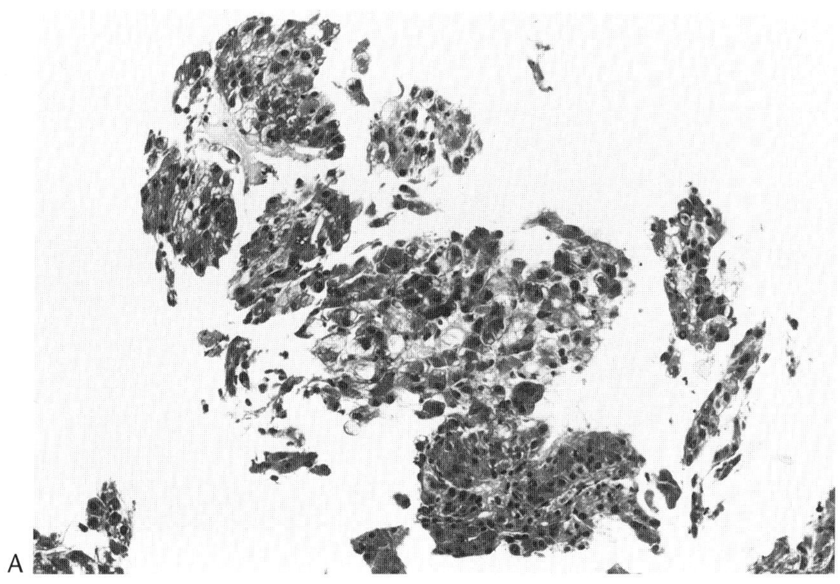

B 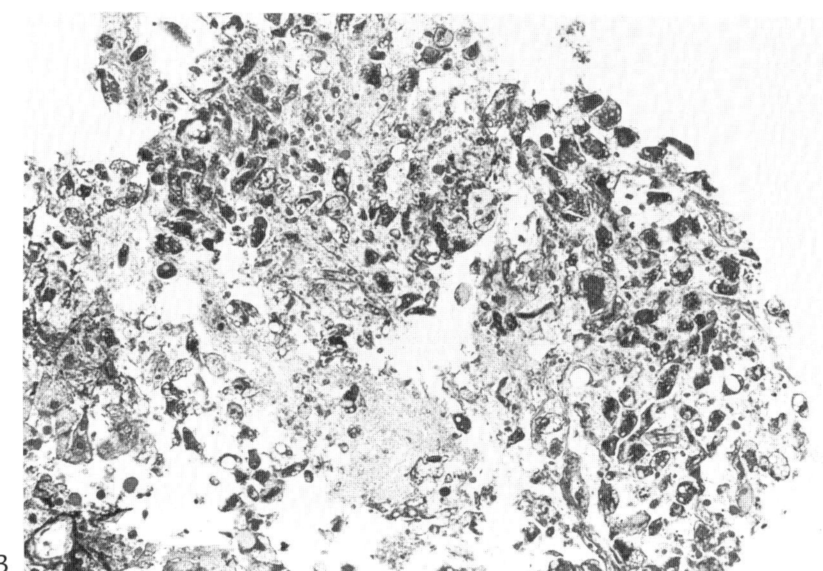

FIGURE 34-4. Liver histology (*A*) before (Edmondson II, H&E, ×33) and (*B*) 3 weeks after (necrosis and degenerative changes of cancer cells, Masson trichrome ×33) proton beam therapy in Case 1. (From Matsuzaki et al.,[74] with permission.)

sis and on the TNM stage of the HCC (Figs. 34-3 to 34-7).

Summary of Proton Beam Radiotherapy

Proton irradiation is a new modality for the treatment of HCC that is safe and effective for local tumor control. Our experience has demonstrated excellent local tumor control for 6 years or longer, as well as maintenance of good quality of life. It could be used even for patients for whom conventional therapies were not available. The only major limitation is that the HCC should be nodular but not diffuse. No serious adverse reactions have been observed.

FUTURE PROSPECTS FOR RADIOTHERAPY OF HCC

Much progress has been made over the past 10 years in efforts to deliver tumoricidal radiation dose to the tumor with an acceptable degree of complications. At present there are three major methods: (1) conformal radiotherapy with a radiosensitizer; (2) radioimmunotherapy; and

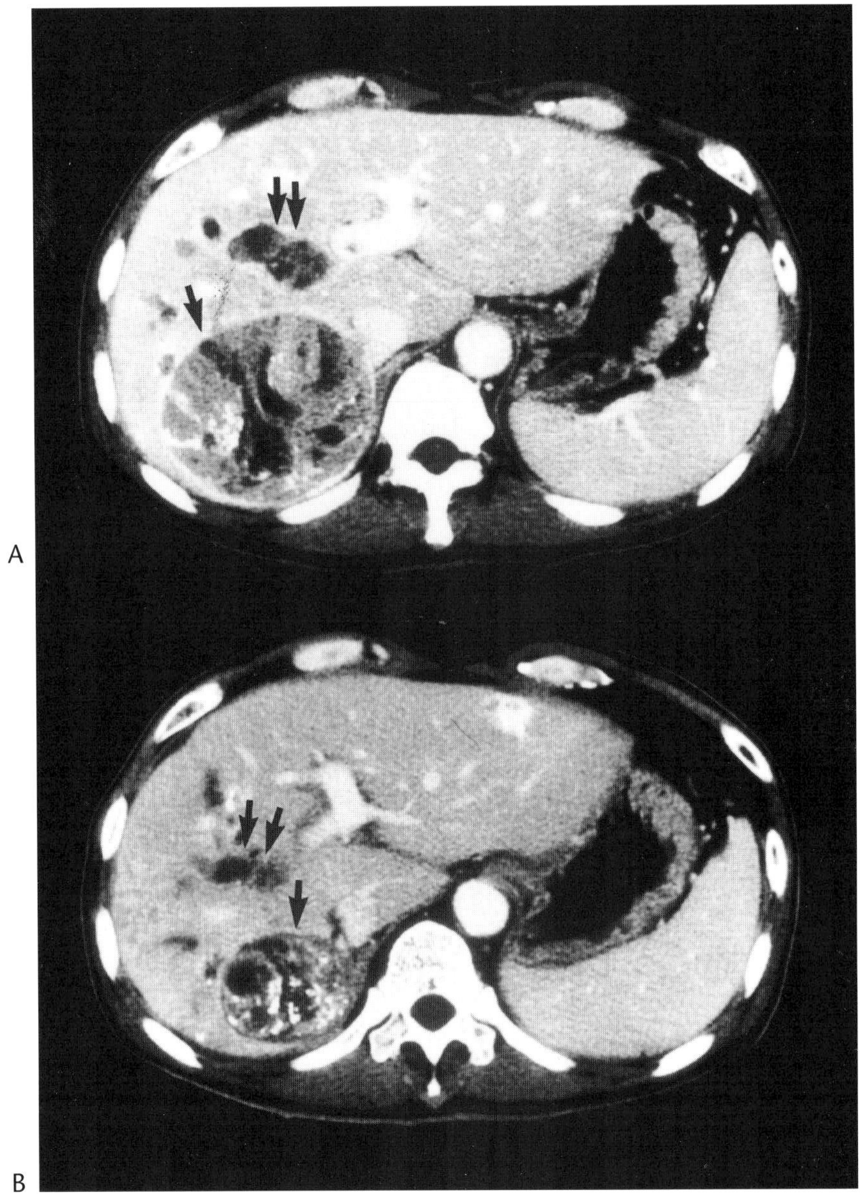

FIGURE 34-5. *Case 2.* A 57-year-old man had multinodular HCC with cirrhosis (Child's grade B) and tumor thrombus in both the portal vein and inferior vena cava. The main tumor measured 6 × 5 cm. Lipiodol embolization was contraindicated because of the risk of provoking hepatic insufficiency. He received proton irradiation in a total dose of 50 Gy, in 13 fractions over 13 days. Radiographic CT images (*A*) before and (*B*) 3 weeks after proton beam therapy in Case 2. Single arrow indicates main tumor. Double arrow indicates portal tumor thrombus. Main tumor, portal, and inferior vena cava tumor thrombi were markedly reduced in size 3 weeks after proton beam therapy. (From Matsuzaki et al.,[74] with permission.)

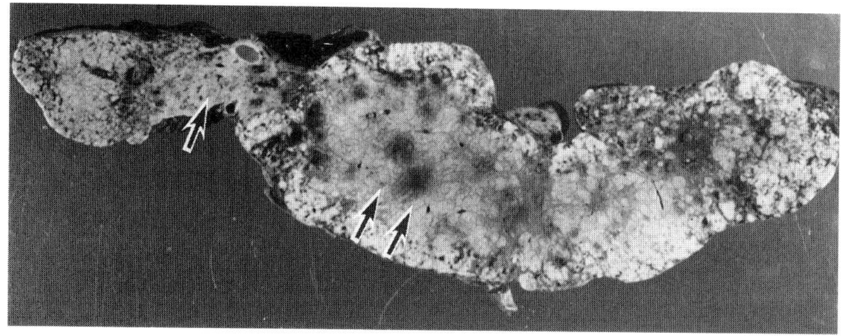

FIGURE 34-6. *Case 3.* A 74-year-old man had two tumors located in the left lateral segment (4 × 4 cm) and right anterior inferior segment (1 × 1 cm). The left tumor was successfully treated by Lipiodol chemoembolization. The avascular right tumor underwent proton irradiation (80.5 Gy, 23 fractions, 45 days). After 6 months, the irradiated tumor disappeared. However, the patient died of heart failure. Autopsy showed the regrowth of the tumor in the left lobe (7 cm), whereas the irradiated right tumor was scarred and degenerated with dense fibrosis without tumor regrowth. No viable cancer cells were observed in this lesion. Single arrow indicates irradiated HCC in the right lobe in Case 3. This irradiated lesion was completely necrotic. Double arrow shows the massive regrown tumor after Lipiodol targeted chemotherapy plus transcatheter arterial embolization (TAE). The regrown tumor in the left lobe treated by successful Lipiodol targeted chemotherapy was classified as Edmondson grade III. (From Matsuzaki et al.,[74] with permission.)

FIGURE 34-7. Histologic findings after proton therapy in Case 3. Proton irradiated lesion in right anterior inferior segment was scarred and consisted of dense fibrosis without tumor regrowth. Hepatocytes were degenerated. (Silver staining, ×13.) (From Matsuzaki et al.,[74] with permission.)

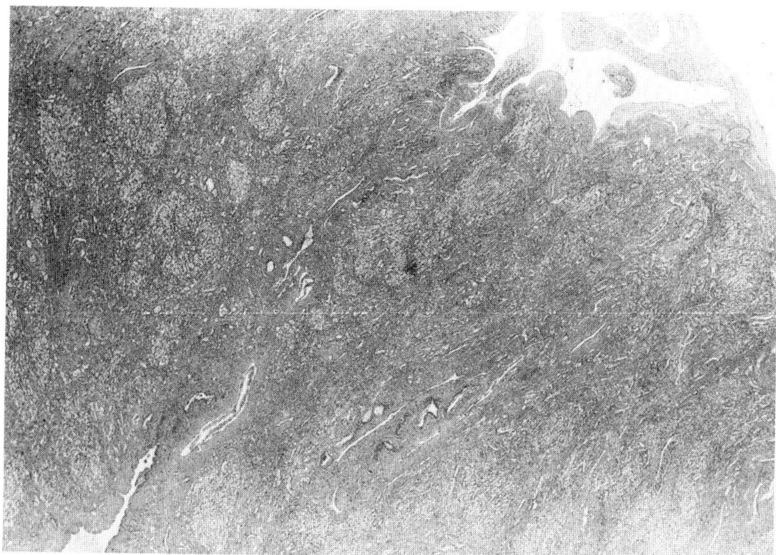

(3) radioembolization (internal radiation with unsealed radioisotopes). In addition, proton irradiation is another new, effective and safe option. Multimodality treatment may be beneficial, and there are reports that unresectable HCCs changed to resectable ones after multimodality treatment. If unresectable HCCs could be controlled for long periods by nonsurgical treatment such as radiation, the survival rate and prognosis would then largely depend on the underlying liver disease, management of which has remarkably improved.

REFERENCES

1. Okuda K, Ohtsuki T, Obata H et al. Natural history of hepatocellular carcinoma and prognosis in relation to treatment. Cancer 1985;56:918–928
2. Ebara M, Ohto M, Shinagawa T et al. Natural history of minute hepatocellular carcinoma smaller than three centimeters complicating cirrhosis: a study in 22 patients. Gastroenterology 1986;90:289–298
3. Venook AP. Treatment of hepatocellular carcinoma: too many options? J Clin Oncol 1994;12:1323–1334
4. Liver Cancer Study Group of Japan. Survey and follow-up study of primary liver cancer in Japan: Report 11. Acta Hepatol. Jpn 1994;14:208–218
5. Ingold J A, Reed GB, Kaplan HS, Bagshaw MA. Radiation hepatitis. Am J Roentgenol 1965;93:200–208
6. Austin-Seymour NM, Chen GTY, Castro JR et al. Dose volume histogram analysis of liver radiation tolerance. Int J Radiat Oncol Biol Phys 1986;12:31–35
7. Jirtle RL, Anscher MS, Alati T. Radiation sensitivity of the liver. Adv Radiat Biol 1990;14:269–311
8. Janjan NA, Cohen E, Adams M et al. Radiation tolerance of the transplanted liver. A histopathologic study in three cases. Am J Clin Oncol 1994;17:129–133
9. Lawrence TS, Robertson JM, Anscher MS et al. Hepatic toxicity resulting from cancer treatment. Int J Radiat Oncol Biol Phys 1995;31:1237–1248
10. Schacter L, Crum E, Spitzer T et al. Fatal radiation hepatitis: a case report and review of the literature. Gynecol Oncol 1986;24:373–380
11. Ohto M, Ebara M, Yoshikama M, Okuda K. Radiation therapy and percutaneous ethanol injection for the treatment of hepatocellular carcinoma. In Okuda K, Ishak KG (eds): Neoplasms of the Liver. Springer-Verlag, Tokyo, 1987, pp. 335–341
12. Matsuura M, Ishikawa A, Nakajima N et al. Radical radiation therapy for hepatocellular carcinoma. Nippon Acta Radiolo 1994;54:628–635
13. Le Pechoux C, Akine Y, Tokita N et al. Case report: hepatocellular carcinoma diagnosed radiologically, treated by transcatheter arterial embolization and limited-field radiotherapy. Br J Radiol 1994;67:591–595
14. Aoki K, Okaaki N, Okada S et al. Radiotherapy for hepatocellular carcinoma: clinicopathological study of seven autopsy cases. Hepatogastroenterology 1994;41:427–431
15. Chen SC, Lian SL, Chang WY. The effect of external radiotherapy in treatment of portal vein invasion in hepatocellular carcinoma. Cancer Chemother Pharmacol 1994;33 (suppl):S124–S127
16. Raoul JL, Guyader D, Bretagne JF et al. Randomized controlled trial for hepatocellular carcinoma with portal vein thrombosis: intra-arterial iodine-131-iodized oil versus medical support. J Nucl Med 1994;35:1782–1787
17. Lawrence TS, Tesser RJ, Ten Haken RK. An application of dose volume histograms to the treatment of intrahepatic malignancies with radiation therapy. Int J Radiat Oncol Biol Phys 1990;19:1041–1047
18. Lawrence TS, Ten Haken RK, Kessler ML et al. The use of 3-D dose volume analysis to predict radiation hepatitis. Int J Radiat Oncol Biol Phys 1992;23:781–788
19. Lawrence TS, Dworzanin LM, Walker-Andrews SC et al. Treatment of cancers involving the liver and porta hepatis with external beam irradiation and intraarterial hepatic fluorodeoxyuridine. Int J Radiat Oncol Biol Phys 1991;20: 555–561
20. Robertson BJM, Lawrence TS, Dworzanin LM et al. Treatment of primary hepatobiliary cancers with conformal radiation therapy and regional chemotherapy. J Clin Oncol 1993; 11:1286–1293
21. Robertson JM, Lawrence TS, Walker S et al. The treatment of colorectal liver metastases with conformal radiation therapy and regional chemotherapy. Int J Radiat Oncol Biol Phys 1995;32:445–450
22. Stillwagon GB, Order SE, Guse C et al. 194 hepatocellular cancers treated by radiation and chemotherapy combination: toxicity and response: A Radiation Oncology Group Study. Int J Radiat Oncol Biol Phys 1989;17:1223–1229
23. Friedman MA, Phillips TL, Hanningan JFJ, Carter SK. Phase III trial of irradiation plus chemotherapy for patients with hepatic metastases and hepatoma. Experience of the Northern California Oncology Group. NCI Monogr 1988;6: 259–264
24. Leibel SA, Pajak TF, Massullo V et al. A comparison of misonidazol sensitized radiation therapy to radiation therapy alone for the palliation of hepatic metastases: results of a Radiation Therapy Oncology Group randomized prospective trial. Int J Radiat Oncol Biol Phys 1987;13:1057–1064
25. Houle S, Yip TK, Shepherd FA et al. Hepatocellular carcinoma: pilot trial of treatment with Y-90 microspheres. Radiology 1989;172:857–860
26. Lau WY, Li AKC. Therapeutic aspects of radioisotopes in hepatobiliary malignancy. Br J Surg 1992;79:711
27. Novell JR, Hilson A, Hobbs KEF. Therapeutic aspects of radio-isotopes in hepatobiliary malignancy. Br J Surg 1991; 78:901–906
28. Order SE, Stillwagon GB, Klein JL et al. Iodine 131 antiferrin, a new treatment modality in hepatoma: a radiation therapy oncology group study. J Clin Oncol 1985;3:1573–1582
29. Tang ZY, Liu KD, Guo YD et al. Tumor imaging and targeting therapy for hepatocellular carcinoma. Preliminary results of experimental and clinical studies. Clin Med J 1986;99: 855–860
30. Liu KD, Tang ZY, Bao YM et al. Radioimmunotherapy for hepatocellular carcinoma(HCC) using ^{131}I-anti-HCC isofer-

ritin IgG: preliminary results of experimental and clinical studies. Int J Rad Oncol Biol Phys 1989;16:319–323

31. Tang ZY, Liu KD, Bao YM et al. Radioimmunotherapy in multimodality treatment of hepatocellular carcinoma with reference to second-look resection. Cancer 1990;65: 211–215
32. Fan Z, Tang Z, Liu K et al. Radioiodinated anti-hepatocellular carcinoma (HCC) ferritin. J Cancer Res Clin Oncol 1992;118:371–376
33. Zeng ZC, Tang ZY, Xie H et al. Radioimmunotherapy for unresectable hepatocellular carcinoma using ^{131}I-Hepma-1mAb: preliminary results. J Cancer Res Clin Oncol 1993; 119:257–259
34. Order SE, Klein JL, Leichner PK et al: ^{90}Yttrium antiferritin: a new therapeutic radiolabeled antibody. Int J Radiat Oncol Biol Phys 1986;12:277–281
35. Order S, Pajak T, Leibel S et al. A randomized prospective trial comparing full dose chemotherapy to ^{131}I-antiferritin: an RTOG study. Int J Radiat Oncol Biol Phys 1991;20: 953–963
36. Nakakuma K, Tashiro S, Uemura K et al. An attempt for increasing effects of hepatic artery ligation for advanced hepatoma. Jap-Deutsche Med Berichte 1979;24:675–682
37. Ohishi H, Uchida H, Yoshimura H et al. Hepatocellular carcinoma detected by iodized oil: use of anticancer agents. Radiology 1985;154:25–29
38. Madsen P, Park C, Thakur M. Dosimetry of Iodine-131 ethiodol in the treatment of hepatoma. J Nucl Med 1988;29: 1038–1044
39. Raoul J, Bourguet P, Bretagne J et al. Hepatic artery injection of I-131-labelled Lipiodol. Part I: Biodistribution study results in patients with hepatocellular carcinoma and liver metastases. Radiology 1988;168:541–545
40. Yoo HS, Park CH, Lee JT et al. Small hepatocellular carcinoma: high dose internal radiation therapy with superselective intra-arterial injection of I-131-labeled Lipiodol. Cancer Chemother Pharmacol 1994;33 (suppl):S128–S133
41. Park CH, Suh JH, Yoo HS et al. Evaluation of intrahepatic ^{131}I-ethiodol on a patient with hepatocellular carcinoma: therapeutic feasibility study. Clin Nucl Med 1986;11: 514–517
42. Kobayashi H, Hidaka H, Kajiya Y et al. Treatment of hepatocellular carcinoma by transarterial injection of anticancer agents in iodized oil suspension or of radioactive iodized oil solution. Acta Radiol Diagn (Stockh) 1986;27:139–147
43. Nakajo M, Kobayashi H, Shimabukuro K et al. Biodistribution and in vivo kinetics of iodine-131-Lipiodol infused via the hepatic artery of patients with hepatic cancer. J Nucl Med 1988;29:1066–1077
44. Yoo HS, Lee JT, Kim KW et al. Nodular hepatocellular carcinoma: treatment with subsegmental intraarterial injection of iodine 131-labeled iodized oil. Cancer 1991;68: 1878–1884
45. Takayasu K, Shima Y, Muramatsu Y et al. Hepatocellular carcinoma: treatment with intraarterial iodized oil with and without chemotherapeutic agents. Radiology 1987;163: 345–351
46. Park CH, Suh JH, Yoo SH et al. Treatment of hepatocellular carcinoma (HCC) with radiolabelled Lipiodol: a preliminary study. Clin Nucl Med 1987;8:1075–1087
47. Novell R, Hilson A, Hobbs K. Ablation of recurrent primary liver cancer using ^{131}I-lipiodol. Postgrad Med J 1991;67: 393–395
48. Bretagne JF, Raoul JL, Bourguet P et al. Hepatic artery injection of I-131-labeled Lipiodol. Radiology 1988;168:547–550
49. Raoul JI, Bretagne JF, Caucanas JP et al. Internal radiation therapy for hepatocellular carcinoma. Results of a French multicenter phase II trial of transarterial injection of iodine-131-labeled Lipiodol. Cancer 1992;69:346–352
50. Maki S, Konno T, Maeda H. Image enhancement in computerized tomography for sensitive diagnosis of liver cancer and semiquantitation of tumor selective drug targeting with oily contrast medium. Cancer 1985;56:751–757
51. Leung WT, Lau S, Ho M et al. Selective internal radiation therapy with intra-arterial iodine-131-Lipiodol in inoperable hepatocellular carcinoma. J Nucl Med 1994;35:1313–1318
52. Levine B, Hoffman H, Freedlander SO. Distribution and effect of colloidal chromic phospate (^{32}P) injected into the hepatic artery and portal vein of dogs and man. Cancer 1957; 57:164–172
53. Kasugai H, Kojima J, Tatsuta M et al. Treatment of hepatocellular carcinoma by transcatheter arterial embolization combined with intraarterial infusion of a mixture of cisplatin and ethiodized oil. Gastroenterology 1989;97:965–971
54. Nakamura H, Hashimoto T, Oi H, Sawada S. Transcatheter oily chemoembolization of hepatocellular carcinoma. Radiology 1989;170:783–786
55. Leung W-T, Lau W-Y, Ho SKW et al. Measuring lung shunting in hepatocellular carcinoma with intrahepatic-arterial technetium-99m macroaggregated albumin. J Nucl Med 1994;35:70–73
56. Yodono H, Saito Y, Saikawa Y et al. Combination chemoembolization therapy for hepatocellular carcinoma: mainly, using cisplatin (CDDP). Cancer Chemother Pharmacol 1989;23 (suppl):S42–S44
57. Yamashita Y, Takahashi M, Koga Y et al. Prognostic factors in the treatment of hepatocellular carcinoma with transcatheter arterial embolization and arterial infusion. Cancer 1991; 67:385–391
58. Kajiya Y, Kobayashi H, Nakajo M. Transarterial internal radiation therapy with I-131 Lipiodol for multifocal hepatocellular carcinoma: immediate and long term results. Cardiovasc Intervent Radiol 1993;16:150–157
59. Novell JR, Hilson AJW. Iodine-131-Lipiodol for hepatocellular carcinoma: the benefits of targetting. J Nucl Med 1994; 35:1318–1319
60. Prinzmetal M, Ornitz Jr EM, Simkin B, Bergman HC. Arteriovenous anastomoses in liver, spleen and lungs. Am J Physiol 1948;152:48–52
61. Gray BN, Anderson JE, Burton MA et al. Regression of liver metastases following treatment with yttrium-90 microspheres. Aust NZ J Surg 1992;62:105–110
62. Lau WY, Leung WT, Ho S et al. Treatment of inoperable hepatocellular carcinoma with intrahepatic arterial yttrium-90 microspheres: a phase I and II study. Br J Cancer 1994; 70:994–999

63. Houle S, Yip TCK, Shepherd FA et al. Hepatocellular carcinoma: pilot trial of treatment with yttrium-90 microspheres. Radiology 1989;172:857–860
64. Shepherd FA, Rostein LE, Houle S et al. A phase I dose escalation trial of yttrium-90 microspheres in the treatment of primary hepatocellular carcinoma. Cancer 1992;70: 2250–2254
65. Yoo HS, Park CH, Suh JH et al. Radioiodinated fatty acid esters in the management of hepatocellular carcinoma: preliminary findings. Cancer Chemother Pharmacol 1989;23 (suppl):S54–S58
66. Rösler H, Triller J, Baer HU et al. Superselective radioembolization of hepatocellular carcinoma: 5-year results of a prospective study. Nucl Med 1994;33:206–214
67. Kanai T, Kawachi K, Matsuzawa H, Inada T. Three-dimensional beam scanning for proton therapy. Nuclear Instruments and Methods 1983;214:491–496
68. Slater JM, Miller DW, Archambeau JO. Development of a hospital-based proton beam treatment center. Int J Radiat Oncol Biol Phys 1988;14:761–775
69. Suit H, Urie M. Proton beams in radiation therapy. J Natl Cancer Inst 1992;84:155–164
70. Particle Radiation Medical Science Center, University of Tsukuba. Collected papers of PARMS (Particle Radiation Medical Science Center) (1980–1989) 1990;1–806
71. Tsujii H, Tsuji H, Inada T et al. Clinical results of fractionated proton therapy. Int J Radiat Oncol Biol Phys 1992;25: 49–60
72. Ohara K, Okumura T, Akisada M et al. Irradiation synchronized respiration gate. Int J Radiat Oncol Biol Phys 1989; 17:853–857
73. Tanaka N, Matsuzaki Y, Chuganji Y et al. Proton irradiation for hepatocellular carcinoma. Lancet 1992;340:1358
74. Matsuzaki Y, Osuga T, Saito Y et al. A new, effective and safe therapeutic option using proton irradiation for hepatocellular carcinoma. Gastroenterology 1994;106:1032–1041
75. Matsuzaki Y, Osuga T Chiba T et al. New, effective treatment using proton irradiation for unresectable hepatocellular carcinoma. Int Med 1995;34:302–304

35

ETHANOL INJECTION FOR THE TREATMENT OF HEPATOCELLULAR CARCINOMA

TITO LIVRAGHI

Percutaneous ethanol injection (PEI) therapy in the treatment of liver tumors was devised independently at Chiba University in Japan and at Vimercate Hospital (Milano) in Italy.[1,2] The grounds for introducing PEI were (1) the good results of previous studies on PEI for the treatment of secondary hyperparathyroidism[3] and on percutaneous interstitial chemotherapy for the treatment of deep-seated abdominal tumors,[4] (2) the ultrasound screening of a cirrhotic population, which led to the detection of an increasing number of small HCCs, and (3) the lack of therapeutic options for these asymptomatic patients because the resectability rate was low.

Ethanol injection for treatment of hepatocellular carcinoma (HCC) acts by diffusing within the neoplastic cells, which causes immediate dehydration of the cytoplasm, with consequent coagulation necrosis followed by fibrous reaction. Within the tumor vessels, PEI induces necrosis of the endothelial cells and platelet aggregation with consequent thrombosis of the small vessels followed by neoplastic tissue ischemia. (This action is limited to the tumor by the fact that the ethanol is infused into the tumor itself.) Two features of HCC favor the toxic action of ethanol: hypervascularization and the difference in consistency between neoplastic and cirrhotic tissue. Since HCC tissue is softer than the surrounding cirrhotic tissue, ethanol diffuses within it easily and selectively and, at the same time, hypervascularization ensures its uniform distribution within the rich network of neoplastic sinusoids.

PEI is usually performed under ultrasound guidance, with a 3.5-MHz convex or sector probes provided with a lateral guide attachment. (When the oblique entry angle is difficult, a 3.5-MHz probe with an incorporated guide permits a perpendicular approach.) Sterile 95% ethanol is administred through either of two types of needle: a 17.7-cm long, 22-gauge spinal needle or, more frequently, a 20-cm long, 21-gauge needle with a closed conical tip and three terminal side holes.

PEI is usually performed in several sessions in an outpatient department or, when HCC is more advanced, in a single session under general anesthesia.[5] The former is used for single HCC less than 4–5-cm in size or multiple HCC with two to three nodules less than 3 cm and for hyperplastic adenomatous nodules.[6] PEI under general anesthesia is used in other presentations provided that HCC, single or multiple, does not exceed 30% to 35% of liver volume, and when there is no neoplastic thrombosis in the main portal branches or in the hepatic veins. Either procedure can be repeated in the event of local recurrence or new lesions.

Patients should fast overnight, as a few develop nausea, although this is rare. Treatment is usually given without sedation and without local anesthesia. Some authors administer standard premedications for analgesia, sedation, and local anesthesia. Local skin preparation with iodized alcohol is applied. During the insertion and withdrawal of the needle, the patient is asked to hold his or her breath; during the injection shallow breathing

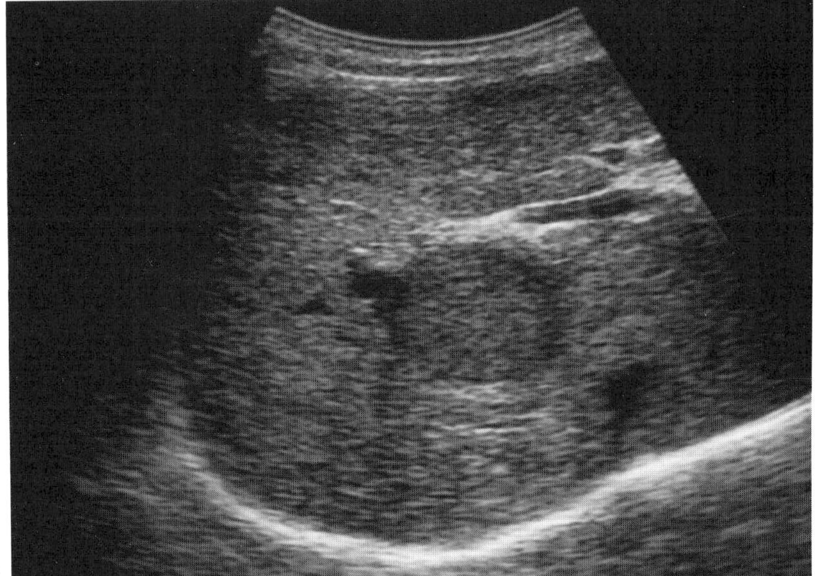
A

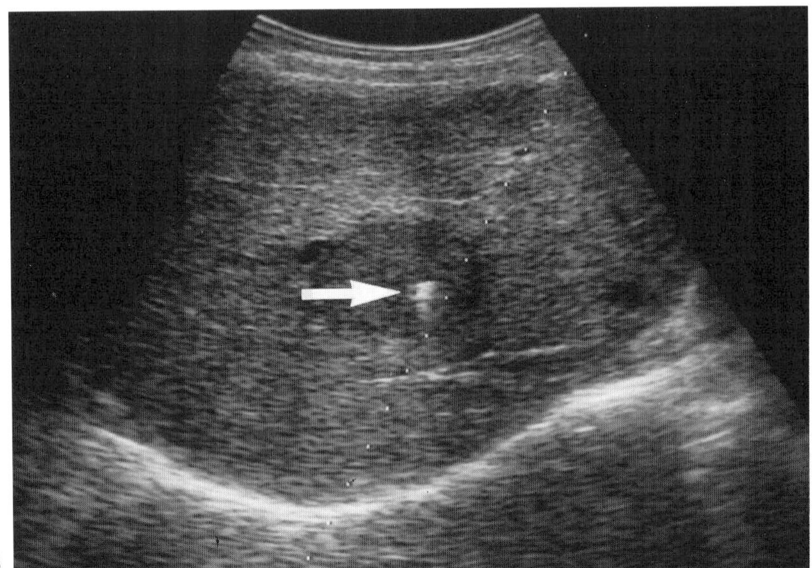
B

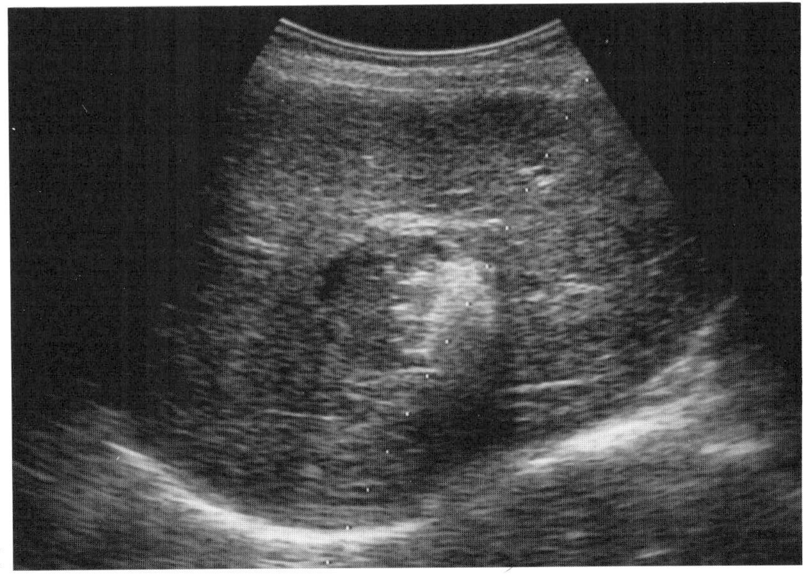
C

FIGURE 35-1. Single HCC, 4.1 cm in diameter, treated with multisession technique (six sessions with nine injections, over 3 weeks). (*A*) Oblique subcostal sonogram, obtained before PEI, shows focal, hypoechoic lesion in right lobe. (*B*) Sonogram shows the 21-gauge multiholed needle tip (arrow) inserted into the lesion, following the electronic puncture line on the monitor. (*C*) Immediately after the injection, the perfused area is clearly seen as a patch of hyperechogenicity. *(Figure continues.)*

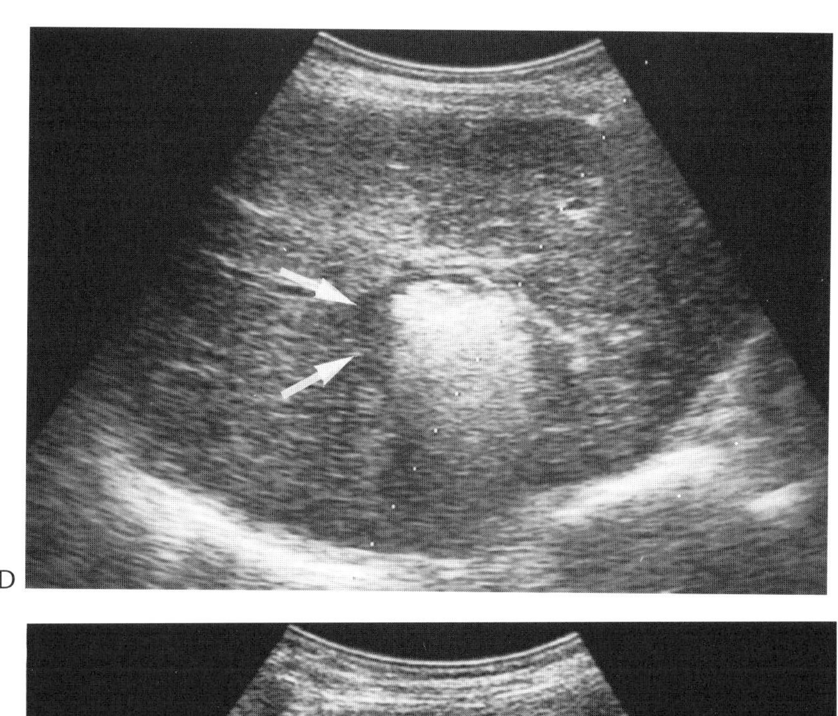
D

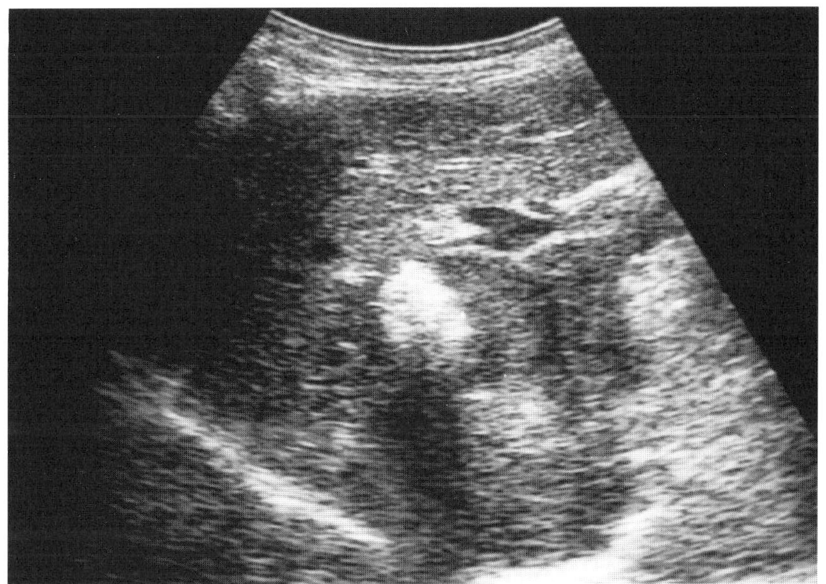
E

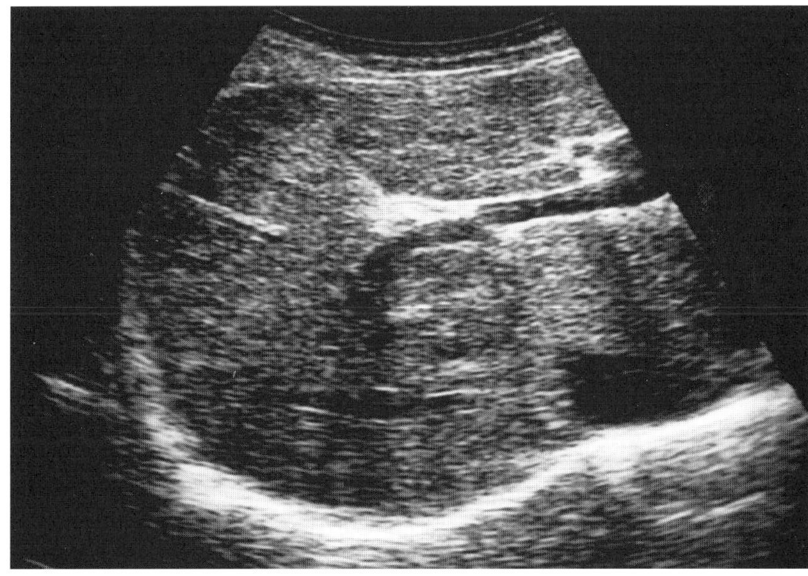
F

FIGURE 35-1 *(Continued).* (*D*) Near end of injection, lesion appears almost completely perfused, except a peripheral semilunar area (arrows). (*E*) At the second session, ethanol is precisely injected into the area considered not to have been treated previously. (*F*) At 6-month follow-up, lesion has become smaller in size and hyperechoic, because of necrotic changes. CT examination showed complete response.

is required. From 1 to 8 ml of ethanol is injected per session, given in one or more injections in different sites in the same session.

The perfused area is clearly seen as a patch of hyperechogenicity (Fig. 35-1). Ethanol is injected slowly and its diffusion checked in real time on the monitor. Ethanol usually spreads within a radius of 2 to 3 cm around the tip of the needle to the periphery of the tumor. Injection is stopped when significant leakage outside the lesion is detected or when diffusion is not clearly visible and then resumed when conditions are right. Leakage is unusual, however, because the surrounding cirrhotic tissue is harder, and ethanol tends to remain within the tumor.

As "alcohol reflux" from the withdrawing needle into adjacent tissue may cause pain, the needle is left inside for 10 to 30 seconds after the injection, especially in superficial lesions, and then withdrawn slowly. If alcohol reflux is appreciated as a rapidly moving hyperechoic line along the needle path, withdrawal is stopped and resumed a few seconds later. In all, each treatment generally takes approximately 15 to 20 minutes, and the patient rests in the waiting room for 1 to 2 hours. Treatment is usually given twice a week. The injection site is chosen before each session to ensure perfusion of areas considered not to have been treated previously. To facilitate this decision, every session is recorded on videotape. Treatment ends when the perfusion of the tumor is considered total. As a rule, using the multiholed needle, lesions smaller than 2 cm are treated in three to four sessions, lesions of 2 to 3.5 cm in four to eight sessions, and lesions of 3.5 to 5 cm in six to twelve sessions. The number of sessions is approximately twice the lesion diameter in centimeters. The total volume is not absolute and should be tailored to the patient.

When treatment is given under general anesthesia ("single session treatment"), no limit is set on the volume of ethanol to be administered.[5] During the procedure, patients receive fructose 1.6 diphosphate, 1,500 mg, and glutathione, 1,200 mg, by intravenous drip with the aim of reducing the systemic effects of alcohol by quickening its metabolism. Care is taken to inject first the deepest portion of the lesion, then followed by the central and finally the superficial portions, the aim being to prevent any initial superficial spillage of ethanol from spoiling the view for subsequent injections (Fig. 35-2). Care is also taken to avoid direct injection of ethanol into the hepatic veins, because too high and too sudden a concentration of ethanol in the blood could lead to cardiopulmonary collapse with prolonged hypoxemia. Treatment ends when the tumor appears entirely hyperechogenic on the monitor.

The time needed for the procedure ranges from 15

FIGURE 35-2. Sonogram, obtained during removal of the needle at the end of injection, shows some reflux of ethanol (arrows) along the needle path; in this case withdrawal is stopped and resumed a few seconds later.

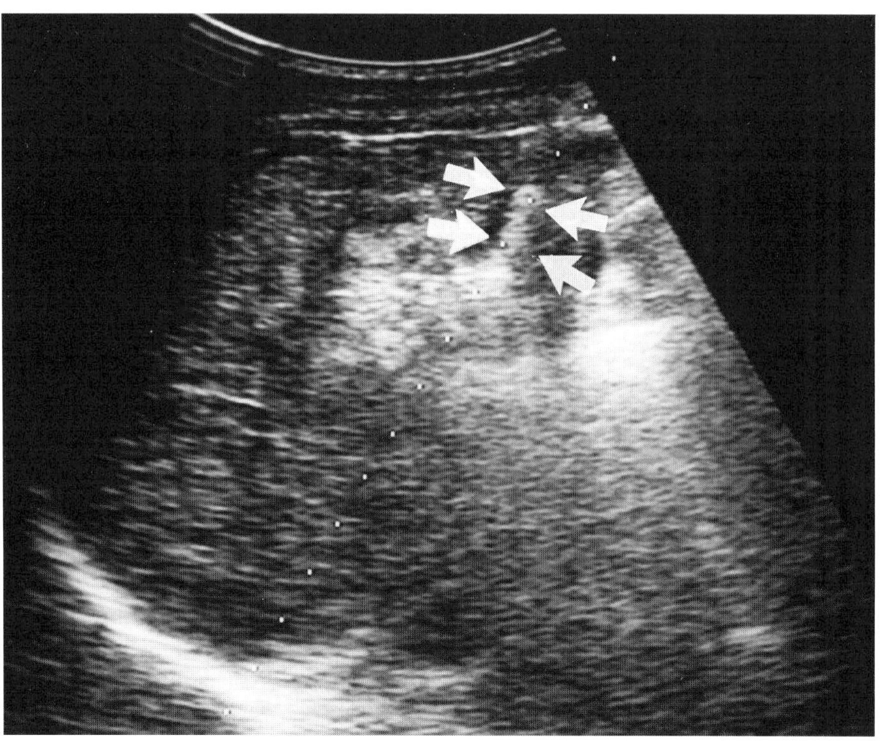

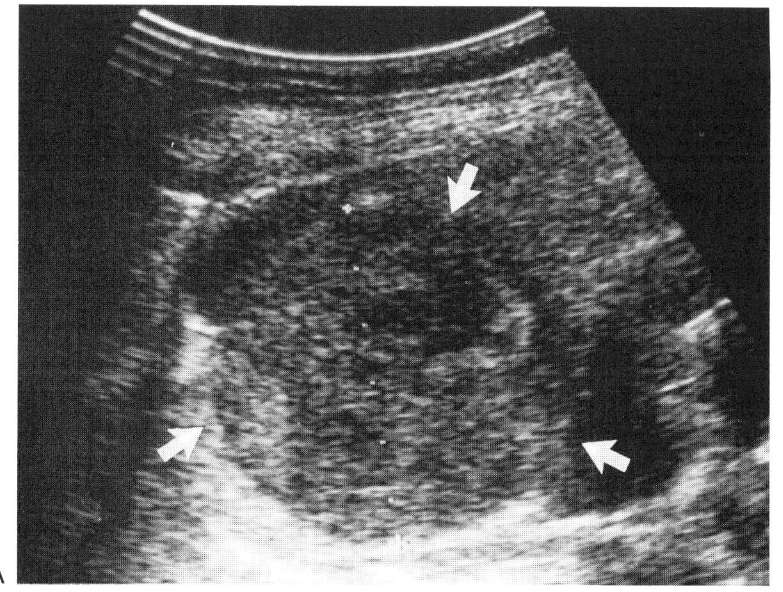
A

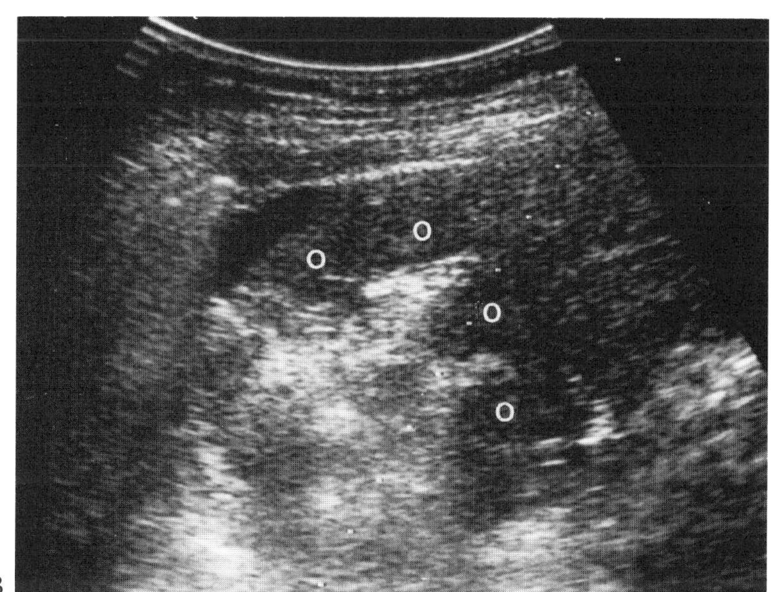
B

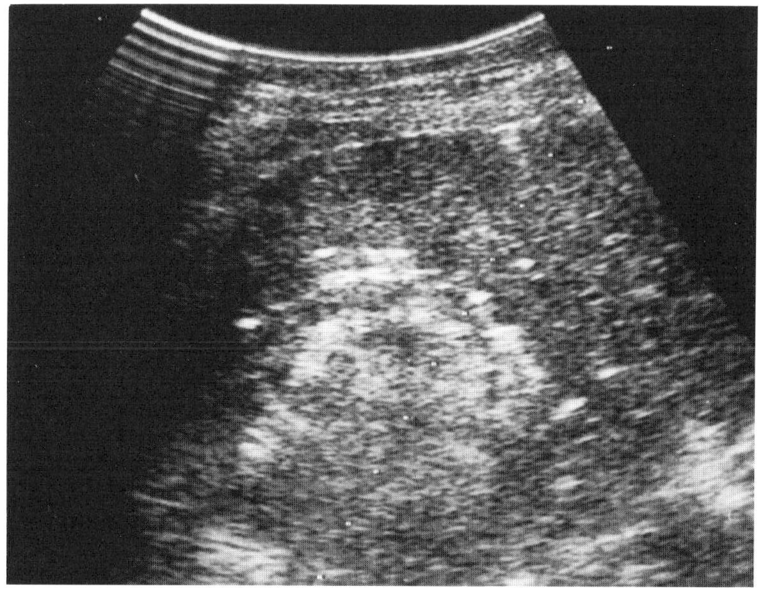
C

FIGURE 35-3. Single HCC, 6.5 cm in diameter, treated with "single session" technique under general anesthesia (55 ml by 17 injections). (*A*) Intercostal sonogram, obtained before PEI, shows focal, isoechoic lesion in right lobe (arrows). (*B*) During the procedure, care is taken to inject first the deepest portion of the lesion, then the central and finally the superficial portions. Sonogram shows ethanol injection at the middle of treatment. Some superficial areas are not yet perfused (circles). (*C*) At the end of treatment, lesion appears homogeneously perfused.

to 50 minutes, depending on the number and size of the lesions. Up to now, the largest total quantity of ethanol injected has been 190 ml with 21 injections in a single tumor 14 cm in diameter. Gas is usually present in the lesion on the days immediately after PEI, particularly when a large amount of ethanol has been injected (Fig. 35-3).

TREATMENT OF PORTAL THROMBOSIS

Treatment of neoplastic portal thrombosis is also possible even for palliation.[7] Ethanol injection is generally performed when the thrombus is located segmentally or subsegmentally, with the aim of stopping its progression along the vessel to the main branches. A one-holed needle is precisely positioned in the thrombus, and the alcohol usually diffuses selectively along it. From 1 to 2 ml is injected per session.

IMAGING MODALITIES

A combination of imaging techniques is used to evaluate the therapeutic response to determine whether any neoplastic tissue persists. These examinations are the same as those used for the initial workup and during the follow-up period. They may include ultrasonography, computerized tomography (CT), magnetic resonance imaging (MRI) and angiography. Patients are evaluated 1 month after PEI and every 4 to 6 months.

We judge the imaging response complete when the CT scans show no areas of enhancement within the lesion, when this finding is confirmed in the follow-up scans, and when the CT and ultrasound scans show no increase in tumor size. Even when the response is complete, the lesions show only a small decrease in size (Fig. 35-5 A-D). On ultrasound scans, all lesions show changes from hypoechogenicity to iso- or hyperechogenicity, and from isoechogenecity or hyperechogenicity to a marbled appearance; however, ultrasound is not sufficiently reliable for recognizing areas that have remained viable (Fig. 35-1).

Color Doppler ultrasonography is useful in the assessment of therapeutic efficacy, demonstrating residual arterial flow within the tumor.[8] Portions of the tumor in which Doppler signals are detected after PEI correspond to the enhancing areas seen on CT or MRI. However, color Doppler should not be used as the final diagnostic test for establishing the outcome of PEI, because it does not detect the new vascularization of small tumors and because bolus CT is more sensitive. Color Doppler is good enough for monitoring the response during the course of PEI treatment, because as long as the signals are still recognizable within the tumor, further treatments should be administered. When no color Doppler signals are found after PEI, further evaluation with CT or MRI is still necessary to rule out false-negative diagnosis.

On MRI, HCC is usually isointense in T_1- and hyperintense in T_2-weighted scans; necrotic tissue shows low signal intensity on T_2-images, whereas viable tissue remains hyperintense (Fig. 35-5B).[9] Contrast-enhanced T_1-weighted images are more accurate than unenhanced images.[10,11] Wedged abnormalities due to hepatic hyperfusion in the arterial phase are commonly seen adjacent to the treated area; it is important to be aware of this abnormality, usually caused by chemical thrombosis of small portal vessels, because it may be misinterpreted as pointing to another pathologic condition.[12]

Angiography is not widely recommended because it is invasive and therefore not often repeatable; however, angiography is reliable for evaluating the efficacy of PEI, because the tumor stain disappears.

TUMOR MARKERS

Assay for α-fetoprotein (AFP) is done before PEI, 1 month after PEI, and every 4 months thereafter. This assay is useful only if AFP is initially elevated (more than 200 mg/ml) and normalizes after PEI. In reality, particularly when HCC is small (less than 5 cm), AFP is not elevated in 60% to 70% of cases.[13,14] When the imaging modalities show a complete response not followed by a large decrease in AFP levels, some undetected or not yet detectable neoplastic tissue is growing elsewhere. Moreover, an increase in AFP levels during the follow-up period suggests a recurrent disease or new lesions.

A relatively new tumor marker is des-γ-carboxy prothrombin (DCP). According to some studies, assays for DCP and AFP combined are more sensitive than AFP alone both to HCC detection[15] and to tumor recurrence after surgery.[16] DCP, therefore, may be useful in the evaluation of the therapeutic efficacy of PEI. We use AFP routinely and resort to DCP when AFP is less than 200 ng/ml.

SIDE EFFECTS AND COMPLICATIONS

Most patients complain of mild pain during or immediately after the injection, but, as a rule, tolerate it and do not discontinue the treatment. Usually pain is confined to the injection site, but sometimes it is felt in the right shoulder or at the epigastric level. Some authors prefer to inject a few milliliters of Xylocaine before withdrawing the needle. Some cases of mild alcohol intoxication have occurred. Fever has occurred, usually after the first sessions when the necrosis of neoplastic tissue is greatest, and lasts several days.

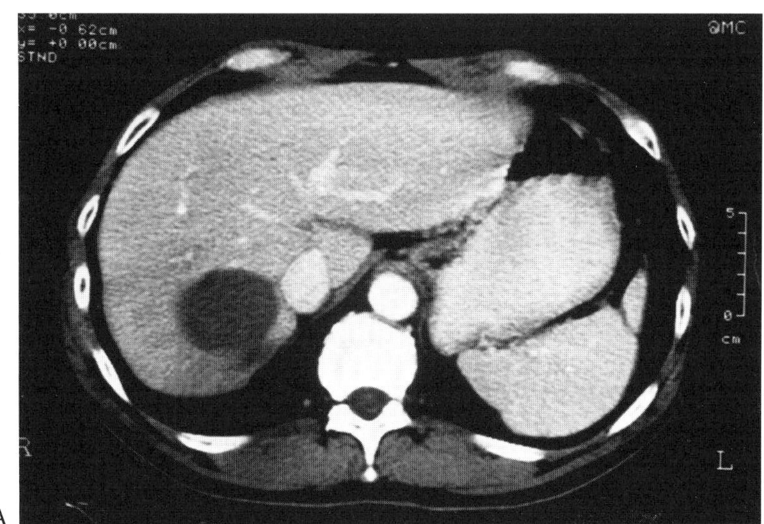

A

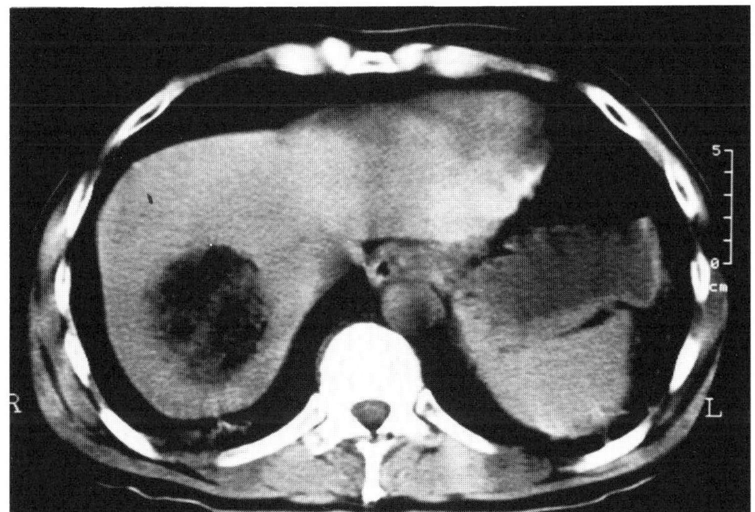

B

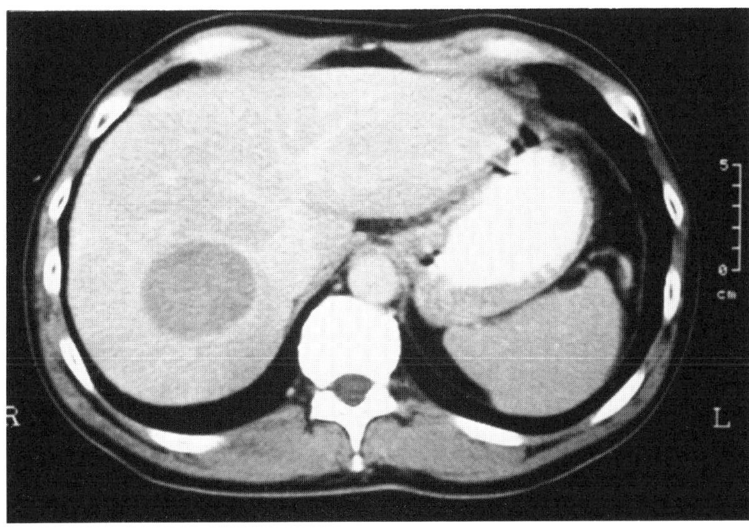

C

FIGURE 35-4. Single HCC, 5.2 cm in diameter, treated with "single session" technique (40 ml by 12 injections). (*A*) Contrast-enhanced CT scan shows lesion with relatively low density (65 H), before PEI. (*B*) Unenhanced CT scan performed 1 day after treatment shows large amount of gas inside and around the tumor. (Density = −240 H). (C) At 1-month follow-up, gas disappeared. Lesion shows diffuse unenhancement (14 H) because of necrotic reaction causing lack of blood supply.

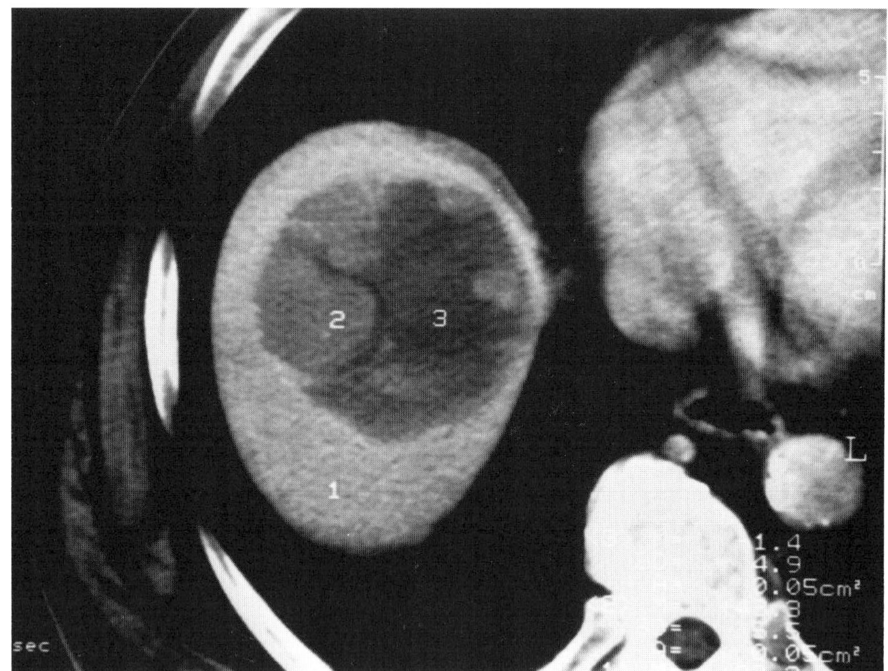

A

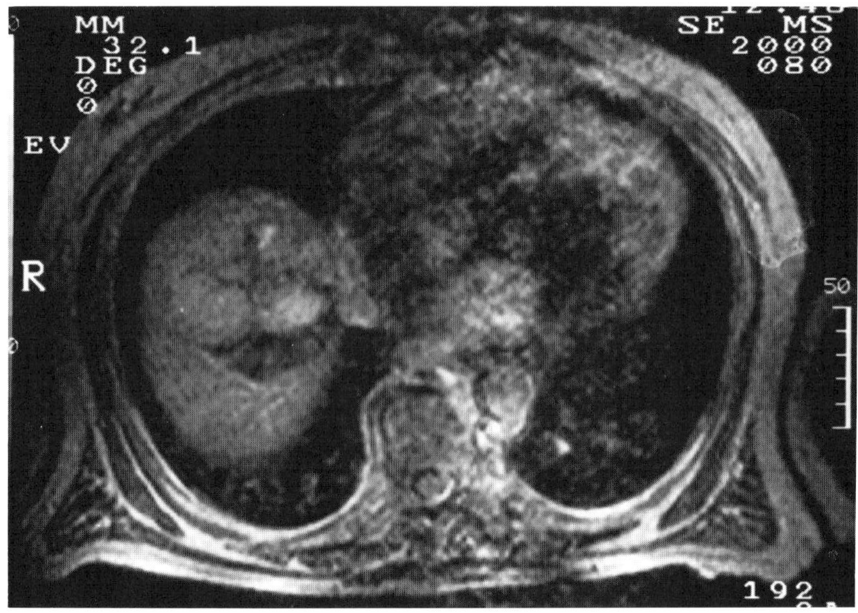

B

FIGURE 35-5. Single HCC 8.1 cm in diameter, treated with two "single session" techniques, because of partial response after the first procedure. (*A*) Contrast-enhanced CT scan obtained 1 month after the first treatment shows partial response. Areas of different density are present inside the tumor. More hypodense areas (no. 3:11 HU) present no enhancement (9 HU on unenhanced CT) and correspond to necrotic changes. More hyperdense areas (no. 2:53 HU) present enhancement (30 HU on unenhanced CT) and correspond to viable neoplastic tissue. Normal tissue around the lesion (no. 1) has density of 92 HU (34 on unenhanced CT). (*B*) T_2-weighted image shows the same pattern, viable tissue being hyperintense and necrotic tissue hypointense. *(Figure continues.)*

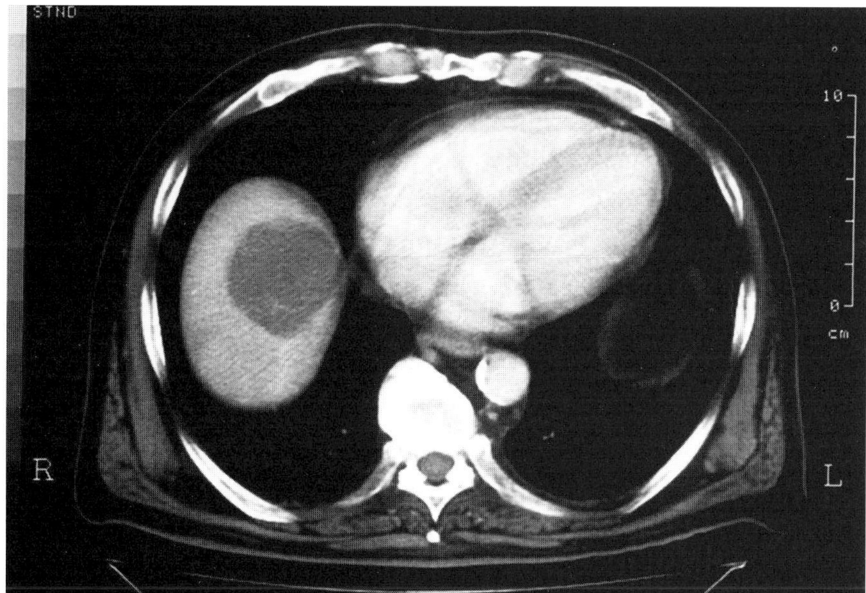

C

D

FIGURE 35-5 *(Continued).* (*C*) CT scan performed 1 month after the second treatment shows complete response. The tumor shows no areas of enhancement. (*D*) Complete response is confirmed on CT scan obtained at 3-year follow-up; the lesion shows only a small decrease in size.

Among 1,574 patients treated by various authors, none died.[17–32] There has been an anedoctal report of one death due to massive area of hepatic necrosis distant from the injection site and to myocardial infarction; however, no direct relation between PEI and myocardial infarction was demonstrated in this case.[33]

Major complications are rare, ranging from 1.3 to 2.4%, and usually are treated conservatively. Additional complications that have been reported include intraperitoneal hemorrhage, right pleural effusion, cholangitis or jaundice secondary to injury of bile ducts, liver abscess, hepatic infarction probably related to reflux of ethanol into portal vein branches, hemobilia, arterioportal shunt, and shock.[34–36] With regard to neoplastic seeding along the needle track, only a few cases are reported, probably because the reflux of alcohol prevents this from happening.[37–41] Mild atrophy, manifested as concavity of the liver surface, or even segmental atrophy can be detected

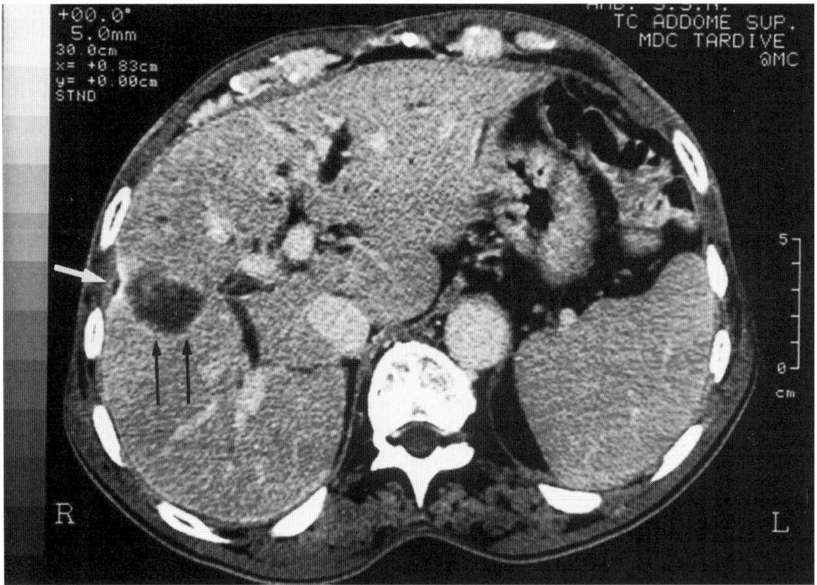

FIGURE 35-6. AT 1-year follow-up, CT scan shows mild atrophy (white arrow) of non-neoplastic parenchyma near the lesion treated (black arrows), manifested as concavity of the liver surface.

with CT, particularly using arterial portography technique (Fig. 35-6). This change is due to a decreased portal blood flow, caused by organized thrombi, in the noncancerous liver parenchyma that surrounds the tumor being treated.[42]

With larger volumes of ethanol per treatment session, when PEI is given under general anesthesia, the complication rate increases. Some cases of alcohol intoxication are observed, but do not require treatment. The highest blood alcohol levels found immediately after treatment were 230 mg/100 ml, returning to normal within 24 hours. Hyperpyrexia always develops in patients who receive more than 50 ml of alcohol. Some transient and variable changes in aminotransferase, bilirubin, blood cells, platelets, hemoglobin, fibrinogen and haptoglobin levels are observed. These changes are due to hepatic necrosis, hemolysis and localized thrombosis. In our series of 103 treatments, one Child's class C patient died of hemorrhage from esophageal varices. Major complications included one hemorrhage requiring transfusion in a large superficially located tumor, one transient renal failure requiring some hemodialysis treatments, and two chemical infarctions of a segment adjacent to the tumor, accompained by pain lasting for some days; minor complications included some modest hemorrhages and some transient liver decompensations. The mortality was thus 0.9% and the complication rate 3.8% (unpublished data).

CONTRAINDICATIONS

Contraindications to PEI include advanced cirrhosis or proneness to severe bleeding. PEI should not be done when prothrombin time is less than 40% or platelets are less than 40,000/mm.[3] Other contraindications include presence of thrombosis in the main portal branches and large or diffuse HCC, although there are some exceptions (Fig. 35-7).

SURVIVAL RATES

The Chiba University group treated 112 patients with PEI, 93 of them with one lesion, 16 with two lesions, and 3 with three lesions, all less than or equal to 3 cm in size. The 1-, 3-, 5-year survival rates were 96, 72, 51% for 60 Child's A patients, 90, 72, 48% for 33 Child's B patients, and 94, 25, 0% for 19 Child's C patients.[20] Our series of 746 patients presented similar results.[31] Others have reported similar survival rates[19,43] (Table 35-1).

The main cause of death among Child's A patients was progression of HCC due to the appearance of new lesions, whereas among Child's C patients it was hepatic failure. The 5-year new lesion rate reported by the Chiba group was 87%. Others have reported 64% to 100%.[19,31,43]

CONCLUSIONS

Rationale

The rationale for using PEI includes the following:

1. The expanding form of the HCC initially shows regional growth, so local therapy such as PEI may be applied.

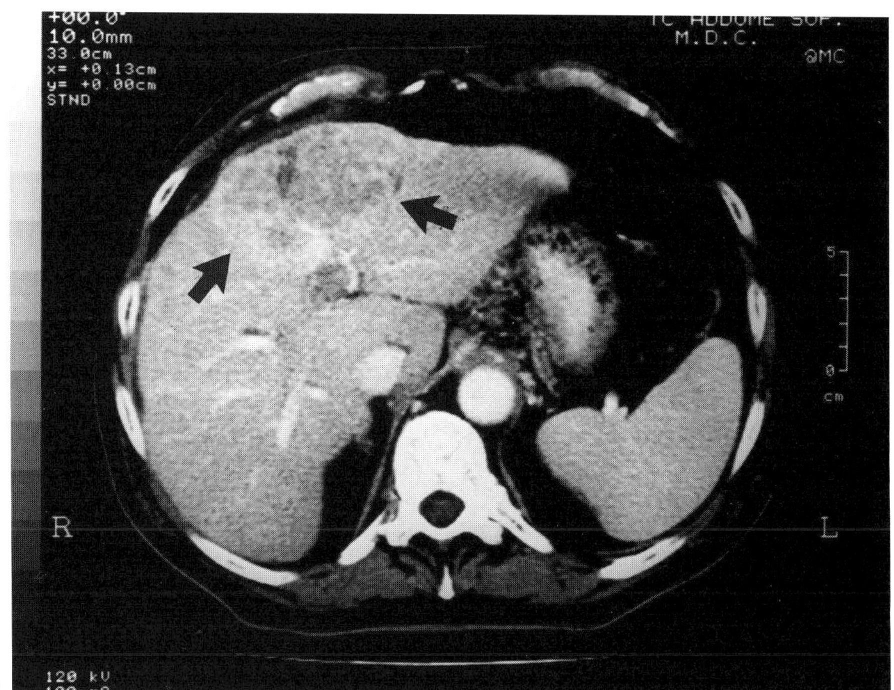

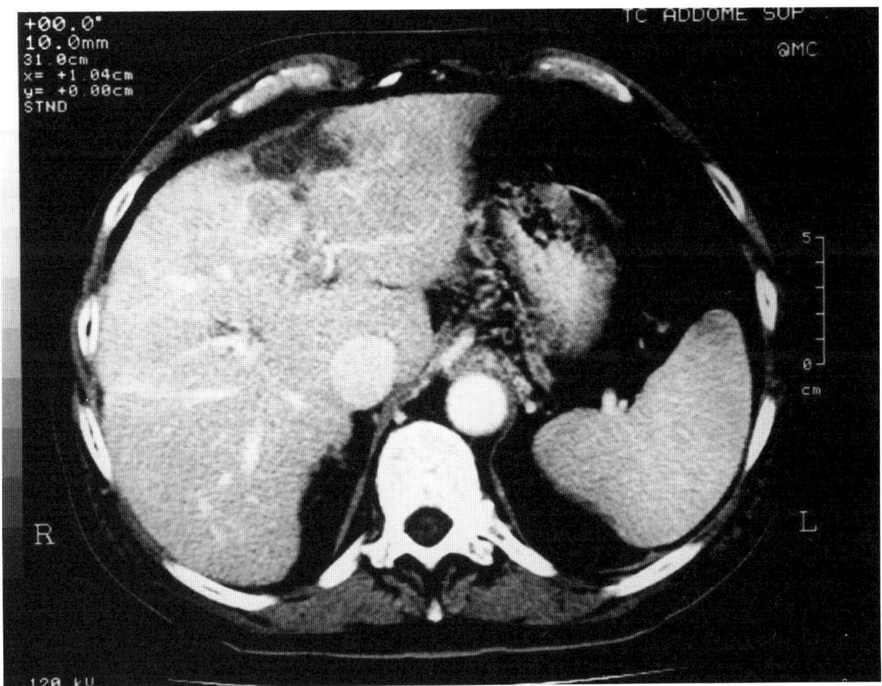

FIGURE 35-7. Large HCC, 12 cm in diameter, treated with "single session" technique. During the years before, this patient was treated with multisession technique for 3 other lesions, smaller in size. (*A*) CT scan obtained before PEI shows infiltrating lesion protruding on hepatic surface (arrows). (*B*) CT scan obtained at 1-year follow-up shows shrinkage and hypodensity of the lesion. AFP dosage decreased from 14,000 to 150 ng/ml.

TABLE 35-1. PEI in HCC: 5-Year Survival Rates

Author	HCC Stage	Size (cm)	Patients (No.)	Child (Class)	1-Year (%)	3-Year (%)	5-Year (%)
Ebara et al.[22]	s–m	≤3	60	A	96	72	51
			33	B	90	72	48
			19	C	94	25	0
Shiina et al.[43]	s–m	≤5	50	A-B-C	87	62	43
Tanikawa[19]	s–m	≤3	217	A-B-C	94	73	48
Livraghi et al.[31]	s	≤5	293	A	98	79	47
	s	≤5	149	B	93	63	29
	s	≤5	20	C	64	0	0
	m	≤3	121	A	94	68	36
	m	≤3	63	B	93	59	0
	s	>5	28	A	96	72	53
	adv	>5	22	A-B-C	90	16	0

Abbreviations: s, single; m, multiple (2 or 3 nodules); adv, single or multiple, with daughter nodules or portal involvement.

2. Ultrasound screening of cirrhotic population allows detection of HCC at its initial stage, when the tumor size is small. In a study of Oka,[44] 82% of the patients had HCC of less than 5 cm when the tumor was detected by ultrasound screening.
3. Ethanol shows sensitive diffusion in HCC, because of the softer consistency and hypervascularity of HCC.
4. PEI carries no risk of loss or of important damage to the remaining parenchyma. In the days following treatment there may be a transient rise in aminotransferase levels but histologic examination has shown no damage to healthy tissue at a distance from the treated lesion.[45] Whether the loss of healthy tissue due to multisegmental resection or the damage to the parenchyma involved in conventional TACE leads to a deterioration of liver function and a hastening of terminal failure is not established but is probable.[46,47]
5. PEI is safe. In all series published to date, comprising 1,574 patients, there were no fatalities and the highest complication rate was 2.4%, most of the complications being treated conservatively. Zero mortality for conventional PEI is in sharp contrast to the mortality for surgery, which, although much lower than it used to be, is nonetheless a factor to be reckoned with. The most authoritative reports put mortality from surgery at 1.4% to 11% and the complication rate at up to 58%. In this connection it should be remembered that patients selected by ultrasound screening are symptom-free and even if not rtreated can expect to live for over a year.[48,49]
6. PEI can easily be repeated when new lesions appear, as they do in the majority of patients followed for 5 years. The new lesions rates in the surgical series range from 75% to 100% and in the PEI series form 64% to 100%. This arises from the multifocal nature of HCC in cirrhotics.[50–52] Thus, the first lesion to show up on the ultrasound scan usually is only the prelude to others and surgery is usually only palliative, not affecting the natural course of the disease. At Chiba University, the new lesions rates of two comparable groups of patients treated by surgery and PEI were the same.[20] As this reflects the natural history of the disease, the patient must be watched closely so that new lesions may be treated as and when they occur and are still small. An advantage of PEI is that the patient is attended by the same operator both for diagnosis and treatment. Moreover, it is now possible to curb the course of the disease by single-session PEI even in some patients who cannot be followed by conventional PEI.
7. PEI is a reproducible procedure in terms of safety and survival.
8. The low cost, the accessibility of the necessary materials, and the easy technique render PEI applicable everywhere.
9. Long-term results for PEI are fairly high. The overall 5-year survival rate in 628 patients with lesions 5 cm or less and compensated cirrhosis was 48%.[31]

Indications

The large number of patients enrolled in ultrasound programs has created a large demand for effective, safe, repeatable, low-cost treatment that can be offered at many centers. PEI substantially meets all these requirement. In the absence of randomized studies, but on the strength of the results reported to date, PEI is indicated for the majority of patients recruited by ultrasound screening, excluding candidates for OLT and, for surgical resection, those selected following the predictive factors established by the Liver Cancer Study Group.[53] In practice, most patients should be managed as follows: early detection of HCC by ultrasound screening, treatment by PEI, follow-up by imaging and tumor markers, and treatment by PEI of any new lesions.

REFERENCES

1. Sugiura N, Takara K, Ohto M et al. Treatment of small hepatocellular carcinoma by percutaneous injection of ethanol into tumor with real-time monitoring. Acta Hepatol Jpn 1983;24:920
2. Livraghi T, Festi D, Monti F et al. US-guided percutaneous alcohol injection of small hepatic and abdominal tumors. Radiology 1986;161:309–312
3. Solbiati L, Giangrande A, De Pra L et al. Percutaneous ethanol injection of parathyroid tumors under US guidance: treatment for secondary hyperparathyroidism. Radiology 1985;155:607–610
4. Livraghi T, Baietta E, Matricardi L et al. Fine needle percutaneous intratumoral chemotherapy under US guidance. Tumori 1986;72:81–87
5. Livraghi T, Vettori C, Torzilli G et al. Percutaneous ethanol injection of hepatic tumors: single-session therapy under general anesthesia. Am J Roentgenol 1993;160:1065–1069
6. Livraghi T, Sangalli G, Vettori C. Adenomatous hyperplastic nodules in the cirrhotic liver: a therapeutic approach. Radiology 1989;170:155–157
7. Livraghi T, Grigioni W, Mazziotti A, et al. Percutaneous ethanol injection of portal thrombosis in hepatocellular carcinoma: a new possible treatment. Tumori 1990;76:394–397
8. Lencioni R, Caramella D, Bartolozzi C. Hepatocellular carcinoma: use of color-Doppler US to evaluate response to treatment with percutaneous ethanol injection. Radiology 1995; 194:113–118
9. Sironi S, Livraghi T, Del Maschio A. Small hepatocellular carcinoma treated with percutaneous ethanol injection: MR imaging findings. Radiology 1991;180:336–336
10. Bartolozzi C, Lencioni R, Caramella D et al. Treatment of hepatocellular carcinoma with percutaneous ethanol injection: evaluation with contrast-enhanced MR imaging. Am J Roentgenol 1994;162:827–832
11. Sironi S, De Cobelli F, Livraghi T et al. Small hepatocellular carcinoma with percutaneous ethanol injection: unenhanced and gadolinium-enhanced MR imaging follow-up. Radiology 1994;192:407–412
12. Ito K, Honjo K, Fujita T et al. Enhanced MR imaging of the liver after ethanol treatment of hepatocellular carcinoma: evaluation of areas of hyperperfusion adjacent to the tumor. Am J Roentgenol 1995;164:1413–1417
13. Chen DS, Sung JL, Sheu JC et al. Serum α-fetoprotein in the early stage of human hepatocellular carcinoma. Gastroenterology 1984;86:1404–1409
14. Livraghi T, Sangalli G, Giordano F et al. 240 hepatocellular carcinomas: ultrasound features, tumor size, cytologic and histologic patterns, serum alpha-fetoprotein and HBsAg. Tumori 1987;73:507–512
15. Brunello F, Marcarino C, Pasquero P. The des-γ-carboxyprothrombin for the diagnosis of hepatocellular carcinoma. Ital J Gastroenterol 1993;25:9–12
16. Weitz IC, Liebman HA. Des-γ-carboxy (abnormal) prothrombin and hepatocellular carcinoma: a critical review. Hepatology 1993;18:990–997
17. Shiina S, Niwa Y. Percutaneous ethanol injection therapy in the treatment of liver neoplasms. In Howard E (ed): Current Techniques in Interventional Radiology Cope C, Philadelphia, 1994, pp. 3.1–3.14
18. Sheu JC, Sung JL, Huang GT et al. Intratumor injection of absolute ethanol under ultrasound guidance for the treatment of small hepatocellular carcinoma. Hepatogastroenterology 1987;34:255–261
19. Tanikawa K. Multidisciplinary treatment of hepatocellular carcinoma. In Tobe T, Kameda H (eds): Primary Liver Cancer in Japan. Springer-Verlag, Tokyo, 1992, pp. 327–334
20. Okuda K. Intratumor ethanol injection. J Surg Oncol 1993; 3(suppl):97–99
21. Kotoh K, Sakai H, Sakamoto S et al. The effect of percutaneous ethanol injection therapy on small solitary hepatocellular carcinoma is comparable to that of hepatectomy. Am J Gastroenterol 1994;89:194–198
22. Seki T, Nonaka T, Kubota Y et al. Ultrasonical guided percutaneous ethanol injection therapy for hepatocellular carcinoma. Am J Gastroenterol 1989;84:1400–1407
23. Borghetti M, Benelli G, Bonardi R. Trattamento mediante alcolizzazione percutanea ecoguidata di piccoli epatocarcinomi. Radiol Med 1991;81:502–509
24. Imari Y, Sakamoto S, Shiomichi S et al. Hepatocellular carcinoma not detected with plain US: treatment with percutaneous ethanol injection under guidance with enhanced US. Radiology 1992;185:497–500
25. Kumada T, Nakano S, Takeda I et al. Treatment of small hepatocellular carcinoma. Cancer Chem Pharmacol 1992; 31(suppl):25–29
26. Vilana R, Bruix J, Bru C et al. Tumor size determines the efficacy of percutaneous ethanol injection for the treatment of small hepatocellular carcinoma. Hepatology 1992;16: 353–357
27. Hisa N, Ohkuma K, Fujikura Y et al. Percutaneous ethanol injection therapy for hepatic tumors. Results and technical considerations. Semin Interv Radiol 1993;10:27–34
28. Redvanly RD, Chezmar JL, Strauss RM et al. Malignant hepatic tumors: safety of high-dose percutaneous ethanol ablation therapy. Radiology 1993;188:283–285
29. Solmi L, Muratori R, Bertoni F, Gandolfi L. Echo-guided percutaneous ethanol injection in small hepatocellular carcinoma: personal experience. Hepatogastroenterology 1993; 40:505–508
30. Onodera H, Ukai K, Nakano N et al. Outcomes of 116 patients with hepatocellular carcinoma. Cancer Chemother Pharmacol 1994;33(suppl):103–108
31. Livraghi T, Giorgio A, Marin G et al. Hepatocellular carcinoma and cirrhosis in 746 patients: long-term results of percutaneous ethanol injection. Radiology 1995;197:101–108
32. Lencioni R, Bartolozzi C, Caramella D et al. Treatment of small hepatocellular carcinoma with percutaneous ethanol injection. Cancer 1995;76:1737–1746

33. Taavitsainen M, Vehmas T, Kauppila R. Fatal liver necrosis following percutaneous ethanol injection for hepatocellular carcinoma. Abdom Imaging 1993;18:357–359

34. De Sio I, Castellano L, Calandra M. Hemobilia following percutaneous ethanol injection for hepatocellular carcinoma in a cirrhotic patient. J Clin Ultrasound 1992;20:621–623

35. Koda M, Okamoto K, Miyoshi Y, Kawasaki H. Hepatic vascular and bile duct injury after ethanol injection therapy for hepatocellular carcinoma. Gastrointest Radiol 1992;17: 167–169

36. Solinas A, Erbella GS, Distrutti E et al. Abscess formation in hepatocellular carcinoma: complications of percutaneous ultrasound-guided ethanol injection. J Clin Ultrasound 1993;21:531–533

37. Cedrone A, Rapaccini GL, Pompili M. Neoplastic seeding complicating percutaneous ethanol injection for treatment of hepatocellular carcinoma. Radiology 1992;183:787–788

38. Goletti O, De Negri F, Pucciarelli M et al. Subcutaneous seeding after percutaneous ethanol injection of liver metastasis. Radiology 1992;183:785–786

39. Zerbey AL, Mueller PR, Dawson SL, Hoover Jr HC. Pleural seeding from hepatocellular carcinoma: a complication of percutaneous alcohol ablation. Radiology 1994;193:81–82

40. Boland GW, Lee MJ, Dawson SL et al. Percutaneous injection of ethanol in a patient with a solitary hepatocellular carcinoma. Am J Roentgenol 1993;161:1071–1077

41. Cardinale L, Castiglione V. Disseminazione neoplastica sottocutanea lungo il tragitto dell'ago. Radiol Med 1995;89: 557–559

42. Yoshikawa J, Matsui O, Kadoya M. Hepatocellular carcinoma: CT appearance of parenchymal changes after percutaneous ethanol injection therapy. Radiology 1995;194: 107–111

43. Shiina S, Tagawa K, Niwa Y et al. Percutaneous ethanol injection therapy for hepatocellular carcinoma: results in 146 patients. Am J Roentgenol 1993;160:1023–1028

44. Oka H, Kurioka N, Kim K et al. Prospective study of early detection of hepatocellular carcinoma in patients with cirrhosis. Hepatology 1990;12:680–687

45. Shiina S, Tagawa K, Unuma T et al. Percutaneous ethanol injection therapy for hepatocellular carcinoma: a histopathologic study. Cancer 1991;68:1524–1530

46. Okuda K, Ohtsuki T, Obata H et al. Natural history of hepatocellular carcinoma and prognosis in relation to treatment. Cancer 1985;56:918–928

47. Groupe d'Etude et de Traitement de Carcinome Hepatocellulaire. A comparison of Lipiodol chemoembolization and conservative treatment for unresectable hepatocellular carcinoma. N Engl J Med 1995;332:1256–1261

48. Ebara M, Ohto M, Sugiura N et al. Percutaneous ethanol injection for the treatment of small hepatocellular carcinoma: study of 95 patients. J Gastroenterol Hepatol 1990; 5:616–626

49. Livraghi T, Bolondi L, Cottone M et al. No treatment, resection and ethanol injection in hepatocellular carcinoma: a retrospective analysis of survival in 391 cirrhotic patients. J Hepatol 1995;22:522–526

50. Adachi E, Maeda T, Matsumata T et al. Risk factors for intrahepatic recurrence in human small carcinoma. Gastroenterology 1995;108:768–775

51. Sheu JC, Huang GT, Chou HC et al. Multiple hepatocellular carcinomas at the early stage have different clonality. Gastroenterology 1993;105:1471–1476

52. Takenaka K, Adachi E, Nishizaki T et al. Possible multicentric occurrence of hepatocellular carcinoma: a clinicopathological study. Hepatology 1994;19:889–894

53. Okuda K. Epidemiology of primary liver cancer. In Tobe T, Kameda H (eds): Primary Liver Cancer in Japan. Springer, Tokyo, 1992, pp. 3–15

54. Bellentani S, Tiribelli C, Saccoccio G et al. Prevalence of chronic disease in the general population of northern Italy: the Dionysos study. Hepatology 1994;20:1442–1449

55. The Liver Cancer Study Group of Japan. Predictive factors for long term prognosis after partial hepatectomy for patients with hepatocellular carcinoma. Cancer 1994;74:2772–2780

36

RESECTION OF HEPATOCELLULAR CARCINOMA

OLIVER F. BATHE
CHARLES H. SCUDAMORE
NADINE R. CARON
ANDREW BUCZKOWSKI

Hepatocellular carcinoma (HCC) is one of the most lethal malignancies in the world and is most prevalent in areas where hepatitis B virus (HBV) is endemic such as East Africa and throughout Asia.[1] In North America, HCC is more commonly associated with alcoholic cirrhosis, especially in Caucasian patients.[2,3] Recently, a strong association between chronic hepatitis C virus (HCV) infection and HCC has been identified.[4]

Generally, the prognosis of HCC is poor. The usual course of an unresected lesion is that of continued, aggressive growth. Pulmonary and skeletal metastases are the most common extranodal sites of involvement at the time of diagnosis; the adrenals, spleen, kidneys, and brain may also be involved at autopsy.[5] The most common causes of death, if the HCC is unresected, are hepatic failure (resulting from replacement of liver parenchyma by tumor cells and/or cirrhosis), gastrointestinal bleeding from varices secondary to cirrhosis and portal hypertension, and progressive cachexia.[6–8] (Table 36-1). In addition, HCCs may rupture, causing fatal intra-abdominal bleeding. Systemic chemotherapy is generally not very effective for HCC, with a very low response rate,[9,10] although initial reports of newer modes of delivery appear promising.[11–13] Data from numerous centers confirm that patients in whom the tumor was successfully treated by resection have a significantly longer survival.[14,15]

The natural history of unresected HCC consists of continued growth with progressive replacement of the liver parenchyma, invasion of intrahepatic and contiguous extrahepatic structure, as well as eventual metastasis to distant sites. The objective of resection is cure, for resection is perhaps the only meaningful chance for cure. Resection also reduces the mass effect of the expanding lesion, preventing compression or invasion of major vascular structures, as well as providing relief from pain. Rarely, when the HCC secretes hormones (classically, erythropoietin[5]), resection also serves to treat the manifestations of this.

In recent years, there have been remarkable advances in the surgical management of HCC. Early diagnosis is becoming more frequent, particularly in those populations subjected to screening programs; a greater proportion of HCCs are resectable on presentation.[16,17] More sophisticated imaging modalities have allowed more accurate preoperative evaluation and staging of tumors. Improved operative techniques have resulted in a great reduction in operative deaths and longer survival.[17–19]

PREOPERATIVE EVALUATION

The objectives of preoperative evaluation of a patient with a liver tumor include diagnosis and localization of the lesion, staging, and determination of resectability.

TABLE 36-1. Causes of Death in Patients With HCC Following Surgical and Nonsurgical Management

				Cause of Death (%)					
Author	Year	Treatment	No. Patients	Hepatic Failure	GI Bleeding	Intra-abdominal Bleeding	Cancer Death (Cachexia)	Others	Unknown
Okuda		Surgical	80	45	13.8	8.8	8.8	7.5	16.3
et al.[6]	1985	Nonsurgical	579	38.5	23.3	13.8	10.9	7.9	5.7
LCSG		Surgical	312	26	9.6	2.2	23.7	9.3	14.1
Japan[7]	1987	Nonsurgical	1679	26.9	20	9.7	27	8.7	4.1
Cottone		Surgical	12	67		33			
et al.[8]	1989	Nonsurgical	25	67	17		8	8	

The patient's ability to tolerate liver resection must be assessed, and this involves evaluation and management of concomitant medical conditions, particularly cirrhosis. If cirrhosis is present, its severity must be determined with respect to functional hepatic reserve. Finally, if ablative therapy is being considered, it is important to delineate the vascular anatomy, determine the presence of hepatic and portal venous thrombosis, and rule out portal hypertension.

History, Physical Examination

Numerous expensive tests can often be obviated by a careful history and an astute physical examination. On physical examination, jaundice should be noted, as should other signs of impaired hepatic function or portal hypertension such as gynecomastia, ascites, spider nevi, caput medusae, splenomegaly, and hepatic encephalopathy. Patients with jaundice secondary to hepatocellular disease often have other clinical features of liver disease. In patients with obstructive jaundice secondary to HCC, the patient usually lacks clinical features of liver failure. Signs of concomitant medical illnesses such as pulmonary disease and congestive heart failure must be noted.

Laboratory Assessment

Abnormalities of coagulation studies must be noted. While mild hyperbilirubinemia is seen in some patients with HCC, more marked hyperbilirubinemia requires more careful scrutiny to differentiate cholestatic and hemolytic causes from hepatocellular causes. If there is any doubt, a cholangiogram should be arranged. A variety of paraneoplastic syndromes such as hypercalcemia, hypoglycemia, and erthrocytosis is found in a few patients.[5]

Approximately 50% to 70% of patients with HCC have α-fetoprotein (AFP) levels that are greater than 200 ng/ml.[20] Levels above 500 ng/ml are virtually diagnostic of HCC,[21] although similar levels have been reported in nonseminomatous germ-cell tumors.[22] Elevated levels have also been reported in gastric cancers, pancreatic cancers, colon cancers, and lung cancers.[22] This is particularly relevant since metastases from these primary sites are included in the differential diagnosis of a liver mass. Since AFP can be elevated in patients with chronic liver disease, its use for evaluating possible HCC may be more specific in patients without HBV infection.[23] Measurements of altered profiles of AFP may be useful in the future for distinguishing chronic liver disease from HCC.[24]

Radiologic Imaging and Endoscopic Evaluation

Radiologic and nuclear imaging studies help establish the origin and nature of any liver lesion and are the mainstay of preoperative staging. Endoscopic evaluation complements these functions. In addition, radiologic studies help to assess for the presence of cirrhosis, fatty infiltration of the liver, ascites, portal hypertension, and concomitant lesions.

ULTRASOUND

Overall, approximately 80% of HCC are seen by ultrasound.[25] Isoechoic HCC may be seen with the aid of selective hepatic artery CO_2 injection.[26] Lesions as small as 5 mm may be seen, and most lesions over 2 cm can be detected.[27] Cirrhosis itself is difficult to diagnose accurately with ultrasound, although ultrasound is excellent for documentation of the presence of ascites and splenomegaly. Echogenic ascites is a sign of hemoperitoneum, which suggests ruptured HCC. Duplex Doppler is useful for detection of hepatic vein and portal vein involvement or thrombosis, as well as vascular sequelae of portal hypertension.

COMPUTED TOMOGRAPHY

Computed tomography (CT) without contrast will detect about 80% of HCCs 1 to 3 cm in diameter,[28] but the appearance is nonspecific. The major limitation with

CT is that small lesions close to the diaphragm and in the left lateral segment and caudate lobe of the liver can be difficult to see. In addition, CT is less effective for detection of involved lymph nodes, in particular portal nodes, and it is poor for detection of micrometastases and peritoneal seeding. Cirrhosis further limits the accuracy of CT,[25] although the typical CT appearance of cirrhosis will often alert the clinician to its presence. CT is also useful in the evaluation of other primary sites within the abdomen, such as the stomach and pancreas.

One of the most sensitive imaging studies for detection and examination of HCC is Lipiodol CT, and its accuracy is comparable to that of intraoperative ultrasound.[29] However, specificity is limited because lesions such as focal nodular hyperplasia, regenerative nodules, and cavernous hemangiomas may also take up Lipiodol.[30]

CT arteriography is useful for preoperative staging when the HCC is known to be vascular, as most HCCs are and when additional vascular tumors are sought. When this is not technically possible, CT arterial portography is favored. CT arterial portography detects 94% of index lesions and 38% of daughter nodules versus 82% and 50%, respectively, with Lipiodol CT.[31]

MAGNETIC RESONANCE IMAGING

Magnetic resonance imaging (MRI) is much more expensive than CT and takes longer to perform. In addition, it is not readily available in some centers. On the other hand, it has excellent contrast resolution and demonstrates vessels well without the aid of contrast medium, making it a useful test in those patients with allergies to contrast material. During pregnancy, when exposure to radiation must be avoided, MRI is also useful. Compared to CT, MRI is better for examination of the pseudocapsule and tumor margins and for detection of portal vein invasion.[32]

ANGIOGRAPHY

Angiography is an important preoperative study because it helps define normal and aberrant anatomy. It may also identify hypervascular lesions too small to be imaged by CT. The patency of the portal venous system can be assessed with the venous phase of the superior mesenteric arteriogram, but false-positive results are possible whenever findings are suggestive of portal venous invasion. An otherwise resectable lesion should not be deemed unresectable because radiographic studies suggest some degree of obstruction of the inferior vena cava. At laparotomy, the vessel is often found to be externally compressed by tumor rather than being directly involved by disease.

OTHER TESTS

^{99m}Tc sulphur colloid scan may be useful in separating focal nodular hyperplasia, hepatic adenoma, and HCC.[33]

Assessment of Functional Hepatic Reserve

In all patients with cirrhosis, the degree of functional impairment of the liver must be quantified. In a patient with a tumor in a normal liver, there is some hypertrophy of the uninvolved liver to compensate for the infiltrative destruction of parenchyma caused by the tumor. In patients with a cirrhotic liver, however, such compensatory hypertrophy is minimal. Further, liver regeneration is impaired in cirrhosis.[34,35] Routine biochemical tests such as total serum bilirubin, serum albumin, and prothrombin time allow identification of a few patients with advanced cirrhosis. However, more sensitive tests are required to identify patients with a more occult impairment of liver function.

The oral glucose tolerance test is used in some centers to assess hepatic reserve. Patients with a parabolic pattern on the tolerance test tend to do better following a liver resection.[36] Measurement of cytochrome a ($+a_3$) in hepatocyte mitochondria (from a liver biopsy) has been reported to reflect hepatic functional reserve and may be predictive of postoperative morbidity and mortality following liver resection.[37] Historically, the bromsulphthalein (BSP) retention test has been used for assessment of hepatocellular reserve; retention rates greater than 30% at 45 minutes indicate that hepatic reserve is insufficient and that resection is contraindicated.[38] This test has been replaced by measurement of indocyanine green (ICG) clearance.[39] CT scan of the liver enables calculation of physical volume of the liver remnant.[49] Liver scintigraphy with technetium-99m diethylenetriamine-pentaacetic acid-galactosyl-human serum albumin (^{99m}Tc-GSA) has been evaluated as a novel method of assessing hepatic functional reserve.[39]

Miyagawa and associates[41] considered the criteria for safe hepatic resection in patients with chronic liver disease to be absence of ascites or ascites that is medically controllable and a serum bilirubin level less than 2.0 mg/dl. In these patients, resection volume was determined by plasma retention rate of ICG at 15 minutes. Their hospital mortality rate of 2.3% attests to the efficacy of this simple approach in selecting patients in whom resection is appropriate.

One of the major problems with currently available methods of assessing hepatic functional reserve is that these are global measurements of hepatic reserve. Unlike in normal livers, in cirrhotic livers the amount of liver resected is not necessarily proportional to the resultant decrease in liver function, for the degree of hepatocyte dysfunction is not uniform in each hepatic segment.[42]

Histologic Confirmation of HCC

While it is tempting to try to obtain a histologic diagnosis of a liver lesion, it must be stressed that biopsy is relatively contraindicated in any candidate for resection, as there is a significant risk of hemorrhage and peritoneal implantation of tumor cells. This is particularly true for tumors situated near the periphery of the liver. Biopsy of tumors situated more deeply in the liver (i.e., at least 1 to 2 cm) may be permissible, but only when done immediately before surgery and when resection includes the needle tract.

Laparoscopy for Staging and Assessment of Resectability

Laparoscopy is a useful investigative tool in the preoperative staging of HCC and aids in formulating a plan of management. Associated cirrhosis and portal hypertension may be discovered during laparoscopy[43–45] that may not be clinically evident or that have not been detected by other imaging modalities. Laparoscopy is also superior to ultrasound or CT in the diagnosis of tumors smaller than 2 cm situated on the surface of the liver, although these may be difficult to differentiate from regenerative nodules. Nodules that are irregular in contour, with a light yellow, dark red, or greenish color, especially those with evidence of neovascularity, are suggestive of HCC.[43,46] In addition, laparoscopy may detect multifocal or satellite tumors and peritoneal metastases not seen by other investigations.[45,47,48] Information obtained at laparoscopy may preclude resection and prevent unnecessary laparotomy in 36% of cases[49] or more.[45] A laparoscopic guided needle biopsy of the lesion may be useful even when resection is not planned or when a satellite lesion needs to be biopsied.

Laparoscopy does have a number of limitations. In patients with portal hypertension, care must be taken to insert the laparoscope away from the umbilicus to avoid injury to engorged portal venous collaterals (caput medusae). Adhesions from previous abdominal operations may preclude visualization of the liver. In addition, the posterior and superior surfaces of the liver, the inferior vena cava, the hepatic veins and the portal structures cannot be assessed. Tumors situated deep in the liver cannot be seen by laparoscopy.

Laparoscopic ultrasonography is a new, potentially useful technique.[50] The entire liver can be assessed, including the posterior and deep portions, and laparoscopic duplex ultrasound allows an accurate assessment of vascular involvement. The ability of this adjunct to prevent unnecessary laparotomy in patients with HCC must still be determined.

CONTRAINDICATIONS

Contraindications to resection (Table 36-2) include severe concomitant medical conditions such as congestive heart failure, ischemic heart disease, chronic lung disease, and renal failure. Advanced age in itself does not preclude resection; survival is not compromised by age following partial hepatectomy.[51–54]

Cirrhotic patients must be thoroughly evaluated as described earlier. The best clinical indicator of whether the patient will tolerate resection is the Child-Pugh classification. Most surgeons would agree that patients with class C cirrhosis are seldom eligible for resection; some surgeons will operate on selected patients with class B cirrhosis, particularly in the case of a small HCC. Acute active hepatitis also generally precludes resection. While

TABLE 36-2. Indications and Contraindications for Resection of Hepatocellular Carcinoma

Indications	Contraindications
Cure	Absolute
Prevent Mass Effect (Palliation)	Refusal of surgery
Progressive jaundice, hepatic dysfunction	Inability to tolerate surgery
Pain	Severe concomitant medical illnesses
Bleeding	Inadequate hepatic reserve for planned resection
Prevent rupture	Bilobar, multicentric disease
Functional tumors	Disseminated disease
Excision for diagnosis	Malignant ascites
? Debulking for potentiation of nonsurgical therapies	Transcelomic spread
	Distant metastases
	Relative
	Invasion of main portal vein
	Invasion of inferior vena cava
	Ruptured HCC
	Acute phase hepatitis
	Refusal of blood products
	When alternative therapies have potential advantages (e.g., transplantation, local ablation)

ascites itself is not a contraindication to resection, care must be taken to rule out malignant ascites. In addition, ascites may be caused by thrombosis of the portal vein and, less often, the hepatic vein, which are contraindications.[5] Bilobar multicentric disease of the liver and distant spread are additional absolute contraindications for resection. Invasion of the main portal vein or inferior vena cava is now considered a relative contraindication. Lymph node involvement and invasion of the biliary tree do not necessarily preclude resection as long as excision with reconstruction is technically feasible. Finally, ruptured HCC may be considered by some to be a relative contraindication for resection, since any surgery would usually be only of a palliative nature.

INTRAOPERATIVE EVALUATION

Following preoperative staging with radiologic imaging and laparoscopy, in about 12% of cases nonresectability is not determined until laparotomy.[49] The relationship of the tumor should be evaluated with respect to the major vessels and contiguous structures. In particular, attachment to the diaphragm may be difficult to detect with preoperative tests. The contralateral lobe of the liver should be examined for additional foci of disease. However, cirrhotic livers have lost their pliability, thus making intraoperative identification of small lesions difficult. For this reason, intraoperative ultrasound is an invaluable tool for detection of additional nodules, particularly in cirrhotics. Intraoperative ultrasound detects 40% to 46% of lesions not seen or palpated at surgery.[55,56] Only lesions smaller than 5 mm are not usually detected by the technique. To increase sensitivity, especially for small, isoechoic lesions, the use of carbon dioxide contrast has been reported to be effective.[57]

RESECTION: TECHNIQUE

Numerous technical advances in liver surgery in recent years have resulted in a steady decline in operative mortality (Table 36-3), and it is now possible to perform major hepatic resections with minimal blood loss. In addition, resections in patients with cirrhosis can now be done with an acceptable degree of safety.

Anatomic Considerations

Segmentally based resections enable complex resections while preserving residual liver tissue. The liver[58] is divided into right and left lobes and further divided into eight segments, based on vascular inflow and bile duct drainage (Fig. 36-1). Each segment is supplied by a sheath containing branches of the hepatic artery and portal vein and a draining bile duct, which enters the middle of the segment. The venous drainage is by hepatic

FIGURE 36-1. Couinaud's segmental hepatic anatomy.

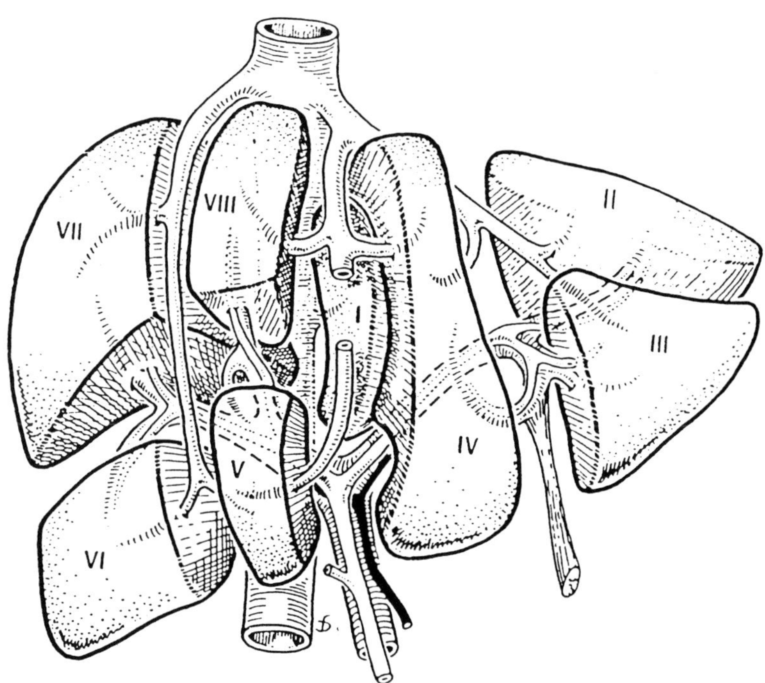

TABLE 36-3. Perioperative Mortality Following Hepatic Resection for HCC

			Before 1987		1987–1991		1992–Present		
Author	Year	No. Patients	% Cirrhosis	% Mortality	% Cirrhosis	% Mortality	% Cirrhosis	% Mortality	
Wu et al.[91]	1980	181	70	8.8					
Kishi et al.[80]	1983	57	39.4	10.5					
Kanematsu et al.[38]	1984	37	100	10.8					Limited resection
Kanematsu et al.[38]	1984	13	100	15.4					Major resection
Okuda et al.[6]	1985	157		3.2					
Lee et al.[67]	1986	109	40.4	2.8					
LCSG of Japan[7]	1987	619		7.9					
Nagao et al.[52]	1987	94		20.2					
Kanematsu et al.[110]	1988	121	80	11.6					
Franco et al.[14]	1990	72			100	6.9			
Nagao et al.[114]	1990	69				10			
LCSG of Japan[20]	1990	2,174				4.1			
Lai et al.[64]	1991	39			84.6	7.7			Small HCC
Hemming et al.[124]	1993	50			26	0.5			All segmental resections
Fan et al.[118]	1994	124					31.5	11.3	
Chen et al.[86]	1994	205					49.8	4.4	
Capusotti et al.[104]	1994	33					100	3	Large HCC
Vauthey et al.[78]	1995	106					33	5.7	
Lai et al.[17]	1995	149	69	21.5					Before 1987
Lai et al.[17]	1995	128			78	14.8			1987–1991
Lai et al.[17]	1995	66					74	6	1992–Present

veins, which tend to run between segmental divisions (Fig. 36-2).

The surgeon must take into account the blood supply of the extrahepatic bile ducts during dissection along the porta hepatis. Extrahepatic bile ducts are supplied by tiny arteries at the 3- and 9-o'clock positions, and a retroportal artery also provides some blood supply in a proportion of the population.[59] This is important to recognize, since circumferential dissection around the bile duct may compromise its blood supply.

Hepatic vascular anomalies are common and should be sought during the preoperative workup. Replaced left or right hepatic arteries may remain uncontrolled by preresection hilar clamping. Hepatic venous drainage is quite variable and may include the presence of several small hepatic veins inferior to the major hepatic veins.

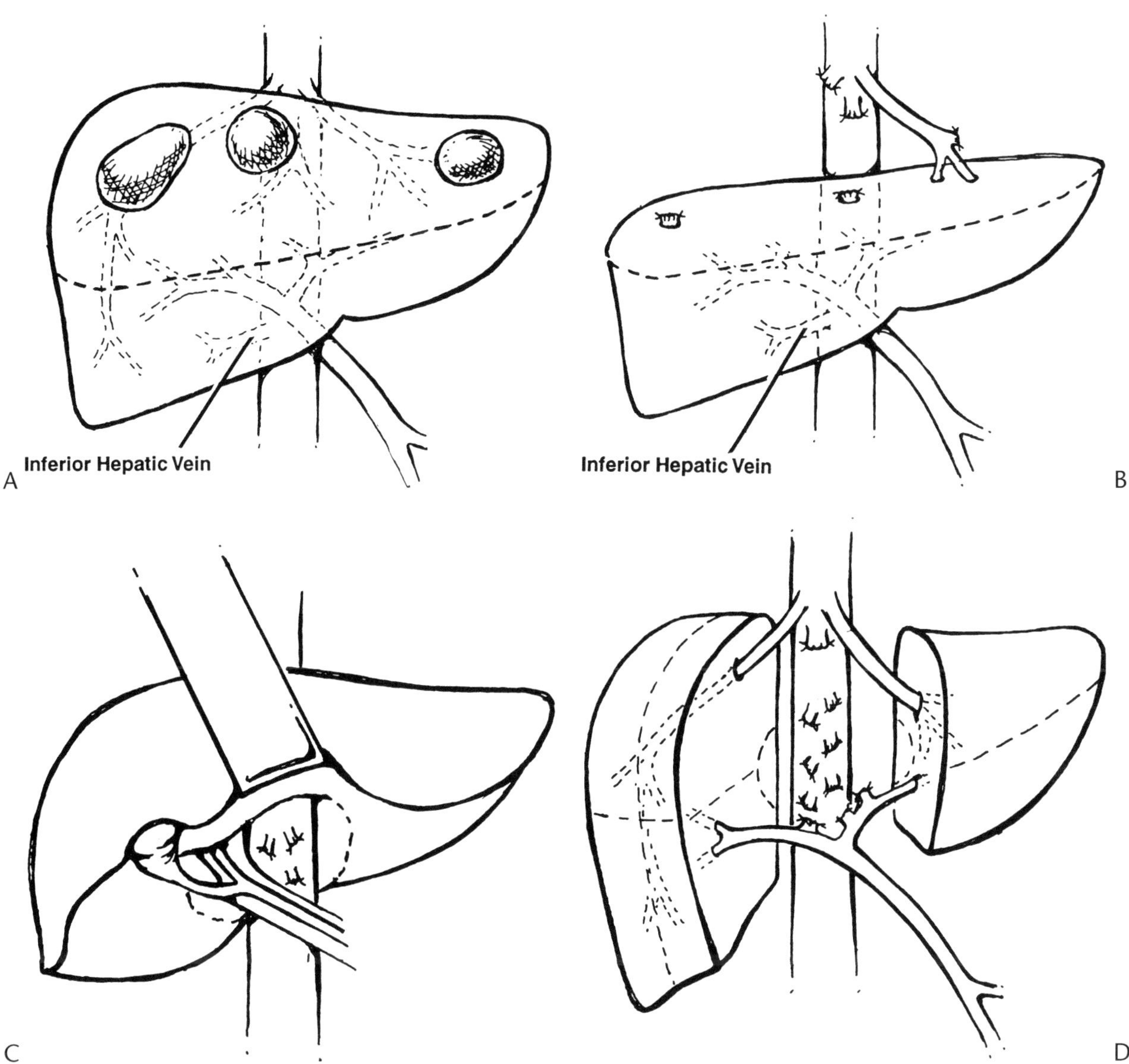

FIGURE 36-2. Examples of some unusual segmentally based resections. Segmentally based resections enable complex resections while preserving residual liver tissue. (*A & B*) Superior hepatic resection, in which the superior segments of both lobes of the liver have been removed. (*C*) Caudate lobe resection. (*D*) Mesohepatic resection.

Knowledge of their presence may prompt more careful parenchymal dissection.

Type of Incision

We routinely use a right subcostal incision with a vertical midline extension as required, often resecting the xiphisternum. This provides excellent access to all relevant structures, including the hepatic veins. Extension of the incision to the left is rarely necessary even for resection of segments 2 and 3. As resection of involved diaphragm can be performed without any additional approach in most of the cases, thoracic extension is extremely seldom needed.

Pre-resection Vascular Control

The development of techniques of vascular inflow occlusion in recent years has led to a significant drop in blood transfusion requirements; a number of techniques have been described. Control of the vasculature can be established as the resection proceeds, or it can be established prior to commencing resection. Pre-resection vascular control can be established by division or occlusion of the vascular structures supplying the segment of liver to be removed, by the Pringle maneuver, or by total vascular isolation. Alternatively, venovenous bypass, as used in transplantation, is an option.

Isolation and clamping of the porta hepatis (the Pringle maneuver) is perhaps the most common method of obtaining vascular control before liver resection. The advantage of this technique is that the surgeon has the freedom to modify the line of resection, ensuring complete removal of the tumor with an adequate margin. Blood loss is effectively reduced.[60] Moreover, the technique is safe, for even the cirrhotic liver can tolerate normothermic ischemia in excess of 60 minutes.[61] Cross-clamp times average approximately 40 minutes, but have approached 90 minutes without untoward consequences (unpublished data). Some have advocated application of the hilar clamp for 15-minute periods and intermittent release of the hilar clamp for 5- to 10-minute periods while compressing the divided liver surface, making liver resection an unhurried procedure.[41] However, it has recently become apparent that reperfusion of ischemic organs may produce a greater degree of injury than the ischemia itself, due to generation of oxygen free radicals and other toxic metabolites.[62] Further, in the vast majority of cases, resection is completed within 60 minutes. We therefore prefer to leave the porta hepatis clamped for the duration of the procedure.

Total vascular isolation for longer than 60 minutes has been shown to be safe[63] and may be useful when performing technically demanding liver resections. In this technique, the inferior vena cava (IVC) is clamped above and below the liver in addition to clamping the porta hepatis. Before performing this maneuver, the patient must be hemodynamically stable and well hydrated with intravenous fluids. The porta hepatis clamp is applied first, followed by the clamp on the IVC below the liver, and then by the clamp on the IVC above the liver. If the patient becomes hemodynamically unstable at any point, the surgeon must assess whether the procedure can be performed using only the Pringle maneuver or whether a venovenous bypass is required (Figs. 36-3 and 36-4)

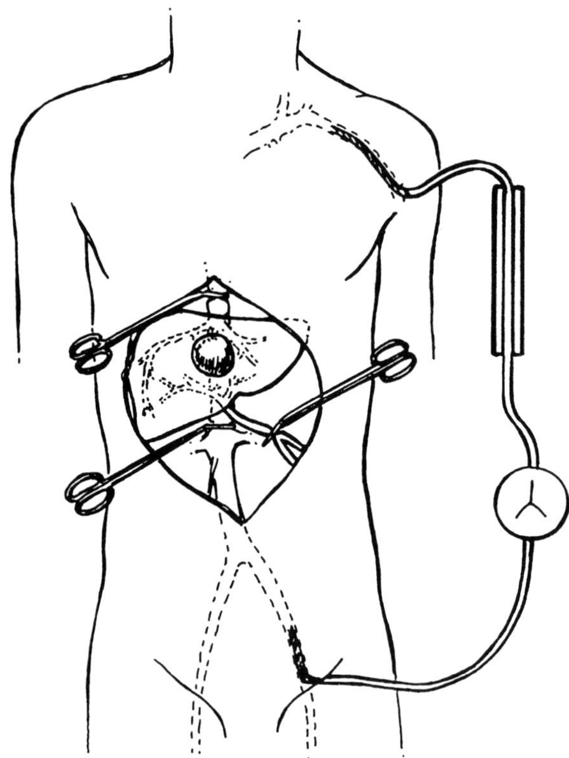

FIGURE 36-3. Venovenous bypass may be useful when performing technically demanding liver resections. Hemodynamic instability is less frequently encountered during venovenous bypass than with total vascular isolation and this technique is therefore preferred to total vascular isolation.

Extent of Resection

The extent of resection to ensure a curative resection remains uncertain. The size of the optimal resection margin is important since the goal of resection is cure, yet the extent of resection is often limited by hepatic functional reserve. A disease-free margin of 1 cm is thought by most to be adequate,[20,40,64,65] but some authors advocate a margin of 2 to 3 cm.[66] Patients with a margin of 1 cm or more have been reported to have a survival benefit over those in whom such a margin could not be secured,[19,67] at least for small HCC.[68] Others have reported that survival is not affected by the status of the resection margin.[65,69–71]

With larger tumors (i.e., larger than 4 to 5 cm), intrahepatic metastases not infrequently develop more than 1 cm away. In the case of limited resection for large HCC, it appears that a macroscopic margin of 0.5 cm is as good as a margin as wide as 2 cm, but surgical treatment in these cases is probably inadequate.[68,69] In patients with normal liver function, a more aggressive resection with margins greater than 2 cm might be beneficial.

Limited hepatic resections (i.e., anatomic or nonanatomic segmental and subsegmental resections) must be considered in patients with a limited hepatic functional reserve or with multiple tumor nodules. In a study by the Liver Cancer Study Group of Japan, of 679 patients with HCC, 83% with cirrhosis, those who had a segmental resection had a significantly better survival rate than those with a massive hepatectomy. However, there was no significant difference in survival between those who had a lobectomy and those who had a segmentectomy.[7] Yamanaka and associates[70] reported that extent of resec-

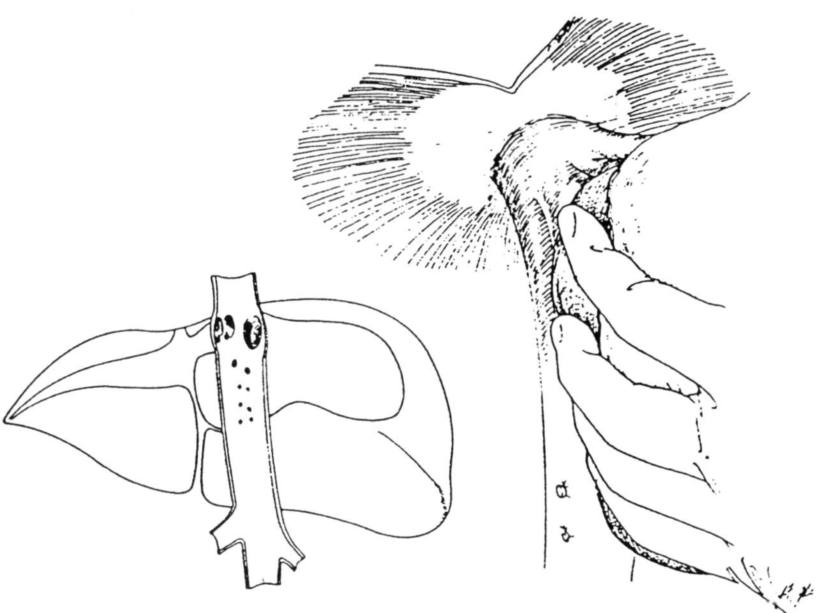

FIGURE 36-4. Smaller hepatic veins draining the caudate lobe or the medial portion of segment VIII are often present. These veins vary in number and enter the IVC inferior to the major hepatic veins. They can not be controlled prior to parenchymal dissection and should be ligated or clipped in continuity as they are encountered during parenchymal transection. (From Foster and Berman,[125] with permission.)

tion is related to long-term survival. Patients treated with hepatic lobectomy had a significantly better 5-year survival rate (84%) than those treated with segmentectomy or subsegmentectomy (50%); those with a wedge resection had the lowest 5-year survival (29%). Masutani et al.[68] compared recurrence rates and survival rates in patients with limited resections (i.e., partial resection and subsegmentectomies) to those who underwent a standard operation (i.e., resection of one or two segments). There was no difference in recurrence rate or in survival rate between the two groups. Further, the pattern of intrahepatic recurrence was similar, with a high proportion of these recurrences occurring in the contralateral lobe. Others have also shown that long-term survival rates after major and limited hepatic resections do not significantly differ.[38,52]

Until more data are available to define the role of limited hepatic resections for cure of HCC, patients with normal livers or with only mild cirrhosis should be subjected to a wider (anatomic) resection. Anatomic lobectomy is usually easier to accomplish than segmental resection and will likely not be followed by significant metabolic consequences in patients with a normal liver. In patients with limited hepatic reserve or multiple tumor nodules, where limited resections are planned, it is likely that achieving an adequate resection margin supersedes the need for achieving anatomic resections.

Use of Intraoperative Ultrasound

Intraoperative ultrasound allows the surgeon to visualize the deep parts of the liver while operating. This enables one to determine the tumor's proximity to important hepatic structures and to identify the landmarks of segmental anatomy. The surgeon can resect the least amount of liver while still obtaining an adequate resection margin.

There are a number of methods of determining the line of resection. Some determine the line of resection by selectively clamping the vascular pedicle feeding the segment(s) to be resected; the line of resection follows the line of color change with liver ischemia. Alternatively, the line of resection can be determined by intraoperative ultrasound definition of segmental anatomy. To identify the area to be resected, injection of indigo carmine into the portal venous branches under ultrasound guidance has been described.[72] The surface of the liver is colored by the injection of the dye to identify the involved segment.

Gouillat and coworkers[73] recently described a technique of ultrasound-guided resection in which insertion of needles under intraoperative ultrasound guidance permits tumor resection, including a free peritumoral margin, while respecting the vessels of the adjacent parenchyma. In this technique, five to seven needles inserted under ultrasound guidance permit delineation of the parenchyma to be resected. Parenchymal transection then proceeds within the defined area following vascular control with the Pringle maneuver, resulting in a nonanatomic resection. An adequate peritumoral margin is possible while avoiding unnecessary and potentially hazardous additional parenchymal excision in the patient with cirrhosis. Gouillat and coworkers[73] routinely use this technique for the resection of small HCC in patients with cirrhosis, in addition to repeat hepatectomies (Fig. 36-5).

SPECIAL CONSIDERATIONS

Despite recent advances, much about the biology of HCC remains to be discovered, and optimization of surgical management is a developing process. Therefore, a number of controversial issues bear discussion.

FIGURE 36-5. Operative procedure of ultrasonically guided resection of HCC, as described by Gouillat, Manganas and Berard.[73] (*A*) To delineate the area to be resected, two to six needles are inserted under ultrasound guidance, at least 1 cm away from the tumor, while respecting the blood supply of the adjacent parenchyma. (*B*) Parenchymal transection is performed along the needles, using an ultrasonic dissector. (From Gouillat et al.,[73] with permission.)

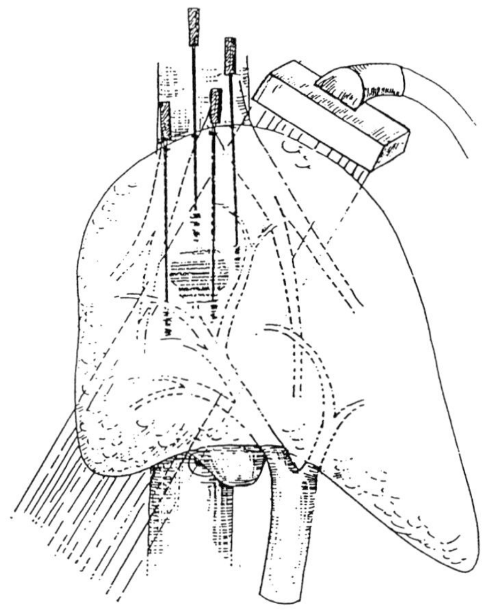

A

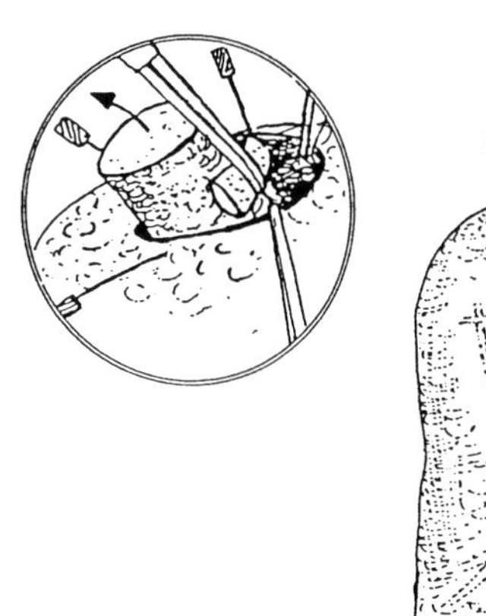

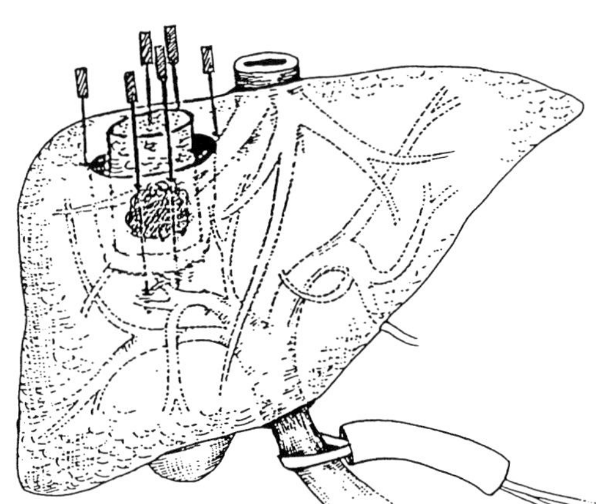

B

Fibrolamellar Variant of HCC

Some studies have shown increased resection rates and better 5-year survival rates for patients with fibrolamellar HCC.[74,75] Some have interpreted this to mean that fibrolamellar HCC is a less aggressive tumor with a favorable prognosis and a high likelihood of cure if resected.[75–77] The overall 5-year survival rate for fibrolamellar HCC is 25% to 36%,[75,76] and up to 63% in patients whose tumors are resected. Nagorney et al.[74] compared 16 patients with fibrolamellar HCC with 55 patients with noncirrhotic nonfibrolamellar HCC and found similar durations of survival. They suggested that better survival rates were related to increased resection rates, since resection rates in patients with fibrolamellar HCC in their series was 75% compared to 49% for noncirrhotic, nonfibrolamellar HCC. A literature survey of patients with fibrolamellar HCC revealed that only 12.5% of patients have survived for 5 years or longer after resection.[74]

It is possible that HCC of the fibrolamellar variant displays such different biologic behavior that stage-for-stage comparison with nonfibrolamellar HCC is of limited value. Fibrolamellar tumors of enormous size are often resectable, sometimes even in the presence of extrahepatic disease. Lymph node metastases are present in approximately 70% of patients with fibrolamellar HCC at the time of presentation,[78,79] suggesting this is an important route of spread. In contrast, lymph node involvement is present in less than 5% of patients with nonfibrolamellar HCC,[67,78,80] although it is much more frequently seen in autopsy series,[5,7] suggesting this does not occur until late in the regular form of HCC. Finally, recurrence is common, and the proportion of these recurrences that have an extrahepatic component is much higher than would be expected in the nonfibrolamellar variant.[79] The biologic behavior of the fibrolamellar variant of HCC, therefore, appears to be quite unlike that of nonfibrolamellar HCC.

Advanced Disease

With the many technical advances in hepatobiliary and vascular surgery, invasion of the main portal vein, IVC, or biliary tract is no longer considered an absolute contraindication for resection. Even the most difficult situation can now be managed by ex vivo hepatic resection followed by auto-transplantation. This technique includes cold perfusion of the organ and its total removal followed by back table resection of the tumor and reimplantation of the liver as in liver transplantation.[81]

VASCULAR INVOLVEMENT

Portal vein invasion is the most important prognostic factor following resection.[19,70,78,82] Some authors believe that involvement of the main portal vein, hepatic veins, or IVC is a contraindication to resection.[83] Portal vein resection and reconstruction are now possible. In addition, anecdotal successes have been reported with combined hepatic resection and removal of portal vein tumor thrombi[84] or resection and reconstruction of the IVC.[85] In 26 patients who had gross involvement of branches of the portal vein, none of the patients survived beyond 3 years; almost 50% survived 1 year.[70] In another report,[20] approximately 55% of patients with main portal vein involvement died within 8 months of resection. Involvement of the first and second branches was associated with approximately 30% and 20% 2-year survivals after resection, respectively. Cure is thus unlikely with patients having involvement of the portal vein and its main tributaries, and extirpation of the tumor under these conditions is only palliative.

OBSTRUCTIVE JAUNDICE SECONDARY TO HCC

Overall, jaundice is present in 10% to 40% of patients with HCC at the time of diagnosis.[5,7,86] The commonest causes of jaundice are the underlying cirrhosis and/or extensive hepatic parenchymal destruction by the tumor.

Obstructive jaundice is seen in 2% to 11.7% of patients with HCC.[5,87,88] Biliary obstruction occurs due to invasion or compression by HCC, involvement of hilar nodes, or hemobilia. In addition, intrabiliary tumor may rarely embolize to cause a more distal common bile duct obstruction. Thus, the ultimate site of duct obstruction may be close to or quite distant from the main tumor mass, depending on the mechanism of obstruction.

Jaundice in the absence of liver disease, a history of intermittent jaundice or biliary colic, biochemical evidence of cholestasis, or bile duct dilatation seen on ultrasound or CT are indications for endoscopic retrograde cholangiopancreatography or, if this fails, a percutaneous transhepatic cholangiogram. A cholangiogram will help differentiate cholestasis from hepatocellular disease in equivocal cases and will determine the level and grade of obstruction.

The ideal treatment is hepatic resection. Even in patients with localized bile duct involvement, successful liver resection with biliary reconstruction has been reported.[89] Unfortunately, most tumors presenting with obstructive jaundice are unsuitable for resection, except fibrolamellar HCC, which has a predilection for biliary involvement. Satisfactory palliation can be achieved with removal of loose tumor debris within the common bile duct and tube decompression or biliary-enteric bypass.[86] A T-tube is easy to insert at the time of common bile duct exploration, but should be avoided. Insertion of a transhepatic tube has several advantages. Transhepatic tubes can be more easily irrigated over a long period and provide better drainage than T-tubes. In addition, properly placed transhepatic tubes can be changed periodically using fluoroscopic guidance when the tubes become occluded.

In a study of 20 patients who presented with obstructive jaundice due to migration of a tumor mass in the biliary tract, drainage alone was associated with a mean survival time of 3.9 months.[86] For those who received drainage followed by transcatheter hepatic arterial embolization, mean survival time was 8.0 months. The two who underwent resection were long-term survivors (one living more than 5 years).[86]

DIAPHRAGMATIC INVASION

Occasionally, a tumor arising from the right lobe extends beyond the confines of the liver and becomes adherent to or invades the overlying diaphragm. In patients with good pulmonary function and in the absence of other contraindications to resection, diaphragmatic involvement is not an absolute contraindication to resection, particularly in the case of fibrolamellar HCC. The appearance of a right diaphragmatic "hump" on chest x-ray has been reported in a majority of patients with diaphragmatic invasion,[90] but the value of diagnostic imaging techniques such as ultrasound for detecting these has been debated.[90,91]

If diaphragmatic involvement has been detected preoperatively, thoracoscopy should be performed to explore the pleural cavity and the thoracic side of the diaphragm. Adherence to lung, pleural spread, malignant effusion, or mediastinal nodal spread precludes resection.[91] In the event that diaphragmatic involvement is discovered during laparotomy, if there are no other contraindications to resection, the diaphragm should be opened 2 to 3 cm away from the adherent tissue to explore the thoracic aspect of the diaphragm, ruling out intrathoracic disease. No attempt should be made to dissect the tumor off the diaphragm because this may cause bleeding, tumor rupture, or contamination of the operative field with malignant cells. The liver and diaphragm should be removed en bloc with a 2 cm margin; up to 50% of the diaphragm can be excised and primarily reconstructed without the need for prosthetic mesh or tissue transfer.[91] In a prospective case-control study, Lau and coworkers[90] found no increase in complication rate or mortality rate following resection of the diaphragm and liver tumor, compared to those who had hepatectomy alone.[90] The survival curves were similar in both groups.

Ruptured HCC

Ruptured HCC has been reported to occur in 3.1% to 14.5% of cases,[17,91–93] and it has been reported to account for approximately 10% of deaths. In Hong Kong, the prevalence of ruptured HCC has fallen dramatically in the last 15 years from 14.5% to 4.5%.[94] Acute abdomen hemoperitoneum, without a history of trauma, should suggest the diagnosis of a ruptured HCC.[95] The mortality rate is high even with successful control of bleeding, due to hepatic decompensation.[96]

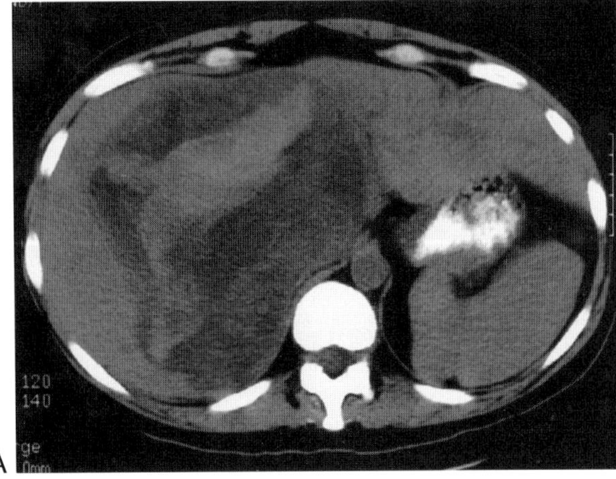

A

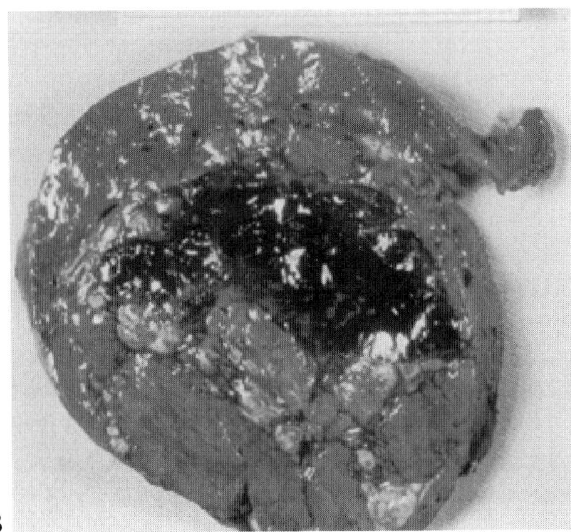

B

FIGURE 36-6. (*A*) CT scan and (*B*) surgical specimen of a giant HCC. As is evident from the CT scan, as the tumor enlarges, tumor necrosis predisposes to contained rupture, which ultimately leads to free rupture. Resection in selected patients results in excellent palliation and sometimes cure.

Abdominal pain and tenderness are the most common manifestations. Hypotension or shock is present in 6.7% to 63.3%.[92–94,96] If the patient is hemodynamically stable enough to tolerate investigation, the diagnosis may be confirmed with CT or ultrasound (Fig. 36-6). Paracentesis positive for blood is seen in 78.6% to 96.8% of cases.[92,93,96] When the diagnosis is made preoperatively, a nonsurgical means of obtaining hemostatic control, such as transcatheter embolization, is preferable.[96,97] Following this, the resectability of the tumor can be assessed in the usual way.

Hepatic resection has been advocated at the time of

initial laparotomy as a means of securing hemostasis and simultaneously removing the cause. The rationale for this is that a staged procedure may compromise the chance for cure, since the spread of tumors after rupture is rapid, and a delay of 2 to 3 weeks may render the tumor unresectable.[92] However, the mortality rate associated with an emergency hepatectomy is high,[92,94] and the situation may predispose to a suboptimal resection of the tumor; there is no beneficial effect on survival.[94] Thus, unless the offending tumor is small and easily removed and there is no cirrhosis in the liver remnant, it is likely better to secure hemostasis and avoid hepatic resection during the initial laparotomy.[94]

Concomitant Gastroesophageal Varices

Esophageal varices were seen in 13% of HCC patients in a North American study.[5] Variceal hemorrhage may be potentiated by portal hypertension, exacerbated by portal venous thrombosis or tumor invasion, or by arterioportal fistulas that occasionally develop with growth of the tumor.[3,98] Further, following resection, the liver remnant must carry the whole of the portal flow, causing the liver to become tense and edematous. This may transiently exacerbate portal hypertension.[99]

A portosystemic shunt procedure done simultaneously with hepatic resection has been advocated. In a study of 10 patients,[100] the in-hospital mortality rate after partial hepatectomy and concomitant distal splenorenal shunt was 10%. Varices were effectively reduced in size and none of the patients had variceal bleeding despite the fact that three had recurrent HCC. Simultaneous transabdominal esophageal transection, gastric devascularization, and/or splenectomy with resection of HCC have also been reported with good results.[52] However, the addition of these procedures to an already major procedure may potentiate the risk of the procedure. Intraoperative hemorrhage and postoperative encephalopathy are potential risks that may be obviated by more conservative measures. Endoscopic sclerotherapy is an acceptable alternative.[101] Endoscopic ligation of varices appears be at least as effective as sclerotherapy and has fewer treatment-related complications.[102]

Recurrent Tumor

The long-term results of resection are not yet satisfactory because of the high rate of recurrence (Table 36-4). Recurrence is the most common cause of death outside of the perioperative period,[71,78,103,104] and the majority of recurrences occur in the liver remnant.[70,105–110]

The pathogenesis of intrahepatic recurrence is poorly understood. It is thought that most recurrences that appear in the liver remnant result from intrahepatic metastases via the portal vein, although nonsynchronous, multifocal tumorigenesis might cause recurrence in some patients, and inadequate resection of the index lesion may be a cause in others. Early recurrence is probably due to pre-existing intrahepatic spread or incomplete removal of the tumor, which becomes manifest 1 to 2 years after surgery.[108,111] Less than 27% of recurrences occur near the resected stump,[108,111] suggesting that incomplete removal of the tumor is responsible for only a minority of recurrences. A multinodular recurrence occurring relatively early probably represents previously undetected satellite lesions that were present at the time of resection of the index lesion.[71,108,111] Late recurrence of cancer (i.e., 3 to 6 years after resection) is probably not due to the presence of occult intrahepatic metastases, but to nonsynchronous multifocal tumorigenesis.[71] Adachi et al.[112] examined cases of resected small HCC without major risk factors for recurrence and showed that the presence of active inflammation was associated with postoperative intrahepatic recurrence. Further, in the cirrhotic liver, recurrence is often in areas of the liver not targeted by ablation of the primary tumor. While these findings suggest that multifocal tumorigenesis in a "fertile field" may be the cause, others have failed to

TABLE 36-4. Cumulative Recurrence Rates of HCC Following Resection

Author	Year	No. Patients	Cumulative Recurrence Rate (%)				
			1 yr	2 yr	3 yr	5 yr	
Hsu et al.[82]	1985	49	16	22			HCC < 5 cm
Kanematsu et al.[110]	1988	73	19	26	33	38	
Nagao et al.[114]	1990	69	56	82			
Ouchi et al.[71]	1993	47			34	40	Intrahepatic only
Chen et al.[108]	1994	205	60	65	77	80	Intrahepatic only
Okada et al.[125]	1994	98	32	62	71		
Capusotti et al.[104]	1994	33	32	64	88		100% cirrhosis, large HCC
Adachi et al.[112]	1995	102	12	38	57	68	Intrahepatic only, small HCC

show a difference in recurrence rates in patients with and without cirrhosis.[108] Reports of intrahepatic recurrence following liver transplantation for HCC, even in the absence of grossly detectable extrahepatic disease,[51,113] suggest that implantation of the liver remnant by circulating tumor cells may play a role in the pathogenesis of intrahepatic recurrence.

Several reports have attempted to evaluate the efficacy of resection of isolated intrahepatic metastases. Survival rates after recurrence were 71%, 42%, and 25% at 1, 2, and 3 years, respectively.[114] In another study, the 1-, 3-, and 5-year cumulative survival rates after re-resection were 88%, 37%, and 37%, respectively. In both studies, these rates were not significantly different than survival rates of patients with no recurrences after hepatic resection.[109] Thus, resection of isolated intrahepatic recurrences appears to be an effective therapy.

The indications and contraindications for resection are essentially the same as for the primary tumor. The preoperative workup and preparation should also be the same as for the primary tumor. Perhaps the most important part of the evaluation, at least in patients with cirrhosis, is assessment of hepatic functional reserve, for tests of functional reserve are often worse on the second resection.[109] Technical difficulties, including severe adhesions or anatomic alterations caused by the previous operation and the limited hepatic reserve, are potential limitations to re-resection.

New modes of therapy for recurrences appear to have promising results. Lai et al.[17] observed a threefold improvement in mean duration of survival in patients with documented recurrent tumors over recent years (10.3 months versus 3.5 months) with Lipiodol-chemoembolization and percutaneous alcohol injection for control of intrahepatic recurrence, as well as resection when indicated. Survival after transcatheter arterial embolization for treatment of recurrences is reportedly of the same magnitude as survival after resection of a primary tumor.[115]

The most frequent site of distant metastasis is the lung. Intra-abdominal metastases, particularly in the adrenal gland, and skeletal metastases are also common.[20] Most extrahepatic metastases are multiple, and they are most frequently associated with an intrahepatic recurrence,[103,107,110] but occasionally a solitary extranodal metastasis is found and extirpation of the lesion may be considered. For an evaluation of surgery for recurrent HCC in extrahepatic sites,[107] 12 patients were found to have an isolated extrahepatic recurrence amenable to resection. Operations included pulmonary wedge resection or lobectomy, excision of abdominal wall metastases, excision of peritoneal metastasis, and gastrointestinal tract resection. All patients received systemic adjuvant chemotherapy. The mean survival after resection of recurrence was 19.7 months. The 1-, 2-, and 5-year survival rates were 92%, 52%, and 26%, respectively. Further recurrence after resection of the extrahepatic recurrence was intrahepatic in the majority of cases (Table 36-5).

Transdiaphragmatic Hepatectomy: A New Approach

Resection of the superior part of the liver (segments VII and VIII) is technically difficult. Additionally, resection of HCC following recurrence may be difficult due to the presence of adhesions and altered anatomy. This makes resection of a recurrent tumor in the superior part of the liver, especially if it is near the confluence of the hepatic veins, potentially hazardous. Finally, cirrhotic patients with portal hypertension are prone to the development of ascites, which may complicate a transabdominal surgical approach. For these reasons, a transthoracic, transdiaphragmatic hepatectomy has recently been described as an alternative approach.[116] The optimal intercostal space for thoracotomy is selected using preoperative ultrasonography, finding the shortest approach to the tumor. A right anterolateral thoracotomy and division of the costal cartilage are performed. Intraoperative transdiaphragmatic ultrasonography aids in selection of the site of division of the diaphragm. Resection of the appropriate segments then proceeds with the use of an ultrasonic dissector, with vascular control. Operative time using the transdiaphragmatic approach was reportedly shorter than in the transabdominal approach, and control of the hepatic veins and inferior vena cava was facilitated by the new approach.

Postoperative Complications

Complication rates following liver resection for HCC are 16% to 52%.[17,78,114,117,118] Some centers have reported decreasing complication rates over recent years.[17,60,119] Complications following liver resection are most likely to occur in patients with cirrhosis, diabetes, chronic obstructive lung disease, and renal insufficiency.[54,120]

With more extensive resections and with liver resection in a cirrhotic patient, blood sugars should be followed closely, monitoring for hypoglycemia.[121] Bleeding may occur from the raw surface of the diaphragm, from the abdominal wall from which collateral vessels supplied the tumor, or from the cut surface of the liver, especially if there is coexisting coagulopathy. Coagulopathy may be due to underlying hepatic dysfunction, to massive blood loss and/or transfusion following a complicated procedure, or due to disseminated intravascular coagulopathy.

Postoperative fever is common and the usual diagnostic workup should be performed. If no cause is found, a low-grade fever (38 °C or less) returns to normal usually within a week or two.[83] Intra-abdominal sepsis is a common problem following hepatic resection, occurring in 3% to 28.6% of cases.[60,122] In any patient with suspected intra-abdominal sepsis, ultrasound and CT are useful in

TABLE 36-5. Survival Rates Following Resection of HCC

Author	Year	No. Patients	% Survival 1 yr	2 yr	3 yr	5 yr	Median Survival (mo)	
Wu et al.[91]	1980	165	55.9	36.8	28.9	16	18.9	
Kanematsu et al.[38]	1984	37	79.9	60.3		32.6		Limited resection, 100% cirrhosis
		13	78.7	67.5		22.5		Major resection, 100% cirrhosis
Okuda et al.[126]	1984	98	62	43	34		19.6	
Hsu et al.[82]	1985	49	95.9	90.8				HCC < 5 cm, excluding operative deaths
		49	63.3	51				HCC > 5 cm, excluding operative deaths
Lee et al.[67]	1986	109	84	72				HCC, excluding operative deaths
Nagao et al.[52]	1987	94	58		33	20		
Kanematsu et al.[114]	1988	107	83		51	26		Excluding operative deaths
Franco et al.[14]	1990	72	68	55	51			100% cirrhosis
LCSG of Japan[20]	1990	2174	67.1		39.6	28.5		
Yamanaka et al.[70]	1990	295	76		44	31		
Ringe et al.[51]	1991	131	67.5	54.4	42.3	35.8	28.7	
Lia et al.[64]	1991	39	59		28	11	18.3	HCC < 5 cm
Ouchi et al.[71]	1993	47	89		65	43		
Suenaga et al.[109]	1994	134	100		88.2	68.1		
Capusotti et al.[104]	1994	33	66	43	37			Large HCC, 100% cirrhosis
Lai et al.[17]	1995	343	60		33	24		(1987–1991)
Vauthey et al.[78]	1995	106				41	26	
Scudamore	Unpublished data	86					22.5	Consecutive series

the detection of fluid collections. In the absence of any persistent uncontrolled focus of contamination, all abscesses should be drained if possible. Pneumonia and pleural effusion are more often seen when a thoracoabdominal incision is used, but all patients are susceptible. The latter may be associated with pulmonary embolism.

A biliary fistula may lead to the skin, to the gastrointestinal tract, or directly into the peritoneum, particularly if there has been bile flow obstruction.[121] Insufficient intraoperative hemostasis or erosion of blood vessels due to localized infection may lead to hemobilia. A diagnostic triad may be seen of biliary colic, obstructive jaundice, and melena and/or hematemesis. Other sources of bleeding should be ruled out.

In the first postoperative days, elevated bilirubin levels are commonly observed, and these normalize within 2 to 3 weeks. The clinician must remain vigilant, however, since a number of more ominous etiologies must be kept in mind. Besides the benign hyperbilirubinemia commonly seen following resection, some other common causes include liver failure, sepsis, hematoma, bile leak, and bile peritonitis. Cholangitis is a less frequent cause. Rarely, hemobilia may be the cause. Jaundice occurring outside of the immediate postoperative period may be secondary to tumor recurrence. Postoperative liver failure in a patient with cirrhosis is usually fatal.[91,118,123]

FOLLOW-UP

Recurrence after resection of HCC is common and may not appear for years. At the British Columbia Cancer Agency, follow-up after resection of primary liver tumors is done every 3 months for the first 2 years, every 6 months for an additional 3 years, and annually thereafter. Follow-up evaluation should invariably include measurement of serum AFP and ultrasound examination of the liver; CT may also be indicated at less frequent intervals.

In some individuals, AFP is the best indicator of recurrent disease. In a study of 41 patients who underwent curative resection of HCC, serum AFP was the first measured abnormality in 34% of patients; ultrasound and CT detected 17% and 2% of recurrences, respectively.

However, in 12% of patients who had an elevated AFP with their initial tumor, no elevation was detected with recurrence.[110] This may have been because the recurrence in this group was actually a de novo neoplasm with different features. Alternatively, it may be that the persistent population of cells composing the recurrent growth is from the original tumor, and these cells have somehow lost their ability to produce AFP. Suenaga et al.[109] reported that serum AFP was normal in 50% of the recurrences they reviewed. Most recurrent HCCs in their series were detected by regular ultrasonographic examination.

For follow-up evaluation after resection of fibrolamellar HCC, measurement of serum AFP is of little use. Frequent ultrasound and CT are the most important follow-up studies for this tumor.[79]

REFERENCES

1. Linsell DA, Higginson J. The geographic pathology of liver cell cancer. In Cameron HM, Linsell DA, Warwich GP (eds): Liver Cell Cancer. Elsevier Scientific, Amsterdam, 1976, p. 2
2. Scudamore CH, Ragaz J, Kluftinger AM, Owen DA. Hepatocellular carcinoma: a comparison of Oriental and Caucasian patients. Am J Surg 1988;155:659–662
3. Nagasue N, Yukaya H, Hamada T et al. The natural history of hepatocellular carcinoma. A study of 100 untreated cases. Cancer 1984;54:1461–1465
4. Haydon GH, Jarvis LM, Simmonds P, Hayes PC. Association between chronic hepatitis C infection and hepatocellular carcinoma. Lancet 1995;345:928–929
5. Ihde DC, Sherlock P, Winawer SJ, Fortner JG. Clinical manifestations of hepatoma. A review of 6 years' experience at a cancer hospital. Am J Med 1974;56:83–91
6. Okuda K, Ohtsuki T, Obata H et al. Natural history of hepatocellular carcinoma and prognosis in relation to treatment. Cancer 1985;56:918–928
7. The Liver Cancer Study Group of Japan. Primary liver cancer in Japan. Sixth Report. Cancer 1987;60:1400–1411
8. Cottone M, Virdone R, Fusco G et al. Asymptomatic hepatocellular carcinoma in Child's A cirrhosis. A comparison of natural history and surgical treatment. Gastroenterology 1989;96:1566–1571
9. Okazaki N. Systemic chemotherapy of hepatocellular carcinoma. In Okuda K, Peters R (eds): Hepatocellular Carcinoma. Wiley, New York, 1976, pp. 469–475
10. Friedman MA. Chemotherapy for patients with hepatocellular carcinoma: prospects and possibilities. In Tabor E, Di Bisceglie A, Purcell R (eds): Etiology, Pathology and Treatment of Hepatocellular Carcinoma. Portfolio, Woodlands, TX, 1991, pp. 287–292
11. Nakamura H, Hashimoto T, Oi H, Sawada S. Transcatheter oily chemoembolization of hepatocellular carcinoma. Radiology 1989;170:783–786
12. Takayasu K, Suzuki M, Uesaka K et al. Hepatic artery embolization for inoperable hepatocellular carcinoma: prognosis and risk factors. Cancer Chemother Pharmacol 1989;23 (suppl):S123–S125
13. Shibata J, Fujiyama S, Sato T et al. Hepatic arterial injection chemotherapy with cisplatin suspended in an oily lymphographic agent for hepatocellular carcinoma. Cancer 1989;64:1586–1589
14. Franco D, Capussotti L, Smadja C et al. Resection of hepatocellular carcinomas. Results in 72 European patients with cirrhosis. Gastroenterology 1990;98:733–738
15. The Liver Cancer Study Group of Japan. Survey and follow-up of primary liver cancer in Japan. Report 9. Acta Hepatol Jpn 1991;32:1138–1147
16. Shanghai Coordinating Group of Research on Liver Cancer. Diagnosis and treatment of primary hepatocellular carcinoma in early stage. Report of 134 cases. Chin Med J 1979;92:801–806
17. Lai ECS, Fan S-T, Chu K-M, Wong J. Hepatic resection for hepatocellular carcinoma: an audit of 343 patients. Ann Surg 1995;221:291–298
18. Okuda K. Primary hepatocellular carcinoma: outcome, prognosis and follow-up. In Terblanche J (ed.): Hepatobiliary Malignancy. Its Multidisciplinary Management. Edward Arnold, London, UK, 1994, pp. 159–168
19. The Liver Cancer Study Group of Japan. Predictive factors for long term prognosis after partial hepatectomy for patients with hepatocellular carcinoma in Japan. Cancer 1994;74:2772–2780
20. The Liver Cancer Study Group of Japan. Primary liver cancer in Japan. Clinicopathologic features and results of surgical treatment. Ann Surg 1990;211:277–287
21. Johnson PJ. Tumour markers in the diagnosis and management of patients with hepatocellular carcinoma. Recent results. Cancer Res 1986;100:68–72
22. Norton JA, Fraker DL. Tumor markers. In Sabiston D (ed.): Textbook of Surgery. The Biological Basis of Modern Surgical Practice. 14th Ed. WB Saunders, Philadelphia, 1991, pp. 491–509
23. Lee HS, Chung YH, Kim CY. Specificities of serum alpha-fetoprotein in HBsAg+ and HBsAg− patients in the diagnosis of hepatocellular carcinoma. Hepatology 1991;14: 68–72
24. Sato Y, Nakata K, Kato Y et al. Early recognition of hepatocellular carcinoma based on altered profiles of alpha-fetoprotein. N Engl J Med 1993;328:1802–1806
25. Miller WJ, Federle MP, Campbell WL. Diagnosis and staging of hepatocellular carcinoma: comparison of CT and sonography in 36 liver transplantation patients. Am J Roentgenol 1991;157:303–306
26. Kudo M, Tomita S, Tochio H, et al. Small hepatocellular carcinoma: diagnosis with US angiography with intraarterial CO_2 microbubbles. Radiology 1992;182:155–160
27. Beningfield SJ. Imaging and differential diagnosis. In Terblanche J (ed.): Hepatobiliary Malignancy. Its Multidisciplinary Management. Edward Arnold, London, 1994, pp. 64–99
28. Takayasu K, Shima Y, Muramatsu Y et al. Angiography of small hepatocellular carcinomas: analysis of 105 resected tumors. Am J Roentgenol 1986;147:525–529

29. Utsunomiya T, Matsumata T, Adachi E et al. Limitations of current preoperative liver imaging techniques for intrahepatic metastatic nodules of hepatocellular carcinoma. Hepatology 1992;16:694–701
30. Jackson JE, Yeung EYC, McCarthy P et al. Case report: Lipidiol retention at the site of liver biopsy; a false positive result in the investigation of hepatocellular carcinoma. Clin Radiol 1989;40:538–540
31. Merine D, Takayasu K, Wakao F. Detection of hepatocellular carcinoma: comparison of CT during arterial portography with CT after intraarterial injection of iodized oil. Radiology 1990;175:707–710
32. Itoh K, Nishimura K, Togashi K et al. Hepatocellular carcinoma: MR imaging. Radiology 1987;164:21–25
33. Rubin AR, Lichtenstein GR, Alvi A. Hepatic scintigraphy in the evaluation of solitary solid liver masses. J Nucl Med 1993;34:697–705
34. Nagasue N, Yukaya H, Ogawa Y et al. Human liver regeneration after major hepatic resection. A study of normal livers and livers with chronic hepatitis and cirrhosis. Ann Surg 1987;206:30–39
35. Chen MF, Hwang TL, Hung CF. Human liver regeneration after major hepatectomy. Ann Surg 1991;213:227–229
36. Ozawa K, Ida T, Yamada T, Honjo I. Significance of glucose tolerance as prognostic sign in hepatectomized patients. Am J Surg 1976;131:541–546
37. Tobe T. Hepatectomy in patients with cirrhotic livers: clinical and basic observations. Surg Annu 1984;16:177–202
38. Kanematsu T, Takenaka K, Matsumata T et al. Limited hepatic resection effective for selected cirrhotic patients with primary liver cancer. Ann Surg 1984;199:51–56
39. Kwon A-H, Ha-Kawa S, Uetsuji S et al. Use of technetium 99m diethylenetriamene-pentaacetic acid-galactosyl-human serum albumin liver scintigraphy in the evaluation of preoperative and postoperative hepatic functional reserve for hepatectomy. Surgery 1995;117:429–434
40. Okamoto E, Kyo A, Yamanaka N et al. Prediction of the safe limits of hepatectomy by combined volumetric and functional measurements in patients with impaired hepatic function. Surgery 1984;95:586–92
41. Miyagawa S, Makuuchi M, Kawasaki S, Kakazu T. Criteria for safe hepatic resection. Am J Surg 1995;169:589–594
42. Takasaki T, Kobayashi S, Suzuki S et al. Predetermining postoperative hepatic function for hepatectomies. Int Surg 1980;65:309–313
43. Nord HJ, Brady PG. Endoscopic diagnosis and therapy of hepatocellular carcinoma. Endoscopy 1993;25:126–130
44. Pagliaro L, Rinaldi F, Craxi A et al. Percutaneous blind biopsy versus laparoscopy with guided biopsy in diagnosis of cirrhosis. A prospective, randomized trial. Dig Dis Sci 1993;28:39–43
45. Babineau TJ, Lewis WD, Jenkins RL et al. Role of staging laparoscopy in treatment of hepatic malignancy. Am J Surg 1994;167:151–155
46. Vilardell F. The value of laparoscopy in the diagnosis of primary cancer of the liver. Endoscopy 1977;9:20–22
47. Fornari F, Rapaccini GL, Cavanna L et al. Diagnosis of hepatic lesions: ultrasonically guided fine needle biopsy or laparoscopy? Gastrointest Endosc 1988;34:231–234
48. Prior C, Kathrein H, Mikuz G, Judmaier G. Differential diagnosis of malignant intrahepatic tumors by ultrasonically guided fine needle aspiration biopsy and by laparoscopic intraoperative biopsy—a comparative study. Acta Cytol 1988;32:892–895
49. Hemming AW, Nagy AG, Scudamore CH, Edelmann K. Laparoscopic staging of intra-abdominal malignancy. Surg Endosc 1995;9:325–328
50. Fornari F, Civardi G, Cavanna L et al. Laparoscopic ultrasonography in the study of liver diseases—preliminary results. Surg Endosc 1989;3:33–37
51. Ringe B, Pichlmayr R, Wittekind C, Tusch G. Surgical treatment of hepatocellular carcinoma: experience with liver resection and transplantation in 198 patients. World J Surg 1991;15:270–285
52. Nagao T, Inoue S, Goto S, et al. Hepatic resection for hepatocellular carcinoma. Clinical features and long-term prognosis. Ann Surg 1987;205:33–40
53. Ezaki T, Yukaya H, Ogawa Y. Evaluation of hepatic resection for hepatocellular carcinoma in the elderly. Br J Surg 1987;74:471–473
54. Sitzmann JV, Greene PS. Perioperative predictors of morbidity following hepatic resection for neoplasm: A multivariate analysis of a single surgeon experience with 105 patients. Ann Surg 1994;219:13–17
55. Sheu JC, Lee CS, Sung JL et al. Intraoperative hepatic ultrasonography—an indispensable procedure in resection of small hepatocellular carcinomas. Surgery 1985;97:97–103
56. Soyer P, Elias D, Zeitoun G et al. Surgical treatment of hepatic metastases: impact of intraoperative sonography. Am J Roentgenol 1993;160:511–514
57. Takada T, Yasuda H, Uchiyama K et al. Contrast-enhanced intraoperative ultrasonography of small hepatocellular carcinomas. Surgery 1990;107:528–532
58. Couinaud CL. Le Foie: Etudes Anatomiques et Chirurgicales. Masson, Paris, 1957
59. Northover JMA, Terblanche J. A new look at the arterial supply of the bile duct in man and its surgical implications. Br J Surg 1979;66:379–384
60. Franco D, Smadja C, Meakins JL et al. Improved early results of elective hepatic resection for liver tumors. One hundred consecutive hepatectomies in cirrhotic and noncirrhotic patients. Arch Surg 1989;124:1033–1037
61. Nagasue N, Yukaya H, Suehiro S, Ogawa Y. Tolerance of the cirrhotic liver to normothermic ischemia. A clinical study of 15 patients. Am J Surg 1984;147:772–775
62. McCord JM. Oxygen-derived free radicals in post-ischemic tissue injury. N Engl J Med 1985;312:159–163
63. Huguet C, Addario-Chieco P, Gavelli A et al. Technique of hepatic vascular exclusion for extensive liver resection. Am J Surg 1992;163:602–605
64. Lai ECS, Ng IOL, You KT et al. Hepatic resection for small hepatocellular carcinoma: the Queen Mary Hospital experience. World J Surg 1991;15:654–659
65. Yamanaka N, Okamoto E. Conditions favoring long-term

survival after hepatectomy for hepatocellular carcinomas. Cancer Chemother Pharmacol 1989;23(suppl):S83–S86

66. Tang ZY, Yu YQ, Zhou XD et al. Surgery of small hepatocellular carcinoma. Analysis of 144 cases. Cancer 1989;64: 536–541
67. Lee CS, Sung JL, Hwang LY et al. Surgical treatment of 109 patients with symptomatic and asymptomatic hepatocellular carcinoma. Surgery 1986;99:481–490
68. Masutani S, Sasaki Y, Imaoka S et al. The prognostic significance of surgical margin in liver resection of patients with hepatocellular carcinoma. Arch Surg 1994;129:1025–1030
69. Yoshida Y, Kanematsu T, Matsumata T et al. Surgical margin and recurrence after resection of hepatocellular carcinoma in patients with cirrhosis. Further evaluation of limited hepatic resection. Ann Surg 1989;209:297–301
70. Yamanaka N, Okamoto E, Toyosaka A et al. Prognostic factors after hepatectomy for hepatocellular carcinomas. A univariate and multivariate analysis. Cancer 1990;65: 1104–1110
71. Ouchi K, Matsubara S, Fukuhara K et al. Recurrence of hepatocellular carcinoma in the liver remnant after hepatic resection. Am J Surg 1993;166:270–273
72. Idezuki Y, Bandai Y. Liver resection in cirrhosis. In Terblanche J (ed.): Hepatobiliary Malignancy. Its Multidisciplinary Management. Edward Arnold, London, 1994, pp. 557–569
73. Gouillat C, Manganas D, Berard P. Ultrasonically guided hepatic tumorectomy. J Am Coll Surg 1995;180:617–618
74. Nagorney DM, Adson MA, Weiland LH et al. Fibrolamellar hepatoma. Am J Surg 1985;149:113–119
75. Wood WJ, Rawlings M, Evans H, Lim CNH. Hepatocellular carcinoma: importance of histologic classification as a prognostic factor. Am J Surg 1988;155:663–666
76. Soreide O, Czemiak A, Bradpiece H et al. Characteristics of fibrolamellar hepatocellular carcinoma. A study of nine cases and a review of the literature. Am J Surg 1986;151: 518–523
77. Berman MM, Libbey NP, Foster JH. Hepatocellular carcinoma. Polygonal cell type with fibrous stroma: an atypical variant with a favorable prognosis. Cancer 1980;46: 1448–1455
78. Vauthey J-N, Klimstra D, Franceschi D et al. Factors affecting long-term outcome after hepatic resection for hepatocellular carcinoma. Am J Surg 1995;169:28–35
79. Stevens WR, Johnson CD, Stephens DH, Nagomey DM. Fibrolamellar hepatocellular carcinoma: stage at presentation and results of aggressive surgical management. Am J Roentgenol 1995;164:1153–1158
80. Kishi K, Shikata T, Hirohashi S et al. Hepatocellular carcinoma. A clinical and pathologic analysis of 57 hepatectomy cases. Cancer 1983;51:542–548
81. Kumada K, Yamaoka Y, Morimoto T et al. Partial autotransplantation of the liver in hepatocellular carcinoma complicating cirrhosis. Br J Surg 1992;79:566–567
82. Hsu HC, Sheu JC, Lin YH et al. Prognostic histologic features of resected small hepatocellular carcinoma (HCC) in Taiwan. A comparison with resected large HCC. Cancer 1985;56:672–680
83. Thompson HH, Tompkins RK, Longmire WP Jr. Major hepatic resection. A 25-year experience. Ann Surg 1983; 197:375–388
84. Kumada K, Ozawa K, Okamoto R et al. Hepatic resection for advanced hepatocellular carcinoma with removal of portal vein tumor thrombi. Surgery 1990;108:821–827
85. Moriura S, Nimura Y, Hayakawa N et al. Combined resection of the inferior vena cava for hepatobiliary and pancreatic malignancies. Hepatogastroenterology 1990;37: 253–255
86. Chen M-F, Jan Y-Y, Jeng L-B et al. Obstructive jaundice secondary to ruptured hepatocellular carcinoma into the common bile duct: surgical experiences of 20 cases. Cancer 1994;73:1335–1340
87. Lee NW, Wong KP, Siu KF, Wong J. Cholangiography in hepatocellular carcinoma with obstructive jaundice. Clin Radiol 1984;35:119–123
88. Okuda K. Clinical aspects of hepatocellular carcinoma–analysis of 134 cases. In Okuda K, Peters RL (eds): Hepatocellular Carcinoma. Wiley, New York, 1976, pp. 387–436
89. Tanoue K, Kanematsu T, Matsumata T et al. Successful surgical treatment of hepatocellular carcinoma invading into biliary tree. HPB Surg 1991;4:237–244
90. Lau WY, Leung KL, Leung TWT et al. Resection of hepatocellular carcinoma with diaphragmatic invasion. Br J Surg 1995;82:264–266
91. Scudamore CH, Shackleton CR, Fache JS et al. Diaphragmatic resection in association with right hepatectomy. Can J Surg 1990;33:21–24
92. Ong GB, Taw JL. Spontaneous rupture of hepatocellular carcinoma. Br Med J 1972;4:146–149
93. Chearanai O, Plengvanit U, Asavanich C et al. Spontaneous rupture of primary hepatoma: report of 63 cases with particular reference to the pathogenesis and rationale treatment by hepatic artery ligation. Cancer 1983;51: 1532–1536
94. Lai ECS, Wu KM, Choi TK et al. Spontaneous ruptured hepatocellular carcinoma. An appraisal of surgical treatment. Ann Surg 1989;210:24–28
95. Lai ECS, Wong J. Surgical management. In Terblanche J (ed.): Hepatobiliary Malignancy. Its Multidisciplinary Management. Edward Arnold, London, 1994, pp. 111–129
96. Miyamoto M, Sudo T, Kuyama T. Spontaneous rupture of hepatocellular carcinoma: a review of 172 Japanese cases. Am J Gastroenterol 1991;86:67–71
97. Chen MF, Jan YY, Lee TY. Transcatheter hepatic arterial embolization followed by hepatic resection for the spontaneous rupture of hepatocellular carcinoma. Cancer 1986; 58:332–335
98. Nagasue N, Inokuchi K, Kobayashi M, Saku M. Hepatoportal arteriovenous fistula in primary carcinoma of the liver. Surg Gynecol Obstet 1977;145:504–508
99. Kanematsu T, Takenaka K, Furuta T et al. Acute portal hypertension associated with liver resection. Analysis of early postoperative death. Arch Surg 1985;120:1303–1305
100. Nagasue N, Yukaya H, Ogawa Y et al. Concurrent treatment of hepatocellular carcinoma and esophageal varices

by hepatic resection and distal splenorenal shunt. Arch Surg 1988;123:509–513

101. Matsumata T, Kanematsu T, Shirabe K et al. Advances in the treatment of hepatocellular carcinoma and concomitant esophageal varices. Hepatogastroenterology 1990;37: 461–464

102. Stiegmann GV, Goff JS, Michaletz-Onody PA et al. Endoscopic sclerotherapy as compared with endoscopic ligation for bleeding esophageal varices. N Engl J Med 1992;326: 1527–1532

103. Lai ECS, Ng IOL, You KT et al. Hepatectomy for large hepatocellular carcinoma: the optimal resection margin. World J Surg 1991;15:141–145

104. Capusotti L, Borgonovo G, Bouzari H et al. Results of major hepatectomy for large primary liver cancer in patients with cirrhosis. Br J Surg 1994;81:427–431

105. Yamamoto J, Kosuge T, Takayama T et al. Perioperative blood transfusion promotes recurrence of hepatocellular carcinoma after hepatectomy. Surgery 1994;115:303–309

106. Takenaka K, Yoshida K, Nishizaki T et al. Postoperative prophylactic lipiodolization reduces the intrahepatic recurrence of hepatocellular carcinoma. Am J Surg 1995;169: 400–404

107. Lo CM, Lai ECS, Fan ST et al. Resection for extrahepatic recurrence of hepatocellular carcinoma. Br J Surg 1994;81: 1019–1021

108. Chen M-F, Hwang T-L, Jeng L-B et al. Postoperative recurrence of hepatocellular carcinoma: two hundred five consecutive patients who underwent hepatic resection in 15 years. Arch Surg 1994;129:738–742

109. Suenaga M, Sugiura H, Kokuba Y et al. Repeated resection for recurrent hepatocellular carcinoma in eighteen cases. Surgery 1994;115:452–457

110. Kanematsu T, Matsumata T, Takenaka K et al. Clinical management of recurrent hepatocellular carcinoma after primary resection. Br J Surg 1988;75:203–206

111. Matsumata T, Kanematsu T, Takenaka K et al. Patterns of intrahepatic recurrence after curative resection of hepatocellular carcinoma. Hepatology 1989;9:457–460

112. Adachi E, Maeda T, Matsumata T et al. Risk factors for intrahepatic recurrence in human small hepatocellular carcinoma. Gastroenterology 1995;108:768–775

113. Schwartz ME, Sung M, Mor E et al. A multidisciplinary approach to hepatocellular carcinoma in patients with cirrhosis. J Am Coll Surg 1995;180:596–603

114. Nagao T, Inoue S, Yoshimi F et al. Postoperative recurrence of hepatocellular carcinoma. Ann Surg 1990;211:28–33

115. Sasaki Y, Imaoka S, Fujita M et al. Regional therapy in the management of intrahepatic recurrence after surgery for hepatoma. Ann Surg 1987;206:40–47

116. Shimada M, Matsumata T, Taketomi A et al. A new approach for liver surgery: transdiaphragmatic hepatectomy for cirrhotic patients with hepatocellular carcinoma. Arch Surg 1995;130:157–160

117. Hemming AW, Scudamore CH, Shackleton CR et al. Indocyanine green clearance as a predictor of successful hepatic resection in cirrhotic patients. Am J Surg 1992;163: 515–518

118. Fan S-T, Lo C-M, Lai ECS et al. Perioperative nutritional support in patients undergoing hepatectomy for hepatocellular carcinoma. N Engl J Med 1994;331:1547–1552

119. Tsao JI, Loftus JP, Nagorney DM et al. Trends in morbidity and mortality of hepatic resection for malignancy: a matched comparative analysis. Ann Surg 1994;220: 199–205

120. Shimada M, Matsumata T, Akazawa K et al. Estimation of risk of major complications after hepatic resection. Am J Surg 1994;167:399–403

121. Akovbiantz A, Schmid M, Schmid E. Postoperative syndromes after liver surgery. Clin Gastroenterol 1979;8: 471–485

122. Pace RF, Blenkharn JI, Edwards WJ et al. Intra-abdominal sepsis after hepatic resection. Ann Surg 1989;209:302–306

123. Tsuzuki T, Ogata Y, Iida S, Shimazu M. Hepatic resection in 125 patients. Arch Surg 1984;119:1025–1032

124. Hemming AW, Scudamore CH, Davidson A, Erb SR. Evaluation of 50 consecutive segmental hepatic resections. Am J Surg 1993;165:621–624

125. Foster JH, Berman MM. Solid Liver Tumors. In: Major Problems in Clinical Surgery. Vol. XXII. WB Saunders, Philadelphia, 1977

126. Okuda K, Obata H, Nakajima Y et al. Prognosis of primary hepatocellular carcinoma. Hepatology 1984;4:3S–6S

37

TRANSPLANTATION FOR LIVER CANCER

KEITH ROLLES

The turning point in the field of clinical liver transplantation was the National Institutes of Health (NIH) Consensus Conference held in Bethesda in 1983.[1] Until that time, only a handful of medical centers in the world regularly performed liver transplantation procedures. During the early years of liver transplantations, all of these centers relied quite heavily on liver cancer patients as candidates for transplantation, as they were found to be more likely to survive the perioperative period than, for instance, patients with advanced cirrhosis. Some patients with secondary malignancy of the liver also received transplants. The main criterion for transplantation in a liver cancer patient at that time was that the liver tumor be unresectable by conventional means, with no evidence of extrahepatic malignant disease.

The introduction of cyclosporine in 1979 and the development of improved perioperative management improved the transplantation prospects for cirrhotic patients whereas the high rate of tumor recurrence seen in transplanted liver cancer patients led to a relative decrease in the numbers of these patients. In Europe, this trend persisted throughout the 1980s and early 1990s; currently only 10% of liver transplant recipients undergo transplantation for liver cancer (Table 37-1).[2] Results have often been good, however (Table 37-2).

TUMOR RECURRENCE AND PRETRANSPLANTATION STAGING

Tumor recurrence rates vary between 11% and 69% (Table 37-2). Notwithstanding the different periods of actual follow-up reported by different authors, the widely varying recurrence rates may also reflect the degree to which pretransplant tumor staging was pursued and the techniques for such staging available at the time. Lipiodol angiography, spiral computed tomography (CT), and magnetic resonance imaging (MRI) are techniques routinely used in many centers today, but these were not available more than a decade ago. Some patients who had tumor recurrence within weeks of transplantation may have had tumor dissemination before transplantation. It is likely that better and more sophisticated preoperative assessment and staging of cancer patients will continue to improve the long-term outlook after transplantation.

INDICATIONS AND CONTRAINDICATIONS

Tumor recurrence is the leading cause of death for patients who have had a transplantation for hepatocellular carcinoma (HCC). The indications for liver transplantation for cancer vary from center to center. In some centers, HCC patients are not considered for transplantation unless under the conditions of specific therapeutic protocols. Penn[3] recommends criteria for transplantation based on the retrospective analysis of the outcome of 637 patients transplanted for primary and metastatic liver malignancies treated in centers throughout the world. Stratification of the data is limited to gross histologic type, tumor recurrence rates, and 2- and 5-year patient survival (Table 37-3). For the entire cohort, the tumor recurrence was 40%, with 81% of deaths from recurrence

TABLE 37-1. Percentage of Liver Transplantations in Europe That Are for Cancer

	Year	Percentage
Prior to	1985	38
	1986	22
	1987	19
	1988	14
	1994	11
	1996	10

(From European Liver Transplant Registry, 1985–96.)

occurring within 2 years of transplantation. The best results were obtained with transplantation for uncommon tumors.

This study did not consider the impact on outcome of the underlying cirrhosis viruses, tumor size, multifocality, or tumor staging. Based on these data, however, Penn recommends that transplantation for hemangiosarcoma and most metastatic tumors, with the exception of those from neuroendocrine primary tumors, is not appropriate. Transplantation for hepatocellular carcinoma and cholangiocarcinoma should be reserved for patients with favorable risk factors, or when combined with well-defined chemotherapy protocols before and after transplantation.

Pichlmayr et al.[4] consider as "favorable" indications for fibrolamellar hepatoma, epithelioid hemangioendothelioma, hepatoblastoma, hepatocellular carcinoma stages 1 and 2, incidental hepatocellular carcinoma in a cirrhotic liver, proximal bile duct carcinoma stages 2 and 3, and metastases from neuroendocrine tumors or from leiomyosarcoma. Borderline indications include some cases of hepatocellular carcinoma, stage III or IV, and some cases of advanced cancer if testing new adjuvant protocols. These views may be viewed as being rather liberal, particularly in view of the growing shortage of liver donors.

On the other hand, the 5-year survival rate of patients currently being transplanted for hepatocellular carcinoma is not significantly different from that of those transplanted for fulminant liver failure, approximately 50% in each group, according to the European Liver Transplant Registry statistics.[2]

Extrahepatic spread, either direct or metastatic, nodal metastases of primary hepatic malignancies, or liver metastases from non-neuroendocrine tumors are contraindications to transplantation.[5] Few would contemplate transplantation for angiosarcoma; for many, leiomyosarcoma, stage III and IV hepatocellular carcinoma, cholangiocarcinoma including Klatskin tumors, and bile duct carcinoma would be considered contraindications.

TUMOR RECURRENCE

McPeake et al.[6] state that post-transplantation tumor recurrence is related to a multiplicity of factors, including (1) clinically and radiologically undetectable micrometastases, (2) cells that escape from the liver during surgical manipulation, (3) the effect of immunosuppression on the natural history of tumor growth, (4) the size of the original tumor, and (5) the number of lesions present in the resected liver (multifocality). In addition, the precise histologic variant of the tumor appears important, and recently it has been postulated that tumor recurrence may be enhanced by down-regulation of oncostatic factors such as angiostatin consequent to removal of the dominant tumor mass.[7]

TABLE 37-2. Liver Transplantation for HCC in Cirrhotic Patients

Authors	No. of Patients	2-Month Mortality (%)	Recurrence (%)	3-Year Survival (%)
O'Grady et al.[28] (Cambridge, UK 1968–1987)	19	32	69	37
Ringe et al.[29] (Hannover 1982–1989)	52	23	36	20
Bismuth et al.[16] (Paris 1980–1989)	60	5	23	49
Iwatsuki et al.[18] (Pittsburgh 1980–1991)	71	15 (3 months)	37	43
Romani et al.[30] (Milan 1985–1991)	19	5	11	80
Tan et al.[27] (London 1988–1991)	15	7	14	63
Mazzaferro et al.[31] (Milan 1991–1994)	48	6	8	75 (4-yr)

TABLE 37-3. Recurrence and Survival Rates for Liver Transplant Recipients Who Were Transplanted for Liver Cancer

Tumor Type	Recurrence (%)	2-Year Survival (%)	5-Year Survival (%)
Incidental[a]	13	57	57
Epithelioid hemangioendothelioma	33	82	43
Hepatoblastoma	33	50	50
Fibrolamellar HCC	39	60	55
Metastatic tumors	59	38	21
HCC	39	30	18
Cholangiocarcinoma	44	30	17
Hemangiosarcoma	64	No survivors after 27.5 months	

[a] Diagnosed only on histologic examination of the excised liver.

MICROMETASTASES AND CIRCULATING TUMOR CELLS: ADJUVANT THERAPY

Micrometastases, including those resulting from cells escaping during surgical manipulation,[8] theoretically would best be treated by perioperative adjuvant therapy. The use of pretransplant systemic chemotherapy, chemoembolization and radiotherapy, followed by intraoperative chemotherapy and postoperative chemotherapy for up to 9 months, appear to have resulted in improved recurrence-free survival posttransplant,[9–14] although these studies had short follow-up periods, and small numbers of patients (some with advanced disease). In contrast, others[6] found no effect of preoperative or postoperative chemotherapy on the incidence or timing of tumor recurrence. Multicenter randomized trials using multimodal adjuvant therapy are needed.

IMMUNOSUPPRESSION AND TUMOR GROWTH

The enhancing effect of immunosuppressive agents on tumor growth and possible early tumor recurrence is a difficult problem because it remains necessary to immunosuppress transplant recipients to prevent graft rejection during the early years post-transplantation.[15]

TUMOR SIZE AND NUMBER

Much more tangible, however, is the relationship between the size of the original tumor, the number of tumor nodules in the resected liver, and the outcome of transplantation, in terms of tumor recurrence and patient survival. Bismuth et al.[16] showed that 83% of patients transplanted for HCCs less than 3 cm in size and with only 1 to 2 tumor nodules had a 3-year tumor-free survival. When looked at independently, tumors smaller than 3 cm fared significantly better than those with tumors larger than 3 cm, and those with 1 to 2 tumor nodules fared better than those with more than 2 nodules. (These patients also received 9 months of post-transplantation chemotherapy with 5 fluorouracil and doxorubicin.) McPeake et al.[6] confirmed that tumor recurrence rates correlate with tumor size and the number of tumor nodules. Patients with single tumors smaller than 4 cm remained tumor-free at rates of 86% and 57% at 1 and 5 years, respectively. Tumors between 4 and 8 cm were associated with a 40% recurrence rate, with 44% 5-year survival. Patients with tumors greater than 8 cm, or multifocal lesions, had a 78% tumor recurrence rate and an 11% 5-year survival rate. In this series, some patients received preoperative chemotherapy or chemoembolization, and some received postoperative chemotherapy on a rather arbitrary basis. Iwatsuki et al.[17] reported significantly better results in patients who received transplants for single tumors less than 5 cm.[18] Recurrence was seen in 7%, compared to 65% in patients with lesions greater than 5 cm. Survival was 71% and 29% at 1 and 5 years, respectively. Schwartz et al.[19] reported no recurrences over a 4-year follow-up of transplantation in 40 cirrhotic patients with hepatocellular carcinomas of 5 cm or less. Of 17 patients with HCCs greater than 5 cm, four developed recurrence (23%). The survival rate for all transplantation patients was 56%.

TRANSPLANTATION VERSUS TUMOR RESECTION

Cancers in the Noncirrhotic Liver and Histologic Variants

Since the surgical treatment of choice for HCC in the noncirrhotic liver is tumor resection, transplantation for HCC in the noncirrhotic liver has been recommended only for large unresectable lesions or multicentric HCC. However, large unresectable lesions and multicentric tumors are associated with high recurrence rates and poor post-transplantation survival and, therefore, should no longer be considered for transplantation, with the exception of fibrolamellar HCC. The results of transplantation for this histologic variant suggest that although ultimately the recurrence rate is not significantly different from nonfibrolamellar HCC, the recurrence-free interval after transplantation is longer, and survival with established recurrence also appears to be longer. A second exception may be the remarkably slow-growing biliary cystadenocarcinoma.

Cancers in the Cirrhotic Liver

Resection of HCCs in cirrhotic livers is usually limited to Child's stage A and B patients. Resections are usually subsegmental and are associated with operative mortality rates from 7% to 20%.[20–22] More extensive resection, involving two or more segments, is associated with an increase in operative mortality, up to 48%.[20] Survival following resection differs markedly for patients with Child's A (56% to 64%) and Child's B (12%)[25,26] stage cirrhosis. Thus, the results with resection in Child's A cirrhosis is comparable to transplantation for similar tumors at 3 years. Recurrence rates following HCC resection are repeatedly reported at more than 50% within 1 to 2 years.[23–26]

Transplantation is generally associated with better survival. Tan et al.[27] reported 1- and 3-year survival rates of 80% and 63%, respectively, in patients receiving transplants and a 15% tumor recurrence rate, compared to 61% at 1 year and 33% at 3 years in tumor resections, with a recurrence rate of 45% for solitary HCCs up to 8 cm in patients with Child's A and B cirrhosis. Bismuth et al.[16] showed overall survival rates for resection at 50% and 47% for transplantation at 3 years. However, the survival rate without tumor recurrence was significantly better for transplantation at 46%, compared to 27% for tumor resection at 3 years. In patients with small (less than 3 cm) uninodular or binodular tumors, transplantation had 83% 3-year recurrence-free survival, compared to 18% for tumor resection. Iwatsuki et al.[18] found similar 1- to 5-year survival rates in resected patients and transplant patients in the Pittsburgh series between 1980 and 1989, with 71% 1-year and 33% 5-year survival for tumor resection, compared to 66% 1-year and 36% 5-year survival for transplantation. Tumor recurrence rates were similar, 43% for transplantation and 50% for tumor resection. However, when hepatocellular carcinoma was associated with cirrhosis, survival rates were significantly better after transplantation.

SUMMARY

Liver transplantation for cancer remains an important option for the treatment of several different types of tumors and particularly for selected cases of HCC. Appropriate case selection criteria are becoming clearer. Tumor types and tumor stages likely to do well or badly are becoming better defined. Tumor recurrence remains the major cause of death after transplantation. However, when resources permit, transplantation appears to be a better option than resection for small hepatocellular carcinomas in cirrhotic livers.

REFERENCES

1. National Institutes of Health Consensus Conference Statement on Liver Transplantation: June 20–23, 1983 Hepatology 1984;4(suppl):1075–1105
2. European Liver Transplant Registry Six Monthly Report, June 1994. European Liver Transplant Association, Villeiuie, Paris
3. Penn I. Hepatic transplantation for primary and metastatic cancers of the liver. Surgery 1991:110;726–734
4. Pichlmayr R, Weimann A, Ringe B. Indications for liver transplantation in hepatobiliary malignancy. Hepatology 1994;20 (suppl):335–405
5. Pichlmayr R. Is there a place for liver grafting in malignancy? Transplant Proc 1988;20(suppl 1):478–482
6. McPeake JR, O'Grady JG, Zaman S et al. Liver transplantation for primary hepatocellular carcinoma: tumor size and number determine outcome. J Hepatol 1993;18:226–234
7. Folkman J. Clinical applications of research on angiogenesis. New Engl J Med 1995;333:1757–1763
8. Kar S, Carr BI. Detection of liver cells in peripheral blood of patients with advanced stage hepatocellular carcinoma. Hepatology 1995;21:403–407
9. Bismuth H, Morino M, Sherlock D et al. Primary treatment of hepatocellular carcinoma by arterial chemoembolisation. Am J Surg 1992;163:387–394
10. Carr BI, Selby R, Madriaga J. Prolonged survival after liver transplantation and cancer chemotherapy for advanced stage hepatocellular carcinoma. Transplant Proc 1993;25: 1128–1129
11. Stone MJ, Klintmalm GBG, Polter D et al. Neoadjuvant chemotherapy and liver transplantation for hepatocellular carcinoma: a pilot study in 20 patients. Gastroenterology 1993;104:196–202
12. Cherqui D, Piedbois P, Pierga P et al. Multimodal adjuvant treatment and liver transplantation for advanced hepatocellular carcinoma. Cancer 1994;73:2721–2726
13. Schwartz ME. Primary hepatocellular carcinoma: transplantation versus resection. Semin Liver Dis 1994;14:135–139
14. Olthoff KM, Rosove MH, Shackleton CR et al. Adjuvant chemotherapy improves survival after liver transplantation for hepatocellular carcinoma. Ann Surg 1995;221: 734–743
15. Yokoyama I, Carr B, Saitsu H et al. Accelerated growth rates of recurrent hepatocellular carcinoma after liver transplantation. Cancer 1991;68:2095–2100
16. Bismuth H, Chiche L, Adam R, et al. Liver resection versus

transplantation for hepatocellular carcinoma in cirrhotic patients. Ann Surg 1993:218;145–151

17. Iwatsuki S, Gordon RD, Shaw BW, Starzl TE. Role of liver transplantation in cancer therapy. Ann Surg 1985;202: 401–407
18. Iwatsuki S, Starzl TE, Sheahan DC et al. Hepatic resection versus transplantation for hepatocellular carcinoma. Ann Surg 1991;214:221–229
19. Schwartz ME, Sung M, Mor E et al. A multidisciplinary approach to hepatocellular carcinoma in patients with cirrhosis. J Am Coll Surg 1995;180:596–603
20. Tsuzuki T, Sugioka A, Heda M et al. Hepatic resection for hepatocellular carcinoma. Surgery 1990;107:511–520
21. Franco D, Capussotti L, Smadja C et al. Resection of hepatocellular carcinomas. Results in 72 European patients with cirrhosis. Gastroenterology 1990;98:733–738
22. Onishi K, Tanabe Y, Ryu M et al. Prognosis of hepatocellular carcinoma smaller than 5 cm in relation to treatment: study of 100 patients. Hepatology 1987;7:1285–1290
23. Nagasue N, Yukaya H, Ogawa Y et al. Clinical experience with 118 resections for hepatocellular carcinoma. Surgery 1986;99:694–701
24. Nagao T, Inoue S, Yoshimi F et al. Postoperative recurrence of hepatocellular carcinoma. Ann Surg 1990;211:28–33
25. Lin TY, Lee CS, Chen KM, Chen CC. Role of surgery in the treatment of primary carcinoma of the liver: a 31 year experience. Br J Surg 1987;74:839–842
26. Kanematsu T, Matsumata T, Takenaka K et al. Clinical management of recurrent hepatocellular carcinoma after primary resection. Br J Surg 1988;75:203–206
27. Tan KC, Rela M, Ryder, SD. Experience of orthotopic liver transplantation and hepatic resection for hepatocellular carcinoma of less than 8 cm in patients with cirrhosis. Br J Surg 1995;82:253–256
28. O'Grady JG, Polson RJ, Rolles K et al. Liver transplantation for malignant disease: results in 93 consecutive patients. Ann Surg 1988;207:373–379
29. Ringe B, Wittekind C, Bechstein WO, Pichlmayr R. The role of liver transplantation in hepatobiliary malignancy: a retrospective analysis of 95 patients with particular regard to tumour stage and recurrence. Ann Surg 1989;209:88–98
30. Romani F, Sansalone CV, Rimold P. Liver transplantation for small HCC in cirrhosis. Transpl Tin 1992;55:215–216
31. Mazzaferro V, Regalia E, Doci R et al. Liver transplantation for the treatment of small hepatocellular carcinomas in patients with cirrhosis. N Engl J Med 1996;14:728–729

38

TREATMENT OF UNRESECTABLE HEPATOCELLULAR CARCINOMA: CYTOREDUCTION BY CHEMOTHERAPY, HEPATIC ARTERY LIGATION, RADIOIMMUNOTHERAPY, AND OTHER METHODS

ZHAO-YOU TANG

Hepatocellular carcinoma (HCC) has surpassed gastric cancer as the leading cancer killer in rural areas of China and ranks second as a cancer killer in the cities in China.[1] Although the 5-year survival rate in the United States was reported gradually increasing from 2% in the 1960s, to 3% to 4% in the 1970s, to 4% to 7% in the 1980s, the dismal overall outcome remains a critical issue.[2] Unquestionable progress has been made in the early detection and resection of small or subclinical HCC.[3–5] Resection of large HCC has also yielded acceptable results in some cases.[6–8] Liver transplantation is thought to be superior to tumor resection for small HCC.[9] Unfortunately, most HCC patients are unresectable.

This work was supported in part by China Medical Board Grant 93-583, "Primary Liver Cancer".

TREATMENT MODALITIES THAT SUBSTANTIALLY IMPROVE HCC SURVIVAL

It is universally accepted that resection of HCC remains the best treatment modality to improve survival. Based on the progress in medical imaging, regional cancer therapies, multimodality combination treatment, and changing concepts in surgical oncology, the role of surgery in the treatment of HCC has become greater.[10]

Analysis of Long-Term Survivors of HCC

The analysis of long-term survivors in our institute revealed that the major source of 5-year survivors from 1960 to 1974 was mainly from resection of large HCCs (91.7%), whereas from 1975 to 1989, small HCC resection surpassed large HCC resection as the leading source of 5-year survivors (54% versus 34.9%). Furthermore, cytoreduction and sequential resection for initially unre-

TABLE 38-1. Analysis of HCC Patients with 5-Year Survival at the Liver Cancer Institute of Shanghai Medical University (1960–1989)

Items	1960–1974	1975–1989	Total
Patients treated	310	1,025	1,335
No. of 5-year survivors	12	200	212
No. of 10-year survivors	8	49	57
Treatment modalities			
Small HCC resection % (n)	8.3 (1/12)	54 (108/200)	51.4 (109/212)
Large HCC resection % (n)	91.7 (11/12)	31.5 (63/200)	34.9 (74/212)
Sequential resection % (n)	0	8.5 (17/200)	8 (17/212)
Palliative surgery % (n)	0	6 (12/200)	5.7 (12/212)

sectable HCC has appeared to be a new and hopeful source of long-term survivors (8.5%), as has palliative surgery (such as hepatic artery ligation and cannulation, cryosurgery, and their combination) (Table 38-1). Of 96 patients surviving at least 5 years, 91 were treated with resection, 5 with cytoreduction and sequential resection.[11] A 5-year survival rate of 14.7% (79 of 539) among patients treated with resection has been reported.[12]

Analysis of survival in different patient groups also indicates that resection of small HCCs yielded a higher 10-year survival compared to resection of larger HCCs (Table 38-2). Among 72 patients who had initially unresectable HCC and were treated by cytoreduction and sequential resection, the long-term survival rate was as high as that for small HCC resection, 62.1% versus 62.9% for 5-year survival, and 45.9% versus 45.7% for 10-year survival.[13]

Analysis of Five-Year Survival in Different Treatment Groups

Analysis of 5-year survival in different treatment groups (Table 38-3) revealed that resection produced the best curative outcome (5-year survival 46.7%; n = 1380), and palliative surgery (including hepatic artery ligation [HAL] and/or hepatic artery cannulation with infusion [HAI], with targeting therapy or radiotherapy, and their combination) ranked second; drug therapy was similar to that for no treatment. Palliative surgery in combination with other therapies was superior to that of palliative surgery alone. Of these, HAL combined with intrahepatic arterial targeting therapy yielded the highest 5-year survival (33.1%), which was mainly a result of a higher sequential resection rate. This suggested that cytoreduction and sequential resection might be an important approach to the treatment of some unresectable HCCs.

TABLE 38-2. Long-Term Survival of Different Patient Groups in Liver Cancer Institute of Shanghai Medical University

Patient Groups	n	% 5-Year Survival	% 10-Year Survival
Small HCC resection	549	62.9	45.7
Non-small HCC resection	831	34.6	26
Curative resection	1,159	52.2	39.6
Palliative resection	221	17.6	—
Sequential resection	72	62.1	45.9

TABLE 38-3. Survival in Different Treatment Groups at the Liver Cancer Institute of Shanghai Medical University (1958–1994)

Treatment Modalities	n	% 3-Year Survival	% 5-Year Survival
Resection	1,380	57	46.7
HAL + targeting therapy	93	42.5	33.1
HAL + HAI	192	26	18.1
Cryosurgery	59	37.7	13.7
HAL + HAI + radiotherapy[a]	71	20.9	11.5
Other regional therapies	48	15.3	10.2
HAI	90	11.9	9.9
Drug therapy	202	0.6	0.6
No treatment	90	4.2	—

Abbreviations: HAL, hepatic artery ligation; HAI, hepatic artery cannulation with infusion of chemotherapy.

[a] Including a few with sequential resection.

STRATEGIES FOR THE TREATMENT OF UNRESECTABLE HCC

The 5-year survival rate for 107 patients with HCCs >5 cm treated by cryosurgery was 22% and in 32 patients with HCCs ≤5 cm it was 48.8%.[14,15] Microwave surgery as regional cancer therapy has been reported.[16,17] In the field of nonsurgical therapies, transcatheter arterial chemoembolization (TACE) was very effective and surpassed radiotherapy as the leading nonsurgical therapy for unresectable HCC. In patients with unresectable HCC (Table 38-4), no 5-year survival occurred from 1958 to 1970, whereas 5-year survival was 7.4% from 1971 to 1982, and 25.7% in 1983 to 1994. Also in 1983 to 1994, 10-year survivors appeared for the first time, which was a result of cytoreduction and sequential resection, as well as advances of palliative surgery.[10]

CYTOREDUCTION AND SEQUENTIAL RESECTION OF UNRESECTABLE HCC

Cytoreduction and sequential resection, which worked for hepatoblastoma,[19] seemed also important as a possible treatment of localized unresectable HCC. With the progress of regional cancer therapies and multimodality treatment, more and more localized unresectable HCCs could be converted to resectable. Few reports of cytoreduction and sequential resection of HCC have appeared.[20–31] In our institute, we have treated patients with unresectable HCC with cytoreduction (including chemotherapy, hepatic artery ligation plus cannulation with infusion, or radioimmunotherapy) followed by resection.[22–31] By the end of 1994, 72 of 633 patients with surgically verified unresectable HCCs have been converted to resectable.[13]

Cytoreduction with median diameter reduced from 10 to 5 cm was mainly a result of multiple combination treatment with HAL, targeting therapy, and fractionated regional radiotherapy. As shown in Table 38-5, this occurred in 45.8% of the 72 patients treated with HAL combined with intrahepatic arterial targeting therapy, 38.9% treated with HAL plus HAI (chemotherapy infusion). It has been repeatedly demonstrated that for cytoreduction, double or triple combination treatment was more effective than any single treatment[24,26,31]

As shown in Table 38-6, the 5-year survival rate of the 72 patients was 62.1%, comparable to that of resection for small HCC (62.9%, n = 549) and much higher than that of the entire series of unresectable HCC. The operative mortality rate was only 1.4% in the 72 patients with sequential resection. A solitary tumor confined to one lobe, without tumor embolus, associated with micronodular cirrhosis, in a patient in whom serum AFP returned to normal level after resection (in patients with α-fetoproteen [AFP]-producing HCC), was associated with longer survival (Table 38-7). The recent advance of TACE has provided a nonsurgical approach for cytoreduction of unresectable HCC, and sequential resection after TACE has also been reported.[32,33]

TABLE 38-4. Improving 5-year Survival of HCC Patients Treated With Palliative Surgery in Different Periods at the Liver Cancer Institute of Shanghai Medical University (1958–1994)

Survival	1958–1970 (%) n = 20	1971–1982 (%) n = 145	1983–1994 (%) n = 367	Total (%) n = 532
1-year	5	35.9	65.8	54.3
3-year	—	12.4	37	27.1
5-year	—	7.4	25.7	18
10-year	—	3.7	18.1	11

TABLE 38-5. Treatment Before Sequential Resection at the Liver Cancer Institute of Shanghai Medical University (1960–1994)

Treatment Modalities	n	%
HAL + Targeting Therapy	33	45.8
HAL + HAI (chemotherapy)	28	38.9
HAL + HAI + radiotherapy	9	12.5
HAI alone	1	1.4
Regional cancer therapy	1	1.4
Total:	72	100

Abbreviations: HAL, hepatic artery ligation; HAI, Hepatic artery cannulation with infusion of chemotherapy.

TABLE 38-6. Survival of Unresectable HCCs and HCCs in Patients Who Received Cytoreduction and Sequential Resection

Survival	% Unresectable HCC[a] n = 663	% Sequential Resection n = 72
1-year	48.9	92.2
3-year	23.8	78
5-year	15.4	62.1
10-year	9.1	45.9

[a] Including 72 patients with sequential resection after shrinkage of tumor by multimodality therapies.

TABLE 38-7. Factors at First Operation Influencing 5-year Survival of HCC Patients After Sequential Resection

Factors		n	5%-Year Survival
No. of HCC nodules	= 1	55	68.8
	> 1	17	53.8
Tumor embolus			
Absent		47	91.4
Present		23	42.3
Tumor(s) involve			
Single lobe		56	76.9
Both lobes or hilium		16	44.2
Cirrhosis			
None		9	100
Micronodular		29	74.5
Macronodular		33	47
AFP after sequential resection	< 200 ng/ml	24	75
	> 200 ng/ml	16	43.8

Abbreviations: AFP, α-fetoprotein.

THE ROLE OF TARGETING TREATMENT IN THE CYTOREDUCTION AND SEQUENTIAL RESECTION OF UNRESECTABLE HCC

For targeting therapy followed by sequential resection, three kinds of targeting therapeutic agents have been used (Table 38-8). In patients with surgically verified HCC, hepatic artery ligation plus intrahepatic targeting therapy yielded the highest sequential resection rate (35.1%) (Table 38-8) when compared to HAL+HAI+radiotherapy (17.6%) or HAL+HAI with chemotherapy (14.6%). Treatment with HAL alone or HAI alone, or regional cancer therapies, rarely resulted in adequate tumor shrinkage to permit sequential resection.

TABLE 38-8. Sequential Resection Rates in Different Treatment Groups at the Liver Cancer Institute of Shanghai Medical University (1960–1994)

Treatment Modalities	n	Sequential Resection n	%
HAL + targeting therapy	94	33	35.1
HAL + HAI + radiotherapy	51	9	17.6
HAL + HAI (chemotherapy)	192	28	14.6
Regional cancer therapies	107	1	0.9
HAL, HAI, or HAE	119	1	0.8
Exploratory surgery only	100	0	0

Abbreviations: HAL, hepatic artery ligation; HAI, hepatic artery cannulation with infusion of chemotherapy; HAE, hepatic artery embolization.

TABLE 38-9. Percentage of Targeting Therapy Involved in Cytoreduction and Sequential Resection in the Different Periods

Period	Sequential Resection (n)	Targeting Therapy n (%)
1978–1983	6	0 (0)
1984–1989	29	14 (43.3)
1990–1994	37	19 (51.4)
Total	72	33 (45.8)

Of the 72 patients treated with sequential resection, 33 were also treated with targeting combination therapy (Table 38-9). In the experimental treatment of nude mice bearing human HCC, radioimmunotherapy combined with chemotherapy and immunotherapy yielded the highest response rate when compared with any one or two of them.[34] The 5-year survival rate was 66.1% for sequential resection with targeting therapy and 57.7% with nontargeting therapy.[28]

INTRAHEPATIC ARTERIAL TARGETING TREATMENT AND FUTURE PROSPECT

The intrahepatic arterial administration of radioimmunotherapeutic agents has proved superior to that of intravenous agents. Multivariate analysis using the Cox model indicated that tumor size and sequential resection were two major factors influencing prognosis, which indicated that targeting combination therapy was inadequate to kill 100% of cancer cells, and therefore sequential resection is needed. A large dose of radioimmunotherapy was not superior to a moderate dose.[35,36] In conclusion, targeting therapy is effective in killing a great number of cancer cells, which is one of the promising approaches in the multimodality treatment of HCC.

REFERENCES

1. Centre for Health Statistics Information, Ministry of Public Health, P.R. China. Selected edition on health statistics of China (1991–1994). Ministry of Public Health, P.R. China, Beijing, 1991, pp.78–79

2. Wingo PA, Tong T, Bolden S. Cancer statistics, 1994. CA 1995;45:8–30
3. Tang ZY. Subclinical Hepatocellular Carcinoma. Springer, Berlin, 1985
4. Tang ZY, Yu YQ, Zhou XD et al. Small hepatocellular carcinoma–three decades' experience. In Jiang SJ, Xiao SD (eds): Proceedings of 1992 Shanghai International Symposium on Gastronenterology. Shanghai Science & Technical Literature Publisher, Shanghai, 1992, pp.52–59
5. Makuuchi M, Kosuge T, Takayama T et al. Surgery of small liver cancers. Semin Surg Oncol 1993;9:298–304
6. Wu MC, Chen H. Hepatectomy for primary liver cancer in 1102 cases. Asian J Surg 1994;17:14–16
7. Lai ECS, Fan ST, Lo CM et al. Hepatic resection for hepatocellular carcinoma. Ann Surg 1995;221:291–298
8. Vauthey JN, Klimstra D, Franceschi D et al. Factors affecting long-term outcome after hepatic resection for hepatocellular carcinoma. Am J Surg 1995;169:28–35
9. Iwatsuki S, Starzl TE. Role of liver transplantation in the treatment of hepatocellular carcinoma. Semin Surg Oncol 1993;9:337–340
10. Tang ZY, Yu YQ, Zhou XD. Evolution of surgery in the treatment of hepatocellular carcinoma from the 1950s to the 1990s. Semin Surg Oncol 1993;9:293–297
11. Du JH, Wang XH, Li XC. Clinical investigation of late treatment results of primary hepatocellular carcinoma. J Hep Bil-Panc Splenic Surg 1995;1:178–180 (in Chinese)
12. Okamoto E, Yamanaka N, Oriyama T et al. Determinants of long-term survival following hepatectomy for hepatocellular carcinoma, with special reference to patients surviving more than 10 years. J Hepatol Biliary Pancreatic Surg 1994;94:1: 107–112
13. Tang ZY, Yu YQ, Zhou XD et al. Cytoreduction and sequential resection for surgically verified unresectable hepatocellular carcinoma–further evaluation with analysis of 72 patients. World J Surg 1995;19:784–789
14. Zhou XD, Tang ZY, Yu YQ et al. The role of cryosurgery in the treatment of hepatic cancer: a report of 113 cases. J Cancer Res Clin Oncol 1993;120:100–102
15. Onik GM, Atkinson D, Zemel R, Weaver ML. Cryosurgery of liver cancer. Semin Surg Oncol 1993;9:309–317
16. Zhou XD, Tang ZY, Yu YQ et al. Microwave surgery in the treatment of hepatocellular carcinoma. Semin Surg Oncol 1993;9:318–322
17. Hamazoe R, Hirooka Y, Ohtani S et al. Intraoperative microwave tissue coagulation as treatment for patients with nonresectable hepatocellular carcinoma. Cancer 1995:75:794–800
18. Yamada R, Kishi K, Sato M et al. Transcatheter arterial chemoembolization (TACE) in the treatment of unresectable liver cancer. World J Surg 1995;19:795–800
19. Reynolds M. Conversion of unresectable to resectable hepatoblastoma and long-term follow-up study. World J Surg 1995;19:814–816
20. Zhang XH, Wu MC, Chen H. Second stage resection for unresectable liver cancer—report of 15 cases. J Hepatol Biliary Pancreatic Surg 1989;1:1–3 (in Chinese)
21. Sitzmann JV, Abrams R. Improved survival for hepatocellular cancer with combination surgery and multimodality treatment. Ann Surg 1993;217:149–155
22. Yu YQ, Tang ZY, Zhou XD et al. Treatment of huge primary liver cancer in stages. Chin J Surg 1983;21:92–93 (in Chinese)
23. Tang ZY, Yu YQ, Zhou XD et al. The changing role of surgery in the treatment of primary liver cancer. Semin Surg Oncol 1986;2:103–112
24. Tang ZY, Yu YQ, Ma ZC et al. Conversion of a surgically verified unresectable to resectable hepatocellular carcinoma—a report of 26 patients with subsequent resection. Chin J Cancer Res 1989;1:41–47
25. Tang ZY, Liu KD, Bao YM et al. Radioimmunotherapy in the multimodality treatment of hepatocellular carcinoma with reference to second-look resection. Cancer 1990;65: 211–215
26. Tang ZY, Yu YQ, Zhou XD et al. Cytoreduction and sequential resection: a hope for unresectable primary liver cancer. J Surg Oncol 1991;47:27–31
27. Tang ZY, Zeng ZX, Liu KD et al. Intrahepatic arterial I-131 antihepatocellular carcinoma (HCC) monoclonal antibody combined with hepatic artery ligation for treatment of unresectable HCC. Antibody Immunoconj Radiophar 1993;6: 167–175
28. Tang ZY, Yu YQ, Zhou XD et al. The role of targeting therapy in cytoreduction and sequential resection of unresectable hepatocellular carcinoma. Chin J Cancer Res 1994;6:24–30
29. Lu JZ, Li BX, Liu KD et al. Alternating chemotherapy and fractionated radiotherapy as a modality for the treatment of primary liver cancer. Chin J Cancer Res 1994;6:69–73
30. Yu YQ, Tang ZY, Zhou XD et al. Resection of huge hepatocellular carcinoma by two stage operation: report of 48 cases. Asian J Surg 1994;17:17–19
31. Tang ZY, Yu YQ, Zhou XD et al. Treatment of unresectable primary liver cancer: with reference to cytoreduction and sequential resection. World J Surg 1995;19:47–52
32. Yu YQ, Xu DB, Zhou XD et al. Experience with liver resection after hepatic arterial chemoembolization for hepatocellular carcinoma. Cancer 1993;71:62–65
33. Elias D, Lasser P, Rougier P et al. Frequency, technical aspects, results and indications of major hepatectomy after prolonged intraarterial chemoembolization for hepatocellular carcinoma. Cancer 1993;71:62–65
34. Bao YM, Tang ZY, Liu KD et al. Radioimmunotherapy combined with chemotherapy and immunotherapy for nude mice bearing human hepatocellular carcinoma. Chin J Oncol 1989;11:245–247 (in Chinese)
35. Liu KD, Tang ZY, Fan Z et al. Radioimmunotherapy in treatment of unresectable hepatoma—a report of 43 cases. Chin J Cancer Res 1994;6:74–78
36. Liu KD, Tang ZY, Lu JZ et al. Long-term results of targeting therapy using radiolabelled antibodies in multimodality treatment of hepatocellular carcinoma (HCC)—an analysis of 75 cases. Acta Acad Med Shanghai 1995;22(suppl):14–18 (in Chinese)

INDEX

Page numbers followed by f *indicate figures; those followed by* t *indicate figures.*